18.50X

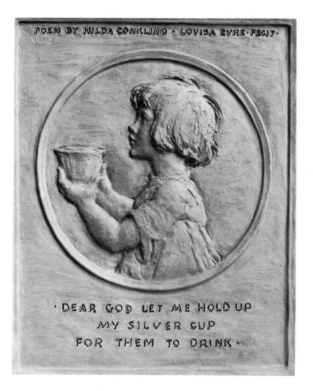

FRONTISPICE BY LOUISA EYRE

The Identifying Symbol of the
Children's Hospital of Philadelphia

Courtesy of Mrs. deLanux, Louisa E. Norton and
Edwards F. Leiper, Jr., Attorney-at-Law

THIRD EDITION

Textbook of PEDIATRIC NURSING

DOROTHY R. MARLOW, R.N., Ed.D.

*Dean and Professor of Pediatric Nursing,
College of Nursing, Villanova University.
(Formerly Associate Professor of Pediatric Nursing, University
of Pennsylvania School of Nursing)*

WITH 572 ILLUSTRATIONS ON 288 FIGURES

W. B. SAUNDERS COMPANY *Philadelphia, London, Toronto*

W. B. Saunders Company: West Washington Square
                           Philadelphia, Pa.   19105

                           12 Dyott Street
                           London W.C. 1

                           1835 Yonge Street
                           Toronto 7, Ontario

Textbook of Pediatric Nursing

Print No.:   3   4   5   6   7   8   9

In Honor

MR. AND MRS. WILLIAM MARLOW

Parents

In Memoriam

MRS. MARGARET M. ADAMS

Teacher, Counselor, and Friend

FOREWORD

A foreword can serve a number of purposes, and it has not been an easy task to decide toward which of these this particular foreword should be directed. Much could be said which primarily would pay tribute to the author. The pages of this book, for example, convey a warmth of feeling for children and an understanding of them seldom achieved in the printed word, and even less often in a textbook. This characteristic is so pervasive it cannot but infect the reader even to the extent of exciting like feelings. The book speaks so clearly for the author, however, in this and in other respects that this purpose was discarded.

These introductory remarks might serve the purpose of orienting the reader to the rich and varied accumulation of knowledge and its systematic organization to be found in these pages. Undoubtedly this volume is rare among texts in the scope and completeness with which the many-faceted aspects of child life are discussed. But this fact, too, will quickly be self-evident, and a second purpose was rejected.

A foreword in the form of a book review offered a highly tempting, if inappropriate, possibility. The unusual features of both the content and its organization demand critical analysis and discussion. A book review would not only misuse the opportunity this foreword offers, but also would probably be of greater interest to the teacher of pediatric nursing than to the student. In any case, it must be left for the columns of the professional journals.

What, then, can this foreword provide? Precisely, because of the nature of this book, the most useful function of a foreword may be a brief guide to the student on how to get the most out of the great deal that it offers. Chapter-by-chapter reading in textbooks is not always fruitful. The student may be searching for general understanding, and specific details are offered—about procedures, about particular situations, or about a group of diseases affecting a particular organ system. Because the information needed is scattered, she may have difficulty bringing together knowledge of people, of their health problems when their defenses fail, and of the kind of nursing care required. She must, however, correlate and integrate this knowledge to give appropriate and helpful nursing care. This difficulty will not be encountered in this text.

Within three consecutive chapters of this book it is possible to acquire a comprehensive picture of the child—his growth and development, his care, and his health problems—at each developmental period. Age and developmental stage are clearly seen as important influences on the occurrence of illness and on its treatment; this fundamental basis for nursing care is obvious. The meaning and significance of illness and hospitalization to the child and to his family are also related to development and make for increased understanding of this problem. The disease conditions commonly found in a given age period become readily apparent, serving not only to sharpen observations, but also to clarify the interrelations between maturation and specific kinds of illnesses.

Read carefully, then, chapter by chapter, for a general understanding of the field of pediatric nursing, for an appreciation of its scope and complexity, for an awareness of the many factors involved in nursing care, and for comprehensive knowledge of the child and his health problems. The possibility for learning does not end here, however. Selected kinds of rereading will be effective in furthering your knowledge and understanding.

Read and study consecutively and carefully each of the chapters on growth, development, and care, in each of the developmental periods. The dynamic process of growth from birth through adolescence emerges, and a text within a text is found. In a similar fashion a text devoted to the health problems of infants and children which are acute or short-term in nature evolves; or one concerned with those problems which require long-term care can be segregated. The presence of several possible texts in one volume makes it relatively easy for you to develop and expand your knowledge of the field on a longitudinal as well as on a cross-sectional basis.

There is another facet of this book to be studied. Nursing is an applied science and of necessity draws heavily upon the basic sciences and other applied sciences for its content. This knowledge is then synthesized and extended to provide a basis for nursing practice. Nursing care practices, general and specific, and the rationale underlying these practices are discussed in some detail throughout this book. You may wish to find another text within a text by delineating those general nursing care practices, together with the supporting knowledge, which can be adapted to a number of age levels and to many disease conditions.

In the final analysis, what you gain from this textbook depends upon you. It cannot give you wisdom, but it offers a foundation for the development of wisdom. It cannot give you understanding of an individual child in the real world of nursing, but it provides the kind of knowledge through which that understanding is made possible. It cannot give you skill in the practice of pediatric nursing, but it offers you the tools with which to work. It cannot give you faith in yourself or in the patients you serve, but it can lead you to the threshold of such faith.

DOROTHY E. JOHNSON, R.N., M.P.H.

Professor of Nursing
University of California
Los Angeles

PREFACE

Advances in child care have been rapid during recent years. Research carried on by disciplines such as psychology, sociology and anthropology has contributed increased understanding of the growth and development of children, the meaning of parent-child relations, the effects of family disruption, and the place of the child and the adolescent in our changing world. Medical research has led to the knowledge of successful methods of prevention and therapy through the use of concepts in the areas of genetics, drugs, advanced surgical techniques and psychiatric care for children.

The role of the pediatric nurse has been influenced by these findings and also by research carried on within the nursing profession itself. In her new role the pediatric nurse is no longer a lone practitioner; she is now a team member working with members of various professions for the welfare of the child and his family. The nurse no longer replaces the mother in the hospitalized child's life; she now helps the mother to provide nursing care for her child when he is well and when he is ill. The nurse no longer sees the child only as the occupant of a hospital bed, but recognizes him as an individual, a member of a family and of the community.

This change in the role of the pediatric nurse places a broader responsibility upon her than she has known before. She must now be cognizant of the contribution she can make as a member of the team in maintaining the integrity of each family, in offering anticipatory guidance, in preventing illness, and in providing skilled nursing care for children when needed. In order for her to assume this role, the pediatric nurse must not only be dedicated to understanding and helping others; she must also be dedicated to understanding herself and her own capabilities, which are of vital importance to the child and family who look to the nurse for understanding in their therapeutic relationship.

In considering the recent research in nursing and related fields, the changing role and responsibilities of the pediatric nurse, and the basic principles of teaching and learning, this textbook has been arranged on an organizational plan based on the growth and development of the child as a basis for his care during health and illness.

In the opening chapters of the book I have attempted to give the student a broad historical perspective of the area of pediatric nursing and a generalized view of the areas of knowledge which must be understood in order to provide care for children today: an overview of the concepts and principles of growth and development, a general discussion of the care of the child when ill and when hospitalized, and a review of the role of the pediatric nurse.

After this general view of content, the remainder of the book is organized into units primarily on the basis of specific growth and development and care of children of various age groups from the neonatal period through adolescence. An understanding of growth and development is vital to the nurse because she is primarily nursing the child, not his disease. After the student has developed an understanding of the healthy child she is led to a consideration of the effect of illness on children in the same age group. Physical and emotional illnesses requiring short-term or immediate care and long-term care are discussed. The various conditions included in each age period have been selected either because they are related to the growth and development process or because their incidence is greatest during that particular age span. Increased emphasis has been placed in this edition on the scientific reasons why certain conditions predominate in each age group. Although many of these conditions may affect children of varying ages in actual life situations, I believe that if students understand the growth and development of children of various ages and the nursing care of a child having a particular condition at one age, they will be able to transfer this knowledge to the care of children of different age groups.

Few conditions have been included for which there is not a discussion of the nursing care to be given in the home or in the hospital, by the mother, the nurse in the hospital, or the public health nurse. Since I have tried to present the nursing care of children so thoroughly, I have purposely not included in this book all the disorders of the pediatric years. On the other hand, I have included some conditions which were not common in the past, but which today because of current research and sociological changes are being seen with increasing frequency. Among others, examples of such conditions include chromosomal anomalies, hypoglycemia, dental problems, minimal cerebral dysfunction, school phobia, drug dependence, and infectious mononucleosis. Discussions of other conditions which are seen less commonly today than in past years, such as rickets, scurvy and acrodynia, have been condensed. However, there has been no reduction in coverage of certain communicable diseases for which newer preventive measures are being found. In the discussion of each condition appropriate concepts such as those related to the areas of nutrition, mental health, prevention of illness, rehabilitation and public health are considered. Details of the pathology of diseases have been included in order to enable the student to understand better the nursing care of children. Further discussion of pathologic processes may be found in the textbooks listed in the references.

In this edition certain additions have been made which I hope will be useful to the student. These include a more detailed history of and an increased emphasis on the care of children, not only in the United States but also throughout the world, changes in the care of the hospitalized child, discussions of the legal aspects of pediatric nursing in various situations, a fuller discussion of genetics and embryology as they relate to the conditions affecting children, newer areas of research being done on the care of mothers and children, the concept of the development of parents necessitated by the growth and development of their child, the care of children whose parents cannot care for them, a description of the changes in the growing child that lead to antisocial behavior, and a broad discussion of the rebellious and impulsive adolescent, the problems of juvenile delinquency and of drug dependence. Further additions to this edition include a table of normal blood values, the most recent schedule for immunizations published by the American Academy of Pediatrics, and the Recommended Daily Dietary Allowances as revised in 1968 by the Food and Nutrition Board of the

National Research Council. New tables of mortality rates of infants, children, and adolescents have also been included. At the same time that I have tried to provide content on the newer forms of therapy utilized in the care of ill and handicapped children based on research, I have attempted to eliminate repetition of content.

In this edition also, greater emphasis has been placed on the role of the nurse in providing emotional support for the child and his parents, both in the hospital and in public health settings. The manner in which the nurse can help the parents support the child in his normal psychological development from birth through adolescence, and the manner in which the nurse herself can support the child in the absence of his parents, are discussed. Suggestions are also given concerning the way the nurse can help the parents prepare their child at various stages in his life for hospitalization and support him when he is physically or emotionally ill. Included also is a deeper and more comprehensive discussion of the nurse's role in helping parents and their child as well as other siblings face crisis situations such as occur in prolonged illness and death. The reactions of the nurse in these situations are also discussed.

I have found that by writing within this organizational framework, by emphasizing the growth and development of children in the family constellation and in various social settings, and by helping students to view parent-child-nurse relations not only through their own eyes but through the eyes of parents and child as well, I can assist students in developing understandings and attitudes which should be beneficial in their work.

The reader will undoubtedly note a change in style in the writing concerning the growth and development of children and that concerning their illnesses. This change has been purposely planned. If one of the purposes of a text such as this is to modify attitudes toward children and parents, then a more informal type of writing is required in the description of the growth and development of children. On the other hand, if knowledge concerning the illnesses of children is to be learned, the student can best absorb the content if it is presented in a clear, brief but comprehensive form.

Pictures illustrating the growth and development of children as well as those illustrating children with various pathologic conditions have been included in this text. A series of illustrations have been included showing the actual steps in the growth and development of one little girl from birth to eight years of age. Pictures of children having various conditions have been included because students may not have the opportunity to care for children having such conditions. After an extensive search of the current literature for colored illustrations of some of the more common illnesses of children, these were found in a German publication, *Frieboes/Schonfeld's Color Atlas of Dermatology*, by J. Kimmig and M. Janner (American edition translated and revised by H. Goldschmidt). I am indeed grateful for being able to share these colored illustrations with students who may not have the opportunity to see these conditions during their experience in pediatric nursing.

The listing of teaching aids and other information and references including publication and periodicals, which have been brought up to date since the second edition, can be found at the end of each chapter. The references given at the ends of chapters have been selected on the basis of their scope of content and their recent publication. For the most part they present, in greater depth than was possible in this text, current and newer knowledge in the medical, nursing and related disciplines. Articles in which original research findings are presented are included because I believe that the beginning student should become ac-quainted with the value of such investigations. At the end of each unit the stu-dent will find Clinical Situations and Guides to Further Study which will serve as a review of the content of the unit. The study questions have been included for the purpose of helping the student bring together the material presented on the care of children in each age group. Some of these questions involve the under-standing of factual material, while others require the student to use judgment in answering situational questions. More cross references than in former editions have also been provided in order to assist the student to understand the content of the clinical area of pediatric nursing.

The material in the text was submitted to physicians, nurses, and other professional persons for their opinions and suggestions. Their appraisals and contributions have helped the author to clarify or expand important areas of content.

Former editions of this textbook, while primarily intended for the use of students preparing to be professional nurses, have also been used by other members of the health team such as physiotherapists and occupational thera-pists among others. Such sharing of knowledge of the area of pediatric nursing by other disciplines will ultimately lead to a closer relationship among health team members interested in the care of children.

Learning by the student comes either through direct experience or through the experience and language of others. The role of the author, as of the teacher, is to bring knowledge to students and to interpret this knowledge in its most intelligible form. Not only must specific knowledge be transmitted, but the author or teacher must also guide the student to other sources of knowledge and to an appreciation of how new knowledge is gained through research.

It has been my hope to make this textbook representative of current thought in the area of pediatric nursing. I will welcome all comments and suggestions from reviewers, teachers and students so that this text can help the nursing stu-dent contribute her best efforts to the care of children and find deep personal satisfaction in working with them and their parents.

Dorothy R. Marlow

ACKNOWLEDGMENTS

Many professional persons—physicians, nurses and members of other disciplines—have contributed their knowledge and support to make the creation of this book possible.

A special tribute should be accorded to those who by their faith in the worthiness of my task encouraged me in my efforts: Dr. Theresa I. Lynch, former Dean of the School of Nursing, University of Pennsylvania; Dr. Mildred L. Montag, Professor of Nursing Education, Teachers College, Columbia University; Dr. Marcia A. Dake, Dean of the College of Nursing, University of Kentucky; Rosemary Johnson, presently a doctoral candidate at the University of California in Los Angeles and former acting Dean, College of Nursing, Arizona State University; and Dr. B. Louise Murray, Associate Professor and Director of Maternal and Child Nursing, School of Nursing, University of Washington.

It is impossible to express adequately the appreciation of the author for the generous assistance of the physicians who contributed to this text:

Mary D. Ames, M.D., Assistant Professor of Clinical Pediatrics, School of Medicine, University of Pennsylvania, and Coordinator of the Department of Rehabilitation, Children's Hospital of Philadelphia

Lester Baker, M.D., Assistant Professor of Pediatrics, School of Medicine, University of Pennsylvania; and Assistant Director of The Clinical Research Center, Children's Hospital of Philadelphia

Mark O. Camp, M.D., Internist, Presbyterian-University of Pennsylvania Medical Center and Taylor Hospital

Harry G. Gianakon, M.D., Child Psychiatrist, The Institute of the Pennsylvania Hospital

Michael B. Gregg, M.D., Assistant Chief, Epidemiology Program, National Communicable Disease Center, Atlanta, Georgia

C. Everett Koop, M.D., Professor of Pediatric Surgery, School of Medicine, University of Pennsylvania, and Surgeon-in-Chief, Children's Hospital of Philadelphia

William J. Rashkind, M.D., Associate Professor of Pediatrics, School of Medicine, University of Pennsylvania, and Director of Cardiovascular Laboratories of the Children's Hospital of Philadelphia

Luis Schut, M.D., Associate in Neurological Surgery, School of Medicine, University of Pennsylvania; Associate in Neurosurgery, Hospital of the University of Pennsylvania and the Graduate Hospital of the University of Pennsylvania; and Chief of Neurosurgery, Children's Hospital of Philadelphia, Veterans Administration Hospital, and Philadelphia General Hospital

The author is indeed grateful to the many members of the nursing profession, educators, graduate practitioners, and students throughout the United

States and Canada, who offered excellent suggestions which have been incorporated in the revision of this textbook.

The author would especially like to express her appreciation to the following:

Evelyn N. Behanna, R.N., M.S., Assistant Professor in Nursing of Children, College of Nursing, Villanova University

Helen T. Coffey, R.N., Supervisor of Medical-Surgical Nursing, Children's Hospital of Philadelphia

Sally Douthwaite, R.N., Health team member in a physician's office

Dorothea Ellis, R.N., formerly Supervisor of the Pediatric Department, Hospital of the University of Pennsylvania

Jessie Glass, R.N., M.P.H., Maternal-Child Health Consultant, Division of Public Health Nursing, Pennsylvania Department of Health

Erna Goulding, R.N., M.A., Associate Director of Nursing, Children's Hospital of Philadelphia

Jacqueline L. Holt, R.N., Ph.D., Associate Professor, Maternal and Child Nursing, School of Nursing, University of Washington

Joan L. Jackson, R.N., B.S., Project Chief Nurse, Rebound Children and Youth Program, Children's Hospital of Philadelphia, Philadelphia Child Guidance Clinic and Children's Bureau

Lutie Clemson Leavell, R.N., M.A., M.S., Professor Emeritus, Teachers College, Columbia University; Consultant, College of Nursing, University of Iowa

Corrine Lewis, R.N., Head Nurse, Baby Surgical Unit, Children's Hospital of Philadelphia

Susan Matern, R.N., M.S., Assistant Professor of Pediatric Nursing, College of Nursing, University of Illinois

Rosemary Rath, R.N., M.S.N., Information and Referral Director, Lehigh County Mental Health and Mental Retardation Program, Allentown, Pennsylvania

Vivian Rhoads, R.N., Supervisor of Medical-Surgical Nursing, Children's Hospital of Philadelphia

Charlotte Spicher, R.N., M.N.Ed., Assistant Professor of Pediatric Nursing, School of Nursing, University of Pittsburgh

Rosemary Sullivan, R.N., Supervisor of Non-Professional Personnel, Children's Hospital of Philadelphia

Margaret M. Wright, R.N., M.S., presently a doctoral candidate at the University of Pennsylvania and formerly Chief Nurse, Mental Retardation Clinical Research Center, Nebraska Psychiatric Institute, University of Nebraska, Omaha

Several other professional persons have also made significant contributions to this book:

Shirley Bonnem, Director, Public Relations Department, Children's Hospital of Philadelphia

Mary Brooks, Coordinator of Children's Activities, Children's Hospital of Philadelphia

Myrtle Feigenberg, A.B., M.S.Ed., Associate Professor of Nursing (Nutrition), College of Nursing, Villanova University

Palmyra Hochgelerent, Hospital School Teacher, Philadelphia Board of Education

Robert A. Israel, Acting Chief, Mortality Statistics Branch, Division of Vital Statistics, Department of Health, Education and Welfare

I should like to express my appreciation also to the authors, publishers and companies who have granted me permission to use their illustrations in this text. I should like to thank the personnel of H. Armstrong Roberts, Photographers; Gilbert and Ring, Medical Photographers; and Mr. Everett H. Shahian and Mr. Don Shenck, Photographers in the Harrisburg, Pennsylvania area for their excellent photographs of children. I should like to express my appreciation especially to those persons responsible for the pictures which introduce the Units of this text: Units I, III, V and VII, Armstrong Roberts; Unit II, The National Foundation–March of Dimes; Unit IV, Gilbert and Ring; and Unit VI, Mr. Don Shenck. I would also like to take this opportunity to thank Mr. Eliot Morse and Mrs. Beatrice Davis of the Library of the College of Physicians and Surgeons, Philadelphia, for their assistance in helping me to obtain resource materials which were helpful in the revision of this text. I would like to thank especially Herr Achim Menge, Georg Thieme Verlag, Stuttgart, Germany, for permission to use the pictures shown on the colored plates in this book.

A special word of appreciation should be extended to Dr. and Mrs. Robert Gens, to Mr. and Mrs. John Haffly and their daughter, Kim, and to the many parents who granted permission for pictures of their children to appear in this book. Although these parents were anxious about the health of their children, they were eager to contribute in this way to the education of nursing students.

Gratitude should also be expressed to Miss Ann C. Preston for her secretarial assistance during the revision of this text.

The author wishes to express warm appreciation to the staff of the W. B. Saunders Company for their fine cooperation. Without their sincere interest and support the revision of this textbook would have been impossible.

I should also like to express my personal appreciation to my parents, Mr. and Mrs. William Marlow, for their endless patience and understanding during the preparation of this book.

DOROTHY R. MARLOW

CONTENTS

UNIT 2 THE NEWBORN

5

6

7

8

14

UNIT 4 THE TODDLER

15

16

17

UNIT 5 THE PRESCHOOL CHILD

18

19

20

UNIT 6 THE SCHOOL CHILD

21

22

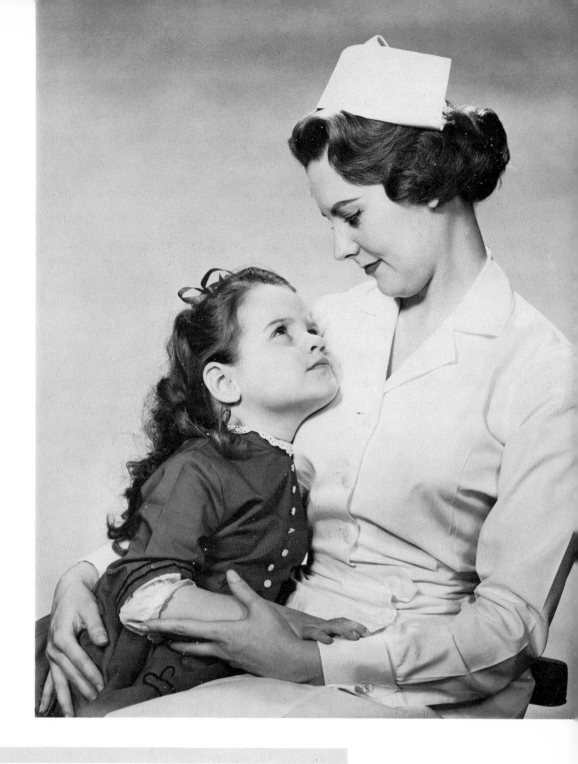

UNIT ONE

INTRODUCTION

1

CHILD CARE THROUGH THE AGES

HISTORY AND PRESENT CONCEPTS OF CHILD CARE

History

The manner in which children have been cared for when well or treated when ill has differed in accordance with how the adult members of society thought of the child, that is, his value for the preservation of the group, their religious beliefs, superstitions, migrations, and what they knew of the causes of illness and its therapy. An understanding of child care since its beginning in time is essential for the nurse so that she may gain an appreciation of the trends leading to our present concepts and practices in relation to children.

The Child in Primitive Societies

Little is known about life in prehistoric times, but child care is believed to have been somewhat like that among cultural groups living today in areas hardly touched by civilization. In such groups persons tend to value a child not for himself, but as a future adult. For this reason his social development according to the customs of the group is of great importance.

In early times primitive groups were nomads who moved constantly in their search for adequate supplies of food and for safety from wild animals and hazardous weather conditions. Such groups, which had to move quickly and frequently for reasons of self-preservation, could not be hampered by sick or weak children. The members of these groups looked favorably on those who were strong and healthy and destroyed those who were not.

When such a society ruled that a malformed or sickly infant would drain the resources of the group, the infant was killed or left behind to die. Sometimes infants were killed simply because they were females who could not contribute as much productive labor to the group as could males. This practice was termed *infanticide*. Probably some infants escaped death, however, because their mothers protected them from the group. Societies then as now were composed of individuals, not all of whom necessarily lived by the rules of the group.

In addition, some primitive peoples believed in superior beings who ruled not only themselves, but also nature and the universe as they knew it. Perhaps, they reasoned, the forces of a storm or a period of prolonged drought was an act of a superior being who was displeased. Perhaps the birth of a deformed infant was also punishment for the previous transgressions of the parents. Such thinking did not cease with the onset of civilization.

Yet we know that the child, even in primitive tribes, had to receive at least a minimum of physical care in order to live. Whether he received also love and affection was dependent on the cultural group in which he lived and on his mother who cared for him.

The Child in Ancient Civilizations

The concept of the importance of the child to his society gradually emerged as each group settled on an area of fertile land instead of wandering in search of food. The child, instead of being a liability, thus slowly became an asset to his society.

Egypt. The early peoples who settled in the valley of the Nile River cared for their children, dressing even their infants in loose clothes and encouraging breast feeding. They encouraged children to learn as well as to participate in outdoor activity. As early as 1500 B.C. treatment for the diseases of childhood was prescribed, different from that given to adults.

Greece and Rome. Physical beauty was considered important to the early inhabitants of Greece; thus the children were reared so that they would have well formed bodies. The importance of the family was stressed in Rome because its function was to raise strong sons to become good warriors who could serve the state.

Hippocrates (460-370 B. C.) in his writings referred frequently to the peculiarities of disease in children. Specific treatment for the illnesses of children as opposed to that given adults was recommended by Celsus, who lived in the first Christian century.

Israel. Among the ancient Jews the hygienic measures prescribed in the Mosaic Law had a great influence on maternal and child care. The Hebrew people recognized the importance of cleanliness and nutrition. They also recognized communicable diseases and made efforts to control them. The religious ceremony of circumcision practiced on male infants also served as a health measure.

Parenthood was honored among the Hebrews, and a large family was considered a sign of God's blessing upon the parents. The greatest disappointment a Hebrew woman could have was to be childless.

The Impact of Christianity on the Care of the Child

Christianity, among other emerging religions, helped to develop a new philosophy of the sanctity of human life. Christianity taught the value of the child as an individual, not merely as a son or daughter who would cherish the parents in their old age and give them grandchildren so that the family might extend for generations to come. Furthermore, since Christianity also taught the protection of the weak by the strong, the care of the ill by the well, the helpless child and the infirm became objects of special consideration. Orphan asylums for dependent children and hospitals for the care of the sick were founded early in the history of the Christian Church.

The Child in Europe

Before the nineteenth century in Europe the life expectancy of human beings was short. Many parents did not live long enough to rear their children in the home. Great epidemics of contagious diseases often swept over the continent. Young men died in war or from injuries sustained while working. Women married early and had large families. The maternal death rate was high. The death rate for the total population was highest in the cities and among the poor.

The result of all these conditions was that there were many orphaned children among the poor of the growing cities. Many infants were taken to boarding homes or *baby farms*. The majority of these children were of illegitimate birth. Frequently, after the initial payment of a fee, there would be no more remuneration forthcoming; therefore it was advantageous to the owner of the "baby farm" to hasten the children's deaths.

Asylums, initially founded for the care of dependent children in A.D. 787, multiplied in number as the demands for such institutions grew. Even though the number of such institutions increased, overcrowding was still a problem. Many children died, owing to their poor condition on admission, to a lack of understanding of the principles of sanitation, nutrition or of housing, to a lack of aseptic technique when needed, and to the extremely poor quality of care which was provided. Because of these unfavorable conditions, it is estimated that half of the infants of the urban poor died before the age of five years.

Probably the darkest period in child care in Great Britain and Western Europe was the beginning years of the Industrial Revolution during the early 1800's. Children as young as six to twelve years of age worked in cotton mills for ten or more hours a day. They often fell asleep at their work, and accidents were common. But since their hands were nearly as skillful as adult hands in tying broken threads, and the cost of their maintenance (if they were apprenticed orphans) and their wages were so low, mill owners employed them in large numbers. Not until the nineteenth century was legislation passed that prohibited the worst evils of child labor.

The Child in the United States

Until the early decades of the twentieth century most children in the United States lived on farms or in small villages. In general this was a healthy life, although children in such areas lacked the medical care and hospital facilities that urban parents could provide. Child labor was never the problem in the United States that it was in Europe; nevertheless the children of the poor were employed in factories and stores where working conditions were unhealthy and hours far too long.

By the middle of the nineteenth century there were large slums in New York and other eastern cities. The people living there were generally from foreign countries, many of them from rural areas and not accustomed to city life. Tenements were overcrowded, unsanitary and in disrepair. Morbidity and mortality rates among infants and children were exceedingly high. Accidents in the tenements and in the streets where the children played were common.

Contaminated milk led to serious intestinal disorders among infants and children. (Dairies and stores which handled milk were not inspected, and milk was not pasteurized.) Milk from tuberculous cows caused many cases of tuberculosis among children.

The condition of neglected, abandoned and ill children aroused public and professional sympathy. The following milestones occurred in this society's effort to improve the lives of these children.

1790. The first orphanage was established and operated at the expense of the public.
1853. The Children's Aid Society of New York was founded to move thousands of homeless children from the streets into foster homes.
1855. The Children's Hospital of Philadelphia was founded, the first hospital dedicated exclusively to the care of children.
1860. Dr. Jacobi in New York established the first children's clinic, where he lectured to medical students on the diseases of childhood.
1875. The Society for the Prevention of Cruelty was organized in New York City.
1880. The Pediatric Section of the American Medical Association was organized.
1888. The American Pediatric Society was organized.
1899. Children's courts came into being, as distinguished from adult courts where all types of criminals appeared.
1909. The White House Conference on the Care of Dependent Children.
1912. The Children's Bureau was established.
1917. The first Federal Child Labor Law was passed (declared unconstitutional after nine months).
1919. The first law for the statewide care of handicapped children.
1919. The White House Conference on Child Welfare Standards.
1930. The White House Conference on Child Health and Protection. *The Children's Charter* was adopted.

1931. The American Academy of Pediatrics was founded.
1940. The White House Conference on Children in a Democracy.
1941. A federal labor law was passed (after other attempts had been made to do so) which could successfully regulate child labor.
1946. The United Nations International Children's Emergency Fund (UNICEF) was created by the United Nations.
1948. The World Health Organization (WHO) was created by the United Nations.
1950. The Midcentury White House Conference on Children and Youth. The *Pledge to Children* was adopted.
1953. The Federal Department of Health, Education, and Welfare was established.
1959. The 14th General Assembly of the United Nations approved the *Declaration of the Rights of the Child.*
1960. The Golden Anniversary White House Conference on Children and Youth.

Two of the most important milestones in the progress toward betterment of life for children were the White House Conferences and the establishment of the Children's Bureau.

The White House Conferences. In 1909 President Theodore Roosevelt called the first White House Conference on the Care of Dependent Children. A similar conference has been held every ten years since that time. As a result of the first conference the United States Children's Bureau was founded, under the jurisdiction of the Department of Labor, since at that time child labor was thought to be the greatest problem of childhood.

The 1919 White House Conference on Standards of Child Welfare marked the culmination of Children's Year. A small group of specialists, laymen and a few foreign visitors met in Washington to discuss the pressing problems of children and youth. After this Conference regional conferences were held to discuss the protection of the health of mothers and their children, the socioeconomic base for child welfare standards, children in need of care, and child labor.

The 1930 White House Conference on Child Health and Protection was called by President Herbert Hoover to study the status of children and to recommend what ought to be done in the future. This Conference produced the *Children's Charter*, which contained nineteen statements concerning what the child needs for his health, education, welfare and protection. This is one of the most important documents in the history of child care.

The 1940 White House Conference on Children in a Democracy followed the great depression. Conference discussions concerned social and economic matters: what children required in a democratic way of life.

The Midcentury White House Conference in 1950 was attended by nearly 6000 delegates from all professions and groups concerned with children. Five hundred of the delegates were young people twelve to twenty-three years of age. The theme of the conference was *A Fair Chance to Achieve a Healthy Personality.* The Children's Bureau subsequently published a booklet entitled *A Healthy Personality for Your Child,* a popular version of the Conference's Fact Finding Digest. The *Pledge to Children* was adopted during this conference.

Pledge to Children

TO YOU, our children, who hold within you our most cherished hopes, we the members of the Midcentury White House Conference on Children and Youth, relying on your full response, make this pledge:

From your earliest infancy we give you our love, so that you may grow with trust in yourself and in others.

We will recognize your worth as a person and we will help you to strengthen your sense of belonging.

We will respect your right to be yourself and at the same time help you to understand the rights of others, so that you may experience cooperative living.

We will help you to develop initiative and imagination, so that you may have the opportunity freely to create.

We will encourage your curiosity and your pride in workmanship, so that you may have the satisfaction that comes from achievement.

We will provide the conditions for wholesome play that will add to your learning, to your social experience, and to your happiness.

We will illustrate by precept and example the value of integrity and the importance of moral courage.

We will encourage you always to seek the truth.

We will provide you with all opportunities possible to develop your own faith in God.

We will open the way for you to enjoy the arts and to use them for deepening your understanding of life.

We will work to rid ourselves of prejudice and discrimination, so that together we may achieve a truly democratic society.

We will work to lift the standard of living and to improve our economic practices, so that you may have the material basis for a full life.

We will provide you with rewarding educational opportunities, so that you may develop your talents and contribute to a better world.

We will protect you against exploitation and undue hazards and help you grow in health and strength.

We will work to conserve and improve family life and, as needed, to provide foster care according to your inherent rights.

We will intensify our search for new knowledge in order to guide you more effectively as you develop your potentialities.

As you grow from child to youth to adult, establishing a family life of your own and accepting larger social responsibilities, we will work with you to improve conditions for all children and youth.

Aware that these promises to you cannot be fully met in a world at war, we ask you to join us in a firm dedication to the building of a world society based on freedom, justice and mutual respect.

SO MAY YOU grow in joy, in faith in God and in man, and in those qualities of vision and of the spirit that will sustain us all and give us new hope for the future.

From the 1950 Midcentury White House Conference on Children and Youth.

The sixth, or Golden Anniversary White House Conference on Children and Youth, was assembled on March 27, 1960. Over 14,000 persons attended this Conference, including about 1400 youths of high school and college age and 500 foreign visitors who were delegates. The purpose of this Conference was to promote opportunities for children and youths to realize their full potential for a creative life in freedom and dignity.

Since the first White House Conference on Children in 1909 progress has been made in advancing and safeguarding the well-being of children in spite of a depression, hot and cold wars, and rapid change. One of the principal contributions of these Conferences has been in keeping the channels of communication open with ideas moving in both directions between the specialists, practitioners, and research workers in children's services and the parents and citizens of this country.

The Children's Bureau.   In 1903 Miss Lillian Wald, who was founder of the Henry Street Settlement in New York City, and Mrs. Florence Kelley of the National Consumer's League saw a need for a Federal organization that would endeavor to improve the conditions of children. They were especially concerned about the high mortality rate, the illegitimacy rate, the orphanages, and child labor among other problems. News of their concern eventually reached President Theodore Roosevelt.

After the meeting of the first White House Conference in 1909 a law was passed in 1912 that established the Children's Bureau. The responsibility of this new Bureau was to investigate and report "upon all matters pertaining to the welfare of children and child life among all classes of our people." [*]

The Children's Bureau is interested in the well-being of all children: the well, the sick and the handicapped. Children from all cultural and racial groups, all socioeconomic levels, whether loved or abused, are the concern of the Bureau.

An important aspect of the work of the Children's Bureau is that of fact-gathering and reporting such statistics as the number of births, the number of children living, with their ages and family incomes, the number of sick or handicapped children, and the number of children of various ages who die. The Bureau is also interested in the number and quality of the people,

---

[*] It's Your Children's Bureau, Children's Bureau, 1964, p. 4.

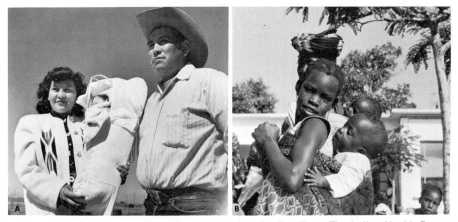

Figure 1–1. Examples of child care. *A,* An American Indian family. (From The Indian Health Program. United States Department of Health, Education, and Welfare, Public Health Service.) *B,* The United Nations Children's Fund,together with the World Health Organization,helps the government to provide care for mothers and children in Dakar, Senegal, French West Africa. (UNICEF photo.)

programs and institutions that help children in the country.

Another aspect of the work of the Children's Bureau is that of setting standards and of building services for children in partnership with states and communities. Such Federal grant-in-aid funds have provided money to help states start new services for children, to develop skilled staffs to work with children and their families, and to make possible demonstration and research projects that have led to better services.

Currently the Federal government is especially interested in preventing the incidence of and improving the services to mentally retarded children, crippled children and juvenile delinquents. The Government is also concerned about children of migratory agricultural workers, those of working mothers, those who are abused or neglected, and those refugees who have no one to care for them.

The Children's Bureau also publishes pamphlets on subjects of interest to the public. The first of these bulletins, *Prenatal Care,* was published for parents in 1913. The bulletin *Infant Care* was published initially in 1914. Many more such pamphlets are listed for students at the ends of the chapters in this text.

To summarize, then, the purposes of the Children's Bureau today are

1. To assemble facts needed to keep the country informed about children and matters adversely affecting their well-being:
2. To recommend measures that will be effective in advancing the wholesome development of children and in preventing and treating the ill effects of adverse conditions:
3. To give technical assistance to citizens and

to voluntary and public agencies in improving the conditions of childhood:

4. To administer the financial aid that the Federal Government appropriates each year to aid the states in building the health and welfare of their children.*

The Children's Bureau is concerned for all children in the United States; however, it also works actively with international organizations such as the United Nations International Children's Emergency Fund, which has as its concern the children of the world.

The Child in the Developing Countries

No one living today can think only in terms of the welfare of the children in his own town, state or country. The speed of modern transport and the exploding world population are bringing the peoples of the world closer together than ever before. Hence health problems which were once the concern of only a small segment of the world's population today potentially threaten the whole world.

Through the international activities of the World Health Organization (WHO), the United Nations International Children's Emergency Fund (UNICEF), and other groups, assistance is being provided to developing countries in their efforts to improve their level of child care.

The World Health Organization. The World Health Organization, established as a specialized agency of the United Nations in 1948, was the first world-wide health organization in history.

---

* It's Your Children's Bureau, Children's Bureau, 1964, pp. 7-8.

DECLARATION OF THE RIGHTS OF THE CHILD
as approved unanimously by the 14th General Assembly of the United Nations, November 20, 1959

WHEREAS the peoples of the United Nations have, in the Charter, reaffirmed their faith in fundamental human rights, and in the dignity and worth of the human person, and have determined to promote social progress and better standards of life in larger freedom,

WHEREAS the United Nations has, in the Universal Declaration of Human Rights, proclaimed that everyone is entitled to all the rights and freedoms set forth therein, without distinction of any kind, such as race, colour, sex, language, religion, political or other opinion, national or social origin, property, birth or other status,

WHEREAS the child, by reason of his physical and mental immaturity, needs special safeguards and care, including appropriate legal protection, before as well as after birth,

WHEREAS the need for such special safeguards has been stated in the Geneva Declaration of the Rights of the Child of 1924, and recognized in the Universal Declaration of Human Rights and in the statutes of specialized agencies and international organizations concerned with the welfare of children,

WHEREAS mankind owes to the child the best it has to give,

NOW THEREFORE

The General Assembly proclaims this Declaration of the Rights of the Child to the end that he may have a happy childhood and enjoy for his own good and for the good of society the rights and freedoms herein set forth, and calls upon parents, upon men and women as individuals and upon voluntary organizations, local authorities and national governments to recognize and strive for the observance of these rights by legislative and other measures progressively taken in accordance with the following principles:

I. The child shall enjoy all the rights set forth in this Declaration. All children, without any exception whatsoever, shall be entitled to these rights, without distinction or discrimination on account of race, colour, sex, language, religion, political or other opinion, national or social origin, property, birth or other status, whether of himself or of his family.

II. The child shall enjoy special protection, and shall be given opportunities and facilities, by law and by other means, to enable him to develop physically, mentally, morally, spiritually and socially in a healthy and normal manner and in conditions of freedom and dignity. In the enactment of laws for this purpose the best interests of the child shall be the paramount consideration.

III. The child shall be entitled from his birth to a name and a nationality.

IV. The child shall enjoy the benefits of social security. He shall be entitled to grow and develop in health; to this end special care and protection shall be provided both to him and to his mother, including adequate prenatal and postnatal care. The child shall have the right to adequate nutrition, housing, recreation and medical services.

V. The child who is physically, mentally, or socially handicapped shall be given the special treatment, education and care required by his particular condition.

VI. The child, for the full and harmonious development of his personality, needs love and understanding. He shall, wherever possible, grow up in the care and under the responsibility of his parents, and in any case in an atmosphere of affection and of moral and material security; a child of tender years shall not, save in exceptional circumstances, be separated from his mother. Society and the public authorities shall have the duty to extend particular care to children without a family and those without adequate means of support. Payment of state and other assistance towards the maintenance of children of large families is desirable.

VII. The child is entitled to receive education, which shall be free and compulsory at least in the elementary stages. He shall be given an education which will promote his general culture, and enable him on a basis of equal opportunity to develop his abilities, his individual judgment and his sense of moral and social responsibility, and to become a useful member of society.

The best interests of the child shall be the guiding principle of those responsible for his education and upbringing; that responsibility lies in the first place with his parents.

The child shall have full opportunity for play and recreation, which should be directed to the same purposes as education; society and the public authorities shall endeavour to promote the enjoyment of this right.

VIII. The child shall in all circumstances be among the first to receive protection and relief.

IX. The child shall be protected against all forms of neglect, cruelty and exploitation. He shall not be the subject of traffic in any form.

The child shall not be admitted to employment before an appropriate minimum age; he shall in no case be caused or permitted to engage in any occupation or employment which would prejudice his health or education or interfere with his physical, mental or moral development.

X. The child shall be protected from practices which may foster racial, religious and any other form of discrimination. He shall be brought up in a spirit of understanding, tolerance, friendship among peoples, peace and universal brotherhood and in full consciousness that his energy and talents should be devoted to the service of his fellowmen.

Courtesy of the 14th General Assembly of the United Nations and of Children, *Vol. 7. United States Department of Health, Education, and Welfare, Social Security Administration, Children's Bureau.*

The headquarters of this organization are in Geneva, Switzerland.

The objective of the World Health Organization is to assist in the attainment by all peoples of the highest possible level of health. To this end this Organization acts as a director and a coordinating authority on international health work, establishes and maintains effective collaboration with governments and other interested groups, furnishes assistance to countries by providing health information, technical, educational and other services, evaluates a country's health problems when requested, stimulates and advances work to eradicate diseases and to prevent injuries, promotes improvement of nutrition, housing, sanitation and other aspects of environmental hygiene, promotes maternal and child health and welfare, and promotes mental health among its many other functions.

More specifically, the present main objectives of the World Health Organization are to control communicable diseases such as malaria, tuberculosis, leprosy, yaws and the venereal diseases on an international scale, to build up public health organizations in countries that have underdeveloped programs, and to educate and train medical and auxiliary personnel in the health fields.

The activities of the World Health Organization prove that nations can work together for an important cause: the improvement of human health.

The United Nations International Children's Emergency Fund. The United Nations created the United Nations International Children's Emergency Fund (UNICEF) in 1946 for the purpose of meeting the emergency needs of children, such as in times of war or other disasters in countries throughout the world. This Organization assists in the child health and welfare programs in more than fifty countries. Aid to a country is given only when requested and on the basis of need without regard to race, creed or political belief.

The United Nations International Children's Emergency Fund is financed by voluntary contributions from governments, from groups and from individuals. In the United States children collect monies for this Organization by participating in the Halloween Trick or Treat effort. Also, the sale of calendars and greeting and Christmas cards by the United Nations International Children's Emergency Fund has provided funds to send medications and food to many ill and impoverished children throughout the world.

The Children of Today in the United States: Trends and Concepts Related to Their Care

Ours is a complex and changing society. Children, as they grow from infancy in a brief span of time, must learn not only to live happily for today, but also to adjust rapidly to the many unexpected events they will face in their tomorrows.

The social forces that are shaping the world now and will have an impact on the future are varied. One characteristic of society today is its emphasis on speed: in its production of goods, in its mode of travel and in its energetic race to conquer space. Also, the total population in the world, as in the United States, is increasing by leaps and bounds; the total population of children is increasing even more rapidly. This poses problems necessitating planning for all types of education, health services and welfare services needed for children of all races and creeds.

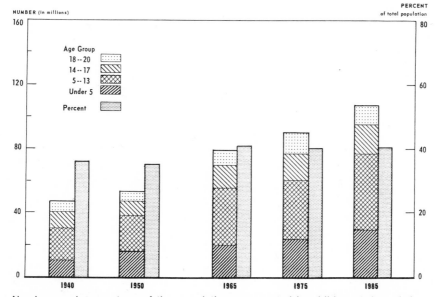

Figure 1-2. Numbers and percentage of the population represented by children and youth from age 0 to 20 years in the United States over a 45-year period. (From Federal Programs Assisting Children and Youth, issued in February 1968 by the Interdepartmental Committee on Children and Youth.)

Typical also of our present society are the uprooting and movement of countless family groups: the migration of families from other lands to our shores, the migration of farm laborers' families to new places of employment, the migration of rural families into the large cities, the migration of middle-class families to the suburbs, and the increase in population of the numbers of urban families that are in the lower income groups.

Partly because of these migrations the *extended family* of a century ago, which included three generations with other relatives living in close geographic proximity, has become fragmented into small *nuclear families* composed of parents, children and perhaps a grandparent. Whereas the extended family was tradition-bound and secure, its members being interdependent one upon the other, today's small family group is largely adrift in a sea of strangers. Attempting to prevent complete disintegration of such small family groups is the responsibility of society's agencies and society as a whole.

Stress has been placed recently on the grinding and binding effects of poverty in our society: poverty of the American Indian, the Negro and the Puerto Rican, as well as the Caucasian in Appalachia and other parts of our country. Federal, state and local governments in the United States are devising ways to break the vicious cause-and-effect circle of poverty at many points. This is essential if all children are to have the opportunity to develop to their greatest potential.

Poverty has as one of its causes the bulldozing of jobs by agricultural mechanization and industrial automation. This increase in mechanization and automation opens new opportunities for technicians and scientists, but results in a dearth of employment for the unskilled labor pool in which some youth without a higher education will stagnate.

Furthermore, the rapid increase in scientific knowledge in the areas of growth and development of children and the causes of illness places the burden especially on the members of the medical profession, who are expected to implement this knowledge with appropriate action. With the current manpower shortage of physicians, nurses and other members of the medical team, adequate implementation for the welfare of all children can hardly be expected to occur.

Federal legislation in the areas of health, welfare and education has snowballed in recent

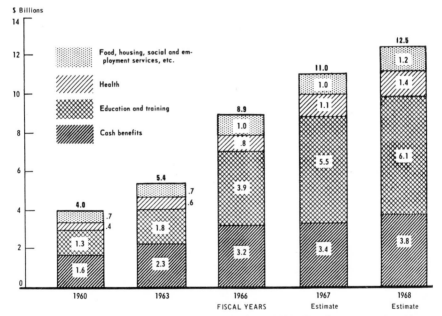

Figure 1-3. Federal expenditures for children and youth since 1960. The figures are based on reports from federal agencies of programs largely for children and young people under 21. Although it shows a steady increase in expenditures during the 1960's, the 1968 figures average less than $153 per child under 21 for the approximately 82 million children in the United States population. In this average, education and training account for $74, and all other programs—including cash benefits and health, nutrition, welfare, employment, housing and other services—account for $79. The 1968 figures are based on the Administration's request for 1968 and not on the much lower congressional appropriation. (From Federal Programs Assisting Children and Youth, issued in February 1968 by the Interdepartmental Committee on Children and Youth.)

years in an attempt to implement some of the results of the Golden Anniversary White House Conference on Children and Youth held in 1960. The federal government has and will continue to expand federally aided programs, will provide even greater support for state services, and will encourage community action on behalf of our children and youth.

In view of these several social forces, the nursing profession has a responsibility with other medical disciplines to create a world in which all children in health and illness will receive optimum care in a secure environment. Some of the ways by which this end can be achieved will be discussed in this text.

The Child in the Community

It is important for the nurse to recognize the great strides that have been made toward the improvement of child care in the community. Such an understanding is essential for her not only as a nurse, but also as a future potential mother and community citizen.

Part of the support which young parents gained from an extended kinship family is now being supplied by federal agencies and privately supported programs. The Children's Bureau has played a vital role in the development of many of these efforts.

One of the most important educational movements in the United States has been the widespread development of programs for culturally deprived children, especially preschoolers. *Project Head Start,* which is sponsored by the Office of Economic Opportunity, has tried to compensate for the cultural deprivation of many thousands of young children between four and six years of age through education and other programs for the disadvantaged. This program was developed because it was recognized that culturally deprived children do poorly in school. As a result of this program, many children's readiness for school and their academic achievement are improved.

In addition, the health goals of Project Head Start are to find and treat existing defects, to assure better health through preventive measures, to educate children and their parents concerning health, and to plan for continuing comprehensive care. Defects of vision and hearing, enlarged or diseased tonsils and adenoids, the presence of allergies, and anemia were found to be the most important problems. Many of the children tested had not been to a dentist, nor had they had adequate immunizations for common childhood diseases. The correction of these problems has not been totally successful. The goals of Project Head Start must be more clearly stated, and more careful community planning

must be done to bring about successful results of these efforts.

Another relatively new project, *Follow Through,* has been initiated for children enrolled in kindergartens and first grades who had been enrolled in Project Head Start and other preschool educational programs. These children will continue to receive special educational attention in the hope of sustaining the intellectual, social and physical gains that had been made by disadvantaged children. This program is administered by the Office of Education with funds provided by the Office of Economic Opportunity.

The *"Rebound" Children and Youth Program,* funded by the Children's Bureau of the United States Department of Health, Education, and Welfare, has as its purposes to find new, effective, yet imaginative ways of meeting the health needs through comprehensive health services of children and youth from disadvantaged families, and to educate, encourage and support their families to become aware of both the health needs of their children and of the resources available. This program has made strides toward achieving these goals in the urban areas where it is in effect.

The Children's Bureau has the responsibility for administering the *Maternity and Infant Care Program,* authorized under the 1963 Maternal and Child Health and Mental Retardation Planning Amendments. This program is concentrating mainly on lowering the incidence of mental retardation caused by prematurity or complications associated with pregnancy. It also provides services to high-risk infants in the form of early treatment to prevent or lighten defects.

During recent years public welfare departments have been attempting to extend the range of services available to children and their families. These services include foster child care, adoption services under public auspices, family counseling, homemaker services, family day care, and protective services for abused or neglected children.

The pressing need of the American Indian and the Alaskan natives for health services has been answered in large part through the efforts of the Division of Indian Health of the United States Public Health Service. This Division is responsible for hospitals, clinics and school health centers. Services provided include public health nursing, dental care, guidance in nutrition, medical social service and special treatment clinics.

Since the Indian population especially is a young one, its most pressing health problems are those of infants and children. The principal health problems of children include accidents, gastrointestinal diseases, tuberculosis and other respiratory diseases, and communicable diseases. The problem of infant and child health is due to the high incidence and severity of infectious disease, the delay in obtaining treatment resulting in secondary complications, and the difficulty in providing preventive medical services. Malnutrition, anemia and poor general environment contribute to the incidence and severity of disease.

Among Alaskan children one of the more prevalent diseases is bronchiectasis. This may be due to repeated inhalation of seal oil during feedings resulting in lipoid pneumonia, frequent lung infections, and bronchiectasis.

Children of migrant farm families are often deprived culturally as well as physically, intellectually and socially. Because of repeated migrations these children have complex needs which can be met only through programs of education, social welfare and medical services.

The initial need of the parents of migrant farm families is for day-care centers where they can leave their children while they work on the farms. The health services provided at these centers depend on local need, interest, professional services and availability of facilities. The common medical needs of these children are for immunizations, improved feeding habits, physical examinations and testing if the children are ill, and correction of problems resulting from ignorance and poverty.

Although most children in the United States are born to citizens of this country, many are being brought into the United States through the process of *intercountry adoptions.* Children who are homeless and face rejection in their native land, such as Korean-Caucasian and Korean-Negro children, may be adopted by American families. Adoption of a child who has probably lacked security in his early life, has lived without one or both of his parents to care for him, places a great responsibility on his new-found parents as he faces a new world, a different language and a very strange culture. Such adopted children can bring added love and joy to a family group if emerging problems are handled with patience and compassion. (The discussion concerning adoption will be presented in Chapter 18.)

School health programs vary, depending on the locale and size of the school. The school nurse may function alone, or she may be a member of the health team consisting of a physician, child psychologist, guidance counselor and social worker. The school nurse's functions may vary from being responsible only for providing first-aid care for children during school hours, to assisting with physical examinations and conducting hearing, vision and tuberculosis screening tests, to checking on immunizations to determine adequacy, to caring for children who have problems such as diabetes or epilepsy, to carrying out sex education programs for children

and sometimes parents as well, to being a health counselor for the families represented by the children in school. The school nurse, then, may be a public health nurse who spends only a brief period of time in the school, or she may be a full-time nurse whose total responsibility is the care of the children enrolled in a particular school.

Camps where normal children may go in the summer for wholesome recreation are located in almost all sections of the country. During the last several years camps have been established also for children having diabetes, cystic fibrosis, orthopedic handicaps, and other conditions. In each camp at least one nurse should be on duty in case of accident or illness. In the camps for the handicapped child, closer medical and nursing supervision is essential for the welfare of the campers.

One of the largest groups of nurses who are active in the community are those employed by public agencies. Since many children having pediatric conditions which required hospitalization a few short years ago are now cared for in the home, public health nurses have a vital role to play in the health of a community's youngest members. Especially needed are nurses who are not only able to give direct care to children, but can also teach such care effectively to the responsible adults in each situation.

Another responsibility which public health nurses assume with other members of the health team is that of implementing the concept of preventive pediatrics. This entails the maintenance of Child Health Conferences (see Chap. 12), immunization against preventable communicable diseases (see Chaps. 12 and 19), education for the prevention of accidents and poisonings (see Chap. 16), case-finding of children evidencing early emotional disturbances so that they can be referred to child guidance clinics or private physicians, and case-finding of children showing signs of physical illness so that they can be referred to the appropriate source for help.

In some communities, centers for the treatment of special conditions have been established, e.g. Poison Control Centers (see Chap. 16), premature infant centers (see Chap. 8), heart centers (see Chaps. 20 and 23) and centers for the diagnosis and treatment of mentally retarded children (see Chap. 20).

Total organized community planning and action are necessary if the needs of all children are to be met. Only by the conscientious effort of persons in many disciplines can optimum physical, emotional, social and spiritual health of all children be achieved.

From the preceeding discussion the student can understand that the nurse has an important role to play in organized community action. She may use her abilities as a health educator, a teacher, a counselor, a research worker, a case finder, and as a compassionate and skilled nurse of the sick.

Parent-Child-Professional Nurse Relations

It is said that the twentieth century is the century of the child. Society realizes that the child is not a miniature adult. His body differs in quality as well as in size from that of an adult. His emotional and intellectual processes and needs are different in degree. These differences make child study a separate discipline in which scientific knowledge in many branches of learning is applied to the care of the child.

The value of the child to society today lies not only in his potential worth as an adult—a parent, a worker in the national economy, a participant in the arts and sciences and in war. The value of the child lies also in his being a child with all the lovable, and sometimes not so lovable, traits of children and the potentially maturing experiences which children, and children alone, provide for parents and all others who care for them. An adult is not mature in the fullest sense of the word until he has developed a capacity for parental love, an unselfish love which finds satisfaction in the happiness of the loved ones. Caring for children can provide an opportunity for adults to develop this form of love.

The care of children day and night, however, can impose too great a strain upon parents and hamper, if not spoil, parent-child relations. When a child is well, a baby-sitter may assist in the care of the child, or if he is old enough he can be taken to nursery school, kindergarten or summer camp.

If the child is ill, a public nurse can come into the home to help the mother with the child's care, or the child can be taken to a hospital for more intensive therapy. *Good mother-child relations are based not on the amount of time they spend together, but rather on the quality of the relation while they are together.*

Few adults working with children are successful in making a child happy unless they themselves find happiness in being with the child. This happiness, however, should not come from their adopting the role of parent substitute. They should provide for the child a sense of security which comes from being with an adult friend who, like mother, does lovingly for the child what he cannot do for himself. The adult who assumes the role of mother to the child, instead of caring for the child only when the mother is unable to provide such care or when she is not present, is not fulfilling the child's real need for the maintenance of close mother-child relations.

The young adult who has known a happy home life and looks forward to marriage, who rates homemaking as of equal value with professional success, is likely to be successful in caring for children. Today there are more parents in professions and more mothers who are professional women than there were a generation ago. Young women today look forward not to the choice between marriage and a profession, but to a combination of marriage and a profession.

One result of the better and more widespread understanding of the emotional life of children is a fuller appreciation of the importance of parent-child-professional woman relations. This, as concerns the nurse, is shown throughout this book.

TEACHING AIDS AND OTHER INFORMATION*

American Academy of Pediatrics
Standards of Child Health Care.

Child Study Association of America
Escalona, S.: Children and the Threat of Nuclear War, 1962.
Weingarten, V.: The Mother Who Works Outside the Home, 1965.

Interdepartmental Committee on Children and Youth
Children in a Changing World (A Book of Charts). Golden Anniversary White House Conference on Children and Youth, 1960.

Project Head Start, Office of Economic Opportunity
Project Head Start, Health Services.

---

* Complete addresses are given in the Appendix.

Public Affairs Pamphlets

Homemaker Services, 1965.

United States Department of Health, Education, and Welfare

Bradbury, C. E.: Five Decades of Action for Children, 1967.
Child Care Arrangements of the Nation's Working Mothers, 1965.
Children in Day Care, with Focus on Health, 1967.
Child Welfare Statistics, 1964, 1965.
Chilman, C. S.: Growing up Poor, 1966.
Cities in Crisis: The Challenge of Change, 1967.
Facts about Children's Bureau Programs, 1965.
Hancock, C. R.: Services under AFDC for Children Who Need Protection, 1965.
Homemaker Service—How It Helps Children, 1967.
Hunt, E. P.: Recent Demographic Trends and Their Effects on Maternal and Child Health Needs
    and Services, 1966.
Interdepartmental Committee on Children and Youth—Seventeenth Year of Work, 1965.
Irelan, L. M.: Low-Income Life Styles, 1966.
It's Your Children's Bureau, 1964.
Kugel, R. B., and Parsons, M. H.: Children of Deprivation, 1967.
Low-Income Families in the Spanish-Surname Population of the Southwest, 1967.
Mental Health of Children, The Child Program of the National Institute of Mental Health, 1966.
Rice, E. P.: Homemaker Service in Maternal and Child Health Programs, 1965.
Services for Children: How Title V of the Social Security Act Benefits Children, 1966.
Some Facts and Figures about Children and Youth, 1966.
The Child Health Act of 1967, December 1967.
The Community Mental Health Center, The Bold New Approach, 1967.

REFERENCES

Publications

Cahill, I. D.: *Child-Rearing Practices in Lower Socioeconomic Ethnic Groups.* New York, Teachers
    College, Columbia University, June, 1966 (Doctoral Dissertation).
Garrison, F. H., and Abt, A. F.: *History of Pediatrics.* Philadelphia, W. B. Saunders Company, 1965.
Ginzberg, E. (Ed.): *The Nation's Children.* 1. The Family and Social Change. New York, Columbia
    University Press, 1960.
Ginzberg, E. (Ed.): *The Nation's Children.* 2. Development and Education. New York, Columbia
    University Press, 1960.
Ginzberg, E. (Ed.): *The Nation's Children.* 3. Problems and Prospects. New York, Columbia Uni-
    versity Press, 1960.
Golden Anniversary White House Conference on Children and Youth, March 27-April 2, 1960: *Con-
    ference Proceedings.* Washington, D.C. Golden Anniversary White House Conference on Chil-
    dren and Youth, Inc., 1960.
Mead, M., and Heyman, K.: *Family.* New York, Macmillan Company, 1965.
Midcentury White House Conference on Children and Youth: *A Healthy Personality for Every Child.*
    Fact Finding Report. Raleigh, N.C., Health Publications Institute, Inc., 1951.
Mid-Decade Conference on Children and Youth: *Children and Youth at Mid-Decade.* Washington,
    D.C., National Committee for Children and Youth, 1967.
Minturn, L., and Lambert, W. W.: *Mothers of Six Cultures.* New York, John Wiley & Sons, 1964.
Neubauer, P. B.: *Children in Collectives: Child-Rearing Aims and Practices in the Kibbutz.* Spring-
    field, Ill. Charles C Thomas, 1965.
UNICEF: *Children of the Developing Countries; A Report by UNICEF.* Cleveland, Ohio, World Pub-
    lishing Company, 1963.
Witmer, H. L., and Kotinsky, R.: *Personality in the Making.* The Fact-Finding Report of the Mid-
    century White House Conference on Children and Youth. New York, Harper and Brothers,
    1952.

Periodicals

Anderson, E. H.: Commitment to Child Health. *Am. J. Nursing,* 67:2076. 1967.
Brewster, B. M.: Extending the Range of Child Welfare Services. *Children,* 12:145, 1965.
Enochs, E. S.: A Report from Abroad; Family and Child Welfare in South Vietnam. *Children,* 13:
    75, 1966.

Ford, L. C., and Silver, H. K.: The Expanded Role of the Nurse in Child Care. *Nursing Outlook,* 15:43, September 1967.

Gans, B.: Some Socio-Economic and Cultural Factors in Western African Paediatrics. *Arch. Dis. Childhood,* 38:1, February 1963.

General Assembly of the United Nations: Declaration of the Rights of the Child. *Children,* 7:74, 1960.

Glasser, P. H., and Navarre, E. L.: The Problems of Families in the AFDC Program. *Children,* 12:151, 1965.

Golden Anniversary White House Conference on Children and Youth. *Am. J. Nursing,* 60:990, 1960.

Kraft, I.: Child Rearing in the Soviet Union. *Children,* 12:235, 1965.

Oettinger, K. B.: A Half Century of Progress for All Children. *Children,* 9:43, 1962.

Oettinger, K. B.: Looking Back and Ahead. *Children,* 12:43, 1965.

Oettinger, K. B.: Youth and Youth Services in England. *Children,* 14:75, 1967.

Schmidt, F., and French, M. I.: White House Conference Followup within the States. *Children,* 9:3, 1962.

Sinclair, A.: The World's Deprived Children. *Children,* 9:84, 1962.

Stearly, S., Noordenbos, A., and Crouch, V.: Pediatric Nurse Practitioner. *Am. J. Nursing,* 67:2083, 1967.

Tieszen, H. R.: A Report from Korea . . . Changes in Services to Children. *Children,* 13:28, 1966.

Who Is To Treat The Whole Family?: *Medical World News,* 8:57, October 27, 1967.

Wiedenbach, E.: Family Nurse Practitioner for Maternal and Child Care. *Nursing Outlook,* 13:50, December 1965.

2

GROWTH AND DEVELOPMENT OF CHILDREN

THE CHILD GROWS WITHIN A FAMILY

Growth and development of the child occur as a result of his hereditary background and the care and love which adults, usually his family, bestow upon him. Although brief mention was made in Chapter 1 of the extended kinship family and its division into smaller nuclear family groups, this concept requires further explanation. More than 200 years ago in this country the child of the pioneers most often grew up within a family which gained its livelihood from the wilderness and from the soil. In such a family several generations lived in the same home or in homes not too distant from each other. The members of the different generations were interdependent upon each other; each family member, no matter how young or old, was recognized as an individual who contributed to the good of all. There was a continuity to life. The young child lived by the rules of his family and of his society. The mores, the values, the traditions were passed from one generation to the next as the children matured.

Although certain members of families remained in rural areas, gradually other family members migrated from the farms to small towns and, as cities grew, moved on to become city dwellers. Over the last few decades some city dwellers have moved out of the congested metropolitan areas and back to the more rural suburbs. This mobility tended to disintegrate the extended families, to submit smaller families and individual family members to a kind of stress unknown to the original, large, self-sufficient family. The stress resulted not only from mobility, but also from the external forces of a changing social and economic order.

The cultural patterns of our present-day society may be defined through broad, overlapping generalizations about contemporary American culture.

The Home

Cultural Patterns: Ethnic Group, Locality, Class, Occupation. There are ethnic groups represented by the few remaining Chinatowns of our large cities, by the Cubans in Florida and by the Puerto Rican and Mexican communities in New York, Chicago and other metropolitan centers, as well as French-Canadian villages in the New England states. The cultural patterns of the middle, southern, eastern and western states differ. Large cities, towns, villages, crossroad neighborhoods and the open country with scattered farms all have characteristic cultural patterns.

In the democratic United States we do not like to speak of people as belonging to an upper, middle or lower class, although there is general recognition that there are class cultures. In general, traits found among college-educated persons are not those of the uneducated.

As professional persons, many nurses are limited in their knowledge of the needs of the poor. The child born into a family of the upper or middle class is, because of the socioeconomic status of his family, likely to have more advantages of good physical care than a child born into a poverty-stricken home. Because of their probable lack of adequate education, parents in the lower-income group are likely not to provide as clean an environment or as adequate care of food substances, with the resulting increased rate of infections and diarrhea, as parents who have had the advantage of better education. Likewise, parents who cannot afford the material advantages of life for their children many times cannot afford adequate medical care for themselves or for their children. Even when they can afford to pay a little for their care, they may be unaware that medical facilities free or at minimal cost are available. Others do not seek assistance even when they know where they can get help at no cost to themselves. The parents and children therefore may suffer from illnesses which could be easily treated if diagnosed early enough. This is not to say that children who do not receive adequate physical care do not receive adequate love. Many times such children during their early years are secure in the knowledge that their parents love them. Unfortunately the effect of poverty on the life of a child may be most intense when he is old enough to venture outside his own home. It is during his years in school that he may compare himself, to his own disadvantage, with others who appear to him to be more fortunate than himself.

Parental characteristics and behavior in general are modeled on those of their group and, specifically, their parents. For instance, physical punishment was characteristically inflicted by immigrants from many countries of Europe, but seldom used among the Chinese or Japanese in places where they retained their native culture. The position of the father and of the mother in the family varies with the customs of the group.

The culture of the ethnic group, the geographic area, urban or rural location, and social class all influence the parents, but are redefined by the *family* itself, that small, closely knit unit of society into which the child is born and in which he is brought up. It is the home culture that is influential in determining the child's growth and development. As he grows older and leaves the home and play group for school and the gang, team, club or clique, home culture is increasingly modified by that of the community.

New Types of Families. In families in which the father is away from home for long periods — e.g. men in the military or maritime service and traveling salesmen — or working in remote areas where it would be impracticable to have their families with them, the mother is likely to be the head of the household. In a modified form the mother as decision maker is found in new settlements on the fringes of large cities. In such families the children rarely see their fathers except on weekends.

The democratic family, in which both parents, and children when they are old enough, participate in making decisions, is the modern type. In this type both parents may work to support the family on a higher level of living than would be possible on the father's salary alone. In an increasing number of youthful marriages the wife works to support or help in the support of the family while her husband finishes his professional education. In former generations a man whose wife worked while he did not was blamed for his behavior and was pitied by her friends. Today it is understood that his education is part of his work — a job which in the long run will provide a standard of living he could not achieve without further preparation.

Another community of young married people has sprung up around military bases. The length of stay at any base is so uncertain that these homes have little of the stability found in civilian community life. But common interests are strong, and such groups are closely knit, often in a town which seldom welcomes them to full participation in its social life.

Young married couples in college or on military bases want children and are willing to make many sacrifices in order to start their families early in marriage. Both parents help in the housekeeping and in the care of the child, fitting their hours of work or study into a schedule which provides for one or the other to be home with the baby throughout the twenty-four hours of the day. When the baby is old enough, he may be placed in a day nursery while his mother is working.

Finally, there are families with a common source of support. Such families are dependent upon some industry and are found in certain sections of many cities. Members of such groups are likely to have many similar social traits.

Incomplete Families. Many children do not live in the type of family built on the love felt between a man and a woman who marry and live to care for their children. There are one-parent families as the result of the death or divorce of a marital partner or as the result of children being born out of wedlock. There are families in which no parents are present in the home, the children being reared by older siblings, grandparents or other relatives. There are children who are cared for by foster parents temporarily or who spend most of their childhood in institutions. Regardless of the relation of the adults to the children, they provide for the young a social and cultural heritage, and a physical climate in which to live. Each member of such a group needs to develop more or less of an understanding of the others and to give and receive love and care from them in order for full development to occur in the individuals and in the group. It is essential for the nurse who seeks to understand the growth and development of any family member, adult or child, to know the identity and role of each member of the group and the interrelation between the individual members.

The Community

The general community pattern of child rearing undoubtedly influences the personality of the older child. He is likely to rate his home, and the way his parents or other adults who care for him treat him, by group standards, and if the home differs widely from the general pattern, he knows it. If all parents inflict physical punishment, the child is apt to accept it as part of the usual parent-child relations. But if he is whipped and yet none of his friends is physically punished, he is likely to blame his parents and feel that they do not love him, that he is abused.

It is in warm home life that the child first learns the meaning of love, of giving up his pleasure because he wants the approval of loving parents. He learns to obey those who are better able than he to understand what should be done in different situations. He transfers this attitude toward authority to his baby-sitter, to neighbors, nursery school workers, nurses and teachers. He adjusts to adult-child relations in a constantly broadening area of social contacts.

THE NURSE'S UNDERSTANDING OF GROWTH AND DEVELOPMENT

The period of growth and development extends from conception to the end of adolescence. It is a complex period during which two cells joined as one normally become a thinking, feeling person who eventually takes his responsible place in society. The nurse should understand this process of growth and development for several reasons.

The nurse must know what to expect of a particular child at any given age and at what age certain types of behavior are likely to emerge in more mature forms. She uses this knowledge to judge each child in terms of norms for specific levels of development. A child may be guided into more mature behavior if the sequence of developmental behavior is understood.

In order for the nurse to help in formulating the plan for total care which the physician and other team members outline for each child, she must know what to expect of different age groups and must know the developmental sequence which occurs throughout childhood and adolescence.

A knowledge of growth and development is important to the nurse so that she may better understand the reason for particular conditions and illnesses which occur in various age groups.

When the nurse has gained experience in applying her study of growth and development in child care, she can teach mothers how to use such knowledge in order that they may help their own children to achieve optimal growth and development.

This chapter, as well as later chapters devoted to growth and development, presents concepts, principles and facts which the nurse should know in order to adapt her care to the needs of children in different age groups. Most ranges of norms for growth and development were established in the past on samples of presumably middle-class Americans. *When average achievement levels are presented for the various age groups, the student must not interpret them as being specific for the development of any one child of a given age. Each achievement may occur normally within a range of time.* The age of a specific achievement given in various tables is usually in the approximate middle of such a range. For example, if the student will refer to page 378, she will note the statement that a toddler walks alone at fourteen months. Actually, the child may normally walk alone at any time in the range between nine and eighteen months of age. The student will probably find it easier to remember specific ages for levels of achievement than trying to remember the limits of ranges within which such achievement can occur.

HEREDITY, EUGENICS AND EUTHENICS

The relatively typical physical pattern of growth and development is influenced by heredity, environment and the child's state of health. The *heredity* of a man and a woman determines that of their children. For this reason the health history of several generations of the families of each of the parents should be studied to determine the hereditary traits likely to exist in the child.

Eugenics is the science that deals with influences that improve inborn or hereditary qualities of the race. Applied eugenics would influence men and women in the selection of marriage partners, helping them to avoid those unions which presumably would produce children below an accepted normal standard and encouraging those which would be likely to produce children above this standard. A few diseases are hereditary, and a tendency to a number of diseases in genetically determined. As has been pointed out, the family history rather than the condition of the child's parents must be studied to determine the probability of a tendency toward a specific disease. Such a study is difficult among the lower-income group, whose health histories are carried by word of mouth, and among some groups whose attitude toward health and illness may be culturally influenced. With the expansion of health work in schools, clinics, public health agencies and occupational health programs, family health histories may become more reliable than they are at present.

Euthenics, in contrast to eugenics, deals with measures to promote health. It concerns itself with healthy intrauterine conditions for the developing fetus and with a wholesome environment not only for children, but also for all age groups.

In hospitals, clinics and public health nursing agencies, mothers as well as students are taught the general principles of child growth and development. They are taught that *each child has a different genetic potentiality for growth and that this potentiality cannot be exceeded, but may be hampered at any stage.* A child who deviates too far from the normal range of height, weight, physical development or behavior should be referred to a physician. The most common cause for concern about a child is a sudden slowing up, not typical for his age, in any aspect of his development. Anticipatory guidance should be given to mothers about changes in the rate of growth and development that can be expected at certain ages.

CHARACTERISTICS OF GROWTH AND DEVELOPMENT

Growth and development are terms often used interchangeably. Each depends upon the other, and in a normal child they parallel each other. But they are not the same. *Growth* refers to an increase in physical size of the whole or any of its parts and can be measured in inches or centimeters and in pounds or kilograms. *Development* refers to progressive increase in skill and capacity of function. The term "maturation" is often used as a synonym for development. *Maturation* has the more limited application, however, of referring to the development of traits carried through the genes. Development is *orderly,* not haphazard; there is a direct relation between each of its stages and the next.

Every child is an individual and should never be considered a typical boy or girl, one unit of a group who are all alike. Each child has his own *rate of growth,* but the *pattern of growth* shows less variability. For example, an infant will be able to sit before he can stand alone. The age at which he as an individual achieves these skills may, as has been mentioned before, occur at any point in a range of time.

Although growth and development – physical, mental, social, emotional and spiritual – proceed at different rates, they are so *interrelated* in the majority of children that the result is a progressive development of the whole child, from infancy to adulthood. Only when growth in any aspect is unusually slow or advanced is this interrelation disturbed so that the child appears abnormal. For example, a boy who at fourteen years of age grows to a height of 6 feet may appear to be physically a man, but emotionally, socially and intellectually he may achieve at a normal pubescent level. Whatever the cause, if a child is notably different from others of his age, he is likely to need help in order to make a good adjustment to home and community life. The child with a long-term illness or a handicap of body or mind also differs from his peers and will need help.

The concept of interrelations in growth is also true for the hospitalized child or one under medical supervision in the home. This is one reason why professional teamwork is important in the care of the ill child. The whole team is needed to foster progression in all areas of development in the hospitalized or home-bound child. Thus the hospital has the school teacher to encourage mental development, and the child care worker (the Play Lady) to create situations in which there may be pleasant social interaction. The psychologist and the psychiatrist help the nurses with the emotional problems of sick children. The dietitian, the physical therapist and all the other members of the team work together, each focusing on a different facet of growth, toward the full development of the whole child. In the home there is the school teacher (visiting teacher), public health nurse, actually all the members of the health team as found in the hospital. Many members of the health team work through the public health nurse. The health team also functions in helping the child make the transition from home to hospital to home.

Stages of Growth and Development

All children go through a normal sequence of growth, but not at the same rate. Nor is the rate the same in all areas. In general, there is a positive correlation between physical growth and mental and emotional development. This may not be true in individual children, of course, and we have learned the danger of attempting to force a child into a standard pattern of growth. There are far too many variations in genetic traits and in the environment to make this possible. The strain upon the child may react upon his personality and even his physical health.

Adults should have a clear understanding of the stages of growth and development so that they can apply their knowledge when caring for children. These stages, listed here, are considered in detail in the chapters on the nursing care of various age groups.

1. Fetal or embryonic—from conception to birth
2. Newborn (neonatal)—from birth to two to four weeks
3. Infancy—from two to four weeks to one year
4. Toddler—from one year to three years
5. Early childhood (preschool)—from three to six years
6. Late childhood (school)—from six to twelve years or puberty
7. Adolescence—from puberty to the beginning of adult life

Norms of Growth

In order to find norms of growth we may study age groups by the *cross-sectional technique* and make a comparison of their average weight, height or other evidence of growth. Consider, for instance, the average height of five-year-olds and of six-year-olds. The difference between these averages is taken as the average growth of a child during his sixth year. In a *longitudinal study* of growth, height and weight of children are followed from birth throughout childhood. Such studies show periods of accelerated growth which correlate with the individual child's stage of maturation. *Spurts of growth* are related to pubescence, which occurs earlier in some children than in others. This acceleration in rate may begin in girls as early as ten years and in others as late as fourteen years; corresponding ages for boys are twelve and sixteen years. An early acceleration in growth is indicative of early puberty. Since the rate slows down a year or two after the onset of puberty, a boy who is late in maturing and ashamed of his small stature and plumpness at thirteen years of age can be told that he is more likely to continue growing than his friend who matured early and is inches taller than he. But a boy who matures early and is shorter than the average for his age is likely to remain short.

The mental, emotional and social aspects of development show the same variations, but are much more influenced by environmental factors than is physical growth. Under conditions of great deprivation, however, as in wartime starvation or prolonged illness or hospitalization, physical growth might be more influenced by environmental factors than mental or emotional development.

Norms or averages of growth must be used with caution, for not only do some children mature early and others late, and thus achieve early or late acceleration in the rate of growth, but also body build and potential height are inherited traits. Because of their heredity some children are short and fat, others of muscular build or medium height, and still others may be tall and slender. Separate norms for each of these three types of body build are of more value than single tables for all children in general.

Study of Growth Patterns

The cross-sectional study of age groups antedated the longitudinal study. From these studies averages were readily compiled. There are disadvantages, however, in their use. These studies did not take into account body build or early and late maturation. At best, in using these schedules, a decision of normality is based on only two gross characteristics: weight and height.

These are inadequate criteria for measuring a child's potential development under existing environmental conditions.

In any consideration of a child's growth the *expected rate of gain* is of greater value than a single measurement taken at any one time. Two examples of growth charts are the *Iowa Growth Charts* and the *Grid-Graph*.

The staff at the University of Iowa produced a series of six charts showing weight-age and height-age for males and females in the age groups of 0 to twelve months, 0 to six years, and five years to eighteen years, based on thousands of observations of children. Figure 2-1 provides an example of an Iowa Growth Chart. The name and birth date of the child are inserted when the record is started. Each time the child is examined, his height and weight are recorded and plotted on the chart. The weight-age is shown in the section at the top of the page, and the height-age at the bottom. The child's progress can be seen in comparison with other children of his height and weight. These forms are easier to use and to read than the more complex Grid-Graph.

In order to measure graphically a child's growth in height and weight, and to record changes in body contours as well, the Grid-Graph was devised. It is based on the assumption that physical development proceeds along regular channels for different body types. The two Grid-Graphs are the Wetzel Grid and the Baby Grid. The Baby Grid is for use with infants from birth to three years, and the other form is for use with children from two to eighteen years of age.

The Baby Grid (Fig. 2-2) is a height-weight gauge of the progress of the individual child.

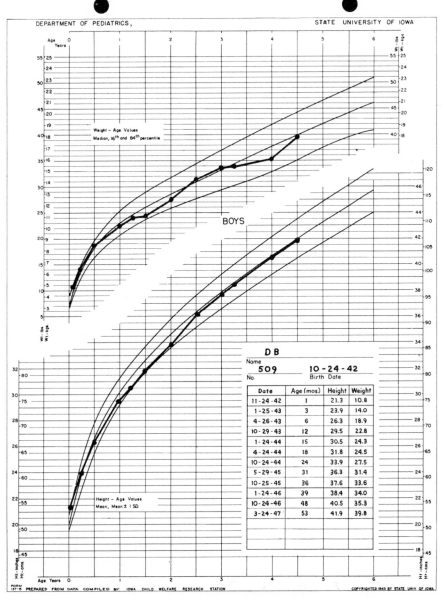

Figure 2-1. Iowa Growth Chart. (From M. E. Breckenridge and M. N. Murphy: *Growth and Development of the Young Child.*)

It has two parts. On the left side of the page is a channel system on which height is plotted against weight. This represents various gradations of build from slender on the right to heavy build on the left. At regular intervals of 10 these channels are crossed by horizontal "developmental level lines," which are actually increment units for development, such as Follows, Smiles, Head Control, through various levels to Speech. On the right side of the page is a grid on which can be plotted developmental levels

against chronologic age with a series of curves or auxodromes which indicate the speed or rate of development for premature, normal and advanced infants. If an infant is healthy and is developing normally, his record will travel channel-wise and will parallel one of the auxodromes. With the use of the Grid it is possible to evaluate how the child is developing in view of his own unique pattern regardless of his physique and growth rate. Thus each child's progress may be predicted from his previous standards, and the

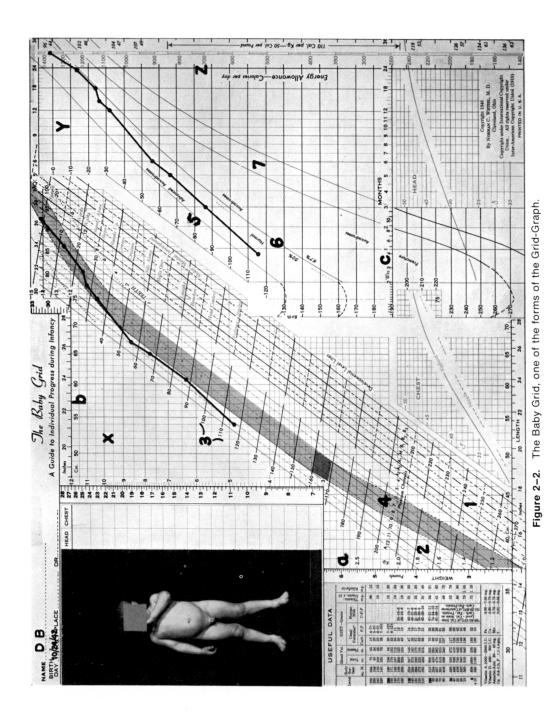

Figure 2–2. The Baby Grid, one of the forms of the Grid-Graph.

physician quickly becomes aware that something is amiss when the growth pattern is distorted. If the infant shifts from one channel to another or lags in his development, he should be examined to determine the cause. The method of use of the Grid for older children is similar to that discussed for the Baby Grid.

The newer tables show more than physical growth and development. These tables include height, weight, number of teeth erupted, carpal bone age, mental age and social age. These criteria can be plotted on a common scale. They show the correlation in measurements of physical and mental growth, i.e. the interrelatedness of growth. In normal growth there is an underlying unity, the presence or lack of which is shown on these graphs.

An adequate clinical history, in addition to the composite chart, is necessary for the proper interpretation of somatic and mental growth. Deviations from the average have no meaning unless factors such as dentition, illness, emotional health and interaction of the social and physical environments are used in interpreting the data.

A newer way by which physical growth patterns can be studied is through the use of *stereophotogrammetry*. Stereophotogrammetry is the production of a contour map of the hills and valleys of the whole human body; thus it is an accurate measurement of physique. This technique is used to measure and understand physiologic differences among people, to observe the growth and development of premature infants and to study the relation between mental retardation and body development. After many children have been measured in this way, a relation may be discovered between the biochemical processes controlling mental development and those controlling body growth.

The *physioprint* is similar in concept except that in this method only the face is measured. This picture is produced by a measured grid projected onto the child's face. The contours, planes, lines and curves of the facial skeletal structure and soft tissues "bend" the pattern on the face into curved lines. This results in a unique contour map of the face, different from anyone else's. The physioprint can register growth changes that can serve as a guide in tooth-straightening and denture-fitting when necessary. It can also aid in the interpretation of family-line transmission of inherited traits.

FACTORS IN GROWTH AND DEVELOPMENT

Growth and development are due not to one factor, but to a combination of many factors, all interdependent.

Heredity and Constitutional Make-up

Embryonic life begins with the cytoplasm and the nucleus of the fertilized ovum, genetically determined by both parents.

Members of families bear physical resemblances, and there is a high degree of correlation of stature with weight among siblings. The rate of growth is more alike among siblings than among unrelated persons. Some children are small not because of endocrine or nutritional disturbances, but because of their genetic constitution. Before evaluating the largeness or smallness of a child, the size of the parents should first be observed.

Racial and National Characteristics

Race

Distinguishing characteristics called racial or subracial developed in prehistoric man. As to height, there are tall and short examples among all races and subraces. Among civilized groups intermarriage has produced mixed racial types.

Nationality. We think of physical characteristics of national groups because the inhabitants of the various nations of Europe tend to be made up of homogeneous subracial groups with specific characteristics. Thus we expect children whose forebears came from the Scandinavian countries to be larger, and those from Sicily to be smaller, than the average American. Yet in America there has been so much intermingling of subracial groups that children with all the typical physical characteristics of any national group are seldom seen.

In studying the changing characteristics of the American people one must consider the influence of immigration. Immigrants frequently established themselves in the United States under conditions of extreme poverty. Their descendants of the second and third generations make up the majority of the middle and upper classes, and the lower-income group is now made up of more recent immigrants.

People from southern and eastern Europe and from Mexico and Cuba predominate among the relatively recent immigrants of the white race. The Puerto Ricans are recent arrivals, and the majority of them hold low-paying jobs. The shortness of stature among these representatives of the white race is a factor in the below-average height of children of the low-income group as compared with children of the middle- and upper-income groups. The latter, as we have noted, came from stock characterized by relatively greater height than the stock from which these more recent immigrants have come. This is not to deny the influence of good diet and of sanitation on children's height, but merely points out that different ethnic groups are likely to have different growth potentials.

Sex

Sex is determined at conception. The male infant is both longer and heavier than the female infant. Boys maintain this superiority until about eleven years of age, when girls, who mature earlier and so reach the period of accelerated growth earlier than boys, are on the average taller than they. Boys, during the prepuberal spurt of growth and thereafter, are again taller than girls. Bone development is more advanced in girls than in boys, as shown in roentgenograms of the wrists of infants and young children. Advance in osseous development is also demonstrated by the earlier eruption of the permanent teeth in girls.

Environment

One example of the influence of environment upon potential height is found among the first and second generations of Japanese in this country. The children are generally taller than their parents because they have had the advantage of better food and living conditions than their parents, who were materially deprived when they came to the United States. A more recent example is that of children whose growth and development were stunted in concentration camps and in poverty-stricken areas in Europe during World War II and who exhibited remarkable improvement upon being removed to better conditions.

Prenatal Environment

Prenatal conditions are part of the environmental climate in which the child develops and should not be forgotten in considering actual development in relation to probable optimal development.

The influence of the intrauterine environment on the child's future development is believed to be great, particularly since the uterus shields the fetus from the full impact of external adverse conditions. On the other hand, the intrauterine environment itself may be substandard. In such a case, if the fetus has reached the stage of viability, early delivery may make it possible to place the infant in a better environment than that of the uterus.

The whole maternal and child care program is changing for the better the environmental influences on the fetus and the young child in the low-income group.

Harmful Prenatal Factors. The prenatal environment is influenced by many factors. The fetus may suffer from nutritional deficiencies when the mother's diet is insufficient in quantity or quality, regardless of her socioeconomic standard of living. There may be mechanical problems due to malposition *in utero.* The mother may suffer from metabolic endocrine disturbances, e.g. diabetes mellitus, which affect the fetus. If it is necessary for the mother to undergo radiation for cancer or other conditions, the infant may be blighted by the treatment. The mother may suffer from an infectious disease during gestation. Rubella (German measles) during the first trimester of pregnancy may lead to abnormal development of the fetus. Other infectious diseases may also affect the fetus, but there is less scientific proof of this. Toxoplasmosis and syphilis during the second and third trimesters adversely influence the fetus. Erythroblastosis fetalis due to Rh incompatibility of the blood types of the mother and the fetus may have a serious influence upon the developing fetus. Commonly, faulty placental implantation or malfunction may lead to nutritional impairment or anoxia. Recent research on smoking has implicated the use of cigarettes by the mother as a possible contributing cause of prematurity. If the mother has had good prenatal care, many of these conditions can be treated, thus ensuring a better prenatal environment for the fetus.

Postnatal Environment

An environment which provides satisfying experiences promotes growth. Since growth and development are interrelated, growth in any one area influences and in turn is influenced by growth in all other areas.

Factors which influence the infant's development are more likely to be of environmental origin than genetic. Among the most important environmental factors are the following.

External Environment. Socioeconomic Status of the Family. The environment in the lower socioeconomic groups is apt to be less favorable than in the middle or upper groups. Parents in unfortunate financial circumstances are less likely to understand the principles of modern scientific child care, they lack money to buy the essentials of health and diet, and often they are unable, unwilling or unsure of how to obtain medical care and hospitalization. Today, however, public health programs and health education programs in schools are gradually assisting such parents to provide better care for their children.

Nutrition. Nutrition is related to both the quantitative and qualitative supply of food elements—proteins, fats, carbohydrates, minerals and vitamins. But the infant's or child's use of a

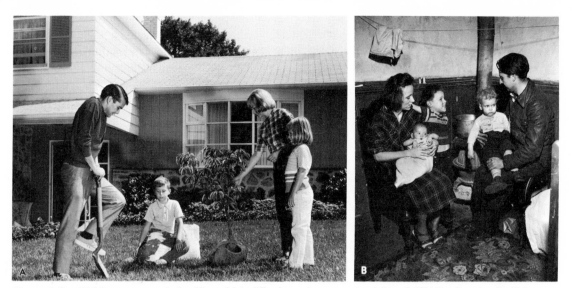

Figure 2–3. Children grow up in families which differ in socioeconomic status. *A*, Middle-class family. *B*, Lower-class family. (H. Armstrong Roberts.)

good diet may be impaired by faulty absorption or assimilation of food substances.

CLIMATE AND SEASON. Climatic variations influence the infant's health. This is not an important direct factor in the United States, since the entire area lies within the temperate zone. Summer heat, however, is important when parents in the lower socioeconomic homes fail to provide adequate refrigeration of food and extermination procedures for flies and other insects. Infants in such families are prone to suffer diarrhea with subsequent dehydration.

The seasons of the year influence growth rates in height and weight, especially in older children. Gains in weight are lowest in spring and early summer and greatest in late summer and autumn. The greatest gains in height among children in the United States occur in the spring.

ILLNESS AND INJURY. Illness and injury, with their accompanying debility and nutritional impairment, have a great influence on weight and some influence on growth.

EXERCISE. Exercise promotes physiologic activity and stimulates muscular development, and fresh air and moderate sunshine favor health and growth. Prolonged exposure to sunshine, especially in extremely warm areas such as the southwestern section of the United States, may cause tissue damage and even more serious consequences if the child is unprotected from the rays of the sun.

ORDINAL POSITION IN THE FAMILY. The child's position in the family is a factor in development for several reasons, among them the following: (1) Children learn from older siblings, and this is an advantage which an only child or the oldest

child lacks. (2) The youngest child may be relatively slow in certain areas of development because he is given little encouragement to express himself. He is the baby and is petted by the whole family. (3) The only child is likely to develop more rapidly along intellectual lines than the average child because he is constantly with adults and is mentally stimulated by their companionship. Like the youngest child of a family, he may be slow in motor development, however, because he has so much done for him. When he is old enough to do things for himself, his parents and other relatives may not permit him to do so.

Internal Environment. INTELLIGENCE. Intelligence is correlated to some degree with physical development; i.e. the child of high intelligence is likely to be better developed than the less gifted child. Intelligence influences mental and social development.

HORMONAL BALANCE. Hormonal balance in the young child is important. Normal secretions of the endocrine glands promote normal growth of the body.

EMOTIONS. Emotional disturbances influence growth, since the disturbed child neither sleeps nor eats as well as one who is happy and contented.

TYPES OF GROWTH AND DEVELOPMENT

Physical Growth

Physical growth includes many things, among them the following.

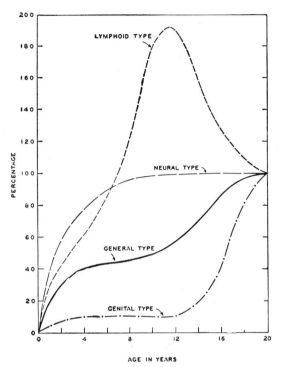

Figure 2-4. Main types of postnatal growth of the various parts and organs of the body. (After Scammon: *The Measurement of the Body in Childhood, The Measurement of Man* University of Minnesota Press.)

Changes in General Body Growth. Changes result from different rates of growth in different parts of the body during the consecutive stages of development. For example, the infant's head size is one fourth of the entire length of the body at birth, whereas the adult's head size is only one eighth of his length. Growth during childhood is primarily linear; growth in adolescence is both linear and in the nature of a filling-out process until adult proportions are reached.

The pattern of general physical growth and types of organic growth are shown in Figure 2-4. From this illustration it can be seen that the rate of growth in general is most rapid during infancy and during puberty and adolescence. The rate of neural growth is most rapid before school age, when it gradually levels off. The rate of growth of lymphoid tissue is rapid until approximately the age of twelve years, when it gradually declines. The rate of genital growth is slow until puberty and adolescence, when it increases rapidly.

Head Circumference. The circumference of the head is important, since it is related to intracranial volume. An increase in circumference permits an estimation of the rate of brain growth.

This measurement has a relatively narrow normal range for a particular age group.

Thoracic Diameter. Chest measurements increase as the child grows and the shape of his chest changes. At birth the transverse and anteroposterior diameters are nearly equal. The transverse diameter increases more rapidly than the anteroposterior diameter; i.e. the width becomes greater than its depth.

Abdominal and Pelvic Measurements. The abdominal circumference is not fixed by the bony cage as is the chest and consequently is affected by the infant's nutritional state, by muscle tone, gaseous distention and even the phase of respiration. The pelvic bicristal diameter (the maximal distance between the external margins of the iliac crests) is not affected by variations in posture and musculature. The pelvic bicristal diameter is a good index of a child's slenderness or stockiness.

Weight. Weight is influenced by all the increments in size and is probably the best gross index of nutrition and growth. There is a wide variation within normal limits for each year of childhood. Excess weight in relation to the height and pelvic diameter is as abnormal as underweight. It may be the result of a glandular deficiency, but is more likely to be due to overeating or to a diet containing too much starch and fat and too little protein.

Height. Yearly increments in height diminish from birth to maturity. The pubescent spurt is the only exception to this downward trend in the rate of growth. There is great variation in the yearly increases in stature among children of the same age. Some children reach adult height in their early teens, but others continue to grow throughout late adolescence. The periods of most rapid growth are infancy and puberty.

Development of Muscular Control

Muscular control does not develop evenly throughout the body. In human beings it follows the spine downward—termed *cephalocaudal*—and in addition proceeds from the *center of the body to the periphery.* The result is that the child holds up his head before he sits. The large muscles of the arms and legs are subject to voluntary control sooner than the fine muscles of the hands and feet. As the child matures, *general movements become specific.* For example, he can use the whole hand before he can pick up a small object with the pincer grasp, i.e. between thumb and forefinger.

There is a normal sequence in the development of manual dexterity and for the stage of locomotion, just as there is for mental development and for emotional and social adequacy. A child should be given the opportunity for learn-

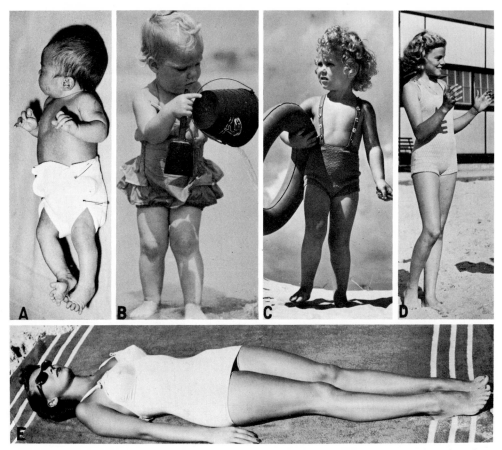

Figure 2–5. Body proportions change during the period of growth. The head size, trunk length and extremity length differ in (A) the newborn, (B) 18-month-old, (C) 3-year-old, (D) 11-year-old and (E) 18-year-old. (H. Armstrong Roberts.)

ing—by either experience or instruction—whenever he is ready to acquire the skill or learn by indirect experience through instruction from others. If these opportunities are presented prematurely and the child is urged to make use of them, he is apt to learn slowly; if too late, he is apt to learn rapidly, but may never acquire the same skill or proficiency he might have had

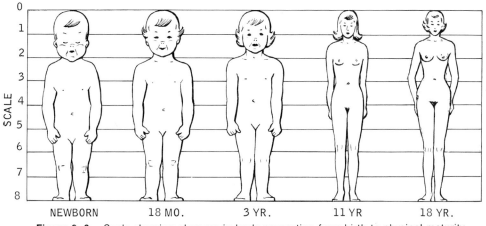

Figure 2–6. Scale showing changes in body proportion from birth to physical maturity.

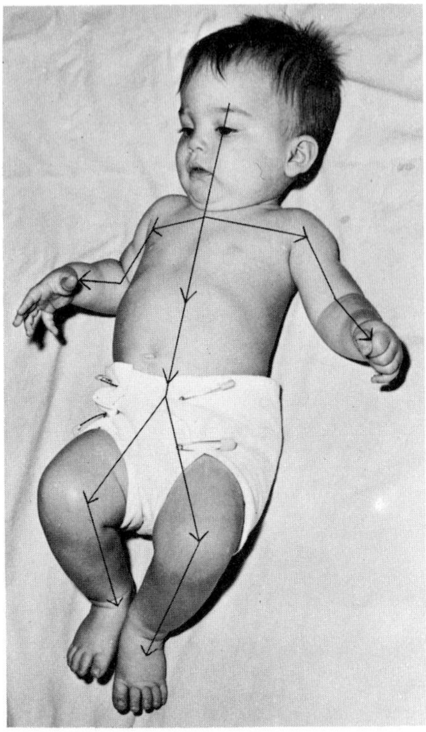

Figure 2-7. The development of muscular control proceeds from head to tail (cephalocaudal) and from the center of the body to the periphery.

if the opportunity for learning had occurred at a more auspicious time. Coincidental acquisition of a skill along with others of his age group is probably more important to a child's personality development than his ultimate proficiency in that particular skill. For example, the child who is physically unable to walk until six years of age has been an atypical child among other children and in his relations with adults. This influence on his personality may be more important than its final effect on his ability to walk, run, dance and perform other activities.

On the other hand, disability during the preschool years may have no permanent effect upon a child. Children often have a remarkable resilience in regard to factors which theoretically would hinder their normal personality development. This is often seen in children who have been denied learning opportunities because of sickness or the stultifying regime of institutional life. An important factor which may determine the effect of a disability on a child is the attitude of the parents and others around him, those *significant persons* who influence his own attitude toward himself and his disability, and his ability to cope with the situation.

Mental Development

Tests of intelligence and mental development have been standardized, much like the standards for growth and development derived from longitudinal and cross-sectional studies in height and weight for children of different ages. There is no foolproof way of measuring the potential development of the genetically carried trait of intelligence, but among children with comparable environmental backgrounds such as those from the middle class the standardized intelligence tests are valuable in predicting capacity for intellectual development. Such tests are used in the school system. They are useful in determining whether achievement is comparable to innate ability.

Mental development depends on numerous factors. It is demonstrated in problem solving and in a general understanding of what to do in a given situation. It is important to let the child solve those problems which he is able to solve by himself and to teach him how to solve problems that are within his ability, but in which he lacks the necessary experience and practice. It is also important to solve for him those problems which are too difficult for him so that the patience of both child and adult will not be affected by his lack of success. By the time the child is a year old he should be in the process of learning decision-making himself and of accepting the decisions of those adults in whose love he feels secure.

The initial problems with which a baby is confronted are physical ones, and he is helped in their solution by the normal reflex actions of his body. The first problem is ingestion of milk. Sucking at the mother's breast and swallowing the milk are processes which require little or no practice to perform successfully. The newborn at the breast for the first time may have difficulty in getting hold of the nipple and may sputter and choke as the colostrum or milk begins to flow. But he soon learns, for he has many opportunities to practice sucking.

An infant learns to want a smiling mother because she does pleasant things for him. An early problem, then, is to make mother smile. He learns not to do those things which make her say in a decisive voice, "No, no," and frown at him.

A small baby is more adept at solving his problems than we are likely to realize, and the behavior which gets him what he wants becomes habitual. Habits can be broken, of course, but the process is difficult for both the infant and the adults about him. He should be helped to the correct solution of a problem, so that he finds pleasure not only in the behavior itself, but also in the social reward of having others pleased with him. Some adults believe that continuous, on-going attention to the infant is "spoiling" him. In reality this is meeting his normal needs and is helping him with his problem-solving efforts. The infant who receives an inadequate amount of real affection must cry to get it because he soon realizes that it is the only way to get attention of any kind. No child is more to be pitied than the crying child. He is robbed of the birthright of children, that of being loved by an increasingly widening circle of adults and accepted in the play groups of his peers.

Thus, although potential mental ability is inherited and fixed at birth, the rate and extent of its development, as measured by any one of the many mental tests, are very much influenced by a child's environment.

Determination of Level of Mental Development

As the structure of the nervous system grows during the prenatal period, rudimentary beginnings of the mind grow with it. As the child develops after birth, changes occur in his mental reactions that show progress from the ability to respond to the simplest stimuli toward functioning in more complex ways. Although mental development is continuous, it may be more rapid in one age period than in another.

Intelligence can be defined as the ability to adjust to new situations, to think abstractly or to profit from experience. Tests of intelligence are of many types. During infancy and early childhood such tests are likely to be of the performance type. The child is asked to manipulate testing materials or to demonstrate his motor ability. Such tests show the general level of intelligence, but do not accurately predict the child's later intellectual attainment.

When the child is able to communicate verbally, verbal intelligence tests may be given; when he is able to write (i.e. in the school age and adolescent groups), individual or group written tests may be used. There is a higher degree of consistency in intelligence test results from the age of five onward than for tests given during the preschool period.

Meaning of the Intelligence Quotient

The intelligence quotient (I.Q.) can be defined as the ratio between the child's chronologic age and his mental age as gained from an intelligence test. The formula for computing the intelligence quotient is as follows:

$$\frac{\text{Mental age}}{\text{Chronologic age}} \times 100 = \text{I.Q.}$$

Since mental maturation is usually reached between the ages of sixteen and twenty-one years, the mental age of the adult cannot be computed in this way. The age of sixteen years has been arbitrarily chosen as the adult's chronologic age. For example, if an adult passed all the questions in the test designed for a twelve-year-old child, his I.Q. would be 75. In the event of a perfect score in the sixteen-year test, his I.Q. would be 100, or normal.

An I.Q. between 90 and 109 is usually considered to be normal or average. The I.Q. of individual children may range above or below this point. Children with an I.Q. of 140 or over are called gifted children, and those with an I.Q. of less than average represent retardation of varying degrees.

Emotional Development

Personality is not a specific attribute, but the quality of any person's total behavior (Woodworth). Two attributes of a healthy personality in adult life are the ability to love and the ability to work.

Stages of Personality Development

Emotional or personality development is a continuous process. In each stage of a child's emotional development there is a central problem which must be solved. These problems are never completely solved, however. If each problem is fairly well solved at the child's particular stage of development, the basis for progress to the next stage is firmly laid. Proper guidance and the solution of the sequence of problems are necessary at each stage of development if functional harmony is to be secured in adult life.

No child succeeds or fails completely in attainment of the goal to be reached at a particular point in his personality development. For example, the child does not learn to trust completely or never to mistrust. Every child leaves the period of infancy with habits of both trust and mistrust. Also, children who achieved a sense of trust initially may have periodic regressions to mistrust when unfortunate circumstances occur later in life. Health of personality is determined by the preponderance of the favorable attitudes and by the kinds of compensations a child develops to take care of his disabilities.

A general, over-all view of the stages in emotional or personality development according to Erik H. Erikson, a psychologist and trained psychoanalyst, is given here. Further discussion will follow in later chapters.

Birth to One Year (Infancy): Sense of Trust. A baby learns to trust the adults who care for him, the mother first, for it is she who is sen-

Table 2–1. *Stages of Personality Development*

STAGE	APPROXIMATE AGE	PSYCHOSOCIAL CRISES	SIGNIFICANT PERSONS	TASKS
Infancy 0–1		Sense of trust vs. mistrust	Maternal person	Getting Tolerating frustration in small doses Recognizing mother as distinct from others and self
Toddler 1–3		Sense of autonomy vs. shame and doubt	Parental persons	Trying out own powers of speech Beginning acceptance of reality vs. pleasure principle
Preschool 3–6		Sense of initiative vs. guilt	Basic family	Questioning Exploring own body and environment Differentiation of sexes
School 6–12		Sense of industry vs. inferiority	Neighborhood School	Learning to win recognition by producing things Exploring, collecting Learning to relate to own sex
Puberty and adolescence . . . . 12–?		Sense of identity vs. identity diffusion	Peer groups and out groups; models of leadership	Moving toward heterosexuality Selecting vocation Beginning separation from family Integrating personality (altruism, etc.)
Late adolescence and young adult . . . . —		Sense of intimacy and solidarity vs. isolation	Partners in friendship, sex, competition, cooperation	Becoming capable of establishing a lasting relationship with a member of the opposite sex Learning to be creative and productive

Based on Erikson: *Childhood and Society.*

sitive to his needs and shows her trust in him.

One Year to Three Years (The Toddler): Sense of Autonomy. The infant develops from a clinging, dependent little creature into a human being with a mind and a will of his own. If a child succeeds in the developmental task of this stage in his maturing process, he will have a degree of self-control not caused by fear, but by his feeling of self-esteem. If he does not succeed, he will doubt his own worth and that of others, and will have a sense of shyness and shame.

Three to Six Years (The Preschool Child): Sense of Initiative. The child at this age wants to learn what he can do for himself. He has an active imagination. He imitates adult behavior and wants to share in their activities. He wants the experience of following his will to the extreme limit. The adult can help prevent the ac-

companying sense of guilt such behavior may bring by imposing necessary limits on undesirable behavior and by providing a climate for exploring new learning experiences which are desirable. The positive, maturing outcome of this force within him is a sense of initiative, delineated by conscience or superego which is developed from parental attitudes and their examples. The negative outcome is a personality overwhelmed by guilt.

Six to Twelve Years (School Age): Sense of Industry. Children in this age group have a strong sense of duty. They want to engage in tasks in their social world which they can carry out successfully, and they want their success to be recognized by adults and by their peers. It is a calm period in which the basis is laid for later responsible citizenship. Society reaches the child directly through the school system and educates him not only in the three R's, but also in the fundamental skills of living in modern society. Children learn skills of workmanship and the ability to cooperate and to play fairly according to the rules. The danger of this period is the development of a sense of inferiority if the parents or the school expects a level of achievement which the child is unable to attain.

Twelve Years (Beginning of Adolescence): Sense of Identity. The sense of identity develops during adolescence. The adolescent wants to clarify who he is and what his role in society is to be. His attitude toward life is, "What will this mean to me?" Success in this period brings self-esteem, an attitude toward the self that is essential to the normal breaking away from dependency upon his parents and to planning for his future. The danger is self-diffusion, for he faces at the time and in his dreams of the future a life full of conflicting desires, possibilities and chances. The childhood sense of belonging because "he always has belonged" is lost in the necessity of changing from childhood dependency to adult responsibility for his own actions and those of others who are dependent upon him. He may, under adverse circumstances, develop a sense of "not-belonging."

Late Adolescence: Sense of Intimacy. After puberty, youths outgrow the "gang age," that age when they find it essential to belong to a group of their own sex and age. Boys are likely to lose interest in scouting, and girls in cliques of their own sex. In adolescence, youth develops a sense of intimacy with individuals of his own and of the opposite sex, and with himself. If a youth is not certain of his identity, he is afraid to have personal relations with others. Success in this period means union with the essence of others and a communion with their own resources. Failure to establish such intimacy results in psychologic isolation — keeping relations with others on a formal basis which lacks warmth. This is likely to result in failure in all the steps in intimacy which lead to selection of a marriage partner ("dating," courtship and engagement) and to satisfaction in marriage.

Evaluation of Emotional Development

Tests of emotional and social development are less concrete than those dealing with physical or mental development. They are more likely to be used in therapy than elsewhere, although they are useful in planning the physical environment and the activities and qualifications of the personnel in institutions dealing with children.

Professional people working with children should be as familiar with these tests as they are with tests of physical growth and development, for a child's environment must be planned to meet all his interrelated needs, physical, mental, emotional and social.

Evaluation devices for measuring emotional or personality development are of several types. Such tests attempt to compare a child's stage of development with that of children of the same age and to show whether he is suffering from some type of personality maladjustment. The results of such tests are not too accurate, since personality is complex and cannot be easily evaluated.

Specific examples of such devices are rating scales, self-appraisal questionnaires, projective techniques such as finger or easel painting, play activities, the Rorschach test, and others. The *Thematic Apperception Test* is one of the most inclusive tests and is frequently used in the diagnosis of generalized anxiety or behavior problems in children.

Social Development

Socialization, or social development, means training a child in the culture of the group. Personality traits can be divided into two classes: social and cultural. *Social traits* are those found in the well adjusted members of every group; they are traits which are necessary to group survival, such as willingness to sacrifice present comfort for future benefit, and, even more important, individual cooperation with group efforts for group benefit. This social characteristic is altruism. Love and consistency in training are necessary in order to socialize a child. Obviously, there are varying degrees of socialization.

Cultural traits are those which vary with the culture of different groups. Child care is a cultural trait in all groups, but the particular way in which a child is cared for is a social trait and is not the same in any two cultures.

A newborn infant is not a social being. This fact may be illustrated by the few authenticated cases of children carried off by wild animals — presumably lactating and capable of carrying a child and keeping it alive. None of these children when found showed the personality characteristics of socialized human beings; they were not socialized according to the definition given above, nor did they behave according to any human culture pattern.

Factors in Social Development

The Play Group. Learning to live happily with adults is quite different from making friends with children of his own age. In general the adult-child relation is one in which the child learns to live within certain restrictions set by loving adults even though at times these restrictions may not be consistently imposed. It is probably a good thing that children do not have perfect parents, nor parents perfect children: family life would be too unrealistic.

Adults do not compete with a child on his own level for the things he wants. When children and adults disagree, it is usually a matter of the adult telling the child to do or not to do something the child does not want to do or is determined to do.

A child who adjusts well with adults may be unable to get along with other children. An only child who has no playmates finds it particularly difficult to learn the give and take of childish play. The teachers in nursery school will help him acquire the technique of getting along with other children. It may be a slow process. The adult who feels that it is easy to make the transition from being the only child in the home to being one among fifteen or twenty others in the nursery school is mistaken. Many nursery school teachers suggest that the child's mother stay with him for the first few days until he has made friends among the other children and thinks of the school as a pleasant place to be in. Eventually he learns to be one of his group, either a leader or a follower, depending on what he can contribute to the group's success in the particular activity in which it is engaged. In the play group or team and even in the gang, leadership springs less from physical superiority—fighting, running, playing ball—than from thinking up interesting activities when the group does not know what to do with itself. The child who can think up activities agreeable to the group, "sell" his ideas to them and lead them to a successful culmination of the project is likely to become their leader.

As a child becomes engrossed in activities with his age group he does not love his parents less, but is less dependent on them for physical care, emotional support and a system of values. He becomes more self-reliant and learns how to use the resources of his group and community resources organized by adults for youth or for all age groups. He is preparing to take the responsibility of marriage and founding a home. Parents become dependent upon him as he matures and as they grow older. He slowly learns to take his place in the economic life of the country and fulfill his role as a citizen.

Summary

Heredity places limits upon development. But as we learn more about a child's needs, we are able to increase the influence of environment. A child needs an environment which provides satisfying experiences. A child desires to repeat happy experiences in which he exercises his growing ability to secure the things he wants and to do the things he strives to perform. Happiness may come only from the satisfaction of having and doing, but even at an early age happiness is likely to be influenced by the approval of other people, as shown in the smiling face, the pleasant sound of the voice and physical caresses.

The child learns most of his fears as he connects unpleasant direct experiences with people and things, or fear is communicated to him by adults or by children who are themselves afraid. Adults may condition him to fear this or that in order to secure obedience. Common examples of this are such warnings as, "The policeman will get you if you do that," or, "You'll get sick and have to go to the doctor or, worse, the hospital if you go without your coat," and the injunction, "You will hurt yourself," often uttered to secure obedience rather than to help the child to learn prudence in his play and to exercise good judgment in new situations.

As far as possible, little children should be shielded from unhealthy sources of anger or undue anger. They need exposure to normal anger. The child and the parent can learn to discuss it and cope with it together. The child learns that it is not he that the parent does not love when the parent becomes angry, but the act of the child. He thus learns that a parent or any other person can love him and at the same time be angry with him for what he has done.

A baby learns at a surprisingly early age the consequences of his behavior in a sequence of acts within a social situation in which he may be the center of attention of both father and mother. When he wants his feeding, he cries for it, and his mother comes and gives it to him. Hunger is a physical need, but its relief is social in the sense that someone must give the baby his feeding. These social experiences are fully as important as experiences with the physical world about him—e.g. that his rattle is fun to suck and that it makes a nice sound when shaken. Both types of experience help a baby to mature mentally, emotionally and socially. Since they involve physical activity and other needs for growth, they serve to further the whole process of maturation.

In her contacts with children the nurse sees the result of all these factors we have considered under physical, mental, emotional and social growth and development. Every child is an individual; no two children are exactly alike. General statements of growth and development must be modified in the light of individual characteristics. But until the nurse knows the child well enough to adapt her care to his individual needs, concepts of growth and development typical of his age group will help her to meet those needs.

Throughout this book general concepts are

developed in relation to the various age groups —from the neonatal through the adolescent period—whose nursing care in health and in disease is under consideration.

PARENTAL ATTITUDES TOWARD GROWTH AND DEVELOPMENT

The old idea of child care was to bring up the child on a strict regimen of food, sleep and play. He was overprotected. The strict routine protected him from accidents and health hazards, but prevented him from acquiring the ability to adapt to life outside of the area controlled by his parents. He could not build up resistance to infection, though infection was prevalent in the society in which he was to take an increasingly active part as he grew out of babyhood into childhood and then adolescence. The overprotected child whose mother claimed that he had never had a cold or sore throat was likely to suffer from a series of severe respiratory infections when he entered school. He did not use good judgment when crossing the street or in climbing or in games which taxed his physical skills. He was apt to be accident-prone when removed from the shelter of his home. He had rigid likes and dislikes for foods and was reluctant to try new dishes. Unless he was in his own bed he could not go to sleep easily or adapt to hours of sleeping other than his accustomed periods. He was indeed geared to a strict regimen which was possible only at home, and was not prepared for even a gradual entry into community life.

Parents were likely to demand that such a child, whom they had allowed little self-direction, should direct himself successfully in school and on the playground. Boys, particularly, were expected to fight their own battles, become leaders in their age group, never come home crying to mother, and in general suddenly change from overprotected, overdirected, obedient little boys in the home to schoolboys who showed ability to get along, if not to lead, in their own age group.

This era of the authoritative, overprotective parent was followed by the trend toward permissiveness. The infant was to be placed on a self-demand schedule of feedings; he was to be offered an unlimited amount of his feeding whenever he was hungry and was to take as little or as much as he desired. The toddler was to choose his own diet from wholesome foods and was never urged to eat. Naps were to be taken when he was sleepy; he was never led, rebelling, to bed. He was never punished. The adult as far as possible permitted him to do what he wanted to do and trusted to the natural consequences of his behavior to show him what was the logical thing to do in problem situations. This attitude was likely to create an inconsiderate child, making heavy demands on the time and patience of his parents. Such a child may be so unaccustomed to discipline of any sort that he is resentful of the necessary restrictions of hospital life.

The newer idea is that the child must be prepared to take his place in the world and to live in a state of workable adjustment with his physical and social environment. He is to be treated as an individual, but as one who has not yet developed to the point at which he can decide what is best for him or recognize the rights of others, and therefore must be subject to parental control or that of the nurse, school teacher or any adult responsible for his care.

As a child grows, parents must learn to view him and themselves differently. Parental attitudes toward a child's growth may be poorly formed because they do not know what to expect of their child and they do not know what his real needs are at various stages of his development. Nurses many times can interpret growth and development to parents and thus alleviate much of their misunderstanding about the process.

Parents are influenced also by the "child" each of them used to be. It is not easy to change each parent's view of his or her own background experiences in childhood. Some parents retain within themselves the children they used to be and see things as though their past home situations still existed. At the same time parents are also looking at the same situations through an accumulation of adult experiences. Parents then see their children as they would a blurred photograph, using a camera which was out of focus. The phases through which a parent progresses as the child grows will be discussed in appropriate chapters throughout this text.

THE NURSE'S ATTITUDES TOWARD GROWTH AND DEVELOPMENT

The attitude of the nurse toward children and the specific manner in which she views child growth and development are dependent, among other things, on the way she herself was reared and on the total knowledge and experiences she has had with children both in her own family and outside of her family. If her own home life was reasonably happy and her experiences with children were satisfying, her attitude toward children in general will probably be a more positive one than if she herself had an unhappy childhood and equally unhappy experiences with other children.

In order to work effectively with children the nurse must become aware of her own thinking in regard to parenthood itself, the role of parents and children, and the family as an institution. The nurse is sometimes inclined to minimize the role of the father in the family constellation and to work only with the mother when planning for the child.

The nurse should also recognize her own cultural attitudes. Many nurses, though able to aid effectively parents and children from the middle class, have difficulty in assisting patients and their parents from the lower socioeconomic groups. This is due to the fact that nurses themselves are primarily middle-class-oriented and have some difficulty in understanding those different from themselves.

In addition the nurse must be perceptive and sensitive to the specific problems of children and their families. In order to develop this sensitivity the nurse must be aware of her own emotional drives so that she can effectively work with mothers of all ages. She should understand her own feelings about authority versus permissiveness so that she can work effectively with the pediatric age group. If the student finds that she is having problems in this area or feels uncomfortable in working with children, she should discuss this matter with her instructor or her counselor. It is unfortunate but usually true that a student who is moody and unhappy caring for children will generally bring unhappiness to the children themselves because of her lack of sensitivity to their needs and their sensitivity to those around them.

The student, finally, must develop a warm and sympathetic yet flexible attitude toward her caring for children. She must realize that in dealing with either normal or problem behavior, a solution based on the child's needs with full recognition of her own feelings about it will usually be most satisfactory, one which will help the child in his movement along the road to maturity and herself in dealing with future problems in this area.

TEACHING AIDS AND OTHER INFORMATION*

American Medical Association

Can Food Make the Difference?
Education of Children for the New Era of Aging.

Child Study Association

Behavior: The Unspoken Language of Children.
Mayer, G., and Hoover, M.: Learning to Love and Let Go; A Guide to Helping Children Become
     Independent, 1965.
Redl, F.: Are Parents Worrying About The Wrong Things?
Wolf, K. M., and Auerbach, A. B.: As Your Child Grows: The First Eighteen Months, 1966.
Wolf, A. W. M., and Dawson, M. C.: What Makes a Good Home?

Mental Health Materials Center

Building Self-Confidence — How Can I Help My Child?
How to Know Your Child.

National Association for Mental Health

What Every Child Needs for Good Mental Health.

National Conference of Christians and Jews

Eagan, J. M.: Rearing Children of Good Will, 1966.

National Society for Crippled Children and Adults, Inc.

Frantzen, J.: Toys . . . The Tools of Children.

Public Affairs Pamphlets

Hunt, J. McV.: What You Should Know about Educational Testing.
Osborne, E.: Democracy Begins in the Home.
Thorman, G., and Neher, J.: Toward Mental Health.
Wolf, A. W. M.: Your Child's Emotional Health.

Ross Laboratories

How to Be a Parent — And Like It.
Seeing Your Children in Focus.
The Phenomena of Early Development.

---

* Complete addresses are given in the Appendix.

United States Department of Health, Education, and Welfare

Hymes, J. L.: A Healthy Personality for Your Child, Reprinted 1966.
Mead, M.: A Creative Life for Your Children, 1962.
Research and Training Programs of the National Institute of Child Health and Human Development, 1965.
Research Relating to Children, Bulletin 20, 1967.
Research Relating to Children, Bulletin 21, 1967.

REFERENCES

Publications

Almy, M. C., Chittenden, E., and Miller, P.: *Young Children's Thinking.* New York, Teachers College, Columbia University Press, 1966.
Babcock, D. E.: *Introduction to Growth, Development and Family Life.* 2nd Ed. Philadelphia, F. A. Davis Company, 1966.
Baldwin, A. L.: *Theories of Child Development.* New York, John Wiley and Sons, 1967.
Bernard, H. W.: *Human Development in Western Culture.* 2nd Ed. Boston, Massachusetts, Allyn & Bacon, Inc., 1966.
Bossard, J. H. S., and Boll, E. S.: *The Sociology of Child Development.* 4th Ed. New York, Harper, 1966
Breckenridge, M. E., and Vincent, E. L.: *Child Development. Physical and Psychologic Growth Through Adolescence.* 5th Ed. Philadelphia, W. B. Saunders Company, 1965.
Child Study Association: *Children of Poverty; Children of Affluence.* New York, Child Study Association, 1967.
Cooper, L. F., Barber, E. M., Mitchell, H. S., and Rynbergen, H. J.: *Nutrition in Health and Disease.* 14th Ed. Philadelphia, J. B. Lippincott Company, 1963.
Dinkmeyer, D. C.: *Child Development: The Emerging Self.* Englewood Cliffs, N.J., Prentice-Hall, 1965.
Duvall, E. M.: *Family Development.* 3rd Ed. Philadelphia, J. B. Lippincott Company, 1967.
Erikson, E. H.: *Childhood and Society.* New York, W. W. Norton and Company, 1964.
Falkner, F. (Ed.): *Human Development.* Philadelphia, W. B. Saunders Company, 1966.
Gesell, A., and Ilg, F. L.: *Child Development.* New York, Harper and Brothers, 1949.
Ginzberg, E. (Ed.): *The Nation's Children.* 2. Development and Education. New York, Columbia University Press, 1960.
Hurlock, E. B.: *Child Development.* 4th ed. New York, McGraw-Hill Book Company, Inc. 1964.
Kagan, J., and Moss, H. A.: *Birth to Maturity: A Study in Psychological Development.* New York, John Wiley and Sons, Inc., 1962.
Kidd, A. H., and Rivoire, J. L. (Eds.): *Perceptual Development in Children.* New York, International Universities Press, 1966.
Landreth, C.: *Early Childhood Behavior and Learning.* 2nd Ed. New York, Alfred A. Knopf, 1967.
Maier, H. W.: *Three Theories of Child Development.* New York, Harper and Row, 1965.
Mussen, P. H., Conger, J. J., and Kagan J. (Eds.): *Readings in Child Development and Personality.* New York, Harper and Row, 1965.
Smart, M. S., and Smart, R. C.: *Children.* New York, Macmillan Company, 1967.
Stott, L. H.: *Child Development.* New York, Holt, Rinehart and Winston, 1967.
Watson, E. H., and Lowrey, G. H.: *Growth and Development of Children.* 5th Ed. Chicago, Yearbook Medical Publishers, Inc., 1967.
Whipple, D. V.: *Dynamics of Development: Euthenic Pediatrics.* New York, McGraw-Hill Book Company, Inc., 1966.
Wickes, F. G.: *The Inner World of Childhood: A Study in Analytic Psychology.* Revised Edition. New York, Appleton-Century, 1966.
Winnicott, D. W.: *The Family and Individual Development.* New York, Basic Books, Inc., 1965.
Witmer, H. L., and Kotinsky, R.: *Personality in the Making.* The Fact-Finding Report of the Mid-century White House Conference on Children and Youth. New York, Harper and Brothers, 1952.

Periodicals

Baumrind, D.: Parental Control and Parental Love. *Children,* 12:230, 1965.
Brody, S.: The Developing Infant. *Children,* 13:158, 1966.
Burchinal, L. G., and Cowhig, J. D.: Rural Youth in an Urban Society, *Children,* 10:167, 1963.
Caldwell, B. M., and Richmond, J. B.: The Impact of Theories of Child Development. *Children,* 9:73, 1962.
Carner, C.: Are We Rejecting Our Creative Children? *Today's Health,* 42:21, February 1964.
Close, K.: Cuban Children away from Home. *Children,* 10:3, 1963,

Close, K.: Giving Babies a Healthy Start in Life. *Children,* 12:179, 1965.

Davis, D. C.: Predicting Tomorrow's Children, *Today's Health,* 46:32, January 1968.

Dittmann, L. L.: A Child's Sense of Trust. *Am. J. Nursing,* 66:91, 1966.

Frankenburg, W. K., and Dodds, J. B.: The Denver Developmental Screening Test. *J. Pediat.,* 71:181, 1967.

Gentry, E., and Paris, L. M.: Tools to Evaluate Child Development, *Am. J. Nursing,* 67:2544, 1967.

Hosely, E.: Culturally Deprived Children in Day Care Programs. *Children,* 10:175, 1963.

Hunt, J. M.: How Children Develop Intellectually. *Children,* 11:83, 1964.

Isler, C.: The Psychological Tests and Their Uses. *RN,* 30:60, May 1967.

Leavitt, S. R., Gofman, H., and Harvin, D.: A Guide to Normal Development in the Child. *Nursing Outlook,* 13:56, September 1965.

Mead, M.: The Changing American Family. *Children,* 10:173, 1963.

Murphy, L. B.: Spontaneous Ways of Learning in Young Children. *Children,* 14:210, 1967.

Olshin, I. J.: Problems in Growth. *Pediat. Clin. N. Amer.,* 15:433, 1968.

Pollak, O.: Some Challenges to the American Family. *Children,* 11:19, 1964.

Rubin, R.: Food and Feeding: A Matrix of Relationships. *Nursing Forum,* VI:195, Spring 1967.

3

ILLNESS AND
THE CHILD

THE DIFFERENCES IN ILLNESS
IN CHILDREN AND ADULTS

The child's body is building up to maximum development rather than being at a plateau of physical fitness or in the stages of decline. The exact age of the peak of the process of bodily repair is not known, but repair does seem to decrease after eighteen to twenty years of age. If the statement that physical adolescence ends with the eruption of the wisdom teeth is correct, this is a concrete example of the last of the building-up process of the teeth. It is true, however, that decay may occur long before this time.

Even though the child is not yet mature, he lacks the reserve forces which the adult has. Such lack is shown in an easily upset electrolyte balance, sudden elevation or lowering of temperature, rapid spread of infection and destruction of body tissue.

The differences in illness in children and adults are based on the anatomic, physiologic and psychologic differences between the immature child and the mature adult.

Anatomic differences between the newborn and the adult are obvious. Size is the outstanding difference; it influences the method and equipment used in caring for the child. A more specific anatomic difference between them is the greater size and weight of the newborn's head when compared with body length and weight. This characteristic, coupled with his immature motor development, makes handling of the infant quite different from that of the older child or adult. Injury can occur to the head of the infant due to falling as a result of the adult's being unable to handle the child properly.

The sutures of the skull in the newborn are not united; the brain is not protected by the skull in the areas of the open fontanels. The infant's bones are neither as firm nor as brittle as those of the older child. Thus, when intracranial pressure develops in the infant, his head simply enlarges as the sutures separate. This is not possible in the adult, who exhibits other indications of increased intracranial pressure.

The normal shape of the head and the chest of the infant can be altered by constant pressure from lying in one position. The parent or the nurse must move the infant frequently so that the child's bones will not become deformed.

In the adult the cardiac sphincter of the stomach is usually fairly tight. In the infant it is more relaxed. This is one of the reasons why vomiting in infancy is so frequent and why so many adults have difficulty vomiting even when they are nauseated.

Certain diseases are influenced by the interaction of anatomic development with physiologic development. An example of such a disease is infection of the middle ear (otitis media), a condition often occurring in young children when they have a sore throat, because the eustachian tube is both shorter and straighter than that of the older child or adult.

The student will find many other examples of disease related to anatomic development of the child throughout the units of this text.

The differences in the *physiologic processes* of the newborn infant and of the older child or adult are less obvious than the anatomic differences. But the physiologic characteristics of an age group are more important in the adaptation of nursing care to needs than are the anatomic ones, since they are subject to greater control by medical and nursing procedures. For example, some blood values of children different from those of adults are shown in Tables 3-1 and 3-2.

Physiologic development influences the little child's susceptibility to certain diseases, the symptoms of disease and the probability of lasting harm. The infant or small child requires a greater caloric and fluid intake in proportion to his weight than does the older child, because of his need to support growth, and to carry on physical activity and basic metabolic functions. Any pathologic condition which causes loss of fluid, e.g. diarrhea or fever, quickly alters the electrolyte balance. Also, when replacing the lost fluids and electrolytes intravenously, the anatomic and physiologic ability of the small child to absorb fluid slowly necessitates careful regulation of the rate of flow. If fluid were injected intravenously into the infant at the same rate it usually is given to the adult, the child would soon have pulmonary edema.

Important among the differences in the occurrence of illness in children and adults is their resistance to disease. The infant derives from his mother a short-lived immunity to certain infectious diseases. Immunization against the contagious diseases he is likely to contact must be given early in infancy, since many of these diseases may be fatal or cause permanent impairment of bodily functions.

In general the symptoms of disease in an infant and in an older child or adult are different, owing to the pathologic state caused by the injurious agents on tissues in different stages of development. It is important in pediatric nursing to learn the cause-effect relation of any pathologic agent to the developmental stage of the child's body, in order to give preventive and curative nursing care and to be prepared for any emergency. For instance, infants and very young children may have convulsions due to the elevation of temperature accompanying the onset of a contagious disease, whereas an older child or adult is likely to have a chill preceding the fever at the onset of an infection.

Mental and emotional reactions to illness differ in various age groups. Both objective signs (those which can be observed) and subjective symptoms (those which cannot be observed and are known only to the person who experiences them) are important in comprehensive nursing. Since the infant and the young child cannot tell how they feel, the nurse is compelled to rely solely on signs. She must know both what to expect and the full meaning of her observations.

The older the child, the more successful he is in communicating symptoms to the nurse. Although an infant cannot tell how he feels, and does not localize pain as an older child will do, he may pull at an aching ear, or cry when some part of his body is moved. Such behavior provides an objective sign of a subjective symptom. These

Table 3-1. *Average Normal Blood Cell Values*

	AT BIRTH	AT 2 DAYS	AT 14 DAYS	AT 3 MONTHS	AT 6 MONTHS	AT 1 YEAR	AT 4 YEARS	AT 8–12 YEARS
Red cells/c.mm. (in millions)	5.1	5.3	5.0	4.3	4.6	4.7	4.8	5.1
White cells/c.mm. (in thousands)	15.0	21.0	11.0	9.5	9.2	9.0	8.0	8.0
Platelets/c.mm. (in thousands)	350.0	400.0	300.0	260.0	250.0	250.0	250.0	250.0
Differential Smears: *Percentages* Polymorphonuclear neutrophils	45	55	36	35	40	40	50-60	60
Eosinophils and basophils	3	5	3	3	3	2	2	2
Lymphocytes	30	20	53	55	51	53	40	30
Monocytes	12	15	8	7	6	5	8	8
Immature white cells	10	5	–	–	–	–	–	–

Adapted from W. E. Nelson: *Textbook of Pediatrics*, 1964.

Table 3–2. *Normal Blood Values*

Base, total fixed cations (Na + K + Ca + Mg)	(Serum)	150–155	mEq./liter
By methods of Hald and Sunderman, normal values tend to be lower		143–150	mEg./liter
Sodium*	(Serum)	136–143	mEq./liter
Potassium*	(Serum)	4.1–5.6	mEq./liter
Calcium*	(Serum)	10–12	mg./100 ml.
Chlorides* (Cl)	(Serum)	98–106	mEq./liter
At birth and during early infancy the plasma (serum) chloride is 6–10 m.Eq./liter higher than that of older infants and children		585–620	mg./100 ml.
ph at 38°C	(Blood, plasma or serum)	7.3–7.45	
The sample must be protected against loss of CO_2 and determination made as soon as possible. Arterial blood in a resting person is about 0.03 pH unit higher than venous blood			
Carbon dioxide content	(Serum from venous blood)	45–70 / 20.3–31.5	vol. per cent / mM./liter
The CO_2 content is lower at birth and rises slightly during the first 4 days of life			
Oxygen saturation	(Whole venous blood)	60–85	per cent
Blood of newborn		30–80	per cent
Hemoglobin			
At birth	(Whole Blood)	17–20	gm./100 ml.
3 months		10.5–12	gm./100 ml.
1 year		11–12.5	gm./100 ml.
5 years		12–13	gm./100 ml.
10.		13–14	gm./100 ml.
Above 10 years		14–16	gm./100 ml.
Methemoglobin	(Whole blood)	0.0–0.3	gm./100 ml.
Premature infants at higher level		(0.4)	
Sugar, fasting			
(Somogyi-Nelson)	(Blood)	60–90	mg./100 ml.
Under fasting conditions capillary or arterial blood and venous blood are nearly the same			
Sugar, fasting arterial (Folin-Wu)	(Blood)	80–120	mg./100 ml.
fasting venous (Folin-Wu)	(Blood)	70–100	mg./100 ml.
Total cholesterol (over 6 yr.)	(Serum)	150–250	mg./100 ml.
Infants		70–125	mg./100 ml.
Newborn		50–100	mg./100 ml.
Bilirubin	(Serum)	0.2–0.8	mg./100 ml.
Higher in newborn		1.0 or more	
Conjugated bilirubin (direct)		0–0.3	mg./100 ml.
Icterus index		4–6	units
Total protein (from nitrogen determination)	(Serum)	6.5–7.5	gm./100 ml.
At birth the protein level is slightly lower			
Nonprotein nitrogen	(Whole blood)	25–40	mg./100 ml.
Urea nitrogen	(Whole blood)	7–15	mg./100 ml.
	(Plasma)	10–17	mg./100 ml.
Creatinine	(Serum)	0.4–1.2	mg./100 ml.
Phenylalanine	(Serum)	0.7–4.0	mg./100 ml.
Prothrombin time (Quick)	(Plasma)	12–15	seconds
Bleeding time		1–3	minutes
Coagulation time (test tube method)		3–9	minutes
Cephalin flocculation	(Serum)	0–1+	units

*In human red blood cells an average concentration of sodium would be about 21 mEq./liter of red blood cells; of potassium about 86 mEq./liter.

The level of calcium in serum is influenced by the concentration of serum protein because part of the calcium is associated with or bound to the protein. Practically all the calcium in blood is in the plasma.

The chloride concentration of whole blood depends largely on the cell volume, since the erythrocyte contains approximately half as much chloride as serum.

Adapted from W. E. Nelson: *Textbook of Pediatrics,* 1964.

signs are important; to learn their meaning is an essential part of pediatric nursing. An older child may use signs of discomfort or pain—whether he feels pain or not—as an attention-getting device. The infant under a year of age does not do this, and behavior indicating pain in a young infant should never be ignored.

The sudden changes in the condition of a sick or injured child, coupled with this inability to express how he feels, mean that the nurse must be constantly on the alert for signs and symptoms of aggravation of or improvement in his condition. She must also be alert for symptoms which may be important to the physician in making a diagnosis or altering a tentative diagnosis.

Appreciation of the psychosomatic influence on diseases peculiar to or occurring in childhood is relatively new. It ties in with advances in the study of child psychology and child psychiatry. In these circumstances the child's emotional state interacts with his physical state to a greater degree than is commonly the case. Charting of physical symptoms means little to the physician in judging the implications of a sudden change in a child's condition unless the nurse also charts his *behavior*. Description of behavior enables the physician to draw conclusions as to the cause of symptoms which may be due to emotional rather than physical factors. Adults verbalize an emotional state as a child does not. Nurses are apt to chart behavior which causes trouble, but not that of a quiet child who has retreated within himself. The latter may be more important than the former, however, in determining the true meaning of a change in symptoms.

A child may face certain critical situations alone with no one to protect him. He may fall and hurt himself when no one is about. A child whose clothing has caught fire may be badly burned while he himself puts out the flames and waits, suffering, for help. But these crises are relatively temporary and evolve out of and merge into other, less fearful situations. Even the injured child cries for his mother and appears to think that with her coming he will feel much better.

But some children, like some adults, do suffer generalized states of anxiety in which a troubled past appears to be ever-present in their consciousness and present pleasures seem only a prelude to unpleasant things to come. But even the most anxious child usually knows that pleasant things sometimes happen. A realistic view includes factors which mitigate the severity of any experience. Children who are too anxious, however, need psychiatric help, in which the nurse plays an important role.

The child's attention span is short but intense. It can be shifted from his bodily discomfort to something pleasant in the environment. Naturally his attention is soon shifted again to his physical condition, and fresh pleasant stimuli should be provided. Above all, he must not be allowed to feel that he is alone in his difficulties. This does not mean that someone must be constantly with him, but rather that he must learn from experience that someone is thinking of him and will come now and then or whenever he cries or calls for help. One advantage for the older children of hospitalization, care in an insititution for convalescent or chronically ill children, or a school for handicapped children, is that he sees others who have problems not too different from his own. An egocentric younger child in such situations not only may gain no support from the presence of other children, but also may fear that what happens to them may happen to him.

Children are apt to plead a physical excuse for not doing things they do not want to do. When a child says that he has a "tummy ache" at school time, but is all right as soon as it is too late to go, he should not be scolded. The adult should view the situation as the child views it and understand that such behavior is meaningful to the child. The important thing is to determine and to resolve any problems the child might be having in relation to school attendance. Children under five or six seldom invent excuses of this kind. With them the problem is to have them report when they do feel physically ill.

Infants and little children are, in general, better patients than adults are because (1) they live in the present, easily forgetting the past and not concerned with the future; (2) their attention span is short; and (3) they are readily interested in other bodily sensations—sights, sounds, a bit of something sweet, the motion of being rocked, or sucking a finger. This apparent transience of discomfort often deceives an inexperienced nurse; she feels that the child's condition is improving. She should, of course, endeavor to amuse the child, but she should not necessarily regard his response as evidence that the cause of pain or discomfort has abated.

TYPES OF ILLNESSES OF CHILDREN

Many specific illnesses such as appendicitis or pneumonia seen in adults are also seen in children. But children, because of their immaturity and the various stages of growth and development through which they pass, are prone to acquire conditions not seen in adult medical practice.

Congenital anomalies such as atresia of the esophagus, imperforate anus or omphalocele, among others, are structural anomalies present at birth, due, it is believed to the faulty interaction between genetic and environmental factors *in utero*. Surgery is now being used successfully to treat anomalies in children who a decade or so ago would have died. Some congenital anomalies such as polycystic kidneys are compatible with life and may not be recognized until childhood or adult life.

Conditions of the newborn such as erythroblastosis fetalis or mucoviscidosis are unknown in adults because the children are either successfully treated prior to adult life, or they die before they reach maturity.

Nutritional disorders are seen more commonly in infancy than later in childhood or adulthood because of the child's rapid growth during the first year of life. Examples of deficiency diseases are rickets and scurvy.

Young children, because of their intense activity, their insatiable curiosity and their immaturity, have more *accidents* such as scalds and falls, and *poisonings* from medications or household solutions than do adults. Lead poisoning from ingestion of lead paint occurs more commonly in the toddler group because of their desire to bite on hard surfaces such as painted crib rails.

Emotional disturbances of children, whether neurotic traits, conduct disorders, psychosomatic disturbances or psychoses, appear to be increasing in incidence among the pediatric age group.

Malignancies, such as leukemia, brain tumor, Wilms's tumor or bone tumor, are seen in children, but they are not as common as in the adult.

Some *illnesses related to the process of growth and development,* such as failure to thrive and acne vulgaris, are seen during the pediatric years.

Infections are extremely frequent causes of concern during childhood, since the infant and the child do not have the immunity to many of them that adults have. Respiratory infections are especially frequent during the years of growth. The child is exposed to many infections when he goes to kindergarten and to school. This is not necessarily unfortunate, since he can thus build up his immunologic defenses against them at an early age.

Diseases and other pathologic states common in children of various age groups are considered in the following chapters. Some of these conditions are acute in one age group and do not extend into other periods of life. Other conditions have their origin during one period and extend into later life. The various conditions found in children are grouped in this book according to the age level when they most commonly occur or when they are of greatest significance to the child and his family.

The student will see that the nursing care of each condition is based on (1) the anatomic, physiologic and psychologic development and the growth factor normal to the age group and on (2) the treatment (preventive or curative) of each disease. This is all the assistance which a textbook can give the student. Adaptation to the needs of the individual child is made at the bedside under the guidance of the instructor.

MORTALITY AND MORBIDITY

Mortality Rates

The older a child becomes, the greater are his chances for survival. The risk of dying on the first day of life is many thousands of times greater than the risk of any day during the school years. Each age group among children is particularly affected by certain factors of a bad environment, is more or less susceptible to certain diseases and is exposed to varying accident hazards. Table 3-3 shows the causes of death

Table 3-3. *Infant Mortality Rates for Leading Causes of Death among Infants: United States, 1956 and 1966*

CAUSE	1956	1966	PERCENT CHANGE
All causes	259.9	237.1	− 8.8
Postnasal causes:			
Postnatal asphyxia and atelectasis	43.4	38.7	− 10.8
Influenza and pneumonia, except pneumonia of newborn	20.7	19.3	− 6.8
Certain infections of early infancy	11.1	9.8	− 11.7
Diseases of the digestive system	10.7	6.6	− 38.3
Ill-defined diseases peculiar to early infancy, including nutritional maladjustment	9.3	28.4	+205.4
Accidents	8.4	8.6	+ 2.4
Infective and parasitic diseases	4.0	3.0	− 25.0
Prenatal and natal causes:			
Immaturity, unqualified	49.3	36.7	− 25.6
Congenital malformations	37.7	33.8	− 10.3
Birth injuries	27.7	19.7	− 28.9

All rates are per 10,000 live births.
Department of Health, Education, and Welfare, United States Public Health Service, National Center for Health Statistics.

during infancy, and Table 3-4 during the remainder of childhood and early adolescence.

The *infant mortality rate* is an expression of the ratio of deaths for infants under one year of age in any given period of time to the number of births during the same period. In other words, it is the number of deaths per 1000 live births. The *neonatal mortality rate* indicates the mortality rate for the first month of life.

The infant mortality rate has declined dramatically since the beginning of this century. In the United States in 1900 it was approximately 200 per 1000 live births. In the first six months of 1967 the infant mortality rate had dropped to an all-time low of 22.9 per 1000 live births. Although this rate is relatively low, the United States still has a higher infant death rate than several other nations. Sweden, for instance, has the lowest infant death rate: 12.4 deaths per 1000 live births.

Although among the Alaskan natives a few years ago the infant mortality rate was 54.8 and among the American Indians was 35.9, still the greatest problem of infant mortality in the United states is concentrated among the nonwhites in big city slums. In some ghetto districts the rate is markedly higher than it is in other areas of the country. If fifty or so of the worst areas were excluded, this country's infant mortality rate would drop abruptly.

The main causes of our failure to have a lower infant death rate are premature birth and inadequate prenatal care. Since lack of prenatal care increases the incidence of prematurity, more emphasis should be given to improved maternity care programs. Such facilities as prenatal clinics must be located in areas accessible to the lower socioeconomic groups.

Years ago the leading cause of death among infants was intestinal disturbances due to bacteria in milk and food. In hot summer weather babies from congested slums suffering from infectious diarrheas filled the pediatric units. Many were not brought to the hospital until they were moribund. Strict control of the production and handling of milk sold by dairies and stores, inspection of food and places in which food was sold or served and the availability of electric refrigeration resulted in a lessening of this once leading cause of infant mortality. Infectious diarrhea still occurs, but it is not as prevalent as it once was.

Another great killer of infants was and still is respiratory infection. Morbidity and mortality from respiratory diseases following contagious diseases have been reduced through immunization programs, which have greatly decreased the incidence and severity of the contagious diseases of childhood. If a respiratory infection does occur, antibiotics are available for use against either a primary or secondary infection. As soon as a substance can be found to stimulate the human body to produce interferon, a protein normally produced by body cells to limit the spread of virus infections, chemicals to control these infections may be used as commonly as antibiotics against bacterial infections.

The principal causes of infant deaths in recent years have been immaturity and other prenatal and natal causes, asphyxia and atelectasis, congenital malformations, birth injuries, influenza and pneumonia, and certain other infections.

During childhood the mortality rates gradually decline so that the total mortality for the period from one through four years of age is greater than that for the period from five through fourteen years of age. The principal causes of deaths of children between one and fourteen years of age in recent years were accidents (except motor vehicle), motor vehicle accidents, malignant neoplasms—including leukemia, influenza, pneumonia and congenital malformations.

Table 3–4. *Death Rates for Leading Causes of Death among Children Aged 1–14: United States, 1956 and 1966*

CAUSE	1956	1966	PERCENT CHANGE
All causes	67.8	57.1	−15.8
Accidents, except motor vehicle	14.9	13.6	− 8.7
Motor vehicle accidents	8.8	10.1	+14.8
Malignant neoplasms	8.4	7.0	−16.7
Influenza and pneumonia, except pneumonia of newborn	6.6	4.5	−31.8
Congenital malformations	6.1	4.9	−19.7
Diseases of heart	1.6	1.0	−37.5
Gastritis, duodenitis, enteritis and colitis	1.4	0.7	−50.0
Symptoms and ill-defined conditions	1.1	1.1	0.0
Meningitis, except meningococcal and tuberculous	1.1	0.8	−27.3
Vascular lesions affecting central nervous system	0.8	0.7	−12.5
All other causes (residual)	16.9	12.7	−24.9

All rates are per 100,000 children aged 1–14.
Department of Health, Education, and Welfare, United States Public Health Service, National Center for Health Statistics.

Morbidity Rates

The *morbidity or illness rates* are, of course, much higher than the mortality rates for children in each age group. According to a Children's Bureau survey as reported in *Illness among Children,* the average boy or girl in the United States has three episodes of acute illness each year. Respiratory conditions are the chief cause of acute illness among children. Approximately one out of five children has at least one chronic condition such as an allergy or respiratory ailment, or some other chronic illness. The rate of illness from chronic conditions increases with age.

As to the hospitalization of children, nonwhite children are hospitalized much less frequently than white children, but when they do go to the hospital, they usually stay longer. As the income of a family increases, the rate of hospitalization of the children increases, but the average length of stay decreases. Rural children are hospitalized less frequently than city children, but they tend to stay longer.

Dental caries is the most common physical defect among school children; however, half of the children under fifteen years of age have never been to a dentist. Even among those receiving dental care, many are not receiving adequate care. Again, children from white, nonfarm, and higher income families receive more dental care than do children from nonwhite, farm, and low-income families.

The drop in the mortality and morbidity rates from contagious diseases in all age groups is proof of the value of research in medicine. Immunization is now possible against many of the former diseases of childhood. One type of infection, however, whose incidence is seemingly on the increase is that caused by *Staphylococcus aureus.* No immunization procedure has yet been found to prevent the spread of infection caused by this organism.

Statistics show that there is a class differential in morbidity and mortality rates among children. The unhygienic environment of children in the low-income groups is reflected in the higher death rate among them as compared with that of children in the middle- or upper-income group in the same age brackets. This is due both to the parent's lack of education in matters pertaining to health and also to their inability to pay for the things that make for good health: adequate diet, good housing, clothing, recreation and adequate medical attention. The health professions must assume the responsibility for educating these parents in the care of their children and the need for medical care when illnesses occur. Medical care and hospitalization are usually provided without charge or at a minimal fee to those who are unable to pay fully for them; however, many do not even today know how or will not take advantage of these opportunities to improve the health of their children.

TEACHING AIDS AND OTHER INFORMATION*

Association for the Aid of Crippled Children

Baumgartner, L., Eliot, M., and Verhoestraete, L.: The Challenge of Fetal Loss, Prematurity, and Infant Mortality.

Canadian Mental Health Association

Suddenly It Happens—Your Child Is Ill.

United States Department of Health, Education, and Welfare

Accidents and Children, 1963.
Changes in Mortality Trends in England and Wales, 1931-1961, 1965.
Infant and Perinatal Mortality in Scotland, 1966.
Infant and Perinatal Mortality in the United States, 1965.
Infant Mortality Trends, United States and Each State, 1930-1964, 1965.
International Comparison of Perinatal and Infant Mortality: The United States and Six West European Countries, 1967.
Mortality of White and Nonwhite Infants in Major U. S. Cities, 1966.
Physician Visits, Interval of Visits and Children's Routine Checkup, United States, July 1963–June 1964, 1965.

---

* Complete addresses are given in the Appendix.

Report of the International Conference on the Perinatal and Infant Mortality Problem of the United States, 1966.

Schiffer, C. G., and Hunt, E. P.: Illness Among Children, 1963.

The Facts of Life and Death, 1968.

REFERENCES

Publications

Catzel, P.: *The Paediatric Prescriber.* 3rd ed. Philadelphia, F. A. Davis Company, 1966.

Conn, H. F. (Ed.): *Current Therapy, 1967.* Philadelphia, W. B. Saunders Company, 1967.

Cooke, R. E., and Levin, S. (Eds.): *The Biologic Basis of Pediatric Practice.* New York, McGraw-Hill Book Company (Blakiston Books), 1968.

Dublin, L. I.: *Factbook on Man: From Birth to Death.* 2nd ed. New York, Macmillan Company, 1965.

Ellis, R. W. B., and Mitchell, R. G.: *Disease in Infancy and Childhood.* 5th ed. Baltimore, Williams & Wilkins Company, 1966.

Fry, J.: *Presenting Symptoms in Childhood.* London, Butterworth and Company, 1962.

Gairdner, D.: *Recent Advances in Paediatrics.* 3rd ed. Boston, Little, Brown and Company, 1965.

Gellis, S. S., and Kagan, B. M. (Eds.): *Current Pediatric Therapy, 1966-67.* Philadelphia, W. B. Saunders Company, 1966.

Gellis, S. S. (Ed.): *The Year Book of Pediatrics — 1966-67.* Chicago, Year Book Medical Publishers, Inc., 1967.

Green, M., and Richmond, J. B.: *Pediatric Diagnosis; Interpretation of Signs and Symptoms in Different Age Periods.* 2nd ed. Philadelphia, W. B. Saunders Company, 1962.

Gustafson, S. R., and Coursin, D. B. (Eds.): *The Pediatric Patient/1967.* Philadelphia, J. B. Lippincott Company, 1967.

Illingworth, R. S.: *Common Symptoms of Disease in Children.* Philadelphia, F. A. Davis Company, 1967.

Kennedy, R. H. (Ed.): *Emergency Care of the Sick and Injured.* Philadelphia, W. B. Saunders Company 1966.

Nelson, W. E. (Ed.): *Textbook of Pediatrics.* 8th ed. Philadelphia, W. B. Saunders Company, 1964.

Shirkey, H. C. (Ed.): *Pediatric Therapy.* 2nd ed. St. Louis, C. V. Mosby Company, 1966.

Silver, H. K., Kempe, C. H., and Bruyn, H. B.: *Handbook of Pediatrics.* 7th ed. Los Altos, California, Lange Medical Publications, 1967.

Stowens, D.: *Pediatric Pathology.* 2nd ed. Baltimore, Williams & Wilkins Company, 1966.

Williamson, B., and Mayon-White, R. M.: *A Handbook of Diseases of Children.* 9th ed. Baltimore, Williams & Wilkins Company, 1964.

Periodicals

Barnard, J.: Your Part in Helping to Reduce Infant Mortality. *RN,* 30:43, November 1967.

Battaglia, F. C., and Lubchenco, L. O.: A Practical Classification of Newborn Infants by Weight and Gestational Age. *J. Pediat.,* 71:159, 1967.

Children Under Pressure: Four Doctor's Views. *Today's Health,* 45:62, September 1967.

Erickson, F.: When 6- to 12-Year Olds Are Ill. *Nursing Outlook,* 13:48, July 1965.

Friedman, R. M.: Interferons and Virus Infections. *Am. J. Nursing,* 68:542, 1968.

Ghosh, S., and Daga, S.: Comparison of Gestational Age and Weight as Standards of Prematurity. *J. Pediat.,* 71:173, 1967.

Graham-Cumming, G.: Prenatal Care and Infant Mortality Among Canadian Indians. *Canad. Nurse,* 63:29, September 1967.

Kang, E. S.: The Genetic Basis of Some Abnormalities in Children. *Children,* 13:60, 1966.

MacQueen, J. C.: Services for Children with Multiple Handicaps. *Children,* 13:55, 1966.

Milio, N.: Values, Social Class, and Community Health Services. *Nursing Research,* 16:26, Winter 1967.

Paulsen, M. G.: Legal Protections against Child Abuse. *Children,* 13:43, 1966.

Pillitteri, A.: Practice in a Pediatric Research Unit. *Am. J. Nursing,* 65:104, August 1965.

Pioneer Surgery Repairs Grotesque Error of Nature. *Medical World News,* 8:29, October 13, 1967.

Selyz, H.: The Stress Syndrome. *Am. J. Nursing,* 65:97, March 1965.

Shapiro, S., and Moriyama, I. M.: International Trends in Infant Mortality and Their Implications for the United States. *Am. J. Pub. Health,* 53:747, 1963.

THE NURSE
AND THE ILL
CHILD

The role of the pediatric nurse has changed during the past several years as research in medicine and its allied sciences has led to improvements in the medical care of children and as research in the social sciences has led to changed views about their psychologic development and needs. In this chapter the emerging role of the pediatric nurse will be explored as a background against which the growth and development of children and their care when ill can be studied.

FACILITIES FOR THE CARE
OF ILL CHILDREN

There are several types of facilities for the care of ill children. These include the pediatric unit in a general hospital or in a children's hospital, the intensive care unit, the pediatric research center, short-term care facilities, long-term care facilities, facilities for the care of ambulatory patients, home care programs, and care of the child at home by a private physician.

The Pediatric Unit

The pediatric unit must be built and furnished to meet the needs of children and of their parents.

Children's needs can be classified under three main headings: adequate provision for care, protection from physical danger, e.g. infection and accidents, and protection from a psychologically threatening environment.

In the pediatric unit the surroundings should be cheerful and the décor scaled to the child's size. Bright colors in addition to the usual pastels can be used. Colored bedspreads remind the child of home. When children are permitted to wear their own clothing rather than hospital gowns, they also tend to feel more as though they were at home. Colorful attire such as pastel dresses worn by nurses in lieu of white uniforms or colorful smocks worn over the uniform tend to brighten the hospital atmosphere as well as to promote better nurse-child-parent relations. Growing plants which can be attended by children provide both color and also an interest for children outside themselves.

In general the pediatric unit should have a smaller number of beds than the usual adult unit, since children need more care than adults. Flexibility of design in the unit is important so that optimum use of space is possible at all times. The hospitalized child should be segregated by care requirements and by age, just as children in the community select their companions when they are well.

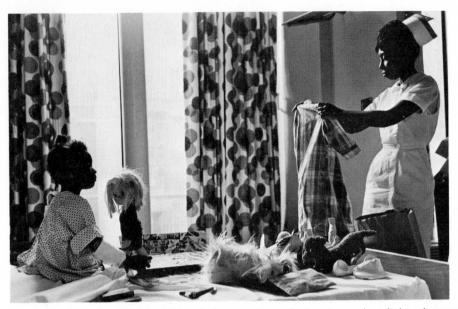

Figure 4–1. Familiar clothing helps the child to feel more at ease in the strange hospital environment. (From "All Rooms Are Private in New Children's Hospital" by William McKillip in *Hospitals*, March 1, 1967.) (Bremen I. Johnson, Director of Bureau Publications, American Hospital Association.)

Each patient unit organized on the basis of age or care requirements should be intimate, informal and small, e.g. having approximately ten beds. The beds should be placed so that the children can relate to both the internal and external environments of the unit. Natural light should be available in patient areas as much as possible.

Each room should have an adjustable hospital bed and an overbed table for meal trays or toys for each child. The hospital bed can be replaced by a bassinet or crib as needed. There should be a bedside cabinet and in addition perhaps a cabinet for favorite toys. Closet space is essential for older children who are permitted to wear their own clothes in the hospital. Each patient area should have facilities for running water. The lavatory should have a gooseneck spout, with either knee or elbow control. The lavatory should be installed near the entrance of the room.

A room containing one bed should be large enough to accommodate two children in an emergency or to accommodate a parent should he request to stay overnight. Such a room could be used also for a critically ill child or for a child who required isolation for a known or suspected infection. Each single bedroom should have a comfortable chair and a wastepaper basket. Each room that is to be used for isolation purposes and for the sickest children should also have an oxygen and a suction outlet. If at all possible, all rooms should have these items for emergency use.

In multiple bedrooms, partitions or cubicles may be installed. Cubicles tend to separate children who otherwise might be able to play together. Cubicles do, however, demarcate areas of potential infection so that isolation precautions can be carried out. They do little to decrease airborne infection. Visitors are encouraged to visit only in their cubicle if there is a question of infection.

If cubicles are used, they should permit visibility of all the children by the nurses. The glass portions of the cubicle walls should be constructed of shatterproof glass in order to make this visibility safely possible.

The nurses' station should be situated centrally within the pediatric unit. Rooms for the sickest patients and young infants should be nearby. Although electronic communications systems should not be installed when human interaction is essential, if one is used, the call system should be one which can be used by younger children. A television monitoring system connected with each room is more desirable than a call system.

A waiting room for parents and friends should be located close to the elevators and stairs. This area should be clearly visible from the nurses' station. The room should be colorfully decorated, soundproofed, and contain comfortable chairs and adequate reading material.

The treatment room and the examination room should be provided in a quiet area of the unit near the entrance. There could be two separate rooms or one quiet, well lighted room which contained all the necessary equipment for examining and treating children. The use

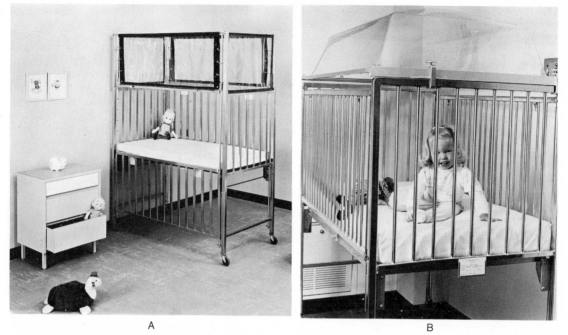

A   B

Figure 4–2. *A*, The sides of the crib should be sufficiently high so that the small child cannot fall when he leans against them. The Springfield crib shown above also has an extension above the crib sides which prevents the active child from falling out of bed. (Hard Manufacturing Company, Box No. 427, Buffalo, New York 14240.) *B*, The Safety Dome Crib Top also prevents the active small child from climbing out of bed. (American Hospital Supply, 2020 Ridge Avenue, Evanston, Illinois 60201.)

of such a room for painful procedures is important so that other children cannot see what is happening to another child. The room should be soundproofed.

Playroom space and a schoolroom are essential for use as therapeutic adjuncts for patients who are ambulatory or convalescent. Children who are well enough can also be taken to these rooms on stretchers or in wheelchairs. The use of these rooms will be discussed later in this chapter.

Meals can be eaten around small tables in the play area or in the center of the pediatric unit. If some children must remain in bed, colorful overbed tables may be used.

Other areas of the pediatric unit include the following: a consultation room providing space to talk privately with parents and children and to demonstrate care necessary after discharge, adequate bathroom facilities for both adults and children, a room which could be utilized for the education of students, and adequate storage space.

Intensive Care Unit or Newborn Intensive Care Unit

Intensive care units or newborn intensive care units for critically ill children or newborns are found in many children's hospitals and large pediatric departments in general hospitals.

Electronic engineering techniques must be specifically adapted to the problems of intensive care for newborns or children. Intensive care necessitates receiving and interpreting continuous information of the physiologic and biochemical status of the children who have conditions predisposing to cardiovascular, respiratory or nervous system collapse. Newborns or children requiring intensive care include, among others, those with congenital anomalies or major illnesses of the newborn, coma, status asthmaticus, severe bronchiolitis and pneumonia, congenital heart disease with failure, and children undergoing major cardiovascular or neurosurgical procedures. Children who are seriously ill from poisoning or trauma are also cared for in the intensive care unit.

Until recently death was defined as the moment when the child stopped breathing. Now the child can be kept alive after the cessation of breathing, after failure of the heart and circulatory system, or even after functional failure of the brain and nervous system. Children can be restored to useful life after temporary failure of one of these vital systems if the gap between changes in his condition and the rapid institution of proper therapy can be minimized.

Through the effective utilization of monitoring devices, comprehensive surveillance of the child's vital systems will enable a medical team to institute supportive treatment, to control the life support system, and to determine when therapy can be discontinued.

Pediatric Research Center

Some children's hospitals have pediatric research centers where little understood diseases are under constant study. Pediatric research centers give nurses a new opportunity to fulfill the basic principles of child care, since the ratio of nurses to patients is high. These centers give children who are able the opportunity to have a schedule much as they followed at home. Careful planning by the nursing staff is necessary to ensure a child's contentment in spite of the painful test procedures that must be done. A dedicated group of nurses working together can minimize the potentially damaging effects of hospitalization.

Facilities for Short-Term Care

Continuity of care for children having short illnesses can be provided through the use of hospital facilities for overnight or short-term observations of children. Such a unit forms a kind of "halfway" house as a means of avoiding prolonged hospitalization while providing care of acute illnesses on a short-term basis.

Facilities for Long-Term Care

Children having handicaps of various kinds may be cared for in long-term hospitals and other facilities instead of at home. Such facilities are important for the care of children whose parents could not provide adequate care and whose homes would not be conducive to a restful, prolonged convalescence, such as in the case of the child having a severe cardiac problem. Available facilities outside the home include public or private hospitals or homes for the convalescent or chronically ill child, residential schools for the handicapped, and summer camps for children having similar diagnoses, such as those having diabetes. Placement of a child into one of these facilities should not be done lightly, since it means taking the child from his parents. But for certain children placement may be a necessity, as will be shown later in this text.

Facilities for the Care of Ambulatory Patients

The pediatric outpatient department can make a real contribution to the hospital because of new medical developments and new social pressures. The outpatient department in many institutions is moving out into the community and toward the concept of a community health service center. The outpatient department today serves not only the indigent, but also persons of all income levels.

Increasing numbers of private physicians use the outpatient department for children having problems needing careful diagnosis and treatment such as those having complex medical or surgical problems or psychologic difficulties. Because of the awareness of the need to avoid the possible trauma of hospitalization, more children having pneumonia, abscesses, urinary or other infections can be treated on an outpatient basis if there is a responsible adult in the home. One of the newer functions of the medical staff in outpatient departments is to trace hereditary conditions and do genetic counseling.

Ambulatory patients should be scheduled carefully and not have to wait in large groups prior to their appointments. Comprehensive high quality services should be made available to all.

Home Care Programs

The home care program in a pediatric unit or children's hospital is a recent innovation, although such programs have existed for the care of elderly or indigent patients. The purposes of the home care program are to prevent or reduce the trauma of hospitalization by shortening the hospital stay and by avoiding the interruption in parent-child relations which hospitalization can produce, to provide for the care of children who can be as well or better treated in their home environments, and to utilize the assistance of appropriate community services as well as hospital facilities for children who no longer need care in the hospital.

In order for the home care program to function well, the child's home environment must be conducive to recovery and there must be someone present in the household competent enough to cooperate with the health team between medical and nursing visits.

Care of the Child at Home by a Private Physician

The mother who cares for her child in the home in cooperation with a private physician, either a pediatrician or a general practitioner, feels more secure if she can contact the physician about any problems she may be having. For this reason many physicians set aside a specific time each day to receive such telephone calls.

The physician, in order to give advice over the telephone, must know the parents well and have faith in their accuracy in describing symptoms. He usually will not have such a relation with a stranger and therefore cannot be expected to assist a parent he does not know.

In order to improve the quality of care given to the children in their practices, some pediatricians have recently employed paramedical personnel, usually a nurse who visits the children in their homes, and a social worker. The nurse may be responsible among other duties for visiting all newborn infants and all infants and children having illnesses in their homes for the purpose of parent education. When the nurse makes a home call, information about the environment of the home and the activities of the family may be added to the child's record. With this type of assistance the pediatrician is able to make more efficient use of his time.

MODERN CONCEPTS IN THE CARE OF HOSPITALIZED CHILDREN

It would be difficult today to find a young adult who had not spent some time in a hospital during his childhood years. Many will remember such experiences with fear and trembling because of the loneliness and pain which they felt at an age when they could not cope with these feelings alone. Needless to say, practices in use in some hospitals today have changed little over the past twenty years, but in others have gone through a period of rapid transition. This has occurred partially because of findings from research in the social sciences, partially because of newer thinking in child psychology, and partially because of social pressure.

Visiting Hours

Many years ago when parents were permitted to visit their hospitalized child only one hour once a month, children were needlessly deprived of parental love. Today many hospitals permit visiting from 2 to 8 P.M. or from early in the morning to bedtime, while other institutions permit visiting at any time during the day or night.

The extent of visiting by the parents should be determined by their need to see the child and, more important, by the child's need for the parents. Some nurses may believe that parental visiting is upsetting to a particular child because he cries when the parent leaves. Nothing could be further from the truth, because such a child is acting normally. If he did not appear upset when the parents left him, the nurses would have need to be concerned. They might believe that such quiet behavior indicated that he had "adjusted" to the hospital routine and the care of nurses when, in reality, he had just given up in despair. A more detailed discussion of this subject will be found in the chapters dealing with illness in the various age groups.

Rooming-In

Parents should never be required to stay at a child's bedside, but neither should they be prohibited from doing this if they so desire.

For parents who stay during the daytime in the pediatric unit, some hospitals provide a comfortable lounge or waiting room where they can relax. In some institutions meals can be served to the parents in the child's room, or they may eat in the hospital's cafeteria or coffee shop.

Mothers of seriously ill children especially may be encouraged to stay in the hospital all night if they desire to do so and facilities are available for their comfort. Fathers may also stay if facilities are made available for them. Various arrangements have been made for parents to stay in the hospital setting. The mother may sleep on a chair, a cot, a folding bed, or a convertible chair in the child's room, if it is large enough. Some hospitals have rooms on the pediatric unit where the mothers may sleep. In case of an emergency they could be easily summoned. Other institutions have a wing of the hospital or a motel type of accommodation for parents and other relatives. In hospitals where no facilities are made for parents to stay they may be directed to accommodations close by in the community.

Some hospitals have *care-by-parent* or *family participation units* where the mother actually lives in the hospital with her child. This method of care has its roots in the Orient, where the whole family becomes involved with the care of the sick. Under this system the child gets attention when he needs it each day from a familiar person, though such care is given under the supervision of the nurse. This is a good setting where nurses can gain experience in communicating nursing skills and explaining procedures to mothers. This should be done, however, without a condescending manner so that all mothers from various backgrounds can learn to nurse their children.

Specifically, the nurses' responsibilities in such a setting are to prepare the parent to meet her child's need in the hospital setting, to help her maintain a schedule similar to the one he had at home, to interpret medical procedures and diagnostic tests that are scheduled, and to do health teaching and anticipatory guidance as necessary. In the family unit the nurse can observe the parents, their skills, attitudes and techniques, and any problems in parent-child relations that may be apparent. The nurse must also observe and evaluate the physical and emotional needs of each mother so that none of them becomes too fatigued by their experience.

Some mothers may be too anxious or guilty or they just may not want to participate in the care of their child in the hospital. Other mothers

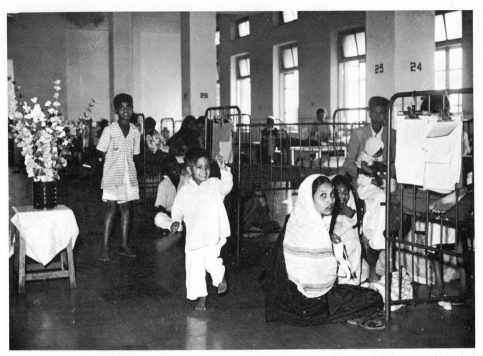

Figure 4–3. Patients in the children's ward enjoy having their parents with them at Sassoon Hospital, Poona, Bombay, India. Although obvious differences exist in the physical environment of this children's unit in India, when compared with children's units in the United States, it meets the needs of children and their parents. (UNICEF Photo by Jack Ling.)

may welcome the opportunity to give their children a sense of security through their presence.

The subject of parents remaining with their children during hospitalization will be discussed in greater detail in the chapters on illness later in this text.

The Health and Nursing Teams

The nurse who cares for children sees her role in terms of her relations with the mother, the child and the family group as a whole. She may be described broadly as not a mother substitute, but as "Mother's friend." In this role the nurse may individually plan for and actually give comprehensive care to children or she may function as a member of a nursing team.

The nurse who is a member of a *nursing team* works closely with one or more professional nurses, nursing students, licensed practical nurses, nurse attendants and others in a joint effort. In order to function as a leader or member of this team, the nurse must understand the comprehensive care of patients assigned to her team and be willing to contribute to their optimum care.

The role of the nurse who cares for children involves not only working with the individual child, his family unit and her nursing team, but also cooperating with members of the broader *health team:* physician, social worker, nutritionist, school teacher, Play Lady, public health nurse, religious counselor and others as the need arises. She fulfills her responsibility as an active participating member of this team, contributing her skills and knowledge to the total effort of the group.

Although the student should know the functions of most of the various members of the health team mentioned above, the functions of the recreation specialist or children activities specialist (Play Lady) and the school teacher may not be so well understood. Both these members of the health team are important adjuncts to total patient care.

The *recreation specialist,* or *children's activities specialist (Play Lady),* has several functions. On the basis of information gleaned about the child she can plan a program for each geared according to her evaluation of his needs. She can also plan group activities when possible to give the children safe outlets for anxieties and hostilities, and can give familiar playthings to children postoperatively in order to reduce their fears. The recreation specialist can plan projects for the children to carry out according to their ages. She can also report on the activities of the children to the medical and nursing staffs.

The functions of the *school teacher* are much the same as they are in classrooms in the community. Further discussion concerning the activities of the recreation specialist and the school teacher will be given later in this chapter and in appropriate chapters throughout this text.

Play and School in the Hospital

The idea of providing opportunities for play and learning activities is certainly not a recent one in institutions, but the practice of providing programs to meet these needs is new in many hospitals.

Play is a child's way of living, his daily "work." It can satisfy needs in the child for his physical, emotional, social and mental development. It is also one of childhood's most effective tools for mastering stress. Play is as essential for the sick child as for the healthy one. The sick child needs it to fill lonely hours and, by expressing his feelings through it, to reduce the trauma caused by hospitalization.

The growth of play and school programs in pediatric units of hospitals is due partly to the improved medical and nursing care which children now receive. Today children recover from their acute illnesses in a shorter time and thus have more time to recover while not on bed rest. Also the current importance placed on the emotional, social and mental aspects of a child's life in the hospital has been due to research in these areas. It is now understood that play can help a child to comprehend intrusive procedures and surgical procedures, and also to express his fantasies, fears and anxieties.

Children can play in areas provided for this purpose or in the center of the pediatric unit. Obviously, if they play where acutely ill children are, they tend to be a disturbing factor in the environment and to be in the way of physicians and other personnel. Hospitals today are either including playrooms in their new buildings or are converting porches or other rooms so that they can be used for this purpose. If no room is available which can be used for this specific purpose, a toy cart can be designed which can be moved from bed to bed.

If a large room and an outdoor area are available for play, some children who are restricted to their beds, stretchers or wheelchairs can be moved so that they can participate in play activities. Certainly the children who cannot be moved should be involved in play activities at their own beds if they are able.

If the student nurse is sincerely interested in providing optimum care for her patients, she will incorporate play into the daily activities of each of her patients and not think of it only when she is assigned for a day or two to the children's activities program.

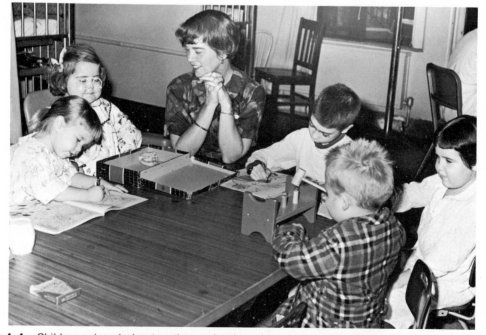

Figure 4–4. Children enjoy playing together under the guidance of the Play Lady. As soon as the child is able to be out of bed, he should be encouraged to play with other children in a group just as if he were at home.

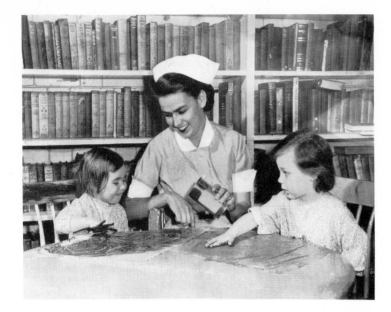

Figure 4–5. The pediatric department can be fun for both the student nurse gaining experience in the care of children and the children themselves. (Johns Hopkins Hospital School of Nursing, Baltimore, Maryland.)

The nurse must consider, when planning activities for any child, his age, his interests, the diagnosis and the limitations imposed upon him by his illness. When the child is acutely ill and unable to play actively with toys, he may enjoy listening to stories. Telling a story instead of reading it draws children into emotional involvement in it. The storyteller can ask questions, insert comments about the individual child and thus make him feel a part of the story itself. If stories about animals or children are told, the child can pretend to be one of the characters and interject his own comments into the narration. Other activities which children on bed rest can do are watching a plant such as a sweet potato vine, a carrot or herbs grow, watching an ant hill or some goldfish in a tank, or a canary or parakeet placed near the bed, or watching supervised television programs.

In the play area children who are permitted out of bed should be free to develop mental, motor and social skills and to express themselves in a variety of art media, such as finger painting or molding with clay. Even in the hospital children enjoy playing with household equipment. They also like equipment peculiar to the hospital which will allow them to work out their feelings about hospitalization.

Children frequently select toys such as doctor or nurse dolls, play syringes and stethoscopes with which they can imitate the activities they see around them. Little girls enjoy constructing paper caps which they wear to make them look like nurses. Old cloth can be used in such play to restrain a doll, to make a doll's sheet, to make bandages or to improvise a sling for a supposedly broken arm. Recently puppets have been used to demonstrate procedures to children who are to be hospitalized. Children enjoy not only seeing "the show," but also playing with the doctor and nurse puppets after it is over. Such activities are therapeutic in that they help the child to work out his feelings about his hospitalization.

Much of the equipment which is of value in the play of normal children is also necessary in the hospital play area, particularly simple craft materials, blocks, puzzles, story books, dolls, doll houses and phonograph records. Children enjoy play telephones because they can pretend that they are calling home. They also enjoy clay, paints, puppets, and pounding boards on which they can express their anger. They enjoy tricycles, carts and wagons through the use of which they develop their large muscles.

Other suggestions for use in the care of a child whose parents cannot or will not communicate with him are surprise boxes made of shoe boxes and filled with various small wrapped toys and cards sent to him in the mail by his nurse. In this way he feels remembered by adults other than his parents.

Children's play areas cannot be kept clean and orderly as judged by adult standards. If the nurses are too concerned about the physical appearance of play areas during playtime, the children feel that the unit personnel do not approve of their play and are likely to enter only half-heartedly into their make-believe, creative work or games.

Children should be taught to take care of their toys which they brought from home or had given them by their parents. They may and indeed should let other children play with them if their social growth is to go forward in the hospital

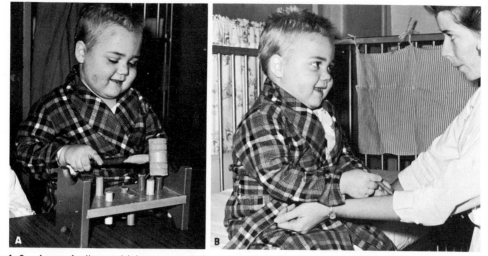

Figure 4–6. Angry feelings which may result from hospitalization can be worked off through the use of (A) a bang board or (B) equipment peculiar to the hospital such as a "play" hypodermic injection for his nurse.

as it normally would in their homes, but a place must be provided where their toys can be safely stored. As a child learns to take care of his own toys he also learns to respect those of other children.

Much can be learned from watching a child play in a relaxed environment. His approach to play and his relation to his peers, parents and other adults should be observed and recorded. Also to be noted are the degree of his activity, his attention span, his ability to tolerate frustration, his verbal ability and his concept formation.

Nurses should have an opportunity to participate in the play program for hospitalized children. In this way they not only learn about children and their play, but also have an opportunity to appreciate the contribution of the recreation specialist or Play Lady to the comprehensive care of their patients.

An important member of the health team in the pediatric unit is the public school teacher, who is generally employed by the local Board of Education, but is released from regular classroom activities to teach hospitalized children. The school teacher works particularly with the children who are in the hospital for relatively long periods of time; however, she will teach any child whose physician recommends this type of activity for him. Even when it is obvious that the child is too ill ever to return to school, keeping up with his class is important to him as a link with the outside world. In some hospitals the teacher teaches at the children's bedsides, while in other institutions the children who are able can be brought together in a classroom set aside for this purpose. The child who is kept busy and feels useful and important, and whose mind is occupied, is a far happier child than one who

is allowed to vegetate. Also, the child who keeps up with his class in their work is able to return to school with his own friends after his hospitalization.

The subjects of play and school for the child will be elaborated upon in subsequent chapters.

THE ROLE OF THE NURSE IN CHILD CARE

Many nurses believe that they can accomplish their mission in child care by providing "mother love" for each child with whom they come in contact. The nurse may believe that her expression of affection, tenderness, warmth and concern will be rewarded by the child's loving her as a mother in return. She may believe that since the parents are not with the child constantly, whether the child is in school or in the hospital, she can replace them in the child's affections.

Love of the parents for a child does not consist only of cuddling, feeding and playing with the infant or child. Love also includes those interactions of parent with child that stimulate growth, perception, curiosity, investigation of the environment, independence, and achievement of age-appropriate tasks. Parental love requires that not only the total dependence of the newborn, but also the increasing independence of the toddler is cause for rejoicing. As the child grows, the parents must be able to encourage further growth and to continue to love the child even though his interests are different from their own. To loving parents the ability of the child to realize his own individual capacities and potential is more important than their own expectations of the child.

Parental love is difficult to achieve. Such a capacity to love is usually based on having had similar experiences in one's own youth. Just as the mature adult finds a sense of achievement and pleasures in his own work, and in his relations with others, so also does he want these same satisfactions for his children. As the mature parent can accept varied feelings relating to anger, love, grief and sex, so also can the child learn through the process of identification.

In our culture such fortunate parents and their children are relatively rare. Many parents today have had serious emotional deprivation in their own early lives, so that in their adult lives they strive for material things to make up for their loss. If such an adult marries another with similar problems, the children of the union may not be able to get much love from their parents because unfortunately they do not have much to give.

But the nurse cannot fill the total need for love in such a child's life. Love results, in the nursing setting, from the mutual effort of the nurse and the child to achieve his recovery. A mutual regard of child and nurse develops after repeated testing of the adult by the child and repeated efforts on the part of the nurse to gain the child's trust. Out of a prolonged interaction as in the instance of a long-term hospitalization, the nurse and the child find the capacity to love. *Love from*

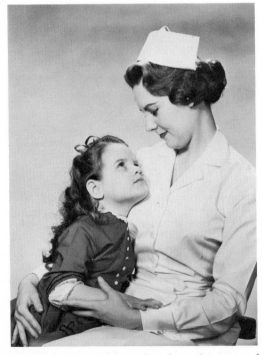

Figure 4–7. The child receives from the nurse affection and a sense of security as well as physical care. (H. Armstrong Roberts.)

the child is the result of the efforts of the nurse and not the initiating force in the relationship. But even then, if the parents have not completely deserted their child, the nurse is still functioning in the role of a *"kind friend"* of his mother's who cares for him when his mother is unable to do so.

Communicating with Parents

If we really want to serve the child well, we first have to communicate in an effective way with the parents, especially the mother. *Communication with the parents should be regarded as a process, the purposes of which are to obtain and to transmit information, to provide an opportunity for them to ventilate their feelings and relieve tension, and to motivate them in the direction of understanding and resolving their own problems.* In order for the nurse to assure effective communication with either parents or children she must have respect for them as human beings, and take into account their needs, problems, fears, customs and cultural backgrounds.

Furthermore, *readiness to learn* is dependent on the parents' present situation. In an acute crisis or a threatening event when they feel insecure, they need to grasp for firm help. At this time they are highly suggestible and will listen to what is discussed. It is important that what is offered has a sound basis, since they will just as easily accept an irrational solution to their problem. Examples of periods in the lives of parents when they need help and guidance in relation to their child are when he is ill or hospitalized and during the difficult periods of his development as during the toilet training period or during adolescence. It is well known that while a slight increase in anxiety or fear is associated with more learning, extreme anxiety has the opposite effect.

In each communication the nurse has with the parents there should be a clearly defined purpose, yet one broad enough to allow for modification as the need arises. For instance, the giving of factual information on health care, feeding, inoculations, and so on, is important; however, the interest of the parent must be ascertained before it is given. If the parent is not interested, little will be gained from such a conference unless the nurse first ascertains what is blocking his interest.

The success of any interview depends primarily on the nurse's ability to establish and maintain a sound interpersonal relation with the parent. The attainment of such a relation is largely based on the nurse's warmth, sensitivity, objectivity and understanding. But speech alone does not transmit depth of interest and feeling. The nurse's physical appearance and movement, such as the neatness and appropriateness of her uniform or clothing, her facial expression, her leaning forward to show interest, her looking directly at the parent to show concern, and the movement of her hands, are vitally important in furthering a good interviewing relation.

Our attitudes and behavior as nurses toward those whom we wish to help have been largely conditioned by our own relations and experience. Among other things, the age and sex of the parent, as well as his physical and personal characteristics, often activate certain feelings and responses which may have no basis of reality in our experience with the particular parent. The nurse may like or dislike a child's parent, not so much because of him as an individual, but because she is attributing to and displacing on him her own feelings which stem from identifying him with someone extremely close, often a parent, brother or sister. The unresolved conflict toward key members of her family is reflected in the way she relates to others in her professional and personal relations. The nurse should be able to recognize and not deny her feelings toward a parent or child, even though she may not know the specific origin of her feelings.

The nurse often represents the same type of figure to the parents as she does to their child. While she can tolerate hostility, guilt and dependency from the child, she finds it more difficult to do so from the parents who are more nearly her own age. The nurse should nevertheless convey her warm acceptance of them and her genuine regard for their feelings. She can provide for the parents a rare opportunity to express their feelings to someone who is understanding and not critical or moralistic. If the nurse finds that she cannot tolerate parental feelings it would be well for her to discuss this problem with her instructor.

There are certain principles which the nurse should be aware of in establishing relations between herself, the parents and their child. If the student has studied these principles before, they will offer a review. If she has not, they should be considered carefully because they will help her in any interview situation she may encounter.

1. *The nurse begins to build a working relationship with the parents and child from her first contact with them, whether it be in their home, in the hospital or in the community.*
2. *The nurse understands that all behavior is meaningful, although the meaning may not always be too clear.*
3. *The nurse accepts the parents and their child exactly as they are.* She should refrain from evaluating actions as "bad" or "wrong" and from passing judgment on other human beings. This does not mean that she is indifferent to ethical values. It simply means that her aim is understanding, and therefore her interest is focused on causation.
4. *The nurse should have empathy for parents and children.* This implies that she appreciates how they feel inwardly, how things are for them, but it does not mean that their feelings or troubles become hers. She would like both parents and children to know that each of their problems is of importance to her and that she is there because she wants to aid them in their solution.
5. *The nurse should be willing to acknowledge the parent's right to his own decisions concerning his children.* Sometimes such decisions may be painful for the nurse to accept.
6. *The nurse permits both parents and child to express negative emotions.* When a parent or child expresses negative feelings, the nurse should be personally secure and not respond subjectively to his statements. Her ability to accept him despite his expression or resentment helps convince him that she truly understands.
7. *The nurse should ask questions which are limited to a single idea or reference.* If her questions are too long or complex, the parent may become confused or ignore the meaning the nurse intended.
8. *The nurse should speak in language that is understandable to the parents.*
9. *The nurse and the physician as well as other members of the health and nursing teams must help the parents and child to feel that there is unity and strength among them.*

Many situations in pediatric nursing require a knowledge by the nurse of interviewing techniques. *A genuine expression of liking and warmth sets the tone for the parents and child and helps them to relax.* Whenever possible, listen and let the parents tell their story, then assist them to explain it more fully. The nondirective method of interviewing can be successful in some nursing situations. The main technique in the nondirective method is to reflect what the parent or child has said, either by asking a question, repeating his last words using a questioning inflection, or by rephrasing what he has said. This method in its pure form limits the nurse to a minimum of verbal activity; however, nonverbal responses in posture or expression can be used.

The principle of the nondirective method may be used when a real conflict is evident such as when discussing the fear of death or of surgery. In such situations superficial reassurance is worthless, because though it may comfort the sympathizer, if offers only temporary relief to the person who is reassured. The nurse can be helpful if she makes a real effort to understand the parent and then to help him identify the reasons for his fears. It is most important to listen, making little comment, and to *be with* the parents or child at such a time.

One caution must be remembered when using the nondirective technique, however. The nurse should not be guilty of probing or leading a parent to say more than he ought to or really wants to say. Such a conference might prove to be dynamite and cause the parent more anxiety than he had prior to it.

In most interviewing situations pauses will occur. The nurse must learn to tolerate pauses with ease. Pauses many times precede a significant turn in the conversation. Perhaps the parent or child would like to say something important and is wondering whether he can really trust the nurse. Perhaps he wants to say something, but finds it difficult to put his concern into words, or he wants to stop talking about a particular topic. Nurses should not be embarrassed by such pauses.

The nurse cannot possibly provide answers or help parents find answers to all the complex problems they and their children struggle with. If she gives them credit for having the capacity to arrive at their own answers, her role will be to help them get a clearer vision of the situation and an awareness of possible alternate decisions and their consequences. *The purpose of the nurse is not to solve problems, but to strengthen the parent's and child's capacity to deal with them. If the situation which either the parent or child presents is beyond the professional competence of the nurse, she should seek help from other members of the health team.*

ADMISSION OF THE CHILD TO THE HOSPITAL

Admission of a child to the hospital can be considered in connection with the activities involved or from the standpoint of the emotional effect upon the child and his family. We shall consider first the emotional effect, because it is often mistakenly accorded less importance than the physical care given the child. The nurse's attitude is probably the most important single factor in the emotional atmosphere during the child's admission (Fig. 4-8).

Hospitalization of children is so common today that we tend to forget its importance as a break in the unity of the family. The feelings of each member of the family must be considered if this break is to result in furthering rather than hindering the emotional and social maturity of all concerned. Although the nurse has the main role in helping the child and his parents adjust to the hospital situation, the entire health team is involved in creating the optimum emotional environment on the child's admission.

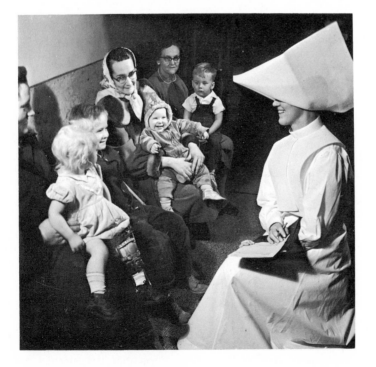

Figure 4-8. The nurse must be understanding of the feelings of parents when she admits their children to the hospital. (William H. Rittase.)

Emotional Reactions on Admission of a Child to the Hospital

Maternal Reaction

A mother whose child has been admitted to the hospital feels not only that he is separated from her, but also that others are taking her place and, furthermore, giving him necessary care which she, with all her intense love for him, cannot give.

Immediate operation is often necessary to save the life of an infant who is born deformed or deviates from the normal, or he may be sent home from the newborn nursery with his mother, for deferred admission to the pediatric unit when he has reached the optimum age for correction of the defect. In general the reaction of parents to such a child at birth is that he presents a threat to all their happy expectations centered around the concept of a normal baby. It is natural that when he is readmitted to the hospital they still feel anxiety, anger, fear, disappointment and possibly guilt (see p. 161 for further discussion).

Anxiety during a child's illness not only interferes with a parent's ability to provide support for the child, but may also be transmitted like an infection to the child himself. The anxious parent can be recognized by his trembling, coarse or wavery voice, restlessness, irritableness, withdrawal or erratic body movements.

When the nurse detects anxiety in the parent, her first task is to identify the causes of the anxiety and to give whatever help she or other members of the health team can to alleviate it.

A mother, particularly with her first child, often feels that his sickness is due to some error she has committed and is her fault. If he was an unwanted baby, she may consider it a punishment for not having had the normal maternal love for the child during her pregnancy and after his birth.

If the parents feel self-blame for the child's illness, the nurse can explain the real cause of illness to them and convey to them her belief that they are competent. If the parents did make an error and the child's illness resulted, the nurse can attempt to convince the parents that a mistake can be made by anyone.

If the parent is anxious because she feels that she is not a competent mother, the nurse can give sincere praise for things she does well in order to increase her self-confidence. Having the mother guide the nurse in details of care as it was done in the home will not only increase the mother's confidence, but will also be reassuring to the child.

If the parents need help with resolving their guilt beyond that which the nurse can give,

they should be referred to another helpful professional person.

Specific Causes of Maternal Anxiety. In addition to her feelings about the illness itself, a mother may be frightened and excited by the new experience of placing her child in the hospital. Among the many factors which increase her anxiety are the following.

1. Fear of the strange environment in the hospital. If the parent is disturbed by the continuing strangeness of the hospital atmosphere, the nurse can try to explain the use of equipment in lay terminology, to make the surroundings more homelike, and to encourage the parents to ask questions which are on their minds. Simple answers to questions asked help to allay anxiety.
2. Fear of separation from the child and fear that the nurses may be unloving or that, because they are able to do so much for him, they will take his love from her. If the mother is anxious because the nurses are giving her child care, the nurse could suggest tactfully that she partially care for the child herself. Such activity would help the mother to cope in a more healthy way with her anxiety.
3. Fear of the unknown and of what will happen to the child immediately and in the future. The life of a handicapped child appears the more difficult because mothers have no clear picture of what it will be like.
4. Fear that the child will suffer.
5. Fear that the condition is infectious and may spread to other members of the family.
6. Fear of unbearable financial obligations incurred through the illness. The social service worker may be able to help with such problems.
7. Fear that society will look upon the illness as a reflection of something wrong with the child's parents.

A mother's anxiety magnifies all other problems. She may enter into long discussions of problems which are extraneous to that of the child's illness. The nurse should accept this as natural and never feel that a mother's dwelling on other difficulties means that she is disinterested in the child.

The majority of mothers want the understanding, sympathetic support which the nurse can give and thereby gain a realistic view of the difficulties which they and the child must face. Some mothers appear withdrawn, however; these are in greater need of help. To assist them to put into words their deep emotion may be too heavy a responsibility for the nurse to undertake. The psychiatrist or psychiatric social worker should be available to guide both the parents in their trouble and the nurse in her contacts with them in order that she may learn to take her place in the mental health program.

The Child's Reaction

Illness or a physical handicap threatens both the physical development of a child and his sense of trust in other people which is important to his emotional development. Sickness causes pain, restraint of movement, long sleepless periods and, in an infant who cannot be fed by mouth, restriction in the fulfillment of his sucking need. When he most needs his mother, he is without her, unless the hospital has provision for her remaining day and night.

Hospitalization is a completely new experience to the infant or young child. When he was taken to the private physician's office or the Child Health Conference, he made friends with physicians and nurses, but he is too young to understand that the hospital personnel are also his friends. Since his mother tends to be anxious, her feeling of fear is communicated to him. What the hospital means to the pediatric patient will depend upon his stage of maturity and upon how accustomed he was to being left with friends of his mother.

Nurse-Child Relations

The needs of the ill child are similar to those of the well child; however, the nurse has a responsibility for meeting part of his needs when he is hospitalized. The child needs to trust those persons responsible for his care. Since he is not able to judge the competencies of the members of the health and nursing teams, he must rely only on his perception of their relations with him. The child must feel that the adults around him know who he is, understand him, and like him as a person, different from the other children. The child needs understanding and physical contact also from his parents. The nurse can help the parents provide the kind of comforting support he needs. Since a child needs to continue to grow and develop while he is a patient, he needs a nurse who is aware of his pattern of behavior at home and can follow it to some degree in the hospital. And last, but not the least important, the child needs to play and come in contact with other children.

The Child's View. The child perceives this relation as one in which he receives from the nurse (1) physical care formerly given by his mother or some other member of the family, (2) new types of care which may be painful and frightening, (3) a sense of security in an adult's affection, and (4) the link with home and mother.

An older child realizes that in addition to the foregoing the nurse teaches him good hygiene and, for girls, is a model of one of the many things they can emulate when grown up. The child may sense, but not clearly perceive, that she teaches him to adapt to his condition, physically and emotionally. He soon learns her relation with his parents and with the physicians and makes use of her contacts with both.

The extent to which nursing care can be given in a homelike setting is a question which each hospital decides in the light of physical resources and available personnel. By homelike physical environment is meant sunlight, color, pictures, music and television, small tables and chairs, toys, wagons, tricycles, and so on. For instance, pink or blue plastic individual bathtubs, floating toys and colored towels and washcloths make the bath more homelike. Food can be served from a self-heated food cart which has been decorated to look like a chuck wagon. The use of a stroller instead of a wheelchair or stretcher to transport the child is another example of the introduction into the hospital setting of compatible equipment and techniques which will connect what of necessity must be strange and cause anxiety in the child with the care he received at home from his mother. Permitting a child to take a doll or other toy to the operating room or to a place where he is to be subjected to diagnostic tests is an evidence of the understanding attitude of nurses and physicians toward his fear.

More important than equipment or methods adapted to children is the rapport between the nurse and the child. Although, ideally, one nurse should give the child all the care he needs during her hours on duty as long as he is in the hospital, realistically this cannot often be done. It is important, therefore, that as few nurses be responsible for the child's care as possible. The child should learn to know "his" nurses and they to know him as a person. If he had a few nurses he knew well, there would be sufficient stability in his relations so that he could accept relief nurses more readily. That nurses wear uniforms and caps which in his view are similar and that they do things for him in much the same way helps him to accept new nurses among those who routinely care for him. A new friend may be pleasant when he knows that the old ones are still there.

The Nurse's View in the Care of the Child. 1. *The nurse perceives her role very much as the child perceives it* because she has defined her role to meet his needs. Some negligent nurses do not live up to the professional role of the nurse, and their influence is soon reflected in a change in the child's definition of the nurse-child relation. His idea that nurses are good to little children may change, and he may think nurses mean, whose role is an authoritative, punitive one, in spite of the physical care they give him according to the best technique.

But to his limited concept of their relations the nurse may add much that the child does not realize.

2. *The nurse guides the hospitalized child to better ways of living.* The nurse should offer opportunities to the child to maintain good habits of hygiene or to improve upon them if possible during the usually short hospital stay. As far as possible, new ways of caring for him, new equipment, new foods in his diet and new concepts of cleanliness should be introduced gradually. Helping the patient to substitute better habits for current ones or harmful ones is so much a part of comprehensive nursing that in this book such habits are taken up in connection with the nursing care of children.

Unfortunately a child may lose good habits while he is in the hospital and regress to infantile ways, or an older child may acquire undesirable habits. A case in point is that of control of urine and stool. A child's physical condition and nervousness due to his strange surroundings may make control difficult for him. But often this is not the cause of a wet and soiled bed. He has cried for a nurse to put him on the "potty" or take him to the toilet. When no one came, he stood holding on to the bars of his crib, crying more loudly, and in the end relieved himself in bed. Nurses know better than to punish or shame a child when this happens. They as well as the parents should realize that he is sick and still almost a baby, but often they do not understand that his emotional state and physical exertion are harmful for him. If nurses are too busy with some important duty, they may think that his needs are not urgent enough. They may consider that it takes less time to change his clothing and his bed when it is convenient than to come at once when he calls. In fact, they may put diapers on a child who has worn pants for months. In consequence, when he wets himself day after day, he ceases to call the nurse and returns to his infantile habit of relieving himself whenever and wherever he feels inclined to do so. He has thus lost a good habit and regressed to earlier behavior.

3. *The nurse perceives her role as a helping person.* Illness and hospitalization cause stress or problems in adjustment for the child and his family. Parents and their children need from the nurse comfort, a source of strength, and knowledge. The nurse therefore must see herself as a helping person who can provide emotional support to those in need. *She must realize that before she can provide support, however, she must first care about her patients sufficiently to earn their confidence.* Only then can she develop a positive emotional relation with the child and his family which is the base for providing such support and strength to them. *The nurse must be aware of the feelings of both parents and chil-dren so that she can respond to them and help strengthen their resources to handle them.*

In the care of the acutely ill child the nurse must recognize anxiety and provide relief from it by patiently listening to complaints, showing concern about the child, and, while providing rest for him, giving him physical care which further indicates her deep interest. *Words alone will not convey to the parents that everything possible is being done to promote the child's recovery.* As the anxiety of the parents is abated, the anxiety of the child will be also, because it is a well known fact that *anxiety is contagious.*

The student nurse may not at first be able to provide the kind or amount of support that children and their parents need. She may be so involved with her own anxiety in having to care for deformed, critically ill or dying children that she may not even perceive the anxiety which surrounds her. *Pediatric nursing requires of the nurse great patience and tenderness, but it also requires great emotional strength in times of stress.*

The student may not be able to handle her overwhelming feelings in her care of children. She may at first attempt to protect herself by building an impenetrable wall between herself and her patients. She may even flee physically from an uncomfortable situation in which she does not permit herself to become emotionally involved. The nurse, to whom parents and children turn for support, thus leaves them at a time when they need her most. If the nurse does not remove herself physically from the situation, she may cut off interaction with patients and their families by utilizing verbal blocks to satisfying communication. She may do this by imposing her own ideas in conversation instead of listening to the ideas of others, by giving weak, false reassurance, by jumping to faulty conclusions, and by changing the subject whenever the topic is uncomfortable for her. Before the student can reassure patients or families she must resolve her own feelings about the care of ill children. She must gain spiritual strength herself and replenish her reservoir of emotional strength before she can help others. Often her instructor or another faculty member can help considerably in achieving these tasks.

In order for the nurse to understand her own feelings and thus be better able to cope with them, she must realize that such feelings do exist, that they exist in every feeling human being. This knowledge may help her learn to use her energy in a more constructive way.

Nurse-Parent Relations

It is a truism that the nurse's relation with the child's parents is based on the fact that they are the parents of the child in her charge. He is the focal point of their relations. Yet the mother may be more in need of the nurse's sympathetic, understanding, permissive guidance than an acutely ill child is of her emotional support. The influence of the mother's attitude upon the child is so great that it is not only for the mother's sake, but also for the child's, that the nurse has a serious responsibility to help the mother. In order to understand how to help mothers the student should be willing to learn from them. She needs to know not only their weaknesses, but also their strengths, and make the most of them in the care the child receives. The student prior to entering nursing is more likely to have had experience solely with children deprived of their mothers' company. But in most cases separation from the mother took place under pleasant auspices, so that neither child nor mother was seriously disturbed. (One or both might have had a moment of concern over what to do without the other. No child likes to be left behind when Mother goes out for the evening, and Mother may have some doubts as to Johnny's being old enough to go to camp. But such partings are chosen, and no great fear is involved.) If the student has had extensive experience as a baby-sitter or camp counselor or has otherwise come in contact with children, she is probably better able to establish rapport with the mother because they have in common a knowledge of children. On this she builds her instruction, drawing from her professional knowledge of sick children.

The mother knows her child far better than the nurse does. The mother may be so intent upon him that she accepts him as the prototype of all children and does not see him against a background of other children; she does not see wherein he is like them or differs from them—his limitations and assets, his potentiality. But even a mother who has a distorted view of her child can teach the nurse many things about him which will help her to understand his behavior. Reliance on the mother as a real help in the adjustment of the child with a chronic condition or severe handicap helps the nurse in her acceptance of his condition. To give the child physical care is usually an emotional relief to the mother and reassures the child in his strange surroundings. The nurse can teach the mother many procedures and ways of caring for the child which she will need to know when she eventually takes him home.

The student knows more about pathology and treatment than the mother does, but what little the mother of a child with a chronic disease or a handicap does know is in direct relation to her child and the care she has given him. Until the nurses have had time to map out a plan of comprehensive nursing for him, the mother may be better able to lift and turn him

so that it does not hurt, to feed him most comfortably or to create a play situation adapted to his likes and limitations. When the student has had time to apply her knowledge to the child, she is able to teach the mother better ways of caring for him. Both the mother and the nurse, then, have much to contribute to each other in applying the principle of quality nursing to the child patient.

The value of a child psychologist with whom nurses can talk over the problems they meet in human relations is generally recognized. These relations are so complex that the guidance of a specialist is often necessary. (This also applies to the nurse's handling of her own emotional problems in the social involvements which constantly occur in the pediatric area.)

It should always be remembered that the child eventually goes home to his family. To bring about changes in habits, however beneficial, which cause strained relations between the child and his parents or friends when he leaves the hospital is of doubtful value. To teach a child not to use indecent words when these same words are part of the neighborhood daily speech is a case in point. To teach a boy not to fight, if his father would punish him if he did not show this ability to care for himself among other boys, would be folly.

A hospitalized child, however, must not be permitted to harm other children even though he may be permitted to do so at home. In this situation *the nurse may condemn the act, but not the child or the teachings of his parents.* One factor in the neurotic disorders of American children stems from the fact that the majority in the low-income group are taught in schools, hospitals and other institutions where the culture of the middle class is held to be the goal of socialization, that their parents' attitudes, beliefs and ways of doing things are not up to standard. Many of the older immigrants and some of the migrants and immigrants of today have come to our cities because they want their children to have advantages they themselves did not have; they want their children to move into a social class above their own. For a son or daughter to maintain the economic and social position of the parents is not the American philosophy. If their children do not surpass them, parents are likely to feel that they did not give their offspring the advantages they should have received.

In spite of this, clashes in the home often arise between parental attitudes and behavior characteristic of a lower class and those middle-class attitudes and characteristics which professional workers are teaching children, not only because they believe in the superiority of middle-class culture, but also because they are preparing the children to move up into the middle class. It is not the child's evidence of his preparation for social mobility which parents resent, but rather the lack of respect for his elders which such teaching is likely to engender. The nurse should help the child to draw a distinction between superficial cultural traits in which he differs from his parents and the fundamental traits which are recognized in all classes as fine and highly desirable. Examples are courage, honesty, fidelity, truthfulness, and self-sacrifice for those one loves.

Parent Education. The discussion of nurse-parent relations leads directly into the matter of parent education. In a broad sense parent education begins in childhood, when the personality of the prospective parent is formed in the home. That is, a child from a stable home in which he participates in good parent-child-sibling relations is being educated for creating such a home when he himself marries and founds a family. In instances of juvenile delinquency or warped personality we constantly hear that the parents are to blame for their children's behavior, but we seldom stop to consider the logic of that conclusion: the parents, too, were once children and therefore were influenced by their own home environment. This is not an acceptance of the fatalistic view whereby the blame for the faults of one generation rests upon the preceding one, and so on back indefinitely. Although personality is strongly set in childhood, it can be altered, albeit with greater difficulty, at any age up to senescence. The nurse, then, must accept the parents' personalities and their attitude toward the child while she guides them to a better understanding of how to help him grow up.

The nurse in any shared nurse-parent learning situation must remember certain basic principles. She must learn first of all what the mother already knows. In other words, the nurse must know the level of the mother's understanding and her background of experience. The nurse must know the mother's resources at home. Does the mother have the equipment she will need or the financial resources to obtain this equipment? The nurse, realizing the mother's problems, must be willing to proceed slowly, allowing time for the mother to absorb what is to be learned. In order to make certain that the mother understands fully, the nurse should either write down what she has said or have the mother repeat what she has learned.

The pediatric nurse's role includes a *demonstration* of physical care and child guidance. That is why it is important that she be prepared to teach the mother. But the nurse's influence on the mother does not always center on physical care and its psychologic components. She demonstrates to the mother how to help the child handle his emotions and also to create or remove stimuli,

increasing those which promote a beneficial response and decreasing those which do not.

Although the nurse has a general background of knowledge and experience, she must recognize her role in her interaction with other professional personnel who give service to the child and his parents. That is, the physician and the child psychiatrist direct the medical and sociopsychologic components of what is demonstrated and taught the parent. The nurse is likely to be the most effective member of the professional group working with the child in the constant application of the plan for parental education; she demostrates, while giving physical care, how to meet the child's emotional needs. She teaches procedures which the parents will have to continue for the child when he returns home—both what to do and its psychologic component.

The nurse helps the mother both physically and emotionally. She guides the mother in her attitude toward the child's condition and in her concept of herself. Parents often blame themselves too much for the afflictions of their children. They should realize that they cannot expect perfection of themselves or of anyone else. They must also realize that child care, like all rationally directed action, is based on a weighing of pros and cons as to what is to be done for the child. Their decision must be based on the probability of the outcome. We can give statistics as to automobile accidents, certain diets and the chances of recovery from specific diseases or injuries, but no one can predict with certainty about a particular child. We often hear a parent say, "We wish we had not consented to the operation." They should be encouraged to believe that they made a wise decision even if, in their particular case, it proved to be wrong.

The Nurse's Responsibilities on the Admission of a Child

The role of the nurse in the admission procedure is complementary to that of the mother and the child. To fill her role she must understand that the mother's behavior is the result of the way the child's sickness and hospitalization appear to her. The mother should never be told not to cry or that she is "really fortunate, because the situation could be worse." Such comments cause a mother to repress her feelings and to be ashamed that she spoke so openly. Repression of anxiety or feelings of guilt or inadequacy causes these feelings to increase, while expression of them diminishes their intensity.

The nurse should never be critical of a mother's attitude however unreasonable it may appear. Such criticism leads to greater tension and possibly to hostility on the mother's part. In order to be helpful the nurse must understand what the illness means to the mother, who may be mis-informed as to the cause, prognosis and necessary treatment.

The following are ways by which the nurse may make the mother feel more secure and calm in the hospital, and the child less restless:

1. The mother should be taken with the child to his bed in the unit or private room. Then she knows where the child is and has a mental pic-ture of his comfortable physical environment. Reducing her anxiety reduces that of the child.

2. The nurse who admits the child should in-troduce herself and the head nurse or team leader to the mother. All names should be clearly pro-nounced. If the child is old enough, he should be introduced to other children of his own age and to the attending personnel.

3. The mother should be given a friendly wel-come and should be seated comfortably. The nurse, even if she has other duties which need her attention, must be unhurried and calm. Her attitude increases the parents' trust in the hos-pital and medical staff which the nurse rep-resents.

4. The admission procedure should be care-fully explained, and all questions asked by the parents should be answered clearly, fully and in a way which will not frighten the mother.

The specific routine of admission is as fol-lows:

1. History of Illnesses. The nurse introduces the mother to the physician who will take the history of the present illness. The child should not be present, for if he is old enough, he will understand and sense his mother's anxiety. Even an infant senses tension and anxiety in his mother.

2. Vital Signs. The nurse takes the vital signs: temperature, pulse, respiration and, if necessary, blood pressure. A temperature reading per rec-tum should be taken last, since it is likely to make the child cry. Crying influences the res-piration and pulse, and an accurate record is not obtained. The blood pressure is taken if ordered by the physician on admission. Since it is dif-ficult to obtain an accurate blood pressure read-ing on an infant or small child, the nurse must be careful to use the correct equipment. A large source of error in taking measurements of blood pressure is the use of a cuff of inappropriate width. The cuff should be about the same width in proportion to the arm circumference as that used for the adult. The width of the arm cuff used on children of various ages follows:

> Newborns—2.5 cm.
> 2 weeks to 1 year—5 cm.
> 1 to 13 years—9 cm.
> Adult—13 cm.

The child should be at rest when the blood pressure reading is made. Excitement, discom-fort, or distrust of the person taking the reading affects the blood pressure so that an accurate reading cannot be made.

The average normal blood pressure readings for children are as follows:

Age	Systolic	Diastolic
Birth	40	—
1 month	80	—
4 years	85	60
8 years	95	62
12 years	108	67
16 years (boys)	118	75
20 years (boys)	120	75

As can be seen from the foregoing blood pres-sure readings, there is a gradual rise in systolic blood pressure in both boys and girls during growth. Diastolic blood pressure rises only slightly over the age span from six to eighteen years. Until the age of fourteen years there seems to be no significant sex difference. After that age the systolic pressure continues to rise in boys, but remains stable in girls. In addition to the age and sex differences in blood pressure readings, there are differences in children who are more mature than others at a given age.

3. Weight. The nurse weighs the child on ad-mission (see p. 276).

4. Examination of the Child. The mother should undress the infant or young child and, if possible, assist with the examination. Every effort should be made by both the physician and the nurse to complete the examination with-out restraining the child; however, the nurse may have to help in restraint of an infant or young child during examination of the head (eyes, ears, nose and mouth). During this part of the examination the nurse holds the child with his back against her chest. Her right hand, placed on his forehead, steadies his head, and her left arm restrains his arms. Sometimes it may be necessary to "mummy" (see p. 301) the body and further restrain the child by leaning over his body while placing her hands on either side of his head.

The nurse should speak to the child and caress him in order that restraint may not be frighten-ing to him or to his mother.

5. Preparation for Procedures. Both the in-fant and the older child should be prepared for treatments and unpleasant procedures, although they cannot understand the implications. This preparation in an infant may be no more than conditioning him to know that an unpleasant procedure is associated with something which brings comfort. We cannot explain the purpose or the procedure of sticking a needle into his arm, but we can make it appear as one of the un-pleasant things which he has learned to accept as part of a pleasant relation with other people.

We talk to him and pet him and let him experience this procedure in a pleasant setting. He should have learned to trust others when unpleasant things are done to him in his routine care (e.g. cleaning his nose). This trust in others carries over from routine care to the unfamiliar experiences in the hospital; he cries from pain, but his fright is decreased. If his mother or a nurse to whom he is accustomed is with him, he applies this generalized experience with unpleasant procedures to this particular incident.

A child in the toddler age group or older should have all procedures which are to be done to him explained in terms he can understand. Listening to the physician's or nurse's heart through the stethoscope is a kind of explanation he understands. Not all procedures can be demonstrated in this way, but the use of such techniques gives the child a basis for understanding the general purpose of examinations and treatments. Picture books and dolls have been used to help a child understand what will be done to him before the examination, treatment or procedure is undertaken. Since verbal explanation may not always be possible, the nurse's presence is needed to provide comfort for the child.

Conference with the Head Nurse or Team Leader

The talk should center on the mother's child and not on children in general. To emphasize this the nurse should speak of the child by name rather than by some general term such as "baby" or "little boy." Such an approach leads up to asking the mother for information about the child which the physicians and nurses need in caring for him. This information should be available to the whole health team. Figure 4-9 gives a suggested outline for obtaining such information, especially after the period of infancy.

The nurse should tell the mother the hours when she will be allowed to visit the child and should explain why it is advisable for the mother to come as often as possible to see him. If a mother seems reluctant to visit frequently, she may be questioned as to the reason, but should not be made to feel guilty about not visiting. If the mother speaks of needing help which the nurse cannot give, arrangements may be made for her to talk with the physician or, with his permission, the social worker.

It should be explained to the mother that during visiting hours she may help in the child's care. There may be little she can do for a critically ill child, but gradually, as she becomes accustomed to his care and as his condition improves, she will be able to do more for him, e.g. giving him the "potty," bathing or feeding him or changing his diaper. Helping in his nursing

care relieves not only the mother's sense of frustration at not being able to do everything for him, but also her sense of guilt if she feels that his sickness was caused by neglect on her part. At the same time she is learning how to give the care he will require after he has gone home.

If the hospital has written policies about visiting hours and regulations as to food, toys, the wearing of gowns and masks, and so on, this should be fully explained to the mother, who should be given a copy of the rules – if the hospital has printed copies – before she leaves the pediatric area.

The mother should remain, if possible, until the child is comfortable. If she has permission from the hospital for unlimited visiting hours of if the child is in a private room, all facilities for her comfort should be explained to her: the location of the washroom, smoking room, lounge, public telephone, and the place where she may sleep and have her meals. In the majority of hospitals only breakfast is served to the mother; for her other meals she may go to the cafeteria or snack-bar. To be away from the child for these short periods gives her a needed change of environment.

If the mother intends to remain with the child during treatments, examinations and the taking of specimens, the purpose of these procedures should be explained to her. Although the parents may participate in the child's care, the nurse must be responsible for the total nursing care. With the mother as an assistant she has an opportunity for health teaching which will affect not only the patient, but also the entire family. It is an ideal situation, for the mother learns through observation and discussion rather than through formal teaching, which is only indirectly related to the individual child.

Nursing Procedures after Admission of a Child

After admission of a child to the hospital the nurse may need to carry out certain procedures, including medical aseptic technique, collection of urine specimens, collection of blood specimens and the giving of medications.

Medical Aseptic Technique. The *purpose* of medical aseptic technique is to prevent transmission of infection from one child to another or to the personnel who care for him. It is the joint responsibility of the medical and nursing staffs to plan the procedures and techniques and to carry out medical aseptic patient care.

Medical aseptic technique is necessary whenever the patient and his belongings are considered contaminated. Those who care for him are considered to be clean when they enter his unit, but to become contaminated when they touch him or his equipment. If only her hands

```
Pediatric Department
Personal History Sheet


Child's name _____     Date of Birth _____
Child's nickname _____     Religion _____
Date of admission_____ Number of previous hospitalizations _____
Does the child know why he is being hospitalized? _____
Has the child been prepared for this admission? _____
How did he react to the preparation? _____
Does he have any special fears about the hospital? Needles? _____
       People in white uniforms? _____ Others?  _____
Names and ages of child's brothers and sisters - _____

Is the child friendly with unfamiliar adults? _____
Is the child friendly with unfamiliar children? _____
Does the child have a pet? _____ Kind_____ Name _____
Have any changes occurred in the child's environment recently? _____
    Birth of sibling (s) _____     Illness in the home _____
    Death of relative _____     Other _____


Eating Habits

How does the child eat? Bottle_____ Cup_____ Spoon _____
Eating schedule _____
Who feeds the child? Adult_____ Child _____
What fluids and solid foods does the child especially enjoy?_____
_____
What fluids and solid foods does the child dislike? _____
_____
Food allergies _____


Sleeping Habits

Usual hour of sleep. Naptime _____     Bedtime _____
Where does the child usually sleep? Crib_____ Junior Bed_____ Adult Bed_____
Does the child sleep alone? _____ If not, with whom does he sleep?_____
Does the child sleep well? _____
Does the child climb out of bed?_____
Does the child have any routines at bedtime? _____ Prayers _____
    Taking a toy to bed_____ Others _____


Toilet Habits

Is the child toilet trained?_____ Bowel movements_____ Urination _____
Terms used for bowel movement_____ Urination_____
What time does the child usually have a daily bowel movement?_____
Does the child wear diapers or panties? _____
Does the child use a toilet chair? _____ Adult toilet? _____
Does the child need assistance with toileting? _____
If the child is taken to the toilet at night, what time is this done?_____
```

Figure 4–9. The Personal History Sheet may be completed by either the mother, the nurse admitting the child to the hospital, the head nurse or the team leader. On another sheet the nurse who admits the child should record her observations of the mother-child relations and their initial adjustment to the hospital. Other personnel who care for the child should make additional comments during the course of the hospital stay.

Personal Care

Does the child need assistance with Bathing _____
                                    Dressing _____
                                    Combing Hair _____
                                    Brushing teeth _____

Play Habits

With whom does the child like to play? Alone _____
                                    With other children _____
                                    With adults _____
What are the child's favorite Games _____
                            Toys _____
Did you bring the child's favorite toy to the hospital? _____

School Activities

Does the child attend Nursery school _____
                    Grade school _____
                    Church school _____
Name of school attended _____
Grade in school _____
Name (s) of favorite friend (s) _____
Name of favorite teacher _____

Special interests

Does the child enjoy any particular Hobbies _____
                                    Radio programs _____
                                    Television programs _____
                                    Books _____

Additional comments which would help make the child's hospital stay as pleasant as possible __
_____
_____
_____

Note : On another sheet the nurse who admits the child should record her observations concerning the mother-child relationship and their initial adjustment to the hospital. Other personnel who care for the child should make additional comments during the course of the hospital stay.

Figure 4–9 (Continued).

touch the patient while the nurse gives him brief nursing care, it is not necessary for her to wear a gown. Only her hands will be contaminated, and she will wash them on leaving the area.

The *isolation unit* is an area, cubicle, room or part of a unit in which one or more patients having the same infectious disease are given care. The furnishings in an isolation unit should be simple, as few as possible for the comfort of the patient and easily cleaned. There should be sufficient equipment for the patient's care, but excess articles should not be kept in the same area. The amount of equipment will depend upon the child's age, the kind of infection and the number of patients isolated in the unit. All furniture, the sink, walls, floor and equipment are considered contaminated in such a unit. The area where the gown is hung is contaminated, but the inside of the gown is kept clean. A damp cloth or a wet mop is used in cleaning the room to prevent organisms from being dispersed in the air. Bedside equipment should be sterilized at regular intervals while the patient is in an isolation unit.

Admission of a patient to an isolation unit involves a number of procedures. It is customary to send the child's clothes home and give the parents instructions as to disinfection or sterilization by airing them, washing them thoroughly or boiling whatever can be sterilized in this way.

Each patient should have his own equipment, such as a thermometer and bathing equipment, in his unit. Toys brought to the hospital with the child should be of the sort that can be easily cleaned; they should be tied to the bed so thay cannot drop to the floor. Care must be taken that the string or tape tying the toys to the crib cannot become twisted around the child's neck.

Visiting an isolated patient is permitted because of the importance of preserving parent-child relations. Parents must observe certain precautions, however, for their own safety and that of the child. They should be given instructions about visiting regulations for such patients. It is a good plan to have these instructions printed in order that parents may read them when they are at home and the initial anxiety over the child's hospitalization is passed.

When parents visit, they must wear isolation gowns, to be discarded after use. (In some hospitals these gowns are sent to the laundry with other contaminated linen; in other hospitals they are not only laundered when necessary, but also autoclaved after use.) The parents must be supervised during visiting hours to prevent their breaking the prescribed hospital technique.

Gown technique is time-consuming, but is one of the most important factors in medical aseptic technique. Anyone who gives direct care involving close contact with a child must wear a gown to protect his clothing from contamination.

The gown must be long enough to cover the nurse's uniform; it should open down the back and be ample enough to lap over the other side.

Some hospitals require that the gown be discarded after each use, but it is more general practice to have it reused for twenty-four hours unless soiled. If it is to be reused, the inside must be kept clean. The gown must be put on, taken off and hung up in a special way in order that the inside does not become contaminated. If the gown is hung inside the contaminated area, it is hung on a hook with the contaminated side out so that persons or equipment nearby will not touch the gown and contaminate the clean inside surface.

Before anyone puts the gown on he must wash his hands thoroughly. The gown is lifted from the hook by grasping the inside near the shoulder seams. The person putting on the gown inserts one arm into a sleeve while still holding the gown with the other hand. The gown is then supported with one hand that is within the sleeve while the other arm is put into the other sleeve. Both hands are uncontaminated, since only the inside of the sleeves and cuffs has been touched. Next, the top backstrings are tied. Then the back edges of the gown are approximated and rolled together, and the lower strings are tied securely so that the gown will not drop upon the patient as the nurse bends over him.

After the nurse has given the child all the necessary care she removes the gown by first untying the strings at the back of the waist. She then washes her hands. She unties the strings at the back of her neck. Next she slips her right hand under the cuff of the left sleeve and pulls it over her left hand, which, remaining in the sleeve, is used to pull the right cuff of the gown over the hand. The right hand, uncontaminated, is withdrawn from the sleeve and used to grasp the clean neck band and support the gown while she withdraws her left hand from the sleeve. Both hands, still uncontaminated, are used to approximate the sides of the neck band. Holding the gown in her left hand, the nurse with her right hand grasps the outside of the shoulder seams and hangs the gown on the hook. The gown must be hung so that both edges are brought together and the top back strings hang free. The neck band and strings can be adjusted with the clean left hand. Both hands can then be used to complete the adjustment of the gown on the hook. The hands and lower forearms must be thoroughly washed before the nurse leaves the unit or touches her uniform.

Mask technique is important, since infectious disease is commonly spread through droplet spray from the nose and mouth, which are also the portals through which respiratory infection is most likely to enter the body. The wearing of masks is a controversial topic, however; some physicians believe masks to be of value, but others believe them to be ineffective. If a mask is worn, it should cover both the nose and the mouth to prevent (1) spreading of organisms present in the spray of the nose and throat of the wearer and (2) inhalation of infectious material in the air about a patient suffering from a respiratory infection. A mask should be worn once, for a period of no longer than one hour, and then discarded, for it is readily contaminated by the constant passage of air through its meshes, which trap bacteria. A mask should never be dropped loosely around the neck and then drawn up into position over the nose and mouth.

Handwashing technique varies in different hospitals both as to the soap or cleansing solution used and the precise procedure. The equipment needed is running water, soap, a nail brush and paper towels, Soap containing hexachlorophene is used in many hospitals. This leaves a film on the skin of adsorbed chemical which has a prolonged antiseptic affect. Repeated use of hexachlorophene soap tends to reduce the normal bacterial flora on the skin surface. It is most effective against gram-positive bacteria. The action of the chemical is reduced when alcohol or water or other soaps which do not contain hexachlorophene are used. The nail brush is kept in a disinfectant near the sink. Paper towels should be available in a suitable container.

The procedure for turning the water on varies with the location of the sink. If it is in the cubicle, the handles of the faucets are usually considered contaminated. If the sink is outside the cubicle, the handles are usually considered clean and must be turned on with paper towels, since the nurse's hands are contaminated. If the water is controlled by a foot pedal, this is always considered contaminated, since it is near the floor.

The hands must be soaped and rinsed three times. If they are grossly contaminated, they must be washed thoroughly or scrubbed with a brush for at least two minutes according to the procedure adopted by the individual hospital staff. The nurse should not give care to isolated patients if she has abrasions on her hands, since she is unable to cleanse them thoroughly. Furthermore, if the patient has an infection which can be contracted through a break in the skin, the nurse might become infected with the organism.

Concurrent disinfection is the destruction of pathogenic organisms carried out continuously while the child is isolated. Such articles as dishes, clothing, bedding and equipment for treatment must be disinfected. Any articles brought into the room which are used by or have touched a patient must be disinfected before being used for another patient. Linens, clothing and eating utensils are sterilized by boiling or autoclaving. Any glass or metal objects which cannot be autoclaved, such as thermometers, must be scrubbed with soap and water and soaked in alcohol or other antiseptic solution, depending on hospital policy. Certain objects such as mechanical equipment which cannot be cleansed by boiling or washing must be exposed to the air and either sunlight or ultraviolet light to kill the surface organisms. The staff in some

hospitals use gas sterilization for equipment which cannot be sterilized otherwise. The need for disinfection of excreta, vomitus and sputum depends on the type of organism causing the illness. Specific directions for disinfection are usually outlined by the hospital and are influenced by sewer facilities in the area.

Terminal disinfection means making the physical environment and the body of the child *clean* so that infection cannot be conveyed to others after he has ceased to be a source of infection.

Collection of Urine Specimens. Urine specimens are usually requested on admission. Collection of such specimens from older children who can cooperate with either the nurse or the mother is relatively easy, but is more difficult from infants.

The collection of urine specimens from infants involves the application of a collecting device to the perineum. In past years the birdseed cup for girls or the test tube for boys was attached to the genitalia. These types of collecting devices were hazardous, since the glass of which they were made could injure the genitalia if the edges were not covered with adhesive tape.

Pediatric urine collectors are now made of clear, pliable, plastic material secured to a sponge ring (Fig. 4-10). After the skin has been cleaned and dried this sponge ring, coated with pressure-sensitive adhesive, is attached firmly around the genitalia. When the child voids, the plastic receptacle can be removed easily. The adhesive surfaces can be pressed together and the specimen sent in the leak-proof bag thus formed to the laboratory.

Since catheterizations are rarely ordered on infants or small children, physicians usually request that a clean urine specimen be obtained. In order to obtain a clean specimen from an infant or small child the genitalia should be cleaned, using cotton balls wet with sterile soap and water and then rinsed with an antiseptic solution. When washing the female genitalia, it is important that a different cotton ball be used for each stroke made from above the clitoris downward to the anus. The strokes should cleanse the meatus first, then move outward to the perineum. After cleaning the genitalia thoroughly, a plastic urine collector should be applied as described above.

To obtain a clean specimen from a preschool or older child who can cooperate, cleanse the genitalia as described above. The female child can sit on a training chair beneath which is a sterile potty or a sterile basin, or she may void into a sterile bedpan. An older boy may void into a sterile urinal or directly into the sterile specimen bottle.

Although a midstream specimen is likely to be cleaner than the urine which is voided initially, such a specimen is difficult to obtain from small

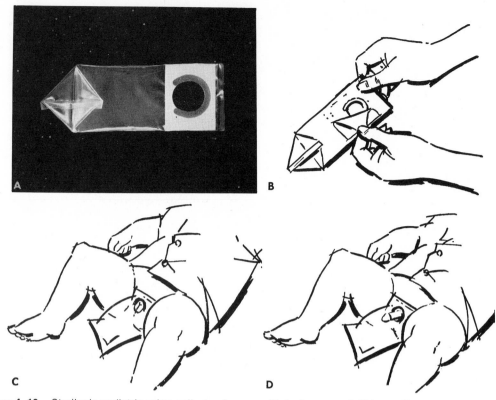

Figure 4–10. Sterilon's pediatric urine collector for use with both sexes. *A*, Urine collector bag. *B*, Removing paper backing exposing adhesive surface. *C*, On the female, the round opening in the bag is placed so as to cover the upper half of the external genitalia. *D*, On the male, the penis is projected through the round opening in the bag. (Courtesy Sterilon Corporation, Buffalo, New York.)

children. If the child is able to cooperate, have him void a small amount into an unsterile container, and then void into a sterile receptacle.

The collection of a continuous or 24-hour urine specimen will be discussed later (see p. 219).

Collection of Blood Specimens. Blood specimens are obtained for various reasons: for determination of the degree of illness, for diagnosis or for evaluation of therapy.

The procedure used for adult patients is used for older children whose veins are large enough and who are able to cooperate after an explanation of the procedure has been given them. In infants and young children whose veins are small only the larger veins may be used, most commonly the femoral or external jugular veins. Since infants and small children cannot understand a verbal explanation, mummy restraint is used, and the procedure is completed as soon as possible. The assistance of the nurse in drawing blood shortens the procedure because the physician can locate the vein with more ease.

The nurse's responsibility is to restrain the child's head during jugular puncture (Fig. 4-11) or the legs during femoral puncture (Fig. 4-12).

After the needle has been removed from the jugular vein, firm pressure should be exerted over the vein for three to five minutes while the child is held in a sitting position. After femoral vein puncture firm pressure should be exerted over the vein, also for three to five minutes, in order to prevent leakage of blood into the subcutaneous tissues. While the infant is restrained, it is important that the nurse make comforting sounds during the procedure and that she hold or rock the infant after the procedure. Small children can be encouraged to play out their anger and frustration caused by the pain of the needle insertion after the procedure has been completed.

Medications. The giving of medications to a child is a serious responsibility. There is even greater need for accuracy in pouring and giving medications than with adult patients. The dose varies with the size and age of the child, and the nurse has no standard dose which she is accustomed to as in giving medication to adult patients. Since the dose is relatively small, a slight mistake in the amount of a drug given makes a greater proportional error in terms of the amount ordered than with the adult dose.

Every hospital has its own method of identi-

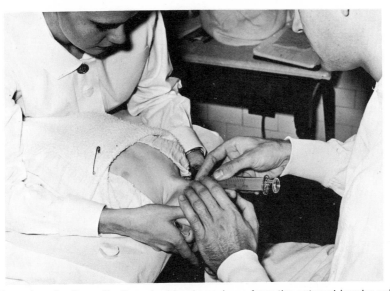

Figure 4-11. Procedure for the collection of a blood specimen from the external jugular vein. The "mummy restraint" (see Figs. 13-5 and 13-6) is used. The child's head is rotated fully to one side and extended partly over the end of the table to stretch the vein. The nurse places the palm of one hand over the occiput, the fingers of the other hand over the bones of the face. The nurse must avoid making pressure over the child's nose or mouth.

fication for patients. Identification is necessary with all patients, but is more difficult with children. The infant cannot give his name, and a small child is likely to give his nickname or only his first name. The nurse must carefully identify a child before giving him medication. Most hospitals use wristbands for identifying children, and the child's name is also marked upon his bed. A double check on the child who is out of bed and old enough to tell is to ask him his name. (The nurse should never say, "Are you Alice White?" but should ask, "What is your name?") The child's name is checked with that on the medicine card, as is done in giving medication to adult patients.

The nurse should give all medications in a way that helps her to establish a constructive relation with the child. To tell a child that a medicine will taste good when it taste bad destroys a child's faith in nurses.

Since the possibility of error is greater in the giving of medication to children than to adults, and since a child's reaction to a dose ordered by the physician is less predictable than an adult's reaction, the nurse must be alert to recognize undesirable effects of the medication given.

DRUG DOSAGE. Since most drugs are put up by drug companies in a convenient form or strength for giving a standard adult dose, children's doses are often computed in terms of fractions of the adult dose on the basis of age or weight. Although the physician prescribes the dosage of medication, the nurse should have a general knowledge of the relation between the customary adult dose and that for children in

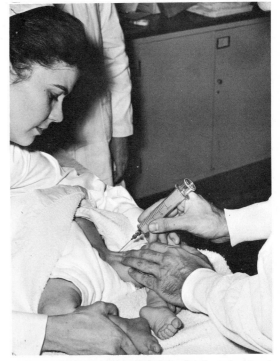

Figure 4-12. Procedure for the collection of a blood specimen from the femoral vein. The "mummy restraint" is used over the upper part of the child's body. The nurse spreads the child's legs apart in a frog position and holds them securely. The infant's genitalia are covered with a diaper.

different age groups from infancy through childhood.

The following rules for calculating drug dosages for children are frequently used:

Fried's Rule (for child less than one year of age)

Infant's dose: $\dfrac{\text{Age in months}}{150} \times$ adult dose

Clark's Rule (for child two years of age or over)

Child's dose: $\dfrac{\text{Adult dose} \times \text{weight in pounds}}{150 \text{ (weight of average adult)}}$

Young's Rule (for child two years of age or over)

Child's dose: $\dfrac{\text{Adult dose} \times \text{age in years}}{\text{Age in years plus } 12}$

Dosages based on the child's weight (Clark's
Rule) give the most accurate results. Many drugs
are calculated entirely on this basis. Some physicians, however, are using a newer method of
determining dosage based on body surface area
because this measurement is believed to be more
closely related than weight to the infant's or
child's metabolism. Although the nurse does not
decide the dosage to be given the child, she must
be alert to amounts of drugs customarily ordered
by the physicians. If an amount ordered seems to
her to be excessive, she should call it to the attention of the physician.

The nurse should know the expected action of
the drug as well as the appropriate dose commonly ordered for a child the size of her patient.
She should also be alert to symptoms of overdosage, since the child usually does not complain,
and report such symptoms at once to the physician so that quick action can be taken to counteract the effects of the drug.

ORAL ADMINISTRATION.   Infants will generally
accept medication put into their mouths, provided it is in a form which they can readily
swallow. A bib should be placed on the infant,
and the medication should be given slowly.
The nurse should raise the infant to a sitting
position or, if this is contraindicated, elevate his
head and shoulders. There is then less danger of
his choking.

The older child, because he is unhappy in the
hospital or has had experience with bad-tasting
medicines, may refuse his medication. There is
no single technique for winning his cooperation.
The nurse must study the situation and find the
best way to get him to take the medication. Her
manner should be positive, firm and kind. When
the nurse gives a child a feeling of support, that
she understands his dislike of the medication
and appreciates cooperation, he is conditioned to
take the medication. She must convey in her
manner rather than in words that he *must take
the medication.* She should never plead or coax.
Children will cooperate more readily if they see
other children taking medicine.

It is a good plan to disguise the taste of a drug

by putting it in cherry syrup, Karo or honey
syrup. Pills should be crushed and the contents
of capsules emptied and mixed with syrup for
children too young to take bulk medication. In
general, medications should not be mixed with
milk or food unless specifically ordered by the
physician, because the child might develop a
serious dislike for that food.

Medication can be given from a medicine glass,
the tip of a teaspoon or a rubber-tipped medicine
dropper. Fluid medications may be sucked
through bright-colored straws.

The nurse should be careful not to let her own
distaste for a drug show in her expression, for the
child will quickly adopt this attitude toward his
medicine from her.

If a child always struggles when medication is
given him and his cooperation cannot be obtained, the nurse should report this to the physician. To struggle may do the child more harm
than to go without his medicine. The nurse
should never hold the child's nose or force the
medication into his mouth, for he may aspirate
the medication. Such action shows that the nurse
is hostile and not helpful to the child.

If the medication is immediately vomited, the
physician should be notified. He may order the
dose to be repeated. Unpleasant-tasting drugs
should not be given around mealtime, for they
may interfere with the child's appetite.

The child old enough to take pills should be
told to place the pill near the back of his tongue
and to drink the water, fruit juice or milk offered
him in order to wash down the pill.

A child who cooperates in taking his medicine should be praised and thereby will know that
his nurse appreciates his help.

INTRAMUSCULAR INJECTIONS.   The giving of
the first intramuscular injection is important,
because on the basis of this experience the child
builds up his attitude toward future injections.
The procedure is the same as for the adult.

If the child is old enough to understand, the
procedure should be explained to him. He should
be allowed to express his fear and resentment of
needles. The child of school age and the adolescent, like the little child, should be allowed to
vent their feelings of dislike or resentment.

Prior to giving an injection the nurse should
spend time with the child and develop a degree of
rapport with him. Then the procedure should be
carried out quickly and gently. It is a good plan
to have a second nurse assist. She supports or restrains the child, or does both. One technique
helpful when giving an intramuscular injection
is to provide a diversionary action by offering the
child something else on which he can fix his
attention. The child could hold someone's hand
and squeeze it when he feels the needle stick, or
he could lie prone and concentrate on pointing
his toes inward. By pointing his toes inward

the gluteal muscles relax and the injection is less painful. Since the injection is painful to some degree, the nurse must help him master his feeling about such necessary forms of treatment.

The upper outer quadrant of the buttocks may be used for injecting medication intramuscularly; however, because serious trauma can result from administering injections incorrectly into the buttocks, many hospitals now recommend the use of the muscle in the anterolateral aspect of the thigh. If the child has sufficiently large muscles on other parts of the body, the injection site should be varied.

After the procedure the nurse should show her approval of the infant or child for his cooperation and hold him for a few minutes so that he does not associate only pain with her ministrations. He may then be given some toy to divert his attention from the experience. If he has been uncooperative, the nurse should not show disapproval. He too should be held and comforted and then given a toy.

An older child may be allowed to select the site for injection, subject to the nurse's approval, and cleanse the area for himself.

INTRAVENOUS ADMINISTRATION. Graduate nurses in some hospitals are permitted to insert medications into bottles of intravenous solutions to be given to children. This procedure requires the utmost care for the safety of the patient.

Usually students, if they are permitted to administer any medication in this way, may give only vitamins. It is essential that the student be aware of the rule regarding this practice in the hospital where she is gaining experience, for her own safety as well as that of the children in her care.

RECTAL ADMINISTRATION. Drugs given by rectum are injected in the same manner as a retention enema. The medication may be mixed with a little water or a small amount of starch solution. It should be given slowly so that all of it is retained. Some medications to be given rectally are also available in suppository form. In explaining this procedure to a young child it can be likened to the experience he has already had of having a rectal temperature taken.

Safety Measures

Accidents are a leading cause of death among infants and small children. Great emphasis should be placed on the prevention of accidents in the hospital, both for the safety of the child while he is there and in order that mothers may have a practical demonstration of how accidents common to little children may be avoided. The following discussion is concerned chiefly with accidents in the hospital, but certain of these also occur in the home.

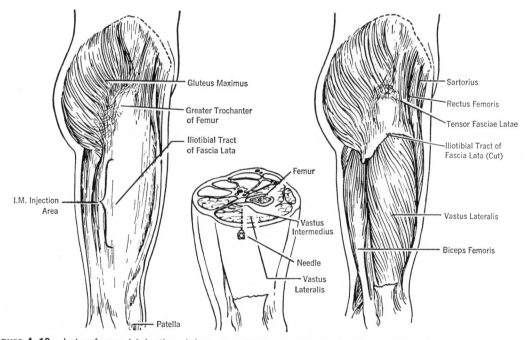

Figure 4–13. Laterofemoral injection. Inject at a right angle into the midarea of the lateral part of the thigh. Do *not* inject into the areas proximal to the knee or hip joints. The superficial location of the lateral femoral cutaneous nerve makes it especially vulnerable to injury; damage due to intramuscular injection has been reported. (M. Pitel and M. Wemett: The Intramuscular Injection. *Am. J. Nursing*, April, 1964, p. 104.)

Many safety measures deal with the construction of the building or unit and are beyond the control of the nurse. Among these are the following:

1. Fireproof, wide stairways.
2. Windows protected by locked screens and window guards and so placed that drafts do not blow upon the children when the windows are open for ventilation.
3. Gates at the entrance to rooms where small children play, so constructed that a child cannot open them or catch his fingers between the door and its frame.

Other measures for children's safety which are directly under the nurse's control are as follows:

1. The catches on the side gates of the crib should be in good condition, and the gates should always be up when the child is in bed. When administering care with the side gate down, the nurse should keep her hand on the infant or little child to prevent his falling, especially if she looks away from him or reaches for an object on the bedside table.
2. Restraints, if used should be applied correctly to prevent constriction of any part of the child's body. The greatest danger is that of strangulation through pressure of a jacket restraint which has slipped out of place and encircled a patient's neck.
3. Medicine cabinets should be locked when not in use, and medications should *never* be left standing on a bedside table.
4. Instruments and solutions should be kept in cabinets or on shelves where children cannot reach them.
5. *Safety pins should be closed* at once when taken from a child's clothing and put out of his reach. An infant or young child tends to put small objects into his mouth.
6. Toys should have rounded rather than sharp edges. They should never be painted with lead paint and should not have small parts which a child could remove and swallow or aspirate. They should never be left on the floor, since a child or a nurse with a child in her arms might trip over them. For the same reason, wet areas on the floors should be dried immediately.
7. Infants and small children should not be allowed to play with tongue depressors or applicators.
8. Electric outlets and fans should be covered when not in use, and the fans should be placed where children cannot reach them.
9. Isolation techniques should be carried out on all children with infectious illnesses. For this to be practicable, adequate facilities must be available for the nurse to wash her hands. She should wash her hands after caring for each child. All other isolation procedures to prevent cross-infection must be rigidly followed. In the children's units of some hospitals ultraviolet rays are used to cut down the number of airborne organisms. The nurse must be aware of symptoms indicating the onset of infectious disease in both the children and herself. Such symptoms should be promptly reported.
10. Nursing bottles should *never* be propped, *nor should feedings be forced* upon a little child. There is danger of aspiration, which may cause pulmonary disease or even sudden death.
11. In giving medication to an infant or a little child who will not cooperate a second nurse is required to assist in gentle restraint. Oily medications should *never* be given orally to a child who is crying, because of the danger of aspiration (see p. 293).
12. Hot-water bottles must always be tightly stoppered and covered before being placed near a child's body or even in the bed with him. The water temperature should not be over 115°F.
13. The bulb of a thermometer should be checked to be certain that it is not cracked. If the temperature is taken rectally, the nurse must hold the thermometer in place so that it will not be dislodged and so that the child will not injure himself if he rolls over.

Discharge From the Hospital

The physician or nurse, or psychiatrist if he was attached to the health team, should tell the parents that it is natural for an infant, or even an older child, when taken home, to show symptoms of a disturbed relation with his parents. He may be more clinging and seek more affection than before hospitalization, but the reverse may also be true, and he may withdraw from or even reject his mother. He may show his need for comfort by sucking his thumb excessively or reverting to behaviorisms which he had outgrown. His mother must accept this regression as the result of the emotional trauma produced by his separation from her and must help him to regain the normal mother-child relations by her unwavering affection.

Discharge of a child from the pediatric unit to his parents' care requires explicit instructions, especially if his mother has not stayed with him during his hospitalization. *These instructions should be given gradually during the hospitalization instead of on the day of discharge, since the mother is usually too excited to com-*

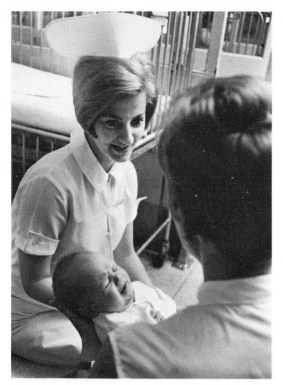

Figure 4–14. Discharge of a child from the pediatric unit to his parents' care requires explicit instructions given during the period of hospitalization. The calm, secure attitude of the nurse helps the mother feel more certain of her own ability to care for the child at home. (Public Relations Department, The Children's Hospital of Philadelphia.)

prehend what she is being told. Important among these are instructions in the use of any specific equipment needed in his care at home, and in the giving of medications; review of the physician's orders; time of the next clinic or physician's appointment; and description of new habits which the child has acquired since his mother last cared for him — e.g. drinking from a cup or eating from a spoon — or new developments in muscular activity. If an infant has learned to roll over, it is important that his mother know it in order to protect him from falling. These new habits change not only the mother's image of her child, but also the way in which she gives him care.

The Role of the Nurse in the Care of the Chronically or Terminally Ill Child and His Family

Earlier in this chapter the general role of the nurse in helping families face the illness and hospitalization of their children was discussed. Usually when a child has a short-term illness with presumably a good outcome, the parents may be anxious, but their anxiety is not that generally felt by parents of a chronically ill child or a child having a terminal illness.

The Care of the Chronically Ill Child

The role of the nurse in helping parents deal with the problem of caring for a chronically ill child such as one having cerebral palsy, poliomyelitis, diabetes, rheumatic fever or some other long-term illness is more complex than that of one caring for an acutely ill child.

Lengthy illness during childhood tends to interfere with the healthy course of the child's development, both physically and emotionally.

The child's need for continuing attention and care makes it extremely difficult for him to achieve his goal in his struggle toward maturity and emotional independence. If the parents are not cognizant of this problem, the child will possibly remain dependent and socially immature. Prolonged illness is likely to prevent the child from developing confidence in his own abilities and a sense of acceptability to his peer group.

Nurses must help parents to understand that they should give the chronically ill child as many of the normal experiences of childhood as possible and by so doing help the child to acquire a positive, healthy attitude toward growing up emotionally and becoming a mature adult. In order to do this successfully parents need to understand the nature of the child's illness, his treatment, and the exact limitations the condition places on the child's activities. Most important, parents and child should understand what the child *can* do as well as what he *cannot* do. Only by exercising his own abilities will the child be able to attain a sense of usefulness and competence.

Parents also should understand how their own reactions to the child's illness, such as great overconcern about his health status, may be a hindrance rather than a help to the child's recovery. Their positive view of his illness will help the child to accept his own limitations and strive to improve his abilities.

The Nurse and the Terminally Ill Child

For most people, even medical and nursing personnel, the phenomenon of death is a very difficult event to face. It is not only difficult for the experienced professional person to face, but it is also difficult to help the nursing student learn in pediatrics to help both the dying child and his grieving parents. Although words can be written on "what you should do in a particular situation," this kind of information is not likely to be of much assistance in an individual practical event in which the student becomes involved. For this reason our discussion of death will concern first the perception of death, then in sequence how the nurse perceives death, what the physician can do, how the parents feel, the meaning of death to a child, and finally the role of the nurse in the care of the terminally ill child and his family.

The Perception of Death. Death is an inevitable and universal experience. But in our American culture, where the emphasis is on life, especially youthful life, the denial of how death occurs is common.

During the education of the nurse, however, death in general is gradually perceived as a natural event in life, one that in many instances is a positive phenomenon in that it relieves the patient of intolerable pain and long-lasting incapacity. Those who are religiously inclined see death as being controlled by a supernatural power, that is in fact "God's will," and that it is the beginning of a new life, whether this includes the idea of eternal reward or punishment or not.

Whether the individual believes that death is a natural event or a supernaturally controlled moment in time, she must still believe that she is able to exert some control in the situation; otherwise the life saving equipment readily available in hospitals would not be used. Even in hospitals controlled by religious groups, nurses tend to believe that God approves their attempt to alleviate discomfort and to prolong life.

Since death itself is an end that comes to all living things, the nurse is bound, in spite of her frequent encounter with the event, in spite of her religious or secular orientation, and in spite of her knowledge of its causes, to have some degree of anxiety about the situation for her patient and for herself. *The fear of death is the most inescapable of all the fears faced by the living.*

The way in which the event of death has been handled in many hospitals has been to remove the dying person, conscious or unconscious, to an area away from other patients. What this means to the conscious patient is that at the very time he needs people around him, he is left alone. Is it any wonder, then, that the older dying child becomes depressed? Do we do this really for the dying patient and his family's comfort, or do we do this because the unit personnel are more comfortable if they cannot see him?

The best way to improve care for the dying patient is to determine the significance of death to the person, whether nurse, physician, parents or child.

The Nursing Student Perceives Death. The attitude of the nursing student toward death is dependent on her culture, age, religion, education, perspective on living, and her own inner security. Because of her youth she has not usually had the experience with life and death that an older person generally has had. Because of her own youth and dreams of a family, the student is especially vulnerable when she sees a family tragedy involving a child. Especially is this difficult in pediatric nursing, where the age of the dying child may not be too far from her own age or possibly from that of one of her siblings. The student may feel as others have felt when caring for a dying child:

"I was panicky. I just knew I couldn't handle the situation alone."

"I prayed that Mary would not die while I was in the room with her. I wanted to run away."

"Jimmy was such a beautiful little boy. I cried until 3 A.M. each day I took care of him."

"After Bridget died I wondered whether I could have done any more for her. I wondered whether I could ever go through this with a child of my own or even if I wanted any children if I might have to face this."

Each student is an individual whose reactions to death are influenced by people and significant events of the past. These influences do not stop even when a young person becomes a graduate nurse. Often a nursing student's or young graduate nurse's first contact with death is clouded by fear and an intense feeling of inadequacy. *It is important, therefore, for the nurse to recognize her own feelings and inadequacies and to work through them sufficiently so that she is able to give care to the dying child and his family.*

Since her own orientation as a nurse is to save life, even an experienced nurse may be ill at ease in talking with and caring for the dying child. Perhaps this is because the individual has never had to face the prospect of "nonbeing" for herself; therefore she is disturbed when she must face it with someone else.

It is possible for the nurse as well as the physician to protect herself from the subject of death by developing a shell around herself, to pretend that death does not occur or that it is not her concern. Some professional persons insulate this shell to the point of callousness. But though this attitude protects the nurse from suffering, it does nothing to help the child and his parents to face the event that is to come.

The first step the nursing student must take is to engage in introspection concerning her beliefs about death and about dying patients. She must understand and perhaps alter her attitude toward the process of dying. To do this the student may need help from her instructor, religious counselor, psychiatrist or another member of the health team. Introspection is difficult and painful, but a necessary part of the educational process. At this time the student must have her religious convictions supported and her reservoir of emotional strength refilled. She must remember that she can and must be helped to understand and handle her own feelings more effectively, for only by so doing can she give emotional support to the child and his parents and share in their grief as a feeling person.

The nurse must be cognizant of the fact that during the process of the child's dying, her closeness to the parents, especially to the mother, involves her in a crisis situation in which her own problems are stimulated by those of the parents. She may become vulnerable as the parent's problems bring to the foreground her own internal conflicts. The nurse in this situation cannot support the mother without having her own needs recognized and met. As long as the nurse is unable to accept her own grief realistically, she will be able to do nothing but inhibit the expression of grief in the parents. But if the nurse can learn to recognize her own underlying feelings rather than negate them, she can get rid of her fears and actually hear what the child and his parents are saying.

Conversation with the dying child and his parents is difficult. The child may be emaciated or disfigured. Some parents are very demanding, and the nurse may respond with anger. Some children are very likable, and the nurse may be grief-stricken by the thought of their deaths.

It is unfortunate when the child's and family's needs are overlooked and the needs of the nurse take precedence. She should appreciate the fact that her attitude is of vital importance in this situation and seek to resolve her own anxieties before entering into this experience.

What the Physician Can Do

Death in an elderly person may be welcomed by the patient and his family because it puts an end to pain and disability. The family is comforted by the knowledge that the person has had a long life and has made some contribution to society. But the death of a child is unacceptable to physicians and everyone else involved. The death of a child from an automobile accident or from a congenital anomaly incompatible with life may come quickly; that from leukemia or a malignant brain tumor usually comes slowly and brings sheer agony not only to the family, but to the entire pediatric unit community as well.

The physician has a responsibility for all his patients to sustain life until he is no longer able to do so. A great deal is currently being written about the problem of when death really occurs for an individual patient. Since this is a textbook for nurses, this question does not have to be explored further here. The important thing is that the nurse know of the research and philosophical exploration currently taking place in this area.

What the physician in addition to his medical therapy does have to do is to decide with the help of other members of the health and nursing teams whether or not the parents and child should be told that death is to be expected. Some physicians believe that parents should be told because it is their right to know what is happening to their child. The physician can tell them about the disease condition affecting their child, that nothing known presently in medical therapy can save their child's life, but that he will be protected from pain and suffering as much as possible. Even when told the truth in this manner, the family must be left with a little ray of hope. Even in malignancy in children there have been just enough unexplained remissions to justify leaving them with a little hope. Usually parents will ask the physician, "How long will he live?" or, "Can he return to school?" The physician can try to answer these questions honestly, but the answers understandably are difficult to formulate.

Most physicians realize the help the religious advisor can give at this time. With the parents' knowledge, they may invite the priest, minister or rabbi to be present during this discussion of their child's illness. For physicians as well as nurses know that if the parents can lean on their religious advisor with confidence, they can support the child better than can the medical and nursing personnel alone.

If an older child asks the physician, "Am I going to die?" this is an even more difficult question to answer than those of the parents. If the child is very stable and mature, some physicians will say, "Yes, but we are not certain when this will be." Children many times can accept this answer better than they can an evasion. If they are old enough to ask this question, they probably have given it a great deal of thought already.

Other physicians believe that the knowledge of death by the parents and the child can only produce more anxiety and that it removes any hope to which they can cling. Actually, no general answer can be given to this question for all families. It is not even clear-cut on many occasions in the instance of an individual family.

How the Parents May Feel

Few human experiences bring with them more suffering to parents than the death of their child. If the parents are told that their child cannot live, they tend to feel limited in their ability to control the situation, and they feel trapped. They are about to lose a loved child and may react stoically or with fear, anger, regression or denial.

Nurses may feel that parents who know the prognosis are being "good" parents when they accept the fact of death gracefully, cause no trouble on the pediatric unit, and are able to provide support for their child. If the family has belief in God, they know that He is omnipotent. Understanding this, they also know that the child's fate is in His hands. Thus they are relieved of their own personal guilt and responsibility.

If the parents lose control, are demanding of the nurses' time, are angry and cry, they are likely to prevent the nurses from performing well with the child and to evoke strong feelings among medical and nursing personnel. Such parents may be avoided at a time when they themselves are most lonely and afraid.

Some parents seem devoid of affect after being told that their child will die. They talk about the coming death with what appears to be a minimum of feeling. At that time they seem to have a lack of emotion, or a dissociation between emotion and mind and body.

Some parents because of their own feelings of guilt and anxiety try to satisfy the child's every whim. They feel that being permissive will prevent frustration in the child and provide a pleasant environment for his last days on earth. Actually, what this behavior really does is to cause the child to regress to an excessively demanding state in which his desires become insatiable. Even the parents eventually react with hostility to such a change in their child. And so a vicious cycle is begun. The parent, knowing of his hostility toward the child, feels increasingly guilty, sets fewer limits on the child's behavior, observes increasing demands by the child, and tries even harder to satisfy these demands. The child, feeling the hostility of the parents, becomes even more insecure and demanding. The child may ultimately suffer more from the hostility of the parents thus engendered than he would have done had consistent limits been set and maintained.

Families after the initial shock may want to know whether they can have a Christmas or a birthday celebration early for the terminally ill child. If the patient is very young without siblings, this may be done. But if he is older and does not know the seriousness of his illness, he may wonder why these celebrations are being held early. Besides, he may be alive when the events naturally occur, and he may be further confused.

If everything medically possible has been done for the child, the physician may ask the parents to help to decide whether to have the child stay in the hospital or to take him home for the remainder of his life. This decision may be based on the presence of other children in the family, the ability of the mother to care for him, and the resources of the family in terms of financial ability and housing. If the child is sent home, the aid of the members of the health team in the community, such as the public health nurse, could be very supportive and helpful to the family.

The Meaning of Death to the Child

As with other aspects of a child's normal growth and development, when he becomes chrono-logically older he changes in his understanding of himself and of the world in which he lives. In like manner he changes his concepts of life and death. Parents cannot really succeed in trying to keep children naive about the fact of death. The best that parents can do is to act naturally in relation to the subject, answer his questions, and thus gradually acquaint the child with this aspect of life.

To a child in the preschool period the idea of death as a physical fact is beyond his level of understanding. A dead person to a small child is one who has gone away as on a trip, but who may eventually return. To a young child, although the dead person he sees may not move, he still lives. Death does not usually frighten a very young child, although if he himself is very ill he may be frightened because of his excessive bleeding or difficult respirations. What frightens him when someone he loves dies is the fact that he has been left alone, that he has been separated from a source of security and love.

Often the young child will have his first real experience with death when a pet dies. At this time he learns that the pet does not return, and he grieves, but in most instances a new pet is obtained and life continues on hardly interrupted.

When the child is about five or six years of age he begins to accept the fact of death, but believes that death has a gradual process to it, that the dead person can return to life, then die again. As in other developmental stages, a child may come to this conclusion earlier or later than five to six years, but it is one stage in his movement toward a mature understanding of the meaning of death.

After they have begun school, children imagine death as being personified in some form. Some children begin to conceptualize death as a person who carries living people off, especially after dark if they are "bad." Some children believe that death is the same thing as a dead person who lies in a coffin. Children between six and nine years believe in general that death is invisible, that no one can really see him until he is carried away himself.

About nine to ten years of age children begin to understand that death is the end-point of the life of the body, that it is inevitable, and that eventually every living thing must die.*

The thoughts of the adolescent concerning death tend to be more varied than those of younger children and are dependent on past memories, degree of belief in a religion, cultural differences, and thoughts of the future.

The way a child views death depends not only on his developmental age, but also on his experiences with death in the past, especially in

---

* M. H. Nagy: The Child's View of Death; in H. Feifel: *The Meaning of Death*. New York, McGraw-Hill Book Company, 1959.

his own immediate family. The meaning of the death of someone close to a child may be varied, depending on his age and relation to the deceased. If a brother or sister dies, the child, no matter what his age, still has his parents on whom to depend. Yet the death of another child affects the parents, who may either turn protectively to the surviving child or children or turn from them in their grief. If the child is older when the sibling dies, he may come to the conclusion that "this may happen to me too, soon, maybe tomorrow or next week." This is a frightening thought for a child of any age. If he also was close to the dead child, he may have guilt feelings about past anger or jealousy toward the dead person or because he failed to do something that would have made him happier when he was alive.

When a parent dies, a real crisis occurs for the child. If the mother dies when the child is very young, he feels frightened by his separation from her. If he is older, he knows that life will never be the same again. If his father dies and his mother must go to work, he suffers not only the loss of his father, but also of his mother, who may be away from him at work part of the day. Also, guilt feelings occur when anyone whom the child loved dies. He may have felt hostile, resentful or jealous at some time toward the deceased. He may even have wished for the removal of the person from his life. When, in effect, his wishes come true, he may feel that what has happened was his fault alone.

The reactions that the child is likely to have concerning the death of someone in the family can be reduced if he knows what is going on and that adults are being honest with him when he asks questions. The decision as to whether or not the child should attend the funeral services depends on his age, the religious custom of the family, and the degree of anxiety which the child shows. Adults should, in general, make an effort to limit expression of their own grief in the child's presence so that their emotion will not be too frightening to the child. But the abilities of the child should be utilized as a contribution to the well-being of the family to whatever extent this is possible.

Children evidence grief in a manner different from that shown by the adult. A child who experiences a deep sense of loss will play actively, "misbehave" by adult standards, or else withdraw. A child should not be reprimanded for his behavior at such a time. This would only tend to increase the burden of guilt he may already feel.

In summary, the way a child views death, especially if he is old enough to know what his illness means, depends on his degree of maturity and the experiences with death he has had in the past.

Opinions vary when the child is terminally ill as to whether or not the child should be told honestly about his own condition and poor prognosis. It is the parents' function with the physician to decide what to tell the child about his condition. It is also the parents' responsibility to decide who should tell the child, whether it be a religious advisor, physician or friend. The important thing for the nurse to know is what information the physician and his parents have decided he should have. Even though the nurse may not agree with what has been told the child, she should respect the wishes of the parents and the physician in this regard and not try to force her beliefs on them. Certainly she should never confuse the child by giving him information he is not able to handle.

The Role of the Nurse in the Care of the Terminally Ill Child and His Parents

The value which society attributes to a person depends on his age, social class, beauty and personality, among other characteristics. A child, therefore, who is just beginning life and has presumably more potential for making a greater contribution to society than an elderly person who "has lived his life" is valued more highly. It should come as no surprise, therefore, that every type of life-prolonging or revival technique is usually utilized to save the life of a child. It should also not come as a surprise that some nurses cannot care for children because they cannot tolerate seeing them die. These nurses have failed to resolve their own feelings, which thus get in the way of helping parents and children in crisis situations.

Death for a young infant such as a premature and for an older child dying with leukemia is different for nurses. The premature infant is not aware of his impending death, while the older child may very well be. This difference changes the way nurses talk, think and act when they are near the patient.

To nurse a child whose death is inevitable and to support the parents is indeed an art and a challenge. First of all the nurse must remember that children who are dying are also still living. She must help them to live their last few days or months to the fullest, to maintain the interests they had before their illness, and to find new ones. The nurse must also remember that children derive security from having reasonable and consistent limits set on their behavior. At a time when the child feels that his body is changing and is undependable, it is especially important that his environment be completely secure.

As was mentioned before, one of the serious problems in the care of the dying child is resolution of the question about how much the parents and the child should be told about the child's condition. If the physician makes this decision alone, many times he does not communicate it to the nurse, who is then left close to the family and the child without knowing how to respond to questions should they arise. A better idea for handling this situation is for the parents, the physician, nurse and other appropriate members of the health team to make the decision together.

The clergy of the family's choosing should be brought into contact with the child and the family as soon as possible if the family wishes to talk with him. The nurse has learned in previous courses the role of the clergy of various religions at the time of death. If the family does not wish to see a religious advisor, the nurse should consider their wishes even though they run counter to her own set of values.

In the past nurses generally emphasized physical care and treatment routines in the care of the dying child and did not provide coordinated consistent psychologic care to him and to his family. After the parents have been told about the seriousness of their child's illness they may bear it quietly and with evidence of inner strength, they may become restless and hostile, or they may become depressed and withdrawn. It is especially difficult for the nurse to help those who are withdrawn. One approach as the parents sit quietly together is for the nurse to say, "This news must disturb you very much." When the parents respond affirmatively to this statement, the nurse can say, "Can you tell me how you feel about it?" If the parents can discuss their feelings, they will probably then be better able to support each other. But the nurse has no right to continue to probe if the parents give an indication that they do not wish to talk. The responsibility of the nurse is to offer her presence, her help, to make her availability known, and to help the parents know that they are not alone. *The helping person's strength at such a time lies in his ability to be able to experience with the parents some of the pain of the tragedy without becoming overwhelmed by it.*

When parents do not express emotion, but seem to accept the child's death too well, the nurse can gently indicate her approval that it is "all right to cry." Such parents need support for their apparent lack of emotion or for the dissociation they feel between mind, action and emotion. The nurse can support them in their apparently unfeeling state by explaining to them that this is nature's protective way so that they can carry on in the face of such a loss. But the nurse should not pressure such parents to cry because by so doing she could destroy the protective mechanism they are using to hold themselves together.

The nurse should not be surprised if the parents of a dying child seem to ignore the child completely and tell her about a past loss. Each such experience a person has had is not lost, but is revived with another impending loss. Especially is this true if the grief work was not completed in the past. The nurse can help such a parent abreact to his past grief so that when the time comes he can grieve about his child with no further need to protect himself from bringing alive old memories.

The grief of parents for a dying child is painful to watch. The nurse should understand the reactions of parents when they cannot leave the child's room as well as when they cannot enter it. She should permit and assist the parents to do any bit of nursing care they wish for their child, but she should also relieve them when they appear to be tired or worn. The parents' attempt to cope with their situation may lead them to provide tender loving care for their child or to rush frantically from task to task in the child's room. They may berate the physicians and nurses or praise their efforts extravagantly. The nurse cannot be disturbed if the mother especially, being another woman, does not react as she expects her to react. Each parent's behavior reflects his attempts to handle his own feelings and as such must be accepted by the nurse.

The nurse in a helping role can give most by furnishing an opportunity for those who are pained to express their anger and fears to someone who will not be devastated by their expressed feelings. The parents should be encouraged to talk about what they want at any particular moment. Nurses should encourage parents to talk about what bothers them so that she can learn what their real concerns may be. She can then help them face the reality of what is taking place. As the parents learn to know the nurse better, they sense the support she can give.

Families need to talk about their child. When they feel lonely and frightened, they want to talk to relatives and friends as well as to physicians and nurses. They must have a chance to be upset so that they can face the reality of what lies ahead. They need to be able to talk with their child if he is old enough to know what is happening. The nurse should be aware of the fact that anticipatory guidance or talking about the impending loss with others helps them to adjust to the impact of the loss itself.

Dying patients, whether adults or children, do not in general want to be left alone. They want frequent contact with another human being. They need the opportunity to talk, to be upset if they know the prognosis. They need to know that someone cares.

The dying child may feel very lonely if his parents do not stay with him constantly. The child therefore needs and wants his nurse to be nearby. Her presence increases his sense of security in the knowledge that she cares.

Knowing this, the nurse should encourage the parents and any other relatives to visit. The problem may then arise that the adults become so upset at the appearance of the child that they leave the room and cannot return because of their own emotion. If they have not told the child that they are leaving, or if they have told him that they would return soon, he may be disturbed by their apparent lack of honesty.

Actually, if the child's visitors cannot control their emotions to some degree, it might be better if they left the room. Adults who have lost their emotional control completely may be very frightening to the child.

Dying children need about the same kind of support as acutely ill children the same age. For example, the greatest fear of the child under five is that of separation from the mother, while the greatest fear of the child from five to nine years is of bodily procedures and mutilation. The older the child, the more likely he is to be concerned about his own death. He will ask questions, and it is the nurse's responsibility to learn exactly what is troubling him. Is he upset because he is in pain, or is it just because he saw his mother crying? Children should know that parents become upset when they are not feeling well and cannot play.

The older child, even though dying, should be treated with dignity and respect as a member of the family group. His opinions should be considered in matters which affect him as an individual, e.g. whether he wants the school teacher to come to see him or whether his younger brother may ride his bicycle while he is in the hospital.

The older child, like the adult, should not be told that he looks better, when he knows that he is very ill. Honesty is important in relations with the child as with the adult.

The child who senses or knows that he is going to die fears going to sleep at night. It is a challenge for the nurse to find nursing measures and appropriate medications to give him needed rest. Night lights and the nurse's looking in on him frequently help the child to feel secure.

Constancy of personnel should be provided so far as possible for the sake of the child and his parents to counteract the feeling of loss and abandonment they may feel. Parents appreciate the same nurses who understand their child being with him. They appreciate honesty in their answers to questions and the opportunity to call at any time to learn how their child is.

In the face of grief many times the questions answered, the directions given to the hospital chapel or local church, the offer to telephone a relative or friend, the touch of a known sympathetic hand, the offer to get coffee, or just the nurse's own presence are all that is required to reassure the parents that the nurse cares.

It is important that the nurse keep the room neat, welcome the family warmly and permit as much visiting as possible. Parents or nurses should not close shades or curtains or talk in whispers in the child's room any more than they should in the room of the adult who is dying.

During the child's terminal illness a place that is comfortable and private for the frightened and grieving family is most important. Provision of such a place gives the family further indication that the nurse understands and cares.

Both the parents and the child should know that the child is getting the best possible care in their situation. The greatest gift the nurse can give to the dying child and his parents is to be with them when words have little meaning. Yet this is not easy for the nurse to do.

When the parents are not told about the prognosis, the nurse is placed in a difficult situation when they or the child asks questions. In this situation it is the nurses who carry the burden of the problem, since physicians are not in frequent contact with the family members. When the child is hospitalized for only a short time and is to be "sent home to die," the problem of questioning is less likely to arise than if the child has a prolonged period of hospitalization. Both the child, if he is older, and the parents then feel more comfortable in questioning the nurse. In this situation the nurse is faced with feelings of frustration, sadness and helplessness.

After the death of the child the nurse usually sees in the hospital setting the first shock wave of disbelief overcome the parents. Then she may see them become gradually aware of what has happened to their child. The nurse rarely sees the restitution which completes the work of mourning, because this occurs over a much longer period of time.

When the nurse tries to help the parents after the death of the child, she should accept whatever behavior they evidence, whether of shock, denial, tearfulness or anger. The danger of grief lies not in how the parents feel, but in their inability to tolerate the feeling, their believing that they should feel or act differently. Keeping feelings hidden at such a time as this does not mean that they will go away. They may burst forth later with surprising impact if they are not worked through.

Nurses many times who cared for a child over a period of time find that after his death they, like the parents, were unable to control their tears. They have sought refuge in linen closets, bathrooms or locker rooms in order to prevent the family from observing their loss of control. Why should not the nurses who worked so closely with a child, giving him the best care they could, also be able to express their deep emotion? Many times parents feel comforted when seeing the nurse cry, because this indicates to them not only that they are not alone in their grief, but also that she as a person was deeply moved by their child's death.

Some parents wish to remain with their child for a while after death or request to see the child if they were not present at the moment of death. Such requests should be honored. The nurse should attempt to tidy the crib or bed and room; however, her most important function is to remain quietly with the parents and to give any support they may need. Sometimes a hand on the parent's shoulder is all that is necessary to help them know that someone cares. After the initial shock has passed, parents appreciate any comments about their ability to care for the child. A nurse's comment, "What wonderful parents you have been," will long be remembered. But many times, simply being with the bereaved parents will give more solace and comfort than the nurse can know.

A first assignment to do postmortem body care on a child can be extremely difficult if two inexperienced students are sent into the room alone. It can be an invaluable experience if an inexperienced student is sent with a mature member of the nursing staff to carry out this procedure.

The question usually arises whether the other children in the hospital unit should be told when a child they know dies. When questions are raised by these children, they are many times told that the critically ill child was transferred to another unit, that he was taken to the operating room, or that he was sent home. Certainly the older children on the unit have further questions about the absent child's condition, but if these questions are brought into the open, the nurses suddenly appear too busy to respond. Although the decision as to what should be done in this situation should be made by the members of the health team on the basis of the number of children involved, their ages, their diagnoses, and their closeness to the dead child among other factors, it is usually the nurse who must eventually answer the question to the children's satisfaction. If the question is not answered adequately, the children learn that death is not a subject that can be easily discussed.

Dying is not only a biological phenomenon, but also a social experience. If the parents and the child do not know the prognosis, they cannot discuss it with others, they cannot say goodbyes, nor can the parents openly plan for ways in which they will handle the situation with other children in the family once the death occurs.

The dying child and his parents present real problems for the nurse caring for them. But if each nurse works out her own religious beliefs and her philosophy and feelings about death, she will be able to provide a human guide to the unknown for the family. She herself will find each situation a challenge in which she can practice the real art and science of her profession.

SUMMARY

Throughout this book is emphasized the importance of the problem which hospitalization presents to a child, and the ways in which hospital personnel and the child's parents can help him to adjust to the situation. There is always the danger to a child's emotional development caused by long-term hospitalization with separation from parents and siblings. To avoid this, infants and young children are being treated whenever possible on an outpatient basis. Antibiotics can easily be given for certain acute infections and in order to limit complications. Outpatient treatment is therefore possible in many cases for which formerly it was necessary to hospitalize the child.

In order to fulfill her role in the total plan of care for every hospitalized child the nurse must think through her own feelings about each family. In some situations a psychiatrist is available to help her, not only so that she may learn how to handle her own emotional problems, but also so that what she does and says will have an immediate and beneficial influence on the parents' attitudes and on the child's condition. Of all the members of the health team, the nurse, by rejection of a child or his parents, would be the most injurious. If she accepts the child, she will learn, while nursing him, to apply her theoretical knowledge and past experience to his care. Having done this, she is in a position to teach the parents.

The mother of a chronically ill child who has been cared for at home can help the nurse in this adaptation of her general knowledge of pediatric nursing to the care of the particular patient. The mother should be considered a member of the health team, the one who works most closely with the nurses.

Pediatric nursing must be adapted to the wide range of development from the newborn infant through adolescence. In order to fulfill her complex role, the nurse must understand the normal physical, emotional, social, mental and spiritual aspects of growth and development of children, and the parent-child relation as background for her care of both the well child and the sick child of varying ages. Each unit of this book deals with a progressively older age group. We must consider the basic characteristics of each group and define the general principles of pediatric nursing to meet their needs. We must then consider the diseases most commonly occurring in each age group and the nursing care involved.

GUIDES TO FURTHER STUDY

1. What is your understanding of the role of the professional nurse in providing care for a sick child? What should be the nurse's relations with the child and with his parents?

2. Make a survey in your community of the types of agencies which provide care for well and for sick children. List them and their specific functions.

3. Study the *Declaration of the Rights of the Child* (p. 8). To what extent do you believe these "rights" are provided for the children in (a) an urban area and (b) a rural area known to you? How are these provided for in these two areas? What conditions in these areas prevent the achievement of any of these goals?

4. Recall a hospitalization experience during childhood. (This may be your own experience or that of a sibling or friend.) Was this a positive or a negative experience? Give specific memories you have about it and propose ways by which they could have been made more pleasant.

5. Define and differentiate clearly between the following terms: (a) growth and development and (b) eugenics and euthenics.

6. Obtain either your own, a sibling's or a friend's "Baby Book." List the steps of growth and development recorded in it. Summarize the principles of growth and development and apply them to this record.

7. Select a well sibling or a friend's child in any of the following age groups: birth to one year, one to three years, three to six years, six to twelve years or twelve to eighteen years. Discuss the growth and development and care of this child with his parents. Define the problems these parents are facing with this child. In class each student will discuss the child she has investigated, highlighting important points about the child's home, type of family, his community, and his physical, emotional, social and mental growth and development, and care.

8. Discuss individually with your own or a friend's grandmother and mother their attitudes about the care of children. State the differences in philosophy or child care practices expressed. What would some of the reasons be for these differences?

9. Immediately after the admission of a child to the hospital, observe the behavior of both the parent and the child. On the basis of specific observations you have made draw conclusions as to the feelings of the parent and the child. What could you as a nurse do to help this parent and child face this situation less anxiously or more positively?

10. What can you observe in the children's area on which you are working that would help a child feel more at home in the hospital setting?

11. Evaluate the unit in which you are working as to its safety for the care of the children. List your findings and make constructive suggestions for its improvement.

12. List the various kinds of personnel in the pediatric unit who provide some type of care or guidance for children and their parents. Differentiate as clearly as you can between the functions of these persons.

13. Children and adults react differently to disease processes. Explain why this is true and what effect this understanding has or will have on the type of care you give to children.

*TEACHING AIDS AND OTHER INFORMATION**

Abbott Laboratories

Parenteral Administration.

American Medical Association

Your Friend, the Doctor.

American Pharmaceutical Association

Usual Doses for Infants and Children, 1965.

Children's Medical and Surgical Center, Johns Hopkins Hospital, Baltimore, Maryland

Dombro, R. H.: Child Life Programs in 91 Pediatric Hospitals in the United States and Canada, 1966.

Child Study Association of America

Wolf, A. W. M.: Helping Your Child to Understand Death.
Arnstein, H.: What to Tell Your Child about Birth, Death, Illness, Divorce and Other Family Crises.

Mental Health Materials Center

Preparing Your Child for the Hospital.

Play Schools Association

Cleverdon, D.: Play in a Hospital.

---

* Complete addresses are given in the Appendix.

Public Affairs Pamphlets

Ogg, E.: When a Family Faces Stress.
Osborn, E.: When You Lose a Loved One.

Ross Laboratories

Hall, E. J., and Bruce, S. J.: Maternal and Child-Health Nursing, 1964.
Your Child Goes to the Hospital.

The Children's Hospital Medical Center, Boston, Mass.

Johnny Goes to the Hospital.

United States Department of Health, Education, and Welfare

Children's Books, 1966, 1967.
Shore, M. F. (Ed.): Red Is the Color of Hurting, 1967.

REFERENCES

Publications

American Academy of Pediatrics: *Care of Children in Hospitals.* Evanston, Ill., American Academy
    of Pediatrics, 1960.
American Academy of Pediatrics: *Standards of Child Health Care.* Evanston, Ill., American Academy
    of Pediatrics, 1967.
Bergmann, T., and Freud, A.: *Children in the Hospital.* New York, International Universities Press,
    1966.
Bermosk, L. S., and Mordan, M. J.: *Interviewing in Nursing.* New York, Macmillan Company, 1964.
Carpenter, K. M., and Stewart, J. M.: *Nursing in a Parent Participation Program. Nursing and the
    Patient's Motivations.* Monogram 19, 1962 Clinical Sessions. New York, American Nurses'
    Association, 1962.
Child Study Association of America: *The Children's Bookshelf; A Guide to Books for and about Chil-
    dren.* New York, Child Study Association, 1965.
Dixon, D. J. W.: *Diets for Sick Children.* Philadelphia, F. A. Davis Company, 1965.
Dovenmuehle, R. H., and others: *Death and Dying: Attitudes of Patient and Doctor.* New York, Group
    for Advancement of Psychiatry, 1965.
Fagin, C. M.: *Effects of Maternal Attendance During Hospitalization on Post-Hospital Behavior of
    Young Children.* Philadelphia, F. A. Davis Company, 1966.
Falconer, M. W., Patterson, H. R., and Gustafson. E. A.: *Current Drug Handbook.* 1968-70. Philadel-
    phia, W. B. Saunders Company, 1968.
Feifel, H. (Ed.): *The Meaning of Death.* New York, Blakiston Division, McGraw-Hill Book Company,
    Inc., 1959.
Flitter, H. H.: *An Introduction to Physics in Nursing.* 5th ed. St. Louis. C. V. Mosby Company, 1967.
Fulton, R.: *Death and Identity.* New York, John Wiley and Sons, 1965.
Geist, H.: *A Child Goes to the Hospital: The Psychological Aspects of a Child Going to the Hospital.*
    Springfield, Ill., Charles C Thomas, 1965.
Geist, H., and Manson, M. P.: *Children Going to the Hospital.* Los Angeles, Western Psychological
    Services, 1965.
Glaser, B. G., and Strauss, A. L.: *Awareness of Dying.* Chicago, Aldine Publishing Company, 1965.
Green, M. M., and Others: *The Concerns of Parents of a Hospitalized Child:* in *Effective Therapeutic
    Communications in Nursing* (Convention Clinical Sessions No. 8) New York, American
    Nurses' Association, 1964, p. 5.
Haller, J. A., Jr., Talbert, J. L, and Dombro, R. H. (Eds.).: *The Hospitalized Child and His Family.*
    Baltimore, Johns Hopkins Press, 1967.
Hamovitch, M. B.: *The Parent and the Fatally Ill Child: A Demonstration of Parent Participation in a
    Hospital Pediatrics Department.* Duarte, California, City of Hope Medical Center, 1964.
Hughes, W. T., Jr.: *Pediatric Procedures.* Philadelphia, W. B. Saunders Company, 1964.
Modell, W.: *Drugs in Current Use 1968.* 14th ed. New York, Springer Publishing Company, Inc., 1968.
Parad, H. J. (Ed.): *Crisis Intervention: Selected Readings.* New York, Family Service Association
    of America, 1965.
Quint, J. C.: *The Nurse and the Dying Patient.* New York, Macmillan Company, 1967.
Rey, M., and Rey, H. A.: *Curious George Goes to the Hospital.* Boston, Houghton Mifflin Company,
    1966.
Robertson, J. (Ed.): *Hospitals and Children.* New York, International Universities Press, 1963.
Vernon, D. T. A., Foley, J. M., Sipowicz, R. R., and Schulman, J. L.: *The Psychological Responses of
    Children to Hospitalization and Illness.* Springfield, Ill., Charles C Thomas, 1965.
Verwoerdt, A.: *Communication with the Fatally Ill.* Springfield, Ill., Charles C Thomas, 1966.

Periodicals

Amend, E. L.: A Parent Education Program in a Children's Hospital. *Nursing Outlook,* 14:53, April 1966.

Amos, A. W.: Establishing A Trust Relationship with Children; in *Exploring Progress in Maternal and Child Health Nursing Practice.* (ANA 1965 Regional Clinical Conferences, No. 3). New York, American Nurses' Association, 1966, p. 9.

Aufhauser, T. R.: Parent Participation in Hospital Care of Children. *Nursing Outlook,* 15:40, January 1967.

Berman, D. C.: Pediatric Nurses as Mothers See Them. *Am. J. Nursing,* 66:2429, 1966.

Bonine, G. N.: Student's Reactions to Children's Deaths. *Am. J. Nursing,* 67:1439, 1967.

Bright, F., and France, Sister M. L.: The Nurse and the Terminally Ill Child. *Nursing Outlook,* 15:39, September 1967.

Cheng, N., Bradshaw, C., and Gentry, B.: A Second Look At Nurses in Color. *Hospitals,* 39:59, June 16, 1965.

Cluster, P. F.: A One-Room School for Hospitalized Children. *Nursing Outlook,* 15:56, August 1967.

Condon, M., and Peters, C.: Family Participation Unit. *Am. J. Nursing,* 68:504, 1968.

Durocher, M. A.: Parent Educator in the Outpatient Department. *Am. J. Nursing,* 65:99, June 1965.

Erickson, F. H.: Helping the Sick Child Maintain Behavioral Control. *Nursing Clin. N. Amer.,* 2:695, 1967.

Folta, J. R.: The Perception of Death. *Nursing Research,* 14:232, 1965.

Ford, L. C., and Silver, H. K.: The Expanded Role of the Nurse in Child Care. *Nursing Outlook,* 15:43, September 1967.

Geis, D. P.: Mother's Perceptions of Care Given Their Dying Children. *Am. J. Nursing,* 65:105, February 1965.

Goodman, J.: A Nurse Is a Heck of a Nice Thing. *Am. J. Nursing,* 67:550, 1967.

Hymovich, D. P.: ABC's of Pediatric Safety. *Am. J. Nursing,* 66:1768, 1966.

Kneisl, C. R.: Thoughtful Care for the Dying. *Am. J. Nursing,* 68:550, 1968.

Live-In Mother's Aid in Hospital Medical Care. *Medical World News,* 8:58, October 27, 1967.

Mahaffy, P. R.: Admission Interviews with Parents. *Am. J. Nursing,* 66:506, 1966.

Manthey, M. E.: A Guide for Interviewing. *Am. J. Nursing,* 67:2088, 1967.

Markowitz, M., and Gordis, L.: A Family Pediatric Clinic at a Community Hospital. *Children,* 14:25, 1967.

McCaffery, M. S.: An Approach to Parent Education. *Nursing Forum,* VI:77, November 1967.

Mercer, L. S.: Touch: Comfort or Threat? *Perspectives in Psychiatric Care,* IV:20, May-June 1966.

Merrow, D. L., and Johnson, B. S.: Perceptions of the Mother's Role with Her Hospitalized Child. *Nursing Research,* 17:155, 1968.

Pillitteri, A.: Practice in a Pediatric Research Unit. *Am. J. Nursing,* 65:104, August 1965.

Pitel, M., and Wemett, M.: The Intramuscular Injection. *Am. J. Nursing,* 64:104, April 1964.

Quint, J. C.: Awareness of Death and the Nurse's Composure. *Nursing Research,* 15:49, 1966.

Quint, J. C., and Others: Improving Nursing Care of the Dying. *Nursing Forum,* VI:368, Fall 1967.

Rakstis, T. J.: How Safe Are Your Child's Toys? *Today's Health,* 45:21, December 1967.

Robischon, P.: The Challenge of Crisis Theory For Nursing. *Nursing Outlook,* 15:28, July 1967.

Rousseau, O.: Mothers Do Help in Pediatrics. *Am. J. Nursing,* 67:798, 1967.

Roy, Sister, M. C.: Role Cues and Mothers of Hospitalized Children. *Nursing Research,* 16:178, 1967.

Seidl, F. W., and Pillitteri, A.: Development of an Attitude Scale on Parent Participation. *Nursing Research,* 16:71, 1967.

Shore, M. F., Geiser, R. L., and Wolman, H. M.: Constructive Uses of a Hospital Experience. *Children,* 12:3, 1965.

Sites for Intramuscular Injection. *J. Pediat.,* 70:158, 1967.

Smith, R. M.: Preparing Children for Surgery. *Hospital Medicine,* 3:68, July 1967.

Stearly, S., Noordenbos, A., and Crouch, V.: Pediatric Nurse Practitioner. *Am. J. Nursing,* 67:2083, 1967.

Townsend, E. H.: Paramedical Personnel in Pediatric Practice. *J. Pediat.,* 68:855, 1966.

VandenBergh, R. L.: Let's Talk about Death: To Overcome Inhibiting Emotions. *Am. J. Nursing,* 66:71, 1966.

Webb, C.: Nursing Support for Your Young Patients' Parents. *RN,* 30:44, February 1967.

Webb, C.: Tactics to Reduce a Child's Fear of Pain. *Am. J. Nursing,* 66:2698, 1966.

Wiedenbach, E.: Family Nurse Practitioner for Maternal and Child Care. *Nursing Outlook,* 13:50, December 1965.

Wu, R.: Explaining Treatments to Young Children. *Am. J. Nursing,* 65:71, July 1965.

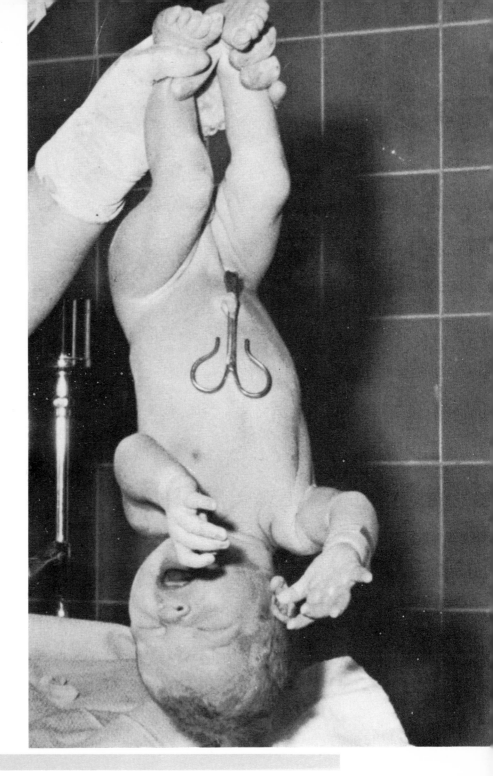

UNIT TWO
THE NEWBORN

5

THE NEWBORN, HIS FAMILY AND THE NURSE

ENVIRONMENT AND DEVELOPMENT OF THE FETUS

The uterus of a healthy woman is perfectly adapted to the needs of the fetus. Her body is the medium which adapts conditions outside her to the developmental immaturity of the fetus. Since her heat-regulating mechanism keeps the temperature within the uterus constant, changes in outdoor or room temperature do not affect the fetus. The amniotic fluid in her uterus acts as a sterile insulating medium in which there is no friction.

The fetus needs oxygen and nutrients in order to live and grow. These are supplied through the blood stream of the prospective mother by way of the placenta and umbilical cord. Through the same route the fetus is relieved of the waste products of metabolism.

The fetus is completely dependent upon the mother for all vital functions because the fetal organs have not developed to the extent that extrauterine life is possible. The lungs are not inflated. The circulatory system is adapted only to intrauterine life; little blood flows through the pulmonary artery, since the foramen ovale and the ductus arteriosus are not closed as they are after birth. The digestive tract cannot reduce

even the simplest foods to the state in which elements can be taken up by the blood stream.

The fetus tends to develop normally even at the expense of the mother. An accident to the woman may involve the fetus. Anything which interferes with the normal transfer of oxygen or nutriment from the maternal blood stream to that of the fetus will jeopardize its safety.

THE NEWBORN

Neonatal Hazards and Preparation

Birth is associated with the most drastic changes that ever befall a person. In extrauterine life all functions undergo a radical change. A sudden adjustment has to be made from a "topsy-turvy aquatic environment" to a so-called sane air existence. After birth the infant must not only continue the vital activities of intrauterine life, but must also initiate other extrauterine processes which his mother performed for him. The normal infant is able to do this, provided he receives essential care. *If the infant is to survive the crucial neonatal period, three conditions are necessary: that he be in good physical condition, that he experience a safe delivery, and that he then receive good care.*

Infant Mortality

Improvement in maternal and infant care has greatly reduced the infant mortality rate in the last twenty-five to thirty years, but the decrease has been slower in the neonatal period than in the remaining months of infancy. From the second to the twelfth month of life less than half as many infants die as between birth and four weeks of age. The highest infant death rate is within the first month of life, and within that month in the first twenty-four hours. The most critical period for the infant is the first hour of life, when the drastic change from intrauterine to extrauterine existence occurs.

The chief cause of death in the neonatal period is *prematurity* (immaturity) (see also Chap. 8). Other causes of death are *congenital malformations* which render it impossible for the infant to establish an independent existence, *birth injuries, asphyxia* and *atelectasis*. All these conditions are discussed in succeeding chapters. Here we should take note that not all the causes of congenital malformations are clearly understood. The number of infants who are kept alive and whose condition is relieved or mitigated by surgery is much higher than it was in the past. Birth injuries are not as common a cause of death as they were even fifteen years ago. An increasing number of prospective mothers are receiving better prenatal care. Difficult deliveries are anticipated and arrangements made for hospitalization of the mothers. Instrumental and operative deliveries are more judicious. The educated nurse-midwife is replacing the experienced but ignorant midwife. For these reasons the percentage of infants injured during delivery has been reduced. Furthermore, more infants are being examined during the first month of their lives by physicians, midwives and nurses after discharge from the nursery. Thus problems arising shortly after birth can be discovered and treated promptly.

Research is currently being done in an attempt to find subtle indicators of fetal distress in order to save infants after birth. One type of research involves taking samples of blood through an amnioscope from the presenting part of the fetus in order to carry out microanalysis to determine the pH of the blood. If the fetus is acidotic, the question arises as to whether immediate delivery is indicated. Another type of research is being done on monitoring of the fetal heart by electronic equipment. This recent diagnostic method traces the progress of the fetus during gestation, labor and delivery. It is particularly valuable during labor contractions when fetal heart tones are not easily detected by auscultation. Still another area of research concerns the deleterious effect of LSD in "psychedelic" doses on the fetus if taken early in the course of pregnancy.

Health and Welfare Measures for Reduction of Infant Mortality. Since 1964, Federal comprehensive care programs for low-income, hard-to-reach groups of mothers and infants at high risk have been in operation. These have represented a major expansion of maternal and child health services beyond that seen in traditional preventive medicine. *There are more than fifty Maternity and Infant Care projects throughout the United States funded by the Children's Bureau for the purpose of improving services to reduce infant mortality and to promote maternal and child health.* More specifically, the goals of these programs include increasing the number of prenatal and postnatal clinics in neighborhoods where they are needed, to provide special services for patients having complications of pregnancy, and to provide hospital care for mothers and infants as needed.

The environment of a pregnant woman influences her health, which in turn creates a healthful or unhealthful environment for the fetus. Unfortunately not all pregnant women can be provided with a healthful environment, but federal, state and local health and welfare programs have made a great difference in the conditions under which the low-income group lives. Since newborn infants are prone to infections, the death rate among them is influenced by good sanitation in the community, cleanliness in the home, fresh air, sunshine, and avoidance of overcrowding in sleeping and living rooms.

Some pregnant women do not go to a physician early in pregnancy, or they pay little attention to his advice. To win them over to a different attitude toward their own health and safety and to create in them a desire for the infant is a challenging task for the nurse.

The young student nurse has a special role in working with these mothers. She is likely to have good rapport with the young prospective mother because as a nurse she is intensely interested in pregnancy, knows well the physical processes that are taking place and, by her own attitude toward health and confidence in the medical advice given, influences the patients in a way different from that in which the older nurse, medical social worker or even the physician influences her.

As long as the infant is well his mother can be taught to give him all the care he needs, and she probably gives it better than anyone else because of her love for him. Some mothers, of course, either do not love their children or are unable to show their love in ways that transmit security to them. The cause for such a situation is often extremely difficult to determine. The mother may be in need of psychiatric treatment. When the mother cannot give her infant the loving care he needs, some other person must be found to serve as a mother-substitute or to supplement the care she gives.

If the baby is not gaining weight as he should or is ill, the professional services of the nurse are needed. Infants have surprising vitality, but little resistance to disease, particularly disease which interferes with electrolyte balance, such as dehydration because of diarrhea, or massive infection with or without a high fever. Mothers must be taught to take the infant's temperature. If it is elevated, he must be seen by a physician, and measures must be taken to prevent the condition from becoming worse.

Clinics, outpatient departments and admitting departments of hospitals, particularly in the low-income areas of large cities, are open twenty-four hours of the day every day in the week. Immediate availability of the physician and the nurse, and hospitalization if necessary, are extremely important.

Even a healthy infant needs a good regimen directed by a physician who examines him at regular intervals. It is often the nurse who welcomes the mother to the physician's office or the Child Health Conferences and helps her to understand the physician's suggestions. Nurses in Child Health Conferences and outpatient departments of hospitals look for signs that the infant is not gaining as he should, has some chronic condition or is in the first stage of an acute disease. They must be particularly skillful in observing symptoms and eliciting information from a mother, since the infant cannot say how he feels.

Health and Welfare programs extend care to individual children, through whom the nurse makes her great contribution to the reduction of infant mortality. Whether the student is having her clinical experience in the pediatric unit or in a public health agency, she is working with individual babies. Only by keeping each one healthy and caring for each one when he is sick or in need of operation will infant morbidity and mortality rates be reduced.

Parental Education

Education for parenthood begins with the general education of the child for responsibilities in family living. Thus one of the best ways to prepare to be a good parent is to grow up in a family having mature parents. More specifically, parental education today begins with the courses which prepare men and women for family life. Such courses are offered in undergraduate and adult education programs. Lectures or conferences for young wives who are pregnant and for their husbands include discussion of the physical and emotional needs of infants and how these needs can best be met. The emotional needs are as important as the physical needs, for lack of affection has an adverse influence on personality development. Among these needs is that

for contact with a soft, warm human body and the slight motion which comes from gentle handling and cuddling in his mother's arms.

Family Responses to the Newborn

The Mother

In caring for the newborn the nurse bases her role on much more than an understanding of his physical attributes. It is her responsibility to help the parents build a happier family life through his coming. In order to do this she must understand the mutual dependency of the mother and her infant.

Mother love is supposed to be the strongest emotional tie between two human beings. The influence of the endocrine glands as they function in the pregnant or lactating mother is evident even among the higher animals. They are gentle in handling their young and are likely to be fiercely protective of them. If all her offspring are taken from a mother, she will become restless, may refuse to eat and may evidence frustration at the blocking of an instinct based on glandular secretion. The human mother has not only this physical basis for her dependency on her infant, but also a love for him which has been developing through the long months of gestation. If she is separated from her baby, she is denied relief from an emotional need based in part on her physical condition.

Up to the child's birth there has been a *symbiotic relation* between the mother and the fetus. A symbiotic relation is one of extreme closeness. Before birth the fetus existed as a parasite within his mother. The two—mother and fetus—were necessary to each other. The fetus could not live unless her body supplied his needs, and she in turn needed the product of conception to complete the physical changes which pregnancy was producing in her. If the fetus should die, the mother would feel emotionally distraught.

Mothers desire to continue this symbiotic relation after the child's birth, and the nurse should recognize the importance of the tie. Modern obstetrical nursing is planned to keep mother and baby together, his bassinet beside her bed. Mothers are urged to nurse their infants, since breast feeding is the closest approach to a symbiotic relation which can be achieved after the birth of the child.

Although the symbiotic relation exists, the nurse must not expect all mothers to hold their newborns comfortably at first. Some mothers will initially touch their infants only with the tips of their fingers. As the mother becomes more comfortable in her role, as her infant gradually responds to her touch, and as their relationship deepens, the mother will eventually be able to hold or enfold her child in her arms. In view of the stages through which the mother must move before being entirely comfortable in caring for her infant, the nurse must not become impatient if the mother does not adjust immediately to the process of breast feeding or rooming-in.

The Father

The family is the strongest social institution in our society. The father has two responsibilities in the family after the birth of his child. His first responsibility is to his wife. The hormonal changes which are inevitable after childbirth produce in many women a state of depression. The mother needs to feel at this time that she is loved so that she in turn can love her infant. The father, therefore, must not only feel love toward his wife, but must also communicate this feeling to her.

The role of the father is honored in many societies. The father, like the mother, has looked forward to having a son or daughter. Half of the child's heredity is transmitted through him, and the infant is as much a continuation of himself as of his wife. He has also the moral obligation to be a provider. In a family the children need the masculine influence as much as they do the feminine. They need a father's affection as they need a mother's. But because of the newborn's immediate need for his mother, the father's role is likely to appear subsidiary and to be taken as a matter of course, and he may feel left out of this most important event in married life.

The modern father is not willing to be left out of all these new activities in the home. He accepts odd chores connected with the baby. He changes

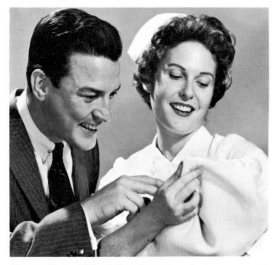

Figure 5–1. This father has already become well acquainted with his child before her discharge from the hospital. (H. Armstrong Roberts.)

diapers, picks his little son up when he cries and cuddles him as successfully as the mother. In this way he reaches the baby's consciousness and lays the basis for affection. As the infant responds, the father becomes increasingly fond of taking an active part in his care. The mother, of course, appreciates this help. So the coming of the baby has strengthened their love for each other through their love for the newborn infant.

The Siblings

The siblings' reaction to the arrival of a new baby in the family is conditioned by their parents' attitude and the number of other members in the family. If the parents encourage the siblings to share in the care of the infant and at the same time provide love and security for them as individuals, the children are less likely to consider the newcomer an intruder in their home. (See Chapter 18 for further discussion of the reaction of siblings to the birth of a child.)

The Newborn's Response to Birth

That giving birth to a child is difficult and even dangerous for the mother is common knowledge, but that even an easy normal birth must be a great strain upon the baby is seldom realized. His body sustains the pressure of the uterine contractions and his head the pressure of the resisting cervix. Although good obstetrical care prevents injury to the infant as well as to the mother and makes his passage through the birth canal less exhausting, birth still remains an anxiety-provoking experience. To this is added the necessity to adapt to life as a separate entity, no longer part of the mother.

As long as the fetus is nurtured through his mother's body, his health and that of his mother are the concern of the obstetrician and the obstetrical nurse. But the infant's health after birth is the concern of the pediatrician and the pediatric nurse.

The World as the Infant Experiences It

Since an infant's senses are not acute and discriminating at birth, the world about him must appear to be "one great, blooming, buzzing confusion." Yet the beginning of personality is there. How far personality at birth determines that of the older child or adult is not known, but it is certain that environmental factors modify personality early in infancy. The infant has two great drives: to be loved and to love. (Although the need to be loved is evident at birth, the drive to love is not manifested until later.) The physical needs of the infant who is loved are sure to be satisfied, but the unloved infant is likely to be neglected. The infant equates the relief of a need with love. Since hunger is an imperative need, it is natural that the infant loves the person who feeds him. Assured of food and cuddling, the infant develops a sense of *trust*. The implication of this is that when the mother holds her baby to her breast while he nurses or when she feeds him from the bottle, she is showing him love in a way that he can sense. The loved, contented baby forms a habit of contentment and does not easily become fretful. Anxiety-arousing stimuli should be kept from him, for a habit of anxiety can be as easily aroused as that of contentment.

Some psychologists believe that the infant is capable of fear and anger at birth. If so, these two emotions are difficult to distinguish. Sudden loss of support or a loud noise will produce a reflex startle reaction, and this is said to be evidence of fear. When he is roaring, we infer that he is angry. In either case he is reacting to a stimulus which he does not like and wants to have stopped. He soon learns that crying will bring someone who will make him comfortable. Since it is generally his mother who does this for him, he soon learns to prefer her to other people. This appears to be the basis of his love for his mother. She responds to his flattering preference for her with endearing attention, and so the cycle of mother-baby, baby-mother love is strengthened. Secure in her care for him, he will accept supplementary care from other people, provided it is *like* that which she gives him.

The child who is cared for by a changing group of people fails to form an affectionate attachment to anyone. He is likely to be very self-centered, and this situation, if continued, is one factor in producing the autistic child.

One principle of child care is that *the infant needs consistent loving care given by one or two people, a minimal amount of anxiety and a maximum amount of contentment.* Only then can the infant learn to adapt to his new environment.

Role of the Professional Nurse

Needs of the Parents

The role of the nurse in caring for the family during the postpartum period must be based not on the needs of the hospital and its staff, but rather on the needs of the parents and their child.

The new family relations which spring from the arrival of the baby are evidenced through all the hours of the day and night, as a new element in the former kinship within the family. The family relations before the first pregnancy were one to one, but with the birth of the first child each member is related to two others.

Neither parent may now expect the entire love and attention of the other. With the second and succeeding births the change in relations becomes more complex (see Fig. 5-2). Note that the father's place in Figure 5-2 is comparable to that of the mother.

The supportive role of the professional nurse in the adjustment of the parents to their new relations to one another and to their child is enacted while giving the mother and her infant physical care. This support gives her role its peculiar significance and makes it more effective than that of the other professional members of the health team. Other team members, of course, give physical help to patients, but it is not characterized by meeting their daily recurrent needs and so is less likely to be helpful in adjustment

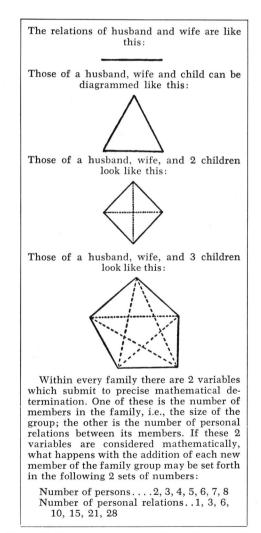

The relations of husband and wife are like this:

Those of a husband, wife and child can be diagrammed like this:

Those of a husband, wife, and 2 children look like this:

Those of a husband, wife, and 3 children look like this:

Within every family there are 2 variables which submit to precise mathematical determination. One of these is the number of members in the family, i.e., the size of the group; the other is the number of personal relations between its members. If these 2 variables are considered mathematically, what happens with the addition of each new member of the family group may be set forth in the following 2 sets of numbers:

Number of persons....2, 3, 4, 5, 6, 7, 8
Number of personal relations..1, 3, 6, 10, 15, 21, 28

Figure 5–2. Bossard's Law of Family Interaction. (J. H. S. Bossard: *The Sociology of Child Development.* Rev. ed. New York, Harper and Brothers.)

to a new situation which involves the minute details of family life.

We are apt to concentrate attention on the mother rather than on the father. This is justified, but both parents (particularly if this is their first child) need help in making all the necessary adjustments involved in childbirth and in the care of the newborn infant. The nurse, more than any other member of the hospital staff, makes the parents feel at home. She is hostess in the hospital and makes the first meeting of the mother and the father, after the birth of their child, emotionally satisfying. The nurse should remember that the mother will be thinking of all that was said and done in this first brief visit until her husband comes again. A satisfying visit promotes tranquil rest; an unsatisfying one, emotional disturbance.

Hospital policies control what the nurse may allow the parents. If the hospital imposes stringent rules as to visiting hours and viewing the infant, this first meeting of husband and wife may be so emotionally unsatisfying that the mother's physical condition is adversely influenced by her disappointment. In any case, however, the nurse's friendly, cordial manner is helpful.

The nurse should accept the mother's dependency needs and not expect from her all the self-care of which she is physically capable. In the early days of ambulation after delivery it is easy for the nurse to forget the emotional effect of childbirth upon a young mother. If the mother is not emotionally ready for the routine self-care customary in the hospital, the nurse should do for her what the mother feels she cannot do for herself. The mother should never be made to feel that she is failing to live up to the nurse's concept of the modern woman who accepts childbirth as a natural process which incapacitates for only a day or two. (Even the most ardent believer in natural childbirth realizes that not all women are capable of carrying it to completion without emotional trauma. This is true also of early self-care.) Nurses should accept and understand the reactions of each mother and plan her care accordingly. When both the physical and the emotional needs of the mother have been met, the mother feels secure in the hospital and can accept the rest she requires before returning to her duties as homemaker. Because of the close emotional union of mother and child, she will not be content unless she knows that the infant, too, is well cared for by the nurses.

The mother should be encouraged to talk over her recent experience in the delivery room and also any matter which worries her about the infant, her own condition or her home. Past experiences are interpreted in the light of the present. If the nurse makes the mother's stay in the hospital as pleasant as possible, the mother's attitude toward future pregnancies and deliveries is likely to be optimistic.

Needs of the Newborn

The basic needs of the newborn are those of any helpless young animal dependent upon its mother, but with these significant differences. He is the most dependent of any young creature for a longer period of time, and yet he is the recipient of the scientific knowledge which only human beings possess and is himself one of the coming generation who will add to this fund of knowledge.

The nurse's knowledge of what is normal in a newborn baby enables her to know what is abnormal. She should observe and appraise the status of the infant when he is brought to the nursery in order that she may report any abnormalities which the physician may have overlooked or which did not appear until after the examination of the baby was completed. *Many potentially dangerous abnormalities of the newborn can be treated before a serious physiologic disturbance results. These require early recognition and diagnosis.*

The newborn is likely to be exhausted by the birth process, and gentle handling to conserve his strength is necessary. His personality is being formed by his experiences even during these first few days of life. Gentleness in caring for him is an expression of love, and makes physical care—his bath and the changing of his diaper—a pleasure to him. He likes skin-to-skin contact. His heat-regulating system is so poorly developed that he needs external warmth. A soft cuddly blanket gives him the feeling of a closed environment of even temperature such as he experienced in the uterus. He needs frequent changes of position, not merely from lying on one side to the other, but also the many minor changes which occur when he is picked up and cuddled.

Self-Demand Schedule. It is believed that the newborn responds to his needs with sleeping when his body needs sleep and with crying when his body needs nourishment. He demands sleep and feedings in accordance with his rhythm of bodily functions, a rhythm which is fairly constant from day to day. *His schedule should be planned in accordance with his demands and will vary with his physical condition.* If he has a fever, he will, of course, want water more frequently, and his sleep will be intermittent. As he matures, the interval between feedings will lengthen and he will take more at each feeding. His periods of wakefulness will be longer, and his total time spent in sleep will be less.

The self-demand schedule must be carried out in a stable environment adapted to the infant's immaturity. This environment is both physical and social. The physical environment must be hygienic, and the social environment such that he learns to associate a feeling of well-being with the care given him.

After the traumatic experience of birth the newborn needs to acquire strength before he will begin to gain in weight and vigor. This is a period of adjustment for him in which the self-demand schedule is particularly important. He should be offered the breast or bottle, but never unduly urged. From the time he enters the nursery his comprehensive nursing care includes meeting both his physical and his emotional needs; otherwise he will not reach and maintain his optimum level of well-being and feel secure in the strange environment of the nursery.

Rooming-in

An environment can be planned which will be suitable for all infants, each of whom requires environmental adaptation to meet his needs. It is extremely difficult to provide this in a nursery where one or two nurses are caring for a large number of infants. Needs are likely to be met at certain fixed times suited to the average infant's schedule for feeding, sleep and periods of placid rest. The nursery schedule is adjusted to administrative and personnel considerations as well as to the needs of the average infant. Many infants are not average, however. Also, a baby's needs vary from day to day. Furthermore, babies need affection shown in ways which are peculiar to the mother-child relation and which no nurse can reproduce in the care of a constantly changing group of babies. Rooming-in is a method which provides for infant, mother and nurse the conditions in which each is most satisfied and can most successfully fulfill his or her role.

Rooming-in is a hospital arrangement whereby the mother has her newborn infant by her bedside and takes as much care of him as her condition permits and she desires. It is a family-centered service in the hospital situation. It is an effort to meet parents' request for more information about the care of the baby, and it gives both the parents and the baby a homelike feeling in the impersonal hospital atmosphere.

The practice of rooming-in gives the young mother an opportunity to become acquainted with her first child and accustomed to his care. It relieves her anxiety as to his welfare in the nursery, where she often hears babies crying and is sure that one of them is hers. It permits the baby's father to hold or feed him or change his diaper. This is a different introduction from standing in the hall and looking through a glass window at a room full of infants while a nurse brings *the one* to the nursery side of the window.

The infant who rooms-in receives more individual attention, for his mother can reach over and pat him, change his position, give him water or replace a wet or soiled diaper. Feeding is promoted because when the mother sees her infant hungry, she is motivated to put him to the breast. If the physician approves of the infant's being on a self-demand schedule, the mother can easily feed him whenever he wants to nurse.

Some mothers, however, do not want the baby's crib beside their bed. They do not want to feed him on a self-demand schedule, nor do they want to give him care. These are likely to be the

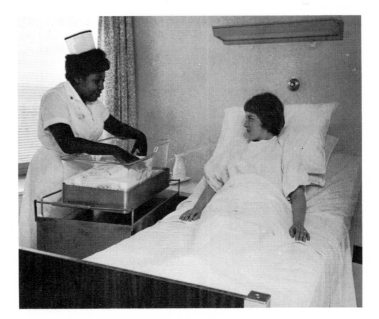

Figure 5–3. Teaching the patient to care for her newborn baby is an important aspect of the rooming-in system. (Courtesy of the Hospital of the Albert Einstein College of Medicine.)

mothers of large families and have been over-worked up to the time of delivery. They are in need of a complete rest and should not be forced to do more for their infants than give them the breast or, if they are bottle-fed, hold them for a few minutes each day.

There are disadvantages to rooming-in from the point of view of both the parents and the hospital. Some mothers are neither physically nor emotionally able to do their part in the room-ing-in care of an infant. The physician may feel that there is danger of infection, although the infectious conditions which the newborn is most likely to contract are those which are carried from infant to infant by the hospital personnel or through the use of improperly sterilized equip-ment. The hospital administrator knows that rooming-in requires more well qualified person-nel and uses more floor space than does the tra-ditional care given to newborns in a central nursery.

For rooming-in to be successful, the staff nurses must have warm, comforting personalities. They must not insist on a rigid plan of nursing care. Rather, they should promote normal relations in the family and help the parents make their own plan for the infant. This they do by sharing with them their own knowledge of child care and giving the parents reassurance in their ability to meet any problems which may arise in the care of the infant.

Modifications of Traditional Maternity Units

Although rooming-in would seem to be the ideal method by which the needs of both newborns and parents could be met, the practice is not widely accepted in this country.

If rooming-in is not practical in the maternity area, the same objectives may be attained in the traditional maternity unit by the following modi-fications in arrangement and in assignment of patients to the nursing personnel.

1. *Individual family units* may be assigned to the nurse for study and the making of a plan of care. She can observe the interpersonal relations within "her family" and plan the care of mother and child with reference to their relation to the father, maternal grandmother or other relatives who visit the patient. In this way she can carry our her supporting role with the family as a whole. If attention is focused on only one mem-ber, the needs of others are likely to be forgotten, and thereby the nurse may create friction within the family which reacts adversely on her patient. Of course if the hospital policy does not permit nurses who are caring for the mothers on the maternity unit to enter the newborn nursery, this family-centered plan of nursing care can-not be carried out. Nevertheless the nurse as-signed to the care of the mother and the nurse caring for the infant may unite as a team in their study of the family and confer on the needs of the family as a whole.

2. Nurses may be helped by the instructors and supervisors to establish a cooperative learn-ing relationship with the infant's parents. Thereby (a) the parents will realize that the nurse is interested in their baby and in their ability to provide good care for him after his discharge from the hospital, and (b) the nurse makes the greatest gain in knowledge and skill from her experience in the nursing care of the infant and his mother.

3. Routines can be made more flexible so that the needs of the individual family may be met through having the nurse use her judgment in the application of hospital regulations. Mothers might be permitted to keep their babies with them for a longer time than is required for feeding. Husbands might be encouraged to talk of their new role of being a father if this is the first child, or of being the father of an increas-ingly large family. The nurse will find that suc-cessful adjustment to the first baby differs in many ways from that to the second and later children.

With the first baby the role of a father is new and at least temporarily appears as the most important of his roles in the many groups to which he belongs. With succeeding children the role of fatherhood is no longer novel and now has the added element of duties and pleasures re-lated to children of different ages and probably sex, and of working with the mother to establish proper sibling relations.

4. Group discussions may be scheduled for mothers in the maternity unit so that their specific needs can be learned and met. Such discussions may be planned by the student nurses under the direction of their instructors.

5. If the mother has had no previous ex-perience, she may be taught to bathe and dress her infant. Even if she is already expert in child care, she may profit by reviewing the hospital technique, and she surely needs to make the acquaintance of her baby in those situations that mean most to him, i.e. in which affection is shown in his direct physical care.

6. Parents may be told of the community resources available in case they need assistance after leaving the hospital.

SHARED LEARNING: NURSE-PARENT EDUCATION

In a narrow interpretation of education, paren-tal education in the hospital is limited to teach-ing mothers to prepare formulas, to bathe their infants and to give them physical care. In a broader sense it is a continuation of the parental education and prenatal courses which the mother has participated in. Such courses give the information needed in making important decisions about the baby, but do not provide ready-made answers to questions about the individual baby in his family setting. It is in the application of what the mothers have already learned that the nurse is most helpful. It is a shared learning experience, for the nurse, like the mother, must apply her knowledge of child care to the individual infant.

If the student nurse has had little experience in caring for infants and if the mother has had several children of her own, it may be that the nurse will learn more from the mother than the mother from her. On the other hand, if the nurse has had considerable experience with children and if this is the mother's first baby, the nurse shares with the mother her greater knowledge.

The nurse should appreciate the mother's level of understanding and background of experience. This will vary with the mother's socioeconomic class and ethnic background and will also depend upon whether this is her first baby and whether she has had experience with the infants of near relatives. The mother may herself be a professional woman working in the area of child care and may be an expert in the daily care of children.

The nurse should know what sort of care will be possible in the home, the equipment available and the level of living which can be maintained. Specific directions should be written down, or if they are given orally, the mother should be asked to repeat what the nurse has said. *Instructions should be given slowly over a period of time; a mother cannot absorb all that she is to learn of child care at one time.* Knowledge and experience should come gradually. If a mother attended prenatal classes, she has already learned much and will learn more from the physicians and nurses in the hospital. The public health nurse will show her the adaptation of all she has learned to the home care of her baby and its application to the immediate situation.

For the student nurse and the young graduate working with the mother as members of the team caring for the child in the hospital, such teaching is a shared learning experience. The expression *shared learning experience* of mother and nurse is often more truly descriptive of their relations than saying that the nurse teaches the patient.

It is simpler to teach the physical care of children than the psychologic care, and this is particularly true of infant care. The tremendous importance of happiness in infancy lies not only in the present, but also in the formation of the child's personality. The mother-child relationship is recognized as the normal center of the baby's emotional development and is therefore most important. Other members of the family and the world outside are likely to influence the infant through their effect upon his mother.

The love of a mother for her child is the great incentive to her for learning how best to care for him. Such love is likely to make her somewhat critical of instruction given in a purely professional way. The nurse's manner should be warm and friendly. She should convince each mother that she is capable of applying the scientific principles of child care.

Recognition of Maternal Dependency Needs

Physical weakness after delivery of a first-born child is likely to increase a woman's feeling of incompetency in the role of mother of an infant who, when she leaves the hospital, will be completely dependent upon her for his care. This brings us to the problem of meeting her dependency needs so that she feels secure and confident that she will receive the help she has a right to expect from her family and the community. If she worries over the future, her relationship with her baby is influenced by her anxiety and ceases to be the happy fulfillment of her pregnancy. This will influence her ability to nurse the baby at the breast, and her insecurity for the baby and herself on leaving the hospital may be communicated to the infant. He is not likely to be a contented, placid baby.

The mother's dependency needs, both physical and emotional, influence her relations with her baby. She needs her husband's understanding love. She needs to know that he loves the baby not only for itself, but also as the common object of their affection, and that the infant strengthens the emotional bond between them. In contrast, the infant may be made the center of emotional conflicts. The presence of other children may be an emotionally sustaining influence on the one hand, but on the other hand may create many problems caused by their jealousy of the attention given the new arrival.

Probably the crucial factor in the situation is how the mother deals with her dependency needs. In the hospital she may resent being asked to undertake more self-care and more care of the baby than she feels able to undertake. At the other extreme there are mothers who are accustomed to denying the existence of their dependency needs. They find even a few days of enforced hospitalization unpleasant and want to go home too early.

Mothers who feel insecure and fear criticism of their care of the baby insist upon rules to follow or depend upon their own mother's advice in all the little day-to-day problems that arise. The mother who finds dependency humiliating may not ask for the help she needs in caring for her baby.

Nurses will find that the mother of a first baby is more likely to feel dependent, whether she acknowledges it or not, than the mother of several healthy children. The baby looks so small and his ways are so different from those of older babies whom she knows that she is afraid he is choking, suffocating or in extreme danger of some sort. Such a mother is apt to feel that his crying is caused by a condition which must be remedied at once. If she is the overdependent type, she will make many demands upon the nurses. If she is accustomed to taking responsibility and denying her dependency needs, she may force herself into the role of the self-reliant, competent mother, but with a feeling that she is not receiving the help to which she is entitled. Neither extreme leads to good mother-child relations. These women need all the help the nurse can give them.

The student in nursing is close in age to many maternity patients and therefore can have a great influence on them. This closeness, which is of potential value, is likely to involve the nurse emotionally in her relations with a young mother and, in so doing, hamper her service to her patient. Young nurses who are married or expect to be married soon may develop a feeling of identity with the mother which hinders rather than helps their nursing care. It is important for them to retain their professional attitude and a degree of objectivity which does not necessarily cause them to be cold or aloof.

The reaction of the mother to childbirth should be considered and her care arranged accordingly. Sending her home from the hospital within a few days after delivery may be necessary. But it is essential that she be given help in the housework and care of the baby. Her own mother or sister or a visiting housekeeper can give her the assistance she needs.

The Unloving Mother

When a mother does not love her baby — as may happen if he is born out of wedlock — the great stimulus to learn to care for him is absent (see Chap. 26). No mother should be urged to keep her child against her wishes. It would probably be far better for both if he were placed in an adoptive home where he could be loved and cherished. Such a mother need not be taught the care of the infant.

There are other mothers who are married, however, who did not want to become pregnant and who feel that the baby interferes with their professional or social life. Many such mothers find that they love the baby dearly when he is put in their arms, but others remain indifferent to him and look upon his care as an unwanted chore. In hospitals where it is the routine for mothers to attend the group discussion meetings and demonstrations of child care these mothers attend with all the others. They are likely to feel guilty that they do not nurture love for the baby and as a result are overpunctilious in learning all the details of his physical care. Later at home, when the public health nurse sees mother and child, the baby's fine physical condition under his mother's care may generate in her a sense of achievement and pride in him which may in turn evoke love.

The unloving mother initially may provoke a negative response on the part of the nurse in the hospital and in the community. It is important, therefore, that each nurse examine her feelings so that she does not stimulate further guilt in the mother by her own attitudes.

TEACHING AIDS AND OTHER INFORMATION*

American Medical Association

A Child in the Family.
Prenatal Care.

American Social Health Association

The Gift of Life.

Child Study Association of America

Auerbach, A. B., and Arnstein, H. S.: Pregnancy and You.
When Parents Get Together: How to Organize a Parent Education Program, 1964.
Wolf, A.W.M., and Dawson, M. C.: What Makes a Good Home?

Public Affairs Pamphlets

Carson, R.: Nine Months to Get Ready: The Importance of Prenatal Care, 1965.
Mace, D. R.: What Makes a Marriage Happy?
Neisser, W., and Neisser, E.: Making the Grade as Dad.

* Complete addresses are given in the Appendix.

Ross Laboratories

Discovering Parenthood, 1962.
Highley, B. L.: Antepartal Nursing Intervention, 1964.
Mother and Baby.
Rubin, R.: Behavioral Definitions in Nursing Therapy, 1964.

United States Department of Health, Education, and Welfare

Infant and Perinatal Mortality in the United States, 1965.
Infant Mortality Trends, United States and Each State, 1930–1964, 1965.
International Comparison of Perinatal and Infant Mortality: The United States and Six Western
European Countries, 1967.
Prenatal Care, 1962.
The Facts of Life and Death: Selected Statistics on the Nation's Health and People, 1965.
The Fateful Months When Life Begins, 1962.
Thomas, M. W.: The Practice of Nurse Mid-Wifery in the United States, 1965.
When Your Baby Is on the Way, 1961 (reprinted 1963).

REFERENCES

Publications

Bernard, J.: *Marriage and Family among Negroes*. Englewood Cliffs, New Jersey, Prentice-Hall,
Inc., 1966.
Bookmiller, M. M., Bowen, G. L., and Carpenter, D.: *Textbook of Obstetrics and Obstetric Nursing*.
5th ed. Philadelphia, W. B. Saunders Company, 1967.
Brim, O. G.: *Education for Child Rearing*. New York, Macmillan Company, 1965.
Chess, S.: *Your Child Is a Person: A Psychological Approach to Parenthood Without Guilt*. New York,
Viking Press, Inc., 1965.
Duvall, E. M.: *Family Development*. 3rd ed. Philadelphia, J. B. Lippincott Company, 1967.
Fitzpatrick, E., Eastman, N.J., and Reeder, S. R.: *Maternity Nursing*. 11th ed. Philadelphia, J. B.
Lippincott Company, 1966.
Gilbert, M. S.: *Biography of the Unborn*. New York, Hafner Publishing Company, 1963.
Goodrich, F. W.: *Preparing for Childbirth; A Manual for Expectant Parents*. Englewood Cliffs, New
Jersey, Prentice-Hall, 1966.
Hamilton, P. M.: *Basic Maternity Nursing*. St. Louis, C. V. Mosby Company, 1967.
Iorio, J.: *Principles of Obstetrics and Gynecology for Nurses*. St. Louis, C. V. Mosby Company, 1967.
Lytle, N. A.: *Maternal Health Nursing; A Book of Readings*. Iowa, William C. Brown Company, 1967.
Malinowski, B.: *The Father in Primitive Psychology*. New York, W. W. Norton, Inc., 1966.
Mead, M., and Heyman, K.: *Family*. New York, Macmillan Company, 1965.
Meaker, S. R.: *Preparing for Motherhood*. 2nd ed. Chicago, Yearbook Medical Publishers, Inc., 1965.
Minturn, L., and Lambert, W. W.: *Mothers of Six Cultures*. New York, John Wiley and Sons, 1964.
Queen, J., and Others: *The Family in Various Cultures*. 3rd ed. Philadelphia, J. B. Lippincott Com-
pany, 1967.
Richardson, S. A., and Guttmacher, A. F. (Eds.): *Childbearing—Its Social and Psychological Aspects*.
Baltimore, Williams & Wilkins Company, 1967.
Robinson, J. F.: *Having a Baby*. 3rd ed. Baltimore, Williams & Wilkins Company, 1966.
Schaefer, G., and Zisowitz, M. L.: *The Expectant Father*. New York, Simon and Schuster, 1964.
Wiedenbach, E.: *Family-Centered Maternity Nursing*. 2nd ed. New York, G. P. Putnam's Sons, Inc.,
1967.
Williams, J. W., and Others: *Obstetrics*. 13th ed. New York, Appleton-Century-Crofts, 1966.
Winnicott, D. W.: *The Family and Individual Development*. New York, Basic Books, 1965.
W. H. O. Technical Report Series No. 331: *The Midwife in Maternity Care*. Report of a W. H. O.
Expert Committee, Geneva, World Health Organization, 1966.
Ziegel, E., and Van Blarcom, C. C.: *Obstetric Nursing*, 5th ed. New York, Macmillan Company, 1964.

Periodicals

Anderson, E. H., and Lesser, A. J.: Maternity Care in the United States: Gains and Gaps. *Am. J.
Nursing,* 66:1539, 1966.
Barnard, J.: Your Part in Helping to Reduce Infant Mortality. *RN,* 30:43, November 1967.
Battaglia, F. C., and Lubchenco, L. O.: A Practical Classification of Newborn Infants by Weight and
Gestational Age. *J. Pediat.,* 71:159, 1967.
Beck, J.: Guarding the Unborn. *Today's Health,* 46:38, January 1968.
Bergin, M. A.: Monitoring The Fetal Heart. *Nurs. Clin. N. Amer.,* 1:559, 1966.
Clark, A. L.: The Beginning Family. *Am. J. Nursing,* 66:802, 1966.

Hilliard, M. E.: New Horizons in Maternity Nursing. *Nursing Outlook,* 15:33, July 1967.

Juzwiak, M.: An Intimate Look at Husband-Coached Childbirth. *RN,* 29:45, December 1966.

Loughlin, B. W.: Pregnancy in the Navajo Culture. *Nursing Outlook,* 13:55, March 1965.

Rubin, R.: Attainment of the Maternal Role: Part I, Processes. *Nursing Research,* 16:237, 1967.

Rubin, R.: Maternal Touch. *Nursing Outlook,* 11:828, 1963.

Rubin, R.: The Family-Child Relationship and Nursing Care. *Nursing Outlook,* 12:36. September 1964.

Saling, E., and Bretscher, J.: pH Values of the Human Fetus During Labor. *Amer. J. Obst. & Gynec.,* 97:906, April 1, 1967.

Schaefer, G.: The Expectant Father. *Nursing Outlook,* 14:46, September 1966.

Stone, A. R.: Cues to Interpersonal Distress Due to Pregnancy. *Am. J. Nursing,* 65:88, November 1965.

Swallow, K. A., and Davis G. H.: 645 Days of Maternity and Infant Care. *Children,* 14:141, 1967.

6

EXAMINATION AND CHARACTER-ISTICS OF THE NEWBORN

Since nurses are assuming increasing responsibilities in relation to newborn infants in that they carry out the routine of physical examination as well as providing them with care in many maternity units, they must understand their physical attributes and functional disturbances. Anatomically, physiologically and psychologically the baby differs from adults and even from older children. His characteristics are those of his age group. Every baby is an individual and should never be regarded as a typical infant, one unit of a group in which all are alike. But averages and *the range of normality should be remembered so that each baby may receive medical care if he deviates too far from the so-called normal.* It is impossible to study the infant except as a living whole; it is essential to understand his physiologic activity, which in turn is strongly influenced by his emotional state.

PHYSIOLOGIC RESILIENCE

Nature provides the fetus and the newborn with a certain physiologic resilience. The normal neonate is relatively indifferent to a range of body temperature from as low as 97 to as high

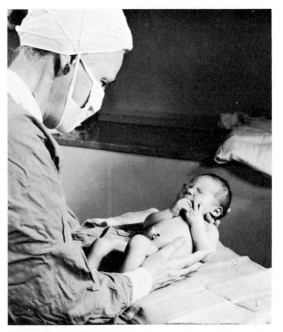

Figure 6–1. The infant is observed for obvious malformations before the detailed examination begins. (Courtesy of Pfizer Laboratories, Brooklyn, New York.)

as 100°F.; in premature infants the body temperature may even drop to 94°. By indifference is meant that the newborn does not seem uncomfortable or show the concomitant signs of low or high temperature which would appear in the adult. The infant has an unstable heat-regulating system, and his body temperature is influenced by the environmental temperature. If the room is cold, so is his body; if he is covered with too many blankets, his body temperature rises. Regulate the temperature about him, and his returns to normal.

The infant is also indifferent to abnormal levels of substances in the blood. The levels usually found in predictable concentration in the blood of normal children are less standardized in the neonate and even more unpredictable in premature infants.

Although the blood glucose level may be low, the usual hypoglycemic reaction of the adult is not seen. The infant shows some departure of the blood hydrogen ion content and carbon dioxide tension from the adult level (see p. 39). There is also an increase in the range of their normal values. The infant can survive without breathing for a relatively longer time than the adult, though there are definite limits to his tolerance for lack of oxygen.

This physiologic resilience has many obvious advantages, and because of it many infants have survived who otherwise would have died. Yet it has one great disadvantage: it conceals or minimizes physical signs of diagnostic value. For instance, infection in the newborn may not be accompanied by fever as it is in older children or adults. In other cases an infant who is moderately dehydrated may have respirations which seem to be barely perceptibly increased, yet he may have a blood pH of 7.2 or even lower without having acidotic Kussmaul respirations. Also, infants do not conform to a pattern in their reactions to drugs; this fact makes it essential that the nurse observe infants carefully for untoward reactions.

All in all, this passive resistance of the infant is an ally. But there are limits to his resistance which cannot be safely overstepped. This is particularly true of the premature infant, who shows few defense mechanisms against unfavorable circumstances.

The first few days of life are normally a time when the infant is in a state of negative balance, e.g. postnatal weight loss, loss of body fluids, and decreases in hemoglobin, calories, nitrogen, sodium chloride and inherited antibodies. There is danger of feeding him too much and too early in an attempt to make up for these losses.

Death on the first day of extrauterine life is not due to wasting of resources. Negative balance is normal, and only harm results from attempting to force it to positive.

LENGTH AND WEIGHT

The length of the average newborn male is 20 inches, or 50 cm.; of the female, 19.6 inches, or 49 cm. The normal range for both sexes is from 19 to $21\frac{1}{2}$ inches, or 47.5 to 53.75 cm.

The weight of the normal newborn also tends to vary. About two thirds of all full-term infants weigh between 2700 and 3850 gm., or between 6 and $8\frac{1}{2}$ pounds. Many infants, of course, weigh more or less than this. The average girl weighs approximately 7 pounds, the average boy approximately $7\frac{1}{2}$ pounds.

During the first few days after birth the infant tends to lose about 6 to 10 ounces, or 5 to 10 per cent of his birth weight. Factors contributing to this initial loss are the withdrawal of hormones originally obtained from the mother, the withholding of water and the loss of feces and urine.

TEMPERATURE, PULSE, RESPIRATION AND BLOOD PRESSURE

The temperature, pulse and respiration of the newborn vary in an unpredictable way. He appears to have a passive resistance or resilience, within a wide range of bodily responses; yet when these limits of tolerance are exceeded, because he lacks the adult's reserve vitality, he may suddenly appear ill. *This need for constant observation is an essential of infant nursing care.* The nurse must learn from experience to recognize the significance of his response to sensations which he cannot let her know about in words or actions, e.g. pushing off the covers if he is too hot.

Temperature

The infant's temperature at birth is slightly higher than his mother's, since the uterus lies deeply insulated within her body. It drops immediately after birth in adjustment to the temperature of the delivery room and then rises to normal within about eight hours. His hands and feet are colder than the rest of his body, since his circulation is poor. This lack of stability, due to underdevelopment of his heat-regulating system, requires that external heat be applied. He is generally wrapped in warm blankets in the delivery room. The nurse who puts him in his crib will have to remember that too much heat for too long will send his temperature above normal.

Pulse

Fetal electrocardiography is used to record electrical impulses of the fetal heart *in utero*. Abnormal intrauterine conditions can thus be diagnosed and evaluated and immediately treated after birth.

A deep flush spreads over the entire body if baby cries hard. Veins on head swell and throb. You will notice no tears as tear ducts do not function as yet.

The skin is thin and dry. You may see veins through it. Fair skin may be rosy-red temporarily. Downy hair is not unusual. Some *vernix caseosa* (white, prenatal skin covering) remains.

Head usually strikes you as being too big for the body. It may be temporarily out of shape — lopsided or elongated — due to pressure before or during birth.

The feet look more complete than they are. X-ray would show only one real bone at the heel. Other bones are now cartilage. Skin often loose and wrinkly.

The trunk may startle you in some normal detail: short neck, small sloping shoulders, swollen breasts, large rounded abdomen, umbilical stump (future navel), slender, narrow pelvis and hips.

Eyes appear dark blue, have a blank stary gaze. You may catch one or both turning or turned to crossed or wall-eyed position. Lids, characteristically, puffy.

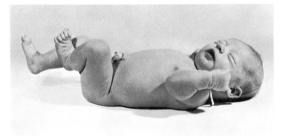

The legs are most often seen drawn up against the abdomen in pre-birth position. Extended legs measure shorter than you'd expect compared to the arms. The knees stay slightly bent and legs are more or less bowed.

Genitals of both sexes will seem large (especially scrotum) in comparison with the scale of, for example, the hands to adult size.

The face will disappoint you unless you expect to see: pudgy cheeks, a broad, flat nose with mere hint of a bridge, receding chin, undersized lower jaw.

Weight unless well above the average of 6 or 7 lbs. will not prepare you for how really tiny newborn is. Top to toe measure: anywhere between 18" to 21".

The hands, if you open them out flat from their characteristic fist position, have: finely lined palms, tissue-paper thin nails, dry, loose fitting skin and deep bracelet creases at wrist.

On the skull you will see or feel the two most obvious soft spots or *fontanels*. One is above the brow, the other close to crown of head in back.

Figure 6–2. What a healthy newborn baby looks like. This unretouched photograph taken 6 hours after birth at Lawrence Memorial Hospital. (From *Baby Talk*, January 1964.)

The infant's pulse is normally irregular, owing to immaturity of the cardiac regulatory center in the medulla. The rate is rapid, around 120 to 150 a minute. Extreme irregularity results from any one of many physical or emotional stimuli. When the infant is startled or cries, his pulse rate not only increases, but also becomes more irregular. Irregularity of rhythm of the pulse may follow that of the respiration.

Respiration

Respiration in the newborn is irregular in depth, rate and rhythm and varies from 35 to 50 per minute. Like the pulse rate, it is readily altered by internal or external stimuli. Normally, respirations are gentle and quiet, rapid and shallow. They can be observed most easily by watching abdominal movement, since respiration in the newborn is carried on largely by the diaphragm and abdominal muscles. Dyspnea or cyanosis may occur suddenly in an infant who is breathing normally. These signs may be the first indication of the presence of a congenital anomaly or other condition from which an infant may suddenly expire if he does not receive adequate care. The nurse should notify the physician if respiration drops below 35 or exceeds 50 per minute when the infant is at rest or if dyspnea or cyanosis occurs.

The normal cry is lusty, frequent and often apparently without cause. If the infant does not cry, he should be stimulated to do so at approximately hourly intervals in order to force expansion of his lungs by the concomitant deep respirations.

Blood Pressure

The blood pressure is characteristically low. It is difficult to determine accurately and may vary with the size of the cuff used (see p. 62).

THE SKIN

The skin of the newborn of the Caucasian race is red or dark pink, in the Negro a reddish black, and in the Mongolian the color of a tea rose. It is soft, covered with lanugo and overlaid with vernix caseosa. There is slight desquamation. Good elasticity or *turgor* is evidence that an infant is in good condition.

Lanugo is a slight downy distribution of fine hair over the body, most evident on the shoulders, back, extremities, forehead and temples. Since lanugo begins to appear on the fetus by about the sixteenth week of gestation and to disappear after the thirty-second week, it is often an evidence of immaturity when present. The premature infant has a heavier showing than the full-term infant. Lanugo tends to disappear during the first weeks of life.

Vernix caseosa is a cheeselike, greasy, yellowish-white substance, sometimes likened to cream cheese or cold cream, which covers the newborn's skin. It consists of secretions from sebaceous glands and epithelial cells. Its distribution over the body is variable, being heavier in the folds of the skin and between the labia. It dries or fades spontaneously and rubs off on the infant's clothing.

Tissue turgor refers to the sensation of fullness derived from the presence of hydrated subcutaneous tissue. Elasticity of the skin is demonstrated when a fold of skin is grasped between the thumb and forefinger. When released, the skin promptly springs back to form the smooth, soft surface of the body.

Observation may reveal the following additional normal findings. *Desquamation* or peeling of the skin occurs during the first two to four weeks of life. Denuded areas may occur where the delicate skin has been rubbed off the nose, knees and elbows because of pressure and erosion on the sheets. The skin of the buttocks needs special care so that it does not become chafed. A wet or soiled diaper should be changed at once.

Transient *rashes* may occur. *Milia* is a condition in which tiny white papillae occur, particularly on the nose and chin, owing to obstruction of the sebaceous glands. These blemishes disappear in a week or two. *Physiologic jaundice* becomes definite between the third and seventh days. It is likely to appear gradually on the second or third day and is seen in the majority of infants (see also p. 105).

There may be marks upon the infant's body. Some are temporary, caused by the trauma of birth; others are due to immaturity, even in the infant born at term; still others are permanent birthmarks. Among the temporary marks are *hemangiomas*, or pink spots, on the upper eye-

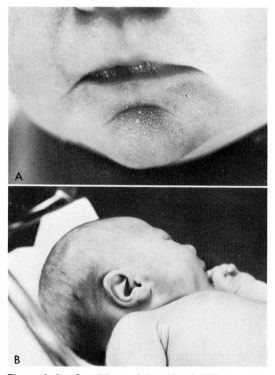

Figure 6–3. Conditions of the skin. *A*, Milia is a condition in which small white papillae occur, especially on the chin and nose. (Courtesy of Mead Johnson Laboratories.) *B*, If forceps were used on the infant's head during delivery, temporary marks may be left on the skin of the face. (Courtesy of Mead Johnson Laboratories.)

lids, between the eyebrows, and on the nose, upper lip or back of the neck. The mother may be reassured that they will disappear spontaneously. If forceps were used during delivery, temporary *forceps marks* may be left upon the part of the body or head where the blades exerted pressure. In a breech delivery there may be edema and extravasation of blood into the tissues of the buttocks and genitals due to trauma to the presenting parts. In fact, there may be *bruising of tissues* on almost any part of the infant's body as he progresses through the birth canal.

Another type of mark which may be present is the so-called *Mongolian spot*. These spots, which are slate colored, usually occur on the buttocks or lower portion of the back of infants whose parents are Negro, Oriental or from the Mediterranean area. They fade during the preschool years without treatment. (See Color Plate I-2.)

By two weeks of age the infant should have the typical rosy, soft, dewy skin which we associate with babies. The sweat glands become active by the end of the second week.

THE HEAD

The head is proportionately large, averaging 34 to 35 cm., or 13.6 to 14 inches, in circumference. The normal limits of head size are 33 to 37 cm., or 13.2 to 14.8 inches. The head is one fourth the total length of the infant. In the adult the length of the head is one eighth of the total height (see Fig. 2-6). The infant's cranium is large and the face relatively small when compared with the adult cranium and face. The jaws are relatively small, and the chin is receding. The circumference of the head equals or exceeds that of the chest or abdomen.

The *fontanels* are openings at the points of union of the skull bones. These should be palpated to determine whether they are open or closed. The anterior fontanel is diamond-shaped and located at the juncture of the two parietal and two frontal bones. It is 2 to 3 cm. or 0.8 to 1.2 inches in width and 3 to 4 cm. or 1.2 to 1.6 inches in length (Fig. 6-5). The posterior fontanel is triangular and located between the occipital and parietal bones. It is much smaller than the anterior fontanel and may be nearly closed. The fontanels bulge when the infant cries or strains or if there is increased pressure within the skull. Increased intracranial pressure may be due to a number of causes, among them hydrocephalus (see p. 214). The anterior fontanel normally closes by the time the infant is twelve to eighteen months old, and the posterior fontanel by the end of the second month.

The bones of the cranium are held together by membranes at the suture lines. During delivery, pressure may mold the head into asymmetrical proportions. In general the head assumes its normal shape by the time the infant is a week old.

Caput succedaneum is swelling or edema of the presenting portion of the scalp and may be localized or fairly extensive. It usually disappears by the third day. (See Figure 6-6.)

Cephalhematoma is an accumulation of blood between the periosteum and a flat skull bone. The collection of blood does not cross a suture line. The mass is soft, irreducible and fluctuating. It does not increase on crying. A cephalhematoma may not be evident during the first few days of life because of the presence of a large caput succedaneum. Aspiration of this sanguineous collection should not be done because of the danger of infection and because the condition usually clears within a few weeks. (See Figure 6-7.)

Face and Neck

The infant's face is expressionless. The ears are flabby until the cartilage calcifies. The neck

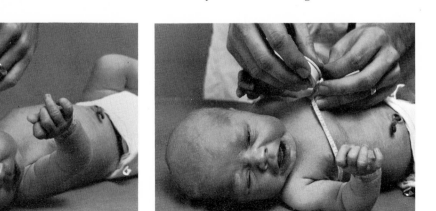

Figure 6–4. The circumferences of the head and chest is measured. In the course of being examined newborns almost invariably protest. (Courtesy of Dr. Charles H. Peete, Jr., and *Baby Talk* Magazine.)

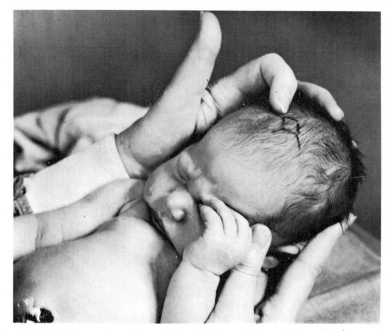

Figure 6–5. The size of the fontanels varies considerably from infant to infant. They are palpated to ascertain their tension. (Courtesy of Pfizer Laboratories, Brooklyn, New York.)

is short and creased. These creases, particularly in a fat infant, are deep and likely to become sore unless carefully cleaned.

In the normal infant it should be possible to turn the head freely from side to side. If there is rigidity, the sternocleidomastoid muscles may have been injured during delivery. When the infant is lying on his back and begins to cry, his head is held in the midline, and both sides of his face are mobile. Absence of symmetry in move-

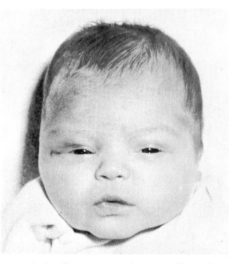

Figure 6–6. Caput succedaneum. Extensive soft tissue swelling of the scalp is evident.

ment or contour is evidence of an abnormality.

The infant who is born with ears like the handles of a loving cup should have plastic surgery performed before he begins school in order to prevent the psychic trauma caused by his being different from other members of his group.

THE CHEST

The chest is bell-shaped and at birth is approximately the same circumference as the abdomen and less than the head. For this reason it appears small. By the time the child is two years old the size of the chest exceeds that of the head, and he begins to take on more nearly adult proportions.

The thorax is almost circular. The anterior and lateral diameters are the same because of the pressure of the arms against the chest wall *in utero*. The infant does not use the thoracic cage in breathing as does the older child or adult; he uses the diaphragm and abdominal muscles to exhale and inhale.

The breasts may be swollen because of hormone activity originating from the mother, and pale milky fluid ("witch's milk") can be expressed. The condition disappears in two to four weeks without treatment, but as long as it lasts the breasts are tender and should be touched only when necessary and then very gently.

The *thymus* is usually proportionately large

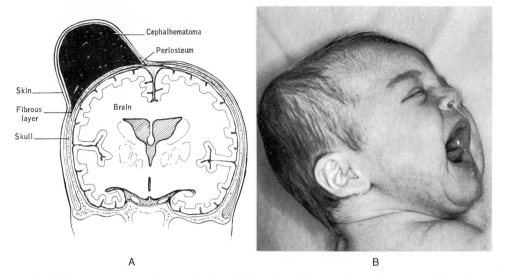

Figure 6–7. Cephalhematoma. *A,* The collection of blood lies between the periosteum and the skull bone. *B,* Cephalhematoma of the right parietal bone.

and triples its weight by the time the child is five years old; it then remains approximately the same size until he is about ten years old, when it begins to decrease. It has been disproved that a large thymus is the cause of respiratory difficulty or sudden death by asphyxia. Usually some other factor is accountable for cyanosis or apnea.

RESPIRATORY SYSTEM

The mechanism of respiration is established before birth, but at birth it undergoes profound changes. Prerespiratory movements begin in the fourth month of gestation. Amniotic fluid may move in and out of the lungs as a result of these tidal movements. Oxygen is, of course, obtained through the placental circulation. The hypoxia resulting from severance of the cord assists in initiating breathing through stimulation of the respiratory center by the accumulation of carbon dioxide. The process of birth and the environmental change also stimulate the respiratory center. The first breath, usually taken within thirty seconds after birth, helps to expand the collapsed lungs, though full expansion does not occur for several days.

CIRCULATORY SYSTEM

At birth sudden changes occur in the circulatory system. The circulatory pattern must change from fetal dependency on the placenta to include the expanding lungs. The functional structures (i.e. foramen ovale and ductus arteriosus) of intrauterine life must be obliterated. The circulation of the pulmonary system is per-

fected, and a short time after birth oxygenated blood flows through the infant's body in the same manner as that of the adult. The foramen ovale (see Fig. 11-6) closes by the third month. The ductus arteriosus is occluded when the infant is from several weeks to four months old. Approximately 2 per cent of newborns have transitory, insignificant heart murmurs caused by blood leaking through openings not yet closed. These murmurs disappear within a few weeks.

The *vascular system* and *heart* are large in the newborn in comparison with their size in adult life. The blood volume of the newborn is about 10 to 12 per cent of his body weight. This percentage is influenced by the amount of blood received from the placenta before clamping of the cord.

Blood

The blood contains a relatively high number of red blood cells and a high hemoglobin level at birth (see Tables 3-1, 3-2). These characteristics are essential to provide adequate oxygenation *in utero* and during the first few postnatal days before the lungs expand fully. Oxygenation improves during the first two weeks of life to the extent that a high red cell count and hemoglobin level are no longer necessary, and hemolysis occurs. There is a continued fall in the red cell count and hemoglobin levels during the first three months of life, resulting in a physiologic anemia.

Physiologic Jaundice (Icterus Neonatorum)

Infants have an excessive amount of bilirubin in the blood at birth. During the first week there is a further breakdown of hemoglobin, thereby increasing the blood bilirubin level. At this time the immature liver cannot excrete bilirubin in sufficient quantities. The result is a jaundice of the skin and sclerae. This occurs in approximately 55 to 70 per cent of all newborns, from two to three days after birth. It increases for a few days and usually disappears by the seventh day. The urine may become dark, and the infant appears sluggish, even showing anorexia. Although the normal bilirubin level is 1.0 mg. per 100 ml. or slightly higher in the newborn, hyperbilirubinemia beyond physiologic levels exists when the total serum bilirubin levels reach 18 to 20 mg. per 100 ml. during the first seven days of life. Continuing jaundice indicates a pathologic condition such as obstruction of the bile ducts, syphilis or erythroblastosis fetalis.

Physiologic Hypoprothrombinemia

During the first few days of life the prothrombin level decreases in all infants. Thus the clotting time is prolonged. This condition is most acute between the second and fifth postnatal days. It can be prevented to a great extent by giving vitamin K to the mother during labor or to the infant after birth. Recovery usually occurs between seven and ten days of age.

GASTROINTESTINAL SYSTEM

Sucking Pads, Mouth and Jaw

The sucking pads are deposits of fatty tissue in the cheeks which persist even when the infant is extremely malnourished. They disappear when sucking is no longer the only way of taking food.

The infant has a receding chin, which trembles at the slightest stimulation, especially if he is startled or whimpers. His tongue is relatively large and protrudes when the mouth is open. The newborn cannot move food from his lips to the pharynx. Later, when food is given, it must be placed at the back of his tongue so that he can swallow it. At two or three months of age salivation occurs. Since the infant has not yet learned to swallow facilely, he may drool.

Esophagus, Stomach and Intestines

The cardiac sphincter is not as well developed as the pyloric sphincter. For this reason the infant should be "bubbled" several times while being fed so that air which he has swallowed may be eructed. (A little milk may come up with the air.) If the air were to remain in the stomach, there would be danger of vomiting or, if it passed into the intestine, of colic.

Occasionally the action of the pyloric valve may not be normal, and regurgitating (the vomiting of food immediately after it has been taken) may be so constant that an infant fails to gain in weight. This pathologic condition will be taken up in Chapter 13.

It is difficult to measure the size of the infant's stomach. The contents are emptied almost immediately into the duodenum. When we look at the infant and the amount of milk he is taking, it is evident that the fluid is leaving the stomach before the feeding is completed. It is likely that at birth the stomach holds from 1 to 2 ounces, at two weeks 3 ounces, at five months 7 ounces and at ten months 10 ounces. The entire formula should be out of the infant's stomach in two and a half to three hours. Digestion is slowed by food high in protein or fat.

The intestinal tract functions as an outlet for amniotic fluid as early as the fifth month of intrauterine life. The normal gastrointestinal tract assumes its function readily after birth. *Meconium,* the first fecal material, is a sticky, odorless material, greenish black to brownish green, which is passed from eight to twenty-four hours after birth.

The nature of the *stools* changes daily in the first week. They are called transitional stools. From the third to the fifth day they are loose, contain mucus and are greenish yellow. After the fifth day the nature of the stools depends on the feeding. The stools of the breast-fed infant are yellow and pasty. The breast-fed infant will normally have from two to four stools a day. The stools of an infant fed on a formula of modified cow's milk are light yellow and hard and are passed once or twice daily. The composition of some commercially prepared formulas is so similar to that of breast milk that it may be difficult to differentiate the stools of infants fed these formulas from those of infants who are breast fed. Later, when the infant is receiving a soft diet, the stools are brown or colored from the kind of food given him.

Abdomen

The umbilical stump begins to shrink and become discolored soon after birth and within a few days turns black (see p. 115). It sloughs off between the sixth and tenth days, but leaves a granulating area which heals in another week. The umbilical cord must be examined closely during the first twenty-four hours after birth and then daily for any trace of bleeding, which should be reported to the physician at once. If bleeding occurs, the cord should be clamped or retied immediately. After the first day there is less danger of bleeding, but signs of infection may appear and should be reported. Extreme care must be taken that this lesion does not become infected, since the blood vessels of the cord and their extension into the abdomen afford a potential portal of entry for organisms until the umbilical wound is completely healed. A bactericidal dye is used in many nurseries to paint the cord stump in order to help prevent infection.

Examination of Internal Organs

In addition to the external examination, three additional tests are necessary to complete the appraisal of the gastrointestinal system of the newborn. These tests are designed to uncover anomalies which prevent normal physiologic processes. *These anomalies, not obvious on general inspection, are of such importance that their early discovery and correction may mean saving the infant's life. Such anomalies include imperforate anus, omphalocele and esophageal atresia.* (see Chapter 10 for further discussion of these conditions.)

Imperforate Anus. In order to test for the presence of this condition, in the absence of a meconium stool, the physician or nurse need only insert into the infant's rectum a thermometer, a gloved finger (since the infant's rectum is very small, it is well to use the index or little finger) or a soft rubber catheter.

Omphalocele. The point of juncture of the umbilical cord with the abdomen should be examined to make certain that a loop of intestine is not protruding into the base of the cord.

Esophageal Atresia. In order to test for the presence of an esophageal atresia, a soft rubber catheter may be passed through the esophagus into the stomach. Any obstruction should be reported immediately, for the infant will be unable to take nourishment. Repair should be made before his condition is weakened by lack of nourishment or before pneumonia develops, owing to aspiration of formula.

These simple tests are not dangerous to the newborn. They may be safely performed by the student nurse under the direction and supervision of the physician or her instructor, if the policy of the agency in which she is gaining experience permits her to do so. The nurse does not, of course, make a diagnosis of a medical condition, but through intelligent observation and description of her findings she is able to inform the physician of conditions which require his consideration.

ANOGENITAL AREA

The infant's buttocks are plump, firm and pink. In the anal region there should be no redness or fissures.

Genitalia

Male Genitalia. The size of the penis and the scrotum varies. The prepuce or foreskin of the penis may adhere to the glans. The testes have usually descended into the scrotum by the eighth month of intrauterine life, but in some cases they remain in the abdomen or the inguinal canal. This condition is commonly known as undescended testes or cryptorchidism (see p. 316).

Female Genitalia. The female genitalia may be slightly swollen, owing to hormone activity originating from the mother. The labia majora are undeveloped, and the exposed labia minora appear large. The vagina exudes a mucous discharge which may occasionally be blood-tinged during the first week. This is also caused by hormones transmitted from mother to infant. The condition should disappear by the second or third week.

Urine

The infant has urine in the bladder at birth and may void immediately or after several hours. In a small percentage of newborns, however, urination may be delayed until the second day. The urine is dilute because of the immaturity of the kidneys and their lack of ability to concentrate. Loss of a large amount of water may result in temporary hemoconcentration. A pink stain may be found on the diaper which is usually due to deposition of uric acid crystals.

SKELETAL STRUCTURE

The bones of the newborn are soft because they are composed chiefly of cartilage in which there is only a small amount of calcium. The skeleton is flexible and the joints are elastic to ensure a safe passage through the birth canal.

The infant's back is normally straight and flat. The lumbar and sacral curves develop later when the infant sits up and begins to stand.

The legs are small, short and bowed or curve outward as the infant lies with his legs abducted and flexed, so that the soles of the feet nearly touch each other. The feet appear to be flat, owing to the presence of the plantar fat pad (a pad of fat in the longitudinal arch of the foot). The legs should be examined to determine whether there is any limitation of movement. The arms, like the legs, are relatively short, and the position of the neonate is often that of the tonic neck reflex (see p. 110). The hands are plump, the fingers relatively short, and the nails are smooth and soft and extend over the finger tips.

The newborn's hands are clenched in little fists. The fingers should be separated and examined. The normal grasping reflex is so strong

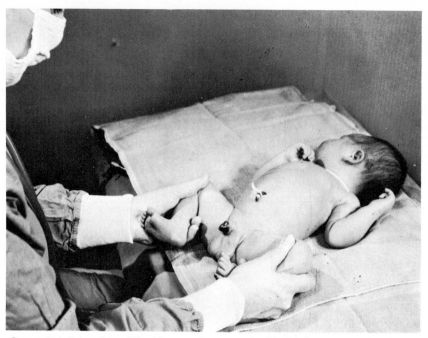

Figure 6–8. Congenital dislocation of the hips may be recognized by testing gross abduction of the thighs and observing for protrusion of the femoral heads. (Courtesy of Pfizer Laboratories, Brooklyn, New York.)

that if an adult's forefingers are placed into the infant's fists, he can be raised from the crib.

Many of the common anomalies of infancy are noted in the extremities (e.g. clubfoot or syndactyly, the latter a union of the fingers or toes). Although these do not interfere with vital functions as do anomalies of the heart, bladder or other internal organs, they are a cause of great anxiety to the parents.

MUSCLES

Muscular contour in the healthy, plump infant is smooth, and his muscles, in spite of their lack of strength and his inability to control them, feel hard and slightly resistant to pressure. The nurse should note whether the infant offers normal resistance to passive movement of his extremities. If he does not, he may be suffering from cerebral injury, narcosis or even shock. If an infant feels limp in the hands of the nurse, the condition should never be mistaken for a mere characteristic of his immaturity.

The movements of the newborn are random and uncoordinated; he wriggles and stretches. When the nurse picks him up, she must support his back and head, for he lacks the muscular strength to hold even his head steady and would slump if placed in a sitting position.

NERVOUS SYSTEM

The nervous system of the newborn is strikingly immature. His bodily functions and responses to stimuli from outside his body are carried on chiefly by the midbrain and reflexes of the spinal cord. The cerebral influence characteristic of even the preschool child is lacking.

As soon as the nerve fibers become myelinated and make the necessary connections with one another, control from the higher cerebral centers begins, and increasingly more complex and purposeful behavior is possible. One can observe the neurologic development from week to week as it proceeds caudally from above.

Reflexes

Certain reflexes are absolutely essential to the infant's life, and many are protective. Among these latter are the *blinking reflex,* which is aroused when the infant is subjected to a bright light, and the *reflexes of coughing* and *sneezing,* which clear the respiratory tract. The *yawn reflex* is in a sense protective, since thereby the infant draws in an added supply of oxygen.

A number of reflex actions are involved in feeding. The *rooting reflex* causes the infant to turn his head toward anything which touches his cheek and is his way of reaching for food. It helps the infant to locate the nipple with his mouth when the breast touches his cheek. The *sucking reflex* provides sucking movements when anything touches the lips. This reflex is normally present at birth and is accompanied by the *swallowing reflex*. The *gagging reflex* comes into play when he has taken more into his mouth than he can successfully swallow. He can also cough if a little of the fluid is "swallowed the wrong way" and enters the trachea.

The infant is not skillful in coordinating all these reflexes and requires help from the mother or nurse. He may have trouble getting the nipple into his mouth, and when he does succeed, the nipple may be under rather than on the tongue. These reflexes essential to successful nursing are absent or underdeveloped in the premature infant, but their absence in the full-term infant would indicate narcosis, brain injury or mental retardation. If the sucking reflex is not stimulated, it ceases to exist.

The *grasp reflex* is present in both hands and feet. An infant will grasp any object put into his hands, hold on briefly and then drop it. At birth he may be able to hold on so securely to an adult's forefinger inserted into his fist that he may be lifted from the crib to a standing position (the "Darwinian reflex"). This grasping action in its reflex form fades. As the infant matures it be-

comes conscious and purposeful and obviously is one which brings him pleasure—shaking his rattle, for instance. Although he cannot grasp with his feet, his toes react to stimulation with an attempt to get hold of the object which touches the sole of the foot or the toes (Fig. 6-9, *A*).

If the infant is held upright around the chest with his feet touching the examination table or crib, he will attempt prancing movements with his legs. This is called the *dancing reflex;* it soon disappears. Not until he is trying to stand and walk does he again make any attempt to move his legs as in prancing, though he gets great fun from kicking as he lies on his back.

The newborn has one great unlearned reaction to strong stimuli: the *startle reflex*. At birth or soon after this reflex is aroused by a sudden loud noise or loss of support. The reaction is a generalized, aimless muscular activity. The startle or *Moro reflex* demonstrates an awareness of equilibrium in the newborn. This reflex can best be elicited when the infant is quiet and without the restraint of clothing. A sudden stimulus such as jarring the table or bassinet will cause the infant to draw up his legs with the soles of the feet turned toward each other and the undersurface of the toes almost touching. The arms assume the embrace position. These move-

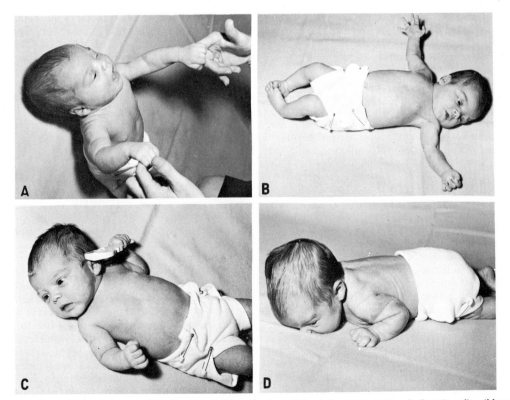

Figure 6–9. Reflexes and motor development of the newborn infant. *A,* Grasp reflex. *B,* Startle reflex (Moro reflex). *C,* Tonic neck reflex. *D,* Lifts head slightly from the bed.

ments, followed by a rather fixed and rigid position, normally are symmmetrical. The Moro reflex is a normal reaction which is strongest during the first eight weeks or so of life; it may persist, but be increasingly difficult to elicit until about the fifth month. In its absence the possibility of brain damage must be considered (Fig. 6-9, *B*).

The *tonic neck reflex* is a postural reflex in which the infant, when lying on his back, turns his head to one side and extends the arm and the leg on the side to which the head is turned at right angles from his body; he flexes the other leg and arm. He may make a fist with both hands. This position has been aptly called the infant's fencing position; it occurs in fetal life by about twenty to twenty-eight weeks of gestation and in the newborn and infant up to about the eighteenth or twentieth week (Fig. 6-9. *C*).

Successful use of the reflex mechanism is evidence of normal functioning of the nervous system. If a reflex is impaired or absent, it may be that the central nervous system has sustained injury. Although it may not be possible to correct the condition, the care of the infant can and must be adapted to his disability. For instance, if he cannot suck, he must be fed by gavage. Certain reflexes present in the newborn disappear as he matures, and the cerebrum exercises greater control over the nervous system. This brings about changes in behavior to which the care given him by the mother or nurse must be adapted.

The Conditioned Reflex. This is the only way by which the infant learns, and it is largely limited to carrying over the satisfaction from feeding to the concomitants of the process. He sees the nurse's or mother's face, although it is blurred for him, and learns to like those who feed him because of their association with the relief of his hunger and the general comfort of being fed.

Motor Activity

The movements of the newborn are rapid, varied and diffuse. Any specific movements he makes are simple reflex actions or are prompted by a reflex action, such as swallowing prompted by the sucking reflex. Although he begins soon after birth to learn about the world through the conditioned reflex, practically all his behavior is still due to reflex response to stimuli. His whole body is likely to be involved in his activity, and his responses appear to be aroused by some generalized state such as hunger, pain or discomfort from lying too long in one position. He does not localize the feeling of pain or hunger.

When the infant feels that something is wrong, he reacts with his whole body and may try out reflex movements which he associates with relief. For instance, although he does not yet connect the breast or the bottle with relief from hunger, he makes sucking movements with his lips and will try to suck anything which comes in contact with them. Specific responses to specific stimuli are an outgrowth of this generalized activity; the useless movements are dropped, and the useful movements which bring him a reward are perfected through practice. This is not due primarily to practice, however, but rather to maturation of his nervous system, muscles, bones and, in fact, his entire body. Maturation does not proceed at the same rate in all the systems of the body, but the general pattern makes possible the typical behavior of infants at certain ages. Naturally they must be given opportunity to try out and practice new responses, or their behavior will be atypical.

At birth the infant can raise his head slightly when lying on his stomach, but not when on his back. If he is pulled to a sitting position, his head falls back, and his spine is curved in a bow from shoulders to hips. At an early age the infant can make crawling movements when on his abdomen and a little later push himself up in his crib by kicking movements.

EMOTIONAL RESPONSES

Signs of emotion in the newborn are extremely difficult to interpret. Probably all that can be said is that two emotional states are evident: in one he lies peacefully, and in the other he appears in discomfort—his face is twisted, and he cries. To this could be added his emotional response to the startle stimulus.

Since vocalization shows his emotion and, increasingly as he grows older, will express *the emotion* he wishes to convey, vocalization is considered under Emotional Responses.

Vocalization

The newborn vocalizes solely by crying, and this he does in response to any discomfort or pain. He is an egocentric little person entirely dependent upon adult care and unable to make his wants known in any other way. His birth cry is the beginning of vocalization and serves two purposes: to supply the blood with sufficient oxygen and to inflate the unexpanded lungs.

If the cry is weak and not sustained, an abnormal condition must be suspected. It should be a lusty cry even with only the stimulation of the birth incident. No one knows whether the birth cry has any connection with discomfort or is a pure reflex evoked by his physiologic needs.

Soon crying is used to express discomfort. If crying brings the infant relief and pleasant sensations from the care given him, he soon learns through the conditioning of this reflex to cry for attention. Even within the first twenty-four hours the cry varies in pitch, intensity and continuity, so that it has meaning to those who are accustomed to caring for infants.

The stimulation to cry comes from the immediate environment or from his own body. He may be hungry, in pain or in need of exercise such as comes from being picked up and moved about. Infants often cry for unknown reasons, and the cause of their discomfort cannot be ascertained. When an infant is neither hungry nor wet, if he stops crying when cuddled, we can infer that this is what he needed, and after being quieted he may be put back in his crib. But the infant who continues to cry while he is being held and petted is probably in distress and should be watched carefully for other symptoms of illness.

Hunger is said to be the most common cause of crying, and this an argument for putting the infant on a self-demand feeding schedule (see p. 124).

The cry is made almost exclusively from vowels produced in the front of the mouth. Soon he makes other sounds which are as important as crying as a forerunner of speech. These sounds are explosive—coos, grunts and gurgles. They probably have no meaning other than that they occur only when he appears contented. But the next stage of vocalization—that of repetition of syllables, as in "ma-ma"—is built upon his practice in phonation.

SPECIAL SENSES

An infant shows by his general discomfort that he can feel pressure, temperature change and pain.

Touch

The sense of touch is the most highly developed of the special senses and is most acute on the lips, tongue, ears and forehead. Failure to grasp the nipple is therefore one indication of brain damage. The normal newborn responds to the touch of the hands of those caring for him from the moment of his birth.

Sight

The eyes are blue or gray at birth, changing to the permanent color in three to six months. Their movements are not coordinated, and both eyes momentarily may turn inward or outward.

It is difficult to know what an infant sees. His eyes are only half open, and the lids are swollen. There may a purulent discharge from the use of silver nitrate (see p. 116). The pupils react to light, and bright lights appear to be unpleasant to the infant.

Recent research has shown that normal full-term newborns do have the capacity to shed tears, although they are usually not obvious until the infant is three to four weeks old.

Hearing

The newborn is deaf until his first cry. To test the hearing of the newborn, a bell may be gently rung (held a little distance from his ear). If he hears it, he will respond with generalized activity of his whole body. The infant normally makes some response to sound from the third to the seventh day, and there is evidence that he hears ordinary sounds before the tenth day. By the fourth week he is likely to react to the voice of his mother or nurse more frequently than to a loud noise.

Taste

The infant's sense of taste is more highly developed than that of sight or hearing. He accepts sweet fluids and resists acid, sour or bitter ones.

Smell

The only evidence of the sense of smell is that many infants appear to smell breast milk and reach for the nipple. There is a wide difference among infants in their apparent ability to smell.

Skin Sensations

Sensations of touch, pressure, temperature and pain are present soon after birth, and at the end of ten days the infant reacts violently to cutaneous irritation.

Organic Sensations

The infant appears to be highly sensitive to organic stimulation, since hunger and thirst are the most common causes of crying. The newborn and the very young infant are not likely to have pain from gas in the intestines, but the infant of a few weeks appears to suffer intensely if his feeding produces colic.

SLEEP

Sleep in the newborn can hardly be distinguished from tranquil rest. The neonate sleeps from fifteen to twenty hours of the day. Short waking periods occur every two hours, but are fewer and shorter during the night, probably because there are fewer external stimuli to arouse him. He is awakened by internal discomfort such as hunger or pain. Hunger is by far the most common cause of an infant's waking before his physiologic need for sleep has been satisfied. As he grows older the length of unbroken periods of sleep and also of wakefulness increases.

IMMUNITY

Antibodies for certain infectious diseases pass through the placenta from mother to infant. Among these antibodies are those of smallpox, mumps, diphtheria and measles if the mother is immune to these diseases. This passive immunity lasts from a few weeks to several months. Little immunity is passed on for chickenpox or pertussis, and young infants may contract these diseases. It is not feasible to immunize very young infants, since they are not sufficiently mature to form antibodies successfully.

If an infant does contract a contagious disease, it is likely to be more severe and to be followed by more complications than in an older child.

TEACHING AIDS AND OTHER INFORMATION*

Public Affairs Pamphlets

Gould, J.: Will My Baby Be Born Normal?

Ross Laboratories

The Phenomena of Early Development, 1962.
Fetal Hemoglobin: Report of the Fifty-Second Ross Conference on Pediatric Research, 1966.

REFERENCES

Publications

Arey, L. B.: *Developmental Anatomy.* 7th ed. Philadelphia, W. B. Saunders Company, 1965.
Avery, M. E.: *The Lung and Its Disorders in the Newborn Infant.* 2nd ed. Philadelphia, W. B. Saunders Company, 1968
Balinsky, B. I.: *An Introduction to Embryology.* 2nd ed Philadelphia, W. B. Saunders Company, 1965.
Barnes, A. C.: *Intra-uterine Development.* Philadelphia, Lea & Febiger, 1967.
Barness, L. A.: *Manual of Pediatric Physical Diagnosis.* 3rd ed. Chicago, Year Book Medical Publishers, Inc., 1966.
Bookmiller, M. M., Bowen, G. L., and Carpenter, D.: *Textbook of Obstetrics and Obstetric Nursing.* 5th ed. Philadelphia, W. B. Saunders Company, 1967.
Cassels, D. E. (Ed): *The Heart and Circulation in the Newborn and Infant.* New York, Grune & Stratton, Inc., 1966.
Craig, W. S.: *Care of the Newly Born Infant.* 3rd ed. Baltimore, Williams & Wilkins Company, 1966.
Davis, M. E., and Rubin, R.: *DeLee's Obstetrics for Nurses.* 18th ed. Philadelphia, W. B. Saunders Company, 1966.
Dawes, G. S.: *Foetal and Neonatal Physiology.* Chicago, Yearbook Medical Publishers, Inc., 1968.
Hurlock, E. B.: *Child Development.* 4th ed New York, McGraw-Hill Book Company, Inc., 1964.
Koop, C. E.: *Emergency Surgery of the Newborn* Clinical Symposia. Ciba Pharmaceutical Products, Inc., Summit, New Jersey, 11:35, 1959.
Williams, P. L., Wendell-Smith, C. P., and Treadgold, S.: *Basic Human Embryology.* Philadelphia, J. B. Lippincott Company, 1966.
World Health Organization, Technical Report Series No. 300: *The Effects of Labour on the Foetus and the Newborn.* Report of a World Health Organization Scientific Group. Geneva, World Health Organization, 1965

Periodicals

Adams, M. M.: Appraisal of the Newborn Infant *Am. J. Nursing,* 55:1336, 1955.
Arnold, H. W., and others: The Newborn: Transition to Extra-Uterine Life. *Am. J. Nursing,* 65:77, October 1965.
Fleming, J. W.: Recognizing the Newborn Addict. *Am. J. Nursing,* 65:83, January 1965.
Hervada, A. R.: Nursery Evaluation of the Newborn *Am. J. Nursing,* 67:1669, 1967.
Klein, D. R.: Prominent Ears in Children. *GP,* 36:126, August 1967.
Mattingly, R. F., and Larks, S. D.: The Fetal Electrocardiogram, *J.A.M.A.,* 183:245, 1963.
Richards, I. D. G., and Roberts, C. J.: The "At Risk" Infant *Lancet,* 2:711, September 30, 1967.
Saling, E., and Bretscher, J.: p^{H} Values of the Human Fetus During Labor. *Am. J. Obst. & Gynec.,* 97:906, 1967.
Wolff, I. S.: When Your Patient Asks: 'Is My Baby Normal?' *RN,* 25:57, April 1962.
Yerushalmy, J.: The Classification of Newborn Infants by Birth Weight and Gestational Age. *J. Pediat.,* 71:164, August 1967.

---

* Complete addresses are given in the Appendix.

CARE OF THE NEWBORN

The family-centered care which the nurse provides for parents and their newborn infants should be based on her understanding of the physical status of the newborn and the emotional reactions of the infant and of his parents to the process of childbirth. The preceding chapter presented the physical and physiologic characteristics of the normal newborn. This chapter is concerned with his care immediately after delivery, in the nursery and after discharge from the hospital.

CARE IN THE DELIVERY ROOM

Immediate care of the newborn includes gentleness and prevention of infection, establishment and maintenance of respiration, care of the umbilical cord, care of the eyes, stabilization of his temperature, identification of the infant and maintaining a record of observations on his condition.

In the delivery room the infant is inspected for any gross anomalies such as spina bifida, cleft lip and cleft palate, imperforate anus, hydrocephalus, birthmarks, or for evidence of shock or birth trauma. Many anomalies are not immediately evident on inspection, however, and these are the concern of the physician and the nurse in the nursery.

Within sixty seconds after the infant's body has been completely born, five objective signs should be evaluated. These are shown on the scoring-system chart developed by Dr. Virginia Apgar (see Table 7-1 and Fig. 7-1) and include heart rate, respiratory effort, muscle tone, reflex irritability, and color. Each of these five signs is an index of the infant's depression or lack of it at birth and is given a score of 0, 1 or 2. The infant is in the best possible condition if his score is 10. If he has a score of 5 to 10, he usually needs no treatment. If his score is 4 or below, the infant's condition must be immediately diagnosed and treatment given. Approximately seventy to ninety infants out of every 100 newborns should receive a score of 7 or above one minute after birth.

The physician and the nurse have several responsibilities in the care of the infant immediately after his birth.

Establishment and Maintenance of Respiration

The infant's respirations must be established and maintained. For this it is necessary that he cry lustily periodically. Full expansion of the lungs provides oxygen for the blood, which until birth was supplied through the placental cir-

Table 7–1. Apgar Scoring Chart

SIGN	0	1	2
Heart rate	Absent	Slow (less than 100)	Greater than 100
Respiratory effort	Absent	Weak cry, hypoventilation	Good strong cry
Muscle tone	Limp	Some flexion of extremities	Well flexed
Reflex irritability: skin stimulation to feet	No response	Some motion	Cry
Color	Blue, pale	Body pink, extremities blue	Completely pink

V. Apgar and others: Evaluation of the Newborn Infant—Second Report. *J.A.M.A.*, *168*:1988, 1958.

culation. Removal of this source of oxygen stimulates respiratory movements within the infant's body, movements which took place in a superficial manner even during intrauterine life. Any infant who does not breathe within thirty seconds after birth is in danger of asphyxia. The need for close observation of the infant and for having everything in readiness for his resuscitation is evident.

Some infants need further stimulation than that provided normally through separation from the mother. Failure to cry may be due to several causes, a common one being obstruction of his air passage with mucus. In order to clear these passages the infant may be held by his feet with the head down and the neck curved backward.

In this position the mucus drains out by gravity. Drainage of mucus may also be facilitated by stroking the neck in the direction of the mouth. This is known as milking the trachea. Respirations may be further stimulated by gently rubbing the infant's back or spanking his buttocks or the soles of his feet. The mucus may be gently wiped from his mouth with the nurse's gloved finger.

If these measures fail, it may be necessary to remove mucus by suction. A soft rubber catheter, no 10 or 12 French, may be used with

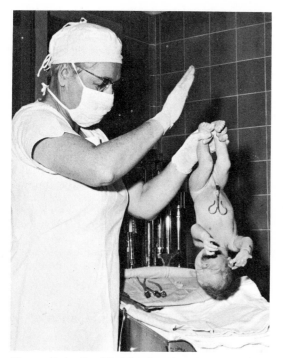

Figure 7–1. Dr. Virginia Apgar, originator of the Apgar score, slaps a baby's feet sharply to determine response to reflex irritability. This normal baby cries lustily. (Courtesy of The National Foundation—March of Dimes.)

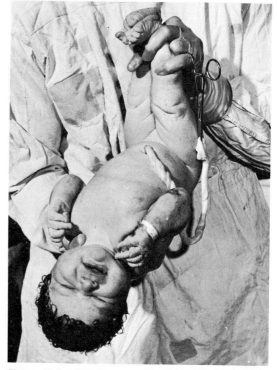

Figure 7–2. Position in which the infant should be held after delivery. If the infant's first breath occurs in the head-up position, respiratory obstruction follows. Note the identification band on the wrist. (From *Resuscitation of the Newborn Infant.* American Academy of Pediatrics.)

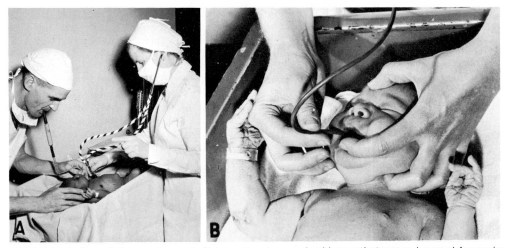

Figure 7–3. Aspiration of the newborn. *A*, DeLee glass trap and rubber catheter may be used for aspiration. Movement of the nurse's finger is the silent method of indicating the heart rate of a newborn. *B*, Method of suctioning the pharynx of a newborn. (From *Resuscitation of the Newborn Infant.* American Academy of Pediatrics.)

a suction appliance, either an electrically powered suction machine or a DeLee mucus trap. (The size of the catheter used may vary, depending on the size of the infant and the procedure adopted by the individual hospital.) When the catheter is in position, gentle suction is made. Suction should not be too vigorous, so as to prevent damage to the mucous membranes. It is important that mucus be removed before the infant draws his first breath in order to prevent him from aspirating it. When as much mucus as possible has been removed, the infant should be placed in the head-down position to induce further drainage unless this is contraindicated.

If the infant does not cry after such resuscitative measures, the physician will clamp the cord, and more drastic means of stimulating the infant to breathe will be used.

After the airway has been cleared, ventilation with oxygen is indicated. If the infant's tongue is lying against the posterior pharyngeal wall, thereby obstructing the airway, a properly placed small pharyngeal airway will correct the obstruction. If the infant still does not breathe adequately, the lungs may be inflated by administering oxygen under controlled intermittent pressure with the use of a snugly fitting mask. Usually pressures of 15 to 20 cm. of water are safe to use. When oxygen is being given, the physician should auscultate the chest to determine whether the gas is entering the lungs.

If the infant's lungs are still not adequately expanded, direct laryngoscopy should be carried out so that any obstructing foreign material can be removed. In some instances positive pressure may be applied by use of a snugly fitting no. 12 French endotracheal tube or by a few short puffs of air at high pressure. In an emergency when no mechanical devices are available, mouth-to-mouth resuscitation using only the air in the operator's mouth may be used. Air forced under too great pressure into the infant's lungs may result in rupture of them. Respiratory stimulants are not used, but a circulatory stimulant may be useful.

Care of the Umbilical Cord

Two clamps are used to compress the cord. They are placed about 2 inches from the abdomen. If possible, this is not done until the cord has stopped pulsating, for the infant will then receive approximately 100 ml. of blood from the placenta, which will provide him with a store of iron and other desirable blood constituents. He will need this iron during the first few months of life when the iron content of his diet tends to be below his needs. But if the mother has been deeply anesthetized, he may evidence signs of depression from passage of the anesthetic or analgesic agent across the placental barrier.

After the cord has been clamped a ligature is tied in a square knot about 1 inch from the abdominal wall. After removal of the clamp the cord should be turned back on itself and tied a second time with the same ligature. Instead of a ligature a clamp which crushes the vessels may be placed on the cord and removed after several hours, or another type of clamp may be left on the cord until it drops off. Some institutions favor the use of a special type of broad rubber band.

There is a difference of opinion as to whether an antiseptic solution and a dressing should be applied to the cord. The custom of the hospital or the physician's order should be followed. Extreme care must be taken that the cord does not become contaminated. The cord is connected with the great blood vessels of the abdomen, through which infection could be carried, with septicemia a likely result.

Care of the Eyes

If the mother has gonorrhea, the infant's eyes may be inoculated with the organism during delivery. If the eyes are not adequately treated at once, ophthalmia neonatorum is likely to develop (see p. 184). A prophylactic treatment against ophthalmia neonatorum is required by legal statute in every state. A germicide must be instilled into the eyes of the newborn shortly after delivery. Silver nitrate has been used for many years. Penicillin, which is a gonococcide, has been used more recently.

If silver nitrate is used, it may be dropped between the eyelids at any time after the head has been delivered until the third stage of labor is completed. The eyelids should be cleansed carefully with a sterile cotton ball moistened with sterile water; wiping should proceed from the nose outward. The lower lid should be pulled down, and 2 drops of a 1 per cent solution of silver nitrate should be instilled into the conjunctival sac. After a minute or two the eyes should be irrigated with warm physiologic salt solution; this washes out the excess silver nitrate and forms a precipitate with the remainder. In about 50 per cent of infants a chemical irritation may result from the silver nitrate. Although within a few hours a profuse discharge may appear in the eyes, there is no permanent ill effect from the treatment and the chemical conjunctivitis.

Penicillin may be administered as a topical application in the form of penicillin ophthalmic ointment or may be given intramuscularly.

Stabilization of Temperature

The temperature of the newborn usually drops immediately after birth, but returns to normal in about eight hours. The temperature in the delivery room is lower than that *in utero*, and this accounts for the drop in the infant's temperature after delivery. To raise his body temperature to normal, he should be wrapped in a warm, sterile cotton flannel blanket immediately after birth.

Identification of the Infant

All infants must be identified in some manner before they are removed from the delivery room.

Several methods are in use, the most common among them being an adhesive label bearing identification information applied to the infant's back, a name bracelet or necklace placed on the wrist or about the neck, identification tapes marked with identification numbers for both the infant and the mother placed about their wrists (see Fig. 7–2), and foot or palm prints of the infant taken while he is still on the delivery table. This last is the most "mistake-proof," but must be carefully done in order to get clear prints. It must be done in conjunction with a form of identification which can be used in caring for the infant.

Baptism

If there is danger of death of the newborn, the majority of Christian parents wish to have their child baptized immediately. This may, of course, take place in the delivery room, but is more likely to be the responsibility of the nurse in the nursery. If the parents are Roman Catholics, a priest should be called if it appears that the infant will live until he arrives. If the parents are Protestant, a minister of their faith should be called. If death is imminent and a priest is not present, the nurse or physician may perform the baptism by pouring water on the infant's forehead while saying, "I baptize you in the name of the Father and of the Son and of the Holy Spirit." The Roman Catholic Church teaches that every fetus and embryo should also be baptized if possible. Conditional baptism can be carried out if it is not certain whether the subject is capable of receiving baptism, by saying, "If you are capable of receiving baptism, I baptize you in the name of the Father and of the Son and of the Holy Spirit." Although it is not essential to repeat the Lord's Prayer or the Apostles' Creed, or both, it is well to do so.

Essentials of Nursing Care

Nursing care is begun in the delivery room immediately after birth and is continued in the nursery or the mother's room if the infant rooms-in with her.

The great need for *gentleness* in caring for the newborn has already been stressed. He has undergone a difficult if not exhausting experience and is now initiating bodily functions for himself which his mother's body performed for him while he was in the uterus. He has been accustomed to his "marine bath," and even the softest fabric is irritating. Being moved about independently is a novel experience after the confinement of the uterus.

Avoidance of infection is imperative. The only

source of infection before birth was through the mother's bloodstream, but now there are many portals of infection. In general his nursing care is that of strict aseptic nursing. Clothing and the linen and blankets for his crib, the gown which the nurse wears, and all equipment used in his care should be surgically clean if not sterile. His bedside equipment is, of course, for his personal use only. The nurse who cares for him should never be on duty if she has a cold, sore throat, loose stools or any septic skin infection. Infection which might be of little consequence in an older child may cause the death of a newborn.

CARE IN THE NURSERY

The newborn, wrapped in a warm receiving blanket, is transferred to the nursery in either a warm crib or the nurse's arms. He is then dressed in a diaper, shirt and gown, and is loosely wrapped in a blanket and placed in a warm crib. If the father has not seen him previously, the infant is shown to him at this time.

One of the newer developments in the care of newborns is to place those born on the same day in a glass-enclosed room. Thus each day a different room is utilized for the new infants. As the newborns are discharged from each room it is cleaned thoroughly. If infection does occur, it is easier to contain in a smaller unit than in a larger nursery area.

General Nursing Procedures

While the newborn remains in the hospital daily care must be provided for him. This is an intermediate step between the care given directly after birth and his care at home. Since many infant deaths occur in the first few days of life, his physical care and the observations made and charted by the nurse are fully as important as those in the first few hours of life.

Only when the nurse is aware of the physical attributes, the physiologic activities and the common functional disorders of the newborn can she appraise the infant put under her care in the nursery. (See Chapter 6 for characteristics and examination of the normal newborn.)

Preliminary Physical Examination

The nurse must observe the infant closely. On his admission or soon after she should appraise his physical status. This appraisal can be accurate only when she knows what is normal and what is abnormal in the newborn. (There is a wide range of individual differences among normal infants.) This knowledge cannot be learned solely in class or from books; it comes only with experience in the care of the newborn. For this reason the student should be particularly careful to query her instructor or supervisor whenever she is in doubt about the significance of variations in an infant's physical state and behavior.

In order for a nurse to apply her knowledge of what is normal to a particular infant, she should know something of his history. She should be congnizant of the mother's age, history of previous and present pregnancies, maternal Rh factor, duration of labor, color of the amniotic fluid and the infant's Apgar score.

The nurse's legal responsibility in the appraisal of the newborn is in part determined by the policy of the agency which employs her and may vary; however, her moral responsibility to provide the best care she can for her patient never varies.

The nurse must remember that the most common signs of infant distress are (1) increased rate or difficulty of respirations, (2) sternal retractions, (3) excessive mucus as when the infant drools or blows bubbles, (4) worried facial expression, (5) cyanosis, (6) abdominal distention or mass, (7) inadequate evacuation of meconium within twenty-four hours after birth, (8) inadequate voiding, (9) vomiting of bile-stained material, (10) unusual jaundice of the skin, and (11) convulsions. It may be that she is responsible for appraisal not only when the infant is brought to the nursery, but also when he is discharged. If so, she should understand the normal maturation which takes place during the first few days of life. She cannot use the same standards of normality for a three-day-old infant that she used during his first hour of extrauterine life.

The role of the professional nurse is being enlarged to include many functions which formerly belonged exclusively to the physician. This is made necessary by (1) the extreme shortage of medical personnel as compared with the increasing demand and (2) the greater competency of the modern professional nurse in assisting the physician by accurate, intelligent observation. Whatever the policy of the hospital, the nurse can best fulfill her responsibility for the infant's complete nursing care by frequent observation of his condition. This is necessary not only for the infant's safety, but also for improvement of her own ability to make discriminating judgments between normal and abnormal states.

In addition to the nurse's appraisal of the infant in order to determine whether problems exist, the nurse may also review parts of the examination with the mother after she is rested so that she will not be worried about characteristics which are normal in the newborn, such as shape of the head or crossed eyes. Such information can prevent or dispel many anxieties which the mother may have.

Continuous Observation

General observation of an infant must be made at frequent intervals during the day and night for evidence of malfunction in vital bodily functions, including respiratory distress.

Respiratory Distress. Respiratory distress is shown by the rate and nature of an infant's respirations, his cry, color and general behavior. If the infant appears to be choking, mucus may be found in the nose or mouth. The air passages may be cleared immediately by placing the infant with his head lower than his body and stroking his neck in the direction of his mouth. If these procedures do not give relief and the physician cannot be reached, the nurse should use an aspirator and provide oxygen if she considers it necessary. To meet such an emergency, equipment for aspiration and oxygen administration should always be kept in the area when newborns are cared for.

Position of the Infant. Because of the possibility of respiratory distress during the first twenty-four hours of life, the foot of the crib or the mattress should be elevated at a 15- to 20-degree angle. The infant should be placed on his side in this head-down position. He should be rotated to the other side every two or three hours.

The infant's bones are soft and molded by pressure. This fact gives us another reason for changing his position frequently, since lying constantly on one side will cause the bones of the skull to be flattened. The shape of the chest is also influenced by the position in which he lies, but seldom to the extent of deformity such as occurs in the skull. Since infants like to face the light and it is essential that they do not lie always upon the same side, the infant's head will be alternately at the "top" or "foot" of the crib.

The newborn should become accustomed to sleeping on his abdomen, but because of the danger of suffocation, he should be placed on his abdomen only when it is possible to watch him closely.

The position in which the infant is held should accord with his level of maturation, particularly that of his neuromuscular system. Even a normal infant cannot hold his head up without support until he is six weeks old. To hold an infant upright in her arms, the nurse should support his head and shoulders with one hand and his buttocks with the other. Her hold upon him should be firm and steady so that he has no fear of loss of support. (Some child psychologists hold that such fear is one of the few fundamental fears of infancy.) An infant enjoys being held, and holding him gives the nurse an opportunity to help him develop a sense of trust in those who care for him.

Temperature. Proper temperature and humidity control must be maintained in the nursery or, if the infant is rooming-in, the mother's room. Room temperature and humidity are important in respiratory considerations, particularly in the newborn infant. During the day the temperature should range from 68 to 76°F., and the humidity from 45 to 55 per cent. The infant's heat-regulating centers are poorly developed, and he reacts quickly to any divergence in temperature of his environment. The air in the room should be fresh, but there must be no drafts. Fresh air usually has sufficient moisture to prevent drying of the mucous membranes of the nose and throat.

The body temperature of the newborn upon admission to the nursery may be subnormal (see p. 100). He should be dressed in dry clothes and external heat applied, if necessary, until his temperature is normal.

If the infant has been delivered in the home, hot-water bottles placed outside the crib covers may be used to provide an accessory heat source.

Since heat perception is poorly developed in the newborn, three precautions in the use of hot-water bottles must be remembered: (1) the temperature of the water must not be over 115°F. (2) The bag must be covered with flannel or a towel and should be checked for leakage before being used. (3) The bag must not be placed upon the infant's chest or abdomen, where its weight might interfere with respiratory movements. Ordinarily three hot-water bottles are used, one under the legs and one on each side of the body. These provide heat for the extremities, where the circulation is poor, without overheating the chest. Hot-water bottles cool quickly and need to be refilled frequently. If three are used, they may be filled in rotation. Electric pads should not be used, for there is always danger of overheating or of shock from faulty connections.

An incubator is the most satisfactory method of applying external heat. The incubator maintains a controlled, uniform temperature. The heat regulator should be set at 80 to 85°F., depending upon the procedure established by the hospital personnel. The infant's temperature must be checked frequently in order that the regulator of the incubator may be adjusted to meet his needs. An infant's temperature responds readily to external heat, and his temperature should be taken every hour until his body heat is established at normal. The average newborn may then be removed from the incubator to his crib, but those who weigh less than average or are debilitated from a difficult delivery may need longer confinement in the incubator.

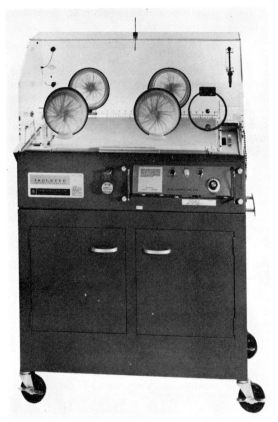

Figure 7–4. Isolette Incubator. The Isolette features an easy-to-clean conditioning chamber, optional humidity and oxygen control, and unequalled isolation through the use of the exclusive microfilter on the outside air adaptor. The infant can be weighed inside the incubator. A "background" air temperature of about 86°F. is maintained by the standard Isolette temperature control. (Courtesy of Air-Shields, Inc., Hatboro, Pennsylvania.)

The amount of clothing and covering an infant needs depends upon the temperature of the room. In general the nursery is kept at a higher temperature than the mother's room, and so the infant who rooms-in will need extra covering. Mothers tend to dress their babies too warmly because they use as their guide the temperature of the infant's hands and feet. Mothers will learn from the nurse that a more accurate way of determining whether an infant is warm or cool is observing the color of his face. If it is flushed, the infant is too warm; if pale or bluish, he is too cool. The mother may feel the arms and legs of the infant, rather than the hands and feet, to check on her observation of the color of his face. She will then have an adequate basis for determining the amount of clothing and covering he needs.

Infants cannot adjust their body temperature to the rapid changes in environmental temperature when they are carried from the nursery through the hall to the mother's room. For this reason they are wrapped in blankets when taken to their mothers.

After the temperature of the newborn has become stabilized it is taken every four hours during the first day and after that twice a day. The temperature may be taken by either the axillary or the rectal method. Each infant should have his own thermometer so as to reduce the possibility of cross-infection in the nursery. If temperatures are routinely taken by rectum, care must be exercised to prevent injury to the rectal mucosa. The thermometer bulb should be examined carefully for imperfections. The infant's legs should be grasped firmly with the nurse's index finger between the ankle bones. The rectal thermometer should be well lubricated and inserted for at least one minute. Some physicians prefer that the infant's temperature be taken by the axillary method. If this is done, the thermometer must be held firmly in the axilla, with the infant's arm pressed against his side, for five minutes or until the mercury stops rising.

Weight. The infant is weighed at birth and each following day at approximately the same time, usually when he is given his morning care. Newborns are usually weighed completely

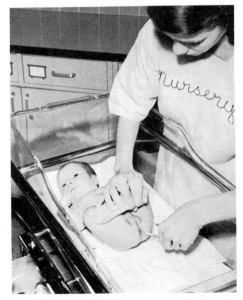

Figure 7–5. The infant's temperature is taken twice a day, rectally. If the infant has a fever, the temperature should be taken every 4 hours. When taking the temperature, the nurse should place her index finger between the infant's ankles and hold the thermometer securely in place. (Davis and Rubin: *DeLee's Obstetrics for Nurses.* 17th ed.)

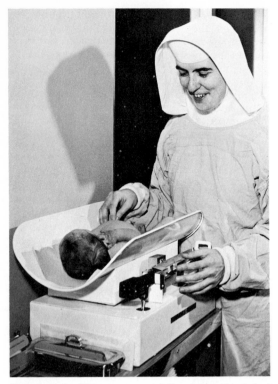

Figure 7-6. The nurse carefully places the infant onto the scoop basket of the scale, which is covered with sterile impervious paper. While weighing the infant, she keeps her hand over the infant's body to protect him from falling. (Fitzgerald Mercy Hospital, Darby, Pa.)

nude in a warm nursery. A fresh sheet of paper or a diaper should be balanced on the scale before he is placed upon it.

If the infant is immature or not in good health or the nursery is not sufficiently warm, he may be weighed, dressed and wrapped in his blanket. Then, when he is undressed for morning care, these articles are weighed and their weight is subtracted from the combined weight of the infant, his clothes and his blanket.

Certain types of incubators contain all necessary equipment, including scales. An infant can then be cared for and weighed without removing him to a cooler atmosphere.

The infant's weight is compared each day with that of the day before. If he loses more than the usual physiologic loss during the first few days or if, after a week, he shows little or no gain in weight, the physician's attention should be called to the weight chart.

Specific Nursing Care

The care of the newborn varies in different hospitals to such an extent that a review of

all the methods used would result in confusion in the mind of the student.

Care of the Skin

Thorough cleansing of the body immediately after delivery is not done, for the vernix caseosa is believed to have a beneficial effect upon the tender skin. The vernix is dissipated in a few days.

The majority of pediatricians accept the theory that the less the skin is handled and abraded by even gentle friction, the better is its condition. Even under this regimen skin irritation may occur in some infants.

The following method is in accordance with modern concepts of child care.

1. Soon after birth the blood on the face and scalp is washed away with a very soft cloth or cotton balls and water.
2. No attempt is made to remove the vernix caseosa, which adheres to the skin and has a protective value. It has been likened to vanishing cream in its softening effect upon the infant's peeling skin.
3. The infant should not be exposed, since he would become chilled. While the nurse is wiping off the amniotic fluid and blood he should be covered with his blanket. The nurse exposes only that part of his body which she is wiping at the moment. In this way his entire body is not uncovered at any time. He is then dressed in a diaper and shirt and loosely wrapped in a fresh blanket.
4. During the first day the vernix caseosa rubs into the skin or comes off on the infant's clothing. On the second day any remnant adhering in the creases of the body may be wiped off with a soft cloth or cotton balls.

Daily Morning Care. The following technique for bathing the infant in the nursery is based on generally accepted principles and is used in many hospitals.

1. His condition is observed at bath time, since he is nude. In bathing him, special attention is given to the condition of the skin, eyes, nose, ears, mouth, umbilicus and genitalia. The bath is a time when the infant is free of restraint from diaper or clothing, and his spontaneous movements may be observed better then than at any other time. Any unusual condition or abnormal movements should be reported.
2. The infant may be washed with a soft cloth or absorbent cotton and clear water. No soap or oil should be used. Recent research has shown that bathing of newborns with hexachlorophene is safe and has value in preventing staphylococcal disease during the first month of life. (This procedure alone, however, will not prevent all infections occurring in the nursery.) A soft dry cloth should be used to dry his face and body and, if cotton was used, to prevent wisps of cotton from clinging to the skin or body orifices.
3. The outer layer of skin normally peels off in minute grainy particles or in fairly large flakes. These areas may be bathed with clear water and dried and have oil applied to them. Cracks in the skin around the wrists and ankles should be cleansed and oiled. It is

often difficult for a mother to believe that these lesions are normal and of no significance. Fortunately they improve readily under proper treatment.

4. Care of the buttocks and genitalia is extremely important. The area should be washed with warm water. In the male infant special attention should be given to the areas of skin contact about the scrotum and the penis. In some institutions a bland soap is used if it is difficult to remove the stool with clear water. There is a difference of opinion as to whether oil should be used on the buttocks. Some physicians believe that its use increases the danger of infection, while others order it to be applied routinely.

5. Talcum powder is usually contraindicated. Some mothers, however, believe that it prevents chafing. Its use, then, with the infant who rooms-in with his mother depends upon her insistence on its value and the policy of the hospital. The harm it may cause to the skin is slight. There is some danger that the mother may shake the can too vigorously and that some of the fine powder particles may drift so that the infant can inhale them. Even the better powders on the market may be irritating to the infant's delicate respiratory tract. Powder accumulated in the folds of skin may become saturated with body secretions. If powder is used with oil, it forms a paste which is likely to retain urine, feces or bodily secretions and prove irritating. Zinc stearate powders should never be used because of their intensely irritating effect upon the respiratory tract. Powders made for infants do not contain zinc stearate, but the ordinary commercial powders may. Powder containing boric acid should never be used because of its poisonous effect on human beings.

6. Other procedures included in the daily morning care are taking the infant's temperature, weighing him, changing the covering on the umbilical cord if one is used or cleaning around the cord stump (see p. 123), changing the sheets and pads of his bed, and cutting his fingernails and toenails if they extend beyond the ends of the fingers and toes. The nails should be cut square, the corners slightly rounded, so that the infant cannot scratch himself.

Skin Irritations. In spite of good care, skin irritations are prone to develop in some infants.

Probably the most common skin irritation after the neonatal period is *miliaria* (prickly heat). It is caused by a superficial bacterial action after excessive sweating during hot weather or fever. The signs are small erythematous papules and vesicles which cause itching. The treatment is cleanliness, washing with warm water and a mild soap, rinsing with clear water and drying thoroughly. Soothing lotions may be used, of which calamine lotion is the most common. It dries the skin as powder does and stays on the irritated area without caking. In general, miliaria is a sign that the infant has been too warmly dressed. Even in hot weather it is not likely to occur in areas freely exposed to the air.

Intertrigo, or chafing, is most often seen in infants with very sensitive skins. It occurs where two surfaces of skin are in contact — behind the ears, in the creases in the neck, axillae and groin and, in the male, under the scrotum — and is particularly likely to occur where there is

moisture from sweat, urine, feces or milk which has dripped into a fold of skin. The condition is also caused by friction, although this is seldom the case in the newborn, whose clothing is soft and whose physical activity is limited.

The manifestations of intertrigo are raw, red, moist areas in the skin folds. The lesions do not itch, and they do not heal by forming a crust or scab. Instead, the area becomes dry and gradually assumes its normal texture and appearance. Prevention lies in cleanliness, particularly in the folds of the skin, and in keeping the skin dry and free from contact with organisms which could cause the area to become infected. The areas may need to be cleansed several times a day if they are soiled or sticky with secretions.

The nurse is not likely to see intertrigo in an infant born in the hospital, but rather in those brought into the hospital by mothers delivered at home and sent to the hospital after a few days because of some complication which required hospital care.

There may be *abrasions* on the heels, knees, toes and elbows from rubbing against the crib linens. These seldom occur in the healthy, well cared for newborn, but are frequent in a neglected, undernourished infant who lies crying and engages in aimless crawling or kicking movements. Such an infant may be brought to the hospital for some illness. The irritated areas should be bandaged lightly and kept scrupulously clean.

Diaper rash is caused by irritation from urine and stool. It is seldom seen in the breast-fed infant, but is common in the infant on a formula. If the stool is irritating and the diaper is not changed immediately, the buttocks may become red, and then shiny and raw. The lesions smart when the infant urinates and are a frequent cause of crying among infants not receiving sufficient care. Treatment consists in exposure of the area to warmth and air by placing a diaper under the infant and laying him on his abdomen with his shirt folded up above the buttocks. The diaper should be changed, of course, whenever it is soiled.

If possible, the area should be exposed to sunlight, but if this cannot be done, the buttocks may be exposed to the warmth of an electric light bulb (25 to 40 watts) placed in a goosenecked lamp. The lamp stands by the crib, and the neck is bent so that the bulb is perhaps 12 to 16 inches from the infant's body. Ointment should not be put upon the skin at the same time the light is used. If the area is raw, the bulb should be farther from the buttocks, for excessive heat will be painful and may cause injury. Great care should be taken that the lamp is secure and the bed clothing in no danger of touching the bulb.

When exposure to sunlight or the use of a lamp

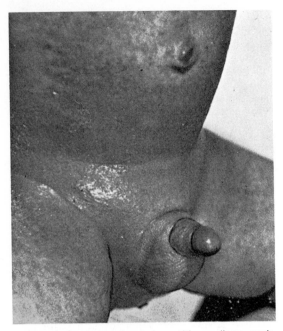

Figure 7–7. Ammoniacal dermatitis or diaper rash. (Courtesy of Dr. Ralph V. Platou and the American Academy of Pediatrics.)

is not practicable or is insufficient therapy, a soothing ointment such as zinc oxide, A and D ointment or methylbenzethonium chloride (Diaparene) will aid the healing process. Diaparene contains a germicide inimical to harmful bacteria which decompose urine in the diaper area and cause irritation.

Diapers which have been improperly washed and rinsed may cause a rash. If diapers are to be washed at home, they should be soaked in cold water, then washed with a mild soap, rinsed thoroughly and, if possible, dried in the sun. One crushed tablet of Diaparene in 2 quarts of water makes an excellent antiseptic terminal rinse for six diapers. This should be poured over the diapers after they have been washed and rinsed. They should soak for a few minutes and then be dried. Commercial laundries do excellent work, and many hospitals as well as private families are using their services.

Cleanliness is the main factor in the prevention of diaper rash. Plastic pants are seldom put on infants, but, when used, may predispose to diaper rash because the diaper is likely not to be changed often enough.

Care of the Eyes, Nose, Ears and Mouth

Care should be given only as necessary to the infant's eyes. Any secretions that have accumulated in the corners should be washed out with a soft washcloth and clear water,

stroking from the inner canthus outward. The eyes should not be irrigated even if there is a discharge unless the physician orders irrigation. If irrigation is prescribed, physiologic salt solution should be used. Boric acid should not be used, since it is harmful when taken internally. Since boric acid solutions are both odorless and colorless, they may be mistaken for water.

Because any severe discharge from the eyes may be evidence of a serious infection, the physician will probably order warm saline irrigations and isolation precautions and send specimens of the discharge to the laboratory for culture. He may prescribe antibiotic drugs or ointment to counteract the infection.

The infant's nose and ears may be cleansed externally by using a twisted cotton cone moistened in water. All excess water should be squeezed out, since it annoys the infant if it drips upon his face. Oil should never be used because of the danger of aspiration with resulting harm to the respiratory tract. No attempt should be made to cleanse the nose or ears internally. Toothpicks or wooden applicator sticks covered with cotton should not be used because of the danger of injury from deep penetration if the infant moves unexpectedly. There is also the risk that the cotton may become loose and lodge in the nose or ear; it will then be necessary for the physician to remove the cotton with instruments.

The mouth should not be cleansed except by offering sterile water between feedings. There is danger of injuring the tissues and thus predisposing to infection.

Care of the Genitalia

The Vulva. The vulva should be cleansed gently with a bland soap and warm water. Some of the vernix caseosa may be removed each day at bath time and when the buttocks are cleansed after passage of a stool. Mothers should be instructed *to cleanse the vulva from the urethra toward the anus,* using a different section of the washcloth with each stroke. With this method there is less likelihood that the urethra will become contaminated with fecal organisms, thereby minimizing the possibility of cystitis due to infection traveling up the urethra to the bladder.

The Penis. In cleansing the penis the foreskin should be retracted, when possible, each day if the infant has not been circumcised. Irritation will result if smegma, a malodorous cheeselike substance, and bacteria are not removed from beneath the foreskin. The cleansing process should be done very gently, and the foreskin should be retracted only as far as it will go without pressure. It must be returned to its normal position immediately afterward to prevent painful paraphimosis due to constriction and edema.

If the foreskin is adherent to the glans during the neonatal period, the physician may postpone retraction. Nevertheless the mother should be taught the procedure so that later, in cleansing the penis, she will be familiar with the technique.

PHIMOSIS. In this condition the foreskin is so tightly hooded over the tip of the glans that it impedes the discharge of urine and predisposes to irritation. The treatment is by circumcision — surgical removal of the foreskin. The operation is performed to prevent infection, to facilitate the discharge of urine and to make the area easier to clean. A written order for the operation must be obtained. The operation is generally done on the first day of life before physiologic hypoprothrombinemia occurs, or on the sixth to the eighth day, at which time the infant has recovered from physiologic hypoprothrombinemia and the bleeding and coagulation times are usually within normal limits.

Although circumcision is a minor operation, the infant needs care after it. The nurse must watch for bleeding. A soothing ointment may be applied to the raw area after the diaper has been changed (some physicians prefer that no diaper be used). Such care should continue until the area is healed.

Care of the Umbilical Cord

During the first twenty-four hours after the infant's admission to the nursery the cord must be observed closely for bleeding. Sometimes the cord contains an excessive amount of Wharton's jelly. When this shrinks, as part of the normal process, a ligature or clamp which was tight becomes loosened, and there is danger of hemorrhage. Normally a clot forms at the end of the cord stump and may prevent bleeding even if the ligature or clamp is loose. But if the clot if dislodged through manipulation, bleeding will occur. To prevent further loss of blood the nurse should apply a sterile hemostatic forceps as far from the abdominal wall as possible. The physician or nurse can then apply another clamp or ligature to the cord, closer to the abdominal wall.

The cord may heal in one of two ways: by dry or moist gangrene. Dry healing is preferred because a dry area is a poor medium for the growth of bacteria. Normally, the umbilical wound is completely healed in a week.

The umbilical area may be cleansed each day with 60 to 70 per cent alcohol, which has a drying effect and promotes antisepsis. Other solutions may be used, depending on the procedure adopted by the hospital personnel. If a cord dressing is used, it should be changed promptly when soiled. If infection develops around the umbilicus, as shown by redness in the area, malodor, or moisture or discharge from the cord, the physician should be notified at once. Treatment of such infection usually consists in frequent applications of an alcohol dressing and an antibiotic applied locally or given systemically, or both.

Inanition or Dehydration Fever

Between the second and fourth days of life the infant may have fever as a result of his low fluid intake with normal fluid loss. His temperature may rise to 102 to 104°F. (38.9 to 40°C.). His skin becomes dry, urine output is decreased, and his face and body show that he has undergone a sudden loss in weight. Treatment consists in increasing the amount of fluid taken, giving water between milk feedings, or in administration of parenteral fluids.

Prevention of Infection

The newborn has little resistance to disease. For this reason all nurses caring for the newborn must understand the importance of aseptic technique. Probably the fundamental rule to be followed by parents and hospital personnel is that they wash their hands thoroughly before handling the infant. In the nursery this is done on entering the room. Antiseptic detergents are better for this purpose than toilet soap, and the hands should be washed under running water. No rings or wrist watch should be worn, since either may be the site of lodgment of bacteria. Even nail polish is forbidden, for it too may be a source of transmission of infection. It is possible for an infant to be orally infected with organisms from his own stool. For this reason the nurse should wash her hands thoroughly after changing his diaper and before feeding him.

In some nurseries all personnel routinely wear masks. Their value is questionable, however. If they are not changed frequently or if they become soiled when adjusted, they are a source of contamination rather than of protection to the infant.

No one who has symptoms of a respiratory, intestinal or skin infection should enter the nursery or rooms where infants are with their mothers; such persons absolutely should have no contact, direct or indirect, with the infants. If the mother acquires an infection, her infant should not be taken to her; if he rooms-in, he should be isolated from her. If she has been in contact with the infant, he should be isolated not only from her, but also from the other infants in the nursery so that he may not be a source of transmission if he has contracted his mother's disease.

Infection is far more likely to be carried by direct contact with an infected person than by indirect contact through contaminated equipment. Nevertheless contaminated equipment is definitely a source of infection. Each infant should have his own personal articles for his bath and other care. These may be kept in his stand or in a drawer underneath the bassinet and taken with him to his mother's room if he is to room-in with her.

An infant in the nursery who shows signs of infection should be isolated at once. The other infants must be closely observed for symptoms of the specific infection which he has contracted. Symptoms of the most common infections are refusal of feedings, frequent loose stools, elevation of temperature, drainage from the umbilicus, and discharges from the eyes or nose. Respiratory infections are first evidenced by a running nose and a rise in temperature. Skin lesions are easily observed when the infant is undressed for morning care or when the diaper is changed.

Records and Birth Registration

The nurse caring for an infant in the nursery is responsible for all notations on his permanent record. When the infant rooms-in, the mother tells the nurse of the care she has given him and her observations on his condition and behavior. This the nurse charts.

In addition to the permanent records, some nurseries have *daily record sheets* which are not permanent records. These are composite tally sheets used for the total nursery population. The auxiliary personnel as well as the nurses record on these sheets the care they have given the infants and their observations, such as morning care, feedings, stool passages and urination. The nurse copies from these temporary daily sheets the notations about each infant onto his individual chart. In some instances she summarizes the information, e.g. the number of stools during the day and the total amount of feeding taken. Important notations commonly included in the nurse's notes on individual permanent records include the following:

The infant's name, day of life, birth weight and daily weight
Observations on his condition: his cry, respirations, temperature, the condition of the cord, mouth, eyes, skin, frequency and nature of stools and urine
The time of feedings and the amount taken and retained; frequency and volume of regurgitation
Medication and treatments given
Execution of all physician's orders, such as administration of oxygen, irrigations, and the like.

The physician, midwife, nurse or attendant who delivers the infant is responsible for the birth registration with the local registrar.

The information necessary for the birth certificate includes the child's name, date and place of birth, names of each of the parents, and other data of local option. This information should be accurate and easily read, since it is filed permanently with the state Bureau of Vital Statistics. Some form of notification of the registration is sent to the parents, who should keep it as proof that the infant's birth has been registered. Proof of birth registration may be important in later life to determine whether a child is of school age, whether a youth is of legal age for employment or voting, or whether a person is old enough for Social Security benefits, and so on.

FEEDING THE NEWBORN INFANT

The infant may be hungry immediately after birth or may show no signs of needing food for the first or even the second day. The nurse should be able to recognize the signs of hunger in the newborn. He becomes restless, cries, moves his head in search of food (the rooting reflex) and makes sucking movements which, bringing no relief, are likely to end in crying.

Usually he goes to sleep for several hours after being fed, wakening when he again needs food or is uncomfortable. The most common causes of crying in a healthy infant are hunger and discomfort from a soiled diaper.

In addition to her responsibility for caring for the infant, the nurse has the responsibility of supporting the mother in her decision as to how to feed her child. This decision may have been made before or after the birth of the infant. Although the nurse should be able to provide information which the mother may request, she should not encourage the mother strongly to feed the infant by either breast or bottle on a rigid schedule or on a self-demand schedule. If she does, she may arouse guilt feelings in the mother if the mother does not or cannot cooperate. For instance, a mother, because the nurse encouraged her to breast-feed her infant on a self-demand routine, tried to do so in order to follow orders. The mother failed in her attempts and felt guilty about her inability to be a "good" mother. Perhaps another mother might have refused to cooperate with the nurse, leading that mother to feel guilty also. The nurse should realize that the bodily contact a mother has with her child in whatever feeding process is used is ultimately of greater importance than the method of feeding used.

Self-Demand Feeding

The infant on a self-demand or self-regulating schedule nurses when he wants food. Then he sleeps until the contractions of an empty stomach waken him. He cries, but when the formula is given him, the muscular contractions cease, and he experiences a pleasant sensation of fullness. If he is fed whenever he is hungry, he will develop a good appetite. Whether he is breast-fed or bottle-fed, he will establish his own rhythm of feeding.

If an infant is on a self-demand feeding schedule, it is particularly necessary for the nurse to recognize signs of hunger in order to satisfy his demand for food, rather than use the bottle to pacify him whenever he cries.

Breast Feeding

Probably the psychologic and emotional factors are more important than the physical factors in helping a mother decide to breast-feed her infant, since satisfactory artificial feedings can be easily obtained.

Some physicians believe that the infant should be put to the breast as soon after delivery as the condition of the mother and of her infant permits. They believe that this early suckling assists in the involution of the uterus, stimulates lactation and also provides emotional satisfaction for both mother and child. Other physicians believe that nursing should be postponed until four to twenty-four hours after birth. This would allow time for the infant's throat to be cleared of mucus and for the infant to sleep after the exertion of birth and of being handled by physicians and nurses in the necessary care after birth. This interval also permits the mother to rest before giving her infant the breast. This first feeding is difficult, for he must learn to take hold of the nipple and to suck.

The typical breast-fed infant is contented, and active in a happy, playful way. After his initial weight loss he should gain from 6 to 8 ounces a week.

If he is underfed, he is likely to be constipated. He may have colic, may vomit, may be irritable and alternate crying with sucking his fingers. Vomiting and colic are also characteristic of the overfed infant. In general, however, the breast-fed infant shows a steady gain in weight and is less prone to intestinal upsets than the infant on an artificial feeding plan.

Advantages to the Mother. The mother as well as the infant benefits from breast feeding. The infant's sucking at the breast promotes involution of the uterus after parturition. Many mothers find great emotional satisfaction in feeding the infant at the breast, for it is the culmination of the symbiotic unity which existed during the infant's intrauterine life. The fact that breast feeding saves time and trouble appeals to some women.

Objections and Contraindications to Breast Feeding. For some women the advantages of breast feeding may be outweighed by other factors. The mother may have conscious or unconscious attitudes toward breast feeding which interfere with her ability to produce milk. She may have negative attitudes resulting from her own upbringing. These may cause her to have an aversion to nursing and the maternal role. Furthermore, her professional education, her outside employment and the rapid pace of present-day society frequently interfere with her ability to relax and make her impatient over the uncertainty of nursing her baby. If the mother works outside the home or has many social engagements, it may be impossible for her to be at home promptly at feeding time, provoking infant distress and discomfort from engorged breasts. In order to provide greater freedom for the mother, to give the father an opportunity to feed the infant and to accustom the infant to a different kind of feeding, an artificial formula may be substituted periodically for a breast feeding.

Another objection which some mothers have to breast feeding is that it ruins the firm contour of their breasts and so makes them look older than they are.

The great contraindication to nursing is *serious illness of the mother.* If she has tuberculosis, her condition may be aggravated by lactation, and her infant would be in grave danger of contracting the disease through intimate contact. A mother may lack the vitality to nurse her infant, owing to some serious complication which developed during pregnancy. For instance, she may be anemic after excessive loss of blood. She may have a chronic disease, e.g. cancer, heart disease or impairment of the kidneys, which is not infectious, but which prevents her undergoing the strain of lactation. Her labor and delivery may have been complicated by an intercurrent illness or emergency operation which requires prolonged convalescence.

If her condition permits breast feeding in the presence of intercurrent infection, her milk may be expressed, boiled and given to the infant. Thus the milk supply will be maintained until she is able to give the infant her breast.

The milk from a *mother addicted to drugs,* e.g. morphine, heroin or codeine, will contain small amounts of the drug. The amount the infant receives may not be enough to hurt him, but it may prove habituating. Penicillin may be passed to an infant through breast milk and produce allergic sensitization.

Menstruation is not a contraindication to breast feeding unless the mother's nutrition is disturbed. *Pregnancy* is a contraindication to breast feeding only because of the strain upon the mother.

Mental illness is not in itself a contraindication to nursing, although grave danger is involved when a small infant is entrusted to a mentally disturbed patient. Since her milk is normal in amount and composition, it may be expressed and given to her child if the procedure does not disturb or aggravate the mother and if there is a probability that her condition will improve to the extent that the infant may safely be put to the breast at some future time.

Local lesions such as cracked nipples, tumors or breast abscess may contraindicate breast feeding. The milk may be manually expressed to relieve the mother's discomfort from engorgement and to maintain breast function so that she can nurse her infant if the local condition is cured. If the milk is not contaminated, it can be given to the infant.

Some mothers have so-called *inverted nipples;* i.e. the nipples do not stand out so that the infant can grasp them with his mouth. A breast shield will help the infant to attain suction and secure the milk, or the milk may be extracted with a breast pump and prepared as a bottle feeding. If a shield is used, a small amount of colostrum or milk may be expressed into it before it is applied, or it may be partially filled with sterile water.

The *infant's condition* may contraindicate breast feeding. He may be too weak to suck, or sucking may exhaust his strength. The premature infant may not only be too weak to suck, but also may lack the necessary reflexes. The infant with a cleft palate or cleft lip is unable to suck, as is the infant with facial nerve paralysis. For such infants the breast milk may be manually expressed and given by medicine dropper.

Erythroblastosis fetalis is not a contraindication to breast feeding, since Rh antibodies in the mother's milk are inactivated in the infant's intestinal tract.

Maternal Personality and Breast Feeding. Studies show that there is a difference between women who want to nurse their infants and those who do not. The desire to breast-feed their infants is common among women who obtain satisfaction in fulfilling the feminine role. They do not feel that childbirth is an ordeal to be feared and consider that wives may lead domestic lives as rewarding as their working husbands. Wanting to breast-feed an infant appears to be closely related to motherly attitudes. Such women are likely to be successful with breast feeding and to be rewarded by the health and vitality of their offspring. Voluntary breast feeding increases their feeling of competency in child care. They are less likely to worry about the child than the mother who has reluctantly consented to breast-feed her infant and lives in fear that her milk supply will not be sufficient to meet his nutritional needs.

Advantages to the Infant. There are many reasons why physicians hold breast feeding to be superior to even an adequate formula properly prepared and given with loving care. The most important arguments for breast feeding from the point of view of the infant's health are as follows:

Breast milk is more easily digested than cow's milk and is designed by nature to satisfy the needs of the human infant just as cow's milk meets the needs of the calf.

Breast milk is available at all times. This fact is important if the infant is to be on a self-demand schedule. Breast feeding can be used to comfort an infant, although this should not be done to excess.

Breast-fed infants have greater immunity to certain childhood diseases. Certain antibacterial and antiviral substances are believed to be transmitted in the milk which increase the infant's resistance to infectious diseases. The extent of this protection has not been proved.

Breast-fed infants are less likely to have gastrointestinal disorders and food allergies in infancy.

Breast-fed infants are less likely to suffer from colds and severe respiratory infections.

Breast-fed infants are less likely to acquire infections in homes where cleanliness is difficult to attain. This is because breast milk is sterile, and the mother's nipples are easily cleaned.

Breast-fed infants enjoy the watchfulness and close contact with their mothers' bodies and can take as much or as little milk as they desire. They can regulate the rapidity of the intake and can never be forced to take more than they want.

Breast-fed infants are less prone to anemia or vitamin deficiency.

Factors in the Supply of Breast Milk. The majority of women who have been delivered of a healthy full-term infant and are themselves in good health are capable of breastfeeding their infants.

Physical factors in the supply of breast milk include (a) an ample diet with an increased protein intake and a sufficient supply of calcium from milk and other sources.

(b) The mother requires an ample supply of vitamins, especially vitamin D, for her needs and also for the baby, since he receives vitamins through her milk.

(c) Her fluid intake should be adequate for her needs, and should supply 16 to 32 ounces of milk for the infant.

(d) The stimulus of the infant's sucking. If the infant does not fully empty the breasts, the remaining milk should be manually expressed (see p. 129).

(e) She needs normal exercise. Housework, if it is not too exhausting, is excellent, but she should also have exercise out of doors every day.

(f) The nursing mother should avoid fatigue. She should have from eight to ten hours of sleep at night and a nap during the day. It must be remembered that her rest is broken by the infant's night feeding.

(g) The amount of milk-producing tissue in the breasts affects the supply. Large breasts may contain a great deal of fat or supporting tissue and an inadequate amount of glandular secreting tissue.

(h) Chemical stimulation by the lactogenic hormones cannot be controlled by any known means, but since the hormones are related to pregnancy, they are in general sufficient in amount.

Psychologic factors in the supply of breast milk are extremely important. The mother needs to feel competent in her capacity to supply the feedings day and night in amounts sufficient to satisfy the infant. She needs to feel secure, happy and relaxed in her family life. Naturally she will become emotionally disturbed at times, and the quantity of her milk will be decreased, but the quality remains unchanged; when she has regained her composure, her breasts will again be full. She should be told that the emotional strain of coming home from the hospital and undertaking the care of the infant may produce a state of tension which will diminish the flow of milk, but that the condition is only temporary.

Secretion and Composition of Breast Milk. The secretions of the mammary glands are under the influence of a lactogenic hormone derived from the pituitary gland and are stimulated through the influence of pregnancy.

The delivery of milk from the breasts is embodied in the milk-ejection or "let-down" reflex. The presence of the infant, his sucking or even his crying causes the release of oxytocin from the posterior portion of the pituitary, which in turn causes the contractile tissue around the alveoli to squeeze the milk into the larger ducts and then to the nipples. If the mother is tense, this reflex will be inhibited and milk present in the breast will not be brought to the nipples.

Colostrum is secreted during the first two to four days after delivery. It is yellow, and thin or watery in consistency. It has more protein and minerals and less fat and carbohydrate than breast milk. It is easily digested and has a mild laxative action.

Mature milk appears two to four days after delivery. By the end of the first month, breast milk is constant in composition and remains so. The amount increases as the infant's need for food increases. By the end of the first week 6 to 10 ounces (180 to 300 cc.) a day is the normal amount of milk for a healthy mother to produce; by the end of the first month, 20 ounces (600 cc.), and later, 30 ounces (900 cc.) a day.

Breast milk is slightly bluish and has a relatively high sugar content. In the infant's stomach, breast milk forms a soft, flocculent curd. If the mother is taking an adequate diet, the vitamin content of her milk is sufficient, or nearly so, for the infant. Mothers should be told that if they take drugs, e.g. opiates, alcohol, belladonna or penicillin, a small amount of the drug will be present in the milk.

Table 7-2 shows the relative composition of

Table 7–2. *Comparison of Human Milk with Whole Cow's Milk*

	HUMAN MILK (PER CENT)	WHOLE COW'S MILK (PER CENT)
Water	87.0 – 88.0	83.0 – 88.0
Protein	1.0 – 1.5	3.2 – 4.1
Lactalbumin	0.7 – 0.8	0.5
Casein	0.4 – 0.5	3.0
Sugar (lactose)	6.5 – 7.5	4.5 – 5.0
Fat	3.5 – 4.0 (More olein and less of the volatile fatty acids)	3.5 – 5.2
Minerals	0.15 – 0.25	0.7 – 0.75
Calcium	0.034 – 0.045	0.122 – 0.179
Iron	0.0001	0.00004
Vitamins (per 100 cc.)		
A	60 – 500 I.U.	80 – 220 I.U.*
D	0.4 – 10.0 I.U.	0.3 – 4.4 I.U.*
C	1.2 – 10.8 mg.	0.9 – 1.4 mg.*
Reaction	Alkaline or amphoteric	Acid or amphoteric
Bacteria	None	Present
Digestion		Less rapidly
Emptying of stomach		Less rapidly
Curd	Soft, flocculent	Hard, large
Calories per fluidounce	20	20

Adapted from W. E. Nelson: *Textbook of Pediatrics.* 8th ed.
*Values are for pasteurized milk.

breast milk and cow's milk. Breast milk has more carbohydrate and less protein than cow's milk, has approximately the same amount of fat and is of equal caloric value.

Technique of Breast Feeding

The mother should be told that the supply of breast milk will be well established by the third or fourth day and only in exceptional cases as late as the fourteenth day. During the latent period before an adequate supply of milk is available, the infant loses weight. This is a normal phenomenon and should not cause the mother anxiety. Glucose water may be given to supply the required amount of fluid.

The usual procedure is to put the infant to the breast immediately after birth or from four to twelve hours after delivery. Those physicians who advise waiting give as their reasons that the infant and his mother should be given time to rest after the birth process and that time should be allowed for mucus to be cleared from the infant's throat before he attempts to suck and swallow milk. The time spent in nursing at the breast and the number of feedings are increased after the first day or two.

Healthy, supple nipples are important in making the feeding time comfortable for the mother. Erect nipples favor ease of sucking. If the nipples are flat, an ointment should be applied with a gentle, rolling motion of the fingers from the outer rim of the nipple to the tip. If the nipples are cracked and painful, they may be lubricated with petrolatum jelly, or a protective nipple shield may be used to minimize the trauma of nursing.

The breasts should be cleansed carefully once a day when the mother takes a shower. No other care of the nipples before or after feeding the infant is usually necessary, although this is a point of controversy among physicians.

The mother's clothing should not be too tight over the breasts. If a little milk tends to exude from the nipples, she should be careful to keep the area and her clothing clean and dry.

The mother should wash her hands thoroughly with soap and water before the infant is put to the breast. She should be in a comfortable position, sitting or lying on her side. Her head should be slightly elevated. In presenting the nipple to the infant and while he is sucking she should support the breast tissue away from his nostrils so that he may breathe easily.

The room should be quiet while the infant nurses, and the mother should not be disturbed in any way. A normal newborn has a "rooting" reflex, so that when anything touches his cheek when he is hungry he turns his cheek in that direction. It is important, therefore, that the nurse not put her hand on the infant's opposite cheek

to try to turn his head toward the breast. If she lets the nipple touch the infant's cheek, he will turn in that direction to suck.

Although the infant obtains 85 to 90 per cent of his feeding in the first five to eight minutes of vigorous sucking, he should be allowed to nurse from ten to twenty minutes. He enjoys this, and the added milk he gets is to his advantage. Since sucking stimulates the secretion of milk, he should nurse from both breasts at each feeding. It is important that the infant grasp the whole nipple within his mouth; otherwise he cannot achieve adequate suction and may gulp air, since the tip of the nipple is so small that he does not close his lips closely around it.

If the milk is not sufficient to meet the infant's needs, complementary feedings of modified cow's milk may be given. It is customary to weigh the infant before and after his feedings if there is doubt about the quantity of breast milk. This, however, is likely to make the mother tense and fearful that she cannot supply his needs. Her anxiety reacts on the physical process of lactation and tends to decrease the supply. Many physicians do not favor complementary feedings because if the infant is completely satisfied, he may not be hungry enough to empty the mother's breasts at the next feeding.

It is not as necessary to bubble the breast-fed infant as it is the bottle-fed one. The infant should be held over the shoulder or seated erect in his mother's lap and gently patted or stroked on the back (see Fig. 7-9). Thereby the air he has swallowed will rise to the top of his stomach and be eructated. It may be advisable with some

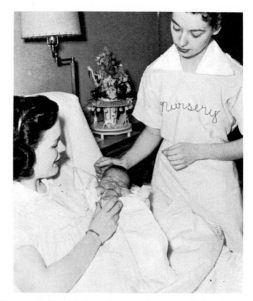

Figure 7–8. Mother learns the art of feeding her baby. (Davis and Rubin: *DeLee's Obstetrics for Nurses.* 17th ed.)

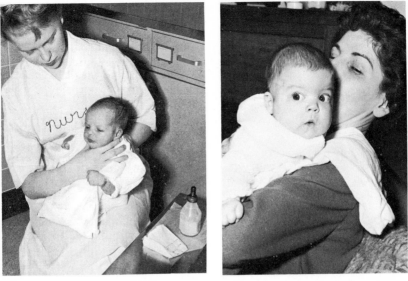

A　　　　　　　　　　　　　　　　　　B

Figure 7–9. Bubbling the baby. *A,* The newborn can be bubbled most satisfactorily in the sitting position while gently leaning over the nurse's arm. This procedure is less likely to contaminate the newborn than if he is held over the shoulder. (Davis and Rubin: *DeLee's Obstetrics for Nurses.* 17th ed.) *B,* The infant can also be bubbled by holding him firmly against the shoulder, supporting his back and head. His back may be patted or rubbed gently in order to help him relax.

infants to do this several times during a feeding and with all infants after the feeding, before laying them in the crib. If the infant's stomach is too full, he may spit up a little milk with each eructation or even after he has been put back in the crib. He may also hiccup. In that case he should be given a little warm water and comforted until the hiccups cease.

Sterile water may be offered between feedings, but it is not necessary for the infant to take it. He should not be urged, for water may interfere with his capacity to finish his next feeding. Giving water is an excellent way to accustom the infant to the rubber nipple so that he will nurse from the bottle in case breast feedings for some reason must be suddenly discontinued. It likewise prepares him to take orange juice in water when the physician orders it.

Infants like to cling to the breast after they have ceased to suck. To remove the infant if he does not voluntarily release the nipple, gentle pressure may be made on his cheeks, or the mother may insert her finger into his mouth. These methods allow air to enter his mouth; suction is then lessened, and he cannot maintain his hold on the nipple. This method is not painful to the mother, nor does it irritate the soft skin covering the nipple.

Rigid feeding schedules are not advisable for the infant. If he is allowed to set his own pace, he will eventually work out a fairly regular demand schedule, and the process is accomplished with little frustration on his or his mother's part.

Manual Expression of Milk. The technique of emptying the breasts when the infant has not done so is as follows:

Grasp the breast with the thumb above and the index finger below the outer edge of the areola. Press the thumb toward the fingers at the base of the nipple with firm, deep pressure. Support the breast with the other fingers. Use a forward stripping movement. Repeat this about thirty times a minute until the breasts are empty; the process usually takes from ten to fifteen minutes. If the milk is to be used for the infant (for instance, if the mother will be away at the next feeding period), it can be kept in a sterile container under refrigeration.

A hand breast pump may be used instead of manual expression. Many mothers find the electric pump superior to the other two methods; however, it is fairly expensive and more likely to be traumatic to the tissues of the breast. It is seldom used in the home.

Wet Nursing and Breast Milk Stations. Wet nurses are rarely used today to provide breast milk for infants other than their own. If they are used, they should have serologic tests and roentgenograms to assure the absence of syphilis and tuberculosis.

Breast milk stations have largely replaced the use of wet nurses in our society. These stations are found in a few of the large cities, but the milk is expensive, and constant supervision of the contributing mothers is necessary to prevent the milk's dilution with cow's milk or water. It is best to have the mothers come to the milk station and express the milk with the electric breast pump.

Breast milk may be pasteurized and kept in sterile containers under refrigeration. It can be frozen and shipped to distant points where it may be thawed and prepared for use as directed by the physician.

Artificial Feeding

Artificial feeding is based on scientific principles of nutrition and sterilization. When breast feeding is not possible and adequate artificial feedings cannot be provided, the morbidity and mortality rates of infants tend to rise.

The following conditions may adversely affect the success of artificial feeding: contaminated cow's milk; a formula not suited to the infant's needs, in either composition or quantity; lack of cleanliness in preparation of the formula and improper refrigeration of the 24-hour supply of feedings; haphazard and irregular feeding; and feeding entrusted to strangers, with implications of lack of interest and affection.

The importance of this last cause is seldom realized and is rather difficult to analyze. An infant becomes accustomed to one person's ways and responds with restlessness on being fed in an unaccustomed way. Some persons believe that the mother responds more quickly to the infant's needs in regulating the flow of milk by tipping the bottle, bubbling him when he needs to expel air, and in general makes the procedure a more personal service adapted to her infant's needs.

In general, for the breast-fed infant the mother-child relation is closer, warmer and more demonstrative of affection. The artificially fed infant, then, may not be likely to feel as contented and secure as the breast-fed infant.

Requirements for Artificial Feeding

Low Bacterial Count of Milk. The fundamental requirement of a satisfactory artificial feeding mixture is that the milk, when taken from the cow, have a low bacterial count. Tuberculosis and undulant fever (brucellosis) can be acquired through milk from infected cows. Dairy herds are screened with the tuberculin test for tuberculosis and the Bang test for brucellosis.

The second requirement is that all milk handlers be free from diseases transmitted through milk, e.g. scarlet fever, streptococcal sore throat, typhoid fever, diphtheria and tuberculosis.

A third requisite is cleanliness in the care of the cows and in the milking process. Most cities require strict inspection of the handling of commercial milk from the dairy to the retail store. The bacterial count and the fat content must conform to certain standards. The milk must be free from preservatives or any injurious substance. It must be pasteurized. Even this clean, pasteurized milk should be pasteurized again or boiled for use in an infant's formula.

Economy and Availability of Milk. In the homes of the low-income group it is necessary that an artificial feeding be inexpensive. This is one reason for the extensive use of sterile evaporated milk. It can be bought in small quantities, and if refrigeration is not available, a small tin can be opened for each feeding. What is not used for the infant can be used by the older children or by adults in their coffee.

Ease of Digestion of Milk. The average infant between four and six months of age can tolerate undiluted cow's milk. For infants under this age the milk is diluted with boiled water. Cow's milk in the infant's stomach forms large, tough curds which can be rendered more digestible by pasteurization, boiling, homogenization, evaporation or the addition of an acid or alkali. In these processes the curd tension is favorably altered.

Nutritional Requirements of Formula for Metabolism and Growth. An *adequate fluid intake* should be 2 to 3 ounces per pound of the expected body weight of the infant, allowance being made for loss of water in urine and stools, by evaporation from the skin and in expired air. The general rule is that a child of one year should take 1000 cc. a day, and an additional 100 cc. should be added for each year of life; e.g. a child of two years should take 1100 cc. of fluid per day.

The protein requirement for growth and for repair of tissue is 1.5 to 2 gm. per pound of body weight. One ounce of cow's milk provides 1 gm. of protein.

The *carbohydrate requirement* in the typical formula for the infant under five months is supplied in the form of Karo or cane sugar. One to $1\frac{1}{2}$ ounces (30 to 45 gm.) is added to the formula. The addition of sugar brings the carbohydrate content of the formula to approximately that of breast milk. For other forms of carbohydrate suitable for use in infant formulas see page 132.

The *caloric requirement* for the infant under three months is approximately 50 calories per pound, and over four months approximately 45 calories per pound, In contrast, the average adult requirement is 20 calories per pound of body weight.

The *basal metabolic needs* are low during the neonatal period. Basal heat production rises rapidly, however, during the first year of life. The caloric requirements for basal metabolic needs are proportionately higher in infancy than at any other time of life. During the neonatal period about 80 calories per kg. of body weight per day are needed to satisfy the infant's nutritional requirements. This amount must be increased rapidly because, although basal metabolic needs do not change, the caloric requirements for growth and energy are much greater in the older infant. Soon a caloric intake of 100 to 130 calories per kg. (45 to 60 calories per pound) of body weight is needed; this requirement remains constant until the age of four months. Caloric needs vary with the infant's activity, his general well-being and his weight gain.

The *fat content* of the formula is not of great importance in the modification of cow's milk and is seldom mentioned in the calculation. Many of the proprietary milks, however, substitute varying proportions of olive, coconut, palm or peanut oil for the butter fat.

Vitamins are usually lacking or in insufficient amount in the artificial feeding. Vitamin A, a fat-soluble vitamin, is needed for growth and for resistance to disease or infection. It, in conjunction with vitamin D, which prevents rickets (see p. 269), is derived from cod liver oil or some form of concentrate. The infant needs approximately 400 International Units of vitamin D each day. Vitamin B complex is needed for optimum health. Vitamin C prevents scurvy (see p. 268). The infant needs 25 to 50 mg. a day. Since vitamin C is easily destroyed in pasteurization of the milk, it must be provided from some other source. Breast-fed infants usually receive a sufficient amount in the mother's milk, though this depends upon her diet. Vitamin C may be supplied by giving the infant 2 ounces of orange juice daily, or ascorbic acid, 25 to 50 mg. a day. One problem that may result from the giving of orange juice is allergy.

In summary, the infant up to six months of age needs approximately 130 to 190 cc. of fluid per kg. (2 to 3 ounces per pound) of body weight per day. The total caloric, protein and fluid needs for the twenty-four hours of the day determine the composition of the formula. The number of feedings decreases as the infant grows older. At one month he will probably be taking five or six feedings. The amount given at each feeding increases as the intervals between feedings lengthen and the infant requires a greater total fluid intake.

Calculation of Formula. The following example may clarify the general statements made about an infant's daily nutritional need and fluid intake.

An infant one month of age weighing 8 pounds requires the following:

Fluid: 2 to 3 ounces per pound of body weight
Total fluid per day: 16 to 24 ounces
Whole cow's milk: $1\frac{1}{2}$ to 2 ounces per pound of body weight. Total amount of milk: 12 to 16 ounces, *or*
Evaporated milk: 1 ounce per pound of body weight
Total amount of milk: 8 ounces

Water: A total of 24 ounces of fluid is required for the formula. Sufficient water is added to the milk to bring the amount of the mixture up to the required 24 ounces: e.g. 16 ounces with evaporated milk, 8 to 12 ounces with whole fresh cow's milk
Calories: 50 calories per pound of body weight
Total caloric requirement: 400 calories per day
Sugar: $\frac{1}{10}$ ounce per pound per day
Volume per feeding: The infant's age in months plus 2 or 3; in this instance, 3 to 4 ounces of formula per feeding
Number of feedings: Total volume of feedings per day (24 ounces) given in 4-ounce feedings results in six feedings per day; given in 3-ounce feedings results in eight feedings per day. During the first six months up to 7 ounces may be given at a feeding. More than 8 ounces is rarely given at a feeding.
Schedule: six feedings (every four hours) of 4 ounces each, or eight feedings (every three hours) of 3 ounces each.

An infant, regardless of his age, is seldom given more than 1 quart of whole milk or one can (13 fluid ounces) of evaporated milk during a 24-hour period because he receives solid food as he needs more nourishment.

Types of Milk and Ingredients for Artificial Feeding

The caloric value of whole cow's milk is 20 calories per ounce.

Certified Milk. This is the purest form of raw milk. It contains less than 10,000 bacteria per cubic centimeter and no pathogens, even before pasteurization. It is produced under special hygienic conditions. All milk containers must be sterilized before use. The personnel who handle the milk must be inspected for evidence of disease which might be transmitted through milk. (Throat cultures are taken, and other tests are made.) Most certified milk sold today is also pasteurized.

Pasteurized Milk. In pasteurization raw milk is heated to 145°F. for thirty minutes. It is then cooled rapidly. In most cities pasteurization of commercial milk is required by law. Pasteurization kills pathogenic organisms, but does not sterilize the milk; it renders harmless *Salmonella typhosa,* tuberculosis bacilli, organisms causing diphtheria and those in the paratyphoid group, and hemolytic streptococci. Pasteurization destroys vitamin C, which is a heat-labile vitamin, and makes the curd in the infant's stomach smaller and softer. Pasteurized milk should be boiled for infant feeding purposes.

Vitamin D-Reinforced Milk. This is whole cow's milk to which has been added vitamin D, which prevents rickets. Milk from cows at pasture contains more vitamin D than that of cows which do not graze on fresh grass. The vitamin D content of milk may be increased by feeding the vitamin to the cow. In practice it is more satisfactory to add the vitamin directly to the milk. This is done in most large commercial dairies and in the production of evaporated milk. The procedure ensures the desired content of vitamin D in all the milk offered for sale.

Homogenized Milk. In homogenized milk the fat globules are broken down and distributed in a state of colloidal suspension throughout the milk. The curd is rendered softer and thus more digestible, and the flavor of the milk is improved. Digestion is thereby aided, since a larger surface area is offered by the smaller fat moieties for interaction with intestinal enzymes (lipase).

Evaporated Milk. This is whole milk from which 60 per cent of the water has been removed. The caloric value is 44 calories (usually considered 40 calories) per ounce. There are 2 gm. of protein per ounce. It is sterile, relatively inexpensive, available in all grocery shops, and can be stored in the home without refrigeration if the can is unopened. Evaporated milk is usually both irradiated and homogenized. It has a fine curd because of homogenization and because the casein has been altered in the evaporation process. To use as whole milk it is only necessary to dilute it with an equal quantity of water.

Condensed Milk. This is evaporated whole milk to which has been added 45 per cent of sugar. The caloric value is approximately 100 calories per ounce. It should not be used for infant feedings since the sugar content is far too high. An infant fed on condensed milk is likely to be pale and fat, have flabby muscles and be subject to diarrhea due to fermentation of the excessive carbohydrate content of his feeding.

Dried Milk. In dried milk the water from skimmed milk has been completely evaporated. Dried milk contains various amounts of fat. It is valuable in the formulas of infants who cannot tolerate the amount of fat present in whole milk. Dried milk produces a fine curd, and any dilution desired can be easily made from the dry powder. It is packed in airtight cans and will keep for months without spoiling; for this reason it is useful in traveling with a baby and under conditions when fresh or evaporated milk is not available. In the drying process vitamin C is destroyed. One ounce by weight or $3\frac{1}{2}$ packed level tablespoonfuls of dried milk mixed with 7 ounces of water gives a mixture having the composition of liquid milk. For infant feeding the powdered milk is mixed with enough cool water to make a paste; to this the desired amount of water is added gradually while the mixture is stirred to prevent the formation of lumps.

Carbohydrates. Carbohydrates are added to the formula to increase its caloric value and improve the flavor, and for their laxative effect. They contain, on the average, 120 calories per ounce. In order to dissolve the carbohydrate it is mixed with a warm fluid.

All types of carbohydrates must be broken down into monosaccharides in the intestinal tract before they can be utilized by the body. The carbohydrates commonly used in infant feedings include the following:

a. Dextrose or glucose. This is easily digested.

b. Sucrose or cane sugar, the cheapest and most convenient form for use in the infant's formula, but with the disadvantage of being too sweet.

c. Lactose or milk sugar. Milk sugar is not sweet to the taste, is similar to the carbohydrate in breast milk and has a laxative value.

d. Dextri-Maltose, a relatively expensive form, but easily digested. This proprietary product consists of a mixture of maltose and dextrins. These are simplified by digestive processes prior to absorption.

e. Karo (corn) syrup, a cheap and easily digested carbohydrate. It should be kept in the refrigerator and carefully covered, since it is a good liquid culture medium for bacteria.

f. Starch, a polysaccharide. It is difficult for the infant to digest unless it is thoroughly cooked (cooking breaks down the starch molecules).

Proprietary Infant Milk Products. These are made by commercial firms and have evaporated milk or dried milk as the base. In some the fat has been removed or replaced, and in others different modifications of the original milk have been made. A few proprietary milks closely resemble breast milk in composition. These preparations are relatively expensive, but have the advantages of convenience, sterility and compactness. The law requires the ingredients to be listed on the container. Usually only boiled water is added to the powdered preparation in order to prepare the formula. Some proprietary formulas are prepared in liquid form in disposable bottles and are ready for immediate use when opened.

Preparation of the Formula

The basic principles in the preparation of the infant's formula relate to cleanliness and accuracy. The formula must be clean and preferably sterile, since it can be a source of infection to the infant. In the milk laboratory of the hospital, personnel should wear gowns and caps, and many hospitals require that they also wear masks. The formula room should not be in the line of traffic of hospital personnel or visitors, nor near the area housing patients. In the home the formula is usually prepared in the kitchen. The mother should wear a clean wash dress or coverall apron.

Equipment. All equipment and ingredients should be ready before preparation of the formula is begun. The ingredients are milk, sterile water and some form of carbohydrate.

BOTTLES. Enough 8-ounce feeding bottles should be provided for the entire twenty-four hours' feedings, and at least one extra bottle to replace any that might be broken. Wide-mouthed bottles are commonly used, since they are more easily and thoroughly cleaned with a brush and the nipple more nearly approaches the form of the mother's nipple. In the hospital each bottle is labeled clearly and accurately with either the infant's name or the type of formula the bottle contains. The formula in the individual feeding bottles should be kept in the refrigerator until feeding time.

NIPPLES. The newborn requires a firm nipple. A nipple which has become flabby from use and repeated sterilization makes sucking difficult for the infant. The aperture in the nipple should be a cross cut, i.e. two 4-mm. incisions in the shape of a cross. Some nipples on the market have this cross cut, but others have the traditional three small holes dispersed in the shape of a triangle. The holes may be enlarged to suit the needs of the infant. Factors determining the size of the holes are the infant's ability to suck (the immature and feeble infant may become exhausted if he has to pull vigorously in order to obtain the milk through tiny holes) and the consistency of the formula.

To enlarge the holes in the nipple, the blunt end of a darning needle is inserted into a cork. The point of the needle is held in a flame until red hot and is then used to puncture the nipple. Since the point is red hot, the rubber melts to form a round aperture. It is better to make three small holes in the shape of a triangle than to make a single hole. The nipple is then placed in cold water to harden the rubber. The flow should be tested before the nipple is used. When the bottle is tipped upside down, milk should drip slowly from the nipple at the rate of one drop per second.

BOTTLE CAPS. Since the nipple must be sterile when it enters the infant's mouth, airtight sterile bottle caps are used. These may be of glass or plastic and are cone-shaped, covering the nipple. They are used if the nipples are put on the bottles when the formula is made. If the sterile nipple is to be put on the bottle just before being given to the infant, a close-fitting rubber or plastic cap may be used to cover the bottle top.

PREPARATION OF FORMULA. There are two general methods used in the preparation of formulas: the aseptic or standard method and the terminal heating method.

Aseptic or Standard Method. The equipment needed to prepare a formula by this method includes the following:

Teakettle or pan
Bottles, nipples, bottle caps
Measuring cup
Pitcher
Measuring tablespoon
Large pan for boiling equipment (covered)
Long-handled spoon
Table knife
Can opener

Funnel
Small pan for boiling nipples and bottle caps (covered)
Tongs
Bottle brush
Small jar with tight lid for storing nipples

The procedure for the preparation of the formula is as follows:

1. Wash all equipment in hot, soapy water and rinse in hot, clear water. Wash the bottles, funnel, nipples and bottle caps with the bottle brush. Squeeze water through the nipple holes to make certain they are open.
2. Place *all* equipment except rubber articles in a covered container and boil for ten minutes.
3. Place nipples and rubber caps, if used, in a covered pan and boil for three minutes.
4. Place nipples in the small, sterile covered jar.
5. Boil water in the teakettle or pan for five minutes. Measure the required amount in the sterile measuring cup and pour into the sterile pitcher.
6. Measure the required amount of sugar or syrup in the measuring tablespoon. Level the contents with a table knife. Add the carbohydrate to the water in the pitcher and stir until dissolved.
7. If canned milk is used, scrub the top of the can with soap and rinse with hot water.
8. Measure the required amount of milk in the measuring cup and pour into the sugar-water mixture. Stir thoroughly with the long-handled spoon.
9. Pour the formula into the sterile bottles through the funnel. Cover the bottles with bottle caps.
10. Place the bottles in a pan of cool water in order to cool them quickly. The water should be as deep as the level of the milk in the bottles. Place the bottles in the refrigerator.
11. When it is time to feed the infant, remove one bottle from the refrigerator. Remove the cap. Remove one nipple from the jar and place it on the bottle. Replace the cover on the jar.
12. Place the bottle in a pan of warm water to take the chill off the formula, and feed it to the infant.

Terminal Heating Method. Terminal heating is now used in many hospitals and homes for all formulas which can tolerate the degree of heat necessary for this form of sterilization. This process produces a bacteriologically safe formula.

The formula is prepared with clean but not sterile technique and poured into thoroughly clean bottles. Nipples are put on the bottles, and caps are placed loosely over the nipples.

In the hospital the bottles are placed in racks and autoclaved for ten minutes at a temperature of 246°F. and 15 pounds' pressure.

For the home a sterilizer may be bought and the hospital technique adapted to its use. The formula should be sterilized for twenty-five minutes at 212°F. The lid of the sterilizer should not be removed until it is cool enough to handle with the bare hand. This is a rough gauge of the time required for the nipples to cool slowly. Under rapid cooling the holes in the nipples tend to become clogged by a thin coagulum which tends to form at the surface. Remove the bottles, tighten the caps, and place them in the refrigerator at a temperature of 40 to 45°F. (4.4 to 7.2°C) until they are to be used.

In many hospitals a commercial formula service is being used instead of having the feedings prepared in a formula laboratory. Mothers can also purchase commercially prepared formulas for use in the home. These may come ready for use, or they may require dilution with sterile water and the use of sterile bottles and nipples. Some formulas may also be purchased in disposable containers with nipples attached. In the home such feedings save mothers time and effort in formula preparation but they do tend to be expensive.

Technique of Bottle Feeding

The nurse or mother should first wash her hands thoroughly with soap and water. The bottle may be placed in a pan of water at a temperature of 120°F. for ten minutes or in an electric thermostat-controlled warmer. To test the temperature and the rate of flow of the milk, the nurse lets a few drops fall on the inner side of her wrist. Warming the feeding to body temperature is not really necessary, however, since infants who have been fed cool milk thrive well.

The nurse checks the name of the infant and that on the bottle before giving the infant his feeding. A mistake in the formula may be as dangerous as a mistake in the giving of medication. She takes a bib and a diaper to the infant's crib and places the bottle on the bedside stand. She changes his diaper and places the soiled one in a pedal-controlled can or on a piece of newspaper or paper towel at the foot of the crib.

After washing her hands again the nurse picks up the infant, wrapped in a blanket if the room is chilly, and sits down in a rocking chair, holding the infant in her lap with his head supported on her left arm. If for any reason the infant cannot be held in the lap, the nurse should sit beside the crib, elevate his head and hold his bottle. The mother may hold the infant in her arms to feed him while she rests in bed during the postpartum period.

A bottle should never be propped on a pad. Propping an infant's bottle may be the severest form of unintentional maternal neglect. An infant is apt to lose his hold on the nipple and be unable to get it in his mouth again; there is also danger that the flow of milk will be too rapid and that the infant might choke. The bottle should be slanted so that the nipple is always filled with fluid; otherwise the infant will suck in air. He may need to be bubbled frequently, and always at the close of the feeding, usually in ten to twenty minutes. After this he should be placed on his right side or prone in his crib. In either of these positions the formula can most easily drain through the pylorus into the intestinal tract.

Any milk left in the bottle should be discarded. The bottle and the nipple are rinsed in cold water. If the infant is in isolation, all equipment should be boiled before being returned to the milk laboratory. The nurse should return to the infant after a few minutes to see whether he has regurgitated or vomited part of his feeding.

The feeding should be charted: the time when given, the amount taken and whether any was regurgitated or vomited. Words which may aid the nurse in charting are eructate, bubble, ruminate, regurgitate and vomit. *Eructate* means to belch. *Bubble* has almost the same meaning, but implies that air is expelled while the nurse is holding the infant upright or is patting or rubbing him on the back. *Rumination* means voluntary or habitual regurgitation of formula into the mouth after it has been swallowed. Such milk may be swallowed again or spit out. An infant who spits out milk may lose a considerable amount of his feeding. *Regurgitate* means to express — "spill over" as it were — a small amount of formula. *Vomiting* means bringing up an appreciable amount of the feeding. If the infant is sick, vomiting may be projectile.

DISCHARGE FROM THE NURSERY

Many pediatricians now recommend that prior to discharge from the nursery all newborn infants be tested for phenylketonuria, galactosemia and fructosemia. The blood test for phenylketonuria should not be performed until the infant has been on milk feedings for twenty-four hours. Any infants who have questionable phenylalanine levels should be retested in four to six weeks. In regard to disorders involving galactose and fructose, the infants should be given feedings with these substances before urine tests are carried out. Infants born into families in which these or other inherited metabolic diseases are known should be carefully evaluated.

CARE AT HOME

Emotional Aspects of Care

After the newborn has been discharged from the hospital his care is primarily the responsibility of the mother. The mother must be lenient with herself at this time, realizing that if she becomes overburdened by her household duties, her care of the infant will not be beneficial for him. At such times she will need some kindly support or temporary relief from the responsibilities of managing her home, by either the father or another member of her family.

An infant in the low-income group is likely to receive as much loving care as one in the high-income group, but he may be cared for by many family members or neighbors, a number of whom may be children who will be awkward in their handling of him. This is in contrast to the more concentrated love and attention which the infant in the middle or upper class receives from a few relatives and friends who are "allowed" to hold him. This difference has an important effect on the emotional development of the child.

The over-all responsibility of the mother for her child is well accepted in our society by all social groups. Not as frequently mentioned, however, is the task of the infant to respond to the mother, at first by smiling, and to communicate his needs to her, whether hunger, thirst or need for contact. Thus the neonate's relation with his mother is truly an interaction. The newborn responds to the mother's stimulation with activities which orient him to his mother. His activities furnish her with cues that then influence her behavior toward him. If the mother sensitively responds to the infant's cues, satisfactory socialization begins. If she does not, a disturbed relation may be begun.

Physical Aspects of Care

Aspects of the infant's care which the mother may possibly want to discuss with the nurse include shelter, room furnishing, bathing, clothing, elimination, sleeping, weighing, taking the temperature, and feeding as well as follow-up care.

Shelter

The nurse does not usually know to what kind of home a newborn infant will be taken on discharge from the hospital. The physical environment of the home of those in the low-income group is likely to be unhygienic, owing to poor neighborhood sanitation, to overcrowding and to parental attitudes toward health. In her experience in public health nursing the student will see many homes in poor neighborhoods and will be aware of the adaptations in child care which must be made under such conditions.

Here we can consider only an ideal home in a good neighborhood. It is important that the sewer and water systems be adequate and the house well built, with equipment for comfort and safety. The infant should have a room of his own. The floor covering and walls should be easy to keep clean; light colors are preferable. Heating and ventilation should be adequate. For the young infant the temperature during the day should be 70 to 75°F., and at night 60 to 65°; for the older child the temperature should be 68 to 70° during the day and 50° at night. There should be no drafts; ventilation can be secured by any of the devices for maintaining fresh air or indirectly from another room. The humidity should be 55 per cent. In winter any device providing for evaporation of water will raise the humidity, such as a humidifier, a receptacle full of water placed on the radiator, or one of the patented devices which fit the radiator.

Room Furnishings

The furnishings should be simple, durable and easily cleaned. Paint in old homes or on old cribs may be a source of lead poisoning if the infant bites the painted surface or puts broken bits of paint-covered plaster from the wall in his mouth.

The infant should have a bed of his own. It is a needless expense to buy a bassinet which is soon outgrown. A better plan is to buy a crib suitable for a child of four or five years. This will give the infant room to roll and creep in as he becomes able to move about and will keep him happy when he wakes and his mother does not come at once. The bars of the crib should be close together and the side gates high enough to prevent his climbing over. The latch should be out of his reach.

The mattress should be firm, but not hard. The cover should be of thin rubber or other waterproof material and large enough to tuck in at the sides and ends. One type of mattress cover is made to cover both sides of the mattress and fastens with a zipper or snaps. A quilted pad large enough to cover the entire mattress is needed, as well as sheets long and wide enough to tuck 12 inches under the mattress at the sides, foot and top. The blankets should be of cotton or wool or a mixture of both. A sleeping bag is good if the infant tends to kick off the covers and the room cannot be kept sufficiently warm. He should not have a pillow until he is old enough to be propped up against it in a corner of his crib. A little infant is no more comfortable with a pillow under his head than without it; he may turn on his abdomen with the danger of suffocating as his face presses against the pillow.

There should be a small chest of drawers for the infant's clothing and personal equipment. As a preschool child he can use the chest and can be taught to put away his own things. There should be chairs for adults, one of them a low rocking chair. When the infant is old enough to sit up, he should have a small chair of his own, low enough for his feet to touch the floor, or the supporting foot rest if it is a high chair. The modern high chair can be lowered so that the infant is on a level with a small table. If the infant is to be left alone, it is safer to have the lower chair. There should also be a shelf for toys, and a playpen raised off the floor.

The infant needs his own bathtub or bathinette. Plastic tubs are light, durable and smooth for the infant's skin. He will need a diaper pail, preferably of the pedal-controlled type, with a closely fitting cover, and later on a toilet seat or training chair. There should be a gate at the door of the nursery, or at the top of the stairs if the family live in a two-story house.

Bathing

The infant is bathed once a day and may be sponged off several times a day during warm weather. The temperature of the room should be 75 to 80°F. Either a bathinette or tub is used. The infant over two months enjoys a bath in the family tub, but the mother may find that stooping tires her. If a tub is used, a bath towel is placed over the bottom. This prevents sliding and adds to the pleasure of the bath. The temperature of the water should be 100 to 105° for the newborn or small infant; for the normal healthy infant it can soon be reduced to 95°. The mother tests the temperature with her elbow or a bath thermometer. Soft towels and a wash cloth are needed.

There should be a bath tray containing the following articles:

Jar of cotton swabs or cotton balls
Dish for soap (soap should be white and unscented)
Bottle or jar of baby oil or lotion
Pin holder
Hair brush and comb
Orange wood stick
Paper bag for waste
Powder (if the mother wants to use it. Cornstarch powder is cheaper than most other powders and is suitable for use on the infant's skin; however, no powder should be used routinely.)
Bland ointment (A and D ointment is effective when necessary on an excoriated diaper area.)

The mother should be taught that there is no set procedure to be followed in bathing the infant, but certain principles must be remembered.

The scalp should be washed once a week. Mothers caring for their first babies may be fearful of washing over the "soft spot," or anterior fontanel. *Cradle cap,* a greasy crust or scale formation on the scalp, often occurs. Treatment of this seborrheic condition is by application of oil or a bland ointment with repeated scalp shampoos until the crust is removed.

The eyes, nose and ears require special attention to prevent injury. The creases of the body must be carefully cleansed and wiped thoroughly. The genitalia and the buttocks are bathed after each stool and, if the infant has a tendency to be chafed, after urinating.

The mother should be given complete directions on the care of the umbilicus before the infant is discharged from the hospital. Usually exposure of the cord to the air promotes rapid healing. There may be a slight bloody discharge from the navel; however, the umbilicus will heal in a few days after separation of the cord. Until the area is completely healed she should not give the infant a tub bath without permission from her physician. Before the infant is discharged the mother may give a demonstration to the nurse to ensure that she (the mother) will not be anxious about her ability to care for the infant at home.

Clothing

Infants today wear very little clothing. Houses are usually comfortably warm in winter, and the less the infant wears in summer, the more comfortable he is. Children outgrow their clothing rapidly, so that it is best to buy only enough for several days' wear and to wash their clothes frequently. All articles of infants' clothing should be soft and nonirritating, simple in design, comfortable, loose for activity, washable, suitable for the weather, easy to put on, absorbent, safe — e.g. no ties around the neck which, if caught in any way, might choke the infant and in any case are uncomfortable — and tailored with safe fastenings to avoid the danger of loose or awkward buttons.

In general, shirts for infants are of cotton knitted material.

Diapers are made of gauze, knitted cotton, bird's eye or cotton flannel. They should be either square — 27 by 27 inches — or oblong — 18 by 36 inches. Many mothers today appreciate the help a commercial diaper service can give, although

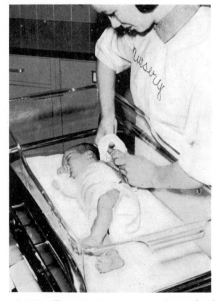

Figure 7–10. The simplest way to dress the infant is to put entire hand through the sleeve, grasp the infant's hand and pull it through gently. (Davis and Rubin: *DeLee's Obstetrics for Nurses.* 17th ed.)

such service tends to be more expensive than caring for the diapers in the home.

To dress the infant, if the shirt is of the slip-over type, it should be gathered in the hands so that it is easily pulled over the infant's head. The double-breasted shirt which ties is more popular, for it is easier to put on, gives double warmth across the chest and does not tear easily. To put the infant's arm through the sleeve, the nurse or mother should put her fingers through the end of the sleeve and put the infant's hand through the armhole. She can then take his fingers in hers and gently pull his hand through the sleeve. The diaper is put on like a pair of pants and pinned at either side to the shirt. The shirt is less likely to tear if it is turned up and the diaper is pinned through the two thicknesses. Turning it up also keeps it clean and dry when the infant voids or has a stool. The diaper should also be pinned securely around the leg openings. For laundering the diapers, see page 122.

Stockings or socks as a rule are used only if the infant's feet are cold, and should be large enough to allow the infant to move his toes without being cramped. If long stockings are used, they are pinned to the diaper, above the knee on the outside of the leg. They are likely to become wet whenever the infant voids. Socks are pretty, but tend to come off when the infant kicks and rubs his legs together.

Bibs are used when the infant is fed. The young infant needs no other clothes, but as he grows older he should be provided with nightgowns, overalls or dresses, sun suits and outdoor clothes for all weather.

Elimination

The breast-fed infant has several stools a day which are soft and rather spongy and may contain a little mucus. They are not likely to chafe him. Their odor is rather aromatic. The stools of the infant fed on cow's milk and cane sugar are yellow and more solid than those of the breast-fed infant. One or two stools a day is normal.

Sleep

The newborn infant sleeps or appears to be sleeping practically all the time he is not feeding. His sleep is light, and there are frequent spontaneous movements of the face and body. He stretches and puckers up his face. When he is only a few weeks old, his sleeping periods are longer and more quiet, but he is also awake and alert for longer periods. This trend continues as he grows out of early infancy.

Weight

Mothers should learn in the hospital how to weigh their infants if they have or intend to have scales at home. Safety factors should be emphasized. The mother should keep one hand over the infant at all times when she is weighing him. She should place the head end of the scale near, but not touching, the wall so that he may not slide out that end. She should hold her hand close enough to his body to prevent his sliding down and over the other end of the scale.

In the home weekly weighings are sufficient. If they are attempted daily, mothers tend to worry about minor fluctuations. Scales are not absolutely necessary, for the infant can be weighed when taken for his check-up to the physician's office or the Child Health Conference (see p. 275). The average infant will gain between 7 and 8 ounces (210 and 240 gm.) each week. Some infants, however, gain 5 to 12 ounces (150 to 360 gm.) a week. If the gain is more or less than this, the mother should notify the physician.

Temperature

Although mothers should be taught how to take the infant's temperature, this should not be considered part of the daily care. The temperature should be taken only when the mother believes that it is not normal.

Feeding

The feeding of the infant should be considered part of the routine activities of daily living in which all the members of the family are engaged. If everyone in the home is to be subordinated to the infant, he is likely to become a disturbing factor. This consciously or unconsciously creates a feeling that he is privileged and influences the emotional relations of parents and siblings toward him and indirectly toward each other. All plans for his care, from the first day in the hospital on, should be made with reference to what is best for him in the family situation.

Feeding time should be pleasant for both the infant and the family. The infant learns to like the one who feeds and cuddles him. The average infant at six weeks of age will smile at his mother when she picks him up and smiles at him. In time he is conditioned to smile because smiling always brings more cuddling and expressions of love from his mother. This is his way of wanting to please her, and it lays the foundation for willingness to do what she wants (obedience), so essential to the willing acceptance of discipline, which in turn leads to self-discipline.

While the mother is in the hospital the nurse should give her (1) a recipe for the formula, (2) a set of instructions, and (3) a demonstration of formula preparation. The mother may be taught either the aseptic technique or the terminal heating method, or both. Teaching may be supplemented by the use of booklets from milk companies; these illustrate the steps by which formulas can be prepared by either method.

Follow-up Care

After discharge the infant should be under continuing medical care.

The mother who has a private physician will put her baby under his care after she and the baby have been discharged from the hospital. But the infant of a mother who is a clinic patient is routinely referred by either the social service department of the hospital or the head nurse (or supervisor) of the obstetrical unit to the public health Child Health Conference in the district in which he lives. The public health agency will be notified of his discharge from the hospital, and a public health nurse will visit in the home to instruct the mother in the adaptation of all she has learned to the home situation. She will check on the equipment for the infant's care and demonstrate his bath and the making of his formula. If further guidance or help which she cannot give is needed, she may refer the mother to The Family Service Society or equivalent agency.

TEACHING AIDS AND OTHER INFORMATION*

American Academy of Pediatrics
Resuscitation of the Newborn Infant.

American Medical Association
A Child in the Family.
Artificial Respiration.

Association for the Aid of Crippled Children
Resuscitation of the Newborn Infant.

Charles Pfizer and Company, J. B. Roerig Division
Infant Feeding Through the Ages.

Evaporated Milk Association
Making Baby's Formula – Aseptic Method.
Making Baby's Formula – Terminal Heat Method.

Mead Johnson Laboratories
Baby Needs Your Help at Feeding Time.
Current Aspects of Infant Nutrition in Daily Practice.

National Society for the Prevention of Blindness, Inc.
Review of Status of State Laws Requiring Use of a Prophylactic in the Eyes of Newborn Infants.

Public Affairs Pamphlets
Carson, R.: Your New Baby.
Riker, A. P.: Breastfeeding.

Ross Laboratories
Breast Feeding.
Formula Preparation Instruction Folders.
Iron in Infancy.

United States Department of Health, Education, and Welfare
Breast Feeding Your Baby, 1965.
Facts About Pasteurization of Milk, 1967.
How to Obtain Birth Certificates, 1966.
Infant Care, 1963. Reprinted 1967.
Minimum Sanitary Standards for Community Infant Formula Services, 1967.
Phenylketonuria: Detection in the Newborn Infant as a Routine Hospital Procedure, 1964.
Rescue Breathing, 1966.
You May Save Time Proving Your Age and Other Birth Facts, 1965.

---

* Complete addresses are given in the Appendix.

REFERENCES

Publications

Abramson, H.: *Resuscitation of the Newborn Infant.* 2nd ed. St. Louis, C. V. Mosby Company, 1966.

American Academy of Pediatrics: *Report of the Committee on the Control of Infectious Diseases.* 14th ed., 1964. Evanston, Ill., American Academy of Pediatrics, 1963.

American Academy of Pediatrics Committee on Fetus and Newborn: *Standards and Recommendations for Hospital Care of Newborn Infants.* Evanston, Ill., American Academy of Pediatrics, 1964.

American Hospital Association: *Procedures and Layout for the Infant Formula Room.* Chicago, American Hospital Association, 1965.

Branin, V. A.: *A Study of Problems Encountered by Twenty-Six Nursing Mothers Following Hospital Discharge;* in *Evaluation of Nursing Intervention* (Convention Clinical Sessions No. 4). New York, American Nurses' Association, 1964, p. 13.

Close, S.: *The Know-How of Infant Feeding.* Baltimore, Williams & Wilkins Company, 1965.

Disbrow, M. A.: *Nursing Intervention as a Factor in Successful Breast Feeding;* in *Evaluation of Nursing Intervention* (Convention Clinical Services No. 4). New York, American Nurses' Association, 1964, p. 5

Feldman, S., and Ellis, H.: *Principles of Resuscitation.* Philadelphia, F. A. Davis Company, 1967.

Fomon, S. J.: *Infant Nutrition.* Philadelphia, W. B. Saunders Company, 1967.

LaLeche League International: *The Womanly Art of Breastfeeding.* Franklin Park, Ill., LaLeche League International, 1963 (Seventh Printing, 1966).

McKendry, J. B. J., and Bailey, J. D.: *The Newborn: A Practical Guide.* Springfield, Ill., Charles C Thomas, 1966.

Mitchell, H. S., and others: *Cooper's Nutrition in Health and Disease.* 15th ed. Philadelphia, J. B. Lippincott Company, 1968.

Special Committee on Infant Mortality of the Medical Society of the County of New York: *Resuscitation of Newborn Infants.* New York, Association for the Aid of Crippled Children.

Periodicals

Adams, M.: Early Concerns of Primigravida Mothers Regarding Infant Care Activities. *Nursing Research,* 12:72, 1963.

Apgar, V., and others: Evaluation of the Newborn Infant—Second Report. *J.A.M.A.,* 168: 1985, 1958.

Barrie, H.: Resuscitation of the Newborn. *Lancet,* 1:650, 1963.

Battaglia, F. C.: Recent Advances in Medicine for Newborn Infants. *J. Pediat.,* 71:748, 1967.

Dyal, L., and Kahrl, J.: When Mothers Breast-Feed. *Am. J. Nursing,* 67:2555, 1967.

Fisch, R. O., and others: The Effect of Excess L-Phenylalanine on Mothers and on Their Breast-Fed Infants. *J. Pediat.,* 71:176, 1967.

Geissler, N. J.: An Instrument Used to Measure Breast Engorgement. *Nursing Research,* 16:130, 1967.

Gezon, H. M., and others: Hexachlorophene Bathing in Early Infancy—Effect on Staphylococcal Disease and Infection. *New England J. Med.,* 270:379, February 20, 1964.

Iffrig, Sr., M. C.: Nursing Care and Success in Breast Feeding. *Nursing Clin. N. Amer.,* 3:345, 1968.

Keitel, H. G.: Preventing Neonatal Diaper Rash. *Am. J. Nursing,* 65:124, May 1965.

Leifer, G.: Rooming-in Despite Postpartal Complications. *Am. J. Nursing,* 67:2114, 1967.

Limaye, R. D., and Hancock, R. A.: Penile Urethral Fistula as a Complication of Circumcision. *J. Pediat.,* 72:105, 1968.

Michelson, A.: Disposable Feeding Bottles. *Nursing Times,* 62:1449, November 4, 1966.

Newton, N., and Newton, M.: Psychologic Aspects of Lactation. *New England J. Med.,* 277:1179, 1967.

Nichols, M. G.: Breast-feeding: A Nurse-mother Discovers Its Joys. *RN,* 50, May 1968.

Rubin, R.: Maternal Touch, *Nursing Outlook,* 11:828, 1963.

Rubin, R.: Food and Feeding: A Matrix of Relationships. *Nursing Forum,* VI: 195, 1967.

Silverman, W. A., and Parke, P. C.: The Newborn: Keep Him Warm. *Am. J. Nursing,* 65:81, October 1965.

Thompson, L. R.: Nursery Infections: Apparent and Inapparent. *Am. J. Nursing,* 65:80, November 1965.

Wiedenbach, E.: Family Nurse Practitioner for Maternal and Child Care. *Nursing Outlook,* 13:50, December 1965.

Yeaworth, R. C.: Students' Attitudes Toward Maternal Role. *Nursing Outlook,* 15:37, July 1967.

8

THE PREMATURE INFANT AND THE POSTMATURE INFANT

PREMATURITY

Premature birth accounts for the highest mortality rate among infants in the first year of life. This is probably the reason why increasing amounts of research have been done during the last twenty-five years on the causes of prematurity and the needs of these infants.

Approximately 10 per cent of all live births are premature. The standard of prematurity should be the number of days of gestation, but this standard correlates with the weight, length and activity of the newborn. Prematures are therefore often defined in terms of weight, length and behavior. *Prematurity* may be defined as the termination of pregnancy in the period from approximately the twenty-eighth to the end of the thirty-seventh week of gestation. Because weight is often indicative of prematurity and physiologic immaturity, a premature infant is considered to be one who weighs 2500 gm. (5 pounds 8 ounces) or less at birth. The length from crown to heel is likely to be close to 18.5 inches (47 cm.). His behavior shows his immaturity: he lacks the normal reflexes and a general ability to carry on vital functions.

Incidence and Causes of Prematurity

In many cases the cause of prematurity is not known, partly because the incidence is highest among the low socioeconomic groups. Prospective mothers in such groups are least likely to have adequate prenatal care, which includes observation and recording of a woman's condition throughout pregnancy. Many of these women are first seen by an obstetrician when they are in labor.

Multiple births are a frequent cause of prematurity; few triplets are carried to term. Toxemia of pregnancy is an important cause, particularly among women not under observation of a clinic obstetrician or their own physician. Antepartum hemorrhage is likely to occur in two important complications of pregnancy: premature separation of the placenta (abruptio placentae) and placenta praevia. Both conditions may contribute to premature birth of the infant. Premature rupture of the membranes invariably causes premature birth.

Among maternal diseases related to premature delivery are (1) those of noninfectious origin – e.g. cardiac disease, diabetes mellitus

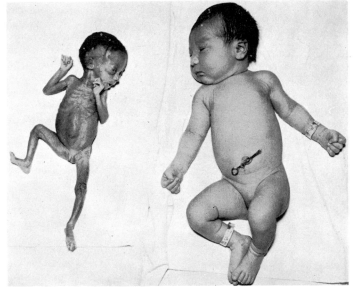

Figure 8–1. The baby on the right is a newborn delivered at term, weighing 3500 gm. The baby on the left is a premature who was born at 26 weeks' gestation and weighed 1100 gm. When this photograph was taken, he weighed 2000 gm. and was 8 weeks old. (Davis and Rubin, *DeLee's Obstetrics for Nurses,* 17th ed.)

and severe sensitization to the Rh blood factor— and (2) those of infectious origin, whether acute or chronic. Chronic maternal malnutrition may also cause premature birth of the infant.

Fetal abnormalities or injury to the mother or fetus, or both, may make it impossible for the infant to be carried to term. Overwork and inadequate diet are important factors in the incidence of premature births in the low socio-economic groups. They are seldom the immediate cause of a premature delivery, but predispose to poor health, if not chronic or acute illness, which interferes with carrying the fetus to term.

Research has shown that premature births occur more frequently among mothers who smoke. With further long-range research perhaps more contributory factors to prematurity will be found.

Prevention of Prematurity

The great preventive measure to reduce the number of premature births is adequate prenatal care for all prospective mothers. Maternal and child health programs—federal, state and local—have provided good obstetrical care for thousands of women who otherwise would have lacked even a minimum of medical supervision during the prenatal period. Maternal care is provided to protect the infant as well as the mother, since *the longer the fetus can be retained in utero, the better are its chances for survival.*

Characteristics of Premature Infants

Physical Characteristics

The premature infant that we see in the incubator is at the same stage of development as the fetus of the same gestational age. The age of viability is commonly said to be seven months. Many premature infants, then, will resemble the fetus of seven months' gestation. The premature infant is adapted to life *in utero.* His immaturity is evident as we look at him. He is small and limp. His skin is thin, wrinkled and red; there is an excess of lanugo and little or no vernix caseosa. His head is relatively large with prominent eyes, soft ears and receding chin. The thorax is less firm than that of the full-term infant. The abdomen protrudes, and the genitalia are small. The extremities are thin, the muscles small. The fingernails and toenails are abnormally soft and short. The subcutaneous tissue is deficient, so that he has a wizened appearance. Extremely small prematures may have a plump appearance because of edema due to a low total serum protein concentration. This is lost, however, in a few days. Engorgement of the breasts, normal in the full-term infant, is absent in the premature, since it is due to hormones from the mother which are passed to the fetus in the late months of gestation. The normal sucking, swallowing and gag reflexes are absent in very immature infants.

Physiologic Handicaps

The nursing care of the premature infant, so far as it differs from that of the normal infant, is based on the physiologic handicaps of immaturity: poor control of body temperature, difficult respiration, inability to handle infections adequately, tendency to hemorrhage and anemia, tendency for rickets to develop, disturbances of nutrition, and impairment of renal function.

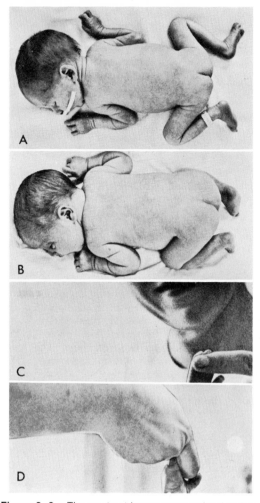

Figure 8–2. The contrast in neuromuscular development and muscle tone between the premature infant
and the normal newborn. In the prone position, *A,*
the premature lies with pelvis flat and legs splayed
out sideways like a frog. *B,* The normal full-term infant
lies with his limbs flexed, pelvis raised and knees
drawn under the abdomen. In the grasp reflex, *C,* the
premature infant grasps the finger weakly, but there
is little muscle tensing. *D,* The normal newborn reinforces the grip when his arm is drawn upwards.
(Courtesy of Mead Johnson and Company.)

Poor Control of Body Temperature. What
was said of the normal newborn's dependency on
the temperature of his environment to maintain
a normal body temperature (p. 118) is even more
important in planning the care of the premature
infant. His nervous system is poorly developed,
and the heat-regulating center in the brain is
immature. The skin surface of the premature is
great in proportion to his weight. He lacks the
insulation of the subcutaneous fat layer, which is
developed in the last month of gestation. His
muscular development being poor, he is inactive.
The metabolic rate is low. If the environment is

too warm he becomes overheated, since his sweating mechanism is underdeveloped. Yet internal
conditions which would cause a fever in a normal infant may be present in the premature
without an elevation of temperature (this often
happens in the dehydrated premature or one with
an infectious condition).

Difficult Respiration. Respirations are difficult and irregular in the premature infant. Since
his lungs are immature, there is incomplete
development of the alveoli and weakness of the
thoracic cage and of the respiratory muscles.
Gaseous exchange is retarded by the immature
alveolar membrane. Then, too, if mucus lodges
in his throat or if a few drops of feeding enter
the trachea, his gag and cough reflexes are too
weak to clear the airway.

CYANOSIS. The premature's tendency to
cyanosis is evidence of inadequate oxygenation
of his arterial blood. This may be due to increased
intracranial pressure from birth trauma, obstruction of the respiratory tract, poor development of the respiratory muscles or some interference with the normal expansion of the lungs.
Abdominal distention may interfere with the
action of the diaphragm.

APNEA. Apnea is a condition of suspended
respiration. It may result from excessive analgesics or anesthetics given the mother during
labor. Expert care during delivery decreases the
danger of birth trauma with resulting cyanosis.
General immaturity of the nervous system and
the respiratory tract is a cause of apnea which
is inherent in the premature infant's condition
and cannot be controlled by the obstetrician,
although modern methods of resuscitation keep
many such infants alive who formerly would
have died at birth.

Inability to Handle Infections Adequately.
The premature infant is very susceptible to
infection, and his ability to handle infection
of any sort is poor because he has poorly developed globulin synthesis, antibody formation
and cellular defense. He does not react to infection with fever or an elevation of the white blood
cell count. He lacks immune substances from his
mother, which are transmitted to the fetus during the last months of gestation.

The immature infant has more avenues for
access of infection than does the normal infant.
His skin and mucous membranes are not as
protective as the more mature skin and membranes of the full-term infant.

Tendency to Hemorrhage and Anemia. The
blood vessels of the premature infant are incompletely developed and therefore more fragile,
the supporting tissue lacks normal elasticity,
and the plasma is hypoprothrombinemic. He
lacks the normal supply of vitamin K. Anemia
results from hemorrhage as with the normal
infant, but the premature suffers more from loss

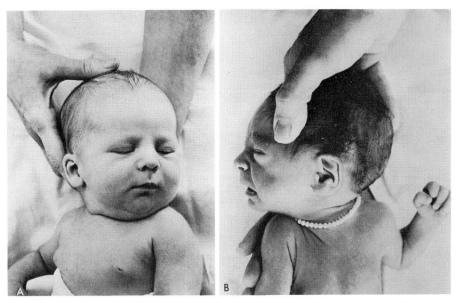

Figure 8–3. Estimation of muscle tone: head rotation. A, In the normal newborn. B, In the premature infant. (Courtesy of Mead Johnson and Company.)

of blood than does the normal infant because he lacks iron and other essential hematogenous factors which the fetus receives during the last months of gestation. His body growth is rapid and therefore requires a greater blood supply. He has an increased proportion of fetal hemoglobin. His red blood cells are easily destroyed, and even a slight loss of blood is of great consequence.

Tendency for Rickets to Develop. The premature infant lacks the calcium, phosphorus and usually the vitamin D normally stored in the body of the full-term infant. Yet his potentially rapid rate of growth requires an ample supply of these minerals, and vitamin D is needed for their utilization. He also lacks the ability to absorb fat-soluble vitamins given in his feedings. The result of these factors is that the premature is more likely to acquire rickets than is the normal infant.

Disturbances of Nutrition. This subject is discussed on page 147.

Impairment of Renal Function. The incomplete development of the kidneys of the premature causes difficulty in concentration of urine, and a proportionately large amount of fluid is lost. He has an unstable acid-base and electrolyte balance.

Care and Treatment of the Premature Infant

Differences in the nursing care of the premature infant from that of the full-term infant are based on the anatomic and physiologic characteristics of prematurity.

CARE IMMEDIATELY AFTER BIRTH

Warmth. The infant is placed in a warm incubator provided with the necessary facilities for increasing environmental oxygen and humidity. Research has shown that premature infants survive best when their body heat loss is reduced.

Initiation of Respirations. The airway should be cleared. Mucus may be removed from the nose and throat by gentle suction. A mucus trap may be used with a no. 8 to 10 French rubber catheter. The infant is placed in a level position or with his head down; this position increases the natural drainage of secretions.

If the infant has hypoxia, he may be given artificial respiration with a mechanical device providing measured positive pressure. If no mechanical device is available, *gentle* mouth-to-mouth insufflation by blowing "puffs" of air through several layers of gauze may be used. Air enriched with oxygen may be given to the infant if an oxygen tube is placed in the operator's mouth. Other more vigorous measures may cause the infant to gasp once or twice, but are not helpful in establishing respiration.

Oxygen Administration. Oxygen should be in readiness if respirations are not established in the first few seconds of life, and later if the infant shows signs of cyanosis. Immediately after birth he may be placed in an atmosphere having an oxygen content of 30 to 40 per cent. To stimulate respiration once it has been established, 95 per cent oxygen and 5 per cent carbon dioxide may be used for short periods only.

Medications. The nurse should know the drugs commonly used in treating conditions usual in premature infants, and such drugs should be in readiness in case of emergency. Epinephrine is given intramuscularly as a cardiovascular stimulant, and caffeine and sodium benzoate is given intramuscularly for respiratory stimulation. To reduce the tendency to bleeding, Menadione (vitamin K) may be given intramuscularly in the lateral aspect of the thigh. Excessive doses are to be avoided, since the drug may cause increased bilirubinemia. Nalorphine hydrochloride (Nalline) should be given intravenously into the umbilical cord to counteract the respiratory depression due to morphine, codeine or other opiates given the mother before delivery and transmitted to the infant via the placenta. If the physician knows that the infant is premature, the mother will probably not receive analgesia.

CARE IN THE NURSERY

The premature infant may be cared for in a premature nursery or in a special area set aside in a newborn intensive care unit (see p. 47). In any such unit all essential diagnostic and therapeutic equipment should be available *immediately* to each infant at any time. In such a unit near each newborn should be equipment for oxygen, compressed air, and suction among others, and outlets for respirators, monitoring devices and infusion pumps. Also readily available should be cardiopulmonary monitoring and resuscitation devices. Research is being done in some institutions on a new electronic monitoring system to prevent mortality and brain damage in premature infants who suddenly stop breathing. In such a unit nurses must be available who can handle both infants and machines in any emergency.

In smaller hospitals having units for newborns an attempt should be made to provide prompt care similar to that given in a larger setting.

Environment. No nurses may enter the premature nursery except those assigned to it. There is usually an isolation nursery for prematures brought to the hospital from other hospitals or from the home.

The infant should be taken from the delivery room to the nursery in a heated carrier. A portable oxygen tank should be available when transporting the infant. The nursery should be isolated from all other units to ensure protection from infection. It should preferably be air conditioned. The humidity of the nursery should not be below 55 or above 65 per cent, the temperature not below 77 or above 90°F. Each infant should have his own incubator or crib.

Good nursing care is essential to the preservation of the premature, and the survival rate is highest where nursing care is adequate in both quantity and quality. Such care must be constant.

Any omission lessens the infant's chance for survival. Nurses caring for premature infants must know the principles on which care of the premature is based and must be skilled in their adaptation to the needs of the individual infant. They must be able to judge his needs at any time and be devoted to providing the best possible care. In no other area of pediatric nursing is the ability to observe and accurately record all symptoms of greater importance. Observations which the nurse should make on the premature infant include quality of respirations, color, sucking ability, activity, cry, and change in his condition such as increased retractions and degree of cyanosis.

Minimal Handling. The nurse should handle a small premature no more than is absolutely necessary and remove him as few times from his incubator or crib as possible. Minimal handling lessens the danger of infection and conserves the infant's strength. Manual skill is also required. Procedures must be carried out with extreme gentleness and precision.

The nurse should accomplish as much as she can in every contact with the infant. Nursing care should be planned around the feeding time. This not only minimizes the danger of infection, but also does not interfere with his rest more than is necessary and tends to keep the concentration of oxygen at the prescribed level in the incubator.

Maintenance of Body Temperature

The premature infant is unable to maintain a stable body temperature. Even minor deviations from the optimum environmental temperature cause a corresponding change in his body temperature. In caring for the premature the danger of his being cold is always stressed. A warm nursery and the use of incubators (see Figs. 7-4, 8-4) make it possible to provide the required environmental heat to maintain each infant's body temperature at 96 to 98°F. (35.5 to 36.5°C.). Ideally, the infant's body temperature should be 98°F., but stability of temperature is more important than maintenance at exactly 98°F. Overheating is as bad for the infant as being cold. The ideal temperature and humidity of the nursery prevent loss of water through the skin and excessive loss through breathing.

Incubators are indicated for infants of 3 pounds or less. If for any reason a premature is placed in the general nursery, the incubator will probably be used until he weighs well over 3 pounds, and even longer if he cannot maintain his temperature, has difficulty in breathing or becomes cyanotic. One great advantage of the incubator is that it can be regulated to meet the needs of the individual infant. In general, the temperature in the incubator should not be over

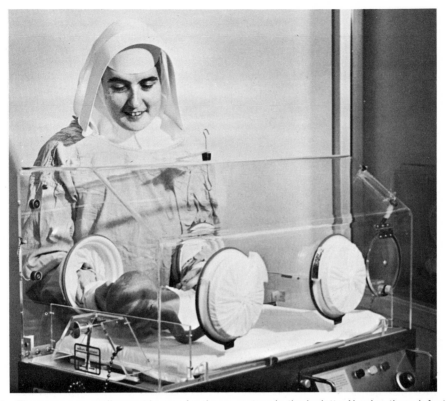

Figure 8–4.   The nurse can easily provide care for the premature in the Isolette. Nursing these infants can be a challenging and rewarding experience. (Fitzgerald Mercy Hospital, Darby, Pa.)

90°F. (32.2°C.); it may be raised or lowered, according to whether the infant requires more or less heat.

Since the objective of applying external heat is to maintain the infant's temperature within a normal range, it is necessary to take his body temperature in order to determine the amount of external heat required. It may be necessary to take the temperature every hour until it is stabilized. The temperature should be taken when the infant is first brought to the nursery. This is done rectally, thereby simultaneously testing for the presence of anal occlusion (see p. 172). After this initial trial the temperature is routinely taken by the axillary method as often as ordered.

Preparation and Use of Incubators.   Types of incubators include, among others, the Armstrong, the Isolette and the heated crib. Each varies from the other in some detail of operation, and the nurse must study the operating instructions provided by the manufacturer.

In the selection of an incubator the points on which it is to be evaluated are (1) easy maintenance of heat and humidity, (2) ease in administration of oxygen, (3) transparent top for easy visibility, and (4) safety alarms to indicate overheating or lack of circulating air.

The incubator should be prepared before the infant arrives. The regulator is set at approximately 90°F. Thereafter it is adjusted so that the infant's temperature is maintained between 96 and 98°F. When the infant is cared for in the Isolette, not only can the temperature of the incubator be regulated by the nurse, but also if an Infant Servo Control Power Unit is attached, the infant himself can act as the Isolette's thermostat. A highly accurate temperature-sensing thermistor is taped directly to the skin of the infant's abdomen. When the infant's abdominal skin temperature changes, the Isolette's heater is turned on or off and the infant's body temperature is stabilized at the desired control point.

The water chamber is filled with sterile distilled water so that the humidity can be increased if necessary. In some instances no increase in humidity is provided. The bed is adjusted as ordered so that the infant's head is level with or slightly lower than his body. The oxygen flow is adjusted and tested every five minutes for concentration, to determine whether it is what the physician ordered. After the concentration has been stabilized it should be rechecked every four hours and the results recorded on the patient's chart. Prematures should be kept in 30 to 40 per cent oxygen only as long as they have symptoms of respiratory distress or cyanosis. The infant may be weighed in the incubator daily or according to the physician's order, depending on his size and condition.

If an incubator is not available, other methods of applying heat must be provided. The most commonly used is the hot-water bottle. The procedure for the use of hot-water bottles has been discussed previously (see p. 118).

Maintenance of Respirations

The respirations of the premature may be rapid, shallow and irregular. The abdominal muscles are used, and there may be some periods of apnea. Gentle suction may be needed to clear the respiratory tract of mucus and other fluid. Stomach lavage may be ordered if the secretions are excessive.

A vaporizer should be used to produce the high humidity necessary for premature infants or those born by cesarean section. This is adjusted to produce a humidity within the incubator of 55 per cent or higher. If the respiratory difficulty is relieved, the vaporizer may be discontinued after twenty-four to thirty-six hours. Routine nebulized water is not necessary and may predispose to skin infections and sepsis. High humidity may be obtained in the home through the use of humidifiers, steam kettles, inhalators, or wet towels placed over a radiator. The towels are kept wet by immersing one end in a pan of water.

Ninety-five per cent oxygen and 5 per cent carbon dioxide may be necessary for thirty to 120 seconds every half-hour to one hour for at least twelve hours to stimulate respirations. It is always necessary to clear the pharynx before giving oxygen and carbon dioxide so that the infant does not aspirate the secretions when he inspires.

The infant should be on his side in the incubator in order to get the maximum amount of air into his lungs. If he is inactive, his position should be changed every one to three hours. If artificial respiration is necessary, it should be given very gently (see p. 182).

When the oxygen concentration in the incubator is above 40 per cent, there is danger of development of retrolental fibroplasia (see p. 150). Several methods may be used to limit the concentration of oxygen to the percentage ordered by the physician. The oxygen flow can be adjusted until analysis shows that the desired concentration has been established. A mixture of 40 per cent oxygen and 60 per cent nitrogen can be used in the incubator; by this means the infant cannot receive more than 40 per cent oxygen, and there will be no danger of retrolental fibroplasia. An oxygen-diluting meter can be used to regulate the concentration of oxygen. This device mixes the air of the room with pure oxygen and can be set to produce any concentration ordered by the physician. It is not, however, a substitute for oxygen analysis (see Fig. 8-5), but keeps the range of concentration within limits.

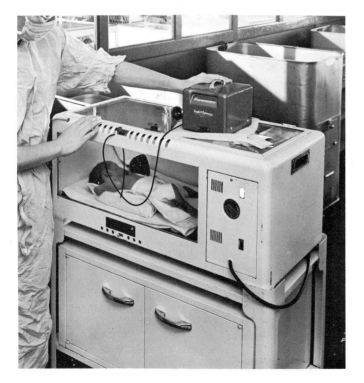

Figure 8–5. Oxygen analyzer. The regulation of oxygen flow does not guarantee that the atmosphere inside the incubator is in accordance with the prescribed atmosphere. The only certain method for determining actual oxygen concentration is to make periodic checks using an oxygen analyzer. (Beckman Scientific and Process Instruments Division, 2500 Fullerton Road, Fullerton, California.)

Oxygen should be given at as low a level as possible in order to afford relief for the infant and should be discontinued as soon as possible.

Charting Oxygen Intake. Each infant's chart should contain a separate oxygen record, which should include (1) the physician's written order for oxygen and its method of administration, (2) the duration of administration, (3) the oxygen concentration, and (4) the infant's response to the concentration and to its duration. The extent of time during which the infant received oxygen must be determined accurately (all interruption in therapy required when caring for the infant must be noted). The oxygen concentration should be analyzed at four-hour intervals, or more frequently if necessary, and charted. The analyzer should be checked periodically against the concentration of oxygen in the air (20.9 per cent oxygen at sea level) and by sampling pure oxygen. If the analyzer provides a correct reading at these extremes, intermediate readings should be reliable. The infant's response, including changes in his color, respirations, pulse, and degree of activity, should be carefully observed and accurately charted.

The danger of giving more oxygen than the infant requires is so well understood that the nurse has a greater responsibility than formerly, when excessive oxygenation was not considered dangerous.

Nutrition

The problem of nutrition in the premature infant is complicated by his difficulty in sucking and in swallowing. Often these reflexes are absent, and he makes no response to stimulation of his lips by a nipple or medicine dropper; food placed in his mouth either runs out or causes him to choke. If he is able to take the feeding or is fed by gavage, the small capacity of his stomach often results in distention and vomiting, which may cause respiratory embarrassment. The gastric acidity is low, and the capacity for absorption of fat is not that of the normal full-term infant. His entire digestive enzyme system is incompletely developed, and he may be unable to handle satisfactorily any type of feeding, even breast milk.

The problem is accentuated by his need for a nutritional intake higher than that of the normal infant, whose weight at birth allows for the initial loss which normally occurs until feeding is established. The premature needs 60 to 80 calories and 3 to 4 gm. of protein per pound of body weight, plus an adequate carbohydrate and liquid intake. Since his ability to absorb fat is poor, skimmed milk rather than whole milk is generally used as the basis for his formula.

Because of the edema present at birth, the premature infant is seldom given a feeding or water by mouth during the first eighteen to twenty-four hours. The initial feeding may be as little as 2 to 4 cc. and may consist solely of a 5 per cent sugar solution. Feedings are slowly increased, and both fat and protein are added to the carbohydrate given in the first few days.

There is no set standard for his feeding; it must be adapted to his individual needs. In general he does not tolerate cow's milk unless the fat and protein content has been altered. If possible, he should be given breast milk, though it may be necessary to dilute it with water. The mother may be able to provide breast milk. If so, it should be expressed manually and given to the infant. The supply is thereby maintained, and the infant may be put to the breast when he is able to suck and swallow adequately.

Mention has been made of breast milk stations where human milk can be bought (see p. 129). Such milk is expensive, however, and it may be difficult to secure a steady supply. Often mothers on the obstetrical unit who have an overabundance of milk will donate the excess to the premature infants in the nursery.

The formula for the premature should be high in protein, low in fat and of average carbohydrate content. Proprietary milks which resemble breast milk in composition are often used.

Methods of Feeding. The method of feeding is extremely important, since there is danger that the infant may aspirate a little of the milk and also since no formula is of advantage unless it is taken and retained. The infant takes so little milk at a feeding that it is generally ordered in cubic centimeters rather than ounces. The warmed feedings are given slowly in small amounts and at frequent intervals. The infant is bubbled frequently. He should never be forced to take the feeding. Underfeeding is less harmful than overfeeding. When feeding a premature in an incubator, he should be held in a semi-sitting position and placed on his right side when he is finished. He should not be permitted to suck longer than twenty minutes at a feeding because he may become too fatigued.

A fixed schedule or an occasional missed feeding may be indicated for weak infants or those whose condition is complicated by vomiting, convulsions, cyanosis or hemorrhage. For an older premature who is gaining weight a flexible schedule is advantageous.

GAVAGE. The infant who is unable to suck or swallow or who becomes fatigued with the effort of nursing or is apt to become cyanotic after feeding by bottle or medicine dropper should be fed by gavage. An indwelling catheter may be used for the infant who cannot suck or swallow. If necessary, mummy restraint may be used (see p. 301).

For gavage feeding the following equipment

is needed: (1) a sterile plastic catheter, no. 5 to 8 French, with a rounded end, (2) the barrel of a glass syringe (sterile), (3) medicine glasses (sterile), (4) sterile water, (5) the warmed formula.

The method of *gavage feeding with an indwelling catheter* (generally inserted by the physician) is as follows:

1. Measure the distance from the bridge of the nose to the lower end of the sternum and place a mark on the catheter.

2. Lubricate the tube with water. Do not use oil, because of the danger of aspiration with subsequent lipoid pneumonia.

3. Insert the catheter through a nostril until the mark is reached.

4. Check for placement of the catheter in the stomach by placing the free end under sterile water in one of the three medicine glasses. If many bubbles rise and then cease, the catheter is in the stomach and the infant is relieved of air which might cause him to vomit during or after the feeding. Bubbles rising periodically, however, are caused by air expelled with each respiration, an indication that the catheter is in the trachea. The infant is then likely to choke and become cyanotic. The tube should be withdrawn at once and reinserted.

Another method to determine the location of the catheter in larger infants and children is by gently aspirating a small amount of stomach contents. This may not be possible in a premature who receives extremely small amounts at each feeding. Only slight suction should be used because of the danger of traumatizing tissue at the end of the catheter. Actually, when gavaging a premature infant, it is relatively difficult to enter the trachea with a gavage tube; however, these tests should be done in order to prevent any possible error.

An additional method to determine the location of the catheter in larger infants and children is by the injection of a small amount of air into the catheter and listening with a stethoscope for its entrance into the stomach. This method should not generally be used for prematures because of the possibility of distention of the infant's stomach with air.

5. When it is certain that the tube is in the stomach, it is taped to the infant's cheek.

6. The barrel of the syringe is connected to the catheter by means of a no. 20 needle which acts as an adaptor.

7. The syringe is held 6 to 8 inches above the infant and the milk poured very slowly into the syringe barrel. No air should precede the milk, and no pressure is used. The milk flows into the infant's stomach by gravity.

8. After the feeding a small amount of sterile water is poured into the syringe to wash out the milk and prevent clogging of the catheter. In a very small infant the amount of sterile water to be used may be ordered by the physician, since overdistention of the stomach may result in vomiting.

9. When the syringe is empty, the catheter may or may not be occluded, depending on the physician's order. Some physicians believe that the tube should be left open, but elevated above the infant's body. If vomiting occurs, the tube acts as a safety valve so that the possibility of aspiration of vomitus is minimized. If the catheter is to be changed, it must be compressed while being withdrawn. This prevents milk from drip-

ping into the pharynx and causing the infant to gag or aspirate it.

10. Place the infant on his right side with a blanket rolled behind him for support.

11. The catheter should be changed at least every four days.

An indwelling catheter is usually thought to be a better procedure to use with small infants than the catheter which is inserted for each feeding.

Gavage feeding without an indwelling catheter differs in several respects from the foregoing procedure. A soft rubber catheter, no. 8 to 10 French, is used. This is passed through the mouth toward the back of the throat. Its location must be tested carefully. The catheter is held in place with the hand near the infant's mouth. The catheter is withdrawn after the feeding and during withdrawal is compressed firmly for the reason given above. Before withdrawal it is a good plan to run sterile water through the catheter at once to clear it of milk and to avoid drippings which might be aspirated.

FEEDING WITH A MEDICINE DROPPER. This method is used for small prematures who have a good swallowing reflex, but cannot suck with sufficient strength to draw the milk through the nipple or cannot swallow rhythmically as they suck. The tip of the medicine dropper is protected with a bit of rubber tubing pulled well over the end of the glass dropper. The soft rubber tubing is less irritating than glass to the delicate mucous membranes of the mouth, and also less dangerous should the tip break. The feeding is given a few drops at a time, with time allowed for the infant to swallow before the bulb is again compressed. If the infant becomes exhausted by this method, he should be fed by gavage until he is stronger.

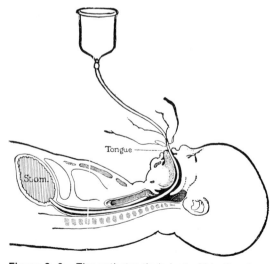

Figure 8–6. The catheter tip is just within the stomach. (Davis and Rubin: *DeLee's Obstetrics for Nurses.* 17th ed.)

BOTTLE FEEDING. Bottle feeding is used with more mature prematures or those with an unusually strong sucking reflex (and adequate ability in swallowing) for their stage of development. There are special nipples on the market for small prematures. If these are not available, a regular nipple which is soft but not flabby may be used. The holes in the nipple should not be so small that the exertion of sucking tires the infant, nor too large, for he might not be able to swallow the milk which fills his mouth as he sucks and as a result might gag or aspirate it. Furthermore, the infant who drains the milk too easily is deprived of the natural satisfaction which sucking brings. The bottle should be held during the entire feeding. Infants large and strong enough to be fed from a bottle also need the closeness and cuddling a mother gives when feeding her child.

Medications

Here are considered only those medications necessary for growth and health.

The premature infant's vitamin requirements are greater than those of the full-term infant, since his antenatal storage of vitamins is incomplete, his growth rate is greater, and the milk given him is small in amount and has been boiled (if he is not breast fed), thereby reducing the vitamin C content. Defective fat absorption reduces the utilization of such fat-soluble vitamins as he receives in his formula. In general he requires 50 mg. a day of vitamin C (this is started as soon as he receives a formula) and 1000 units a day of vitamin D, which is given him within two weeks after birth.

Iron must be added to his intake by about two months of age, but may be given earlier with the hope that he can utilize it if his hemoglobin level is under 8 gm. or if he has lost blood. In general, iron is not well utilized until the second or third month of life.

Prevention of Infection

Gastrointestinal Infections. Infections of the gastrointestinal tract are common in premature infants and are most likely to be caused by contaminated nipples, bottles or other things used in feeding.

Skin Infections. Infections can find entrance through slight trauma to the skin. Some skin infections are transmitted by contact, however; such infections are likely to be transmitted from infant to infant, if equipment is shared in common or if the nurses fail to wash their hands thoroughly after care of each infant. Skin infections may also be contracted from linen which has not been sterilized before use.

BATHING THE INFANT. The incidence of staphylococcal epidemics in nurseries can be reduced through the use of hexachlorophene in soap or solution form. In bathing the premature the nurse should wet her hands, take one teaspoonful of this lotion and work it into a lather. She should apply the lather over all the baby's body, cleansing the diaper area last. She should be careful not to get any lather into the infant's eyes. The lather should then be removed with sterile cotton and water and the infant patted dry with a soft towel.

Respiratory Infections. Organisms that cause respiratory infections are likely to be carried to an infant by the personnel who care for him. The staff caring for prematures should wear gowns and possibly caps. In some hospitals masks are also required, but in other hospitals are considered unnecessary. If one is worn, it should be adjusted properly and changed at least every half hour. A mask should never be used for the purpose of allowing a person having a respiratory infection to enter the nursery.

Organisms causing respiratory infections may be carried by the air from infant to infant. For these reasons each infant should be in strict isolation, and any infant showing signs of a respiratory infection should be removed from the nursery.

In the majority of hospitals airborne organisms are prevented from drifting into the premature nursery, when the door is opened, by an antechamber between the main hall and the nursery.

General Suggestions for Prevention of Infection. No nurse should ever touch a premature unless she has thoroughly cleaned her fingernails and washed her hands and arms to the elbow with ample hexachlorophene soap and running water. Rings and watches must never be worn in the nursery.

Each infant should have his own equipment. All other equipment used for the infants and for their examination should be kept in the nursery, and traffic there should be kept at a minimum.

Supplies such as linens, blankets and cotton should be sterile when brought into the nursery and as far as possible sterile when used in the care of the infants. The outer wrapping of all such equipment should be removed before being brought to the nursery, in an area set aside for the purpose.

Nurses caring for a premature infant who exhibits evidence of infection must not care for the well prematures in the nursery.

There should be no dry dusting or sweeping in the nursery. A damp mopping should be done daily with a clean mop, hot water and a cleansing powder. The daily dusting should be done with a damp cloth.

Treatment of Infections. The premature infant has an unpredictable response to many antibiotics. Doses of medication suitable for infants can cause untoward reactions in a premature who cannot detoxify or excrete them at a rate expected for his size. More research must be done to determine effective yet safe dosages for these infants in order to prevent deaths from toxic levels of drugs.

Diseases of the Premature Infant

The ability to observe and describe symptoms so that the physician has an accurate and reliable account of an infant's symptoms and behavior is one of the chief distinguishing characteristics of the professional nurse. *Important among the observations which a nurse should make of the premature infants under her care are (1) nature of the cry, respirations, color, activity, condition of the skin and umbilicus, and bladder and bowel function; (2) stability of body temperature under slight variations of external environmental conditions; (3) response to feedings in relation to the method used, the swallowing and sucking reflexes, the amount taken and retained and the activity of the infant during feeding; (4) symptoms of unfavorable response to the environment; (5) symptoms of illness, knowledge of which is necessary to the physician's diagnosis and treatment, especially of serious conditions likely to occur in the premature.*

Retrolental Fibroplasia

History. The condition was diagnosed and the cause discovered within the last thirty years. The condition is peculiar to infants under 1500 gm. in weight and of gestational age of six to seven months.

Incidence. Retrolental fibroplasia is the chief cause of neonatal blindness and has re-placed ophthalmia neonatorum as the most common cause of blindness in children. It occurs in the smaller, less mature infants more frequently than in the larger and more fully developed prematures. The condition involves both eyes and may produce complete or almost complete blindness. The effects are not immediately apparent, but can be detected by the physician when the infant is several weeks or months of age.

Etiology. The cause of this condition is oxygen poisoning, the oxygen acting upon the primitive vasculature of the eyes. A high concentration of oxygen causes spasm of the retinal vessels; this leads to exudation of blood and serum through the walls of these vessels.

Pathology. The retinal veins dilate and become tortuous. There is hemorrhage with exudate into the retina, and finally separation of the retina from the inner surface of the eye occurs. Some of these changes may regress, but in other instances they continue until the retina detaches and floats forward in the eye. Eventually the retina may become atrophic, a completely detached and useless fibrotic mass (Fig. 8–7). Some light perception may be present, but the child has no useful vision. Glaucoma may occur in the late stage of the disease, and corneal opacities may result.

Diagnosis. Routine ophthalmoscopic examinations of premature infants should be made so that the condition may be detected early. Such examinations should be begun in the nursery.

Prevention. Oxygen therapy should be given only when an infant is in immediate need of oxygen, and then only in the lowest concentration which will satisfy his need. The concentration should never exceed 40 per cent unless it is needed as a lifesaving measure. Even in this situation oxygen should be discontinued as soon

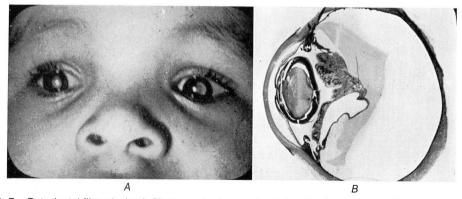

A   B

Figure 8–7. Retrolental fibroplasia. *A,* Photograph of eyes of an infant to show the complete white opacification of the tissues behind the pupil. This is the end-stage of retrolental fibroplasia. *B,* Sagittal section of an eye removed from this child. One sees the entire retina detached and pulled forward toward the lens and a band of scar tissue encircling the posterior aspect of the lens. The whole disorganized mass makes up the retrolental eschar. (From the collection of Dr. Arnall Patz, Baltimore.) (Schaffer: *Diseases of the Newborn.*)

as possible. Physicians order oxygen by concentration rather than by rate of flow. The nurse must check the oxygen concentration in the incubator and adjust the flow so that it does not exceed 40 per cent unless ordered. This requires that an accurate oxygen analyzer be part of the standard equipment of every nursery (see Fig. 8–5). Frequent analysis of oxygen concentration is necessary even if oxygen-limiting devices are used on the incubator.

If the infant's condition is such that he should have a higher oxygen concentration, the exact concentration should be ordered by the physician and not given on the judgment of the nurse, except in dire emergency (the pediatric staff may be asked for routine orders to cover such emergencies). Oxygen therapy should be discontinued as soon as there is no further need for it.

There is no obvious contraindication to the use of oxygen therapy in infants over 5 pounds, but such infants seldom need it, since their respiratory and circulatory systems are more completely developed.

Pulmonary Hyaline Membrane

Incidence. This condition is found in about 50 per cent of premature infants who die within a few days after birth. It seldom occurs in full-term infants, but may develop in infants whose mothers have diabetes or in infants delivered by cesarean section.

Pathology. A membrane is deposited along the walls of the bronchioles, the alveoli and the alveolar ducts.

Etiology. The membrane has been thought to be due to inhalation of amniotic fluid, or it may be formed from extravasated blood or edema fluid.

Course. Respirations are normal for the first two or three hours after birth. Then dyspnea develops. There is retraction of the ribs and lower portion of the sternum. The infant becomes cyanotic, and his rapid, grunting respirations give evidence of his difficulty in breathing. Although death may occur, improvement may come about rapidly if the infant survives for several days.

Prevention and Treatment. Prevention involves many of the factors already mentioned in the delivery and care of the newborn. Cesarean section should be avoided if possible. Mucus and amniotic fluid should be aspirated from the respiratory tract, and the gastric contents from the stomach. If the infant shows signs of difficult breathing, the oxygen content in his environment should be increased and the humidity raised. Research is being done on the use of hyperbaric oxygenation in the treatment of these

infants. Secondary infections are prevented by the use of antibiotics. If an infant has respiratory distress, he should be given nothing by mouth because of the danger of aspiration.

Nursing Care. The nursing care is that of the premature or normal newborn, but with added precautions against aspiration of feeding and with closer observation for a change in condition. The obstetrical nurse rather than the pediatric nurse aids in prevention by good prenatal care and immediate care after birth while the infant is still in the delivery room.

Vomiting

The most common causes of vomiting are overfeeding or too rapid feeding. The preventive, therefore, is reduction of the intake and slow feeding. If the infant's condition permits of his being held for his feeding, he may be bubbled several times during the feeding and before he is put back in his incubator. Abdominal distention not only causes vomiting, but also hinders respiration because of elevation of the diaphragm. Congenital malformation of the esophagus hampers the swallowing of milk, and that taken into the mouth is ejected. Increased intracranial pressure is a serious cause of vomiting, which may be projectile.

The nurse should chart not only the amount, color and nature of the feeding vomited, but also the conditions under which vomiting occurred. This will aid the physician in his diagnosis and may also indicate defective feeding technique on the part of the nurse which she will be anxious to correct.

Diarrhea

A premature infant normally has four or five stools a day. Increased frequency or loose stools are serious in the premature, since he needs all the nutriment of his feeding for metabolism and growth; also he cannot easily tolerate excessive fluid loss. Because of the low tolerance of his gastrointestinal tract for fat, the fat content of his feeding may be the cause of the diarrhea, or overfeeding may be responsible.

Diarrhea in infancy may occur with either an enteral or parenteral infection. The physician should be notified at once and the infant placed on strict isolation so that the infection—if that is the cause of the diarrhea—is not transmitted to other infants in the nursery. Vomiting often accompanies diarrhea and should be carefully observed and charted, since these observations will help the physician in making his diagnosis and planning therapy. Diarrhea can cause death of the premature infant quickly, and therefore immediate therapy is necessary.

Dehydration

Dehydration is more important in infancy than in childhood and even more serious in the premature than in the normal infant. In the premature, dehydration is certain to follow an inadequate fluid intake. It has already been noted that diarrhea and vomiting cause dehydration.

Jaundice

Jaundice in the premature, as in the full-term infant, may be physiologic, i.e. due to bilirubinemia in the early postnatal period. Physiologic jaundice is of no great importance, but jaundice which persists or becomes excessive is indicative of some serious condition, such as erythroblastosis fetalis, congenital anomaly or obstruction of the bile ducts, congenital toxoplasmosis or septicemia. The nursing care is that of the condition causing the jaundice.

Pallor

Pallor accompanies shock and hemorrhage. It is often seen in infants who fail to breathe at birth and may be a symptom of intracranial injury.

Convulsions

One reason why premature infants should be under constant observation is the danger of convulsions. The accompanying anoxia and stress threaten his welfare. The nurse must be there to render care. A description of the convulsion may assist the physician to arrive at a diagnosis and correct the cause if correction is possible. A convulsion may be a symptom of intracranial hemorrhage or of a congenital cerebral defect, or may be the result of prolonged anoxia. It may be caused by hypoglycemia or hypocalcemia or an overwhelming bacteremia.

Prognosis in Prematurity

The premature's chances of survival are much less than those of the full-term infant. Twelve to 20 per cent of prematurely born infants die. About half of all deaths in the first month of life occur in infants classified as prematures. The smaller the infant, the less are his chances of survival. About half of the deaths in the premature group occur on the first day of life.

Causes of Death. Immaturity itself is the fundamental cause of the high death rate among premature infants. Only a small number of those who weigh less than 1000 gm. survive. Respiratory failure is responsible for many deaths. Birth injury such as intracranial hemorrhage with resulting damage to brain tissue may cause immediate death. Congenital malformations may make vital physiologic functions impossible. Infection, as already noted, is far more likely to be fatal to the premature than to the full-term infant, since the premature can neither combat the infection nor withstand its systemic effects. Also, the cause of the prematurity, if known, may affect the ultimate prognosis.

Factors Favoring Survival. Favorable prognostic signs in the premature are a birth weight of more than 1500 gm., good muscle tone and normal respiratory activity. If the infant is not cyanotic and exhibits an active response to stimulation, his immediate condition is likely to be good. When the gag and swallowing reflexes are present, he will be able to take his feedings with less danger of aspirating fluid. The importance of stabilization of body temperature has been shown. Absence of other serious conditions is additionally hopeful.

Parental Problems Due to Prematurity

The birth of a premature infant presents a crisis for the family. Usually, unless the mother has expected a multiple birth and knows that the infants may be premature, she has no warning and is therefore not prepared for the event. After a fast trip to the hospital following the onset of labor, she is usually treated with some degree of apprehension and is rushed to the delivery room to give birth to her infant without anesthesia.

The mother may or may not see her infant before he is placed in the incubator. If she does see him, his unattractive appearance may startle her.

Although the parents may have many questions after the birth, physicians and nurses often avoid answering them directly because they do not want to arouse either false hope or despair. The parents may sense the air of suspense concerning the infant's condition with resulting anxiety and fear. Furthermore, when the mother is ready for discharge, she must leave her frail infant in the nursery until he weighs 5 or $5\frac{1}{2}$ pounds. This may mean separation from the parents for weeks or months.

As with other crisis situations, parents should be helped to confront their problem realistically instead of trying to pretend that it does not exist. Ways to help such parents include the physician's discussing frankly the infant's condition with them, having both parents speak of their fears for the infant, and having nurses who understand the degree of anxiety such parents feel. Also, friends can function in a beneficial way if they are willing to help with necessary tasks and if, instead of sending the usual "get well" cards, they send wishes that indicate their concern for the infant's survival.

The mother who is told realistically what chances for life her infant has may not be comforted, nor is she necessarily made less anxious, but she is probably less frightened about the future than the mother who is afraid to ask the question, "Will my baby live?"

Many mothers of premature infants try to blame someone or something for this unfortunate event, even though the real cause of the prematurity may not be known. An individual mother may blame an older child because he asked to be lifted up, her husband because he did not carry the groceries or the laundry for her, or the physician or the nurse for some imagined failure in therapy. The process of blaming is one way to avoid facing the truth and does not contribute to coming out of this crisis strengthened.

If the infant dies, the parents should be helped to mourn and not merely be told that they should forget about him and have another child. Unfortunately such advice has been too freely given. (See page 73 for a discussion of the ways nurses can help the parents of a dying child.)

If the infant lives, the parents need an opportunity to learn to care for him before he is discharged from the nursery. They need encouragement in learning to handle a small, delicate infant, although by the time he is discharged he is almost the size of a normal newborn. In many hospitals areas are set aside where parents can attend demonstrations of the care of the infant, including bathing, dressing, methods of formula preparation and feeding techniques. As they practice these techniques, they gain confidence in their own abilities and have less anxiety over the infant's care.

The nurse should also emphasize the protective care of the infant in the home environment. She should stress principles of safety and hygiene throughout all her teaching. She should also give anticipatory counselling about the infant's probable growth and development even though the physician will also follow the child's growth in the future.

If the mother is a clinic patient whose infant will be followed up by a public health nurse and will attend the Child Health Conference, she should meet the nurse who will visit her home and should be made familiar with the help which will be given her. The public health nurse should visit the home before the infant's discharge to evaluate the setting and to make suggestions as to how conditions may be improved for the infant's welfare. She should make suggestions as to his physical environment, including the equipment needed in his care, and should evaluate the mother's feelings about the infant. The public health nurse should also visit the family after the infant's discharge from the hospital in order to give necessary guidance and assistance.

Mothers in the middle class have probably read a great deal about premature infants and may have studied their characteristics and care in college classes on child development. These mothers understand the theory of premature care, but need help in putting it into practice. Since they are not likely to be clinic patients and to receive the routine help of a public health nurse, they are in even greater need of an opportunity to care for the infant while he is still in the hospital.

Mothers of premature infants often worry for fear that the infant will not develop normally and will be mentally retarded, frail and small. This is not wholly so, and the nurse may tell the mother that studies of children born prematurely show that by and large they develop more rapidly than infants born at term, and that if age were dated from the time of conception rather than from birth, prematures are frequently on a par with infants born at term. Any lag in development of the premature in comparison with term infants tends to decrease with age and at the end of several years to become indistinguishable.

In early infancy the premature may appear backward in motor control, less so in sensory acuity, but still not up to the level of the normal infant. Prematurity does not influence intelligence, but emotional and social behavior is likely to be less mature than in children born at term. Some premature infants tend to develop undesirable behavior patterns. They may be overdependent and are likely to be negativistic. This is largely due to the overprotective attitude of his parents in infancy and to later pressure upon him to catch up with other children of his age. He is confused by the change of attitude and finds it difficult to adjust to the new demands made upon him.

Probably helping the mother to feel secure in her ability to care for the premature is the most important factor in forming good mother-child relations. If such a relation exists, a mother is not afraid to correct the child. She should let the child experience the minimal frustrations that occur in daily life and develop early independence.

POSTMATURITY

The infant who remains in the uterus from one to three weeks or more after the expected date of delivery is classified as postmature. About 5 per cent of newborn infants are born postmaturely.

Characteristics of Postmature Infants. The postmature infant has the behavior and appearance of an infant from one to three weeks of age. He is more mature, mentally alert and thinner than the normal newborn infant. His nails and scalp hair are longer than those of a full-term infant, and he has no lanugo or vernix caseosa on his skin. His skin may be peeling and appear to have the consistency of parchment. These infants generally do not exceed 23 inches in length.

Treatment. Labor may be induced before the cervix is soft, but such treatment may pose a greater risk than postmaturity. Cesarean section may be done on older women having their first infants, especially if the fetus shows signs of distress.

Prognosis. Among infants born three or more weeks after the expected date the mortality rate is likely to be two to three times greater than that among infants born at term.

Placental Dysfunction Syndrome

One possible cause of postmaturity is the placental dysfunction syndrome. In this con-dition the placenta does not function adequately in the nutritional and oxygen exchange between mother and fetus. As a result the fetus does not grow properly.

Etiology. The etiology of placental dysfunction syndrome may be toxemia of pregnancy, syphilis, advanced maternal age or an unknown cause.

Clinical Manifestations. Evidences of fetal distress appear as a result of oxygen lack *in utero.* The vernix, umbilical cord, skin and nails absorb bile pigment from the released meconium. In mild degrees the nails and vernix are stained green. In more severe forms they are stained bright yellow. In infants who do not live, lanugo hairs and evidences of meconium can be found in the finer branches of the bronchial tree, probably due to the vigorous respiratory efforts of the fetus resulting from hypoxia.

Treatment and **nursing care** of these infants center on their respiratory difficulties.

Prognosis. If the newborn lives for the first forty-eight hours, his chances for survival are good.

TEACHING AIDS AND OTHER INFORMATION*

Association for the Aid of Crippled Children

Baumgartner, L., Eliot, M., and Verhoestraete, L.: The Challenge of Fetal Loss, Prematurity, and Infant Mortality.

National Society for the Prevention of Blindness, Inc.

Prevent Retrolental Fibroplasia in Premature Infants with Oxygen Control.

Ross Laboratories

Your Premature Infant.

United States Department of Health, Education, and Welfare

Weight at Birth and Cause of Death in the Neonatal Period, United States, Early 1950, 1965.
Weight at Birth and Survival of the Newborn, by Age of Mother and Total-Birth Order, United States, Early 1950, 1965.
Weight at Birth and Survival of the Newborn by Geographic Divisions and Urban and Rural Areas, United States, Early 1950, 1965.
Your Premature Baby, 1963.

REFERENCES

Publications

American Academy of Pediatrics Committee on Fetus and Newborn: *Standards and Recommendations for Hospital Care of Newborn Infants.* Evanston, Ill., American Academy of Pediatrics, 1964.
Avery, M. E.: *The Lung and Its Disorders in the Newborn Infant.* 2nd ed. Philadelphia, W. B. Saunders Company, 1968.
Babson, S. G., and Benson, R. C.: *Primer on Prematurity and High-Risk Pregnancy.* St. Louis, C. V. Mosby Company, 1966.

*Complete addresses are given in the Appendix.

Bookmiller, M. M., Bowen, G. L., and Carpenter, D.: *Textbook of Obstetrics and Obstetric Nursing.* 5th ed. Philadelphia, W. B. Saunders Company, 1967.

Craig, W. S.: *Care of the Newly Born Infant.* 3rd ed. Baltimore, Williams & Wilkins Company, 1966.

Crosse, V. M.: *The Premature Baby.* 6th ed. Boston, Little, Brown and Company, 1966.

Davis, M. E., and Rubin, R.: *DeLee's Obstetrics for Nurses.* 18th ed. Philadelphia, W. B. Saunders Company, 1966.

Drillien, C. M.: *Growth and Development of the Prematurely Born Infant.* Baltimore, Williams & Wilkins Company, 1964.

Haselkorn, F. (Ed.): *Mothers-at-Risk: The Role of Social Work in Prevention of Morbidity in Infants of Socially Disadvantaged Mothers.* Garden City, New York, Adelphi University School of Social Work, 1966.

Liebman, S. D., and Gellis, S. S. (Eds.): *The Pediatrician's Ophthalmology.* St. Louis, C. V. Mosby Company, 1966.

Leifer, G.: *Principles and Techniques in Pediatric Nursing,* Philadelphia, W. B. Saunders Company, 1965.

Pittinger, C. B.: *Hyperbaric Oxygenation.* Springfield, Ill., Charles C Thomas, 1966.

Schaffer, A. J.: *Diseases of the Newborn.* 2nd ed. Philadelphia, W. B. Saunders Company, 1965.

Silverman, W. A.: *Dunham's Premature Infants.* 3rd ed. New York, Harper and Brothers, 1961 (Second Printing, 1964).

Willson, J. R., Beecham, C. T., and Carrington, E. R.: *Obstetrics and Gynecology,* 3rd ed. St. Louis, C. V. Mosby Company, 1966.

Periodicals

Bettering The Odds for Survival. *Medical World News,* 9:42, March 1, 1968.

Boxall, J. F.: Are Premature Infants No Longer Individuals? *Nursing Times,* 62:421, March 25, 1966.

Callon, H. F.: The Premature Infant's Nurse. *Am. J. Nursing,* 63:103, February 1963.

Cook, C. D., and Cochran, W. D.: The Respiratory Distress Syndrome of Newborn Infants. *New England J. Med.,* 270:673, 1964.

Cort, R. L.: Clinical Observations in Newborn Premature Infants. *Arch. Dis. Childhood,* 37:53, February 1962.

Davidson, M., and others: Feeding Studies in Low-Birth-Weight Infants. *J. Pediat.,* 70:695, May 1967.

Drug Hazards to the Premature. *J.A.M.A.,* 203:26, January 29, 1968.

Flatter, P. A.: Hazards of Oxygen Therapy. *Am. J. Nursing,* 68:80, 1968.

Ghosh, S., and Daga, S.: Comparison of Gestational Age and Weight as Standards of Prematurity. *J. Pediat.,* 71:173, 1967.

Gore, G. V.: Retrolental Fibroplasia and I.Q. *New Outlook for the Blind,* 60:10:305, December 1966.

Gorten, M. K., and Cross, E. R.: Iron Metabolism in Premature Infants. *J. Pediat.,* 64:509, 1964.

Hargrove, C. S.: Hyaline Membrane Disease. *RN,* 30:78, February 1967.

Irwin, T.: High-Risk Care Saves Lives and Minds. *Today's Health,* 46:42, January 1968.

Isler, C.: Help for the Victims of Retrolental Fibroplasia. *RN,* 30:37, August 1967.

Lowenfeld, B.: The Impact of Retrolental Fibroplasia. *New Outlook for the Blind,* 57:402, 1963.

Oski, F. A., and Barness, L. A.: Vitamin E Deficiency: A Previously Unrecognized Cause of Hemolytic Anemia in the Premature Infant. *J. Pediat.* 70:211, 1967.

New Parameters in Neonatal Growth — Cell Number and Cell Size. *J. Pediat.,* 71:459, 1967.

Rose, P. A.: The High Risk Mother-Infant Dyad — A Challenge for Nursing? *Nursing Forum,* VI:94, November 1967.

Slatin, M.: Extra Protection for High-Risk Mothers and Babies. *Am. J. Nursing,* 67:1241, 1967.

"Vulnerable" Mothers, Infants Aided by Pilot Program. *Today's Health,* 46:45, January 1968.

9

THE IMPORTANCE OF HEREDITY AND ENVIRONMENT IN DISEASES OF CHILDREN

Whether a newborn or older child is healthy or has a hereditary disease or a congenital disease or anomaly depends on many factors, which can be grouped under the main headings of *heredity* and *environment.* These are discussed broadly in Chapter 2; however, the student must have a more specific knowledge of their influence if she is to understand the causes of many of the diseases of children. This chapter is therefore a brief review of the theory of genetics learned earlier in the student's educational experience.

HEREDITY

The term *heredity* means the transmission of potential traits from the parents to their children. The life of each child begins with a fertilized egg or *zygote* composed of cytoplasm and a nucleus. Within the nucleus there are genes on the chromosomes. Many defects found in children can be traced to abnormalities of the chromosomes and genes; however, even if the components of the zygote are normal, a child may have abnormalities due to an injurious *environment in utero.*

Chromosomes are threadlike structures which carry the genes. In the human being each sperm and each egg carry a set of twenty-three chromosomes, twenty-two of which are somatic chromosomes, numbered from 1 to 22 in order of decreasing size, plus one sex chromosome. After the egg and the sperm have united at conception, the fertilized egg contains forty-four autosomes (twenty-two pairs) and two sex chromosomes. Many of these chromosomes can be identified under the microscope by their shape. Each chromosome in the egg can be matched with one in the sperm cell except for those that determine the sex of the individual. These consist of two large X chromosomes in the female and one large X and a smaller Y chromosome in the male.

The *karyotype* shows the chromosome constitution of the normal human somatic cell or a photographic representation of the human chromosomes arranged in pairs or groups in the order of descending size or position of the centromere or constricted area which joins the two chromatids of any metaphase chromosome.

Chromosomes are composed of nucleic acid and protein. Chemically speaking, the genes within the chromosome are composed of nucleic acid, of the type known as deoxyribonucleic acid (DNA). *DNA* is now generally accepted as being the storehouse of genetic information. Some evidence seems to indicate that genes, the units of heredity, are actually segments of DNA and that possibly many thousands of genes exist in each DNA molecule. The structure of a DNA molecule is like a rope ladder which has been twisted around itself or is in the form of a double helix.

Deoxyribonucleic acid plays an important role in determining hereditary characteristics. Each gene carries instruction about a particular trait or characteristic of the organism. Like the chromosomes, the genes are also paired. A pair of genes may carry the same or different instructions. For a *particular trait,* if the two members of a pair of genes carry similar instructions, the person is said to be *homozygous*. If the two members carry different instructions, the person is said to be *heterozygous*. In this situation the trait that results is determined by one member of the pairs of genes. This gene is then *dominant*. The gene whose trait is not manifested is *recessive*.

Dominant abnormal traits are relatively rare, but when they do occur, the person is usually heterozygous. This person has one dominant pathologic gene and one recessive normal gene for the trait under discussion. If such a person marries someone who is free of this trait and has two normal recessive genes, there is statistically a 50 per cent chance of their offspring having or not having this trait. If one of the unaffected children marries a normal person, none of their children will be affected, but if one of the affected children marries a normal person, the possibilities are that half of their children will carry the trait on their gene. Examples of pathologic conditions discussed in this text which may be inherited as dominant traits include osteogenesis imperfecta, sicklemia and thalassemia minor. In some instances a dominant trait may skip a generation, or the transmitting person may carry the anomaly without clinical manifestations.

If a person who has an abnormal recessive gene paired with a normal dominant gene marries a person who has two normal genes for the

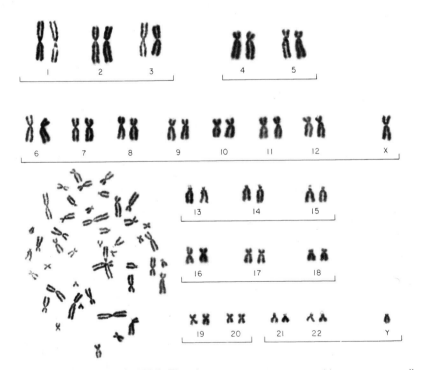

Figure 9–1. Normal male karyotype (× 2200). The chromosomes are arranged in groups according to size. The approximate length of chromosome number 1 is 7 microns. The somatic cell from which the karyotype was structured is also shown. (From A. G. Bearn; in P. B. Beeson and W. McDermott (Eds.): Cecil-Loeb *Textbook of Medicin.* 12th ed.)

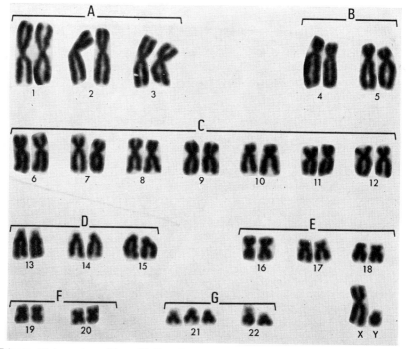

Figure 9–2. Trisomy 21 karyotype. (From Walker, Carr, Sergovich, Barr and Soltan: *J. Ment. Defic. Res.,* 7:150-163, 1963.)

trait discussed, the children will be normal. If that heterozygous person marries another heterozygous person, however, each child would have one chance out of four to be homozygous for the trait, i.e. affected by the pathologic trait. Half of the children of such a union would be heterozygous for the trait, like their parents; they would seem normal, but would carry the pathologic gene. On the other hand, if two persons marry, both of whom are homozygous and have an abnormal recessive trait, all their children will be abnormal.

Pathologic conditions which may show autosomal recessive inheritance include Tay-Sachs disease, mucoviscidosis, galactosemia, phenylketonuria, sickle cell anemia and thalassemia major. These clinical conditions may also result from genes which have undergone mutation.

Mutation causing abnormal gene development is a process which is not completely understood. *Mutation* means a fundamental change in the structure of a gene which results in the transmission of a trait different from that normally carried by the gene. Research has been done on high-energy radiation as one cause of mutations. Such radiation can come from cosmic rays, radium, x-rays and isotopes. We do not know exactly how much radiation a human being can be exposed to safely. Heat and some chemicals have also been found to be mutagenic agents.

Mutations can change the genetic constitu-

tion of the child so that body function is changed. These have been termed *inborn errors of metabolism.* Such mutations produce biochemical disorders (resulting from a deficiency of an essential body chemical), which are evidenced in anomalies of metabolism. Many structures of the body can be affected. In some conditions only a single known enzyme is affected. In other conditions the defect has not yet been identified, so that it is classified by the deficiency of some normal product which should be present or by the abnormal product which accumulates in the body.

Inborn errors of metabolism do not produce symptoms which can be recognized at birth. Examples of such conditions are agamma-globulinemia (a manifestation of a defect in plasma protein metabolism—immunoproteins) and phenylketonuria (a manifestation of a defect in metabolism and transport of an amino acid—phenylalanine). These conditions will be discussed in Chapter 14.

Certain characteristics such as color blindness and certain diseases such as hemophilia are sex-linked. As was mentioned above, in males the sex chromosomes are unequal in size, the X chromosome being large and the Y chromosome small. The X chromosome carries many genes. The Y chromosome is concerned only with maleness. The X chromosome of the male therefore has genes which are not matched with those of the Y chromosome. If a gene located in the X chromosome of the male is not normal, it

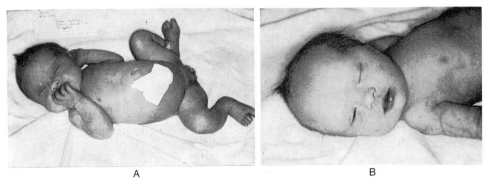

A   B

Figure 9–3. A, Over-all view of mongoloid infant made on the second day of life. General hypotonia is suggested by the relaxed appearance in what appears to be an awkward position. B, Head and face of the infant show the round, short skull, well developed epicanthus, slanting of lid slits upward from within outward, and shallow orbits. (Schaffer: *Diseases of the Newborn.*)

can become evident even if it is recessive. Thus the X chromosome of the female passes the characteristic to the next generation of male children. This is the reason why certain hereditary pathologic traits such as that for hemophilia A may be seen in the males of the family and only rarely in the females.

Some genes lead to congenital defects which are incompatible with life. These defects may cause death *in utero* or soon after birth.

Recently anomalies have been associated with abnormal size and configuration of chromosomes and abnormal chromosome counts rather than with alterations of specific genes. Sometimes during cell formation two chromosomes fail to separate at cell division. The nucleus of one daughter cell has one more and the other one less than the normal number of chromosomes. This process is termed *nondisjunction.* There is apparently no cause for most cases of non-

disjunction; however, they seem to occur more often in the cells of older parents.

When an extra representative of any chromosome is present *(trisomy),* a number of abnormal traits characteristic of that chromosome will appear. When this germ cell unites with a normal one at the time of fertilization, the embryo that results will have an abnormal chromosome count. If the embryo survives, it will have various congenital defects. Probably the best known example of trisomy is Down's syndrome (mongolism), in which there are usually forty-seven chromosomes, with an extra chromosome number 21. This condition may be called trisomy 21. A few children have this chromosomal material arranged not as a separate chromosome, but as a *translocation* of the long arm of the twenty-first chromosome onto either a chromosome of the D group (13-15) or another chromosome of the G group (21-22). (See Figure 11-27, page 221).

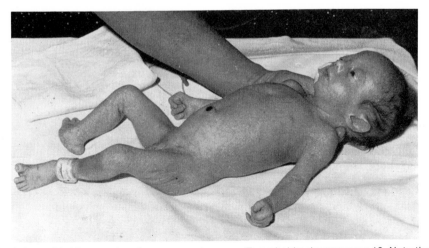

Figure 9–4. Infant with trisomy of a chromosome in group E, probably chromosome 18. Note the overlapping fingers, rocker-bottom feet, simplified patterns of the ear, and dorsiflexion of the big toe. (Courtesy of D. H. Carr, in Thompson and Thompson: *Genetics in Medicine.*)

Two other conditions besides Down's syndrome are caused by chromosomal abnormalities. These are the trisomy 16-18 syndrome and the trisomy 13-15 syndrome. Since they occur very rarely, they will be discussed no further in this text. With further research in this area more chromosomal defects will be found associated with clinical abnormalities.

ENVIRONMENT

The geneticist is intensely interested in the environment of the embryo and the fetus because it is difficult to distinguish between the influences of heredity and those of environment. Prenatal development takes place within the shelter of the uterus; however, various influences—infectious, endocrine, mechanical, nutritional, irradiation and chemical agents—may affect the growing organism.

The organism is most vulnerable to injury during the first trimester *(embryonic period)* of pregnancy, when the principal organ systems of the body are forming. During the *fetal period,* or the last six months of pregnancy, when the fetus is growing, injury may occur, but major anomalies do not result.

Infections such as rubella and toxoplasmosis may cause congenital anomalies in the embryo during the first trimester of pregnancy. Although rubella is usually a mild disease, the virus may penetrate the placental barrier and damage the developing embryonic tissue. It is important, therefore, that each woman should develop immunity to this disease before childbearing age. This means that exposure should be planned so that immunity can be obtained. If a woman is not immune and contracts rubella in the first eight weeks of her pregnancy, the chance of her producing a grossly defective infant is one in three or four. Problems associated with congenital rubella include cardiac lesions, microcephaly, brain damage, eye disorders and deafness.

Infections occurring later in the prenatal period produce clinical manifestations similar to those which would be seen after birth. The spirochete causing syphilis can infect a fetus before it is born. The mother should be adequately treated with penicillin before the birth of her child. Abnormal endocrine factors, such as exist in the diabetic mother, may influence the development of the embryo. Mechanical injury due to pressure from outside the mother's body may result in the death of the embryo or fetus. Positional defects due to pressure from the uterus or a portion of his own body may deform the jaw, face or legs of the growing organism.

The mother's nutritional state is important, since the fetus requires adequate nutrition. Without it, either death *in utero* or deformity may result. Experience with infants born in concentration camps during World War II and in areas where the level of living is down to little more than the maintenance level has shown the deleterious influence of poor maternal nutrition upon the fetus. Nevertheless the fetus tends to be nourished at the expense of the mother's body.

Irradiation of a pregnant woman's abdomen may cause malformations of the embryo, especially if it is done very early in the course of pregnancy. X-ray examination of the abdomen of any woman of childbearing age should be done only during the first two weeks after a regular menstrual period. Research is being done on the effect on the children of irradiation of fathers near the time of conception.

Injury to the fetus from the use of chemicals by the mother has had wide publicity. Drugs found to be teratogenic include thalidomide, which causes defects of the limbs mainly, but may also cause deformities of the heart, kidneys and blood vessels.

There is some question also as to whether LSD and other hallucinogenic drugs may cause abnormalities. Current research shows that potentially all drugs can cross the placenta, but many variables determine whether a drug has a teratogenic or a depressant effect on the fetus. The nurse should caution all pregnant women with whom she comes in contact to take *no* medications except those prescribed for her by her physician.

In summary, it may be stated that most congenital deformities are the result of the interaction between genetic and environmental factors, and that often more than one anomaly may occur in the same fetus. There may be abnormal development of any part of the body or of any organ.

HEREDITARY AND CONGENITAL DISEASES AND ANOMALIES

It has been noted that *hereditary diseases* and a tendency to certain diseases are fixed at the time of conception. In contrast, *congenital disease* is acquired while the infant is *in utero.* Congenital disease, then, is subject to preventive medicine. Prenatal care of the prospective mother is not only for her sake, but also for the health of the fetus.

Congenital deformities or anomalies are extremely important, since many of them permanently disable a child. The influence of anomalies upon the child's personality cannot be disregarded; many of them limit his social life and activities of daily living.

Congenital anomalies are structural anomalies present at birth. They may be obvious on examination of the newborn, or they may be defects of histologic structure.

One of the reasons why more deaths occur in the first month than during the remaining months of the first year of life is that many congenital abnormalities are compatible with intrauterine life, but not with extrauterine life. Approximately 15 per cent of deaths in the neonatal period are caused by such gross malformations.

The application of medical knowledge to the prevention of congenital malformations has not changed the incidence to any great extent, and the problem remains one of the most important in the field of preventive medicine.

Parents' and Nurse's Reaction to an Imperfect Infant, and How the Nurse Can Help the Parents With This Problem

Parental education should include the possibility of giving birth to an imperfect infant. In a class with other prospective parents, husbands and wives together can consider this possibility objectively. If their first knowledge on the subject comes when their child is born with a disease or an anomaly, it is difficult for them to maintain an objective point of view. Men and women of marriageable age should know that prevention begins with conception, i.e. impregnation of the ovum by a spermatozoon, neither of which carries genes causing hereditary abnormality. Once the ovum has been impregnated, medical care is no longer centered on the unfortunate combination of disease- or abnormality-bearing genes which might have been avoided, but rather on the developing fetus.

Parents have an aversion to the idea of something inherent in themselves which has been or could be transmitted to their children. Primitive people were not alone in their belief that a congenital malformation or illness was punishment for wrongdoing. Even modern parents, when told that their child has a congenital anomaly, will many times respond with some such statement as, "What did I do wrong during my pregnancy?" "What did my husband do wrong in the past?" "What have we ever done to others to deserve this?" "What great sin did we commit that our child has to suffer so much?"

When a defect is discovered in a newborn infant, the physician is responsible for telling the parents the sad news. After the parents have been told that an imperfect infant has been born, it is only natural that they evidence disappointment, grief, and despair. The perfect infant they had anticipated was born an imperfect human being.

In the instance of discovery of a defect in a newborn, the parents need to be helped to stay with their responsibility. They, especially the father initially, need help in making necessary decisions, such as when surgery is necessary immediately after birth. As a matter of fact, although exceptions may be made, depending on the individual mother, father and physician, the mother should be helped to see her infant and care for him if possible so that the period of separation of mother and child is minimized. Some physicians believe that a mother should be protected from seeing her malformed infant for several days after his birth. In this situation, if the child dies, the mother will have to mourn for him on the basis of fantasy and not reality.

Most parents feel some degree of guilt and blame others or feel self-blame for their infant's condition. If the mother can be helped to see that an abnormal condition in her infant is not her fault, nor that of her husband, and that the physician is not to blame, she is more likely to accept the condition realistically and adjust to the infant's needs.

When parents continue to assume their responsibilities to satisfy their needs to be mothers and fathers, nurses should encourage them, because this is how they learn to know their child as a person. If the parents are truly involved, their despair or guilt may turn toward more adequate problem-solving.

When a hereditary disease is discovered later in the child's life it must be discussed in an honest, matter-of-fact manner. The nurse should have some knowledge of what has been discussed so that she can support and assist the parents in the most appropriate way.

After the immediate action on the problem the members of the health team, including the nurse, must help the parents to face the situation realistically so that they do not go shopping around for a magical cure. The parents must be helped to plan for therapy, if anything can be done about the problem, to capitalize on the child's assets, and to become familiar with the patterns of growth and development of such children. In order to help the parents in this way, the nurse should know the therapy that can be carried out in the various types of malformations and conditions, and their eventual prognoses.

The nurse should help the mother discuss her feelings about her ill infant, whether of guilt, embarrassment, anger or fear, but she should not probe for information. If the mother wishes to talk, the nurse should demonstrate nonverbal and verbal acceptance and understanding by her support and warmth.

After the mother's discharge and prior to the infant's discharge from the hospital, especially if the mother has been unable to accept his problem, the public health nurse may encourage her to return to the nursery to see her infant. If such a mother can then express her feelings, she may be better able to mother her baby in spite of what the future may hold.

The nurse can help parents create positive yet realistic attitudes toward their defective child. They must be helped to rid themselves of guilt feelings in order to prevent their treating the child too permissively. If they do not help him toward whatever degree of maturity and independence he is capable of, they will be failing in their responsibility of preparing him for life.

Parents, also, if their guilt feelings are intense, may so focus their attention on the defective child that the normal children in the family are not given the emotional care they need for healthy development. It may also be true that the mother focuses so much attention on the child that the father feels neglected.

The attitude which parents develop toward their imperfect child will in many ways be the attitude his siblings, peers, relatives and other members of the community will develop toward him. If a misfortune is accepted as a part of life, the manner of life may have to be changed accordingly, but in most situations the child can still learn to enjoy his areas of normality to the fullest as an individual and as a community member.

Since some malformed infants require prolonged care and training, the nurse should be cognizant of the care facilities and the financial resources available in her community and state which can assist such parents and their children. She should learn the ways these children can be referred to such sources of help.

Much of the information learned in Chapter 4 concerning the manner by which a nurse can comfort and further assist the parents when their child is dying can be utilized when a child is born with a hereditary or congenital disease or anomaly.

The nurse who cares for an imperfect infant faces several challenges. The physical aspects of the infant's care may be complex. The specific care of these infants will be discussed in later chapters in this text.

The nurse in addition to the parents may be emotionally disturbed by the infant who has a hereditary or congenital disease or anomaly. Before she can be of support to the family of the child she must be aware of her own feelings. The nurse's feelings about the various conditions of the newborn involve her attitude toward both the affected infant and his parents. Her attitude also may be complicated by imagining how she would feel if the infant were her own.

If the student has difficulty in handling her feelings comfortably, she should seek the guidance of her instructor so that she can achieve a positive, helping relationship with the parents and a less stressful experience for herself in providing care for the child.

Great strides have been made in genetics, not all of which can be included in this text. The student is referred to the references at the end of this chapter for further explanation of specific areas of interest.

Genetic Counseling

Many young married couples are concerned about the advisability of having a child if the one they had was not normal, or more children if there is a family history of a disease or anomaly. Often the probabilities of offspring being affected by hereditary diseases or transmitting them in the future to their children can be predicted through a thorough study of the parents' family histories and genetic make-ups. Parents want to find out precisely what the disease may be, how their child can be treated or cured, and whether it is in fact a familial disease which will occur in other children of the family living or yet unborn.

The nurse is in no position to give advice on this subject. She can, however, cooperate by sharing information concerning the family with another member of the health team such as a physician who knows the couple well or a genetic specialist who can help them to consider all the factors involved. Even a geneticist would find it difficult to tell a couple exactly what to do about having a child or more children, but he could tell them what their chances might be of having a child with a defect.

The nurse who has been supportive of parents in their time of crisis, whether at the time of the death of one or more of their children, possibly due to mucoviscidosis or some other problem, may be sought once again for support in forming a decision as to whether they should have more children. As was mentioned previously, although she is not qualified to counsel in this area, she can support them in the decision they have made after discussion with the physician or geneticist.

The area of genetic counseling may indeed play a large part in the efforts of preventive medicine in the future. The nurse as a member of the health team will have a role to play in assisting other health team members in their work.

THE COLLABORATIVE PROJECT

In order to try to determine why one out of five pregnancies fails to produce a healthy, living child, why so many mentally retarded or otherwise congenitally defective children are born, and why so many of these have mental or physical handicaps caused by damage to the nervous system, fifteen of the leading medical centers in the United States, in cooperation with the Public Health Service's National Institute of Neurologic Diseases and Blindness, are carrying out what is known as the *Collaborative Project on Cerebral Palsy, Mental Retardation, and Other Neurological and Sensory Disorders of Infancy and Childhood.* The purpose of this Collaborative Project is to try to determine the roles played by heredity, environment, psychologic aspects, sickness or accident of the mother, and other factors occurring before, during or after birth in producing defects of the child. Some 50,000 mothers and their children are to be studied in the project. These mothers are examined, observed and interviewed at routine intervals. The results are recorded along with data concerning pregnancy, labor and delivery, and the growth and development of the child from birth through school age.

Although the main focus of this study is on neurologic and sensory disorders, other related areas are being studied, such as growth and development noted above. Some diseases in children, such as inborn errors of metabolism (phenylketonuria among others) that cause toxic effects on the brain producing certain types of mental retardation, have only recently been discovered. It is hoped that other causes of defects in children will be discovered in the years to come as a result of this Collaborative Project.

TEACHING AIDS AND OTHER INFORMATION*

The National Foundation–March of Dimes

Birth Defects—Social and Emotional Problems.
Birth Defects; The Tragedy and the Hope.
Chemistry, Chromosomes, and Congenital Anomalies.
Corner, G. W.: Congenital Malformations: The Problem and the Task.
Genes in Families and in Populations.
The Riddle of the Chromosomes.

United States Department of Health, Education, and Welfare

Genetics and the Epidemiology of Chronic Diseases.
The Fateful Months When Life Begins: A Nationwide Collaborative Mother-Child Study.

REFERENCES

Publications

Arey, L. B.: *Developmental Anatomy.* 7th ed. Philadelphia, W. B. Saunders Company, 1965.
Balinsky, B. I.: *An Introduction to Embryology.* 2nd ed. Philadelphia, W. B. Saunders Company, 1965.
Barnes, A. C.: *Intra-Uterine Development.* Philadelphia, Lea & Febiger, 1968.
Chipman, S. S., and others: *Research Methodology and Needs in Perinatal Studies.* Springfield, Ill., Charles C Thomas, 1966.
Crew, F. A.: *The Foundations of Genetics.* New York, Pergamon Press, Inc., 1966.
Hsia, D. Y.: *Medical Genetics.* Chicago, Year Book Medical Publishers, Inc., 1966.
Knudson, A. G.: *Genetics and Disease.* New York, McGraw-Hill Book Company, Inc., 1965.
Reed, S. C.: *Counseling in Medical Genetics.* 2nd ed. Philadelphia, W. B. Saunders Company, 1963.
Roberts, J. A. F.: *An Introduction to Medical Genetics.* 4th ed. New York, Oxford University Press, 1967.
Rubin, A. (Ed.): *Handbook of Congenital Malformations.* Philadelphia, W. B. Saunders Company, 1967.
Scheinfeld, A.: *Your Heredity and Environment.* Philadelphia, J. B. Lippincott Company, 1965.
Smith, A.: *Genetics in Medicine.* Baltimore, Williams & Wilkins Company, 1966.
Thompson, J. S., and Thompson, M. W.: *Genetics in Medicine.* Philadelphia, W. B. Saunders Company, 1966.
Valentine, G. H.: *The Chromosome Disorders.* Philadelphia, J. B. Lippincott Company, 1966.
Williams, P. L., Wendell-Smith, C. P., and Treadgold, S.: *Basic Human Embryology,* Philadelphia, J. B. Lippincott Company, 1966.

Periodicals

Apgar, V.: Drugs in Pregnancy, *Am. J. Nursing,* 65:104, March 1965.
Boggs, T. R., Hardy, J. B., and Frazier, T. M.: Correlation of Neonatal Serum Total Bilirubin Concentrations and Developmental Status at Age Eight Months. (A Preliminary Report from the Collaborative Project) *J. Pediat.,* 71:553, October 1967.

* Complete addresses are given in the Appendix.

Davis, D. C.: Predicting Tomorrow's Children. *Today's Health,* 46:32, January 1968.

Douglas, G. W.: Rubella in Pregnancy, *Am. J. Nursing,* 66:2664, 1966.

Gerald, P. S., and others: A Ring D Chromosome and Anomalous Inheritance of Haptoglobin Type. *J. Pediat.,* 70:172, 1967.

Hall, J. G., and Hecht, F.: The Autosomal Trisomies. *Am. J. Nursing,* 64:87, November 1964.

Hillsman, G. M.: Genetics and the Nurse. *Nursing Outlook,* 14:34, January 1966.

Juberg, R. C.: Heredity Counseling. *Nursing Outlook,* 14:28, January 1966.

Kang, E. S.: The Genetic Basis of Some Abnormalities in Children. *Children,* 13:60, 1966.

McGavin, D. D. M., and others: The Cri-du-Chat Syndrome with an Apparently Normal Karyotype. *Lancet,* 2(7511):326, Aug. 12, 1967.

Murphy, E. A.: The Rationale of Genetic Counseling. *J. Pediat.,* 72:121, 1968.

Owens, C.: Parents' Reactions to Defective Babies. *Am. J. Nursing,* 64:83, November 1964.

Poland, B. J.: Study of Developmental Anomalies in the Spontaneously Aborted Fetus. *Am. J. Obst. & Gynec.,* 100:501, 1968.

Rorke, L. B., and Spiro, A. J.: Cerebral Lesions in Congenital Rubella Syndrome. *J. Pediat.,* 70:243, 1967.

Secrest, H. P.: Nurses and the Collaborative Perinatal Research Project. *Nursing Research,* 15:159, 1966.

Selye, H.: The Stress Syndrome. *Am. J. Nursing,* 65:97, March 1965.

Singer, D. B., and others: Pathology of the Congenital Rubella Syndrome. *J. Pediat.,* 71:665, 1967.

Winick, M.: Birth Defects: What Is Being Done About Them? *Nursing Outlook,* 14:43, January 1966.

Wood, J. W., and others: Mental Retardation in Children Exposed in Utero to the Atomic Bombs in Hiroshima and Nagasaki. *Am. J. Pub. Health,* 57:1381, 1967.

Zellweger, H., McDonald, J. S., and Abbo, G.: Is Lysergic-Acid Diethylamide a Teratogen? *Lancet* 2(7525):1066, November 18, 1967.

10

CONDITIONS OF THE NEWBORN REQUIRING IMMEDIATE OR SHORT-TERM CARE

In order to provide care to the newborn infant the nurse must understand the several kinds of illnesses he may have. These include congenital diseases, congenital anomalies, birth injuries, respiratory conditions, and infections. For the sake of clarity the various conditions included in each of these classifications will be divided into those which require immediate or short-term care, discussed in the present chapter, and those which require long-term care, to be discussed in Chapter 11.

CONGENITAL DISEASES

Hemolytic Disease of the Newborn (Erythroblastosis Fetalis)

Hemolytic disease of the fetus or newborn includes a number of hemolytic processes.

Etiology. Hemolytic disease is due to the development of an isohemagglutinin in the maternal serum, the result of incompatibility of parental genetic factors. Antibodies traverse the placenta and produce agglutination of the infant's red blood cells. The two most important hemolytic diseases are due to isoimmunization to (1) the Rh factor and (2) to A or B substances.

Hemolytic Disease Due to Rh Incompatibility

There are three blood combinations which are always compatible, i.e. when the Rh factors of the blood of each parent are such that an infant-mother sensitization cannot arise. These are (1) when both parents are positive, (2) when both are negative, and (3) when the mother is Rh-positive and the father is Rh-negative. Erythroblastosis fetalis occurs when the mother is Rh-negative and the father—and therefore the fetus also—Rh-positive. About 15 per cent of the white population are Rh-negative and 85 per cent positive. Very few Asian or Negro women are Rh-negative.

Etiology. Erythroblastosis fetalis does not

always occur in the infant born of an Rh-incompatible mating, because of the vagaries of maternal sensitization, paternal heterozygosity and small families. The first child is less apt to be affected than are later ones. The reason for this is that the mother who produces antibodies easily will begin to do so in response to the stimulus of the first fetus. The titer is further stimulated by succeeding pregnancies.

Rh isoimmunization evidently results from a relatively large transplacental hemorrhage at delivery or, probably more often, from sometimes undetectable bleeding which occurs at any time during pregnancy. All Rh-negative women are at risk because even when their postpartum blood specimens contain no Rh-positive fetal erythrocytes, Rh immunization can still take place. Sensitization may also result if the mother has had a transfusion or an injection of Rh-positive blood cells. These anti-Rh agglutinins are carried from the mother's blood across the placenta into the bloodstream of the fetus and destroy the fetal erythrocytes by their specific reaction with the Rh-positive cells.

Clinical Manifestations. The vernix caseosa is often yellowish; in some cases there may be severe edema (*hydrops fetalis*). Jaundice appears on the first day, and there is progressive anemia due to the severe hemolysis. Enlargement of the liver and the spleen is common. In severe cases the central nervous system may be affected, as evidenced by opisthotonos, spasticity, abnormal Moro reflex, inactivity, and anorexia present from the third to the fifth day after birth. Under such circumstances kernicterus (jaundice of the basal ganglia) may be present.

Laboratory Findings. The mother's blood is found to be Rh-negative and the infant's Rh-positive. The Coombs test result on the infant is positive. His blood picture shows anemia with an increased number of nucleated red blood cells. The indirect serum bilirubin level is increased. The anti-Rh titer of the mother's blood is elevated.

In order to determine how ill an infant of an Rh-negative mother is, the physician can do an amniocentesis by injecting a needle into a pregnant uterus and withdrawing from the amniotic sac a few drops of amber fluid. A spectrophotometric analysis of the bilirubin concentration of this amniotic fluid can determine the diagnosis or degree of illness of the fetus. Therapy is aimed at inducing birth early and carrying out an exchange transfusion.

Course. In severe hemolytic disease the infant may be born dead or may die within the first few days of life. On the other hand, with prompt therapy complete recovery is the rule.

Kernicterus sometimes follows severe hemolytic disease of the newborn. The symptoms may appear within the first week of life or months later.

The more important symptoms are noted above. Such sequelae, it is believed, can be avoided through the use of exchange transfusions when the serum bilirubin threatens to rise above a critical level of 20 mg. per 100 ml. If the infant survives, there may be central nervous system damage.

Treatment. The infant should receive an exchange transfusion with fresh Rh-negative blood which is compatible with the mother's serum by the indirect Coombs test. This should be done as soon as possible after delivery and repeated later if necessary.

Exchange Transfusion. A polyethylene catheter is inserted into the umbilical or other large vein. Small amounts (approximately 10 to 20 ml. at a time) of the newborn's blood are withdrawn and equal amounts of Rh-negative blood injected. This process is continued until most of the newborn's blood has been replaced; approximately 500 ml. of blood are generally used in this procedure. Antibiotics are given after transfusion to prevent infection. Repeated small transfusions may be necessary later.

If the infant is too young for an emergency delivery and an exchange transfusion is indicated, the physician can administer an intrauterine transfusion into the abdomen of the unborn child. The position of the needle in the abdomen of the fetus is checked by x-ray to determine its location. Since transfused blood survives only temporarily, repeated transfusions may be necessary.

The degree of anxiety which the mother feels during the intrauterine transfusion may be great because of the research nature of the procedure. The nurses caring for the patient must share her hope that the fetus will survive and strive to support her confidence in her physician. Many pregnant women complain of backache during the procedure because they must lie on a hard x-ray table for a long time. Comfort measures such as backrubs to reduce the strain should be carried out. Waiting for the birth of the infant produces further anxiety in the mother. She may believe that he has died if he simply stops kicking. The nurse must be supportive until the infant is actually born and the outcome of the procedure is known.

Prevention. Prevention begins in the prenatal period. All pregnant women should have their blood typed. Any woman who is Rh-negative should have her antibody titer ascertained after the thirty-sixth week. Thus in the event of a rising titer a tentative diagnosis can be made even before the birth of the child. If the newborn infant is Rh-positive, if the Coombs test result is positive, and if the infant exhibits a rapidly rising bilirubin level, treatment is indicated.

Currently physicians are doing research in an attempt to eradicate erythroblastosis fetalis.

They are giving a special anti-Rh immuno-globulin intramuscularly to Rh-negative mothers within three days after delivering their first Rh-incompatible infant so that they will not develop the antibodies that will destroy Rh-positive blood. This vaccine is a highly concentrated solution of Rh antibodies obtained from Rh-negative persons who have been sensitized to the Rh factor. Later, when the blood of these mothers was tested, it was found to lack anti-Rh-positive antibodies. Each mother was thus passively protected against incompatibility with a future Rh-positive fetus. Unfortunately the vaccine is not effective on Rh-negative mothers who have already developed their own active antibodies by having given birth to an Rh-positive infant.

Hemolytic Disease Due to ABO Incompatibility

Etiology. The etiologic process is the same as in Rh incompatibility. Clinical manifestations of hemolytic disease are more commonly due to ABO incompatibility than to Rh incompatibility. In ABO incompatibility the difficulty is caused by the presence of the blood group A or B factors.

Hemolytic disease due to A or B incompatibility is not usually anticipated unless there is a history of this problem among previous children in the family.

Course. A or B isoimmune disease of the newborn is usually mild and may even pass unnoticed. It should be treated, however, if signs are well developed.

Clinical Manifestations. Mild jaundice appears during the first thirty-six hours of life. On physical examination the physician may find enlargement of both the liver and the spleen. Central nervous system complications are rare. There is little or no edema.

Treatment. The majority of affected infants need no treatment, but an exchange transfusion (using group O blood of appropriate Rh type) may be needed if the infant's serum bilirubin level approaches 20 mg. per 100 ml. Treatment is aimed at the prevention of kernicterus.

Nursing Care in Hemolytic Disease of the Newborn. Skillful nursing is needed. An incubator to maintain the infant's temperature should be in readiness, as well as oxygen in case he becomes cyanotic. Preparation for exchange transfusion should be made when it is known that the birth of a possible erythroblastotic infant is expected or as soon as possible after it has been proved that the infant needs an exchange transfusion. His condition must be closely watched during and after treatment, and special attention must be paid to respirations, pulse, temperature and evidence of increasing lethargy. At all times the nurse should watch for and report to the physician the following symptoms: increasing jaundice, pigmentation of urine, edema, cyanosis, convulsions, and changes in any of the vital signs. She should change the lethargic infant's position frequently to prevent atelectasis and infection. If kernicterus is present, however, the infant should be handled as little as possible, since movement is likely to result in increased spasms. Because the infant is weak and may have difficulty in sucking, a soft nipple with a large hole should be given him, or he should be fed with a medicine dropper. These infants may be breast fed, since it is doubtful whether agglutinins in the breast milk would affect their circulating erythrocytes to a great extent.

Hemorrhagic Disease of the Newborn

Etiology. This disease is due to a deficiency of prothrombin resulting from either immaturity of the liver or a deficiency of vitamin K. Vitamin K, which is ordinarily elaborated by bacterial action within the intestinal tract during later life, is lacking in the sterile newborn. It is essential to the formation of prothrombin by the liver.

Clinical Manifestations. There is bleeding from the skin, retina, conjunctiva, mucous membranes, umbilical wound or viscera. The infant may have tar-colored stools, owing to blood in the fecal matter, or hematemesis (vomiting of bright red blood). Such bleeding may occur with or without trauma and is most likely to appear between the second and fifth days of life, when the available prothrombin is at the lowest level (see Physiologic Hypoprothrombinemia, p. 106).

Laboratory Findings. The prothrombin time is prolonged; the coagulation time may be normal or prolonged.

Treatment. Vitamin K is given intramuscularly once or repeated as necessary. The effect is much slower, however, than if the vitamin is given intravenously. A transfusion of fresh, matched whole blood may be given. If the bleeding is from accessible bleeding areas, pressure dressings may be applied with topical application of anticoagulants (thrombin or fibrin foam).

Prevention. The mother may be given synthetic water-soluble vitamin K intravenously or intramuscularly four to twelve hours before delivery, or she may take it daily by mouth for several days before the beginning of labor is expected. This will help to correct maternal hypoprothrombinemia due to poor diet and thus may help to raise the prothrombin level of the infant at the time of birth. Direct administration of vitamin K to the full-term infant is more effective than administration to the mother before delivery. Vitamin K may be given intramuscularly to the infant immediately after birth or orally if there is any bleeding. Large doses of vitamin K have been found to be conducive to the development of hyperbilirubinemia.

Nursing Care. The nursing care is that of the normal or premature newborn, with special care in handling to avoid the slightest danger of trauma and resulting bleeding. The nurse must observe these infants even more carefully than others for evidence of bleeding from the umbilical wound or gastrointestinal tract, as shown by tar-colored blood in the stool or bright red blood in the vomitus.

CONGENITAL ANOMALIES

Emergency Surgery and the Newborn

Several of the congenital anomalies seen in newborns can be corrected by surgery immediately or soon after birth. The normal newborn is an excellent surgical risk during the first forty-eight hours of life, but the mortality rate rises rapidly when the infant is more than seventy-two hours old. After this period several factors make operation more dangerous. The most important of these factors are (1) changes in fluid and electrolyte balance, (2) the normal breakdown of the red blood cells, and (3) the lessening of the infant's physiologic reserve, i.e. all the elements necessary for carrying on the vital functions, which he received through the placenta while still *in utero.*

Transportation of the Newborn to the Hospital

Newborns delivered in the home or in a hospital in which surgery is not done on this young age group must be transferred to a hospital or medical center where adequate personnel and facilities for therapy are available. All too often the infant is simply wrapped in a blanket and transferred in a vehicle in which no emergency equipment is available.

The newborn should be transferred in an ambulance which has a portable incubator with oxygen available in order to maintain his body temperature and the oxygen level in his blood. Equipment for suctioning should also be available in case of the need for removal of secretions.

The person responsible for the transfer of the newborn should be medically oriented and aware of the observations to be made and the appropriate treatment to be given in case of an emergency. For instance, the nurse or other skilled attendant should prevent the torsion of an omphalocele and prevent the aspiration of fluid by suctioning of the esophagus or stomach when a diagnosis of esophageal atresia or intestinal obstruction has been made. Other observations and methods of therapy will be discussed under the various appropriate diagnoses in this chapter.

Preparation for Surgery

On arrival at the hospital or medical center the newborn requiring immediate surgery should be cared for in an area where emergency equipment and experienced personnel are available such as in a newborn intensive care unit (see pp. 47 and 144). The same care exerted when transporting the infant from hospital to hospital should be taken when transporting him from his crib or incubator to the x-ray department or operating room.

Preoperative preparation gives diminishing returns if it is prolonged. Opaque material should not be used in establishing the diagnosis of atresia of the esophagus or upper intestinal obstruction because of the possibility of aspiration of fluid into the lungs with resulting pneumonia. Blood chemistry studies, if done at all, should be done by microtechniques to prevent depletion of blood volume. The newborn should be handled as little as possible. He should be hydrated, but surgery should not be postponed beyond the second day of life.

Extremely small doses of preoperative medication will prevent secretions from accumulating in the respiratory tract, and emptying the stomach of gastric contents will prevent vomiting with the danger of aspiration of vomitus. An environment with a high oxygen content is required so that the infant may not become exhausted by his efforts to have a sufficient intake.

To be successful, surgery of the newborn requires early diagnosis, minimal preparation and an expert team, including a surgeon, a pediatrician, a radiologist and an anesthesiologist who are experienced in working with infants, and nurses who are thoroughly accustomed to nursing the newborn who undergoes operation.

Physiologic Problems in Surgery of the Newborn

There are many problems in surgery of the newborn which make it a specialty for surgeons and nurses alike. The newborn does not show gradually increasing signs of loss of blood as do older children and adults. Because of the elasticity of his blood vessels, the infant may show no danger signs until he suddenly goes into shock. Then he is pulseless, and the blood pressure is low and the skin mottled. Because of this characteristic response of the newborn undergoing operation, hemorrhage must be anticipated and blood given before his condition is serious. It is difficult to give the correct amount of blood when he is in shock, since too much fluid given then may cause pulmonary edema.

Other problems include an unstable weight status, diminution of certain aspects of renal function, labile control of body temperature, and a response to a lack of oxygen by increased respirations which, if allowed to continue, may result in exhaustion and death.

Nursing Care of the Newborn
After Surgery

Infants have a remarkable resilience; on the other hand, they lack the physiologic reserve which older children have. If all goes well, an infant's recovery is rapid, but if complications arise, a state of emergency exists which may develop with little warning.

Since the condition of the newborn postoperatively may change very rapidly, the nurse must check his condition frequently, especially his temperature, the quality of his respirations and color, and the presence of bleeding among other observations, and assume the responsibility for carrying out lifesaving procedures in the absence of the physician.

The most crucial period after surgery of the newborn is the first hour postoperatively. He must be assisted to maintain his body temperature between 97 and 99°F. by the use of an incubator, to recover from anesthesia, and to maintain the patency of his small airway by positioning of his head and by suctioning of secretions from his nasopharynx. High humidity is usually maintained in the incubator in order to dilute secretions in the nasopharynx and to compensate for fluid lost because of a rapid respiratory rate. Oxygen is also usually given to newborns postoperatively in approximately 40 per cent concentration; however, higher concentrations may be given as necessary.

The newborn may die quickly from exhaustion unless his nursing care is planned to protect him from unnecessary external stimuli. Such care as the changing of dressings, the administration of medications and the taking of vital signs should be planned to be done together so that the infant does not have to be disturbed repeatedly.

The newborn postsurgical patient should be turned from side to side without disturbing him more than necessary; however, he should be prevented from assuming any position which would constrict his diaphragmatic movements on respiration. The nurse should also observe the newborn carefully to prevent constriction of any dressings which might hinder respirations.

Fluid balance is maintained initially by the intravenous route. Intravenous solutions, electrolyte solutions and medications are given very slowly. Intravenous fluids are ordered in drops per minute as well as in cubic centimeters per hour in order to prevent too much fluid being given too rapidly. (See page 299 for further discussion of intravenous therapy.) The site of the needle insertion or of the cutdown should be inspected frequently for leakage. The infant should be weighed within his incubator if possible in order to determine whether adequate or more than adequate fluids are being given.

The nurse is responsible for observing gastrostomy or chest tubes, catheters and intravenous tubing to determine their adequate functioning. If the newborn is fed by gastrostomy tube, it should never be clamped for fear of regurgitation through the esophagus and aspiration into the lungs, and for the purpose of relieving gaseous distention. After feedings the end of the tube should be elevated approximately 6 inches or at a height determined by the physician. The purpose of elevating the open-ended tube is so that, should the stomach contract, the contents could be easily expelled. Depending on the procedure used in the individual hospital, the gastrostomy tube should be irrigated with a small amount of saline solution prior to feedings. (See page 147 for the procedure of feeding by gavage.)

When oral feedings are begun, a small amount of glucose water may be given. The nurse must observe the infant carefully to determine whether he has adequate sucking and swallowing reflexes. If suctioning is indicated, it should be done promptly.

Since the newborn has an inadequate cough reflex and thus cannot clear the nasopharynx, the danger of vomiting with aspiration into the lungs is ever present. In order to prevent this he may have constant suction drainage from his stomach established, or his head may be placed lower than his body and turned to the side so that secretions and vomitus can drain from his mouth. If aspiration does occur, endotracheal suctioning must be instituted promptly.

As the newborn shows progress he is gradually removed from his incubator and given decreasing concentrations of oxygen until he can live comfortably and safely in a bassinet in the stable temperature of the newborn unit.

The emotional support which the parents of a malformed newborn need has already been discussed on page 161. The student should review this subject in order to obtain a more complete view of total family care.

The care of the postoperative newborn is an exceedingly important area of pediatric nursing. The details of nursing care of infants having various conditions will be discussed when the conditions are described.

Conditions Which May Require
Surgical Correction

Congenital Laryngeal Stridor

Noisy respiration—a crowing sound on inspiration—is a condition which may be due to a number of factors. The physician will determine the cause of the stridor, and the treatment is based upon his findings. No therapy may be required, or immediate treatment may be necessary if the child is to survive. The nursing care will be based upon the plan of treatment outlined by the physician.

Etiology. Laryngeal stridor lasting after the first few days of life is due to some abnormal condition in or around the larynx which may be located by laryngoscopy (Fig. 10-1). The most common cause is flabbiness of the epiglottis and the supraglottic aperture. Other causes include epiglottal redundancy, relaxation of the laryngeal wall, absence of the rings of the trachea, deformity of the vocal cords, or a web which partially occludes the larynx. In the older infant or child, stridor may be caused by laryngeal infection (see p. 402), tetany (p. 324) or a foreign body in the larynx (p. 292).

Clinical Manifestations, Diagnosis and Treatment. The main diagnostic symptom is noisy breathing, often with a crowing sound on inspiration. This is most noticeable when the infant cries, and is present at birth or shortly thereafter. This symptom may be accompanied by mild or severe intercostal and supraclavicular retractions. The infant may become cyanotic and dyspneic.

Treatment is based on correction of the underlying cause. For mild stridor there is no specific therapy, but for severe stridor operation may be necessary. If the infant appears unable to take in sufficient oxygen on inspiration, an emergency tracheotomy (see p. 406) may be done. Such an operation may be only a step toward further corrective surgery. For deformity of the larynx, laryngoplasty may be necessary.

Course and Prognosis. If the condition is uncorrected, constant retractions of the thorax may cause deformity, since the bones readily bend under pressure. If the infant has difficulty in nursing, he may not take sufficient nourishment, and malnutrition may result. Naturally a respiratory infection increases the difficulty and may cause a mild chronic condition to become severe.

The mild, simple form of congenital laryngeal stridor usually subsides by the time the infant is six to eighteen months old. The child does not become cyanotic, and he shows no symptoms other than his noisy breathing. But the *prognosis* in congenital stridor due to some malformation of the larynx will depend upon the cause.

Nursing Care. Feeding may be a problem, since any interference in breathing makes sucking difficult. The infant will have to be fed slowly, stopping frequently for him to breathe unimpeded by nursing. The respiratory process is more imperative than his desire for food, and so he will stop to breathe without the hindrance

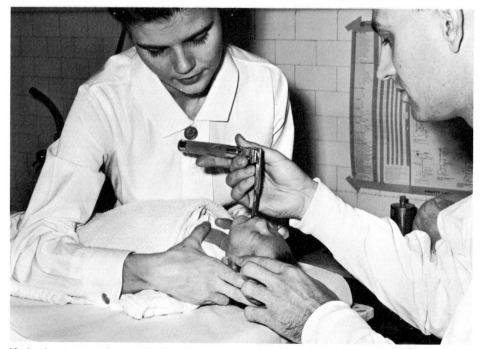

Figure 10–1. Laryngoscopic examination. A mummy restraint is applied, and a small blanket roll is placed under the infant's neck. Note the position of the nurse's hands in holding the infant's head.

of sucking. This does not mean that his hunger is satisfied. The nurse should wait a few moments and then offer him the nipple again. If he appears to have difficulty in swallowing the milk, the nurse should remove the nipple from his mouth at once. A small nipple will probably give the best results. The size of the hole in the nipple should be carefully chosen to give the rate of flow which the infant finds easiest to handle. All infants, of course, should be held when fed and never left with the bottle propped on a pad, but with these infants it is imperative that they be held in the correct position and the bottle supported at the proper angle.

The mother should have ample opportunity to become accustomed to the infant's noisy breathing before she leaves the hospital; otherwise she has no standard by which to judge whether his condition becomes worse. The difficulty in breathing is likely to increase if a respiratory infection develops or if the infant aspirates a little of his feeding or in some other way undergoes an added strain on his already inadequate breathing. The mother should give the infant his bottle with the nurse beside her to show her the proper technique. The nurse should call her attention to the infant's reaction to too rapid feeding or failure to withdraw the nipple from his mouth if he appears unable to take the milk. If he is a breast-fed infant, the mother will have had ample opportunity to learn the technique of feeding him before she takes him home.

Since a respiratory infection increases the infant's breathing problem, it is important that he be kept from every source of respiratory infection. He should be kept warm, dry, and away from drafts at all times. Raising the humidity in his environment is helpful.

Choanal Atresia

Choanal atresia is a congenital obstruction of the posterior nares at the entrance to the nasopharynx. The obstruction is usually caused by a membrane, but in rare cases by a bony growth. The condition may be unilateral or bilateral.

Clinical Manifestations, Diagnosis and Treatment. The *symptoms* of bilateral obstruction are mouth-breathing and, since the infant cannot suck and breathe at the same time, difficulty in taking his feedings. There may be dyspnea because he cannot obtain enough oxygen when breathing through his mouth. If the obstruction is unilateral, the infant may do well unless infection occurs and persists on the side opposite the obstruction.

The *diagnosis* is confirmed by passing a sound, probe or soft rubber catheter up the nostril until it meets the obstruction.

Bilateral atresia should be relieved as early as possible, since it is one cause of asphyxia of the newborn. By using a nasoscope the physician is able to pierce the obstruction if it is membranous. A bony obstruction requires extensive operation. Unilateral choanal atresia need not be corrected until the infant is in optimum condition.

Nursing Care. There is little in the nursing care of these infants which is specifically directed toward relief of their condition. The nostrils should be kept clean. Feeding the infant is difficult, since he has trouble in breathing and sucking at the same time, and since there is danger of aspiration of the formula. The precautions and techniques are similar to those outlined in the nursing care of the infant with congenital laryngeal stridor.

Conditions Incompatible with Life, but Amenable to Surgical Correction

There are several congenital anomalies of the gastrointestinal tract which, though incompatible with life, may be corrected by surgical treatment. These anomalies are imperforate anus, atresia of the esophagus, omphalocele, diaphragmatic hernia and intestinal obstruction. These lesions are often associated with other congenital anomalies and are also seen in premature infants. Early diagnosis and treatment are essential in saving life. Operation immediately after birth is indicated when the infant has a diaphragmatic hernia or a large omphalocele.

The difficulties of surgery of the gastrointestinal tract in the newborn increase hour by hour. The infant swallows air, and the gastrointestinal tract becomes distended. He becomes progressively more exhausted because of his increased respiratory rate and is less able to withstand operation.

Three procedures were outlined under Examination of Internal Organs (p. 107) which nurses may carry out to determine the presence of anomalies which require immediate treatment. The nurse should report her findings to the physician, who would then check the symptoms and determine the treatment to be given.

In addition, the nurse should observe an infant closely for four important signs which indicate the possibility of a lesion incompatible with life. These signs are cyanosis, vomiting, absence of stools, and abdominal distention.

Cyanosis is indicative of many conditions. Those we are concerned with here are diaphragmatic hernia and atresia of the esophagus. *Vomiting* of bile-stained material is a sign of intestinal obstruction. An infant with a diaphragmatic hernia may have repetitive vomiting. In atresia of the esophagus there is immediate vomiting of the undigested formula. *Absence of stools* is the characteristic sign of any form of intestinal

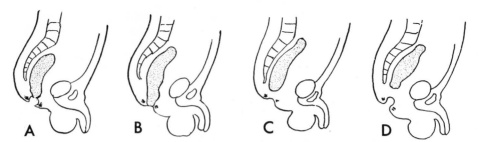

Figure 10–2. Diagrammatic illustration of 4 types of congenital anorectal malformation. (From P. Hanley and M. O. Hines, in *Christopher's Minor Surgery.* 8th ed., edited by Ochsner and DeBakey.)

obstruction, as is *abdominal distention*. Although these four signs may be seen in the normal newborn, they should be reported promptly to the physician in order to lead to early diagnosis and treatment of conditions incompatible with life, but amenable to surgical correction.

Imperforate Anus

Incidence and Etiology. This is the most common congenital anomaly of the newborn which is incompatible with life. In the eighth week of embryonic life the membrane which separates the rectum from the anus normally is absorbed, and thus a continuous canal is formed whose outlet is the anus. If this membrane is not absorbed and union does not take place, an imperforate anus results. A fistula between the rectum and the vagina, perineum or fourchet in the female, or the urinary tract, scrotum or perineum in the male, is likely to be formed when the infant has an imperforate anus.

Diagnosis. The diagnosis is made when (1) no anal opening is found on cursory examination of the infant in the delivery room; (2) the physician or nurse cannot insert a small finger or thermometer into the infant's rectum; (3) there is no meconium stool; and (4) later abdominal distention occurs. In the presence of these signs the distance between the closed end of the rectum and the anal dimple is ascertained by x-ray examination. The infant cries, and the

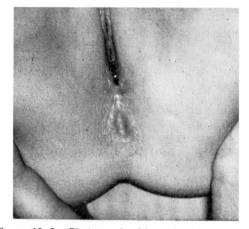

Figure 10–3. Photograph of imperforate anus, type III (Fig. 10–2, *C*). (From P. Hanley and M. O. Hines, in *Christopher's Minor Surgery.* 8th ed., edited by Ochsner and DeBakey.)

air which he swallows goes only to the closed end of the rectum. In order to force air down through the bowel, the infant is held upside down or on his side with his knees pushed against the abdomen. An opaque object is placed at the anal dimple, and the roentgenogram thus shows the distance of the rectum from the anus.

Obstruction in a male infant must be relieved at once, for the stool cannot be passed, but an emergency is not so likely in a female, since a

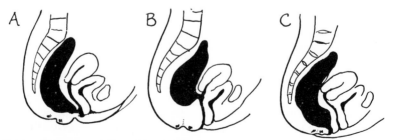

Figure 10–4. Schematic representation of imperforate anus, type III (Fig. 10–2, *C*), with associated fistula in the female. *A,* Low rectovaginal. *B,* High rectovaginal. *C,* Rectoperineal. (From P. Hanley and M. O. Hines, in *Christopher's Minor Surgery.* 8th ed., edited by Ochsner and DeBakey.)

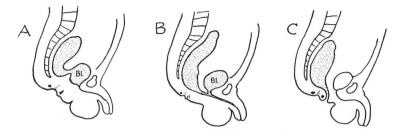

Figure 10–5. Diagrammatic representation of imperforate anus, type III (Fig. 10–2, *C*), with associated fistula in the male. *A,* Rectovesical. *B,* Rectourethral. *C,* Rectoperineal. (From P. Hanley and M. O. Hines, in *Christopher's Minor Surgery.* 8th ed., edited by Oschsner and DeBakey.)

fistula probably exists into the vagina, perineum or fourchet. The outlet of the fistula is easily found on inspection. The urine should be watched for flecks of meconium.

Treatment. The surgical procedure depends upon the type of anomaly. The anal defect may be such that the opening is covered by a thin membrane through which meconium can be seen. In this case the physician is able to perforate the membrane with a blunt instrument, and no further treatment is required. If the distance between the anal dimple and the blind end of the colon is not more than 1.5 cm., correction is made through the perineum, but if the distance is greater than 1.5 cm., a colostomy is performed while awaiting definitive operation, or the colon is brought down through the anal dimple by an abdominal-perineal procedure. If the anus is normal, but the closed end of the rectum ends in a blind pouch a few centimeters from the sphincter, the condition, called *atresia of the rectum,* must be surgically corrected as would any other colonic obstruction.

Nursing Care. One of the most important characteristics of the professional nurse is her ability for intelligent interpretation of meaningful observations. The detection of imperforate anus is a case in point. In her appraisal in the nursery the nurse should observe the newborn for the indications of imperforate anus mentioned previously and report promptly those found.

After the diagnosis of occlusion has been made the physician may order gastric suction. If operation is to be done, there may be no specific preoperative preparation. Postoperatively, if the operation has involved only the anal area, that site should be kept dry and clean. If a colostomy has been made, the skin around the wound must be kept clean. The infant's skin is more readily irritated than that of the older child or adult, and cleanliness is very important. Aluminum paste or zinc oxide ointment is used to protect the skin. If the skin breaks down, karaya gum powder may be sprinkled liberally on the area. The paste which is formed should be allowed to adhere to the skin for several days. When it comes off, the

skin beneath is healed. The adhesive straps with ties which hold the colostomy dressing in place should be adjusted so that they remain clean and so that the dressing may be easily changed. An abdominal binder or a folded diaper (pinned around the abdomen) may be used instead of adhesive tape to prevent breakdown of the skin. If surgery for this condition is not successful, the child may become a rectal cripple unable to control the seepage of feces from his rectum. This condition, depending on its severity, causes social problems as he grows older in that he may not be acceptable to his peer group who have been successfully bowel trained.

Atresia of the Esophagus

Incidence, Pathology, Clinical Manifestations and Diagnosis. Among the obstructive anomalies of the gastrointestinal tract in the newborn, this condition ranks second (imperforate anus holding first place). The esophagus, instead of being an open tube from the throat to the stomach, is closed at some point. A fistula is common between the trachea and the esophagus. In approximately 80 per cent of these newborns the esophageal atresia is proximal and the tracheo-esophageal fistula is distal.

At birth the infant has excessive mucus in the nasopharynx and therefore is cyanotic. When the mucus is withdrawn by aspiration and oxygen is given, the difficulty in breathing subsides, and the infant acquires the normal pink of the newborn. But as the secretions in the nasopharynx accumulate, he again becomes cyanotic. Nurses who care for newborns either in the delivery room or in the nursery should recognize this typical behavior and report the presence of excess mucus *immediately!* If this condition is suspected, the infant should not be fed until he is thoroughly examined and the patency of the esophagus determined.

If a soft no. 8 rubber catheter cannot be passed through the infant's nose and down the esophagus, it is probably blocked by the area of atresia. An x-ray film shows the tip of the catheter coiled

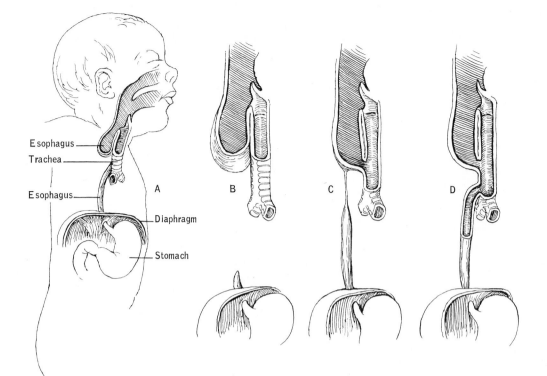

Figure 10–6. Atresia of the esophagus. *A,* Most common form. The upper esophagus ends in a blind pouch. The lower esophagus communicates with the trachea. *B,* The upper esophagus ends in a blind pouch. The lower segment does not communicate with the trachea. *C,* The upper esophagus ends in the trachea. A cordlike connection with the lower esophagus may or may not be present. *D,* Both upper and lower portions of the esophagus connect with the trachea.

back upon itself in a dilated esophageal pouch. *No radiopaque substance should be instilled into the esophagus because of the danger of the infant's aspirating it.* If the infant has a tracheo-esophageal fistula, the roentgenogram will show air in the gastrointestinal tract.

If the newborn's condition is not recognized and he is fed, the nurse will note that the first mouthful goes down, but since the fluid can go no farther than the atretic area, the second is immediately expelled through the nose as well as the mouth. The infant chokes, sneezes, coughs and shows his discomfort by generalized movement. He is likely to aspirate some of the feeding, and pneumonia results. If he has a distal tracheo-esophageal fistula, the stomach contents may be vomited into the tracheobronchial tree.

Treatment. Immediate operation is necessary. Depending upon the type of atresia, the following operations are performed: (*a*) An end-to-end anastomosis of the upper and lower segments of the esophagus is done and the fistula ligated. (*b*) If there is no lower portion of the esophagus or if the distance between the lower and upper esophageal pouches is too great for anastomosis, a cervical esophagostomy is performed, and later a colon transplant is done.

In some premature infants and in infants having severe pneumonia a double-lumen polyethylene catheter is passed into the esophagus and attached to a pump so that sump drainage can be collected. The catheter is attached to the nose with adhesive tape. A gastrostomy is then made, and the infant is fed through a tube inserted into the stomach. An end-to-end anastomosis is carried out when the infant has gained weight and has been cured of his pneumonia. If an end-to-end anastomosis is not possible, an operation is performed in which either the right or transverse portion of the colon is brought into the chest to join the upper normal portion of the esophagus with the stomach. If a stricture occurs at the site of the anastomosis, it can be dilated later. The chance of survival depends upon the age, weight and general condition of the infant and upon whether other anomalies are present.

Nursing Care. It is advisable to place the infant in an incubator where he can be kept warm and is protected from infection. He should also be in an environment of high humidity, since this will tend to liquefy the thick mucous secretions which accumulate in the trachea. The nurse should observe the infant's respirations constantly to determine the need for

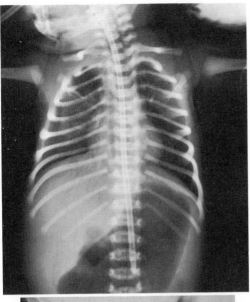

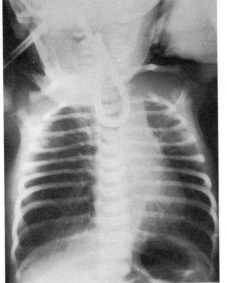

Figure 10–7. Atresia of the esophagus. *A,* Newborn with catheter passed through normal esophagus into stomach. *B,* Newborn with esophageal atresia, showing catheter coiled back in blocked esophagus. (Courtesy of Radiology Dept., Children's Hospital, Philadelphia.)

aspiration of secretions. The physician will perform tracheal aspirations if necessary, but the nurse may do nasopharyngeal aspirations. Tracheotomy may be necessary if respiratory difficulty persists (see p. 406).

If a gastrostomy has been done, feedings are begun several hours after operation. The feeding may be given by slow drip (by gravity) from an infusion bottle or by gastrostomy tube, according to the following procedure.

Gastrostomy Feeding and Care. The equipment for feeding includes a tray on which are the warm formula, a sterile funnel or Asepto syringe and a sterile nipple filled with sterile cotton.

Attach the funnel or syringe to the gastrostomy tube and fill with the formula before the clamp is removed. This will prevent air from being forced into the stomach. The funnel or syringe is then elevated to allow the fluid to run slowly into the stomach. Force should never be used. Since up to this time the stomach has not received food, distention by introducing air or feeding too rapidly must be avoided.

Some physicians prefer that for infants under one year the gastrostomy tube remain open at all times, but elevated above the infant's body. If vomiting then occurs, the tube provides a safety valve.

The infant fed through a gastrostomy tube should be given the opportunity to satisfy his need for sucking. He is given a sterile nipple filled with sterile cotton to suck on while the milk is running into the stomach through the gastrostomy tube. Sucking on the nipple provides him with a normal pleasure, and he relaxes while being fed. This facilitates the flow of milk. When the feeding is finished, the infant should be held quietly in the nurse's arms.

The care of the skin around the gastrostomy is exceedingly important. This area must be kept clean and protected with aluminum paste or zinc oxide ointment. To prevent displacing the tube when the dressings are changed, the inner side of the adhesive strap which holds the dressing in place should be covered with a second strip so that the part of the tape which extends over the dressing will not stick to it. The adhesive straps can then be tied together over the dressing.

The use of antibiotics will depend on the type of organism cultured from the cut end of the tracheo-esophageal fistula. As in other conditions involving the gastrointestinal tract, blood or plasma is given as necessary, and fluids are administered parenterally. There should be a minimum of salt content in these fluids so that the tissues do not become edematous. Depending on the infant's condition, feedings may be given by mouth, or through a tube into the esophagus or through a gastrostomy, if that operation has been performed, for two to three days after operation. Feeding by mouth should be done as soon as it is safe to do so, for fluid passing through the esophagus lessens the danger of a stricture which will require dilation.

The psychologic needs of these infants for sucking and warmth and comfort from body contact must be met so far as is possible. They are in the hospital for a relatively long time and might easily become typical hospitalized children, emotionally starved, though physically well cared for.

Omphalocele

Incidence and Diagnosis. An omphalocele is a herniation of abdominal viscera at the point where the umbilical cord connects with the abdomen. The defect occurs from the sixth to the tenth week of intrauterine life. The sac which covers the hernia is composed of transparent avascular membrane.

The *diagnosis* is made by inspection. Although the omphalocele is easily seen, it is sometimes so small that it appears to be part of the normal umbilical cord.

Clinical Manifestations, Treatment and Prognosis. On examination of a large omphalocele the mass of abdominal viscera seems to be greater than the size of the abdominal cavity into which the viscera must be placed.

The *treatment* is immediate operation—replacement of viscera into the abdomen and closure of the abdominal wall—before the bowel is expanded by swallowed air and before the sac dries or is contaminated by bacteria. Even if it is protected by a sterile dressing, the sac may become infected by airborne bacteria. The operation may be done in one or two stages. Owing to the difficulties just noted, plus the fact that the condition is often only one of several anomalies, the mortality rate is relatively high even with expert care.

With tremendously large omphaloceles some surgeons are postponing operation and instead are painting the area with Mercurochrome, which produces an eschar that eventually converts the omphalocele into a large ventral hernia.

Diaphragmatic Hernia

Incidence, Pathology, Clinical Manifestations and Diagnosis. Although this condition is reported today more frequently than it was in the past, this may be due not to an increase in the number of infants born with the anomaly, but rather to earlier and more accurate diagnosis.

A diaphragmatic hernia is more common on the left side. The lesion ranges from a slight to an extensive protrusion of the abdominal viscera through an opening in the diaphragm into the thoracic cavity.

The *symptoms* form a characteristic clinical picture, and the diagnosis can often be made in the delivery room if the lesion is extensive. On the other hand, in less severe states no symptoms may appear until later. The symptoms are severe respiratory difficulty, often with resulting cyanosis; a relatively large chest; failure of the affected side of the chest to expand as does the unaffected side; and a relatively small abdomen. When the herniated bowel fills with gas, all these symptoms increase in severity. Obviously no breath sounds are heard in the side of the defect when the lung is collapsed by abdominal viscera.

The *diagnosis* is made by physical examination and confirmed by roentgenograms of the chest. These show air from the intestinal tract in that part of the bowel which has protruded into the

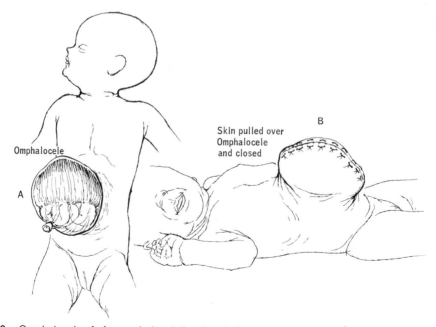

Omphalocele

Skin pulled over
Omphalocele
and closed

A

B

Figure 10–8. Omphalocele. *A*, An omphalocele is a herniation of the abdominal viscera at the umbilicus. *B*, The skin is closed over the omphalocele.

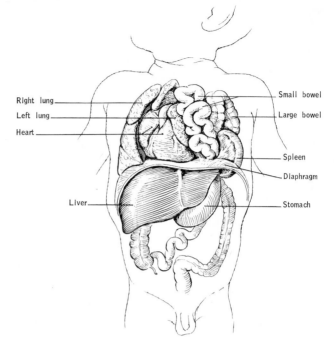

Figure 10–9. Diaphragmatic hernia. The abdominal viscera have herniated into the thorax. The thoracic viscera have been displaced and compressed.

hernia and is pressing against the organs of the chest.

Treatment, Prognosis and Nursing Care. Immediate operation is indicated. Gastric suction is used to remove secretions and swallowed air from the stomach and the intestinal tract. The operation consists in replacing the abdominal viscera in the abdominal cavity and in repair of the diaphragmatic defect. The lung on the affected side will then fill with air, and normal breathing will occur. If operation is not done immediately, the *prognosis* is very poor: the infant will probably die within the first month of life.

Postoperative *nursing care* is extremely important. Gastric suction is used to prevent abdominal distention immediately after operation. Transfusions of plasma or whole blood are given when necessary, and fluids are given intravenously until the infant can take them by mouth without abdominal distention. Feedings may be given by gavage on the second or third postoperative day. When fed by gavage, the infant is not so likely to swallow air as he is when sucking.

Intestinal Obstruction

Etiology. Intestinal obstruction in the newborn may result from a number of conditions— congenital atresia or stenosis of the intestine, malrotation of the colon with volvulus of the midgut, internal hernias, peritoneal bands, meconium ileus or Hirschsprung's disease (p. 334).

CONGENITAL ATRESIA OR STENOSIS OF THE INTESTINE. This condition is due to an arrest in development during the second and third months of intrauterine life. Stenosis (a narrowed lumen) may occur when the intestine develops from a solid structure into a hollow tube. In the course of normal development the diameter of this tube is sufficient throughout its length for the intestines to perform their physiologic functions, but in stenosis at one point only a minute passage is open. In atresia (no lumen) the intestinal tube is completely occluded at one or more points. The intestine may be divided into separate segments connected, in some cases, with fibrous bands.

MALROTATION OF THE COLON WITH VOLVULUS. During the tenth week of embryonic development the emerging ileocecal structure normally rotates so that the cecum lies in the lower right quadrant of the abdomen and is fixed there by the mesentery. If this process does not occur, the colon may remain in the right upper quadrant. Here an abnormal membrane may obstruct the duodenum. This obstructing band is one of the most significant findings in malrotation. A more serious complication is volvulus of the midgut, which happens because of lack of mesenteric attachment. The freely mobile loops of small intestine twist on themselves, produce obstruction and may go on to necrosis from lack of blood supply.

INTERNAL HERNIAS AND OBSTRUCTION CAUSED BY PERITONEAL BANDS. Internal hernias are caused by a loop of bowel slipping out of the normal position and becoming caught in a defective area of the mesentery or becoming compressed between bands of the peritoneum. In either case intestinal obstruction occurs.

MECONIUM ILEUS. This condition may occur in infants born with mucoviscidosis (cystic fibrosis) (see p. 328). The infant lacks the enzymes normally supplied by the pancreas and discharged into the intestinal tract. While the infant is still *in utero* this deficiency causes the meconium to be more sticky than is normal. It is of a putty-like consistency which causes it to adhere to the mucosa of the intestinal wall, and obstruction results. Fortunately, less than 10 per cent of newborns suffering from cystic fibrosis have meconium ileus.

Clinical Manifestations. The three main symptoms of intestinal obstruction are (1) absence of stools. If the infant has no stool within four hours after birth, examination for the presence of meconium may be made by inserting a gloved finger into the anus. If no indication of meconium is found, a colonic irrigation with not more than 10 ml. of physiologic saline solution may be ordered. (2) Vomitus stained with bile is diagnostic of intestinal obstruction, though obstruction may produce nonbile-stained vomitus as well. (3) Abdominal distention is a symptom of intestinal obstruction, though it may be physiologic in a normal child until meconium is passed. All infants have these symptoms to a degree, but the presence of two of these manifestations should suggest investigation.

The higher the obstruction, the earlier the symptoms appear, and the earlier can the diagnosis be made and treatment instituted. For this reason the lowest mortality rate is among infants with high obstruction.

Diagnosis. The decisive factor in the diagnosis is the roentgenogram, which shows the presence or absence of obstruction.

Treatment. The treatment is surgical. The majority of operations performed upon the newborn are for intestinal obstruction. The mortality rate is relatively high, but lowest among those cases in which the diagnosis is made early and relief is obtained before the infant's condition has degenerated.

Nursing Care. It is the nurse who is most likely to observe the main symptoms of intestinal obstruction in the newborn infant. She observes readily whatever has meaning for her. That is why the pathology and etiology of this condition have been given in somewhat extensive detail.

BIRTH INJURIES

This is an inclusive term embracing both avoidable and unavoidable trauma at birth and also permanent damage occurring soon after birth.

Intracranial Hemorrhage

Etiology, Incidence and Diagnosis. Trauma to the cranium is especially apt to occur when the infant's head is large in proportion to the size of the mother's pelvic outlet, when labor is prolonged and during a breech presentation or a precipitate delivery. It may also be seen in newborns with hemorrhagic disease. The two common types of hemorrhage are *subdural* and *subarachnoid.* Hemorrhage may extend into the ventricles or the brain substance itself.

Intracranial hemorrhage is the most common and severe type of birth injury. It occurs more frequently in premature than in full-term infants.

Diagnosis is based on a history of difficult delivery and an increase in cerebrospinal fluid pressure. The presence of a few blood cells in the cerebrospinal fluid is not of particular diagnostic value, because a minute amount of bleeding into the cerebrospinal fluid may be normal in the newborn.

Clinical Manifestations, Treatment, Prevention and Prognosis. Intracranial hemorrhage may be evident at birth or may be diagnosed later in an infant apparently normal at birth. The nurse may observe somnolence or limpness in the infant, or irritability and restlessness. Opisthotonos may be present, the Moro reflex absent, muscular twitchings and convulsions may occur, and the cry may be high-pitched and shrill. Cardiac and respiratory functions may be abnormal with resulting pallor and cyanosis. The temperature may be even less stable than that of the normal newborn. The fontanels may bulge if the increase in intracranial pressure is great. Paralysis may appear in a few days.

The results of *treatment* may be quite satisfactory. The infant needs warmth and rest and may be placed in an incubator where oxygen is available if needed. His head should be elevated. Hemorrhage may be controlled by the administration of vitamin K. The physician may order a sedative such as phenobarbital to control the convulsions. Prophylactic antibiotics are given. If a subdural hematoma is present, it is generally treated as described on page 352.

As with many other birth injuries, better obstetrical care is the best *preventive.*

In the majority of cases the *prognosis* is good, and the child may completely recover. Other infants may show mental retardation or a tendency to convulsions or may be handicapped by cerebral palsy. Those who do not survive usually die within the first three days after delivery.

Nursing Care. These infants are generally placed in incubators. Since the sucking and swallowing reflexes are weak or absent, the infant must be fed with great care. If he vomits after feedings, he should be placed on his abdomen or on his right side with a rolled blanket at his back, unless the physician has ordered that this is not to be done. In this position, drainage from the stomach to the duodenum is favored, and vomiting may be decreased. The infant must be observed for increased intracranial pressure and for convulsions (see p. 351).

Medications such as sedatives, vitamins or prophylactic antibiotics may be given orally or by injection. The nurse may assist the physician with treatments such as spinal punctures or aspiration of a subdural hemorrhage.

Peripheral Nerve Injuries

Brachial Plexus Palsy (Erb-Duchenne Paralysis)

Etiology and Clinical Manifestations. Brachial plexus palsy is a paralysis of the upper arm. The cause is trauma involving the fifth and sixth cervical spinal nerves or their trunks. The injury results from pulling the infant's shoulder away from the head during delivery. The arm on the affected side is adducted, extended and internally rotated with pronation of the forearm. The hands and fingers are not affected. The arm cannot voluntarily be abducted from the shoulder or externally rotated, and the forearm cannot be supinated. The Moro reflex is absent on the affected side, and there may be sensory loss on the lateral portion of the arm.

Treatment. The arm should be immobilized in a position of maximal relaxation, i.e. abducted and rotated externally with the elbow flexed. Later an airplane splint may be used to keep the arm in this position. To prevent contraction deformity, the physiotherapist may manipulate

and massage the arm gently. In persistent cases neuroplasty may be necessary.

Nursing Care. The arm is to be immobilized as the physician may order. In general a clove hitch restraint is used. The equipment needed for this is (1) a strip of gauze bandage 2 inches wide and 1½ yards long, and (2) cotton wadding covered with gauze, cut to 2 inches wide and long enough to encircle the infant's wrist.

To apply the restraint, spread the gauze strip out on the bed with one end toward the nearer side of the bed. In the middle of the strip make a figure of eight, as shown in Figure 10-11. Place the gauze wadding around the infant's wrist. Place circles of restraint around the padding on the wrist. Pull the ends of the bandage to the desired tightness. Tie the ends of the gauze to the bedsprings at the head of the bed so that the arm is elevated to the proper angle. Care must be exercised to prevent cutting off the circulation and yet have the bandage tight enough not to slip over the infant's hand.

The fingers and the hand should be observed for coldness or discoloration and the skin under the restraint for signs of irritation. These infants need even more love and affection than the normal infant does.

Prognosis. The prognosis usually cannot be determined for several months. If the paralysis is due to edema and hemorrhage around nerve fibers with no laceration, the prognosis is good. If laceration of the nerve has occurred, operation must usually be considered.

Facial Nerve Paralysis

Etiology, Clinical Manifestations and Prognosis. Facial nerve paralysis results from pressure over the facial nerve in front of the ear. This pressure may have occurred during labor or may have been due to the use of forceps during delivery. The paralysis is generally unilateral. When the infant cries, movement is observed

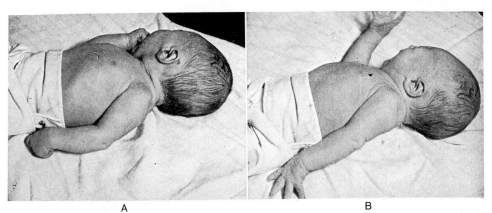

A   B

Figure 10–10. Brachial plexus palsy of the left arm. *A,* The arm at rest. *B,* Asymmetric response to Moro reflex. (R. J. McKay, Jr., and C. A. Smith in W. E. Nelson: *Textbook of Pediatrics.* 8th ed.)

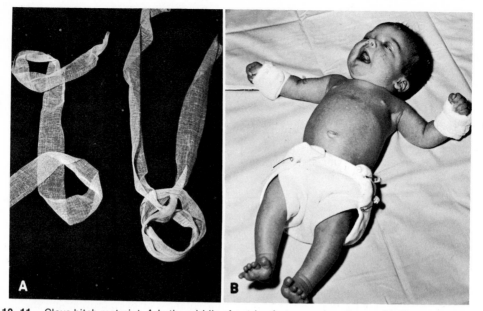

Figure 10–11. Clove hitch restraint. *A,* In the middle of a strip of gauze make a figure of 8. Place one loop over the other. *B,* Place the restraint over the wadding wrapped around the wrist (or ankles). Pull the gauze restraint securely, but not tightly enough to cut off the circulation. The response of this infant, namely crying, is the typical response to restraint. When the clove hitch restraint is used on an infant having brachial plexus palsy, the affected arm should be elevated and the ends of the gauze tied to the head of the crib.

on only one side of his face. The mouth is drawn to that side. The eye on the affected side is partially open. If the nerve is only injured by pressure, recovery can be expected in a few weeks; if the nerve is torn, however, neuroplasty may be required.

Nursing Care. The nurse must be patient when feeding the infant, since sucking may be difficult for him. The physician will order care of the exposed eye. If a shield is applied, it

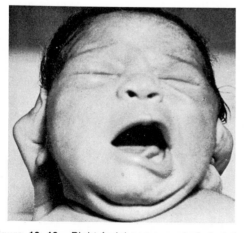

Figure 10–12. Right facial nerve paralysis in infant delivered without forceps. (Davis and Rubin: *DeLee's Obstetrics for Nurses.* 17th ed.)

may be necessary to restrain the infant's arms so that he does not pull it off. He can be held and cuddled like a normal infant.

Injuries to Bones

Etiology and Types of Fractures. Although the newborn's bones bend easily on pressure, as when traction is applied during delivery, a fracture may occur. Fractures occur mainly in the skull, clavicle or long bones.

Fractures of the skull are of two types: (a) linear fractures, the more common type, do not produce symptoms and require no treatment; (b) depressed fractures appear as a dent in the infant's head. Treatment is by early operation, which prevents injury to the cortex due to prolonged pressure.

Fracture of the clavicle is the most common fracture of the newborn. It may occur when delivery of the shoulder is difficult. The infant fails to raise his arm on the affected side, and the Moro reflex is possible only with elevation of the unaffected arm. The infant may be able to raise his arm, however, if the fracture is of the greenstick type, which is common in infants and little children. The prognosis in either type of fracture is excellent. Treatment is by immobilization of the arm and the shoulder on the affected side.

Fractures of the long bones of the arms or legs, unless of the green-stick type, prevent the infant from moving the limb. The treatment of a fracture of the humerus is strapping the arm to the chest and later placing it in an airplane splint or shell cast. For a fracture of the femur the leg is placed in Buck's extension (see p. 424). Splints are used for immobilizing other bones of the extremities. Excessive callus formation is likely to accompany rapid healing.

Nursing Care. Nursing care of these infants includes maintenance of good body alignment, splint or cast care (see p. 231) and prevention of pressure areas. Care has to be adapted to the position in which they must lie or the part of the body which is immobilized. Demonstrations of affection for the infant must also be adapted to his condition. The infant in traction cannot be fed at the breast, but his mother's milk may be expressed and given him. In this way the supply of breast milk will be maintained, because the infant is likely to have a longer hospital stay than is customary.

Injury to the Sternocleidomastoid Muscle

Etiology, Pathology and Treatment. About two weeks after birth, or even earlier, a small, firm mass may be noted in the midportion of the sternocleidomastoid muscle. This may be caused by a small hematoma resulting from injury or may be a fibromatous malformation in the muscle itself. The injury generally, but not always, results in *torticollis* (wryneck), a condition in which the head inclines to one side. The majority of these tumors resolve under treatment before the infant is one year old.

Treatment lies in gently extending the neck so that the face is in the opposite direction. The mother can be taught to turn the infant's head to the normal position and flex the neck toward the unaffected side. This may be done as often as twenty-five times twice or three times a day. If the condition is present when the child is two years old, operation may be required.

Nursing Care. Nursing care must be adapted to the limitation of movement of the infant. The nurse should talk to the infant and should cuddle him before and after the exercise.

RESPIRATORY CONDITIONS

Respiratory distress in the newborn may be due to a number of causes, but for a better understanding of the nursing problems of these infants two main groups of pathologic conditions which seriously interfere with normal respiration will be considered. (1) Failure of the respiratory center of the central nervous system may be due to anoxia, intracranial hemorrhage, anomaly, trauma or narcosis. (2) The second group includes peripheral respiratory difficulty (alveolar exchange of oxygen and carbon dioxide) due to atelectasis, hyaline membrane syndrome, pneumonia or aspiration pneumonia. Conditions not discussed in this chapter are treated elsewhere (see Index).

Anoxia of the Newborn

Types, Incidence and Etiology. Anoxia of the newborn is a condition in which his organs, especially the brain, receive much less oxygen than they need for optimum functioning. Anoxia is not a clinical entity in itself. Some of its causes are known, but others have not yet been identified. Anoxia is an important cause of perinatal death or lasting damage to the tissue of the central nervous system. Cerebral palsy may result or mental retardation be evident later in life.

Fetal anoxia may be due to any cause which limits the oxygen supplied by way of the maternal and fetal circulations from reaching the brain of the fetus. Causes include systemic conditions of the mother such as poor oxygenation of the blood due to cardiac failure or low blood pressure. Anoxia may also be caused by conditions of the uterus and the placenta which impede the maternal fetal circulation or by physical obstruction to adequate circulation due to a knot or kink in the umbilical cord.

Postnatal anoxia may be due to any cause which limits the supply of oxygen or renders the cells unable to use the oxygen available. This is the case, for example, if an overdose of barbiturates has been given. During severe shock, oxygen is not sent to the cells in adequate amounts. Even obstruction of the air passages by mucus may drastically diminish the supply of oxygen reaching the brain. Lasting causes of anoxia include severe anemia due to hemorrhage or hemolytic disease, poorly oxygenated blood due to a cyanotic type of congenital heart disease, or inadequate pulmonary ventilation due to malformation of the lungs.

Clinical Manifestations. It is extremely important that the nurse know the signs of both fetal anoxia and anoxia in the newborn. Fetal anoxia is evidenced by an increase in activity of the fetus followed by diminution. The fetal heart beat slows and weakens. When fetal anoxia is present, the infant is delivered immediately in order to save his life.

Symptoms of anoxia in the newborn include signs of yellow, meconium-stained amniotic fluid and yellowish vernix caseosa, pallor or cyanosis (even duskiness of the skin), lack of muscle tone, and variable heart beat.

Treatment. The treatment depends upon the stage of the anoxia and the cause of the condition. Mechanical techniques include mouth-to-mouth insufflation, administration of oxygen by moderate pressure (20 to 30 cm. of water for less than 0.2 second) or through an intratracheal catheter, and the use of "seesaw" respirators. Artificial respiration is of no value unless some expansion of the lungs has taken place. Nalorphine hydrochloride (Nalline) may be given intravenously to reverse respiratory depression due to narcotics given to the mother.

The method of *artificial respiration* for infants and small children advocated by the American Red Cross is as follows:

Clear the child's mouth of any foreign matter.

Place the child on his back, and use the middle finger of each hand to lift the lower jaw from beneath and behind so that it juts out. Hold the jaw in that position with one hand. Place your mouth over the child's mouth and nose, making a reasonably leak-proof seal, and breathe into the child smoothly and steadily until you observe the chest rise. As you start this action, move your free hand to the child's abdomen, between the navel and the ribs. Apply continuous moderate pressure to the abdomen to prevent the stomach from filling with air. When the lungs are inflated, remove your lips from the child's mouth and nose and allow the lungs to empty. Repeat this cycle, keeping one hand beneath the jaw and the other hand pressing on the stomach at all times. The rate should be about 20 cycles per minute. After every 20 cycles rest long enough to take a deep breath.

Carbon dioxide should not be given before spontaneous respiration occurs. Stimulants frequently used include caffeine and sodium benzoate given intramuscularly. After the immediate emergency 5 per cent carbon dioxide and 95 per cent oxygen may be given for one-half minute to two minutes every half-hour to two hours in order to stimulate deeper respirations.

Infants with respiratory distress should be wrapped in a warm blanket or placed in an incubator. Aspiration to remove mucus from the throat is a routine procedure.

Nursing care is the same as that of atelectasis (see below).

Prevention. Preventive measures applying to the management of labor include reduction of analgesia and anesthesia and administration of oxygen during the second stage of labor. Preventive measures applying to the care of the infant include maintenance of an open airway, administration of oxygen as needed, provision of skin stimulation and keeping the infant warm.

Atelectasis

The lungs are collapsed in fetal life, and the fetus receives oxygen through the maternal circulation. After birth, with the infant's first breath, the lungs normally expand to a variable degree. It may be days or weeks before full expansion takes place.

Atelectasis—collapse or imperfect expansion of lung tissue which carries air—is found in greater or less degree in almost all infants dying soon after delivery. The condition may be either primary or secondary. In *primary* atelectasis the alveoli fail to expand initially. This is common in premature infants and in full-term infants who have suffered brain injury. In *secondary* atelectasis the alveoli collapse after they have once been expanded by air; this may occur when the infant has pulmonary disease.

Clinical Manifestations. The symptoms are irregular, rapid, shallow respirations accompanied by a respiratory grunt and flaring of the nostrils. The skin is mottled. Cyanosis may be persistent or intermittent; it decreases if the infant cries or is given oxygen. There are intercostal and suprasternal retractions. Fine rales may be heard. On auscultation of the chest poor respiratory exchange is evident. X-ray films reveal increased density which may be present throughout both lungs.

Treatment. By bronchoscopy the physician determines whether any obstruction is present and removes it if possible. Oxygen may be given so that the open areas of the lungs will have a sufficient supply. The environmental humidity is raised in order that secretions may be liquefied and that the infant may be able to cough up the material. The physician may order 5 per cent carbon dioxide, and 95 per cent oxygen to be given in order to stimulate respirations. Caffeine

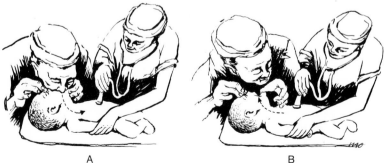

A   B

Figure 10–13. Mouth-to-mouth insufflation. *A,* Air is breathed into the infant's lungs. *B,* The lungs are allowed to empty. The stethoscope is placed over the abdomen in order to determine whether air is being forced into the stomach.

and sodium benzoate may be given intra- muscularly. The infant's skin may be stimulated in order to induce crying. His position should be changed every hour or two to provide opportunity for collapsed areas to expand. Antibiotics are given for persistent atelectasis in order to prevent secondary infections. The fundamental treatment is directed toward the underlying condition.

Course, Prognosis and Prevention. The *course* is difficult to predict. Even with early diagnosis and treatment the *prognosis* is poor and death not infrequent. *Prevention* of atelectasis in the infant includes prenatal care of the mother. Premature labor or a difficult delivery in which intracranial hemorrhage occurs is the cause in many cases. Fetal or neonatal anoxia is evidently a predisposing factor, as are pneumonia and hyaline membrane disease.

Nursing Care. The nurse should keep in mind the infants under her care who are likely to have atelectasis, such as those who were born prematurely or by cesarean section, those whose mothers had problems during pregnancy, and those who have had intracranial injury or are sick from pneumonia or other respiratory conditions. The nurse must observe these infants closely to detect the first symptoms of distress and also to give an accurate description of their condition to the physician. These infants should be kept warm, preferably in incubators where oxygen can easily be given and the humidity raised. It may be necessary to aspirate the upper respiratory tract if the infant's nose and throat appear to be clogged with mucus. Thy physician may also order aspiration of the gastric contents in order to prevent aspiration of vomitus should vomiting occur. The infant must be fed slowly and with great care, and the physician may order gavage feedings. All possible measures to prevent abdominal distention must be taken.

The nursing care should be planned so that the infant is disturbed as little as possible; there is more than the usual need for gentle handling. Every precaution should be taken to prevent infection, since even a simple respiratory infection may prove fatal.

Pneumonia

Incidence and Pathology. Pneumonia is responsible for approximately 10 per cent of neonatal deaths. The disease may accompany an infection which is not of the respiratory tract. Pneumonia in the newborn and the older infant is usually bronchopneumonic rather than lobar.

Etiology. Organisms which may cause pneumonia in the infant are not the same as those responsible for the disease in older children and adults. In the newborn, pneumonia may be due to bacteria or viruses. The chief causative agents in pneumonia occurring within the first few weeks of life are coliform organisms, enterococci, Klebsiella, Pseudomonas, Proteus, Salmonella and Staphylococcus.

The causes of pneumonia in the newborn are connected with the birth process as well as with contact with infection after birth. During delivery, infection may come from aspiration of infected amniotic fluid or vaginal secretions. Infection may be carried to the respiratory tract by way of the bloodstream. After birth the infectious organism is most commonly acquired through contact with the mother or with a nurse who has a cold. Although slight respiratory infections in the newborn do not always result in pneumonia, the danger is so great that no one with even a simple cold should care for him. Skin infections caused by a staphylococcus are also a cause of pneumonia in the newborn, whose resistance to any type of infection is low.

Clinical Manifestations. The first sign of pneumonia in the newborn is rapid respiration, which may reach 80 per minute, more than the nurse can count with accuracy. Respiratory distress is evident in flaring of the nostrils. The infant appears listless, is pale or cyanotic, and has a temperature higher or lower than normal. He is likely to refuse his feedings and suffers from abdominal distention.

Treatment. In general the plan of treatment includes chemotherapeutic agents against the common organisms causing pneumonia in infancy. Bacitracin or an antistaphylococcal synthetic penicillin may be used in the treatment of staphylococcal infections. If the exact causative organism can be isolated through laboratory tests, treatment can be made more specific. Oxygen is routinely used to relieve the respiratory distress.

Aspiration Pneumonia

The first *symptom* of aspiration pneumonia is generally an attack of coughing or, since the cough reflex of the newborn is imperfect, of choking. The usual symptoms of pneumonia are likely to follow within a short time. *Prevention* lies in careful feeding of infants and is therefore the responsibility of the mother and the nurse.

One advantage of breast feeding is that aspiration is not too likely. The newborn has not learned the technique of correlating sucking and swallowing. If the flow of milk is too rapid for him to swallow, he can pull away from the breast more readily than from a bottle held in a nurse's hand. The size of the hole in the nipple is important, and the nurse should be sensitive to the infant's need to swallow what he has in his mouth before more flows in.

If the infant chokes on the feeding and is in

immediate danger, the emergency measure is to suspend him by his feet. This permits aspirated milk to drain from the lungs. (For artificial respiration see page 182). After feeding, the infant should not be placed on his back, but on his right side or abdomen so that if he vomits, the material will drain from the mouth.

Treatments which disturb the infant emotionally or physiologically, e.g. puncture of the jugular or femoral veins, should be done two hours or more after feedings.

INFECTIONS

Organisms Causing Infection Before Birth

Certain infections may be passed from the mother to the child either before or during birth. These include ophthalmia neonatorum, thrush, congenital syphilis, toxoplasmosis and cytomegalic inclusion disease.

Ophthalmia Neonatorum (Gonorrheal Conjunctivitis)

Etiology. The causative organism, *Neisseria gonorrhoeae* (a gram-negative, coffee bean-shaped diplococcus), is found in a smear or culture taken from the purulent exudate from the eye.

The newborn acquires the infection during the birth process by direct contact with infected material in the vagina of the mother. The condition is to be reported to the Board of Health as a contagious disease.

Clinical Manifestations. The onset is usually within two or three days after birth, but symptoms may appear earlier. There is redness and swelling of the lids and a profuse, purulent discharge.

Complications. The common complication is corneal ulceration with resulting opacity and partial or complete loss of vision. The extent of the handicap depends on the duration and severity of the untreated condition.

Treatment. Penicillin is the preferred drug, but erythromycin, a tetracycline or chloramphenicol may be administered topically and systemically. The infant is kept in strict isolation. Symptomatic therapy consists in removing the discharge thoroughly with irrigations, usually of physiologic saline solution.

Prognosis. Excellent results are obtained with treatment. Ophthalmia neonatorum was formerly the greatest cause of blindness in infancy, but today the incidence is slight.

Nursing Care. It is difficult to instill drops into the eyes of a newborn infant at the time of delivery. The nurse must be absolutely sure that the drops are instilled within the eyelids. The medication may cause a slight irritation and redness of the eyes and the lids for a few days.

The infant's arms must be restrained so that he does not rub his eyes. If only one eye is affected, a shield is placed over the other one to protect it from infection. The purulent discharge is removed by frequent irrigations. When irrigations are done, the infant should be restrained in mummy fashion (see p. 301), and a second nurse should steady his head. As in all eye irrigations, the fluid should be warmed to body temperature, and the flow should be directed from the inner canthus outward. The nurse must be extremely careful that no drop of the return flow splashes into her own eyes as she leans over the infant.

Prevention. The prophylactic measure is to keep the mother free of infection. If the mother does not come under the care of a physician until the time of delivery, however, instillation of silver nitrate or penicillin safeguards the infant. State laws require prophylactic treatment of all infants at birth even though there is no reason to believe that a particular newborn is infected (see p. 116).

Thrush (Oral Moniliasis)

Etiology and Mode of Transmission. The causative agent of this infection is *Candida (Monilia) albicans.* The organism is normally present in the vagina of the mother, and is a saprophyte in the mouth of older children and adults. Thrush is a fungus infection; the spores grow on the delicate tissue of the buccal mucosa, producing mycelia. The infant may become infected from improperly sterilized nipples or the breast of his mother.

Clinical Manifestations. The mouth of the infant who has thrush contains white patches which resemble milk curds. They are different

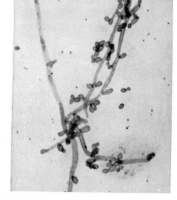

Figure 10–14. Candida in scrapings of thrush. (Pillsbury, Shelley and Kligman: *Cutaneous Medicine.*)

from milk curds, however, in that they are difficult to remove from the mucous membrane and, when removed, leave a bleeding area. These pearly-white, elevated lesions, which occur on the tongue margin, inside the lips and cheeks and on the hard palate, are painless. If the infection is localized in the mouth, the systemic symptoms tend to be mild, although the infant has anorexia. Esophagogastritis or pneumonitis may develop, however, as a result of invasion by the infective organism. (Color Plate I-1.)

Treatment and Prognosis. Nystatin is effective in the *treatment* of these lesions and may be applied locally with a soft swab. (It will not hurt the infant to swallow whatever is left in his mouth). Aqueous gentian violet, 1 per cent solution, or 1:1000 aqueous solution of benzalkonium chloride (Zephiran) may be used. These latter drugs are only moderately effective.

The *prognosis* in general is very good, recovery taking place in three or four days.

Nursing Care. Preventive nursing is based on absolute cleanliness of all articles which enter the infant's mouth: the mother's nipples, or the rubber nipples used in artificial feeding. Applicators used in the infant's mouth should be sterile. An older infant's toys and pacifiers must be clean.

To prevent the spread of thrush, the infant should have his own feeding equipment, which should be sterilized before being returned to the milk laboratory. It may be difficult to coax an infant to take enough nourishment. If the nipple irritates his mouth, a medicine dropper may be used.

If the physician orders the infant's mouth to be swabbed with gentian violet, the mother should be warned of the purple discoloration, since the dye produces a startling effect.

Congenital Syphilis (Lues)

Etiology and Description. The causative agent of syphilis is a spirochete, *Treponema pallidum.* Congenital syphilis and childhood syphilis will be considered here.

Congenital syphilis and acquired syphilis have been greatly reduced in incidence throughout most of the United States; however, their incidence has begun to rise again in the past few years. The mode of transmission to the fetus is by direct inoculation into the blood stream through the placenta during the latter half of pregnancy. Thus the disease is beyond the primary stage when the infant is born.

Clinical Manifestations. Although a variety of other conditions have symptoms similar to those of syphilis, a typical combination of symptoms points to the diagnosis of syphilis. The symptoms may be divided into two groups: those which appear early and those which appear later in the course of the disease.

EARLY SYMPTOMS. The more severe the infection, the earlier will the symptoms be apparent; in general they appear before the sixth week. Characteristic symptoms are as follows: (1) a persistent rhinitis, which has been given the name of "snuffles." This is a profuse mucopurulent nasal discharge, which may be blood-tinged and is irritating to the upper lip. The lip may become excoriated from the discharge. (2) There is a rash, heaviest over the back, buttocks and thighs, and involving the palms and soles. (3) There may be bleeding ulcerations and moist lesions of the mucous membranes of the mouth, lips, anus and genitalia. (4) The infant is anemic. (5) There may be osteochondritis or periostitis, or both, of the bones. (6) Pseudoparalysis or pathologic fractures may be present. (7) The liver and the spleen are enlarged. (8) There may be chorioretinitis with later atrophy of the optic nerve.

LATER SYMPTOMS. Later clinical manifestations are as follows: (1) destruction of the bones of the nose, so-called saddle nose, in which the nose dips slightly beyond the bridge and rises again toward the tip; (2) a periostitis of the tibiae in which these bones develop a sharp forward curve, a condition called saber shins. (3) The deciduous teeth are normal, but the central incisors of the permanent teeth are peg-shaped with a characteristic Gothic-shaped notch, so-called Hutchinson's teeth (Fig. 10-15, *D*). (4) The lesions of early syphilis around the mouth and nose become linear fissures which form radiating scars on healing (rhagades). (5) Interstitial keratitis may develop when the child is six to twelve years old. Photophobia, lacrimation, general discomfort and impairment of vision are symptoms of this condition. (6) Neurosyphilis, manifestations of which may appear at any time from one to ten years of age. The symptoms are hemiplegia, spastic paralysis and mental retardation. The child is slow in talking and is irritable and restless.

Diagnosis. The diagnosis is confirmed by serologic tests. A Wassermann reaction may be determined at any time, or blood may be obtained from the cord at delivery. Blood tests, however, are less accurate in providing proof of the presence of syphilis in the newborn than later in life. When the infant is six months of age, positive serologic results are more indicative of a syphilitic infection. A second test should be done, however, before the diagnosis is confirmed even at this age if no other manifestations of the disease are evident. Scrapings from moist lesions may show *Treponema pallidum* (darkfield examination is done on the scrapings).

Prognosis. Prompt treatment. of early congenital syphilis will usually result in a cure and in normal growth and development. Although late congenital syphilis may be cured,

A   B

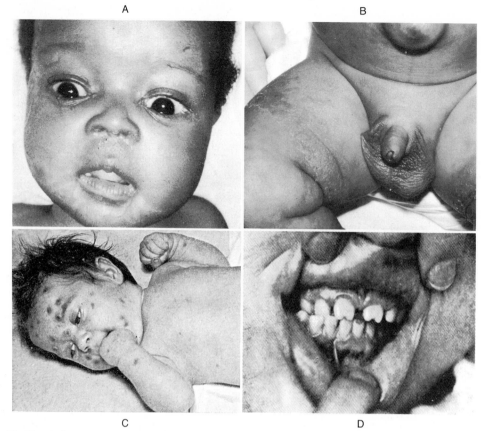

C   D

Figure 10–15. *A,* Congenital syphilis. This infant has "snuffles." (Courtesy of Dr. Ralph V. Platou and the American Academy of Pediatrics.) *B,* Rash of congenital syphilis on thighs. (Courtesy of Luis Schut, M.D.) *C,* Maculopapular eruption of congenital syphilis. (Katharine Dodd in W. E. Nelson: *Textbook of Pediatrics.* 8th ed.) *D,* Hutchinson's teeth in congenital syphilis in a boy 10 years of age. (Katharine Dodd in W. E. Nelson: *Textbook of Pediatrics,* 8th ed.)

the pathologic changes will remain for life.

Prevention. A serologic test is required in most parts of the United States before marriage or during pregnancy. This is probably the greatest preventive measure against congenital syphilis. Case finding in adults is furthered by the requirement of physical examinations in many types of work and in the armed services. The almost universal custom of prenatal care during pregnancy has increased the opportunity for early treatment of syphilis if a woman is found to have the disease. Cure may then be effected before the infant is born. Even later treatment may prevent syphilis in the infant or mitigate his condition.

Treatment. For early syphilis any of the penicillins may be given by injection. If the patient is sensitive to penicillin, erythromycin or tetracycline may be given. Follow-up serologic tests should be done on both the infant and the mother.

Nursing Care. Basic to the nursing care is the danger of transmission of the disease. Al-

though the organism dies rapidly on exposure, it may be transmitted by direct or indirect contact. The organisms are found in the skin lesions and the nasal discharge of the host and invade the body of another through a break in the mucous membranes or skin. In many hospitals, nurses caring for infectious syphilitic infants are required to wear rubber gloves and a gown. During the infectious period no pin should be used in the infant's clothing because of the possibility of the nurse sticking herself with a contaminated pin. Diapers should be tied in place temporarily. After a few days of treatment the infant is probably no longer infectious.

Feeding is made difficult by the presence of snuffles. The nose should be cleansed of discharge before the bottle or breast is offered. The upper lip should be kept clean, and cold cream should be applied to prevent excoriation from the irritating nasal discharge. Careful handling of the infant is necessary, for bone lesions cause him pain on movement. If the nurse is caring for an older child who shows signs of photophobia due to interstitial keratitis, she should darken the room for his comfort; if he is old enough, he may wear dark glasses.

Congenital syphilis represents a failure in finding a syphilitic infection in an antepartal patient; therefore public health nurses are stressing the need of prenatal care, including serologic examinations, treatment if necessary and follow-up study on infants on whom treatment has been started.

Toxoplasmosis

Incidence, Etiology and Transmission. This is an uncommon disease of the central nervous system. The causative organism is the *Toxoplasma gondii,* which is considered to be a protozoon. The severe infantile form occurs when the fetus acquires the infection *in utero.* The fetus may be prematurely born, stillborn or born at term. The disease may also be acquired after birth.

Clinical Manifestations, Prognosis and Treatment. Evidence of chorioretinitis (inflammation of the choroid and of the retina) may be detected in the eyegrounds. Cerebral calcifications may be present. Hydrocephalus (see p. 214) or microcephalia (see p. 220) may occur. Psychomotor retardation and convulsions are also symptoms. During the acute stage, symptoms of encephalitis may appear. The organism may be isolated from cerebrospinal fluid or from other tissues of the body.

In the infantile form the *prognosis* is poor. Although active congenital toxoplasmosis may cause death in days or weeks, the illness may regress, leaving one or more of the various disabilities mentioned above.

The use of pyrimethamine (Daraprim), which is a folic acid antagonist, and sulfadiazine as a combined *treatment* shows promising results. When these drugs are used, frequent leukocyte counts must be made, since both may produce leukopenia.

Nursing Care. The nursing care is based on the relief of symptoms. The child is made as comfortable as possible. The nurse should keep in mind both the symptoms and the possible complications so that she may give an accurate account to the physician.

Cytomegalic Inclusion Disease (Salivary Gland Virus Disease)

Incidence, Etiology and Transmission. This condition is a generalized illness caused by a salivary gland virus which occurs almost exclusively in newborns. The occurrence of symptoms with this disease is unusual, although salivary gland virus causes symptomatic human infection frequently. Transplacental transmission occurs, resulting in infection of the newborn.

Clinical Manifestations, Prognosis and Treatment. Symptoms may be mild with recovery or severe, leading to a rapidly fatal disease. In severely affected infants, hepatosplenomegaly, purpura, jaundice and signs of central nervous system involvement may be present. The child may have convulsions, microcephalia, hydrocephalus and chorioretinitis. If the infant survives, permanent neurologic sequelae such as mental retardation occur. Clinically, this condition resembles toxoplasmosis. The only treatment known at present is to support the patient and to keep him as comfortable as possible.

Organisms Causing Infection after Birth

Any pathogenic bacteria or virus may cause infection in the newborn. The chief organisms affecting the newborn are coliform organisms and *Staphylococcus aureus*; others include enterococci, Klebsiella, Pseudomonas, Salmonella and Proteus.

Types of Infections. The most common types of infection occurring in the nursery are septicemia, pneumonia and skin and umbilical infections. Diarrhea is still a common infection, although its incidence has been reduced in this country.

Clinical Manifestations and Treatment. It is extremely difficult for the nurse to recognize infection in the newborn, since his reactions to it may be so general that infection is not suspected. This is one reason why the nurse should report anything slightly abnormal even in an apparently "normal" newborn. The pediatrician makes his diagnosis by appraising the significance of every factor in the total clinical picture.

Signs indicating that something is wrong with an infant include cyanosis, convulsions, listlessness, anorexia, vomiting, jaundice and diarrhea. Fever may or may not be an indication of infection, since it may be the result of keeping the infant too warm. Absence of fever has little diagnostic significance, since the newborn may not react to even a massive infection with an elevation of temperature. The difficulties in making a diagnosis of infection are even greater in the premature than in the normal newborn. Laboratory studies and x-ray examination may be necessary.

If a specific infecting organism is found, *treatment* is mainly by administration of the appropriate chemotherapeutic agent; if a specific organism is unknown, an agent effective against a number of organisms is given.

Infections Caused by Escherichia Coli

Escherichia coli is the most common cause of serious infection of the newborn and is capable of producing a number of pathologic conditions, among them septicemia, pneumonia, meningitis and diarrhea. Neomycin is commonly used for intestinal infections; kanamycin, for systemic infections.

Infections Caused by Staphylococcus Aureus

Etiology, Onset, Types, and Modes of Entry. *Staphylococcus aureus* is a gram-positive organism which under the microscope appears in clumps. It is second only to *Escherichia coli* as a cause of infection in the newborn. Unfortunately the incidence of this type of infection in newborn nurseries is increasing. Many strains of the organism appear to be resistant to the majority of known chemotherapeutic agents.

The initial infection usually occurs while the infant is in the hospital, but may appear weeks or months later. This is one of the many reasons why all infants should be under the care of a private physician or be visited by a public health nurse and taken regularly to a Child Health Conference or clinic. An infection of this type acquired while the infant is in the nursery is likely to spread to other infants even though the customary isolation technique has been followed.

If the infant is breast-fed, the mother may acquire mastitis due to infection of the nipple from the organisms in his mouth. An infant may also infect other members of the family if he is discharged before the infection has been recognized and treated.

The primary infection with *Staphylococcus aureus* is commonly but not always of the skin. It may be an infection of the nasopharynx or of the cord stump carried from one infant to another. Pneumonia, septicemia or enteritis may represent infection with *Staphylococcus aureus*. Osteomyelitis or meningitis may be a complication of septicemia. A leaking meningocele or a circumcision wound may also be the site of an infection.

SOURCES OF INFECTION IN THE NURSERY. Pathogens may be brought into the nursery by the nurses caring for the infants or by other personnel. The mother also is a possible source of infection to her child. Infection is spread readily from one infant to others.

Treatment and Prevention. Systemic *therapy* requires giving an antibiotic effective against the specific organism infecting the infant. The drugs include bacitracin or one of the antistaphylococcal synthetic penicillins. Indiscriminate use of prophylactic antibiotics should not be condoned, because this will only result in the emergence of more resistant strains of bacteria. Skin lesions in general are treated by bathing the infant with a soap or a detergent containing hexachlorophene. Bacitracin ointment may be applied to the skin lesions, but in some cases it

may be necessary to drain the lesions surgically.

Prevention is as important as treatment. No one with a skin infection should enter the nursery or the rooms occupied by the mothers. A mother who becomes infected should be isolated, and her child, if there is any reason to believe that his contact with her may have caused him to become infected, should be isolated from other infants in the nursery.

Every infant in the nursery should have his individual equipment, and all personnel caring for the infants should use soap or a detergent containing hexachlorophene when washing their hands. Personnel should be aware also that the anterior nares are the main reservoir in carriers of *Staphylococcus aureus*. (See page 123 for the advisability of wearing masks when caring for infants.) Infants may be bathed with soap or a detergent containing hexachlorophene to lessen the chance of skin infection, and the umbilical cord stump may be routinely painted daily with bactericidal dyes. The nursery must not be overcrowded, for then it is almost impossible to maintain isolation technique.

If an epidemic starts, certain measures are routine. New patients are isolated. Rigid isolation technique is enforced. Another nursery should be opened for newborns delivered after the epidemic started and therefore not exposed to the infection in the contaminated nursery. Contaminated equipment should be thoroughly scrubbed with soap and water and sterilized if possible. The floor and walls should be cleaned and aired, curtains and furnishings washed. Nose and throat cultures should be taken of all nurses and other personnel who have cared for the infants in the infected nursery. It is imperative that each nursery have its own staff of nurses. As a preventive measure, an antibiotic effective against the particular strain of staphylococcus responsible for the original epidemic may be given to each infant in the clean nursery from his admission until discharge.

If these drastic measures are carried out for three weeks, the epidemic will probably come to an end. Such an epidemic is one of the most serious which may occur in a nursery for newborns.

Impetigo of the Newborn

Etiology, Incidence and Transmission (Color Plate 1-4). The causative organism may be staphylococci or streptococci. These organisms invade the superficial layers of the skin. The condition occurs more readily in the newborn than in older children and adults because their resistance is lower. Impetigo may be carried from one infant to another in the nursery.

Clinical Manifestations, Treatment, Prognosis and Nursing Care. The first symptomatic lesions are erythematous papules. Then super-

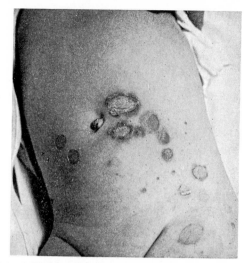

Figure 10-16. Impetigo neonatorum. (R. J. McKay, Jr., and C. A. Smith in W. E. Nelson: *Textbook of Pediatrics.* 8th ed.)

ficial vesicles containing fluid appear. The covering of these vesicles is loose and wrinkled. The fluid soon becomes purulent, and an area of erythema develops around each vesicle. The pustule ruptures, and crusts may develop, although this is more common in older children than in the newborn. The lesions usually occur on moist surfaces or body creases, and last from one to two weeks. Constitutional symptoms are rare.

Treatment consists in removing the epidermis with alcohol sponges and exposing the denuded areas to dry heat. Affected areas may also be treated by washing with soap containing hexachlorophene. Bacitracin or neomycin ointment may be applied locally. Systemic antibiotic therapy may be necessary.

Impetigo of the newborn was formerly a dangerous infection which led to sepsis and pemphigus, but today, with antibiotic treatment, the *prognosis* is good. Superficial lesions heal without scarring, although more extensive, deeper lesions may leave scars. Strict isolation technique should prevent the occurrence of impetigo in the nursery.

Furunculosis

Etiology, Incidence, Pathology and Clinical Manifestations. Staphylococci are, in general, the pathogenic organisms which cause furunculosis. Although the condition may occur at any time during childhood, it is most frequent and most dangerous in malnourished newborn infants. Furuncles are most likely to occur on the head, but may appear on the back or the back of the extremities.

Furunculosis is an infection of the sebaceous glands or hair follicles. The furuncle soon develops into a red, pointed or rounded lump. In a few days it softens, and a core is formed. When a number of such lesions are present, the condition is called *furunculosis.* The infant seldom shows systemic symptoms. In extreme cases, however, anorexia and toxemia may occur.

Treatment. Antibiotic therapy depends upon the specific organism causing the condition. This can be found through an epidemiologic survey of the family. A neomycin-bacitracin ointment may be applied in the nostrils, under the fingernails and around the perianal area to help prevent spread of the infection. The infant should be bathed daily, using soap containing hexachlorophene or a similar antiseptic to prevent spread of the infection. Hot compresses may be ordered to further maturation of the furuncle and, after it has opened spontaneously or been incised, to further drainage.

The diet should be low in carbohydrate and high in vitamin content. A sufficient fluid intake is necessary, and the electrolyte balance must be maintained.

Nursing Care. Aseptic nursing technique in the nursery is the best preventive of furunculosis. Particularly in hot weather the infant's position should be changed so that all surfaces of the skin are exposed in rotation to the air.

If furunculosis develops in an infant in the nursery, he should be removed and isolated elsewhere. With the first sign of the lesion the area should be cleansed with care. If the lesion is on the scalp, the area around the furuncle should be shaved. The nurse will carry out the physician's orders for treatment. The infant must not be allowed to rub the area; arm restraints (see Fig. 11-5) should be applied if necessary. The nurse should be careful that she herself does not become infected; the slightest scratch or abrasion on her hand may easily be a point of entrance for the organism.

Epidemic Diarrhea

Etiology, Incidence and Transmission. In the newborn no single organism has been identified which is invariably the cause of epidemic diarrhea, though severe epidemics have been cause by virulent strains of *E. coli* bacilli or by viruses producing respiratory infections in adults. Diarrhea is a highly contagious disease easily carried from one infant to another. An infant who acquires the condition should be taken from the nursery and isolated elsewhere.

An infant may contract the disease through a contaminated formula or from the hands of his mother or nurse who themselves carry the organism, but are without clinical symptoms, since they have the adult's resistance to the infection. The importance of this source of infection is seldom realized. It is impossible to sterilize human hands completely, and even careful washing may not eliminate the risk of carrying the pathogenic organism to the infant.

Clinical Manifestation, Treatment and Course. The main *symptom* is frequent watery stools, which are likely to be expelled with considerable force. The infant has abdominal distention; he may refuse his feedings or, if he takes them, vomit. As a rule there is elevation of the temperature. The weight loss is largely due to loss of fluid, which may be extremely rapid. Loss of fluids results in electrolyte imbalance and dehydration. Acidosis may result.

The *treatment* is similar to that given infants with diarrhea (see p. 297). The obstetric unit should be closed unless all new cases can be cared for in other quarters by nurses who have not been in contact with the infants suffering from this infectious condition. If the cause of the infection is the enteropathic strain of the colon bacillus, neomycin may be ordered and given orally. Fluids and electrolytes are given parenterally to supplement or replace the oral intake.

The disease must be reported to the health authorities because of its infectiousness. The *course* is severe, and the mortality rate may be as high as 25 to 40 per cent of affected infants.

Nursing Care. Nursing care is both preventive and supportive. Rules and regulations safeguarding infants from all sources of infection are an administrative responsibility, but conscientious application of these regulations in the direct care of infants is the function of the nurse. It is she who will see the first loose stool and note the presence of mucus in it, observe the infant's refusal of part or all of his feeding—probably vomiting what he has taken—and note his rise in temperature. The pathologic organism must be isolated in the laboratory examination of a stool specimen before the diagnosis of infectious diarrhea is made, but measures to protect the other infants in the nursery must be taken as soon as infection is suspected. In the majority of hospitals the nurse has a standing order to place an infected infant in isolation even before the physician has made his diagnosis and given her written orders to do so.

The probable treatment which the physician will order has been outlined. All but the parenteral administration of fluids is carried out by the nurse. Few infants having medical conditions require such constant attention as those suffering from epidemic diarrhea.

Prevention of excoriated buttocks is an immediate problem in the nursing care. The diaper must be changed frequently. If the room is warm enough, it is advisable not to diaper the infant, but rather to place a pad made of folded diapers under his buttocks and leave him uncovered. If the temperature of the room requires application of heat, a cradle with an electric light bulb in the top may be placed over his body and covered with a sheet. Care must be taken that the sheet does not touch the bulb, since it might be scorched and become ignited.

In some hospitals the diapers from an infected infant are soaked in a disinfectant before being sent to the laundry, or they may be placed in a container marked for special care in the laundry.

For additional care of infants with diarrhea, see page 298.

Umbilical Infection

Etiology, Clinical Manifestations, Complications, Treatment, Prevention and Nursing Care. Umbilical infection is usually due to *Escherichia coli* or staphylococci, but may be due to other pyogenic organisms. The *symptoms* are redness and moisture of the stump of the cord. These symptoms may be slight or severe, but in no case should they be disregarded. In severe cases there may be a characteristically foul odor from the stump. The condition may clear up without systemic effects. But if the causative organism is one of the pus-producing type, septicemia may develop. Infection by the tetanus bacillus is less common, but produces a higher mortality rate (see p. 192).

Treatment consists in the administration of a broad-spectrum antibiotic immediately. Cultures with antibiotic sensitivities should be obtained. Some physicians recommend hexachlorophene baths and the application of triple dye to the umbilical area. If an abscess forms, incision and drainage become necessary.

Prevention of the infection is discussed on pages 115 and 123.

This is another condition in which close, intelligent observation of the infant by the nurse is of the utmost importance. The responsibility for noting the first signs of infection rests with her.

Early recognition and treatment may prevent serious, if not fatal, systemic complications. As with any infection, the infant should be isolated and, preferably, removed from the nursery.

Sepsis Neonatorum

Etiology, Clinical Manifestations and Treatment. Sepsis neonatorum may be caused by any pathogenic organism which has entered the bloodstream. The portal of entry may be through the skin, mucous membranes, respiratory or gastrointestinal tract, umbilicus, or circumcision or other wound. The infection may occur prenatally, during delivery or postnatally.

The *symptoms* and signs may appear suddenly after an insidious onset, the infant at first appearing only restless or listless with anorexia and poor weight gain. Later there is evidence of dehydration and emaciation. There may be vomiting and diarrhea. The infant's temperature and white blood cell count may be elevated, depressed or normal. Convulsions may or may not be present. Signs of jaundice may appear. On examination the spleen and the liver may be found enlarged. The majority of these symptoms are so variable that the diagnosis is made upon the general picture and the laboratory findings, particularly the blood culture and nasopharyngeal culture.

Immediate *treatment* consists in administration of large doses of broad-spectrum antibiotics. After the laboratory blood examination has proved the specific organism causing the septic condition the specific antibiotic is given. Symptomatic therapy is carried out from the onset of the disease. The infant is isolated. He may be placed in an incubator so that he can be more easily observed and so that the temperature, humidity, and oxygen administration can be regulated accurately. Fluids may be administered parenterally, and a blood transfusion may be necessary. Oxygen is given as the need arises.

Prognosis and Course. If the condition is recognized early and treatment is instituted at once, the mortality rate is low. The probability of death increases as the untreated condition becomes more severe. The nidus of the infection should be sought; it may be in the meninges, the perineum or elsewhere. The organism in the bloodstream may cause secondary infection in almost any part of the body. If meningitis develops, convulsions may ensue. If the infant survives, hydrocephalus may result. Characteristic signs of damage to brain cells may be evident as the child grows older (mental retardation).

Prevention and Nursing Care. *Prevention* lies in aseptic technique during delivery and in the technique which has already been outlined for the prevention of infection among infants in the nursery. Personnel caring for newborn infants must be exceptionally conscientious in reporting any infection, however slight, in their own bodies. In a modern hospital where good technique prevails it is probable that bacteria in the nose and throat of some member of the hospital personnel who comes in close contact with the infants are the greatest potential source of danger to them.

The preventive *nursing care* which has already been described in relation to infectious conditions applies in the care of infants suffering from sepsis neonatorum. Again, accurate observation and prompt reporting are of tremendous importance. From the discussion of signs and symptoms it is evident that the condition at the onset may easily be considered only a minor ailment and may go untreated until grave symptoms develop and the probability of complete cure is slight.

Tetanus Neonatorum

Etiology, Incidence and Incubation Period. The causative organism is the tetanus bacillus (*Clostridium tetani*), an anaerobic, spore-forming, gram-positive bacillus. Entrance into the bloodstream of the newborn is through the umbilical wound. Tetanus is most unlikely to occur in a well regulated hospital, since the natural environment of the organism is in the soil. In children and adults the organism enters the bloodstream through a deep puncture of the skin and underlying tissue. Since infants and children today receive antitetanus injections with the other types of early immunization, the incidence of tetanus among them is low.

Tetanus cannot be transmitted through contact; it must enter the body through a break in the skin. It develops only where it is not exposed to the air. Isolation of the infant is not necessary, but it may be carried out to protect the child from other infections.

Tetanus of the newborn is extremely rare in the United States, but occurs in other countries where the hands of the attendant at delivery (untrained midwife, neighbor or one of the family) are contaminated and a contaminated knife is used to cut the cord.

The *incubation period* is five days to several weeks. The shorter the period of incubation, the greater is the probability of a fatal outcome. In the average hospital in the United States an infant is not in the nursery more than five days, and if the condition were to occur, it would probably be after the infant had been sent home. Again we see the need of follow-up of all infants who are not under the care of a private physician.

Clinical Manifestations. The symptoms which accompany tetanus neonatorum are produced by the toxic effects on the nervous system of the exotoxin of the tetanus bacillus. The infant is irritable and restless; he cannot open his mouth or suck because of *trismus,* or tetanic spasm of the muscles of the jaw, and has great difficulty in swallowing. The facial expression is drawn and anxious. A symptom of diagnostic importance is stiffness of the neck. Painful muscular contractions or convulsions recur periodically. *Opisthotonos,* with the head drawn back and the back arched, occurs as a result of contraction of the strongest muscles in the body. As a result of spasms of the facial muscles a fixed expression, or *risus sardonicus,* may be seen. Tactile or auditory stimuli may induce convulsions. The temperature may be elevated, rising to 104°F. (40°C.). The white blood cell count is 8000 to 12,000, and there is a slight increase in the cerebrospinal fluid pressure.

Treatment, Prevention and Nursing Care. Adequate *treatment* and nursing care cannot be given unless a nurse is with the child at all times. Tetanus antitoxin is given to neutralize the free toxin in the body and around the site of the infection. Before administration of the antitoxin the infant's sensitivity to horse serum should be tested in order to prevent a serum reaction.

Measures to control convulsions are essential. Sufficient doses of sedatives are given to keep the infant relaxed and semiconscious. The level of sedation should be kept constant. Stimulation or unnecessary handling should be reduced to a minimum.

Nursing care should be planned around the periods when medication or necessary treatment is given. Secretions in the nasopharynx should be aspirated. Oxygen administration may be necessary. Oxygen and carbon dioxide may be ordered to stimulate respirations. The equipment for tracheotomy should be ready for immediate use if needed. (For care of a child having a tracheotomy see page 406.) Since the infant is heavily sedated and unable to suck or swallow, it is necessary to feed him by gavage. Fluids will probably be administered parenterally. An intake and output chart must be kept.

Prevention of tetanus neonatorum lies in the use of sterile instruments to cut the cord and adequate care of the cord during the neonatal period. For prevention of tetanus in the infant, see page 278.

Prognosis. The prognosis is very poor, the mortality rate being up to 50 per cent of the cases. Death is usually due to respiratory failure, exhaustion or a complicating aspiration pneumonia. If the infant survives, however, recovery is complete.

TEACHING AIDS AND OTHER INFORMATION*

American Academy of Pediatrics
Resuscitation of the Newborn Infant.

American Medical Association
Artificial Respiration.

National Society for the Prevention of Blindness, Inc.
Review of Status of State Laws Requiring Use of a Prophylactic in the Eyes of Newborn Infants.

Ross Laboratories
Intrauterine Transfusion and Erythroblastosis Fetalis: Report of the Fifty-Third Ross Conference on Pediatric Research, 1966.
Problems in Neonatal Surgery: Report of the Forty-Ninth Ross Conference on Pediatric Research, 1965.

The National Foundation – March of Dimes
Birth Defects – Social and Emotional Problems.
Birth Defects; The Tragedy and the Hope.

United States Department of Health, Education, and Welfare
Blood and the Rh Factor, 1966.
Rescue Breathing, 1966.

REFERENCES

Publications
Abramson, H. (Ed.): *Resuscitation of the Newborn Infant and Related Emergency Procedures – Principles and Practice.* 2nd ed. St. Louis, C. V. Mosby Company, 1966.
American Academy of Pediatrics: *Report of the Committee on the Control of Infectious Diseases.* 14th ed., 1964. Evanston, Ill., American Academy of Pediatrics, 1963.
American Public Health Association: *Control of Infectious Diseases in General Hospitals.* New York, American Public Health Association, 1967.
Avery, M. E.: *The Lung and Its Disorders in the Newborn Infant.* 2nd ed. Philadelphia, W. B. Saunders Company, 1968.

---

* Complete addresses are given in the Appendix.

Conn, H. F. (Ed.): *1968 Current Therapy.* Philadelphia, W. B. Saunders Company, 1968.

Feldman, S., and Ellis, H.: *Principles of Resuscitation.* Philadelphia, F. A. Davis Company, 1967.

Rubin, A. (Ed.): *Handbook of Congenital Malformations.* Philadelphia, W. B. Saunders Company, 1967.

Schaffer, A. J.: *Diseases of the Newborn.* 2nd ed. Philadelphia, W. B. Saunders Company, 1965.

Silverthorne, N., and others: *Principal Infectious Diseases of Childhood.* 2nd ed. Springfield, Ill., Charles C Thomas, 1966.

Smith, C. H.: *Blood Diseases of Infancy and Childhood.* 2nd ed. St. Louis, C. V. Mosby Company, 1966.

Smithells, R. W.: *Early Diagnosis of Congenital Abnormalities.* Philadelphia, F. A. Davis Company, 1964.

White, R. R.: *Atlas of Pediatric Surgery.* New York, Blakiston Division, McGraw-Hill Book Company, Inc., 1965.

Williams, R. E. O., and others: *Hospital Infection; Causes and Prevention.* 2nd ed. Chicago, Year Book Medical Publishers, Inc., 1966.

Periodicals

Adriani, J.: Anesthesia for Infants and Children. *Am. J. Nursing,* 64:107, August 1964.

American Heart Association: Closed-Chest Method of Cardiopulmonary Resuscitation. *Am. J. Nursing,* 65:105, May 1965.

Battaglia, F. C.: Recent Advances in Medicine for Newborn Infants. *J. Pediat.,* 71:748, 1967.

Buchanan-Davidson, D. J.: Erythroblastosis Neonatorum. *Am. J. Nursing,* 64:110, April 1964.

Douglas, G. W.: Rubella in Pregnancy. *Am. J. Nursing,* 66:2664, 1966.

Freda, V. J., and Robertson, J. G.: Amniotic Fluid Analysis in Rh Iso-Immunization. *Am. J. Nursing,* 65:64, August 1965.

Freda, V. J., and others: Suppression of the Primary Rh Immune Response with Passive Rh I & G Immunoglobulin; and A Landmark in Medical Progress: Prevention of Rh Sensitization (Edit.). *New Eng. J. Med.,* 277:622, 1036, November 9, 1967.

Glynn, E. M.: Nursing Support During Intra-Uterine Transfusions. *Am. J. Nursing,* 65:72, August 1965.

Goulding, E. I., and Koop, C. E.: The Newborn: His Response to Surgery. *Am. J. Nursing,* 65:84, October 1965.

Hoffmann, F. D., and Herweg, J. C.: Status of Serological Testing for Congenital Syphilis. *J. Pediat.,* 71:686, November 1967.

Koop, C. E.: Clinical Advances in Pediatric Surgery. *Pediat. Clin. N. Amer.,* 11:33, 1964.

Lin-Fu, J. S.: New Hope for Babies of Rh Negative Mothers. *Children,* 16:23, January-February 1969.

Marden, P. M., Smith, D. W., and McDonald, M. J.: Congenital Anomalies in the Newborn Infant, Including Minor Variations. *J. Pediat.,* 64:357, 1964.

Martin, L. W., and others: Nursing Care of Infants with Esophageal Anomalies. *Am. J. Nursing,* 66:2463, 1966.

Owens, C.: Parents' Reactions to Defective Babies. *Am. J. Nursing,* 64:83, November 1964.

Queenan, J. T.: Intra-Uterine Transfusion for Erythroblastosis Fetalis. *Am. J. Nursing,* 65:68, August 1965.

Rhea, J. W., and others: Effect of Hyperbaric Oxygenation on Neonatal Tetanus. *J. Pediat.,* 71:33, July 1967.

Stenchever, M. A., and Cibils, L. A.: Management of the Rh-Sensitized Patient. *Am. J. Obst. Gynec.,* 100:554, February 15, 1968.

Thompson, L. R.: Nursery Infections: Apparent and Inapparent. *Am. J. Nursing,* 65:80, November 1965.

Winchester, J. H.: Rescuing Newborns with Minisurgery. *Today's Health,* 46:52, January 1968.

11

CONDITIONS OF THE NEWBORN REQUIRING LONG-TERM CARE

CONGENITAL DEFORMITIES

Several congenital anomalies require care over a period of weeks, months or years. Long-term conditions such as inborn errors of metabolism, which are not usually diagnosed during the first few days of life, will be discussed in later chapters. For many of the anomalies discussed in this chapter, surgery early in life is the treatment of choice. The risk to life must be considered in relation to the probable advantage to the child of operation. It is difficult for parents to be objective in making the decision for or against surgical treatment. Before operation is undertaken the parents should be convinced that their decision is right, that the probable benefit justifies the risk. Then, if the child should die, they do not blame themselves for permitting the operation.

Surgical correction may be necessary later. The treatment and nursing care of some of these children will be discussed in chapters dealing with children of the age group in which correction of the anomaly is generally made.

Skin Lesions

Nevi

Nevi in the newborn are of two types: (a) the vascular group, due to hyperplasia of blood or lymph vessels; (b) nonvascular nevi, caused by an overgrowth of connective or epidermal tissue. In either type the defect probably originates in the germ plasm. The hereditary factor is apparently important.

Nevus Vasculosus. The nevus vasculosus, commonly called a birthmark, is composed entirely of blood vessels. These marks are likely to be flat and to appear on the back of the head. No treatment is required, since the majority disappear spontaneously.

The so-called *port-wine mark* is a flat, irregularly shaped mark often found on the side of the face. It is light pink in the newborn, but later becomes deep purple. It is due to a malformation of superficial capillaries and does not respond too well to local treatment. It may be removed by surgery or irradiation only by an

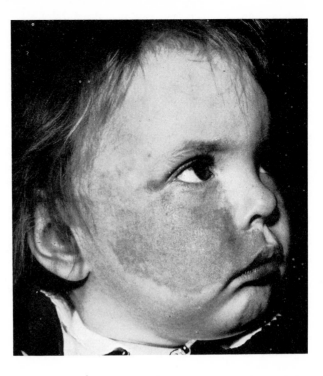

Figure 11–1. Nevus flammeus, or port-wine stain, present at birth. (Pillsbury, Shelley and Kligman: *Manual of Cutaneous Medicine.*)

expert in this kind of treatment. A small or faint lesion which appears to be similar to these marks on the face may appear on the nape of the neck, bridge of the nose or on the eyelids. These lesions, unlike those of the face, disappear without treatment.

The so-called *strawberry mark* is a slightly raised, bright red to deep purple nevus which may disappear spontaneously. These marks may be removed by applying carbon dioxide snow or dry ice over the area. Such treatments may be given at intervals of three to four weeks. After each treatment zinc oxide or another bland ointment should be applied to the area. The area should be covered with a dressing which should be changed daily. Radium therapy is also effective, but must be given only by an expert in this kind of treatment.

A *cavernous hemangioma* is formed by large

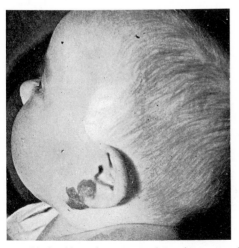

Figure 11–2. Vascular nevus (strawberry mark). (C. F. Burgoon, Jr., and C. S. Wright in W. E. Nelson: *Textbook of Pediatrics.* 8th ed.)

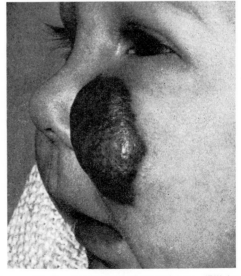

Figure 11–3. Cavernous hemangioma. (Pillsbury, Shelley and Kligman: *A Manual of Cutaneous Medicine.*)

sinus-like blood vessels. These lesions are cystic, deep-lying vascular anomalies that are blue or purple. Treatment is by irradiation (x-ray or radium), injection of a sclerosing solution, or surgery. Treatment should be begun early, since the lesions tend to grow larger as the child grows. There is also the possibility of severe hemorrhage if some trauma causes the lesion to bleed.

Pigmented Nevi. These lesions vary in size and color from harmless freckles to dark hairy nevi. Although such lesions are rarely malignant, the child should be kept from irritating the area. Although such nevi do not grow rapidly, they develop in proportion to the child's growth and therefore become increasingly more difficult to remove. If they are large, dark and on the face, they may cause both parents and child the emotional trauma likely to accompany any conspicuous disfigurement.

TREATMENT. The most satisfactory treatment of pigmented nevi is by surgical excision, including a portion of the nearby normal skin. Nevi on parts of the body where constant irritation of the skin occurs must be observed at regular intervals and removed if changes in size or nature occur. Operation must be done if they appear to be growing at a disproportionately greater rate than the body skin. If only the cosmetic effect is the concern of the physician and the parents, the time for removal makes little difference. In general, however, it is advisable that operation be done during the first year of life or in the early school years.

Gastrointestinal System

Cleft Lip and Cleft Palate

Etiology, Pathology and Incidence. The terms "cleft lip" and "cleft palate" describe the condition. The cause is a failure of union of the embryonic structures of the face. Fusion of the maxillary and premaxillary processes normally occurs between the fifth and eighth weeks of intrauterine life. The palatal processes fuse about one month later. Failure of fusion results in the typical cleft lip and cleft palate.

This partial or complete nonunion may involve more than the palatal bone and the upper lip. It may affect the maxilla, premaxilla and tissues of the soft palate and uvula. All these defects or any combination of them may occur. The abnormality appears to run in families and therefore to be influenced by heredity, but other factors may be involved. The condition is often one of several anomalies in the infant.

The *incidence* of cleft lip or cleft palate is about one in 800 of the population.

Psychologic Trauma. To learn that their newborn infant suffers this abnormality is a great shock to the parents—less so, however, if some relative on either side of the family lines has had a successful repair of the same condition. A sympathetic, tactful nurse can do a great deal to relieve their distress. She may show them "before and after operation" pictures of infants who had this deformity. These pictures may relieve parents of some of their anxiety about the appearance of their own infant.

Cleft Lip

Incidence and Pathology. Cleft lip is one of the most frequently occurring congenital anomalies. It is more common in males than in females.

The defect is due to incomplete fusion of the central processes with one or both of the lateral processes from which the area around the upper jaw, lip and nose is formed. If the fissure is unilateral, it is generally below the center of one of the nostrils; if bilateral, beneath both nostrils. The extent of the defect varies from a slight indentation to an open cleft. The incomplete cleft

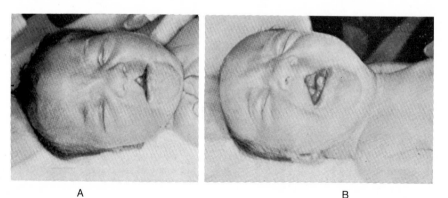

A   B

Figure 11–4. *A*, Midline cleft of the lip. *B*, Same child with mouth open to reveal the midline cleft of the palate. (Schaffer: Diseases of the Newborn. 2nd ed.)

may be little more than a notching of the vermilion border of the lip, but on the other hand may extend to the nostril. The complete cleft usually involves the alveolus to some degree, and the ala (the flap of flesh forming the side of the nostril) is displaced toward the side. The floor of the nares and even the gum in which the upper teeth are set may also be deformed.

Treatment and Prognosis. Plastic surgery should be done for the child's comfort as well as the cosmetic effect. In the mild incomplete type the child is not hampered by the deformity, and correction may be done at any time when he is in good condition. With complete cleft lip, repair should be made as soon as the child's condition permits, since the deformity interferes with feeding. The infant also becomes accustomed to breathing through his mouth, with the result that the mucous membrane becomes dry and cracked, and infection is more likely. In the rapidly growing structure of the infant's face the cleft prevents normal development. The psychologic effect upon the parents, even if they try to be objective in their attitude toward the child's deformity, is likely to hinder the usual face-to-face cuddling which infants normally receive. If they show him to friends, he may not receive the warm greeting which adults normally give to perfect, healthy infants and which the infant needs so as to develop his trust in others.

The *prognosis,* when repair is made by a competent plastic surgeon, is very good. The operation is usually done when the infant is one or two months old. At that time he should be free from infection and gaining weight. Postoperatively a Band-aid may be used to hold the suture line together. In many hospitals a *Logan bar* is used to prevent stretching of the wound postoperatively when the infant cries. (A Logan bar is a wire bow placed over the wound with each end taped to the cheek on which it rests.)

Preoperative Nursing Care. While the infant is at home the nurse should encourage the mother to treat him as if he were a normal infant. He should not be overprotected and certainly never rejected. The mother should not keep him from relatives and friends who will eventually accept him as a normal infant. She must realize, however, that the first impression of a child so disfigured is startling, and allow others to become accustomed to his appearance before expecting from them the normal reaction to an infant.

She should have explained to her that the infant's difficulty in feeding is due to the fact that he cannot create a vacuum in his mouth and so is unable to suck. A soft nipple with a relatively large hole, a special type of nipple or a rubber-tipped medicine dropper may be used to feed him, although in extreme cases gavage may be necessary. The mother can be taught whatever procedure is appropriate for her child. If a soft nipple is used, the infant should be assisted in sucking with a biting type of movement. In feeding with the dropper the rubber tip should be put on the top and to the side of the tongue and as far back in the mouth as is practical. He should be bubbled frequently, for he swallows more air than the infant nursing from the breast or the bottle.

Some physicians believe that the infant's hands should be restrained when he is not being held if he shows any tendency to irritate the cleft lip. With a small infant it is usually sufficient to pull the sleeves of the shirt down over the hands and to pin the edge of each sleeve to the diaper. Because of his need for sucking pleasure, some physicians recommend the use of a pacifier by such infants. The older infant's hands may be restrained by using the clove hitch restraint (see p. 180), or elbow restraints (Fig. 11-5) only if absolutely necessary.

Because of mouth-breathing the lips are dry, and it is important to prevent cracks or fissures through which infection may enter. The area should be kept clean, and water should be given after feedings to rinse out the mouth. The mother or nurse should also watch for signs of respiratory distress or gastrointestinal disturbance. Every precaution should be taken to protect him from infection. The routine care of an infant must be taught the mother, since the infant will be at home until he is old enough for operation.

Postoperative Nursing Care. The infant will require close observation to keep the airway open. He is accustomed to mouth-breathing, which may be difficult postoperatively. The nurse should report to the physician if the tissues of the tongue or mouth or the lining of the nostrils is swollen from surgery. A laryngoscope, endotracheal tube and suction apparatus should be ready for use if necessary.

The solution to be used for cleansing the nostril and the incision should be ordered by the physician. The nurse should cleanse the suture line frequently and with great care. The lip should be patted, not wiped. If a crust forms, a scar is likely to result; if a suture is pulled or sloughs out, the suture line will not be even.

The infant should receive the routine nursing care needed by all infants; he should be kept comfortable, warm and dry. He should be kept from crying, for even with the Band-aid or Logan bar, crying puts some strain on the suture line. His mother should be encouraged to stay and comfort the infant so that he will not cry. He can be held and carried about. He should be given the feeding to which he is accustomed.

If a medicine dropper is used, it should be inserted in the corner of the mouth so as not to touch the area about the suture line. He should be fed slowly and in a sitting position. He should be

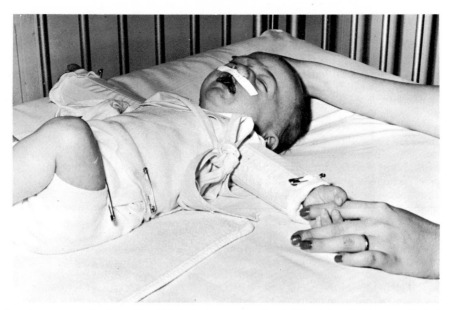

Figure 11-5. Appearance of a 2-month-old infant after repair of a cleft lip. A Band-aid is used to hold the suture line together. Elbow restraints prevent the infant from rubbing his face. The mother remained with this child throughout his hospitalization.

bubbled frequently both for relief of air which he has swallowed and for its general comforting effect. Water should be given to cleanse the mouth of milk after the feeding. As with any infant, water should be given between feedings.

If the hands must be restrained to prevent the infant from rubbing his face, normal movement is prevented. To improve the circulation and make the infant more comfortable, the arms should be released, first one and then the other. Since the infant cannot suck, he should be held and cuddled frequently to provide emotional satisfaction.

The infant should never be placed upon his abdomen, or even upon his side if there is a likelihood that he may roll over on his face. In the lateral position he is less likely to aspirate mucus or regurgitated milk. His position should be changed frequently to lessen the danger of hypostatic pneumonia. If it is impossible to support him on his side, or if his position is changed and he lies upon his back, he may be held in the desired position by bands about the wrists fastened with the clove hitch restraint (see p. 180).

The adhesive anchoring the Band-aid or Logan bar, if these are used, should be kept clean and dry and be replaced if it loosens.

After approximately two weeks, when the lip is completely healed, bottle or breast feeding may be resumed. Only an infant with an incomplete cleft can nurse, and therefore few of these infants are breast-fed satisfactorily. For a breast-fed infant, however, the mother should express her milk before and during the postoperative period when the infant is unable to suck.

Cleft Palate

Incidence, Etiology, Pathology and Clinical Manifestations. Unlike cleft lip, which occurs more frequently among boys than girls, cleft palate is more common in girls than in boys. Although it is often associated with cleft lip, the two anomalies are not always simultaneously present. Cleft palate is more serious than cleft lip. It interferes more with the infant's feeding and breathing and is far more difficult to repair.

The fissure may involve only the soft palate or may extend into the nose and also the hard palate. The cleft is in the midline of the soft palate and on one or both sides of the hard palate, and of course is longitudinal. The cleft forms a passageway between the nasopharynx and the nose. This passageway causes part of the difficulty in feeding and is a factor in susceptibility to infection.

The infant is unable to suck well, and even if he tries to suck, part of the feeding may be expelled through the nose.

As soon as the child has enough teeth to hold a dental speech appliance in place, one can be made to fit the deformity. If the cleft is not repaired before the child learns to talk, and if a dental speech appliance is not used, the guttural tone produced by the deformity may become habitual and persist after repair of the cleft has made normal speech possible.

Instructions to the Mother on Discharge of the Infant from the Nursery. As with the infant with cleft lip, the parents of a child with cleft palate are apt either to overprotect him or emotionally reject him. While he is still in the nursery the mother should be taught how to care for him, and he should become accustomed to her feeding him.

The *nutritional problem* is immediate. An adequate fluid intake is necessary to prevent dehydration. The mother should be taught how to feed the infant with a soft nipple having holes large enough to permit the milk to drop into the infant's mouth without sucking, or with a special nipple with a flange that covers the defect in the cleft palate so that the infant can suck. The infant may also be fed with a medicine dropper. Some physicians recommend the use of a Brecht feeder; however, there is a danger in using it because the feeding may be expressed too rapidly into his mouth and the infant may choke. Gavage should be used as a last resort. The infant should be held in an upright position in order to facilitate swallowing the feeding without regurgitation through the nose or without aspirating it. He should be bubbled frequently. Later on, perhaps when several months old, he may be fed with a spoon or may learn to take his milk from a cup.

The infant's mouth is easily infected. Some physicians believe that until he is old enough to cooperate, his arms must be restrained to prevent him from sucking his fingers or otherwise irritating the cleft. Other physicians and those interested in early childhood development believe that if the infant can be observed frequently, restraints should not be used, since they prevent him from exploring his world and his own body. If the infant is not permitted to explore and discover himself, he will have missed a sensory stage which is almost impossible to make up later. The mouth should be kept clean at all times, and for this purpose the physician may order a mild antiseptic. Feedings should be followed by a little water to rinse out the mouth.

Unless these infants are under the care of a private physician, it is essential that they be taken to a cleft palate clinic or a pediatric clinic at regular intervals in order to determine the proper time for operation. Repair may be attempted when the infant is as young as eighteen months or two years old, or may be postponed until he is five years old. The optimum time for operation depends upon the condition of the child. When operation is delayed, the surgeon may use to advantage the normal structural changes which take place in the palate during growth in the preschool years. On the other hand, if correction of the defect is not made before the child has learned to talk, he may retain his guttural speech.

The care of a child having a cleft palate requires the services of a cleft plate health team, the members of which are listed on page 428, where the care of a toddler having cleft palate repair is discussed.

Circulatory System

Changes Occurring in the Circulatory System at Birth. With the severing of the umbilical cord there is increased pressure from the incoming blood in the left side of the heart. This eventually causes the foramen ovale to close. In fetal life much of the pulmonary arterial blood passed through the ductus arteriosus to the aorta. At birth the muscles in the wall of the ductus arteriosus constrict, although complete closure may not occur until the second or third month of life. The heart has less work after than before birth, since placental circulation has been replaced by that of extrauterine life.

Congenital Heart Disease

Etiology, Diagnosis and Types of Cardiac Defects. The heart is completely developed in the first eight weeks of intrauterine life. One or several anomalies may result from maldevelopment of the heart or great blood vessels leading to and from the heart with the result that the infant is born with congenital heart disease. Such defects may be hereditary, e.g. those caused by defects inherent in the genes or germ plasm. They may be caused by vitamin deficiency or viral infection such as rubella (German measles) occurring during the first trimester of pregnancy. Anomalies of the bones, especially of the spine, may affect the development of the blood vessels in the embryo. Fetal intracardiac disease is possible. After birth there may be failure of obliteration of the ductus arteriosus or foramen ovale.

The *diagnosis* is based on the health history of the mother during pregnancy and on the characteristics of congenital heart disease in the infant. The signs and symptoms of congenital heart disease include abnormal murmurs, varying degrees of cyanosis and dyspnea, and in later months or years generalized poor development and clubbing of the fingers and toes. The infant is weak and often irritable.

The diagnosis is confirmed when radiographic examination shows divergence of the heart from its normal position and contour. Such an examination repeated at intervals of several months may reflect continued changes in the structure of the heart as the infant's body develops. Examination with barium given by mouth may show indentation of the esophagus by the aorta and other vessels.

By *electrocardiography* variations in the normal electrical potentials of the different parts of the heart can be noted. The electrocardiogram shows

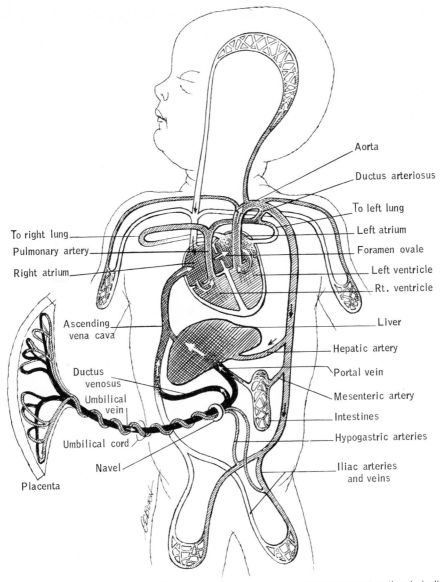

Figure 11–6. Diagrammatic illustration of fetal circulation. The degree of oxygen saturation is indicated by the blackness of the vessels.

the condition of the muscular structure of the heart.

For *angiocardiography* the child is usually anesthetized, and radiopaque material is injected into a peripheral vein; its course through the heart chambers appears on a succession of x-ray pictures taken at rapid intervals. Abnormal communications between the chambers of the heart are also evident. *Selective angiocardiography* is being used more than venous angiocardiography because it is a more satisfactory method of determining specific heart

defects. The radiopaque catheter is moved into the heart chambers themselves, and the contrast material is injected into specific areas. The structure of the heart can thus be more clearly seen by roentgenogram.

Cine-angiocardiography is the process by which motion pictures can be taken of successive images seen on the fluoroscopic screen. Because of improved techniques angiocardiography and cine-angiocardiography are now considered by many to be part of the cardiac catheterization technique.

Cardiac catheterization is done under either general or local anesthesia. If local anesthesia is used, the infant should be under heavy sedation. The physician who catheterizes the heart must be supported by a well trained team of assistants accustomed to working with him. A small radiopaque catheter is inserted into a large vein of an arm or leg and pushed into the right atrium. With the tip of the catheter the physician can examine the heart minutely for anomalies of structure, often found in the right ventricle and the pulmonary artery. He is able to determine the blood pressure within the heart itself, and samples of blood can be taken to determine the exact degree of oxygenation. This procedure is not without risk; hence the nurse should be careful how she reassures the parents of a very ill child who is having this study done.

Congenital defects in cardiac structure may be classified in two groups: (1) *acyanotic* heart disease, in which the infant is not cyanotic, and (2) *cyanotic* heart disease, in which the infant shows varying degrees of cyanosis.

A detailed approach to the treatment and care of children having congenital cardiac disease will be discussed under the condition tetralogy of Fallot, one type of cyanotic heart disease.

ACYANOTIC TYPES OF CONGENITAL HEART DISEASE

In acyanotic congenital heart disease either there is no abnormal communication between the pulmonary and systemic circulations or, if such a connection is present, the pressure forces the blood from the arterial to the venous side. The peripheral blood is therefore oxygenated as in a normal infant, and cyanosis does not result. If the anomaly is such that venous blood eventually mixes with arterial blood when the heart weakens, cyanosis may result.

Coarctation of the Aorta

Types, Clinical Manifestations and Diagnosis. There are two types of coarctation. In the *infantile* or *preductal* type there is a constriction between the subclavian artery and the ductus (Fig. 11-7). This condition can be corrected by surgery. The *postductal* type consists of a constriction at or distal to the ductus arteriosus. The symptoms in this type depend upon the degree of coarctation. Blood pressure is higher than normal in the upper part of the body, resulting in headache, dizziness, epistaxis, and later cerebrovascular accidents. Blood pressure in the legs is relatively low, resulting in absence or diminution of femoral pulses.

The *diagnosis* is based on the reversal of normal blood pressure relations in the arms and legs and is confirmed by x-ray study. In older children the roentgenogram may show enlargement of the heart which was not evident during routine examination of the newborn, together with notching of the ribs due to enlarged collateral vessels.

Treatment and Prognosis. Surgical repair consists in cutting out the narrowed portion of the aorta, with anastomosis of the ends. In some cases a graft of transplanted aorta is inserted where the narrowing is so extensive that removal with anastomosis is not practical.

If the infant's condition is such that the physician believes that he can live until he has reached the preferred age for correction, operation is postponed until the child is from eight to fifteen years old. Operation should be performed at this age rather than during early childhood because the segment used as a graft will not grow as does the aorta. The shorter the time after operation before maximum growth of the child is reached, the less is the danger from difference in the rate of growth between the graft and the main structure of the aorta.

The *prognosis* is dependent upon the success of surgery. If the operation is successful, life expectancy should be normal.

Aortic Stenosis

In this condition blood cannot pass freely from the left ventricle to the systemic circulation because of stenosis of the aorta. The degree of constriction varies from so mild that the child is asymptomatic to so severe that it causes dizziness and can lead to sudden death. This normally can be surgically corrected (using the open-heart technique) by dividing the stenotic valves of the aorta or dilating the constricting aortic ring.

Patent Ductus Arteriosus

Etiology, Incidence and Clinical Manifestations. The ductus arteriosus (Fig. 11-8) normally closes shortly after birth. If the ductus remains open, blood under pressure from the aorta is shunted into the pulmonary artery, since the blood pressure in that vessel is less than in the systemic circulation. As a result, oxygenated blood recirculates through the pulmonary circulation. This may lead to increased vascular pressure in the pulmonary tree and diminished blood flow in the aorta.

Patent ductus arteriosus is one of the most common cardiac anomalies. It is frequently the only cardiovascular anomaly, but may occur in conjunction with other cardiac defects. It is almost twice as frequent in female infants as in male ones.

The *symptoms* of patent ductus arteriosus in the infant are usually so slight that the con-

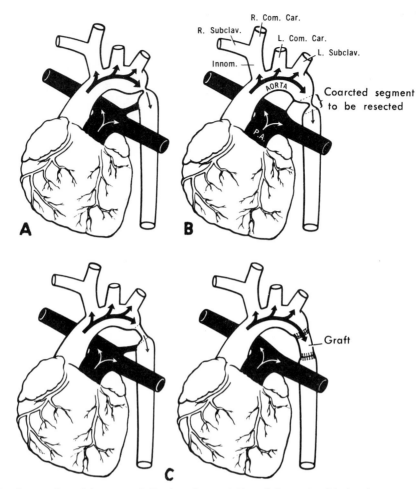

Figure 11–7. Coarctation of the aorta. *A,* Preductal coarctation of the aorta with the ductus arteriosus open or closed. *B,* Postductal coarctation of the aorta with the ductus arteriosus closed. *C,* Longer areas of constriction, where anastomosis of aortic segments is not feasible, require the use of a graft to bridge the gap. (From *Diagnosis of Congenital Cardiac Defects in General Practice.* Heart Association of Southeastern Pennsylvania and American Heart Association.)

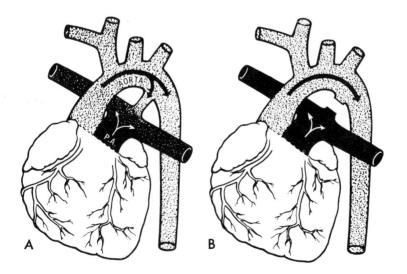

Figure 11–8. Patent ductus arteriosus. *A,* Relation of ductus arteriosus to great vessels. *B,* Ductus arteriosus transected (as shown here) or ligated. (From *Diagnosis of Congenital Cardiac Defects in General Practice.* Heart Association of Southeastern Pennsylvania and American Heart Association.)

dition is not discovered at the initial examination, but is found during a routine examination later. As the child grows older and is more active, the characteristic symptoms appear. He is likely to show progressively greater dyspnea on exertion. Examination may reveal a malfunctioning left ventricle or congestive heart failure. Progression of the lesion is due to the strain upon the heart of pumping blood which passes a second time through the pulmonary circulation while at the same time supplying adequate systemic circulation for an active infant or child. It is easy to prevent overexertion in an infant, but far more difficult to limit the activities of a growing child without overprotecting him and building up the very qualities which may make for a handicapped child disliked by his playmates.

If the ductus is large and much blood from the aorta is shunted into the pulmonary circulation, there may be retardation in growth.

Physical signs include increased pulse pressure, sometimes felt when taking the radial pulse. Pulsations are of the water-hammer type. A cardiac thrill in the second left interspace is usually present; this may radiate over a larger area of the chest. There is the classic *machinery murmur,* continuous from systole into diastole. The electrocardiogram usually shows no abnormality, but roentgenograms show a vigorously pulsating pulmonary artery and increased pulmonary vascularity. The heart may be normal in size, but is more likely to be enlarged.

Diagnosis, Treatment and Prognosis. The *diagnosis* is made on the clinical symptoms and signs of a machinery murmur of the heart and a low diastolic blood pressure. Cardiac catheterization (see p. 201) shows a normal or increased pressure, roentgenograms show the shadow of the pulmonary artery to be larger than normal, and angiocardiography shows the ductus arteriosus.

The *treatment* is surgical, by division and ligation of the ductus, preferably when the child is about three years of age. If necessary, however, operation may be done earlier if the child is in serious difficulty. After the repair the heart becomes normal in size, murmurs disappear, and there is a general improvement in the child's condition.

With modern surgery done by a skilled specialist, the *prognosis* is excellent. The surgical mortality rate in the uncomplicated condition during childhood is extremely low. Without repair subacute bacterial endocarditis or cardiac failure may develop as the child leads the less sheltered and more strenuous life of the school-age group.

Dextrocardia

In this condition the heart is in the right side of the chest. This may occur with or without reversal of the other organs. Although the heart may be normal, associated anomalies often complicate the condition. If no other anomalies are present, no treatment is necessary, and the prognosis is excellent.

Double Aortic Arch

Infants and children with this defect may have respiratory symptoms or dysphagia, or both. These symptoms, beginning in the first year of life, arise from compression by the branches of the aorta on the trachea or esophagus, or both. This is due to the persistence of embryologic vascular precursors of the aorta and stem branches. The infant, in an effort to find relief, will hold his head in an extended position. The diagnosis is made on x-ray examination, which shows constriction of the esophagus by the aorta. Constriction or deviation of the trachea can also be seen. The treatment is surgical, and the prognosis is excellent.

Interatrial Septal Defect

This is one of the more common congenital anomalies. The incidence is higher among girls than among boys. There is a communication between the left and right atria. Since oxygenated blood in the left atrium is under the higher pressure, it is forced through the defect in the separating wall into the right atrium. Such an arterial-venous shunt does not produce cyanosis. Terminally, however, or with heart failure, if a reversal of flow occurs, cyanosis may become evident.

The *diagnosis* is made on the basis of the roentgenogram and the electrocardiogram. The heart is enlarged, and there is congestion of the pulmonary circulation. On auscultation a loud murmur is heard in the area of the pulmonary artery.

The *treatment* is surgical repair of the defect. The edges of the opening are pulled together and sutured, or the opening is occluded by a plastic patch placed over the aperture. This operation may be done with the aid of the heart-lung machine. Without operation the life expectancy is only thirty-five years.

Interventricular Septal Defect

This anomaly consists of an opening between the right and left ventricles. The condition may be slight or severe.

In the *mild form* the defect is so slight that only a small amount of oxygenated blood passes from the left to the right ventricle. It is a common congenital defect. The heart is seldom enlarged, and the only clinical finding is a murmur accompanying the heart beat. The treatment is by surgical closure of the opening. Since the ventricle must be entered, the heart-lung machine must be used in order to enable the surgeon to reach the defect. In this condition subacute bacterial endocarditis may develop at the site.

In the *severe form* there is a large opening in the septum, and oxygenated blood in greater amount passes from the left to the right ventricle. The result may be pulmonary hypertension. The symptoms include cardiac failure, a tendency to pneumonia and retarded growth. The diagnosis is made from the roentgenogram and the electrocardiogram. The treatment is by surgical closure of the defect. The heart is opened, and the edges of the septal opening are drawn together, or a plastic patch is placed over the opening. This kind of operation involves the use of a cardiac bypass by means of the heart-lung machine. Without operation the prognosis is poor.

If pulmonary hypertension with a ventricular septal defect becomes so severe that the predominant shunting of blood is reversed, the child is cyanotic and the condition is inoperable. This phenomenon is known as the *Eisenmenger complex.* A technique currently used to prevent the development of the Eisenmenger complex is banding of the pulmonary artery. This is usually done on the infant with a ventricular septal defect prior to the development of irreversible pulmonary hypertension. A piece of Teflon tape is sutured circumferentially around the pulmonary artery to decrease the pulmonary blood flow.

Pulmonic Stenosis

Although these constrictions may exist in newborn infants, symptoms may not be present for several years. Cardiac failure may occur, and the prognosis is generally poor. Treatment is surgical, by valvulotomy or mechanical dilatation of the passage through which blood must pass from the heart into the respective vessels.

CYANOTIC TYPES OF CONGENITAL HEART DISEASE

The common cause of the congenital cyanotic types of heart disease is a communication between the pulmonary and systemic circulations through which venous (unoxygenated) blood enters the systemic circulatory system. Cyanosis may be seen at birth or may not be apparent until later, commonly during the first year of life; it tends to increase as the child grows older.

Polycythemia (an increase in the number of red blood cells per milliliter of blood) results from the need of the tissues of the body for an adequate supply of oxygen. The symptoms vary in degree with the extent and nature of the anomaly. In general, there is clubbing of the fingers and toes, retarded growth and shortness of breath on exer-

tion. If the blood, thickened by an abnormal concentration of red blood cells, clots in the blood vessels, further complications result.

Tetralogy of Fallot

Incidence and Pathology. This is the most common type of cyanotic congenital heart disease which is compatible with continued existence into childhood. Pathologically, there are four associated anomalies: (1) funnel-like or valvular pulmonic stenosis, (2) interventricular septal defect, (3) dextroposition of the aorta, and (4) hypertrophy of the right ventricle.

Pulmonary stenosis restricts the flow of blood from the heart to the lungs; the right ventricle hypertrophies and facilitates venoarterial shunting. Dextroposition of the aorta also leads to venoarterial shunting. Since cyanosis is dependent upon the absolute concentration of reduced hemoglobin in the capillary circulation, it is evident that in the systemic circulation, containing a rich admixture of venous blood from the start, this value is almost invariably surpassed, and cyanosis is thus clinically manifest.

Clinical Manifestations and Diagnosis. The arterial blood is not normally saturated with oxygen, and as a result the skin is not the natural pink, but has a bluish tint. The fingers and toes become clubbed and have a purplish hue, since the capillaries are distended with poorly oxygenated blood. The condition worsens during even the first year of life. The body's reaction to the inadequate supply of oxygen is an increased production of red blood cells (polycythemia).

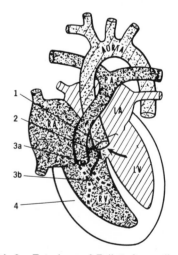

Figure 11–9. Tetralogy of Fallot. Anomalies include (*1)* overriding aorta, (*2)* high ventricular septal defect, (*3a*) valvular pulmonary stenosis and (*3b*) infundibular pulmonary stenosis, and (*4*) hypertrophy of right ventricle. (From *Diagnosis of Congenital Cardiac Defects in General Practice.* Heart Association of Southeastern Pennsylvania and American Heart Association.)

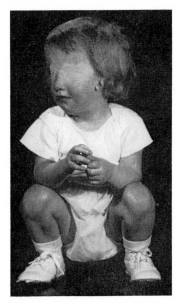

Figure 11–10. Tetrology of Fallot. Child squatting. (Nadas: *Pediatric Cardiology.* 2nd ed.)

The child's general condition is poor. His growth is retarded; exercise causes severe dyspnea. In order to relieve the strain of standing, he favors the *squatting position*. This behavior has diagnostic value. Although he may be of normal intelligence, the poor supply of oxygen to the brain is likely to produce mental retardation, syncope or convulsions. The child is apt to be emotionally unstable, irritable and overdependent upon others. His parents, concerned over his physical condition, are likely to avoid discipline to prevent frustration, since they do not want him to become excited or cry. The child realizes that if he cries, he will get his way and so is apt to become the typical spoiled child.

The *diagnosis,* based on the symptoms, is confirmed by radiographic examination of the heart, which shows the enlarged chamber on the right side, the decrease in size of the pulmonary artery and reduced blood flow through the lungs. The unusual shape of the heart has led to its being called the wooden shoe or *boot-shaped heart* (*coeur en sabot*). The child should be allowed to handle the diagnostic equipment before examination so that the procedures will be less frightening to him. If he is to take barium, the addition of chocolate to the mixture may make it look and taste like the chocolate milk to which he is accustomed. Laboratory findings show the decreased oxygen saturation of the blood, and exercise tolerance tests prove the child's tendency to extreme dyspnea.

Instructions to the Mother. On the mother rests the responsibility for giving the child good care until the time when operation is to be performed. Both physical and mental hygiene must be considered. Provision for normal growth and development is essential, but requires constant good judgment so that the child is neither overprotected nor allowed an independence in which he overtaxes his weakened heart. This program is easy to carry out while the infant is still so young that he accepts his mother's plan for all his activities of daily living.

During this period the infant becomes ac-

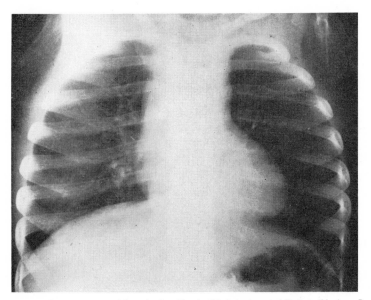

Figure 11–11. *Coeur en sabot* contour of heart of patient with tetralogy of Fallot. (Nadas: *Pediatric Cardiology.* 2nd ed.)

customed to limitation of activities without overdependence on others. He also learns to trust others to give him the help he needs. Overfatigue should be avoided, and certainly he should never be urged to exertion beyond his tolerance. It may be difficult for the entire family and those adults he contacts outside the family circle to carry out such a regimen with a young child whose handicap is not visible, but it is in this period that the foundation for a strong, happy personality is made.

The child should never acquire the feeling of undue importance which is apt to develop in one who feels that his heart condition makes him a special child who must always have his own way and be given first consideration. The influence upon the other children in the family must be considered. Although his needs may be more important than their pleasures, his pleasure is not to be gained at the expense of their constant inconvenience. He should lead as normal a life as is compatible with his welfare, but learn to accept frustration and the inevitable restrictions which his condition imposes on his activity and social relations. He cannot do all that other children do.

The physician will discuss with the parents the influence of cyanosis upon the child's intelligence. If he is retarded, the parents are apt to attribute the retardation entirely to his physical condition, forgetting that low intelligence may be due to a number of factors. To lead as normal a life as is compatible with his condition is the best way to realize to the full his potential mental capacity. The experiences which develop the normal child, but in which he cannot participate, should be replaced by experiences of comparable learning value. His toys should be light and easily handled. He should learn that a ball rolls, though he may not be able to creep after it

for any length of time. He may not creep up a flight of stairs, but he may go up one or two steps. He should be carried about more than the average child is and should be allowed to handle everything within the nursery. Picture books are valuable. He can pat-a-cake to slow music. Overexcitement is as taxing for him as overactivity. As he grows older he must learn not to compete in games requiring agility and strength. As a rule, competitive games are too exciting for these children. Even the very little child can learn that fun does not necessarily come through getting ahead of someone else.

If the mother proves her ability to give good care and to observe signs of a worsening in his condition, he may not need frequent visits to the physician. But if she is unable to judge his condition and to give him the care he requires, he should be seen regularly by the family physician or pediatrician. If he has been referred from the hospital to the children's clinic, he should be under the observation of the pediatrician there and should be visited by the public health nurse. He should be seen by his physician before even minor surgery is done. The danger is not only from the anesthetic—often minor surgery would not require the use of an anesthetic—but also from the possibility of infection. Prophylactic antibiotic medication may be indicated.

Treatment and Prognosis.   The treatment is surgical, and may be corrective or merely palliative. Without operation the life expectancy of the child is almost always shortened. Operation is postponed as a rule until the child is three years of age or even older, but if his condition is critical, operation may be done upon the infant.

Palliative surgery does not correct the deformity. An artificial ductus is made which connects the systemic circulation with the pulmonary artery. This allows for greater blood flow to the

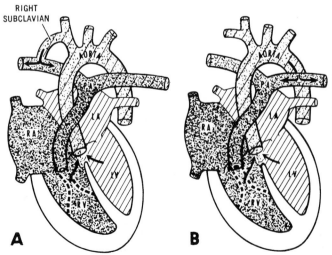

RIGHT
SUBCLAVIAN

A   **B**

Figure 11–12.   Tetralogy of Fallot. *A,* Volume of blood to lungs increased by joining right subclavian to right pulmonary artery (end-to-side anastomosis—Blalock procedure). *B,* Volume of blood to lungs increased by creating stoma between left pulmonary artery and aorta (side-to-side anastomosis—Potts procedure). (From *Diagnosis of Congenital Cardiac Defects in General Practice.* Heart Association of Southeastern Pennsylvania and American Heart Association.)

lungs, which in turn results in increased oxygenation of the blood in the left side of the heart and ultimately in the systemic circulation. In the Blalock-Taussig operation an anastomosis is made between the subclavian artery and the pulmonary artery. In the Potts operation a side-to-side anastomosis of the pulmonary artery and the aorta is made.

Corrective surgery is undertaken frequently today. With the use of the heart-lung machine it is possible to resect the pulmonic stenosis and close the ventricular septal defect. The risk of such surgery is no longer as high as it formerly was, because of improved techniques.

Pulmonic Stenosis with Patent Foramen Ovale

In this condition venous blood from the right atrium is shunted to the left atrium with resulting cyanosis. Clinically, the condition may simulate the tetralogy of Fallot. Treatment is by surgical valvulotomy of the stenosed pulmonary valve with or without closure of the septal defect. The prognosis after repair is good.

Transposition of the Great Vessels

Incidence and Pathology. The incidence of this condition is almost as high as that of tetralogy of Fallot. In this anomaly the aorta has its origin in the right ventricle, and the pulmonary artery has its origin in the left ventricle. Because of this the aorta carries unoxygenated blood to the systemic circulation, and the pulmonary circuit carries oxygenated blood back to the lungs. An infant can survive initially only if an associated defect such as an atrial or ventricular septal defect or a patent ductus arteriosus is present.

Clinical Manifestations and Diagnosis. An infant born with transposition of the great vessels may not be too cyanotic at birth because of the patent ductus arteriosus, but may become extremely cyanotic soon after birth. Such an infant is likely to be dyspneic and unable to suck. Later growth is severely retarded, and there is clubbing of the fingers and toes. The diagnosis is made by cardiac catheterization and related roentgenograms. Laboratory findings include an elevated hematocrit value and polycythemia.

Treatment and Prognosis. As a result of recent research into the treatment of this condition, more infants live today than ever before. Palliative treatment is aimed at achieving adequate mixing of oxygenated and unoxygenated blood. This can be accomplished by removing the atrial septum and can enable the infant to survive until corrective surgery can be done.

One palliative nonsurgical technique currently used is the Rashkind-Miller procedure. This involves passing a double-lumen cardiac catheter with a sharp point on the tip and an inflatable balloon just behind the tip through the femoral vein to the right atrium. The sharp tip of the catheter pierces the septum into the left atrium. The ballon is then inflated with a dye so that the right size can be determined. When the balloon is pulled back to the right atrium, it leaves a septal defect, allowing the unoxygenated and oxygenated blood to mix. This procedure is repeated until the filled ballon can be drawn without resistance from the left to the right atrium. After this procedure the infant's color improves, and heart failure, if present, disappears.

The second and corrective stage of this therapy is done when the child is between eighteen months and three or four years of age with the aid of the cardiopulmonary bypass machine. This complex Mustard procedure is one by which total correction of the transposition can be obtained.

The *prognosis* of infants having transposition of the great vessels has been greatly improved since the discovery of these new procedures. If the condition is recognized early enough, most children can be ultimately cured.

Nursing Care. The nurse caring for the newborn in the nursery should recognize the infant having this condition, although cyanosis may not be too severe because of the patent ductus arteriosus. She should, however, recognize the increasing dyspnea and the infant's inability to suck. These newborns have increased secretions, though not as profuse as the child having atresia of the esophagus. The sooner newborns having this condition have their palliative operation, the better are their chances for life. It is therefore extremely important for the nurse to report her observations as soon as they are made.

There are other rare cardiac anomalies nearly all of which are surgically correctible at present.

NURSING CARE IN CONGENITAL HEART DISEASE

The nursing care of infants and children with congenital anomalies of the cardiovascular system is extremely important. What is done for the child is, of course, dependent upon the treatment outlined by the physician and involves difficult procedures and nursing skills.

The nurse should become familiar with the parents' reaction to being told that their child has a congenital cardiac condition, and she should learn how to reassure them without minimizing the danger of the defective heart. She should teach the parents how to care for the child in the interval between his leaving the newborn nursery and his re-entrance into the hospital for operation. What has been said about the care of the child with the tetralogy of Fallot may also be applied to other types of congenital heart disease.

Congestive Heart Failure

Clinical Manifestations. The nurse should be aware of the fact that infants, like adults, having severe cardiac problems may suffer congestive heart failure. The first indication of this problem occurs when the mother or nurse notices that the infant does not feed as well as he did. He may tire easily when he sucks and may fail to gain weight. If permitted to rest after every ounce or two of formula, he may have a sufficient intake of nutrients.

Other indications of congestive heart failure may be a weak cry, cyanotic or pale color, edema, rapid heart beat and rapid respirations which may be accompanied by an expiratory grunt, suprasternal retractions, and flaring of the alae nasi. On x-ray films the heart may appear enlarged.

Treatment and Nursing Care. *Therapy* for an infant having congestive heart failure includes the use of digitalis, diuretics if edema is present, and oxygen. When pulmonary edema is present, any superimposed infection should be treated appropriately. Salt may need to be restricted in the infant's diet in order to prevent the retention of excess fluid. A low-salt formula may be ordered. As the infant recovers he may be graduated to a moderately low sodium preparation. Morphine sulfate may be given for its beneficial effect in pulmonary edema.

Treatment begins with digitalization. The dose is estimated according to body weight and is adjusted according to the infant's response. The use of maintenance doses of digitalis is necessary unless the cause for the failure is completely corrected. If it is continued, the amount given must be adjusted upward as the child gains weight. Toxicity may occur in infancy and is especially to be feared, since there are few warning symptoms prior to ventricular fibrillation, or heart block itself occurs. Treatment consists in stopping the medication until signs of toxicity are gone and then resuming the drug, if necessary at a lower dosage.

The infant in congestive heart failure needs more rest than the normal child. He should have small frequent feedings higher than average in calories. Some physicians recommend the use of a pacifier to keep him happy and content.

An infant having this condition is most comfortable in a sitting position or when held over his mother's or nurse's shoulder. A special cardiac chair (see Fig. 11-13) may be utilized especially to advantage if the infant has rapid, labored respirations.

Any condition complicating congestive heart failure such as infection, anemia or electrolyte imbalance should be promptly treated.

See page 161 for the discussion of the parent's reaction to an infant having a congenital anomaly.

The nursing care of a preschool child undergoing surgical correction of a cardiac anomaly is discussed on page 513.

Central Nervous System

Spina Bifida

Incidence and Types. Spina bifida is a malformation of the spine in which the posterior portion of the laminae of the vertebrae fails to close. It may occur in almost any area of the

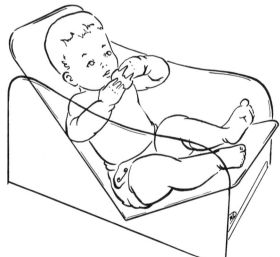

Figure 11-13. Cardiac chair. Children, particularly babies, with pulmonary congestion, seem more comfortable in the sitting position. (Nadas: *Pediatric Cardiology.* 2nd ed.)

spine, but is most common in the lumbosacral region. It is the most common developmental defect of the central nervous system, occurring in about one out of 1000 newborn infants.

Three types are discussed: (1) spina bifida occulta, in which the spinal cord and meninges are normal, the defect being only of the vertebrae; (2) meningocele, in which the meninges protrude through the opening in the spinal canal; and (3) meningomyelocele, in which both the spinal cord and the meninges protrude through the defect in the bony rings of the spinal canal. Meningomyelocele is the most serious type.

Spina Bifida Occulta

Clinical Manifestations, Diagnosis and Treatment. The majority of patients have no symptoms. Some may have a dimple in the skin or a growth of hair over the malformed vertebra. If the condition is suspected from these signs or upon physical examination, a roentgenogram will rule out or confirm the diagnosis. There is no need for treatment unless neurologic symptoms indicate that the defect is greater than was thought. If there is a possibility that the spinal cord may be involved in the defect, surgical treatment is indicated.

Meningocele

Clinical Manifestation, Diagnosis, Treatment and Prognosis. On examination the newborn infant is found to have a defect in the spinal column large enough for the meninges to protrude through the opening. The defect is usually in the center line. There is generally no evidence of weakness of the legs, for the infant stretches and kicks in a normal manner, or of lack of sphincter control, though this is difficult to ascertain in the newborn.

The *prognosis* is excellent. Surgical correction is done on these defects. Hydrocephalus may be an associated finding or may be aggravated after operation for a meningocele.

Meningomyelocele

Clinical Manifestations, Diagnosis, Treatment and Prognosis. In this condition an imperfectly developed segment of the spinal cord, as well as the meninges, protrudes through the spina bifida. The round, fluctuating bulge resembles that of the meningocele and is usually located in the lumbosacral region. There may be a minimal weakness to a complete flaccid paralysis of the legs and absence of sensation in the feet. The

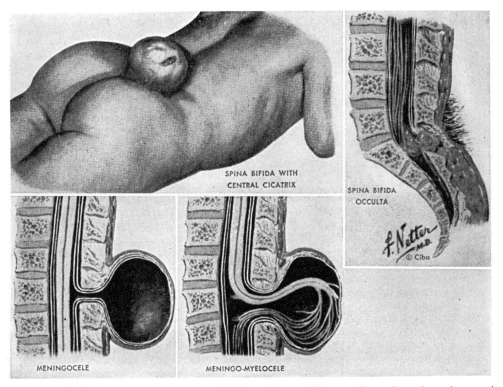

Figure 11–14. Diagrammatic representation of types of spina bifida, meningocele and meningomyelocele. (Copyright, The Ciba Collection of Medical Illustrations, by Frank H. Netter, M.D.)

feet may be clubbed. Bowel and bladder functioning require careful evaluation.

The objectives of *treatment* and nursing care are to prevent infection of the sac and to help restore function orthopedically and urologically.

Operation removes a cosmetically unacceptable deformity, prevents infection and in many instances improves the neurologic deficit, since traction is removed from the nerve pathways. Although, in the past, operation for meningomyelocele was postponed in order to cure any infection present, currently correction is done as early as possible, preferably in the first twenty-four hours of life. The reason for this early correction is that some newborns appear to have a degree of motor ability in the legs at birth which decreases soon after birth. Early operation is advocated therefore to prevent further deterioration of neural tissue.

Usually clinically silent, the *Arnold-Chiari syndrome* is a congenital malformation of the occipitocervical region, with displacement of the cerebellar tonsils and adjacent structures into a funnel-shaped enlargement of the upper cervical canal and swelling and displacement of the medulla against the upper portion of the spinal cord. The defect originates between the sixteenth and twentieth weeks of fetal life. This syndrome may occur in children having lumbosacral spina bifida with meningomyelocele. The medulla and part of the cerebellum are pulled into the foramen magnum because the cord is attached at the site of the defect in the spine. The result may be an acute obstruction to the flow of cerebrospinal fluid, and hence hydrocephalus may follow repair of a meningomyelocele.

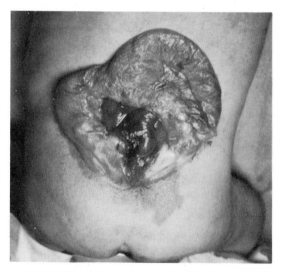

Figure 11–15. Meningomyelocele. (Courtesy of Luis Schut, M.D.)

The symptoms are the result of complete or partial block of the flow of cerebrospinal fluid. In infants clinical manifestations include a running nose (sometimes confused with an upper respiratory tract infection) and crowing respirations. The nurse must observe these manifestations because immediate relief of pressure is indicated. In older children, manifestations include stiff neck, headache and dizziness. When the child is old enough to walk or talk, his gait is unsteady and his speech impaired.

Surgery is the only known treatment for the Arnold-Chiari syndrome.

Nursing Care in Meningocele and Meningomyelocele

Preoperative Nursing Care. Until the operation is performed, the newborn should be kept flat on his abdomen with a single layer of sterile petrolatum gauze or a Telfa pad saturated with Varidase solution over the lesion. No diaper should be applied. The object of care is to prevent breaking the meningocele sac; therefore no pressure is to be put upon it.

If for some reason the neurosurgeon prefers to wait to operate on the lesion, preoperative nursing care is that of a normal infant so far as it can be given while protecting the sac from pressure, injury or infection. To decrease the danger of infection of the area from urine and feces, the genitalia and buttocks must be kept scrupulously clean. The infant should not be diapered if the meningocele is in the lower portion of the spine. If the covering of the sac is infected or thin, some physicians order Varidase solution to drip on the area. The infant is placed in bed, and a meningocele apron is applied (Fig. 11-16). This is done by taping an oblong piece of plastic sheeting below the defect. The larger portion of the piece of plastic should be in the direction of the child's head. Either Scotch tape or masking tape should be used to hold it in place. The piece of plastic should then be folded back on itself and taped again to the skin so that it covers the buttocks and shields the defect from feces. It is customary in some hospitals to place the infant on a Bradford frame with the cover divided so that urine and stool may pass between the sections of the frame.

USE OF A BRADFORD FRAME. The frame is covered as follows:

Canvas covers the head and foot areas of the frame, and foam rubber is placed between the covers. The open area between the covered head and foot sections of the frame is provided for the purpose of drainage of urine and feces away from the body. The covers are stretched tightly over the frame to prevent sagging from the weight of the infant's body. Plastic covers are placed over the top and bottom sections of the divided canvas frame cover. A sheet is put tightly over each section of

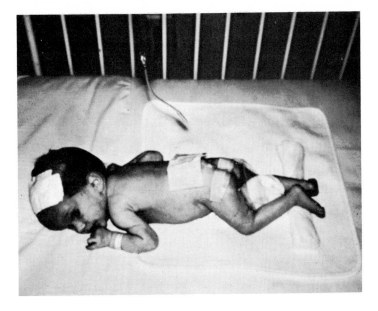

Figure 11–16. Meningomyelocele. The meningocele apron is in place, and Varidase solution drips slowly onto the sac. (Courtesy of Dr. Eugene B. Spitz.)

the frame. The frame is then placed on blocks to elevate it slightly from the bed.

Since the infant is incontinent, sheets of plastic are draped over the top and bottom edges of the opening in the frame cover to permit urine and feces to drain into a bedpan placed below the opening. Folded diapers are placed over the plastic and under the infant so that the plastic does not irritate the skin.

Fixation in the correct position is important. Ankle restraints, using a clove hitch restraint, are applied. The child is not to be placed on his back, since such position would cause pressure on the sac. If the surgeon permits, the child should be supported in the side position with a rolled blanket or pillow behind the head and the buttocks. The pillow or blanket behind the buttocks must be protected from fecal staining by a plastic cover. If the infant is unable to move his legs, foam rubber pads covered with soft cloth may be placed between the legs to prevent pressure on the skin of the knees and ankles. The infant's position should be checked at least every hour.

To prevent deformity of the feet when the infant is placed on his abdomen, the ankles should be supported with foam rubber pads so that the toes do not rest upon the bed. To prevent injury from rubbing the skin of the elbows, face and knees, a mild ointment such as A & D ointment or zinc oxide may be used. To prevent chafing of the knees, ankles, toes and sides of the heels, should the infant move his legs back and forth on the sheet, it is a good plan to use long stockings, but since he has no diaper to which they may be pinned, it is difficult to keep them on his legs.

To change the frame covers or bed, the child may be placed on his abdomen or side in a baby carriage. If the physician permits, the nurse, aide or mother during visiting hours may hold the child to prevent complications arising from constant lying on the frame.

Antibiotics may be used if infection is suspected.

In addition to the danger of infection of the sac, the bladder of an infant having a meningomyelocele may also become infected. According to the urologist's evaluation, the infant's bladder may need to be credéd if the sphincter is tight and urine is retained. The nurse, or the mother when the child is at home, is responsible for emptying the infant's bladder every two hours during the day and once at night. Pressure should be applied firmly but gently, beginning in the umbilical area and slowly progressing under the symphysis pubis and toward the anus. The mother should be helped to learn this procedure as early as possible. She should practice under supervision until she feels secure. As the child grows, his urine may be expressed less frequently. If he has normal intelligence, by the time he is three or four years of age he should be able to assume part of the responsibility for doing this procedure himself.

The infant may be transferred directly from the nursery to the pediatric unit. If he is taken home before his readmission to the hospital for operation, his parents will care for him. The father can make a substitute for the Bradford frame, and the mother can cover it as described above. She can carry out the essential features of nursing care and will have more time to hold the infant than do hospital personnel. Both parents should be shown how to hold him without causing pressure upon the sac.

The infant should be held for his feedings, if the physician permits. He may be held in the normal feeding position with the nurse's elbow rotated to avoid touching the sac. If the sac is large, he can be held on the shoulder, his mother's or the nurse's hands supporting him above and below the sac, while a second person, standing behind her, holds the bottle to his mouth. He cannot be bubbled like the normal infant, but the feeding should be stopped and the nipple withdrawn from his mouth several times during the feeding so that he may rest and air be expelled. If the lesion is in the lumbosacral area, he may be gently rubbed between the shoulders; this has a soothing effect and may aid in expulsion of air. These infants can also be fed lying on the side on the nurse's or mother's lap.

Contamination of the sac can be prevented by covering it with sterile gauze or a sterile towel when the infant is removed from bed.

If the physician believes that the infant should not be removed from the frame or bed for feeding, the restraints may be loosened and the infant turned slightly on the side. The nurse or mother should elevate his head slightly with her hand when feeding him. She should offer substitute pleasure for that of being held for his feeding, such as stroking his skin or singing to him.

One of the most essential functions of the nurse is observation and accurate reporting of the behavior of these infants, as well as of signs and symptoms directly connected with their condition. She should record activity of the legs and the degree of continence, noting whether there is retention of urine or fecal impaction. All the vital signs should be taken and recorded with extreme care.

Postoperative Nursing Care. The goal of surgical treatment is closure of the surface defect while preserving all functioning nervous tissue.

The nurse is responsible for observing and reporting all signs and symptoms of the infant's condition. Temperature, pulse and respiration must be taken frequently. Symptoms of shock must be anticipated and an incubator be in readiness for use. If an incubator is not available, a heat cradle may be placed over the infant. Since he may have respiratory difficulty, oxygen should be kept near his bed. Abdominal distention caused by paralytic ileus or distention of the bladder follows most spinal cord surgery and should be reported immediately.

The physician may request that the circumference of the infant's head be measured frequently in order to determine whether hydrocephalus follows repair of the meningomyelocele.

The surgical dressing should be kept clean and dry by the use of a meningocele apron.

Casts applied to the child's legs should be positioned properly and handled carefully (see p. 231).

Nutrition is important. Postoperatively, some surgeons prefer to have the infant fed in as natural a position as possible, while others prefer to have him fed in bed until the operative site is completely healed. If the infant is fed in the prone position in bed, his head should be slightly elevated either with the nurse's hand or by elevating the top end of the frame if one is used. The nipple should be withdrawn several times during the feeding to allow the infant to rest and to facilitate expulsion of air. Gavage feeding may be necessary (see p. 147).

All the foregoing suggestions for postoperative care are subject, of course, to the physician's orders.

Postoperative Habilitation. *Habilitation* of the child is necessary after operation. Functional improvement of the legs and bowel and bladder function will require a long time and diligent care. Habilitation emphasizes constructive use of the normal parts of the body and minimizes the disabilities, making the child as self-helpful as is possible in the activities of daily living. Although the child is to be taught activities which render him less dependent on others, he must also learn to accept help which normal children do not need. The adult must make an attempt to help the child keep up with the appropriate growth and development sequence for his age.

Incontinence after infancy creates social problems. The child should be taken to the toilet at the time he usually has a bowel movement. A suppository may be used until he establishes regularity. The child may need a special diet to avoid constipation. If he can achieve regularity of stool, he will be more socially acceptable. Regularity of urination is of even more importance. Mechanical means for making pressure on the urethra may be used to prevent incontinence. If he cannot urinate, his bladder will need to be emptied by the Credé method (i.e. pressed upon periodically to expel urine), as it was prior to operation. A child of three or four years can be taught to Credé his own bladder by blowing up a party balloon as he bends over and presses on his bladder. His mother can then do Credé for residual urine. A distended bladder must be prevented, since it is more subject to infection. Reflux from a distended bladder may result in hydroureter and hydronephrosis with resulting kidney damage. For all these reasons a schedule of toileting should be instituted.

Follow-up care by a urologist is necessary. Some urologists have attempted by surgical means to form a substitute bladder by transplanting the ureters into the sigmoid colon. Unfortunately, ascending infection often followed this procedure. More recently a section of the ileum has been isolated, and the remaining portions have been anastomosed. One end of the

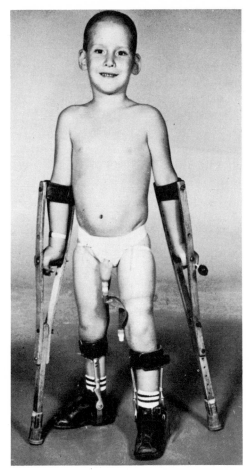

Figure 11–17. Hill Pediatric Male Urinal (Davol).

isolated segment of ileum has been closed and the other end brought to the surface of the abdomen. The ureters have then been transplanted into this substitute bladder. An ileostomy bag, if fitted carefully over the stoma, receives the urine and prevents leakage.

Although his legs may be totally or partially paralyzed, the infant can be taken about in a stroller and later can learn to use a wheelchair and possibly to walk with braces and crutches. If the physician elects to use braces on the child, currently the belief is that heavy bracing should be used first, gradually reducing their weight as the child grows. The parents can be taught by the physiotherapist to exercise the child's legs appropriately.

Care must be taken to prevent obesity or malnutrition and secondary contractions or other deformities. Any infection that occurs should be promptly treated with antibiotics. If the child is normal mentally, he can become a socially useful member of society.

Encephalocele

An encephalocele is a protrusion of brain substance through a congenital defect in the skull. It occurs through a failure of the bones of the fetal skull to unite in the normal manner. It is commonly found in the midline and in the occipital or parietal area, although it may also be found in the frontal bone, the orbit of the eye or in the nose.

Clinical Manifestations, Diagnosis, Treatment, Prognosis and Nursing Care. The *symptoms* depend upon the degree of involvement of

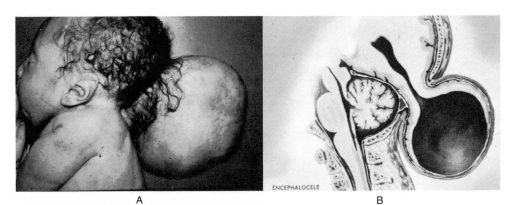

A   B

Figure 11–18. Encephalocele. *A,* Occipital Encephalocele (Courtesy Luis Schut, M.D.) *B,* Diagrammatic representation. (Copyright, The Ciba Collection of Medical Illustrations, by Frank H. Netter, M.D.)

the nervous tissue and upon the location of the defect. The diagnostic evidence is a sac or hernia into which the meninges, cerebrospinal fluid or cerebral tissue has entered. Roentgenograms show the defect in the skull. Early surgical repair is indicated.

The *prognosis* depends upon the extent and location of the encephalocele. If it ruptures, there is danger of meningitis.

The *nursing care* is that of a normal infant, plus relief of symptoms and extreme caution in handling the infant. It is essential that no pressure be brought upon the sac and that it be not injured in any way.

Hydrocephalus

Hydrocephalus is due to inadequate absorption of cerebrospinal fluid, with a corresponding increase of fluid under pressure within the intracranial cavity, or to obstruction within the ventricular system. To understand this process it would be well to review the formation, flow and absorption of cerebrospinal fluid (see Fig. 11-19).

Cerebrospinal fluid is formed by the choroid plexus of the four ventricles and by filtration from capillaries. It passes from the lateral ventricles by way of the foramina of Monro into the third ventricle. From the third ventricle it flows through the aqueduct of Sylvius into the fourth ventricle, and then into the cisterna of the subarachnoid space by way of the foramina of Luschka and the foramen of Magendie. From there it passes under the base of the brain and up over the convexity into the cortical sulci until it is finally absorbed into the venous sinuses by way of the arachnoid villi. It flows along the tissue spaces of the sheaths of all the cranial and spinal nerves and is taken up by the vascular system. Normally the amount absorbed equals that secreted (Fig. 11-19).

Etiology. The obstruction in the flow of cerebrospinal fluid may be due to one of several causes. There may be congenital maldevelopment of the ventricular foramina, neoplasm may be present, or a fibrous residue of meningitis may occlude the reabsorptive surfaces. Hemorrhage from trauma may cause hydrocephalus in the young infant.

The accumulation of fluid in the ventricles generally enlarges the infant's skull, since the sutures are not closed, and the bones are soft and yielding under pressure. The cranial enlargement tends to decrease the pressure upon the brain.

Treatment should be started as soon as the clinical manifestations are observed, before damage to the brain itself occurs. Several shunting procedures are now in use: e.g. ventriculovenostomy (shunting from the ventricle through the internal jugular vein to the right atrium of the heart), ventriculoperitoneostomy, ventriculoureterostomy and lumbar subarachnoid peritoneostomy.

The *prognosis* is dependent to a great extent on the promptness of treatment and the kind of operation performed.

Communicating Hydrocephalus

Etiology. In communicating hydrocephalus there is a normal communication between the ventricles and the subarachnoid space at the base of the brain. There may, however, be adhesions between the meninges at the base of the brain, meningeal hemorrhage or a congenital defect in the brain, which prevents the absorption of cerebrospinal fluid. Hydrocephalus may occur after a successful operation for meningocele.

Clinical Manifestations, Diagnosis and Treatment. The obvious *symptom* is an increase in size of the infant's head because of excessive amounts of cerebrospinal fluid. The fluid which is not absorbed in the subarachnoid space accumulates, compressing the brain and distending cranial cavity. The sutures fail to close, and the bones of the skull become thin.

There is an excess of spinal fluid outside the brain. The convolutions of the brain are flattened and atrophied. Usually, however, the pressure of the fluid does not enlarge the head as much as in noncommunicating hydrocephalus, because the brain atrophies, and this increases the space which the fluid may fill without enlargement of the skull. The fontanels are tense and widened. The child tends to be irritable and to have anorexia.

The *diagnosis* is confirmed by puncture of the fontanels, and ventriculography may be used.

The *treatment* is surgical. Sometimes spontaneously a balance may rarely occur in the young child between the secretion of fluid and its absorption. Operation, however, should be performed as early as possible to prevent damage to the brain. Since the difficulty is mostly mechanical, corrective measures are aimed at forming an outlet for the surplus fluid.

Noncommunicating Hydrocephalus

Etiology and Pathology. In noncommunicating hydrocephalus, which is more important than the communicating type, there is a block between the ventricular and subarachnoid systems. Such a block may be partial or complete. It may have begun in the latter months of intrauterine life. Mechanical causes include tumor, hemorrhages or anomalous development of the pathway. A mechanical block may result from

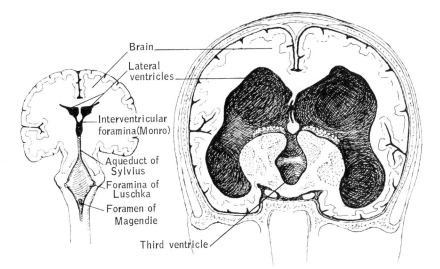

Brain
Lateral ventricles
Interventricular foramina(Monro)
Aqueduct of Sylvius
Foramina of Luschka
Foramen of Magendie
Third ventricle

Figure 11–19. Noncommunicating hydrocephalus. *A,* Diagrammatic representation of brain showing sites of possible obstruction of cerebrospinal fluid. *B,* Diagrammatic representation of brain showing dilatation of lateral and third ventricles of brain.

absence of an aqueduct or stenosis or obstruction by exudate or a blood clot. The foramina of Magendie and Luschka may be occluded.

Fluid distends the ventricles. There is a gradual thinning of the brain substance, which is compressed between the distended ventricles and the expanding skull. The bones of the cranium become thin, the fontanels large and the sutures separated.

Clinical Manifestations and Diagnosis. In the congenital type of noncommunicating hydrocephalus the infant may die *in utero,* or a cesarean section may be done to deliver the child.

After birth an increase in size of the head is noticeable. The fontanels widen instead of narrowing and are tense. Irritability, anorexia and vomiting occur. The infant becomes increasingly helpless and less able to raise his head. The neck muscles are underdeveloped from lack of use. Affect and normal responses may be diminished. Nystagmus or convergent strabismus may be present. There is possibly some interference with sight. The eyes seem to be pushed downward and protrude slightly. The sclerae are visible above the iris, since the upper lids are retracted by the taut skin over the bulging forehead. The scalp is shiny, and the veins are dilated.

The muscle tone of the extremities is frequently abnormal. As the child's condition deteriorates, his body becomes emaciated, often weighing less than the head. The cry is high-pitched and shrill. Convulsions may occur. These infants have little resistance to infection; therefore the administration of antibiotics may be necessary.

Operation may be indicated to prevent further enlargement of the head and to facilitate nursing care of a child with massive enlargement.

Symptoms in hydrocephalus due to infection, e.g. that resulting from meningeal inflammation, develop slowly or are clinically unrecognized. The bones yield to pressure as

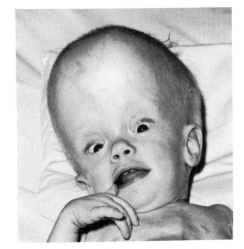

Figure 11–20. Noncommunicating hydrocephalus. The infant is helpless and lethargic. Strabismus is present. The "sunset sign" of the eyes is obvious. The scalp veins are dilated. A covered pad of sponge rubber is kept under the infant's head. A blanket roll is kept under his shoulders.

in the congenital type. The course is progressive.

Diagnostic tests are done to indicate the site of the obstruction. The head is measured daily to compare its growth with that of the normal child. By ventricular puncture the presence of excess fluid and the approximate thickness of the cortex are determined. *Ventriculograms* or *pneumoencephalograms* using small amounts of air are helpful in establishing a diagnosis.

Treatment and Prognosis. Since the causes of noncommunicating hydrocephalus are mechanical, *treatment* must be surgical.

Modern surgery bypasses the point of obstruction by attempting to shunt the cerebrospinal fluid to another area where it will be absorbed and finally excreted.

Probably the most common treatment now in use for hydrocephalus is a shunt from one lateral ventricle into the circulating blood by way of the internal jugular vein to the right atrium of the heart or the superior vena cava just proximal to it. A valve has been invented which prevents blood from flowing back into the ventricles, but allows the cerebrospinal fluid, when under pressure, to enter the circulation. Several complications can follow this procedure, such as thrombosis of the jugular vein, obstruction of the valve or sepsis. The tube must be replaced at intervals with the further possibility of infection.

In the ventriculoperitoneal shunt a tube is run from the ventricle to the peritoneum. An omentectomy is done to prevent blocking of the end of the tube.

In spinal ureterostomy the effectiveness of the tube is not influenced by the child's growth, but when a ventriculoureterostomy is done, longer tubes must be inserted as the child grows. In both spinal ureterostomy and ventriculoureterostomy it is necessary to remove one kidney in order to insert the tube into the ureter.

A problem in the management of children having a ureterostomy is the loss of great quantities of salt in the fluid passed through the shunt. Massive sodium depletion may result. Infection reaching the cerebrospinal fluid from the bladder by way of the shunt is combated by the use of antibiotics.

In the Torkildsen operation (ventriculocisternostomy) a tube is run from the lateral ventricle to the cistern of the fourth ventricle.

The *prognosis* in the past was poor, but with newer surgical techniques excellent results have been obtained. If the brain is not seriously malformed at the time of operation, mental function may not be impaired. Motor function is retarded if the child cannot lift his head and move as a child would normally do. In many cases there is neurologic impairment. Death may occur from extreme malnutrition or intercurrent infection.

Nursing Care. The hydrocephalic infant may be admitted to the hospital for diagnosis before operation is undertaken. The nursing care will include assisting with a number of tests. The basic care of the child admitted for diagnosis is that of the child admitted for operation.

PREOPERATIVE CARE. With early diagnosis of the enlarging head, treatment is given before nursing care becomes difficult. The nurse is responsible for observing the degree of irritability and changing vital signs. She should report such changes promptly. She must also provide

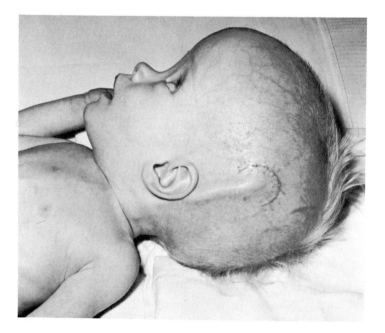

Figure 11–21. A hydrocephalic infant on whom was done a ventriculoperitoneal shunt. Note the presence of the tube as it emerges from the skull and passes under the skin of the scalp and the chest.

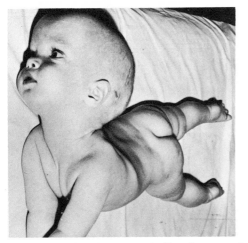

Figure 11–22. Opisthotonos resulting from meningitis in a hydrocephalic infant.

care for the child who exhibits the manifestations of anorexia and vomiting.

Nursing care presents many difficulties. The children may be unable to raise or even move the head, brain damage may have delayed their mental development, and malnutrition may have resulted from inadequate food intake and frequent vomiting.

These infants must be kept clean and dry, especially in the area around the creases of the neck where perspiration and vomitus may collect.

To maintain nutrition, the feeding schedule should be arranged to avoid vomiting; i.e. the intervals between feeding should be those ordered by the physician, and all necessary care should be given *before* a feeding so as to avoid moving the infant after he has been fed. He should be held for his feedings. Since the head is heavy, the nurse should rest her arm upon a pad placed over the arm of her chair, or upon the mattress of the crib if it is low enough for her to do so. If the head is very large, the infant cannot be bubbled. The bottle should be taken from his lips several times during the feeding, and his head and shoulders be slightly elevated (if the physician permits) while he is gently rubbed between the shoulders. When he is returned to his crib, he should be placed on his side to prevent aspiration of vomitus.

The infant's position should be changed frequently to prevent hypostatic pneumonia and to lessen the danger of pressure areas. These lesions are likely to appear on the head and ears unless every precaution is taken to prevent them. A pad of lamb's wool or sponge rubber should be placed under his head. A full-length sponge rubber mattress or an alternating pressure mattress is excellent. If pressure areas develop, great care must be taken to prevent infection, which, in the infant's debilitated condition, might result in septicemia.

When the child is lifted from his crib, his head must be carefully supported in order to prevent trauma. In changing his position in bed, the weight of the head should be borne in the palm of the nurse's hand, thereby freeing her other hand to move the body. It is essential that head and body be rotated together, bringing no strain upon the neck. To lift the infant, the nurse leans over the crib, places her arm under his head and adjusts the head agianst her chest. She then raises him with her other arm supporting his body, as with a normal infant.

If a spinal puncture is to be done for diagnostic purposes, the nurse gives the usual assistance to the physician. The equipment needed

Figure 11–23. Restraint of a child for a lumbar puncture. The nurse places one hand behind the child's neck and the other under his buttocks. By resting her body gently on the infant's body and by applying pressure on the neck and legs, she can thus round his back and keep it parallel with the side of the treatment table.

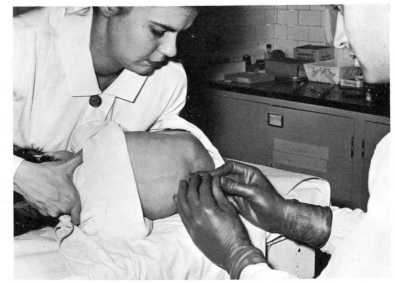

is the same as that for the procedure on an adult. The nurse's most important responsibility in assisting with the procedure is restraint of the patient in such a way that his back is rounded and parallel with the side of the treatment table. With a small infant the nurse may place one hand behind his neck and the other hand over the buttocks and bend his back to the desired extent. To restrain an older infant or child, she may place one hand behind his neck or one arm around his neck and grasp his legs, and place her other arm around the buttocks and grasp his hands. By putting pressure on the neck and legs she can bend the child's body as necessary. An older child can be restrained with a sheet folded lengthwise in the same way as can an uncooperative adult.

The nurse's responsibilities in assisting with a ventricular tap are to apply a mummy restraint and to hold the head securely, because the needle is inserted through brain tissue. After the tap the nurse must watch for signs of shock and for leaking of fluid through the tap holes.

The parents should have constant contact with the neurosurgeon. All diagnostic procedures should be explained to them, and they should be encouraged to help with the infant's care while he is in the hospital.

POSTOPERATIVE CARE. The temperature, pulse and respiration should be taken every fifteen minutes until the infant is reactive; blood pressure readings, if ordered, are taken at the same time (a small blood pressure cuff is needed). Signs of increased intracranial pressure are irritability, bulging of the fontanel, lethargy, vomiting, elevated systolic blood pressure, widened pulse pressure, slowing or a change in the pulse and respiration rates, or change in body temperature.

Recording of the vital signs may be ordered hourly for several days. If the temperature is elevated, sponging with tepid water, and aspirin may be ordered, and the infant should be clothed only in his diaper.

Fluids are given intravenously slowly in quantities proportionate to weight until the infant can be fed orally. If they are given too rapidly, there is danger of circulatory overload and cardiac failure.

Mucus from the nose and throat should be aspirated whenever necessary to prevent difficulty in breathing and the danger of aspiration of mucus. As in the care of every hydrocephalic infant, there is danger of pressure areas developing on parts of the scalp which support the weight of the head. Cotton may be placed behind the ears, and over the ears under the head dressing. The child should be turned at least every two hours.

The elevation of the infant's head and his general position depend upon the amount of fluid draining through the tube used to shunt fluid from the ventricular system to another site—atrium, peritoneal cavity or ureter. The nurse should record her observations of the bulging or tenseness of the fontanel. The physician will direct the elevation of the head and shoulders and the general position of the infant so as to increase or decrease the rate of drainage. If the fontanel becomes depressed too rapidly, a subdural hematoma may develop. If the anterior fontanel is depressed, the infant should be placed flat in bed with the head slightly lower than the body. When the tenseness of the anterior fontanel is normal, his head should be slightly elevated or flat.

If a spinal ureterostomy or ventriculoureterostomy has been done, a 24-hour urine specimen must be collected to determine the amount of fluid and electrolytes being excreted from the body.

The infant may be placed in a mobile metabolic crib (see Fig. 11-24). Accurate urine collections may be obtained by the use of this device from children from birth to two years of age. The infant lies on a nonirritant, nonwettable nylon mesh hammock which is held taut between stainless steel rods. This "bed" is suspended in a transparent box made of heavy duty acrylic plastic. The front of the box is hinged to allow easy access to the infant. The top of the box is open to allow for ventilation. The urine from the child

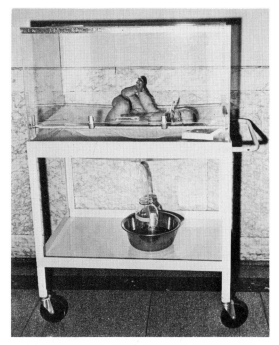

Figure 11–24. The mobile metabolic crib. (Courtesy of Lester Baker, M.D., and Charles W. Thomas Plastics, Inc., 4540 Worth Street, Phila., Pa.)

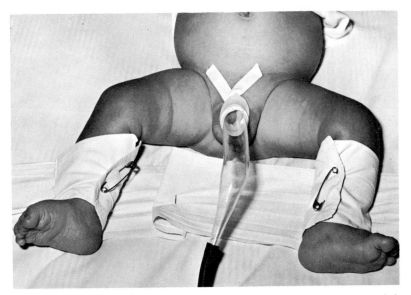

Figure 11–25. Procedure to be used for the collection of a 24-hour urine specimen from an infant boy. The collecting tube is held in place by adhesive tape. The ankle or extremity restraint is used to restrain the infant's legs. Note how the restraint is pinned in the middle in order to make it smaller.

passes through the mesh to a collecting bottle below. The stools, unless of a diarrheal consistency, remain on the nylon mesh. The infant requires no restraint when urine is collected in this manner.

If a metabolic crib is not available, The following techniques may be used:

For the male infant a plastic funnel-shaped tube is used. It is applied to the genitalia by means of a binder with a hole through which the narrow end of the funnel protrudes. A flange around the rim of the appliance prevents it from slipping through the hole. If such a binder is not available, a finger cot can be attached to the collecting receptacle with adhesive tape, and the other end of the finger cot can be cut and attached to the penis and lower portion of the abdomen with tape (Fig. 11-25). A plastic or rubber tube is attached to the open end of the funnel, which drains into a bottle attached to the bottom of the infant's crib.

For the female infant a specimen halter may be used to which is attached a plastic ring. Plastic tubing may be attached to the ring (Fig. 11-26). The other end of the plastic tubing is placed in the drainage bottle attached to the bottom of the infant's crib.

A device similar to the one used for the collection of a single specimen of urine (see p. 68) can be used for the continuous collection of urine if it is attached to a container at the foot of the bed.

The infant is restrained on the back by abdominal and ankle restraints. Such restraints (Fig. 11-26) are made of double-thickness muslin with ties at both ends to tie on the springs of the bed. The abdominal restraint has a flap of double-thickness muslin stitched to its center. This flap may be pinned around the infant's abdomen. The ankle or extremity restraint has two smaller flaps sewn to it. These flaps may be pinned securely around the ankles or wrists. If this restraint

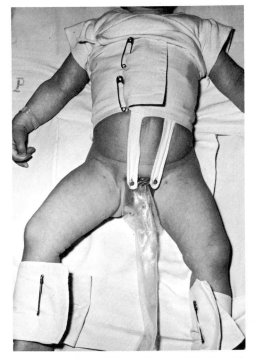

Figure 11–26. Procedure to be used for the collection of a 24-hour urine specimen from an infant girl. A specimen halter to which is snapped a plastic ring and tubing is used. The other end of the plastic tubing is placed in the drainage bottle attached to the bottom of the infant's crib. The abdominal and extremity restraints are used to restrain the infant adequately.

is too large, a tuck can be pinned in the center (Fig. 11-25).

The head of the crib should be slightly elevated if the infant's condition permits, to prevent a backflow of urine. The genitalia should be cleansed frequently to prevent excoriation. The restraints should be removed frequently, and passive exercise should be given to the legs and arms if the child cannot move himself. The nurse should not leave him until the restraints are again in position.

The physician usually orders sodium chloride to replace the amount lost through a ureteral shunt.

If a peritoneostomy (ventriculoperitoneal shunt) has been performed, the infant immediately postoperatively is given nothing by mouth. Abdominal distention is handled with a nasogastric tube which may be connected to mechanical suction. Irrigation of the tube may be necessary. The drainage is measured, and the amount and color are charted.

The infant's mouth becomes dry, and mouth care is required four times a day. As soon as the child can tolerate them, clear fluids are given orally. The milk formula is introduced gradually, and later solid foods, suitable to the age of the infant, are given. A high protein diet should be offered.

The nurse should closely observe and report to the physician any of the following: signs of infection, tenseness of the anterior fontanel (an indication of inadequate drainage of the cerebrospinal fluid), vomiting (an indication of increased intracranial pressure or intolerance of diet), signs of dehydration such as loss of skin turgor, convulsions (duration, where initiated, all parts of the body involved and the type of movements), the vital signs, coldness or clamminess of the infant's body, pallor or mottled condition of the skin, the state of consciousness, movements or signs of paralysis, the kind of drainage from the incision, and the degree of restlessness and irritability of the child.

Teaching the Parent Before Discharge of the Infant.
The importance of the mother's understanding the care she is to give her infant, and important conditions she should watch for and report to the physician, cannot be overestimated. She should be instructed in a way which will not increase her anxiety. She may be told of the success other mothers have had in caring for infants such as hers. This will help her to gain confidence in her ability to give the infant the care he needs. To understand the operation which was performed is a basis for understanding the reason for the care she is taught and for following instructions exactly. She should understand the signs of increased intracranial pressure and of dehydration and their importance. With the surgeon's guidance the nurse may suggest exercises to the mother which will

help to strengthen the infant's muscles so that he will learn to lift his head.

If the mother cared for the child before operation, she is probably skillful in handling him, but she must learn the problems which may arise in relation to the shunt. She should know the danger signals of too rapid drainage and should watch for them.

If the child is completely helpless and cannot move his body, there is always danger of pressure areas not only on the head, but also on the body. In hot weather the danger of such lesions is increased. Methods of prevention can be taught to the mother. The infant should lead as normal a life as possible. He should be given toys, and should be taken about in a baby carriage or stroller whenever possible.

Microcephalia (Microcephaly)

Etiology, Clinical Manifestations and Treatment.
Microcephalia is a relatively uncommon congenital anomaly. It is accompanied by mental deficiency. It is easily recognized at birth by the smallness of the skull. Growth of the skull is largely dependent upon development of the brain. Arrested brain growth is the cause of microcephalia and may be due to hereditary factors, toxoplasmosis, German measles during pregnancy, or irradiation of the mother during the second or third month of pregnancy.

The *symptoms* are the small skull (less in volume and in circumference than normal in relation to the body build of the infant) and severe mental retardation.

There is no *treatment* for this condition. Habilitation should be attempted to whatever extent is possible.

Down's Syndrome (Mongolism)

Incidence, Etiology, Clinical Manifestations, Treatment and Prognosis.
This condition occurs most frequently in the Caucasian race, although it sometimes appears among Negroes. The *incidence* is the same among all socioeconomic classes and both sexes.

The *cause* has only recently been discovered. There are three known causes of mongolism, all of which are associated with chromosomal abnormalities (see p. 159). The most common chromosomal abnormality in mongolism is trisomy of chromosome 21. This occurs once in every 600 births. The total chromosome count, instead of the normal forty-six, is forty-seven. This type of mongolism is rarely familial, but usually occurs in children born to older women. The other causes of Down's syndrome—translocation of chromosome material or mosaicism—are rare.

The *signs* may be recognized at birth, but

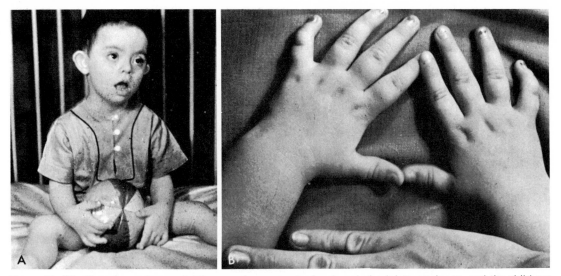

Figure 11–27. Down's syndrome. *A,* The muscles are underdeveloped, the joints are loose, and the child can assume unusual positions comfortably for prolonged periods. *B,* The hands are short and thick, and the little finger is curved. (Courtesy of Dr. Ralph V. Platou and the American Academy of Pediatrics.)

not all need to be present in order for the diagnosis to be made. The infant's physiognomy resembles that of an Oriental. The head is relatively small, the occiput flat and the face round. The eyes are set close together and slant slightly upward. The palpebral fissures (the openings between the eyelids) are narrow. The nose is flat, and the tongue protrudes. These children breathe through the mouth and may drool. Eruption of the teeth is delayed. The hands are short and thick, the little finger is curved, and the creases of the palms and the prints of the feet are unlike those of a normal infant. There is a wide space between the first and second toes. The muscles are underdeveloped, the joints loose, and the child can assume unusual positions. Growth and development are slow; mental development seldom reaches beyond that of the average child of five to seven years of age. Associated anomalies are frequent, among them congenital deformities of the heart. Chronic myelogenous leukemia has been found to be about twenty times as frequent in the mongoloid population as in the normal population.

These children are seldom destructive, but are restless, inattentive and happy-go-lucky. They are often considered "cute" by strangers who do not understand their condition and are encouraged to show off their ability to assume unnatural positions.

Such children need continuous health care and supervision. They have little resistance to infection and may die early of an intercurrent infection. Modern drug therapy has prolonged their life expectancy to some extent.

Although there is no *treatment* for the con-dition, habilitation is important. These children may or may not be difficult to train. They respond to training by copying techniques shown to them repeatedly in a consistent manner. In adolescence vocational training may be considered. Some communities have organized classes so that these children can be trained to the limit of their abilities.

It is difficult for the parents to accept the child's condition. This is especially true if he is the only child of older parents. If the infant is the child of young parents, they may be afraid to have other children. In any event the parents need help from professional persons in understanding the child's limitations and in planning his life to make the most of his capacities and to give him a happy childhood.

Many community resources are available to help the parents of children having Down's syndrome to meet the short- and long-term problems presented by these children. The nurse should be cognizant of the specific resources available for them in the community in which she is employed.

Cri du Chat Syndrome

This newly discovered and apparently rare syndrome is believed to be due to an abnormality of the number 5 chromosome. It is so named because the newborns affected have an unusual cry that resembles the meowing of a cat. They have poor sucking reflexes and peculiarly formed faces. They fail to thrive physically and undergo severe mental retardation.

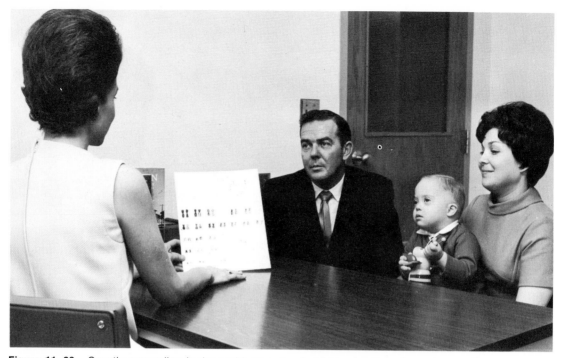

Figure 11–28. Genetic counseling is done with parents of child having Down's syndrome. (Courtesy of The National Foundation–March of Dimes.)

For further discussion of the care of the mentally retarded child, see page 526.

Genitourinary System

Obstruction of the Urinary Tract

Etiology, Clinical Manifestations and Diagnosis. Obstruction to the flow of urine is important because of the back pressure produced above the level of the obstruction. The back pressure of accumulated urine causes the tract to become distended proximal to the point of obstruction. This may lead to stasis, hydroureter, hydronephrosis, possible infection and death due to renal insufficiency.

The *symptoms* are obstruction while voiding, dribbling, bladder distention or the presence of an abdominal mass. Infection of the urinary tract results in fever, chills, pyuria and convulsions. If there is eventual loss of kidney function with uremia, death results.

A number of tests are used to determine the location of the obstruction. It may be in the upper or lower urinary tract, above the bladder or below it. The symptoms are not always indicative of the site of the obstruction.

Diagnostic tests include catheterization immediately after voiding to determine the amount of residual urine. Intravenous urography is used to visualize the urinary tract and to measure renal excretory function. Cystoscopic examination and retrograde pyelography may be performed. The blood urea nitrogen level and phenolsulfonphthalein excretion rate may be determined to measure renal function.

Obstruction of the Lower Urinary Tract

Pathology and Clinical Manifestations. Causes of lower urinary tract obstructions include urethral valves (filamentous valves that obstruct urinary flow are most commonly found in boys), urethral diaphragm or congenital narrowing of the urethra, obstruction of the neck of the bladder (the most common site of obstruction), severe phimosis (obstructive phimosis is rare), neuromuscular dysfunction such as is found in association with cord injury and meningomyelocele, and meatal stricture.

All these obstructions result in dilatation and hypertrophy of the bladder. Residual urine is constantly present. The ureters dilate and become tortuous from the back pressure of urine which cannot pass into the distended bladder. Later the renal pelves enlarge from pressure of urine which cannot pass down into the distended ureters. Destruction of kidney tissue inevitably results.

The *signs* and *symptoms* are abnormalities of urination, a palpable, distended bladder and possibly distended ureters and kidneys. Infection of the urinary tract may be frequent.

Obstruction of the Upper Urinary Tract

Upper urinary tract obstructions are usually unilateral. The bladder is not involved. There is no problem of urination unless an infection occurs. Anomalies involving the ureters are the most common anomalies of the urinary tract.

The following *types* occur: obstruction or stricture of a ureter, congenital absence of one ureter, duplication of the ureter of one kidney, pressure of an aberrant blood vessel which blocks drainage through the ureter, neoplasm, calculi or an inflammatory stricture.

Clinical Manifestations. Often there are no symptoms, or there may be vague symptoms such as failure to grow normally, hypertension, fever, bacteriuria, pyuria or a mass in the abdomen.

Treatment of Upper and Lower Obstructions. The bladder is emptied by gradual decompression through an indwelling catheter. If the obstruction can be relieved by surgical means, operation is attempted in spite of the reduced renal function. Infections should be eradicated with appropriate chemotherapeutic medications. Little can be done for chronic renal insufficiency, manifested by progressive renal dysfunction. Death results from renal failure.

Course and Prognosis. Untreated obstruction results in renal insufficiency. If operation can remove the obstruction, improvement may result, and the child may live for many years.

Patent Urachus

Etiology and Pathology. Patent urachus is due to persistence of the embryonic connection of the umbilicus with the bladder. Occasionally the urachus may persist, and urine is discharged through the umbilicus after birth. Often there is also an obstruction of the urinary tract below the bladder. Many times there is only a cyst at the upper end of the tract, extraperitoneally under the umbilicus.

Clinical Manifestations and Treatment. When the entire urachus is present, urine dribbles from the umbilical region. When a urachal cyst is present, there is a deep midline swelling below the umbilicus.

If the urachus is patent, the tract should be obliterated surgically. Urachal cysts should be removed before they become infected. If they do become infected, they should be drained surgically before removal. Appropriate antibiotics are given for infection.

Congenital Cystic (Polycystic) Kidneys

Etiology, Pathology, Clinical Manifestations and Treatment. The *cause* is unkown. The infantile form is probably transmitted as a mendelian recessive trait. The renal tissue is filled with cysts of varying sizes. The kidneys are enlarged and, when exposed at operation or autopsy, have a spongy appearance. The renal pelves and calices are distorted because of the amount of surrounding tissue. The condition is rarely unilateral. Other anomalies may also occur, e.g. hydrocephalus, polydactylism or cardiac malformations.

The *clinical findings* depend upon the location of the cysts. On palpation both kidneys (less frequently only one) are found to be enlarged. There is increasing renal insufficiency and, as a result, hypertension and signs of congestive cardiac failure. There may be severe growth retardation. Laboratory findings show recurrent bacteriuria, hematuria, proteinuria and elevated blood nonprotein nitrogen levels. X-ray films (urograms) show enlargement of the kidney and deformity of the calices and pelves.

There is no specific *treatment*. Supportive and palliative measures may be used to combat renal acidosis and insufficiency. Surgical drainage of large cysts may be done when they interfere with renal function.

The *prognosis* depends upon the type and severity of the interference with function. In severe types the infant dies *in utero*. Among infants living at birth renal function decreases over the years. In less severe cases, although the first symptom may appear in childhood, the condition may not become too evident until adult life.

Wilms's Tumor

Incidence, Clinical Manifestations and Diagnosis. Wilms's tumor is a highly malignant embryonal adenosarcoma of the kidney. It develops from abnormal tissue in the embryo, beginning to grow before or after the infant is born. It is one of the most frequent types of neoplasm occurring during infancy or the toddler age. It is commonly unilateral, but may be bilateral.

There are seldom *symptoms* other than a mass in the abdomen which is usually discovered by the physician in a routine examination of the child, or the mother may notice the mass while bathing him or changing his diaper.

After the diagnosis has been made the physician and the mother must be careful not to palpate the infant's abdomen, since handling might favor metastasis. The tumor extends through the kidney capsule or renal vein and then spreads to other areas of the body by way of the circulatory system. The late symptoms are anemia and cachexia.

The *diagnosis* is confirmed by intravenous pyelography, which shows the distortion and displacement of the pelvis of the kidney.

Prognosis, Treatment and Nursing Care. The condition without treatment is always fatal. With adequate treatment the prognosis today is not as hopeless as it once was. The tumor tends to produce pulmonary metastases via the renal vein and venous circulation to the right side of the heart and thence through the pulmonary artery to the lungs.

The *treatment* is surgical extirpation with x-ray irradiation before and/or after surgery. Operation should be done immediately after the diagnosis has been made. Actinomycin D is given preoperatively and postoperatively to a child having Wilms's tumor.

The *nursing care* is that of the normal infant, with special attention to nutrition. The specific danger in care is manipulating the abdominal wall inadvertently, as in bathing the infant or when fondling him, and thereby increasing the danger of metastasis. The mother should be cautioned against this, and in the hospital a sign should be placed on the infant's crib or on his abdomen—"Do not palpate abdomen."

Exstrophy of the Bladder

Pathology and Clinical Manifestations. Complete exstrophy is an extensive anomaly. The lower urinary tract—i.e. the entire bladder to the external urethral meatus—is exposed and may be without ventral covering. The defect in the male infant may be accompanied by a short penis, epispadias, undescended testes or an inguinal hernia. In the female infant the clitoris may be cleft, the labia separated and the vagina absent. In either sex the rectus muscles below the umbilicus are separated, and the pubic rami are not joined.

In complete exstrophy the posterior bladder lining is exposed and appears bright red through the fissure in the abdominal wall. The condition is more common in boys than in girls.

The defect is obvious at birth. Urine seeps onto the abdominal wall from the abnormal ureteral outlets. This causes a constant odor of urine and excoriation of the surrounding skin. There may be ulceration of the mucosa of the bladder. The separation of the pubic rami causes a waddling gait when the child learns to walk.

Treatment, Complications and Prognosis. If the exstrophy is not complete, the abdominal and bladder walls may be closed by plastic surgery. Even complete exstrophy has been corrected by plastic surgery with excellent results. The child then voids normally. In the majority of

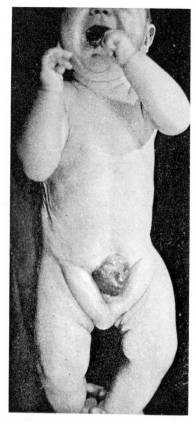

Figure 11–29. Exstrophy of the bladder. Five-month-old infant with exstrophy of the bladder and bilateral indirect inguinal hernias. The association of these 2 conditions is common. (Gross: *The Surgery of Infancy and Childhood.*)

cases of complete exstrophy, however, the ureters are transplanted into the sigmoid (lower colon). Urine is then passed with stool from the anus. Plastic repair of the bladder, abdominal wall and external genitalia may be done. When the child is old enough to have control of his bowel movements, he learns to retain the urine in the colon by tightening the sphincter muscle. He is given antibiotics to combat infection. The waddling gait is improved by a brace which corrects the deformity of the pelvic girdle or by surgery.

If the ureters are transplanted to the colon, hydronephrosis and hydroureter may result from back pressure originating at the site of the ureteral anastomosis. An ascending infection, usually caused by the colon bacillus, may result in pyelonephritis. Before operation there is danger of infection around the area where the skin is constantly irritated by urine.

The *prognosis* depends upon the injury done to the kidneys by the back pressure of urine for which there is no adequate outlet, and upon whether the child has suffered severe or chronic infection of the urinary tract. Even if there is no infection of the kidney, these children may have a chronic disturbance of the body chemistry, since the bowel surface may absorb secretory products from the urine when the ureters are transplanted to the sigmoid.

Parent Teaching Before Discharge of the Infant from the Nursery. It is important that the parents be taught the general care of these infants. Good hygiene is necessary so that the infants may be in optimum condition to withstand an infection of the skin or kidney and, later, surgical correction of the anomaly. The nurse should understand the mother's distress over her child's condition and appreciate that his care may be a task which she cannot immediately undertake. The nurse's acceptance of the child's condition is as important in teaching the mother as are the procedures in the care of the anomaly.

The mother may not have sufficient self-control to cleanse the area around the exposed bladder until she has become accustomed to the sight of the defect. If she is to be taught before she leaves the obstetrical unit, she should be fully recovered from parturition. If she is not ready for his care, it would be better to keep him in the hospital for a few days and have the public health nurse instruct her after he has been sent home. The mother should learn to keep the bladder area very clean and to apply sterile petrolatum gauze over it in order to prevent infection and possible ulceration. A bland ointment may be applied around the bladder area in order to protect the skin from draining urine. The diaper should be changed frequently for the infant's comfort and to prevent the odor of urine, which will embarrass the mother when she shows him to her friends. Stool should be removed immediately so that it does not contaminate the bladder mucosa. The infant's clothing should be light so as to avoid pressure on the exposed bladder.

Nursing Care. *Preoperative* nursing care includes the care outlined above to be taught the mother. If the infant is not a newborn in the nursery, but an older infant admitted to the pediatric unit for tests or operation, the mother may be able to give good hints on his care. This will ensure the continuity of care which makes the transition from home to hospital less disturbing for the infant. If operation is to be done when the child is old enough to understand that he is to undergo surgery, he should be emotionally prepared for the experience. The parents must be psychologically ready for operation to be done before it is undertaken. It is helpful to both the parents and the child to allow the mother to help with his care in the children's unit.

If a urine specimen is needed, it is collected from the opening in the bladder with a medicine dropper, or the child may be held over an emesis basin in such a position as to allow urine to drip into the basin.

Postoperative care is that of any surgical patient. The dressings must be kept clean and dry. If the child is old enough to establish control of the anal sphincter muscle, he should be taught to hold the muscle tight to prevent seepage of urine. There will be some soiling of his clothes while he is acquiring this control. He should never be made to feel ashamed of "accidents." Control will be acquired more readily if he is not too anxious about his condition.

Hypospadias

Etiology, Treatment and Prognosis. Hypospadias is a congenital malformation in which the urethra, in the male, opens on the lower surface of the penis just behind the glans, in the body of the penis or on the perineum; rarely, in the female, the urethra opens into the vagina. In the male associated congenital *chordee* is a cordlike anomaly which extends from the scrotum up the penis and pulls it downward in an arc. Urination with the penis in the normal elevated position is impossible.

The *treatment* is by plastic surgery. If the anomaly is slight, no treatment is given, since only severe forms interfere with procreation.

The child's parents are likely to be overconcerned about his condition. If it is severe, the

Figure 11–30. Anomalies of the male genitals. *A,* Hypospadias, showing in one drawing a composite of the common locations of the deformity. *B,* Hypospadias of a severe degree in a false hermaphrodite. *C,* Epispadias. (From Arey: *Developmental Anatomy.* 6th ed.)

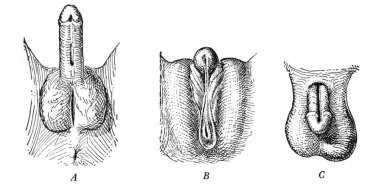

A   *B*   *C*

anomaly should be repaired before the child is of school age so that he will not be embarrassed when voiding before his peers. In both sexes the problem with which the parents and child need help is chiefly psychological.

Epispadias

In this anomaly the urethra opens upon the dorsal surface of the penis. The urethra may lie just behind the glans or, in conjunction with exstrophy of the bladder, extend the whole length of the penis.

The treatment is surgical. The emotional and psychologic problems involved are the same as those in hypospadias.

Intersexuality

Parents feel guilty about the birth of a child whose sex is not easily determined. Intersexuality is an extremely disturbing anomaly, although its influence on physical health is slight. If there is any question about the sex of the child because of the lack of distinctive genitalia, the newborn should have an exploratory examination to determine the gonadal sex. This should be done before the parents announce the child's sex to their friends and information for the birth certificate is given. The social role of the boy is different from that of the girl; clothing, activities and the pronominal references of speech all set off one sex from the other. It is psychologically harmful to both parents and the child if the infant believed to be of one sex is later found to be of the other. All psychologic identifications have been made in terms of the sex originally determined by the physician.

Parents, and the child when he is old enough, need to understand the anatomic problems involved and the treatment which should be given. The treatment, depending upon the causes of the problem, may be surgical or medical. They need support from professional people who consider the problem objectively, without the morbid curiosity and pity which friends and relatives may show. A child with such a problem needs help at school in adjustment to his peer group. It is advisable to have the child under the supervision of the guidance clinic. Parents, even the most understanding ones, cannot judge the depth of such a child's emotional problems.

Three types of intersexuality will be discussed: pseudohermaphroditism in the female, pseudohermaphroditism in the male, and hermaphroditism.

Pseudohermaphroditism in the Female (Congenital Adrenal Hyperplasia)

Etiology, Clinical Manifestations, Diagnosis and Treatment. Female pseudohermaphrodi-

tism is the most common problem in intersexuality or sexual differentiation. It is due to an inability to synthesize hydrocortisone from its precursors. The deficiency of hydrocortisone results eventually in adrenocortical hyperplasia and overproduction of androgens. Increased androgenic—i.e. producing male characteristics —steriod secretion by the fetal adrenal cortex causes masculinization of the external genitalia in the female infant. Recently more cases have been seen in infants born of mothers treated with steroids during pregnancy than have occurred spontaneously.

The *clinical findings* are enlargement of the phallus or clitoris, fusion of the labia resembling a bifid scrotum, and hypospadias. Such infants have a cervix and a uterus and the female chromosomal pattern.

The *diagnosis* may be made by exploration and biopsy of the gonads during the neonatal period or by assay of steroid excretion products in the urine.

In spite of the anomalous external genitalia, these children should be reared as girls. If the child is given hydrocortisone, the production of corticotropin will be inhibited and the production of androgens reduced. Infants who do not have adrenal hyperplasia require no treatment other than corrective plastic surgery. Correction should be undertaken between the ages of eighteen months and four years.

If the diagnosis is made in infancy and plastic surgery is performed in the toddler or preschool age, the *prognosis* is very good.

Pseudohermaphroditism in the Male

Etiology and Treatment. There are several types of this condition, but all such infants are chromosomal males. One type is caused by gonadal dysgenesis. These are infants whose testes were damaged early in fetal life, resulting in feminization of the fetus. Another type is characterized by normal female external genitalia, but testes, not ovaries, internally. In this type the testes should be removed and the child reared as a girl. At the usual time for puberty the child should be given estrogens to compensate for those normally produced by the ovaries of the female. In still another type the genitalia are predominantly masculine or ambiguous. Such children masculinize at puberty. Any structures not of the male sex should be removed surgically.

True Hermaphroditism

True hermaphroditism is rare. The clinical findings show both ovarian and testicular tissue in the same infant. The chromosomal sex may be male or female. True hermaphroditism must be excluded in all infants showing intersexuality

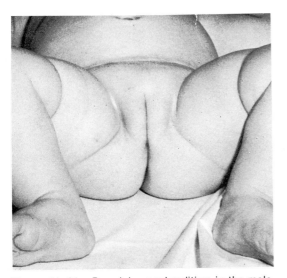

Figure 11–31. Pseudohermaphroditism in the male. View of torso of 1-month-old infant showing normal female configuration. A swelling can be seen in the right inguinal region. At operation this proved to be a testis which had herniated into the inguinal canal. The external genitalia appear to be made up of completely normal female labia, clitoris, vulva and vagina. Skin biopsy revealed the male chromosomal pattern. At laparotomy no female internal organs were found. (Gaspar, Kimber and Berkaw, in A.M.A. *J. Dis. Child.*, Vol. 91, with the permission of the authors.)

except those with congenital adrenal hyperplasia. The treatment is the same as for male pseudohermaphroditism.

Orthopedic Anomalies

As recently as twenty years ago children with minor orthopedic deformities were hospitalized for months. Today, with the recognition of the psychologic importance of the separation of the child from his mother, such children are treated largely on an outpatient basis. They are admitted to the hospital only for application of a cast or for operation and are cared for at home between admissions. This places increased responsibility upon the nurse to help the mother understand the care of the child.

Clubfoot

Clubfoot is a foot which has been twisted out of shape or position *in utero* and cannot be moved to an overcorrected position. An infant may appear to have this deformity because of the fetal position of comfort *in utero*. Unlike true clubfoot, however, his foot can be moved to a correct or even overcorrected position and made normal by simple exercises. In such a case before the mother is given the infant to nurse or fondle, she should be told that the defect is only temporary.

Incidence, Etiology, Diagnosis, Pathology and Types. True clubfoot is one of the most common orthopedic deformities. Several theories have been advanced to explain the *etiology*. The condition may be due to a defect in the ovum, a familial tendency or arrested growth. It may be a paralytic deformity occurring in conjunction with meningomyelocele. Not all cases of clubfoot in older children are congenital in origin. The defect may have been caused by injury or poliomyelitis.

The *diagnosis* of the specific type of clubfoot (several types are recognized) depends upon the anomaly in the individual child. The *pathology* varies from slight changes in the structure of the foot to abnormalities in the bones of both the foot and the leg.

The two most common types of clubfoot are talipes equinovarus and talipes calcaneovalgus. Both types are usually bilateral. In *talipes equinovarus* the foot is fixed in plantar flexion and deviates medially; i.e. the heel is elevated. The child walks on the toes and outer border of the foot. More than 95 per cent of the cases of congenital clubfoot are of this type. In *talipes calcaneovalgus* the foot is dorsiflexed and deviates laterally; i.e. the heel is turned outward, and the anterior part of the foot is elevated on the outer border. The child walks on the outwardly turned heel and the inner border of the foot.

Treatment and Nursing Care. *Treatment* should be started as soon as possible. Delay makes correction more difficult, since the bones and muscles of the leg develop abnormally, and the tendons will be shortened. In infancy, treatment is usually conservative. It may consist in manipulation, the application of a cast to hold the foot in a corrected position, or use of a wedged cast. The advantage of a wedged cast is that a position of greater correction can be achieved and that the cast need not be changed. A Denis Browne splint is often used for infants under one year of age. The appliance is made of two foot plates attached to a cross bar. When the splint is fitted to the shoes, varying positions of angulation of the feet may be maintained by set screws. As the child kicks, he automatically moves his feet into a corrected position.

If conservative measures fail, correction to as near a normal position as possible may be done under anesthesia and a cast applied. Surgery on the tendons and bones may be done in early childhood, and the leg and foot placed in a cast.

Most of the nursing care of children having club feet is given by the mother at home. When the child is admitted to the hospital, the usual method of applying a cast is followed. A plaster of Paris bandage is closely fitted over stockinet or wadding extending from below the knee to the toes. In the Kite method of correction the cast is wedged. When the child returns to the pedia-

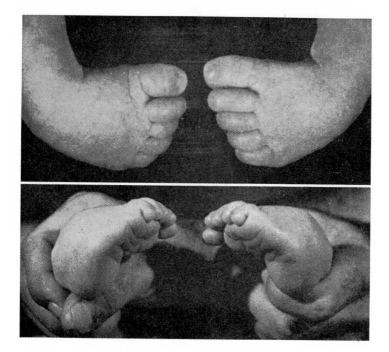

Figure 11–32. Congenital club-feet. (From W. R. Miller: *J. Pediat.*, Vol. 51.)

tric unit after application of a cast, the nurse should observe for areas of pressure and should note the condition of the skin around the edges of the cast, the circulation in the toes as shown by color and temperature, the child's ability to move his toes, and any sign of discomfort. If pressure areas develop or if the circulation is impaired, the cast is split to relieve the pressure or is removed. The nurse may put adhesive petals around the edges of the cast to prevent the plaster from irritating the skin.

Children are mischievous and are likely to slip small particles of food or anything else under the edge of the cast. It requires close observation to prevent a child from doing this, but prevention is essential, since such particles may cause irritation and possibly infection. No powder or oil should be put on the skin beneath the cast. Neither will add to the child's comfort, and both may cause irritation.

If manipulation is used to place the foot in a corrected position and a cast is applied, the child should remain in bed for twenty-four hours with the leg and the foot elevated on pillows or in a sling which supports the cast evenly. Elevation prevents swelling of the foot and leg and also constriction of the circulation.

If the child has undergone operation and a cast has been applied, upon his return to the pediatric unit the nurse must watch for evidence of impairment of circulation or sensation and bleeding, i.e. for discoloration of the cast over the wound, and report these observations to the physician. After operation it is necessary to change the cast about every three weeks in order

to bring the foot gradually into normal position and ensure permanent correction. When the cast is no longer needed, exercises and special orthopedic shoes may be required.

Instructions to the Mother. Before the infant is discharged from the nursery the nurse should discuss with the mother the necessity of taking the infant regularly to the clinic or to her private physician. Mothers are naturally distressed at the discomfort of corrective measures. They may need encouragement to follow treatment through until all possible correction has been made and the surgeon has discharged the child. If the mother is to manipulate the foot, she should be taught by the physician and supervised in her practice until she can do so correctly.

If the child is sent home from the pediatric unit in a cast, the mother should understand that after the position of the foot has been corrected, as shown by roentgenograms, the cast will be removed and the foot manipulated. If she has not already been taught how to do this, the physician will show her the procedure, and she should practice under his supervision or that of the nurse. The mother should be told that eventually the child will be fitted with shoes designed to correct a clubfoot and will learn to walk, but that it may be necessary for him to wear a splint on the leg and the foot at night.

After manipulation or surgery and the application of a cast the mother should be told that it will be necessary to bring the child back to the surgeon for examination over a period of months. Often parents believe that operation will correct the condition without further ado.

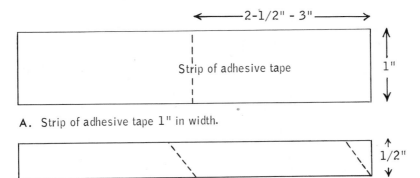

A. Strip of adhesive tape 1" in width.

B. Strip of adhesive folded in half with the adhesive side out. Cuts are made as indicated by the broken lines approximately every 2-1/2 " to 3" apart. Petals may be longer depending on the thickness of the cast.

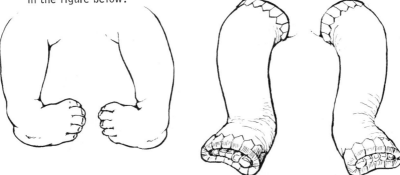

C. Completed petal. Petals are placed over the edge of the cast as shown in the figure below.

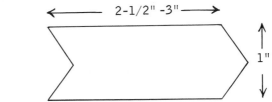

D. Bilateral talipes equinovarus before and after application of the plaster casts. Adhesive petals have been placed around the ends of the casts.

Figure 11–33. Method of applying adhesive petals around the edges of a cast to prevent the plaster from irritating the skin.

If the family is financially unable to bear the expense of frequent changes of cast, special shoes and possibly surgery, the parents should be referred to the medical social worker. Often an apparent lack of interest in returning for necessary treatment of the child may be due to financial difficulty in meeting the cost of his care.

Prognosis. The prognosis depends to a great extent upon the age of the child when treatment was begun. If the deformity is corrected in infancy, there is usually a good functional result, although the shape of the foot is not always normal in severely affected children.

Dislocation of the Hip

Etiology, Incidence and Diagnosis. Congenital dislocations of the hip are believed to be due to lack of embryonic development of the joint. Although this seems to be true, the cause is not entirely clear. It has been suggested that heredity is a factor.

Newborn infants seldom have a complete dislocation of the hip. Rather, the head of the femur does not lie entirely within the shallow acetabulum. When the child begins to walk, weight bearing may convert this condition to a true dislocation.

The anomaly is more frequent among girls than among boys, the ratio being seven to one.

This is one of the congenital anomalies which may not be discovered in the neonate, but may be found during the regular monthly examinations which every infant should have.

The initial *diagnosis* is based upon the following symptoms, which become apparent during the first or second month of life. The first and most reliable sign is limitation in abduction of the leg on the affected side. When the infant is lying on his back with knees and hips flexed, the normal hip joint permits the femur to be abducted until the knee almost touches the table at an angle of 90 degrees. With dislocation, abduction on the affected side is limited to no more than 45 degrees.

Pathology, Clinical Manifestations of Complete Dislocation, and Treatment. The early sign of dislocation of the hip is a shallow and extremely oblique acetabulum. The head of the femur on the affected side tends to be smaller than normal, and the ossification centers are delayed in appearance. Evidence of true dislocation is found on the roentgenogram, which shows lateral and upward dislocation of the head of the femur in relation to the acetabulum.

Signs and symptoms of complete dislocation are shortening of the leg and asymmetry of the gluteal skin folds, limited ability to abduct the leg and, when the child begins to walk, a characteristic limp. *Trendelenburg's sign* is present: lowering of the normal hip when the child is stood upon the affected leg and raises the normal leg.

If the dislocation is bilateral, the gait will be waddling and lordosis will be evident. The child is likely to be late in walking.

Treatment should be started as soon as the diagnosis is made. Delay prolongs treatment and may result in conversion of a partial to a complete dislocation. The objective of treatment is to place the head of the femur within the acetabulum and by constant pressure to enlarge and deepen the socket with ultimate correction of the dislocation. This is achieved in the young infant by placing a pillow between his thighs, thereby keeping the knees in a froglike position. The pillow should be protected by a plastic covering over the infant's diaper or under the cotton

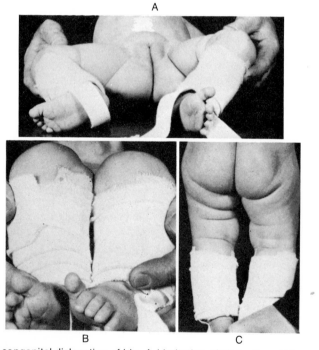

A

B   C

Figure 11–34.   Bilateral congenital dislocation of hip. *A,* Limitation of abduction of hip as seen in dislocation and dysplasia but also in coxa vara and positional contractures. The left hip will not abduct as much as the right. For cases with bilateral limitation a symmetrical decrease in abduction may be difficult to detect. *B,* The Galeazzi sign, valuable in detecting dislocation of the hip with upward displacement. The asymmetrical level of the knees when the infant is on a flat, hard table indicates either displacement or shortening of one femur. *C,* The asymmetry of gluteal folds and the adduction of the involved hip. These are physical signs which raise the suspicion of dysplasia or dislocation. (J. Cohen, in The Biologic Basis of Pediatric Practice, edited by R. E. Cooke, published by The Blakiston Division, McGraw-Hill Book Co., New York, 1968.)

pillow cover. The Fredjka splint is a more elegant modification and is easier to maintain in position. With the older child a stiff, shell-like cast may be used which spreads his legs apart and forces the head of the femur into the acetabulum. Complete casts are not used during the first few months of life, but, when applied, will be maintained for six to nine months.

If operation is performed, an open reduction of the dislocation or repair of the defect in the acetabular shelf is done. A cast is applied after operation to hold the head of the femur in the corrected position, i.e. fitted into the socket of the acetabulum.

Nursing Care. In general a child is admitted to the hospital for application of a cast. If a cast is used, it encircles the waist and extends down to the toes. The cast holds the leg in an abducted position. In bilateral dislocation both legs are abducted and held in position by the cast.

When the child returns to the unit after having his cast applied he should be placed on a mattress covered with water-repellent material. Boards should be placed under the mattress to prevent it from sagging. The child's head should be slightly higher than his feet so that urine and stool will not soil the cast. This can be accomplished by supporting the child's head, back and each leg with rubber-covered pillows. If the pillows are arranged properly, the heels will not rest on the mattress, and the upper part of his body will be higher than the buttocks. In order to prevent soiling the cast when a bedpan is used, a piece of plastic is tucked under the front and back edges of the opening around the buttocks and genitalia. The fracture bedpan is then slipped beneath the buttocks with the ends of the plastic strips hanging into the pan. For urination unaccompanied by stool, a male or female urinal is more convenient and comfortable than the bedpan.

After application of the cast a child who is not toilet-trained may be placed on a Bradford frame (see p. 210). This helps to keep the cast clean. If ponies or blocks are used under the head of the frame, they should be placed under the child's shoulders, never directly under the head. Lower blocks should balance the ponies, and the corners of the frame should be tied to the bed to prevent its slipping. Pillows should be placed at the sides of the frame to support the child's arms. A restraining jacket and ankle restraints are used to maintain the child's position and to prevent his falling.

The cast may be painted with white shoe polish or shellac according to the procedure adopted by the hospital. The skin around the edge of the cast is in danger of becoming excoriated. To prevent this the edges should be smoothed or lined with a waterproof material (see p. 229). "Petals" of waterproof adhesive tape, moleskin, or pieces of polyethylene plastic drapes or other substance are placed around the openings of the cast to protect the plaster and the stockinet lining from soiling and to prevent bits of plaster from cracking off and slipping under the cast.

The perineum should be kept clean. The nurse should wash the skin under the edge of the cast whenever necessary and dry it *thoroughly.* Neither oil nor powder should be used on the skin under the cast. The opening around the buttocks and genitalia should be covered with plastic material taped in place. If a diaper is necessary, it should be small and changed as soon as it is soiled.

The nurse should watch closely for signs of impaired circulation such as discoloration or cyanosis, impaired movement, loss of sensation, edema or temperature change in the toes. She should also watch for evidence of discomfort. These indications of poor circulation are generally caused by pressure of a cast which fits too closely over some area of the extremity.

If operation has been done, the nurse should watch for bleeding, and if there is evidence of hemorrhage, she should report it to the physician.

The small child who has nothing else to entertain him is likely to put bits of food or small articles under the cast. The nurse should have frequent physical contact with the child. She should give him toys too large to be used in this way and should watch him closely when he has food in his hands. She should also investigate the area under the cast to make certain that no excoriations or foreign material is present.

A hospital for acutely ill patients may have a special unit for convalescent and chronically ill children. If the child cannot be sent home, he may be placed here. Every effort should be made to give children who are not sent home as normal a life as is possible in an institution. Many of the suggestions outlined below for the mother to follow are applicable to the care of the institutionalized child. Carts built for crippled children, adult wheelchairs with the back dropped and the foot raised level with the seat or kiddie cars may be provided for children able to use them.

Guidance of the Mother After the Child's Discharge from the Hospital. Children with long-continued disabilities should lead as normal a life as possible. They should be given the means to help themselves in habilitation in all the daily life activities. A large plaster cast which holds the legs in frog position is unsightly and difficult to fit into clothing, furniture or equipment made for normal children. Practical ideas in use in many convalescent units will help the mother care for her child. Wide flaring pants extending down to the ankles may be used to cover the cast. These are made of attractive material and worn with a jacket of the same or a contrasting color. In such an outfit the child feels dressed up.

A home-made substitute serves the same purpose as the Bradford frame. It will resemble a sling in which the child's legs can extend over the edges. The canvas sling is suspended from a wooden frame. Another appliance which can be used is a stroller made of wood with openings for the legs on either side. The base must be large so that the stroller does not tip. Casters put at the corners should be large enough to permit pushing the stroller easily.

A wooden cart is often used in hospitals and convalescent units. It resembles a long wooden box mounted on a chassis which has large wheels at the top and small wheels, which pivot, at the bottom. The cart can be pushed like a baby carriage, and the child can turn the cart so that he can look this way or that by revolving the large wheels. The cart will hold a Bradford frame the width of the child's body, but support must be provided for the legs, which extend over the side of the cart. If the child has control of urination and defecation, he may be laid upon the mattress in the cart rather than upon a Bradford frame.

Any appliance made by the parents or any technique used in his care should be checked by the physician to ensure the child's safety and to protect the cast from cracking.

If the parents take the child home before the cast is completely dry, they must be taught how to inspect the cast for cracks, dents or breaks, how to observe the extremity and skin around the edges of the cast for signs of infection and pressure, and how to keep the cast clean.

These are long-drawn out cases, and the final result is uncertain. All that has been said previously about the psychologic management of handicapped children should be applied in the care of these children, whether at home, in a convalescent unit or in a hospital. Since the child will be readmitted to the hospital many times during the course of treatment, a good working relation between nurses and parents is essential or, in the clinic situation, among the parents, hospital and public health nurses and medical social service worker.

Osteogenesis Imperfecta

Etiology, Incidence, Diagnosis and Clinical Manifestations. The congenital form of osteogenesis imperfecta is rare. It is recessive in inheritance and is characterized by ribbon-like bone shadows with numerous fractures. Fractures may occur *in utero* or during the process of birth. Minor trauma just from a change of position can result in relatively painless fractures of the bones. Many of these children are dwarfed because of multiple fractures of the long bones and compression fractures of the vertebral bodies.

Children with this condition have blue scleras.
Treatment and Nursing Care. Orthopedic management may help these children, but the condition cannot be cured. They should be kept in a state of good nutrition. They should be handled gently in order to prevent further fractures.

Developmental Anomalies of the Extremities

Congenital anomalies of the extremities vary in severity from a slight defect of one extremity to an absence of a functional limb. *Polydactyly,* the presence of more than the ordinary number of digits, may be inherited as a dominant trait. *Syndactyly,* a partial or complete fusion of fingers or toes, may involve only skin, or the bones themselves may be fused. These conditions can usually be corrected by surgery.

In more severely affected infants there may be an absence of a part or all of any of the four limbs. Within the past few years such deformities became publicized because of the effect of the drug thalidomide on the embryo. The habilitation of such children is complex, involving skeletal, neuromuscular, psychologic, social and intellectual factors. The successful treatment of such a child involves the whole medical team, including pediatrician, orthopedist, psychiatrist, psychologist, prosthetist, social worker, occupational therapist, physiotherapist, nurses, and

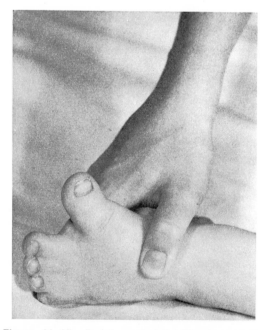

Figure 11–35. Pedal syndactyly. (Courtesy of Dr. Frank Mayfield. From Caffey and Silverman, in L. E. Holt, R. McIntosh and H. L. Barnett: *Pediatrics.* 13th ed. New York, Appleton-Century-Crofts, 1962.)

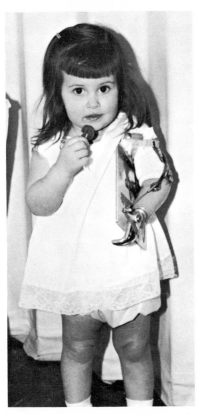

Figure 11–36. This little girl appears to have adjusted well to her prosthesis. She is able to carry a story book under her deformed arm. (M. I. Lineberger: *Nursing Outlook,* January 1959, p. 28.)

other professional persons as needed. The parents and the child himself are of great importance in therapy if the objectives of habilitation are to be achieved.

In order for this comprehensive therapy to be successful these children must be well motivated to learn how to use the usual prosthetic devices or the newer externally powered prostheses necessary for them to achieve independence.

If the parents see other children with amputations who are adjusted to their prostheses, they will be more likely to accept such treatment for their own child. How a parent reacts to the prosthesis often determines to a large degree how useful it will be, since the child generally adopts the attitude of his parents.

The accepted method of treatment today is to fit the child *early* with a functioning prosthesis, because this leads to more normal development and less atrophy of the parts of limbs present, and to greater patient and parent acceptance of the prosthesis. The nurse must learn how to help her patient manipulate his own prosthetic devices, since there are too many types of prostheses to be discussed here.

A congenital limb deficiency has a profound effect on the life of the afflicted child and his parents. Even professional persons may have to control their reactions to a seriously deformed child. The parents of such newborns must be told the truth about their child as soon as possible after birth even though this is a difficult thing to do. Because medical and nursing personnel may not invite further communication about such anomalies, the parents may, in addition to their feelings of guilt, feel rejected, hopeless and helpless.

The parents and the child should be accepted by the medical team and helped to verbalize their feelings about their disappointment. They should be told about the use of prosthetic devices early so that they are realistic in their hopes for the child. With support and guidance the parents ultimately should be able to discuss the disability realistically, to accept the child's need for both independence and dependence, and to free themselves from self-blame so that they can help the child to accept his own difference from other children. When the child asks about his deformity, the parents should give a simple, truthful answer such as, "You were born like that." Later he will need more detailed answers to his questions and further help with his problems. If the parents receive help with their own problems, they will be in a better position to help their child through his difficulties. If the parents' attitude toward the deformity is one of acceptance that it exists, but that it does not bar the child from living, the child and his friends will adopt this attitude also.

Special clincs have been established throughout the country for children having developmental anomalies of their extremities; however, not all states have them. The goal of every clinic for children having amputations is the same: to fit and train the child as early in his life as possible.

CLINICAL SITUATIONS

Mr. and Mrs. Jamison had moved into a moderately low-income housing area a short time before their first child, Joan, was born. Mr. Jamison planned to attend college while his nineteen-year-old wife looked forward to caring for her infant. Since Mrs. Jamison knew few people in her new community and since she had no previous experience with children, the public health nurse was asked to visit Mrs. Jamison and her five-day-old infant on their first day home from the hospital. Mrs. Jamison asked several questions.

1. "I have read about 'demand feedings' for babies. Why are these important?"
   a. "The more often you feed Joan, the better her nutritional status will be."
   b. "If you give Joan feedings every four hours, she will quickly learn correct eating habits."

c. "If you feed Joan when she is hungry, you will be meeting her individual needs."

d. "If you feed Joan frequently, you will not have to adhere to a rigid schedule and to plan your other household responsibilities around it."

2. "I am concerned because Joan's breasts are swollen a little even though the doctor said this was normal. What could I do about this?"

a. "All newborn infant girls have breast changes to a degree. It is nothing to worry about."

b. "Be certain to ask your doctor again about these changes. They may be important."

c. "Some newborn infants respond in this way because of hormone activity originating from the mother. No treatment is necessary."

d. "Fortunately few infants have this congenital condition. Be certain that you express the secretion from the breasts so that the swelling is reduced."

3. "Sometimes when I feed Joan her bottle, she has 'air on her stomach' and vomits a little formula when I place her in her crib. How can I prevent this?"

a. "Do not give her all the formula the doctor recommended because she is obviously eating too much."

b. "Bubble her frequently during her feeding and especially after she has finished eating. Then place her in bed on her right side."

c. "Bubble her frequently during her feeding and especially after she has finished eating. Then place her in bed on her left side."

d. "Bubble her frequently during her feeding and prop her against a pillow in the corner of her crib so that it will be mechanically more difficult for her to vomit."

4. "I am concerned about Joan's bowel movements. Do you think they are normal?" The nurse should know that the stool of a normal six-day-old formula-fed baby should be

a. Greenish-black, sticky in consistency, and odorless.

b. Hard in consistency and almost white.

c. Yellow, putty-like to hard in consistency.

d. Yellow, soft in consistency.

5. The nurse should know in discussing infant feeding with mothers that breast milk in comparison with cow's milk per volume contains

a. More carbohydrate, less protein.

b. More carbohydrate, more fat.

c. More carbohydrate, more protein.

d. More calories per ounce.

6. When the nurse was examining Joan, she realized that the infant should be referred to the physician if she had the following manifestations:

a. Positive rooting reflex and positive sucking reflex.

b. Positive grasping reflex and negative Chvostek's sign.

c. Negative startle reflex and negative tonic neck reflex.

d. Positive tonic neck reflex and positive swallowing reflex.

7. The nurse tested Joan's Moro reflex. A normal baby would respond by

a. Sudden, generalized, symmetrical movement with the arms thrown outward in an embrace position and the legs drawn up together.

b. Rapid movement of the arm and leg on the side where the nurse stimulated her.

c. Slow, generalized, random activity of the whole body followed by a rigid positioning of the extremities.

d. Rapid movement of all the extremities, but with no fixed pattern.

Mr. and Mrs. Basito had a five-year-old daughter, Dolores, when Juan was born prematurely in the emergency room of their local hospital. Since both parents had to work because of financial problems, Mrs. Basito had not had time to visit the clinic for prenatal care. At birth Juan weighed 4 pounds 1 ounce. He was admitted to the pediatric unit and placed in an incubator.

8. The nurse regulated the temperature of the incubator on the basis of

a. The environmental temperature of the unit.

b. The temperature of the infant's extremities.

c. The set temperature of 88°F. for all prematures.

d. The infant's body temperature.

9. Juan had a period of apnea about three hours after delivery. The nurse, in order to stimulate his respirations since no mechanical resuscitator had been brought to his unit,

a. Held him by his ankles with his head down and spanked him.

b. Plunged the infant alternately into a bath basin of warm, then a basin of cool water.

c. Carefully suctioned the infant, then gently carried out mouth-to-mouth insufflation.

d. Gently suctioned the infant, then applied rhythmic pressure to his chest.

10. Oxygen was ordered for Juan in the usual concentration. The nurse should realize that in order to prevent retrolental fibroplasia she should

a. Maintain a constant level of oxygen concentration less than 40 per cent in the incubator.

b. Give at least 70 per cent oxygen to prevent this condition.

c. Open the arm holes of the incubator in order to mix the oxygen with room air to prevent too high a concentration.

d. Use an oxygen analyzer once a day to check the concentration of oxygen in the incubator.

11. A few hours after delivery Juan's skin began to be increasingly jaundiced. His bilirubin level was found to be near the critical level. A diagnosis of erythroblastosis fetalis was made. The nurse should realize that

a. His mother was Rh-positive, his father Rh-negative.

b. Both parents were Rh-negative.

c. Both parents were Rh-positive.

d. His mother was Rh-negative, his father Rh-positive.

12. An important reason why one or more exchange transfusions are done on an infant having erythroblastosis fetalis is to prevent

a. Hemorrhagic disease of the newborn.

b. Kernicterus.

c. Ophthalmia neonatorum.

d. Toxoplasmosis.

13. When Mrs. Basito was discharged from the hospital, she came to the pediatric unit to visit her son.

She became emotionally disturbed when she saw the nurse feeding Juan by gavage even though the physician had told her he was doing well. The nurse could explain the reason for this procedure and reassure her by saying

a. "I am feeding Juan this way in order to prevent infecting his mouth with a rubber nipple, since he has very little resistance to infection."

b. "Although Juan is gaining weight well, we do not want to tire him by having him suck on a nipple."

c. "Juan is more likely to vomit and inhale his formula if we feed him by nipple."

d. "I am very busy. This is the quickest way I can feed Juan and be certain that he gets all his formula."

14. When Juan weighed 7 pounds, the physician discharged him from the hospital. Before discharge the nurse demonstrated the physical care he would need at home. In view of the total family situation, which comment by the mother should alert the nurse to the mother's need for further guidance?

a. "Dolores, his sister, is so anxious to help me take care of the baby."

b. "Poor Juan. I have caused him so much trouble. I will never let anything happen to him again."

c. "He is such a beautiful baby! All my neighbors will want him when they see him."

d. "My husband wanted a son so much. He has prayed each night that he would live."

Tommy Walker, who had a unilateral cleft lip, was admitted to the pediatric unit from the newborn nursery because his mother was emotionally unable to care for him at home. Mrs. Walker had previously had two infants who died at birth. Both she and her husband were distraught over Tommy's obvious defect.

15. The nurse could best help Tommy's parents adjust to their situation on admission by

a. Placing him in a crib where other parents and children could not see him.

b. Explaining that Tommy's deformity is really mild in comparison with others she has seen.

c. Agreeing with the parents that Tommy's deformity is difficult for her to accept also.

d. Treating Tommy as a normal infant and at the same time accepting the parent's feelings of disappointment.

16. After operation on the cleft lip Tommy's parents were delighted with the results. On his tenth postoperative day his mother asked for permission to hold her baby and to try to feed him. The nurse explained that

a. The mother could hold Tommy on her lap and feed him with a rubber-tipped medicine dropper if she did not touch the area around the suture line.

b. Tommy should lie flat in bed during his feeding because of the possibility of injury to his lip.

c. Only nurses were permitted to feed babies while they were hospitalized.

d. Tommy would have to be fed by gavage for at least a few more days and that the mother would have to wait until the baby was discharged to care for him.

17. Tommy's mother asked several questions about the skin of a newborn infant. The nurse should realize that only one of the following characteristics is found in all normal infants

a. Mongolian spots.

b. Miliaria.

c. Intertrigo.

d. Good turgor.

18. Since Tommy was Mrs. Walker's first living infant, she asked the nurse several questions about his care after discharge from the hospital. She asked, "Should Tommy's mouth be wiped out each morning when I bathe him?"

a. "Yes, in order to clean away milk curds."

b. "No, you will probably gag the baby and cause vomiting."

c. "Yes, cleanse the mouth with a cotton swab moistened with boric acid solution in order to prevent thrush."

d. "No, a baby's mouth should not be cleansed except by rinsing after feedings with boiled water."

19. "How can diaper rash be prevented?"

a. "Powder the buttocks thoroughly, particularly in the creases, when you change Tommy's diaper."

b. "Wash his buttocks with a mild soap and water and dry thoroughly whenever you change his diaper."

c. "Wipe the buttocks with a dry swab and oil well when he is soiled."

d. "When you change his diaper, wipe the buttocks with oil and powder in the creases well."

GUIDES FOR FURTHER STUDY

1. Make a list of questions asked by mothers of newborns who have been admitted to the pediatric unit for treatment of congenital anomalies. Discuss your answers to these questions in seminar.

2. List the specific differences between fetal and postnatal circulation. If expected changes do not occur at or after birth, which congenital heart lesions would result? What clinical manifestations of these conditions could you observe?

3. Observe a group of normal newborns for common traits and for individual differences in relation to sleep, i.e. bodily movements, facial grimaces, sucking activity and reactions to hunger. Discuss your observations in seminar.

4. Discuss in seminar differences in practices of various religious and cultural groups in relation to the care of newborns.

5. Help an individual mother plan a 24-hour program of care for a normal newborn infant. What difficulties were encountered?

6. A newborn having a meningomyelocele is being discharged from the nursery. He will be admitted to the pediatric unit of another hospital in two weeks for operation. Help the mother plan a program of care for this infant at home. During your discussion note the mother's attitude toward this infant. What could you do or recommend in addition to helping her plan for his physical care that would assist her in adjusting emotionally to this situation?

TEACHING AIDS AND OTHER INFORMATION*

American Medical Association

Vascular Birthmarks and Your Child.

Association for the Aid of Crippled Children

The Child with Brain Damage.
The Child with Spina Bifida.

National Association for Retarded Children, Inc.

A New Dimension of Love.
Centerwall, S. A., and Centerwall, W. R.: A Study of Children with Mongolism Reared in the Home
     Compared to Those Reared Away from the Home.

National Society for Crippled Children and Adults, Inc.

Lewis, R. S.: The Brain Injured Child (The Perceptually Handicapped).
McDonald, E. T.: Bright Promise.
Sugar, M., and Ames, M. D.: The Child with Spina Bifida Cystica; His Medical Problem and Habil-
     itation.

The Children's Hospital Medical Center, Boston, Mass.

Birthmarks.

The National Foundation-March of Dimes

Birth Defects—Social and Emotional Problems.
Birth Defects; The Tragedy and the Hope.
Chromosome 21 and Its Association with Down's Syndrome.

United States Department of Health, Education, and Welfare

Childhood Disorders of the Brain and Nervous System.
Dittmann, L.: The Mentally Retarded Child at Home, A Manual for Parents, 1959 (reprinted 1964).
Inborn (Congenital) Heart Defects, 1964.
Mongolism (Down's Syndrome): Hope Through Research, 1968.
Research Explores Cleft Palate, 1966.
Spina Bifida—A Birth Defect: Hope Through Research, 1968.
The Cat Cry Syndrome, 1965.
The Child with a Cleft Palate, 1953 (reprinted 1963).
The Child with Central Nervous System Deficit, 1965.
The Mongoloid Baby, 1960 (reprinted 1964).
The Thalidomide Story, 1965.

REFERENCES

Publications

Birch, H. G. (Ed.): *Brain Damage in Children: The Biological and Social Aspects.* Baltimore, Williams
     & Wilkins Company, 1964.
Blakeslee, B. (Ed.): *The Limb-Deficient Child.* Berkeley and Los Angeles, University of California
     Press, 1963.
Buck, P. S., and Zarfoss, G. T.: *The Gifts They Bring; Our Debt to the Mentally Retarded.* Don Mills,
     Ontario, Longmans Canada Ltd., 1965.
Carter, C. H.: *Handbook of Mental Retardation Syndromes.* Springfield, Ill., Charles C Thomas, 1966.
Cassels, D. E.: *The Heart and Circulation in the Newborn and Infant.* New York, Grune & Stratton,
     Inc., 1966.
de Gutierrez-Mahoney, C. G., and Carini, E.: *Neurological and Neurosurgical Nursing.* 4th ed. St.
     Louis, C. V. Mosby Company, 1965.
Ferguson, A. B.: *Orthopaedic Surgery in Infancy and Childhood.* 3rd ed. Baltimore, Williams &
     Wilkins Company, 1968.
French, E. L., and Scott, J. C.: *How You Can Help Your Retarded Child: A Manual for Parents.* Phil-
     adelphia, J. B. Lippincott Company, 1967.

---

* Complete addresses are given in the Appendix.

Keith, J. D., Rowe, R. D., and Vlad, P.: *Heart Disease in Infancy and Childhood.* 2nd ed. New York, Macmillan Company, 1967.

Larson, C. B., and Gould, M.: *Calderwood's Orthopedic Nursing.* 6th ed. St. Louis, C. V. Mosby Company, 1965.

Lewis, G. M., and Wheeler, C. E.: *Practical Dermatology for Medical Students and General Practitioners.* 3rd ed. Philadelphia, W. B. Saunders Company, 1966.

Morley, M. E.: *Cleft Palate and Speech.* 6th ed. Baltimore, Williams & Wilkins Company, 1965.

Nadas, A.: *Pediatric Cardiology.* 2nd ed. Philadelphia, W. B. Saunders Company, 1963.

Robinson, S., Abrams, H., and Kaplan, H.: *Congenital Heart Disease.* 2nd ed. New York, The Blakiston Division, McGraw-Hill Book Company, Inc., 1965.

Rubin, A. (Ed.): *Handbook of Congenital Malformations.* Philadelphia, W. B. Saunders Company, 1967.

Schaffer, A. J.: *Diseases of the Newborn.* 2nd ed. Philadelphia, W. B. Saunders Company, 1965.

Periodicals

Apgar, V.: Drugs in Pregnancy. *Am. J. Nursing,* 65:104, March 1965.

Arey, J. B.: Abdominal Masses in Infants and Children. *Pediat. Clin. N. Amer.,* 10:665, 1963.

Atkinson, H. C.: Care of the Child with Cleft Lip and Palate. *Am. J. Nursing,* 67:1889, 1967.

Carter, C. H.: Unpredictability of Mental Development in Down's Syndrome. *South Med. J.,* 60:834, 1967.

Etheridge, J. E.: Hypoglycemia and the Central Nervous System. *Pediat. Clin. N. Amer.,* 14:865, 1967.

Goulding, E. I., and Koop, C. E.: The Newborn: His Response to Surgery. *Am. J. Nursing,* 65:84, October 1965.

Kallaus, J.: The Child with Cleft Lip and Palate: The Mother in the Maternity Unit. *Am. J. Nursing,* 65:120, April 1965.

Kane, H. A.: Recent Advances in Pediatric Cardiology. *Pediat. Clin. N. Amer.,* 15:345, 1968.

Linde, L. M., and others: Growth in Children with Congenital Heart Disease. *J. Pediat.,* 70:413, 1967.

Linde, L. M., and others: Mental Development in Congenital Heart Disease. *J. Pediat.,* 71:198, 1967.

MacQueen, J. C.: Services for Children with Multiple Handicaps. *Children,* 13:55, 1966.

McDermott, M. M.: The Child with Cleft Lip and Palate: On the Pediatric Ward. *Am. J. Nursing,* 65:122, April 1965.

McNamara, D. G.: Acyanotic Congenital Heart Disease. *Pediat. Clin. N. Amer.,* 11:295, 1964.

Melicow, M. M.: Ambiguous Genitalia in Neonates and Infants. *Hospital Medicine,* 3:48, November 1967.

Moore, M. L.: Care of the Hydrocephalic Child. *RN,* 29:79, November 1966.

Paine, R. S.: Hydrocephalus. *Pediat. Clin. N. Amer.,* 14:779, 1967.

Pidgeon, V.: The Infant with Congenital Heart Disease. *Am. J. Nursing,* 67:290, 1967.

Pump Drains Excess Cranial Fluid. *Medical World News,* 8:66, October 6, 1967.

Rashkind, W. J., and Miller, W. W.: Creation of An Arterial Septal Defect Without Thoracotomy. *J.A.M.A.,* 196:991, 1966.

Ripley, I. L.: The Child with Cleft Lip and Palate: Through His Years of Growth. *Am. J. Nursing,* 65:124, April 1965.

Singer, D. B., and others: Pathology of the Congenital Rubella Syndrome. *J. Pediat.,* 71:665, 1967.

Soules, B. J.: Thalidomide Victims in a Rehabilitation Center. *Am. J. Nursing,* 66:2023, 1966.

Steele, S.: The Nurse's Role in the Rehabilitation of Children with Meningomyelocele. *Nursing Forum,* VI:104, November 1967.

Stone, N. W.: Family Factors in Willingness to Place the Mongoloid Child. *Am. J. Ment. Defic.,* 72:16, July 1967.

Vermooten, V.: Congenital Abnormalities of the Kidney. *Hospital Medicine,* 3:57, July 1967.

When Knife is Gentler than the Hand. *Medical World News,* 8:74, December 1, 1967.

Whitmore, W. F.: Wilms's Tumor and Neuroblastoma. *Am. J. Nursing,* 68:527, 1968.

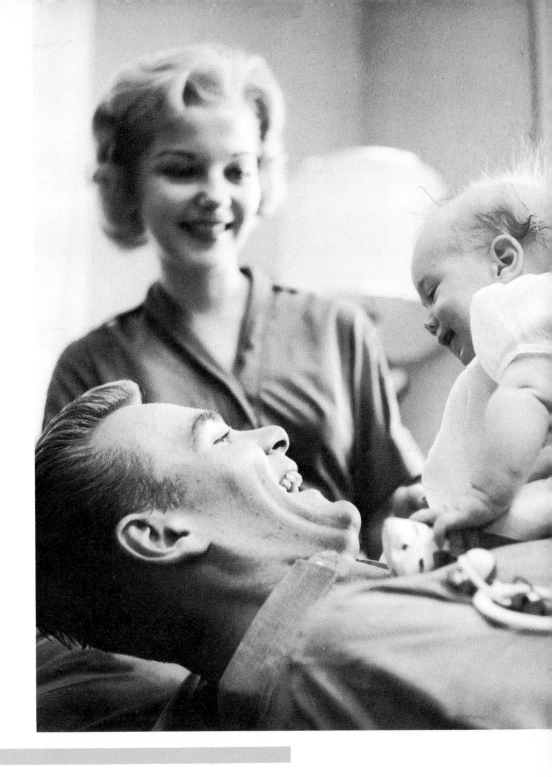

UNIT THREE

THE INFANT

12

THE NORMAL INFANT: GROWTH, DEVELOPMENT AND CARE DURING THE FIRST YEAR

The care and development of the infant throughout the first year of life will be considered in this unit. As with the newborn, his emotional and physical status and his needs in health and in sickness will be discussed.

Just as growth and development occur in the child, so also must the process of development occur in his parents as they keep pace with his natural maturation. During the first year of an infant's life the parents must learn the cues, what the child is trying to tell them, and then act on their observations. They must learn to observe their infant's behavior and to act toward fulfilling his needs. Some parents unfortunately are not prepared to undergo the emotional development needed in relation to their child's development. These are the parents who particularly need help in understanding the usual steps in a child's development. Nurses many times can interpret this process to parents and

thus alleviate much of their misunderstanding.

Parents also need help in becoming more flexible and adaptable in meeting their child's needs. Parents are influenced by the child each of them was in the past. It is not easy to change each parent's view of his or her own background experiences. Some parents retain within themselves the children they used to be and see things as though their past home situations still existed. At the same time they are also looking at the same events through an accumulation of adult experiences. Parents then see their children as they would a blurred photograph, using a camera which is out of focus. The phases through which a parent should progress as the child grows will be discussed in appropriate chapters throughout this text.

Stress must be placed on the fact that spontaneity and enjoyment of the infant by the adult are probably of greater significance than the specific procedures used in his care. If the parent or the nurse is particularly harassed and over-burdened, her care will not be beneficial for the infant. At such times some kindly support or temporary relief from the pressure may be necessary.

OVERVIEW OF THE INFANT'S EMOTIONAL DEVELOPMENT

The nurse should understand a child's developmental needs and should know how to respond to them so that he may continue to grow emotionally and physically while he is in the hospital as he would at home. This is particularly important with infants and young children because separation from their parents, in itself, produces problems with which they need help.

Sense of Trust

As was stated earlier (see p. 29), different components of the healthy personality develop at various periods in the process of growing up. The first of these, and probably the most important, is the *sense of trust,* which normally develops in the first year of life. It is, of course, strengthened or weakened by experiences after that age, but the foundation is laid in infancy. If this sense of trust in others is not learned, the reverse, a *sense of mistrust,* is acquired. This tendency will be increasingly difficult to change as the infant enters childhood. A distrustful child is not friendly, and his attitude evokes a similar response in adults and other children.

During the first year the infant is completely dependent upon his mother or someone who is a temporary substitute for her such as his father, siblings, baby-sitters or grandmothers. His preference will probably be for his mother.

The infant's earliest approach to life is *incorporative,* as shown in his wanting to put everything into his mouth, to make it a part of himself. If this need is satisfied, he has laid the foundation for *giving* as well as *receiving.*

Turning to his mother or her substitute for comfort and love is the first evidence of an infant's desire to *turn outward* for pleasure. His interest is no longer solely in physical sensations which he himself produces (sucking his fingers, sucking at the breast or on the nipple of his bottle, kicking, stretching, and the like) or which someone provides for him (the comfort of having his diaper changed or his warm bath). The growing infant learns very slowly that *people* give care which he enjoys and so learns to turn to them for relief of tensions.

The sense of trust does not develop independently of other aspects of growth. Initially it is based on consistently similar events such as the occurrence of hunger and the receiving of the proper feeding. If the feedings are not sufficient or are improperly given, the infant will begin to establish a sense of mistrust. Trust is an integral part of his total development. An infant learns to trust others through the relief of his basic needs; i.e. he learns to trust those who give him pleasant sensations. The young infant does not differentiate his body from that of others who handle him. He likes the warm feeding in his mouth, but does not differentiate his mother's hand upon the bottle from his own fingers. Later, when he has learned the limits of his body and knows in a vague way that he is a separate organism, he will respond to his mother's presence. *He has learned to associate her care and caresses with her.* He smiles and coos when he sees her, for he knows that something pleasant will happen to him. He has learned to trust his mother and has laid the foundation for trusting other people.

If, however, someone speaks to him in a harsh tone or is sudden and spasmodic in his movements, the infant is frightened. He has received his first lesson in *mistrusting* others. If this happens often, he is likely to grow uneasy and apprehensive. This may happen especially if the infant's parents are under considerable tension and anxiety in their marital relations. If such is the case, they may need marriage counseling or psychiatric care in order to prevent later severe mental illness characterized by mistrust in their child. *The sense of trust is indeed the cornerstone of a wholesome personality.*

During the first six months of life the infant wants to *receive all* that has to him a connotation of pleasure. He is not ready to give or even forego pleasure. When at six weeks of age he smiles at his mother, it is not to give her pleasure, but because he feels comfortable. He smiles in his sleep and when alone. In imitation of his mother he smiles when she smiles. Later he learns that she smiles when he smiles and coos and that a smiling mother does pleasant things for him.

During the second six months the infant learns to *bite.* The first teeth erupt between the fifth and seventh months, and he quickly learns to use them. His playful putting of everything available into his mouth becomes a drive to have something between his gums on which he can bite.

As he develops he becomes increasingly aware of himself as a separate organism. His mother, thinking that he is now more sturdy and less dependent upon her, is likely to leave him more to himself while she resumes activities which she enjoyed before his birth. If she intends to continue with a profession or employment outside the home, she wants to accustom the infant gradually to her absence. She leaves him alone while she does her housework. Although she has always done this, the infant while very young slept the greater part of the time, but now is awake and alone.

A crisis occurs at this time, for he is no longer a passive recipient of attention from other people; he is becoming an active person in his social environment and is also seeking control over his physical environment. The crisis develops around the adjustment which mother and infant make to their changed relations. The infant's successful adjustment depends less on the amount of time his mother now spends with him than on the *quality* of their relations during his first six months and while the crisis is being resolved. Another factor in his adjustment is the continuity of care from other members of the family which formerly supplemented that of his mother.

NEEDS DURING THE FIRST YEAR

Although the infant's need to put everything into his mouth and later to bite was given priority among his essential needs because of its great psychologic importance, he has five other needs which must be met if he is to learn to trust the people about him: *feeding, sucking pleasure, warmth and comfort, both love and security,* and *sensory stimulation.*

Need for Feeding

The infant's world is small. He has no sense of time and lives entirely in the moment. The only rhythms he knows are those set up by his physiologic mechanism. He experiences hunger, which produces tension. He soon learns that people around him can satisfy this need and reduce his tension—make him comfortable—and that this is done with varying emotional attitudes on their part. This is a time for showing him love and affection.

Nurses are often criticized for the professionally unemotional attitude they show when feeding hospitalized infants. This is unfortunate, since infants sense a lack of warmth and spontaneity. We have also noted that breast feeding is more emotionally satisfying for the infant than bottle feeding if the mother sincerely desires to breast-feed him. The mother's attitude or that of her substitute is expressed in voice, touch and handling the infant while he is nursing. He associates this attitude with being fed and later on with food. Unfortunately even the mother's attitude is not always one of pleasure in caring for the child she loves. If she employs someone else to care for him, he will probably be kindly treated, but no one else would be likely to show the affection which a loving mother would give and which the infant needs. Today, when many

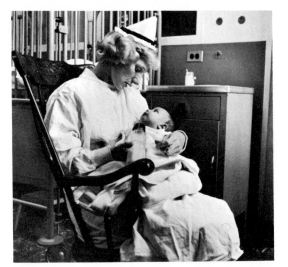

Figure 12–1. When feeding the hospitalized infant, the nurse gives him, in addition to food and sucking pleasure, warmth, comfort and a feeling of security. (Courtesy St. Luke's Hospital, New York City.)

young mothers want a career outside the home, affectionate infant feeding is one of the main problems of child care.

Need for Sucking Pleasure

The infant's habit of putting fingers and toys into his mouth is closely allied to his pleasure in sucking. The need for sucking, however, is quite apart from the need for food. He thoroughly enjoys the act of sucking, and if he does not have the opportunity for it, tension results. Giving him something to suck on relieves the tension, and he promptly relaxes. Being put to the breast or held lovingly with the nipple of his bottle between his lips and the milk in his mouth is his first experience of love and comfort. The intensity of the sucking urge varies and is an example of individual differences in children.

During the second six months he may bite upon the nipple. If he is at the breast, this hurts his mother even if his teeth have not erupted. She may think of weaning him. If this is done and he is taught to drink from a cup before he has outgrown the need for sucking, he will suck upon anything else he can use for the purpose. If he wants to bite, he should be given a piece of toast or a suitable toy. He may, however, continue to bite the nipple. If the infant is breast-fed, the mother may use a shield for protection. The intensity of the urge to find satisfaction through sucking and biting gradually decreases as other gratifications become available.

Need for Warmth and Comfort

An infant enjoys the warmth and softness of his mother's body when held in her arms. He has a real hunger for this pleasant experience. He enjoys rhythmic rocking, being handled and the comfort of having his position changed.

Need for Love and Security

Just as the infant becomes hungry, is fed and becomes relaxed, repeating the rhythm over and over, so he needs a rhythm of attention shown in bathing him, riding in the stroller, being played with, being cuddled close to his mother's body and being put to sleep. Throughout these activities of daily living he needs a feeling of security, of being wanted and loved. Infants are not consciously apprehensive about the future, but their daily care is the basis for either serenity or a tenseness which in an adult we would call apprehension or generalized anxiety.

Need for Sensory Stimulation

Infants need to be stimulated by a change of environment, by a change in position, by contact with various textures of materials, by sights and sounds and by human contact. If they do not receive such stimulation in their daily care, they will not grow and develop normally. The need for sensory stimulation can be met by a loving mother who takes her infant with her as she moves through her daily routine, who talks and sings to him as she cuddles him, and who gradually introduces him to wider and more varied learning experiences and activities.

Methods of Meeting the Needs

Meeting the infant's needs is an interrelated process which begins immediately after birth. The infant's communication with the outside world is normally through his mother.

Breast feeding meets many needs simultaneously. The infant is held close to his mother and has the comfort of taking as little or as much as he wants. Many physicians believe that the breast can be given to comfort the infant even if he is not hungry.

If the infant is bottle-fed, he should be held in the same position as the infant at the breast. If the mother accepts the idea of a self-demand schedule (see p. 124), the infant will establish his own feeding rhythm. The holes in the nipple should be of such a size that two or more hours of sucking a day are required for him to take his entire feeding. Bottles should never be propped, because propping does not fulfill the basic needs of an infant.

If his basic needs are met, an infant cannot be spoiled in early infancy. His mother should go to him if he is uncomfortable—wet, cold or tired of lying in the same position. Spoiling does

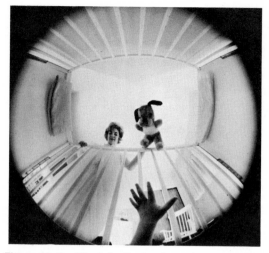

Figure 12–2. The infant's view from the center of his world. (Courtesy of Mr. Jack Tinney and *Baby Talk Magazine,* April 1967.)

not result from his being kept comfortable, and he needs pleasant experiences in order to trust others.

When the infant has developed to the stage at which he identifies his mother and others who care for him as separate beings, he does not want to be left alone. He needs to have someone look into his room and speak to him frequently until he learns that temporary absence does not mean that the friends in whose presence he feels secure are permanently gone. If he has to endure long periods of separation, he may become chronically afraid that he will be left alone. (The family dog is a poor substitute for human companionship, but better than inanimate toys). During this period the infant may become very shy and appear insecure and afraid of the world. Sympathetic adults must accept this lack of friendliness and, without forcing their attentions upon him, win his trust.

In early infancy the child cannot express his wants, and his mother must anticipate his needs. Later he will convey his wants through movements and sounds. Development of speech is primarily determined by his stage of mental growth and his need to communicate with others. But an important factor, often overlooked, is his mother's response to his coos and babbling. The smiling and cooing of the infant are enormously rewarding to the mother. If she responds by talking to him, showing her appreciation of his achievement in one way or another, he will continue to vocalize and will speak at an early age.

In summary, the infant will learn to adapt to his world by having his needs met initially. First of all he will cry to indicate his need for food. The mother will offer her breast or a bottle feeding to meet his need. If later the infant cries again, but the mother produces no feeding, the infant feels great discomfort because of his hunger and the fact that his crying produced no response. In turn the infant will evolve a new behavioral response. He will either suck his fingers and ultimately go to sleep or he will cry with rage. The infant thus learns to adapt to his world and in time to control his environment through a change in his behavior.

Although the very young infant needs maximum pleasure and minimum discomfort, the older infant needs small doses of anxiety to learn how to handle frustrations and be prepared for the usual problems every child must meet. If he has not been overprotected, everyday experiences are likely to provide all the frustration he requires to build up his ability to handle successfully the activities of daily living.

Frustration of Needs

Some infantile responses persist in adult life, but are modified by the culture of the group. Probably the adult fondness for biting into crisp food and for chewing gum is an infantile pleasure carried over into adult life.

If the child's need for food is not met, he may exhibit anxiety shown by overeating or not eating enough.

If his need for love and security is not met, the child may doubt his own ability to influence his environment and become insecure in his personal world. He may not be able to take the next steps in personality development. If he does not learn

to trust others, he does not merely remain neutral toward them, but rather is likely to be unable to make and hold friends, for he mistrusts them as he learned to mistrust those who cared for him in his early infancy.

If the infant does not receive sensory stimulation, he probably will not develop normally intellectually. He needs perceptual experience early in life in order to prevent growth failure and serious behavioral abnormalities.

OVERVIEW OF PHYSICAL GROWTH AND DEVELOPMENT

Principles of Growth and Development

Chapter 2 dealt with the general principles of growth and development. These might be summarized as follows.

Development of the human organism is a *continuous process* which begins before birth, each stage being dependent upon the preceding stages. A specific example of this would be the development of human dentition (Fig. 12-3).

An infant is usually born without teeth. Already, however, he has twenty deciduous (primary) teeth in his mandible and maxilla, some of which began to calcify *in utero*. Eruption of the primary teeth begins at approximately seven months postnatally (see Fig. 12-3). For some infants, teething brings no discomfort, for others it is a painful experience. It does not, however, cause a high fever, diarrhea or other serious upset, though the infant's fluid intake may de-

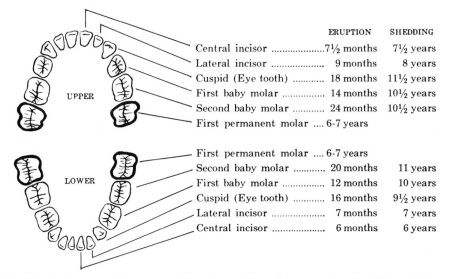

	ERUPTION	SHEDDING
Central incisor	7½ months	7½ years
Lateral incisor	9 months	8 years
Cuspid (Eye tooth)	18 months	11½ years
First baby molar	14 months	10½ years
Second baby molar	24 months	10½ years
First permanent molar	6-7 years	
First permanent molar	6-7 years	
Second baby molar	20 months	11 years
First baby molar	12 months	10 years
Cuspid (Eye tooth)	16 months	9½ years
Lateral incisor	7 months	7 years
Central incisor	6 months	6 years

Figure 12-3. The development of human dentition is a continuous process from the fifth month *in utero* to maturity. (Courtesy of Niles Newton, Ph.D., and *Baby Talk Magazine*, November 1967.)

crease slightly, and if he does not eat well, he may have a slight electrolyte imbalance and sleep poorly. The permanent teeth begin to form soon after birth. These erupt when the deciduous teeth are shed, usually about age six or seven. The eruption of the last permanent teeth, the third molars, indicates the approximate time of cessation of growth.

The term *developmental sequence* means that these changes are specific, progressive and orderly and lead eventually to maturity. All children progress through similar steps, but the age at which each child achieves these steps varies, since achievement depends upon his inherent maturational capacity interacting with his physical and social environment. It is especially important for nurses to observe *individual differences* in order to meet adequately the needs of each child.

The different areas of growth are *interrelated.* All types of growth and development—physical, mental, emotional, social and spiritual—proceed together and in various ways affect each other in the normal advance toward maturity.

Three principles should be stressed in motor development. (*a*) Muscular development is *cephalocaudal,** i.e. proceeding from the head to the feet. The result is that the child acquires the ability to control his neck muscles before those of his legs and feet. (*b*) The development of muscular control is also from *proximal to distal;* i.e. development begins near the body and progresses outward to the extremities. (*c*) The two preceding principles operate in conjunction with development from *general to specific* movement. Muscles controlling gross movements are in general the large muscles proximal to the body. The child uses the larger muscles of the upper arms and legs before he has control of the muscles of the hands and feet, fingers and toes. The infant waves his arms and kicks long before he is able to control the muscles of his fingers in handling anything. Children hold their toys, roll over and sit up before they are able to pick up a crumb as an adult would do.

Tests of motor ability are used as intelligence tests in the young infant, since a child of subnormal mentality is late in sitting, standing, walking and achieving control of the arms and hands in any but gross movements.

Basic Factors in Development

Development results from two basic factors: maturation and learning.

---

* From *kephalos,* Greek for head, and *cauda,* Latin for tail, so called because of the location of the nerve cells of the central nervous system which control muscular activity. Tail is here the equivalent of the lower part of the spinal cord.

Maturation refers to the inborn, genetically transmitted capacity for development. This capacity normally covers all areas of development.

Learning is the result of experience, experimentation and training. The test of learning is whether it changes behavior. The ability to learn is highly dependent upon the inborn capacity for mental development. If the potential capacity for learning is poor, i.e. if the child has low intelligence rating or quotient (I.Q.), he will find learning difficult. The child learns from experience that the floor is hard when he falls upon it and that strained fruit tastes good when he is given a spoonful. Later on he learns by experimentation to open and close the door and the easiest way to creep up stairs.

When he has matured to a higher level, he will learn partially from the experience of others, both by observing them and by listening to what they tell him. He has learned that adults know much more than he does and that what they say —in earnest, not in jest—is true. When his mother tells him that the stove is hot and will burn his hand if he touches it, he believes her and usually does not experiment to find out. From a child who describes his stay in a hospital he learns what hospitalization may be like. When he goes to school, he will learn from the experience of men since man was first upon this earth.

Maturation and learning are interrelated. No learning takes place unless the child is mature enough to be able to understand, and change his behavior. If he is forced beyond his capacity to learn, unfavorable attitudes may be established which may later retard learning in that area. *The child who is not given opportunity to learn by experience and from others at the optimum time— that period in his development when he is best able to learn the particular task—is hindered in the learning process.* An adult in charge of a child for even a short period should consider his interest in learning, his perseverance in carrying out the activity over a period of time, and his progress.

For example, if a mother places her month-old infant in a sitting position in a corner of the crib, he will probably fall over because his muscles are not mature enough to support him in that position. He may be thoroughly frightened by the experience of having lost his balance and fallen. If, however, a mother observes her older infant repeatedly trying to pull himself to a sitting position even though he falls over many times, she should recognize his eagerness to learn and should help him until he is able to sit without support. Thereby she will have helped him in his development by assisting him at the right time and in the right way.

In summary, the effectiveness of teaching or learning depends upon the child's maturity.

His maturity, on the other hand, when tested by his behavior, will be greatly influenced by his opportunities to learn.

Levels and Achievements in Growth and Development

It is important for the student to review the overall principles of emotional and physical development in order to understand the specific growth levels and range of achievements typical of infants during their development month by month.

The behavior of infants as it changes with development has been the subject of much research. As was mentioned before, each achievement of a child may occur normally within a range of time. The age for specific achievements given in various tables in this book (see Table 12-1 and Figures 12-4 through 12-16 on pp. 247 through 259) is usually the average age of children in such a range. These schedules will probably not be typical of many infants whom the student knows, because they are *averages* and therefore do not necessarily apply to any one infant. Few infants are the average for their age in all areas covered by these schedules. Furthermore, there are great individual differences among infants. These schedules will, however, provide a kind of yardstick with which the student can determine in a general way whether individual infants she is caring for are developing according to the usual pattern.

PLAY

Purpose. Infants learn many things through play. In play they practice motor skills, acquire control of the body and gain in general coordination of movements and specific coordination of hand-eye movements. Infants learn to relate to objects and to people, to express their feelings and to work off frustrations through play. *Play, then, is all-important in the development of the child's personality*; it occupies almost all his waking hours.

(Text continued on page 260.)

Table 12–1. *Average Achievement Levels of Infants, 1 Month to 1 Year*

1 MONTH

Physical
    Weight: 8 pounds. Gains about 5 to 7 ounces weekly during first 6 months of life
    Height: Gains approximately 1 inch a month for the first 6 months
    Pulse: 120–150
    Respirations: 30–60
Motor Control (Figs. 12-4, 12-5)
    Head sags when supported. May lift head from time to time when he is held against his mother's shoulder
    Makes crawling movements when prone on a flat surface
    Lifts head intermittently, though unsteadily, when in prone position. Cervical curve begins to develop as the infant learns
        to hold his head erect
    Can turn his head to the side when prone
    Can push with feet against a hard surface to move himself forward
    Has "dance" reflex when held upright with feet touching the bed or examining table
    Shows a well developed tonic neck reflex (head turned to one side, the arm extended on the same side and the other arm
        flexed to his shoulder)
    Holds hands in fists. Does not reach with hands. Can grasp an object placed in his hand, but drops it immediately
Vision
    Stares indefinitely at his surroundings and apparently notices faces and bright objects, but only if they are in his line
        of vision. Activity diminishes when he regards a human face
    Can follow an object to the midline of vision
Vocalization and Socialization
    Utters small throaty sounds
    Smiles indefinitely
    Shows a vague and indirect regard of faces and bright objects
    Cries when hungry or uncomfortable

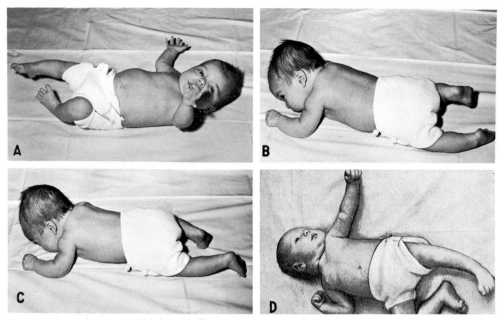

Figure 12–4. The one-month-old infant. *A*, Shows random, generalized activity in response to stimulation. *B*, Makes crawling movements when prone on a flat surface. Pushes with toes. Holds hands in fists. *C*, Lifts head from the bed a short distance. Can turn head to the side when prone. *D*, Has a well developed tonic neck reflex.

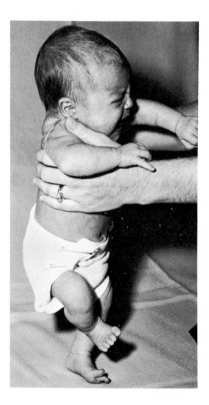

Figure 12–5. The one-month-old infant has a "dance" reflex when held upright with feet touching the bed or examining table.

Table 12–1. *Average Achievement Levels of Infants, 1 Month to 1 Year*
(Continued)

2 MONTHS

Physical
  Posterior fontanel closed
Motor Control (Fig. 12-6)
  Can hold head erect in midposition. Can lift head and chest a short distance above bed or table when lying on his abdomen
  Tonic neck and Moro reflexes are fading
  Can turn from side to back
  Can hold a rattle for a brief time
Vision
  Can follow a moving light or object with his eyes
Vocalization and Socialization
  Shows a "social smile" in response to another's smile. This is the beginning of social behavior. It may not appear until the third month
  Has learned that by crying he will get attention. His crying becomes differentiated; the sound of his crying varies with the reason for crying, e.g. hunger, sleepiness or pain
  Pays attention to the speaking voice

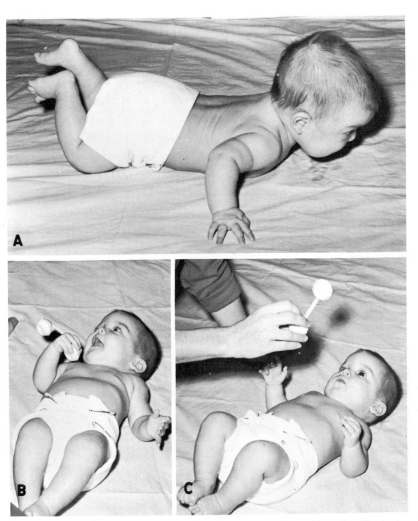

Figure 12–6. The 2-month-old infant. *A,* Can hold the head erect in midposition. Can lift the head and chest a short distance above the bed or table when lying on abdomen. *B,* Can hold a rattle for a brief period. *C,* Can follow a moving object with eyes.

Table 12–1. *Average Achievement Levels of Infants, 1 Month to 1 Year*
(Continued)

3 MONTHS

Physical
  Weight: 12 – 13 pounds
Motor Control (Fig. 12-7)
  Holds his hands up in front of him and stares at them
  Plays with hands and fingers
  Reaches for shiny objects, but misses them
  Can carry hand or object to mouth at will
  Holds head erect and steady. Raises chest, usually supported on forearms
  Has lost the walking or dancing reflex
  Grasping reflex has weakened
  Sits, back rounded, knees flexed when supported
Vision
  Shows binocular coordination (vertical and horizontal vision) when an object is moved from right to left and up and
    down in front of his face
  Turns eyes to an object in his marginal field of vision
  Voluntarily winks at objects which threaten his eyes
Vocalization and Socialization
  Laughs aloud and shows pleasure in making sounds
  Cries less
  Smiles in response to mother's face

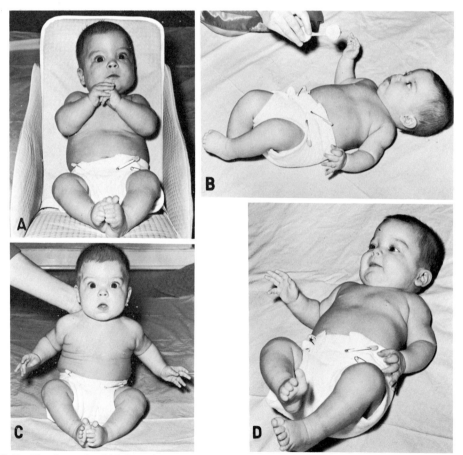

Figure 12–7. The 3-month-old infant. *A,* Holds hands up in front and plays with fingers. *B,* Reaches for a shiny object, but misses it. *C,* Sits with support, back rounded, knees flexed. *D,* Smiles in response to mother's face and laughs aloud.

4 MONTHS

Physical
  Weight: Between 13 and 14 pounds
  Drools between 3 and 4 months of age. This indicates the appearance of saliva. He does not know how to swallow saliva, which therefore runs from his mouth
Motor Control (Fig. 12-8)
  Symmetrical body postures predominate
  Holds head steady when in sitting position
  Lifts head and shoulders at a 90-degree angle when on abdomen and looks around
  Tries to roll over. Can turn from back to side
  Thumb apposition in grasping occurs between third and fourth months
  Holds hands predominantly open. Activates arms at sight of preferred toy
  Sits with adequate support and enjoys being propped up
  Tonic neck reflex has disappeared
  Sustains portion of own weight
Vision
  Recognizes familiar objects
  Stares at rattle placed in his hand and takes it to his mouth
  Follows moving objects well. Even the most difficult types of eye movements are present
  Arms are activated on sight of dangling toy
Vocalization and Socialization
  Laughs aloud and smiles in response to smiles of others
  Initiates social play by smiling
  Vocalizes socially; i.e. he coos and gurgles when talked to
  He does not cry when scolded. He is very "talkative"
  "Talking" and crying follow each other quickly
  Shows evidence of wanting social attention and of increasing interest in other members of the family
  Enjoys having people with him

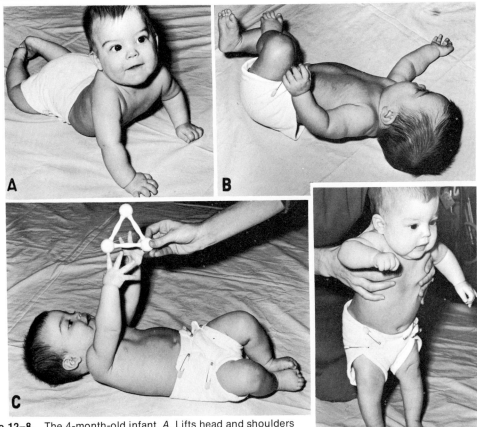

Figure 12–8. The 4-month-old infant. *A*, Lifts head and shoulders at a 90-degree angle when on abdomen and looks around. Can hold head steady. Is increasingly aware of surroundings. Is socially inclined. *B*, May roll from back to side. *C*, Grasps for a toy with whole hand. Has symmetrical body posture predominantly. Holds head in midline. Can open and close hands on rattle. Can coordinate hands and eyes sufficiently to reach and grasp on sight. *D*, Sustains part of own weight when held.

Table 12–1.   *Average Achievement Levels of Infants, 1 Month to 1 Year*
(Continued)

---

5 MONTHS

Physical
    Weight: Twice the birth weight (15 – 16 pounds)
Motor Control (Fig. 12-9)
    Sits with slight support. Holds back straight when pulled to sitting position
    Can use thumb in partial apposition to fingers more skillfully
    Can balance head well
    Reaches for objects which are beyond his grasp. Grasps objects independently of direct stimulation of the palm of the
      hand (partial grasp). Grasps with the whole hand. Accepts an object handed to him
    Has completely lost the Moro reflex
Vocalization and Socialization
    Vocalizes his displeasure when a desired object is taken from him

---

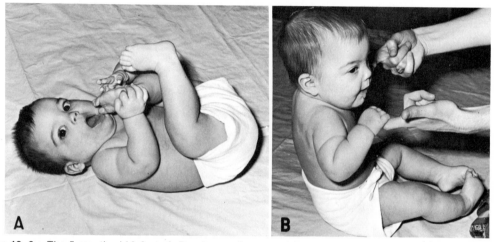

Figure 12–9. The 5-month-old infant. *A,* Reaches and grasps objects with the whole hand and carries them to mouth. *B,* Holds back straight when pulled to a sitting position. Continues to drool.

---

6 MONTHS

Physical
    Gains about 3 to 5 ounces weekly during the second 6 months of life
    Grows about ½ inch a month
    May be teething
Motor Control (Fig. 12-10)
    Sits momentarily without support if placed in a favorable leaning position
    Grasps with simultaneous flexion of fingers
    Retains transient hold on 2 blocks, one in either hand
    Pulls himself up to a sitting position
    Completely turns over from stomach to stomach with rest periods during the complete turn. This ability is important
      in protecting him from falling out of bed
    Springs up and down when sitting
    Bangs with object held in his hand, rattle or spoon
    Hitches. Hitching is locomotion backward when in a sitting position. Movement of the body is aided by use of his arms
      and hands. This ability is usually present by the sixth month
Vocalization and Socialization
    Babbles from the third to the eighth month
    Vocalizes several well defined syllables. Actively vocalizes pleasure with crowing or cooing. Babbling is not linked with
      specific objects, people or situations
    Cries easily on slight provocation (change of position or withdrawal of a toy)
    Thrashes arms and legs when frustrated
    Begins to recognize strangers (fifth to sixth month)

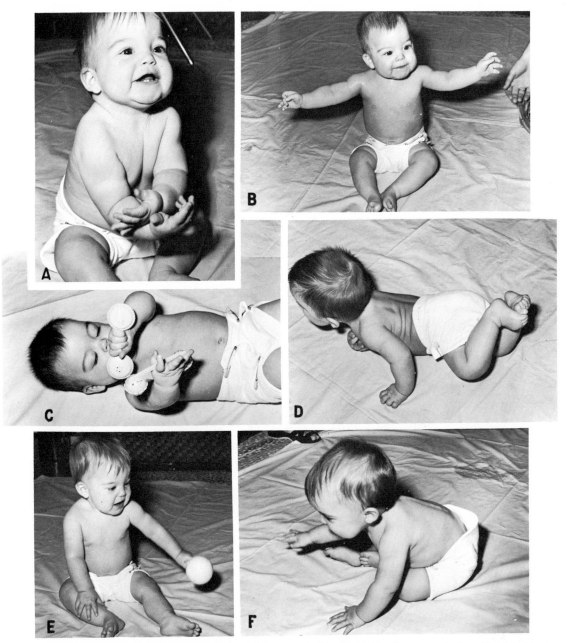

Figure 12–10.   The 6-month-old infant. *A,* Has 2 lower central incisors. *B,* Sits momentarily without support. Holds arms out for balance. *C,* Retains transient hold on 2 objects. Grasps with flexion of fingers. *D,* Turns completely over. *E,* Bangs with a rattle held in hand. Balances well by leaning forward slightly on one or both hands. *F,* Can hitch. Moves backward in a sitting position by using arms and hands to push.

Table 12–1.   *Average Achievement Levels of Infants, 1 Month to 1 Year*
(Continued)

---

7 MONTHS

Motor Control (Fig. 12-11)
    When lying down, lifts head as if he were trying to sit up
    Sits briefly, leaning forward on his hands. Control of trunk is more advanced
    Plays with his feet and puts them in his mouth
    Bounces actively when held in a standing position
    Can approach a toy and grasp it with one hand
    Can transfer a toy from one hand to the other with varying degrees of success
    Rolls more easily from back to stomach
Vocalization and Socialization
    Vocalizes his eagerness
    Vocalizes "m-m-m" when crying
    Makes polysyllabic vowel sounds
    Emotional development, 7 to 8 months: Shows fear of strangers.
    Emotional instability shown by easy and quick changes from crying to laughing

---

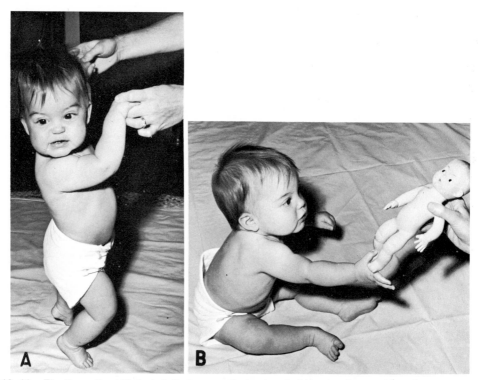

Figure 12–11.   The 7-month-old infant. *A*, Bounces actively when held in standing position. Can support a larger portion of own weight for a longer time. *B*, Can approach a toy and grasp it with one hand.

Table 12–1.   *Average Achievement Levels of Infants, 1 Month to 1 Year (Continued)*

8 MONTHS

Motor Control (Fig. 12-12)
  Sits alone steadily
  Complete thumb apposition
  Hand-eye coordination is perfected to the point that random reaching and grasping no longer persist
Vocalization and Socialization
  Greets strangers with coy or bashful behavior, turning away, hanging his head, crying or even screaming, and refuses
    to play with strangers or even accept toys from them
  Shows nervousness with strangers
  Emotional development: "Eight months' anxiety," to be distinguished from anaclitic depression (see p. 262), occurs
    between the sixth and eighth months as a result of the child's increased capacity for discriminating between friend
    and stranger
  Affection or love of family group appears
  Emotional instability still shown by easy changes from laughing to crying
  Stretches arm to loved adult as in invitation to come

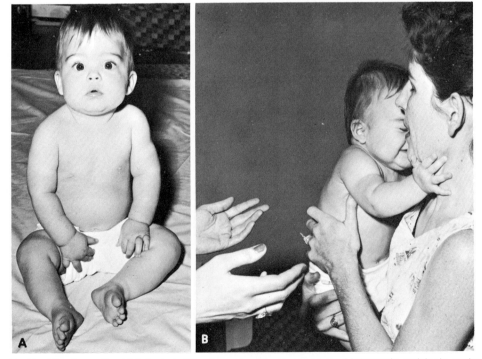

Figure 12–12.   The 8-month-old infant. *A,* Sits alone steadily. Has increased interest in activity in environment. *B,* "Eight months' anxiety." Greets stranger by turning away and crying.

Table 12–1. *Average Achievement Levels of Infants, 1 Month to 1 Year (Continued)*

9 MONTHS

Motor Control (Fig. 12-13)

Shows good coordination and sits alone

Holds his bottle with good hand-mouth coordination. Can put the nipple in and out of his mouth at will

Preference for the use of one hand is marked

Crawls instead of hitching. Crawling may be seen as early as the fourth month; the average age is about nine months. In crawling the infant is prone, his abdomen touching the floor, his head and shoulders supported with the weight borne on the elbows. The body is pulled along by the movement of the arms while the legs drag. The leg movements may resemble swimming or kicking movements

Creeps. This is a more advanced type of locomotion than crawling. The trunk is carried above the floor, but parallel to it. The infant uses both his hands and knees in propelling himself forward. Not all infants follow this pattern of hitching, crawling and creeping. Different children stress different means of locomotion and may even skip a stage. (This is particularly likely if an infant is sick or for some other reason is unable to practice moving about)

Raises himself to a sitting position. Requires help to pull self to feet

Vocalization and Socialization

Shows the beginning of imitative expression. Sounds stand for things to him. Says "Da-da" or some such expression

Responds to adult anger. Cries when scolded

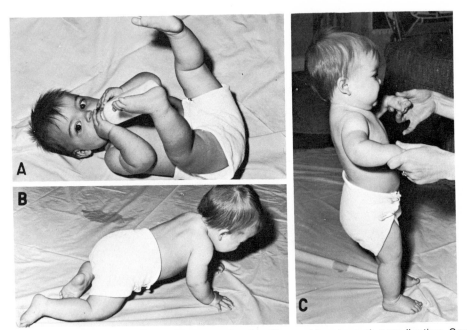

Figure 12–13. The 9-month-old infant. *A,* Holds own bottle with good hand-mouth coordination. Can put the nipple in and out of mouth at will. *B,* Can creep. Carries trunk above the floor, but parallel to it. Uses both hands and knees in propelling self forward. *C,* Can pull self to feet if assisted.

Table 12–1.   *Average Achievement Levels of Infants, 1 Month to 1 Year*
(Continued)

10 MONTHS

Motor Control (Fig. 12-14)
  Sits steadily for an indefinite time. Does not enjoy lying down unless he is sleepy
  Makes early stepping movements when held
  Pulls himself to his feet, holding to the crib rail or similar support. (This is a good time to begin the use of the play pen
    or yard)
  Creeps and cruises about very well. (Cruising is walking sideways while holding on to a supporting object with both
    hands)
  Can pick up objects fairly well and pokes them with his fingers
  Feeds himself a cracker or some such food which he can hold in his hand
  Is able crudely to release a toy
  Can bring his hands together
Vocalization and Socialization
  Says one or two words and imitates an adult's inflection
  Pays attention to his name
  Plays simple games as bye-bye and pat-a-cake (motor control is such that he can bring his hands together) and peek-a-boo

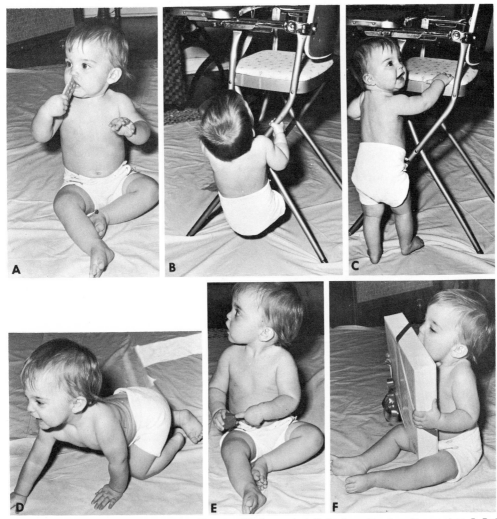

Figure 12–14.   The 10-month-old infant. *A,* Sits steadily for an indefinite time. Feeds self a cracker. *B,* Pulls self to feet, holding on to legs of chair or similar support. *C,* Cruises or walks sideways around furniture while holding on to supporting object with both hands. *D,* Creeps well. *E,* Can pick up objects fairly well and pokes them with finger. *F,* Plays peek-a-boo over top of box.

Table 12–1. *Average Achievement Levels of Infants, 1 Month to 1 Year*
(Continued)

11 MONTHS

Motor Control (Fig. 12-15)
  Stands erect with the help of his mother's hand or supporting himself by holding on to some object as the side of his
    play yard

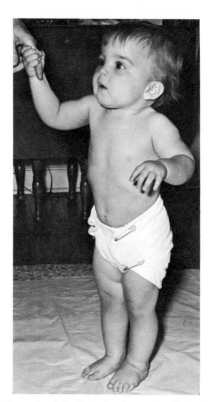

Figure 12–15.   The 11-month-old infant stands erect with the help of mother's hand.

12 MONTHS

Physical
  Weight: Three times his birth weight (21 – 22 pounds)
  Height: 29 inches
  Head and chest are equal in circumference
  Has 6 teeth
  Pulse: 100 – 140 per minute
  Respirations: 20 – 40 per minute
Motor Control (Fig. 12-16)
  Stands for a moment alone, or possibly longer
  Walks with help. Cruises, walking sideways around chairs or from chair to chair, holding on with one hand
  Lumbar curve and the compensating dorsal curve develop as he learns to walk
  Can sit down from standing position without help
  Holds a crayon adaptively to make a stroke and can mark on a piece of paper
  Can pick up small bits of food and transfer them to his mouth. Can drink from a cup and eat from a spoon, but requires
    help. He likes to eat with his fingers
  Cooperates in dressing; e.g. he can put his arm through a sleeve. Can take off his socks

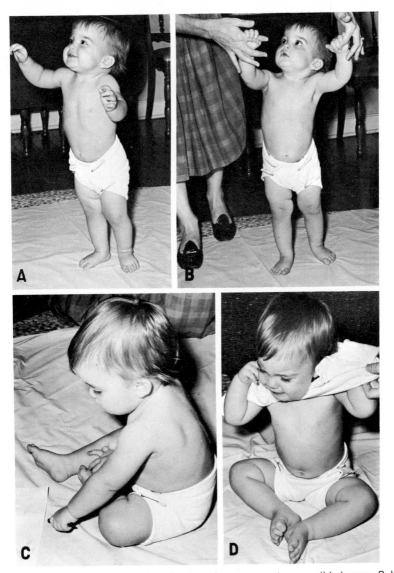

Figure 12–16. The 12-month-old infant. *A,* Stands alone for a moment or possibly longer. *B,* Walks with help. *C,* Holds a crayon adaptively to make a stroke and can mark on a piece of paper. *D,* Cooperates in dressing. Puts arm through sleeve.

Vocalization and Socialization

Can say 2 words besides "Mama" and "Dada"

Slow vocabulary growth, as a rule, owing to his interest in walking

Knows his own name

Uses expressive jargon. Communicates with himself and those around him

Inhibits simple acts on command. Recognizes the meaning of "No, no"

Shows jealousy, affection, anger and other emotions. He may cry for affection. He loves an audience, and will repeat a performance which brings a response. Crying is more often associated with irritation or frustration than it formerly was. Stiffens in resistance

Loves rhythms

Still egocentric, concerned only with himself

Learning to play with things and to amuse himself with his own movements and the sounds he can make begins in infancy. Later on in childhood he learns to play with other children. This, it is said, lays the foundation for adult ability to work well with others.

Although the general purposes of play are the same for all infants, each discovers how to use a particular toy or game for his own purposes. Thus play is an individual matter. Not all children learn in the same way from playing, because play is a result of each infant's or little child's need at the time. For this reason, play should be self-directed. Adults, through their interest in a child's development, are apt to overdirect his play activity.

Selection of Play Materials. The variety of toys generally listed as suitable for children of any age group is based on the assumption of normal growth and development. The nurse, knowing the characteristics of growth and development of each age level, will select from the toys suitable for the age group the ones best adapted to a particular child's needs, for he may be advanced or retarded for his age.

Selection is important, for toys have many functions; i.e. toys help children to learn different things in different ways. An essential factor in the selection of a toy is that it be safe for the child's use. This, in general, depends on his level of growth and development, but varies with his physical condition and other characteristics. Some children are more cautious than others. This may be due to slow or rapid development, but also to specific experiences from which a child has learned to be careful when trying out a new use for toys. It is never safe to give toys designed for older children to infants. For instance, the small plastic parts which an older boy uses in building a toy car would not be suitable for an infant, for he would put them into his mouth and might easily swallow or even aspirate them.

Toys should be washable, durable, easily handled, not too heavy, and smooth with rounded edges and no sharp points. Children enjoy gaily colored toys. If the toy is painted, it should be with nonlead paint. The size of the toy should be appropriate to the use the child will make of it. An infant's toy should be well constructed. For instance, a rattle should be one the infant cannot break when he bangs it against the rail of his crib. If it broke, he might pick up and swallow some of the pebbles it contained.

A toy should be one with many uses for the child. It is difficult to predict to what uses he may put it, and his creative ability should be encouraged. But safety factors must be considered. Blocks are meant for building, but the infant may throw them. For this reason they should be made of some rubberlike substance so that he can hurt neither himself nor another child. These he can place together, clap together or toss as he happens to fancy. Cuddly toys can be used in many ways besides being cuddled at bedtime. They can be dropped, dragged along or sat upon. Many adults do not understand that the infant may use a toy for its express purpose and also for whatever other use he desires. They bring pressure upon the child to use a toy as an older child would do or even to watch them use it, withholding the toy if the child grasps for it.

Suggested toys include large wooden beads and spools strung on a cord or shoe string, rattles, soft toys (not fuzzy) of different shapes, balls and large or small blocks.

Play Responses During Infancy. Toys to be used during the first year must be very simple. The infant's attention span is short.

BIRTH TO FIVE MONTHS. An early type of motor play is for exercise, but it is also thoroughly enjoyable to the infant. He reaches for objects and attempts to turn from back to side. He kicks, wiggles and plays with his hands.

FIVE TO EIGHT MONTHS. At this age the infant still finds pleasure in motor activity for its own sake. He plays with his feet, bounces his body, shakes his head, leans against objects when learning to sit, grasps at anything he can reach and moves on the floor or in his play yard by hitching. He usually plays contentedly by himself during the first six months. By seven months he enjoys company, but is still happy playing alone with his toys. He likes to explore his hands and feet and talks to himself. He enjoys his bath when free from the restraint of clothing and can move his body easily.

EIGHT TO TEN MONTHS. Motor activity is still the infant's chief source of play. He kicks his legs. Now that he can sit alone he likes to lean over the side of his carriage or the arm of his chair. He plays with his toes and rolls with ease. He crawls, creeps or pulls himself into a sitting position and stretches to get toys which are out of his reach. He transfers a toy from one hand to the other and puts the toy into his mouth. He has learned where the toy goes when he drops it over the edge of the crib or the tray when he is sitting in his high chair, and looks down at it.

TEN TO ELEVEN MONTHS. The child still plays alone for relatively long periods, but lets the family know when he wants their company or the stimulus of having another toy. His play is becoming more highly developed. He plays in a sitting position, creeps about, pokes objects with his fingers and enjoys pulling himself up to a standing position.

TWELVE MONTHS. Now the child plays with several toys, picking them up and dropping them. He can grasp a ball and let it go, and will take or give a toy on request or gesture. He greatly enjoys walking with help.

EFFECTS OF SEPARATION FROM PARENTS

Factors in Development of the Child. *It may be said that the kind of person the infant will become depends in part upon the characteristics of his parents, their relations to each other, and the emotional atmosphere of the home in general.* Their attitude toward the infant is of fundamental importance. *He may receive from them a feeling of love and peace or anxiety and insecurity.*

Among the significant developments in psychiatry in recent years has been the increasing awareness that the kind of parental care given during infancy and early childhood is of great importance to the child's future mental and physical health.

During infancy and early childhood he should have an intimate, warm and continuous relationship with his mother or permanent mother-substitute in whom he finds happiness. In such a situation the basis for mental ill health characterized by excessive anxiety and feelings of guilt is not likely to develop.

Maternal Deprivation. *Maternal deprivation is the term used for an infant's lack of this warm relationship.* The condition occurs when the mother cannot give loving care even though the infant lives with her, or when the child is removed from his mother's care, is hospitalized or institutionalized, or remains in the home while she is absent.

There are various degrees of deprivation. In a situation of *incomplete* or *partial deprivation* the infant or young child may show acute anxiety, at the same time experiencing an excessive need for love and affection. In *complete* or *total deprivation* the infant may become incapable of forming normal relations with others.

Since the infant learns to know his mother as a person when five or six months old and to recognize and fear strangers when seven to eight months old, he should have his mother or a permanent substitute to care for him and be near him during his first year.

Although deprivation during infancy is serious, the effects of deprivation differ according as it occurs in the first or the second half of the first year.

DEPRIVATION IN THE FIRST SIX MONTHS. Infants of this age have inadequate psychic and physical development to adjust to an impersonal sort of care given by a succession of kindly, competent persons who do not love them as they would their own infants. Infants deprived of maternal care by their own mothers or by an adequate mother-substitute lack all that goes with love and seldom receive sufficient stimulation to promote normal development. In foundling homes they become emotionally isolated from adults,

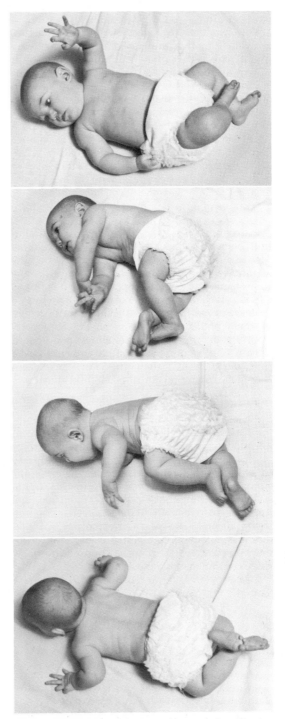

Figure 12–17. An early type of motor play. The infant turns well from back to abdomen. (Courtesy of Lew Merrim and *Baby Talk Magazine*, June 1967.)

and their activity is likely to be restricted. They generally show signs of retarded mental development even if they receive the best possible physical care.

The result of such care in foundling homes is evident in the infant's behavior. The young infant may cry a great deal. He may not gain weight as he should, and his motor development is likely to be poor, since he is seldom handled or taken from his crib. Gradually he will refuse contact with adults. He will lose weight, and his sleep pattern will be altered. He will develop a rigid facial expression. He has poor resistance and is liable to contract infections readily. After a few months he will become completely passive and eventually appear retarded. He may make bizarre finger movements. The incidence of marasmus and the death rate are relatively high among these children.

Prevention of maternal deprivation in foundling homes is almost impossible. Foster home care should be provided in the earliest months of infancy, and the child should remain in the same home with his loving, permanent mother-substitute. If foster home care is impossible, a permanent mother-substitute should be provided in the foundling home. She should be chosen from among the nursing personnel and should have a limited number of infants to care for so that she can give them individual attention. She must communicate to each child that he is loved and wanted.

An infant hospitalized because of a congenital deformity or illness may exhibit the same symptoms as the infant in a foundling home if warm, affectionate care is not provided. Such care is often more difficult to provide in a hospital than in a foundling home because of the constant change in the nursing personnel (both nursing students and auxiliary personnel) and also because the more acutely ill infants need more than their proportionate share of attention. An adequate, stable graduate nurse staff is essential on the pediatric unit if these children are to receive continuous loving care.

DEPRIVATION DURING THE SECOND SIX MONTHS. This is the period when *anaclitic depression* occurs. It results from a change in the infant's life, from the warm relations with his mother and family to a situation in which he is one of a group of infants who do not receive continuous loving care from their mothers.

The result is that the infants become depressed, cry a great deal and look sad, and are withdrawn in their relations with adults caring for them. This is in decided contrast to their previous happy, outgoing behavior. They may refuse to eat and may lose weight. They will cling to a doll or a blanket brought from home. The last stage of detachment is evidenced by the child's delay in response to the mother when she visits him,

by his establishing superficial positive relations with other adults, and by his increased auto-erotic behavior. If deprivation continues more than three months, the constant crying subsides. The sad expression is replaced by a rigid facial expression. They may suffer anorexia and sleep disturbances. It may become difficult and eventually impossible for nurses to establish contact with them.

If the child is restored to his mother within three months, recovery may be rapid. If deprivation continues, recovery becomes increasingly difficult and less likely to be complete.

PREVENTION OF ANACLITIC DEPRESSION. After six months of age the normal infant takes the initiative and seeks adult contact. He needs room where he can creep and cruise around unrestrainedly. He needs space for motor activity and for investigation of his environment. Above all, he needs the continuous warm affection of a mothering person who gives him individual attention. If these two requirements are fulfilled, he may continue to be an essentially normal infant; otherwise he will probably become depressed and unloving.

Summary and Conclusions. Reactions of infants to maternal deprivation can be classified into three time-sequence stages: protest (crying), despair (quiet and subdued behavior) and denial (even of the mother). After the mother reappears the child may continue to be withdrawn, to have altered sleeping or eating patterns, to cling to the mother and to be afraid of strangers. Although damage to the child due to maternal deprivation may be severe, recently some question has been raised about the effects of deprivation being irreversible in later years. Certainly not every deprived child has grown up to be a delinquent or an unloving adult or has had the serious personality problems formerly blamed on maternal deprivation early in life.

Although the probable results of extreme deprivation are those which have just been described, some infants who have lacked their mother's love for any of a number of reasons appear to suffer little permanent personality damage. The reasons for this are not clearly understood but may depend upon the age of the child, length of separation, the parent-child relation before separation, the care of the child by other adults during separation, and the stress of the illness itself. It must be remembered that each infant's environment is influenced by his characteristics. Though it should not be so, a pretty child who was friendly before separation from his mother is apt to evoke a warm response from those who care for him. His life is likely to be different from that of the child who, on entrance to the institution, did not respond to the friendly advances of the personnel. The personnel of an institution are human and likely to be very different in their treatment of the likable and unlikable infants.

To fulfill the function of her profession, every nurse should provide the kind of warm, loving care which children need to prevent them from suffering the effects of maternal deprivation. The specific nursing practices which may help to prevent the occurrence of maternal deprivation include frequent body contacts with the child, continuity in contact with the child of a few nursing personnel, genuine interest of these personnel in the child, provision for a variety of sensory stimuli for him, and finally the establishment of the nurse as a friend to the mother, a friend who can serve as a bridge between her and her child.

Foundlings and Adoptions. In the foregoing discussion the term "foundling home" was used. A *foundling* is an infant abandoned by its parents and found by others. Such infants in general are adopted, since the demand for infants eligible for adoption exceeds the supply. Although time must elapse between the finding of an infant and his legal adoption, he may be given temporarily to the future adoptive parents through a legally approved organization. Adoptive parents, as a rule, want to take the infant when he is only a few weeks old. Thus few foundlings, if they are normal infants, remain in institutions.

Homes for infants retain the word "foundling," since they were incorporated when in fact they did care for foundlings and because they still receive infants deserted by their parents and care for them until adopted. In general, the infants and children in these homes are illegitimate children whose mothers surrendered them to the institutions at birth and who are there only until adopted. Infants who are in a children's home for a long time are those whose parents are unable to care for them or are not considered by the court to be able to provide a suitable home for them. Such children generally come from homes where both the physical and the social conditions are poor, though the mothers might have had loving relations with the infants. It is these infants, rather than foundlings, who constitute the great problem of the institutionalized child.

Aid for dependent children under the Social Security Act has resulted in relatively few infants and children being institutionalized because of the death of one or both parents.

INFANT CARE

Daily Care

Every infant and every other member of the family—mother, father and siblings—have their individual needs. The plan for the infant's care must take into consideration ways of adjusting all these common and conflicting needs. Parents should not feel that they must give up their whole lives for their infant. If they do, their care may ultimately lack spontaneity and warmth.

The natural rhythms of a normal infant and of the particular infant must be considered. These rhythms will change as he grows older. His pattern of sleeping and waking and his periods of playful exercise will alter. The parents have schedules which their activities require them to follow and with which the infant's schedule is interrelated. Both parents should plan to spend some time with the infant in the evening, and this requires a corresponding arrangement of his periods of sleep.

If the mother does her own housework and is not employed outside the home, she is able to spend considerable time with the baby, at periods which best fit into her schedule. But if she works outside the home, it may be necessary to adapt his schedule to the hours when she is free to be with him. If there are siblings in the home, her activities must be adapted to their needs also. She and her husband should spend some time with the siblings without the infant being present to distract the parents' attention from the other children. This is important in the prevention of sibling jealousy of the infant and in their acceptance of their status as older than he. Older siblings should realize that they are given prerogatives he does not receive, just as he receives attentions not given them.

As the infant shifts to having three meals a day with nourishment such as orange juice between meals, he may gradually be included in the family group at meal times.

Since an infant is not old enough to tell how he feels, his mother should watch for signs and symptoms of discomfort and illness. The infant's color is a good indication of his condition. His eyes should be clear and bright. When tired, he should fall asleep without fretting.

There is no set pattern of daily care for all infants, since their needs vary from month to month, and the family situation of each differs from that of the others.

Carrying the Infant

The technique of carrying the infant is based on his anatomic structure and motor ability. His head is large in proportion to his body, and he is unable to hold his head erect without support until he is about three months old. The shoulders and back must be supported at first because of weakness. If the student remembers these two facts, lifting and carrying the infant will be comfortable and safe for him and easy for her. Different techniques for carrying infants have been given descriptive titles, such as the *cradle technique* and the *football hold*. Each technique has its special use.

The *cradle technique* is commonly used in lifting, turning and carrying the infant. The nurse or mother grasps his feet with her right hand (in order not to press

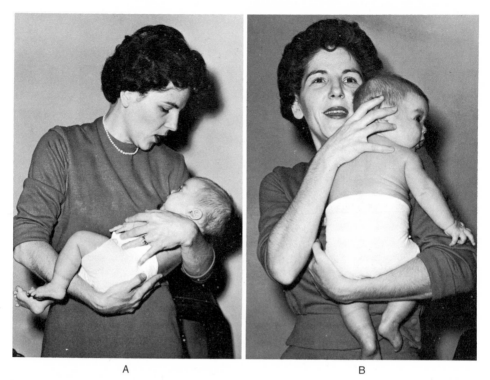

A   B

Figure 12–18. *A,* A modified cradle position. The young infant's head and back must be supported adequately. *B,* The infant may be held upright against the shoulder. The head must be supported until the infant is able to do so by himself.

the ankle bones together she keeps her index finger between the ankles), slides her left hand and arm under the infant's back, giving support to the buttocks, back and head. She then brings her right hand up and under the buttocks, while she moves her left arm and hand up to give greater support to the head, shoulders and back. She then raises the infant so that he is cradled in her arms, his body against her chest.

If the nurse or mother holds him in an upright position, on her shoulder, her left forearm is under his but-tocks, his body pressed against her chest and shoulder and his cheek resting slightly over her shoulder. Support for his back and head is given with her other hand. If for a moment she must use her right hand, as in opening a door, she should bend her body backward so that his body is pressed against hers by gravity and he lies there without a sense of loss of support.

The *football hold* is useful in washing the infant's head over a basin or making the crib while holding the infant. His hips are supported in the bend of the

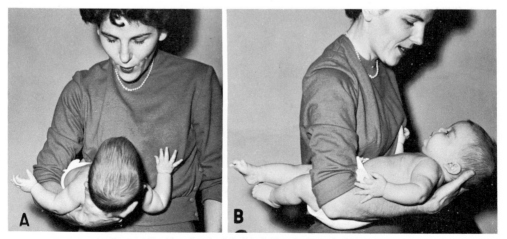

Figure 12–19. Football hold. *A,* Front view. *B,* Side view.

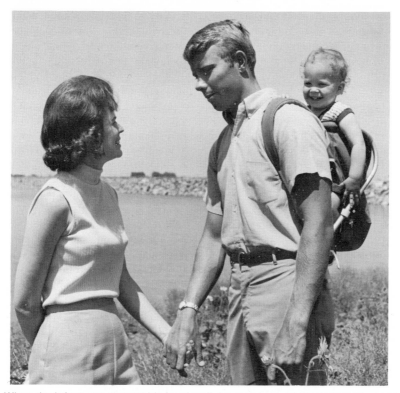

Figure 12–20.   When the infant can support his head well, he may be carried comfortably on his parent's back. (Courtesy of M. S. Hansson, Gerry Designs, Inc., Boulder, Colorado.)

nurse's or mother's arm, with the forearm and hand supporting his back and head. This frees her other hand and is therefore a convenient way of carrying an infant.

As the infant grows older and is able to support his head, the parents may take him with them outdoors in a sling (see Fig. 12-20). This type of transportation of the infant permits the parents greater freedom for shopping or participating in outdoor activities.

Bathing

The purpose of the bath is not only cleanliness, but also to give the infant a chance to exercise without clothing and, if he is put in a tub of water, to kick and splash. It is a time for mother or nurse to talk to him and play with him. It provides her with an opportunity to note his growth and development and to observe his body for evidence of rash or chafing.

The time for the bath can be whenever the mother or nurse finds it most convenient. The bath should not be given within one hour after the infant has been fed, however. It should have a regular place in the day's schedule of care and should never be given when the mother is tired or the infant fretful. The modern father bathes the infant now and then in order to learn to know him better and to give him the same sense of being loved and cared for by his father that he has from his mother.

For the procedure of the bath, see page 136. The infant may have a sponge bath in bed or be bathed in a tub. A tub-stand combination constructed for the purpose of infant bathing may be used if the parents can afford it. The tub cover has straps which buckle over the infant's chest so that the mother can change the infant's diaper and wash his buttocks without fear of his falling. When using this equipment, the mother may have difficulty in transferring the infant from the table to the tub. The equipment for bathing the infant should be conveniently near and everything required in readiness so that the mother will not have to leave him.

Safety factors must be kept in mind when bathing the infant; precautions to safeguard him and to avoid fear are necessary. An infant or little child should never be left alone in a tub of water even if he is old enough to sit up and hold on to the sides of the tub. It is not safe to give him a powder can to play with even if it appears to be empty, for he may inhale a little of the powder left in the bottom of the can if he shakes it vigorously.

It is important that the infant learn to like his bath. If he is immersed in the tub too quickly or does not feel that he is held securely, he may stiffen and appear startled. If this happens, he may acquire an adverse attitude toward his bath. The nurse or mother should place him in the tub very gently. She should hold him with his head and shoulders on her forearm and her hand grasping his opposite arm. He should not be soaped too liberally, since it is then difficult to retain a firm hold upon his body and limbs. He would be frightened if he were allowed to slip or if his face were covered with water.

Clothing

Various kinds of sleeping garments are used for infants. Many mothers like to put a night-gown on the infant when he is old enough to kick the covers off. If the gown is open at the bottom and all down the back, the sides should be folded so that he does not lie upon the gown and wet it when he voids. If there is a drawstring through the hem and the gown is partially closed at the back, the drawstring can be tightened so that the gown covers his feet, but he must have room to kick unrestrainedly. As he grows older and becomes more active, he needs pajamas or sleepers with feet. The two-piece type saves laundry and time, since it is necessary to change only the lower half when he soils the garment.

A sleeping bag or garment made of blanket material like a loose, long, full-sleeved kimono with the bottom sewed up and closed with a zipper in front is useful for keeping the infant covered. It should be large enough for him to move freely within it. The neck should be loose so as not to bind him when he turns.

When the infant learns to creep or move around freely, his clothes should be loose in the crotch and the armholes. Overalls will protect his legs when he creeps. They should be open in the crotch so that the diaper may be easily changed. Sun-suits are excellent in summer weather.

Shoes should be soft until the child walks. They are needed only to protect his feet when he crawls or creeps. If the floor covering is warm, smooth and clean, he should be allowed to go barefoot. Crawling and creeping exercise the foot muscles. Socks are worn with the shoes and should be at least $\frac{1}{2}$ inch longer than his feet. Infants' feet grow quickly, and unless the socks are ample in size when bought, they will soon be too small. They should not be used if they cramp the child's toes.

Fresh Air and Sunshine

The infant should be outdoors as much as possible. He should be dressed according to the weather. When the day is warm enough, an infant of three or four weeks may be given a brief sun bath. Such baths are desirable even if he is outdoors a great deal and is kept in a sunny room when indoors, since ultraviolet rays are de-stroyed by window glass, clothing and the dust and smoke in the atmosphere. The infant's first exposure to the sun should be for only three to five minutes, and only the face and hands should be exposed. Both the time of exposure and the area exposed are gradually increased until the skin of the body and limbs is pigmented. Sun baths should be given before 11 a.m. or after 3 p.m. The infant should be placed with his feet away from the sun and his eyes and head protected from the glare. Deep burning is harmful to the child. The objective of sun baths is to acquire an even tan. While having his sun baths he should continue to take vitamin D.

Exercise

An infant gets exercise in a number of ways. He is active at bath time. Mere change of position is a form of exercise. When he is old enough to turn over — and later play in his play yard — his clothes should not restrict his movements. He should have toys which encourage movement.

Sleep

The greater part of a young infant's time is spent in sleep. Currently research is being done on the amount of REM (rapid eye movement) sleep which an infant obtains as evidenced by his grimacing, sucking, and squirming activity during apparent sleep. The infant needs rest for his rapid growth and his energy output. The amount of sleep he takes depends upon his needs, which vary from day to day. If he is given the opportunity, he will develop his own schedule.

The position in which an infant is placed for sleep is important. As soon as he can move his head from side to side to prevent his nose from being pressed against the surface on which he lies, it is safe to place him on either his back or his abdomen. The danger of sleeping on his back is that he may vomit and aspirate fluid. In general, lying on his side is preferred for comfort and safety.

Signs of increasing maturity in relation to sleep are a reduction in the total sleeping time and longer intervals between sleeping periods. Although each infant varies from any standard or norm, eighteen to twenty hours of sleep a day is typical during the first few months of life. At three months the usual amount of sleep in a 24-hour period is about sixteen hours. He will often sleep throughout the night. At six months the average amount of sleep is about twelve hours at night and three to four hours during the day. The number of naps and their length vary with the individual infant. At one year of age he sleeps about fourteen hours out of the twenty-four. At this age he is fearful of leaving his mother and of being deserted by her.

He should not be put to bed and immediately left alone in the dark. A soft light is often used to make the situation more familiar. A child of this age should have one or two naps a day.

Promotion of Sleep, and Care After Wakening. Overstimulation should be avoided before bedtime. The infant should be dry and comfortable. He may need to keep a favorite toy with him to hold so that he feels secure while he goes to sleep. Quieting activities should be provided, such as rocking him or singing to him.

The environment should be suited to his needs, one of which is a room of his own. Twilight is preferable to either a bright light or darkness. The light, even if dimmed, should not shine directly in his eyes.

The temperature of the room should be such that the infant is neither chilled nor overheated. A suitable temperature in the day would be 70 to 75°F. and at night 60 to 65°F. The room should be well ventilated, but there must be no drafts. Screens should be used to cut off unavoidable drafts, but blankets should not be hung over the sides of the crib, since they may fall on the infant and smother him.

The mattress should be firm and completely covered with heavy plastic material. A small piece of light plastic material should not be used under the sheet. Should the infant pull the sheet from the bed, he might be covered with the plastic, which could cut off his supply of air. Pillows are not used, since there is danger of his burying his face in one or having it fall on his face. In either case he might be suffocated. He should lie on a flat surface, since this is best for his bone development.

After the infant has wakened, the window shades should be pulled so that the room is light. The older infant should have his face washed to give him a feeling of freshness.

Safety Measures

Importance of Accident Prevention. Since accidents are a principal cause of death of infants and children of all ages, great emphasis should be placed on accident prevention. Nurses and mothers must consider the child's interests and the hazards resulting from the activities into which his interests lead him. The protection and education needed by each sex and age group are then adapted to the prevention of accidents to which they are most liable. Health education during the prenatal period and while mothers are in the obstetrical unit should be constructive, not listing all possible dangers to which a child might be subjected, but emphasizing reasonable precautions against the hazards he is likely to encounter in the near future. Accident prevention education should be given slowly to parents and to children.

It may sound ridiculous to speak of teaching accident prevention to an infant. What is meant, of course, is merely that he becomes accustomed to the safety measures which are used in his care. He learns by observing his mother's actions what behavior of his displeases her, such as behavior which may lead to his harm. As he passes from the toddler into the preschool age simple explanations can be given. He should learn to exercise caution, because he may be hurt if he does not. A certain degree of fear of being hurt is normal and is the logical reason for caution. Health hazards tend to lessen as the child goes to school and later enters adolescence, but accident hazards increase. Accident prevention is taught in the schoolroom and on playgrounds. Accidents common to each age group will be mentioned in this text in their appropriate place.

Specific Safety Measures. Safety factors during the bath, in relation to toys or clothes and in the selection of furniture have already been discussed.

The sides of the crib should always be raised and secure when the infant is in it unattended. The crib should have narrow spaces between the rungs so that the infant's head, arms or legs cannot be caught between them. The infant's bed should not be placed near a radiator, since he may burn his hand if he touches it when reaching through the bars of his crib. It should also be out of range of windows with venetian blinds, since the infant may become fatally entangled in a dangling cord. Safety pins should always be closed and removed from the crib; they should never be stuck in the mattress or left in a receptacle or cake of soap (soap is sometimes used to lubricate the point of a safety pin so that it goes through the thick layers of diaper more readily).

Since an infant puts everything within reach into his mouth, small articles should not be left in his crib or close to his chair. Articles which frequently are aspirated are beads, coins, peanuts, and the like. Even an infant too young to roll may move himself upward by pushing with his feet. For this reason he should never be left unprotected on a bed or a stand. If the mother or nurse must reach for some equipment, she must keep one hand on the infant.

All toys and infant furniture should carry a guarantee that no paint containing lead or other poisonous substance was used. The infant might ingest such substances when he licks and chews his toys or the bars of his play yard or crib.

Guard rails or gates at the top and bottom of steps will prevent serious falls when the infant begins to creep. When the infant is old enough to creep on the floor, all electrical outlets which he can reach should be covered. Tablecloths which hang over the edge of the table should not be used, since the toddler or even the infant who creeps about will pull on them. This will carry anything on the table, e.g. hot foods, over the edge, possibly spilling the contents upon the child, or hitting him as they fall. An adult with a baby in arms should not walk on a slippery floor or where toys or other small articles have been left on the floor. It is difficult to regain balance after stumbling with an infant in one's arms.

Infants living in highly populated metropolitan areas are many times the victims of rats. Rats attack infants especially when they are sleeping and may bite or chew the face, fingers or toes. Prevention lies in the elimination of rats from the area.

INFANT FEEDING AND NUTRITION

Feeding of the newborn was discussed in Chapter 7. The infant will continue to feed from the breast or bottle until he is weaned, at which time he will learn to drink from a cup. Mothers who breast-feed their infants may want to give them experience in the use of a bottle, giving them water, a formula or orange juice in this way. If an emergency arises and breast feeding must be discontinued, his acceptance of the bottle is helpful both to him and to those who care for him.

Table 12-2 gives the nutritional requirements of infants under one year of age.

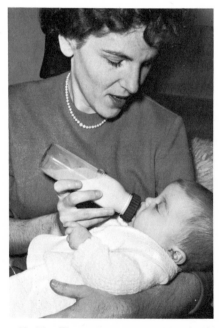

Figure 12–21. The mother may want to give her infant experience in sucking from a bottle even though it is usually breast-fed.

Addition of Other Foods and Substances to the Diet

The age at which additional foods are added to the infant's diet depends on the physician and on the infant's mother. Some infants enjoy the addition of foods such as strained meats, fruits, vegetables and cereal before they are a month of age even though at first they may have difficulty swallowing them. Infants should in general be given solid foods before the age of three to four months in order to make their diets more nutritionally complete and to become accustomed at an early age to various tastes and textures of food. Infants under five to six months of age accept new foods easily, but after that age they may begin to resist new tastes and textures.

Specific substances to be added early are water, vitamin C, vitamin D, iron and possibly sodium fluoride.

Water. Newborn infants learn to drink water —boiled for safety—from a bottle. This is given them between feedings because they need more fluid than is supplied in either breast milk or their formula. The infant's thirst should determine the amount of water he takes. In the home the mother should prepare freshly boiled water daily. The water is put in 4-ounce sterile nursing bottles. When the infant is about five months old, some of the daily supply of boiled water should be kept in a sterile covered container and may be offered from a cup; this, however, is supplementary to the use of the bottle until he learns to drink from the cup. Some pediatricians believe that when the infant is about four months old he may be given unboiled water if the water supply in his community is considered safe.

Vitamin C. The infant requires a minimum of 35 mg. of vitamin C daily to prevent scurvy. The addition of vitamin C is particularly important for the bottle-fed infant, since this vitamin is destroyed by heating the milk in the formula. Vitamin C is usually given also to breast-fed infants to assure an adequate supply (the mother's intake of this vitamin may be insufficient, in which case the infant will not receive enough to meet his needs).

The physician will order orange juice, tomato juice, or ascorbic acid in tablet form to satisfy the need of the infant for vitamin C, beginning by about two weeks of age. Some physicians seem to prefer the use of ascorbic acid in tablet form to fulfill the infant's need.

When orange juice is used, it is customary to begin with $\frac{1}{2}$ tablespoonful of strained fresh juice diluted with an equal quantity of water. This is increased slowly until 2 or 3 ounces of juice and a small amount of water are given daily at two months of age. Frozen orange juice may be used and diluted with boiled, cooled water according to the directions on the can.

Table 12–2. *Recommended Daily Dietary Allowances for Infants 0 to 12 Months of Age*

	0–2 MONTHS WT.–4 KG. (9 POUNDS) HT.–55 CM. (22 INCHES)	2–6 MONTHS WT.–7 KG. (15 POUNDS) HT.–63 CM. (25 INCHES)	6–12 MONTHS WT.–9 KG. (20 POUNDS) HT.–72 CM. (28 INCHES)
K calories	kg. × 120	kg. × 110	kg. × 100
Protein	kg. × 2.2 gm.[a]	kg. × 2.0 gm.[a]	kg. × 1.8 gm.[a]
Fat-soluble vitamins			
Vitamin A activity	1500 I.U.	1500 I.U.	1500 I.U.
Vitamin D	400 I.U.	400 I.U.	400 I.U.
Vitamin E activity	5 I.U.	5 I.U.	5 I.U.
Water-soluble vitamins			
Ascorbic acid	35 mg.	35 mg.	35 mg.
Folacin[b]	0.05 mg.	0.05 mg.	0.1 mg.
Niacin equivalents[c]	5 mg.	7 mg.	8 mg.
Riboflavin	0.4 mg.	0.5 mg.	0.6 mg.
Thiamine	0.2 mg.	0.4 mg.	0.5 mg.
Vitamin B_6	0.2 mg.	0.3 mg.	0.4 mg.
Vitamin B_{12}	1.0 μg	1.5 μg	2.0 μg
Minerals			
Calcium	0.4 gm.	0.5 gm.	0.6 gm.
Phosphorus	0.2 gm.	0.4 gm.	0.5 gm.
Iodine	25 μg	40 μg	45 μg
Iron	6 mg.	10 mg.	15 mg.
Magnesium	40 mg.	60 mg.	70 mg.

[a] Assumes protein equivalent to human milk. For proteins not 100 per cent utilized, factors should be increased proportionately.

[b] The folacin allowances refer to dietary sources as determined by *Lactobacillus casei* assay. Pure forms of folacin may be effective in doses less than ¼ of the RDA.

[c] Niacin equivalents include dietary sources of the vitamin itself plus 1 mg. equivalent for each 60 mg. of dietary tryptophan.

From the Food and Nutrition Board, National Academy of Sciences–National Research Council: Recommended Daily Dietary Allowances (1968).

In teaching mothers how to give orange juice to their infants the following precautions should be stressed: (1) the orange juice should not be boiled or have hot water added to it, since vitamin C is easily destroyed by heat. It is also destroyed through prolonged contact with the air or a utensil containing copper (e.g. a bowl). (2) To mothers of a low socioeconomic group and possibly to those of low intelligence it should be explained that orange-flavored drinks (orange soda and the like) usually contain no fresh orange juice and may contain ingredients harmful to the infant. It is also necessary to stress the need for cleanliness throughout the procedure of preparing and giving the orange juice.

If the mother prefers to use *tomato juice,* the infant must be given twice the amount of fresh orange juice prescribed by the physician. The tomato juice should be given in an equal amount of water. Since a small infant cannot take much fluid in addition to his formula, tomato juice is not given until he is five or six months old.

Ascorbic acid in tablet form may be given in addition to the orange juice until the infant is old enough to take willingly the required amount a day, or the physician may order it if an infant cannot tolerate orange juice. Ascorbic acid tablets must be crushed and dissolved in boiled, cooled water before being given to the infant.

Vitamin D. This vitamin is added to the diet when the infant is about two weeks old; in general, 400 International Units are required per day. Vitamin D helps the infant to make use of the calcium he receives in his milk; in this respect it is a substitute for sunshine or is needed in addition to sunshine. As was mentioned on page 131, Vitamin D-reinforced whole milk or evaporated milk is available commercially. Many other preparations containing vitamin D are also available, such as cod liver oil and concentrates and other fish liver oil concentrates. The amount of these substances to be given to the infant depends on the physician's order. Vitamin D preparations vary so much in potency that the physician's order should be followed carefully.

Plain cod liver oil is used less frequently than formerly. Usually ¼ teaspoonful is given at first and increased to 1 or 2 teaspoonfuls.

The way in which it is given is important. It is given cold. The mouth of the bottle should be wiped to remove all the old oil. No displeasure or disgust should be shown while giving this medication, since the infant will copy the attitude toward the oil from the adult who gives it. The infant's head should be elevated and the infant should be held in a sitting position when he is given the medication by dropper or spoon, in order to prevent aspiration (see p. 293). Preparations containing oil should never be given while the infant is crying.

The usual dose of vitamin D concentrates is 5 to 10 drops a day.

Some vitamin D preparations can be given in milk, but the infant may not take all the milk and therefore will not ingest the full dose of the

269

vitamin. It is not feasible to put any oily substance into the formula because (1) the oil adheres to the glass, and (2) since oil rises to the top when the feeding bottle is inverted, the infant sucks the oil through the nipple only at the close of the feeding.

Mothers should be cautioned against increasing the amount of vitamin ordered. Hypervitaminosis may result.

Iron. Although normal newborn infants have an extra supply of iron at birth, they need additional amounts to meet their requirements during growth, especially after the first few months of life. In the usual infant diet one half or more of the total daily intake of iron is provided by iron-enriched cereals. For premature infants dietary iron is inadequate for their rapid growth, so supplemental iron should be given (p. 149).

Fluorides. The effect of fluoride in drinking water is to strengthen calcification of forming dental tissues and thus to make the enamel of the teeth more resistant to decay. In many cities the fluoride content of the water supplies is adjusted to adequate levels in order to improve the dental health of the children in the community. For infants who do not receive adequate fluorides in their drinking water the daily administration of a solution of sodium fluoride or a vitamin preparation containing fluoride is recommended. The usual dose prescribed by a physician for an infant is approximately 0.5 mg. of sodium fluoride each day. As the child grows older the dosage should be increased, and the substance may be given in tablet form. A fluoride preparation can also be applied to erupted teeth to prevent cavity formation.

Addition of Solid Foods

Foods Which Infants Like. The infant will take solid foods which he likes more readily than those which he dislikes. In general, infants like bland foods which are *slightly* sweet, sour or salty. They do not like bitter foods or those strongly sour or salty. An infant's preference for texture and consistency of food varies according to his age. Naturally the newborn infant likes only liquid food. An infant a few weeks old likes food which feels smooth (puréed food). When his teeth are coming through, he likes foods on which he can chew, such as teething biscuits, zwieback or chopped foods. The shift from puréed to chopped foods should be a gradual one. Chopped foods ("junior foods") can be started from six to nine months, depending upon the infant's ability to chew.

Infants prefer food at moderate temperatures. An infant may be frightened by food either too hot or too cold and may refuse it when it is offered him again.

Method of Introduction. The infant's reaction to his first solid food is to make sucking movements with his tongue which cause the food to be pushed out of his mouth. It must be remembered that the infant has to learn the method of smoothly transferring solid food from the front of the mouth to the pharynx. The nurse should explain to the young mother that this reaction is to be expected.

An infant's introduction to solid food should be a pleasant experience. The infant should be held securely in the same position as for taking his formula from the bottle, but his head and shoulders should be raised slightly more than in bottle feeding. A bib is necessary, since he will spit out the food and make his fingers sticky by putting them into his mouth. The food should be smooth and thin. Cereal should be diluted with the formula; fruit or a vegetable, with boiled water.

A small serving (1 teaspoonful) is all that an infant will take at first. A small spoon should be used. (Do not use a spoon with a curved handle; it is awkward in an adult's hand.) The food should be placed on the back of the infant's tongue, but no pressure should be exerted, since that would cause him to gag. New foods should be introduced one at a time. A new food should be offered before his formula or a food to which he is accustomed. The infant should not be hurried, coaxed or allowed to linger. Thirty minutes is long enough for a feeding. If he has not taken the food at the end of that time, the feeding should be discontinued and another attempt made the next day. Medication should not be mixed with the food unless the physician specifically orders that this be done.

Many mothers and nurses become anxious when teaching an infant to take solid food. The feeder should be calm, patient, gentle, and pleasant in her approach to the infant. He is then more likely to take the food than if he is scolded or coaxed. He should never be held tightly in an effort to control his hands, nor be forced to eat. Such measures make him antagonistic to the feeding process. If the nurse or mother is giving the infant foods which are distasteful to her, she should not show any evidence of her dislike. The infant is likely to imitate her reaction to the food. If he wants to touch the food, he should be allowed to do so. Touching is one of his methods of learning. His hands, of course, should be washed both before and after his feeding.

Just as physicians vary as to the time for starting solid foods, so they vary as to which food should be given first. Traditionally, cereal has been the first food to be given.

Cereal. Early administration of cereal was formerly advised because it contains iron. A young infant needs iron since he does not receive a sufficient quantity of it in breast milk or his formula. But cereal, unless it is enriched, does not contain as much iron as some puréed foods; hence many physicians order other foods before cereal is started.

Cereals which are ready-prepared for infant use may be given, or the infant's portion may be taken from that prepared for the family breakfast. Dry cereals, however, are not suitable for infants. Cereals especially prepared for infants are more finely divided and easily digested than those for the family table. If the cereal cooked for the family is to be used for the infant, his serving should be cooked longer in order to break the starch or polysaccharide down to the simpler forms of carbohydrate—disaccharide or monosaccharide—which the infant can more readily digest. (It is best to use a double boiler to cook cereals so that the cereal does not stick to the bottom of the pan.) Cereals prepared for the infant should not be sweetened.

A variety of cereals should be given so that the infant may learn to accept a variety of tastes. It is well to begin with a teaspoonful of cereal once a day. This may be increased gradually until at six or seven months he will take from 2 to 5 tablespoonfuls a day.

As the infant grows older he may be given a baked or boiled potato in place of his cereal. The potato can be mashed with a fork and moistened with a little boiled milk or water.

Fruits. Fresh fruits (e.g. apples, peaches, apricots) should be stewed and put through a sieve. No sugar should be added. Banana can be given raw, mashed to a pulp with a spoon. The fruit should be thoroughly ripe. The giving of fruit should be started with 1 teaspoonful, and the amount gradually increased until the infant is getting 3 or 4 tablespoonfuls a day. Several kinds of fruit should be tried so that he learns to like a variety.

Vegetables. As with fruit, the infant should be given only a teaspoonful at first, with an increase until he is taking 2 to 4 tablespoonfuls. The vegetables should be steamed or cooked in as little water as possible in order to retain their mineral and vitamin content. Vegetables, when first introduced, should be put through a sieve. The infant should be given green and yellow vegetables which have a bland taste and contain necessary vitamins. Later, when he is teething, he should be given coarsely mashed or chopped vegetables. Peas, carrots or string beans may be included in the diet, and should be cooked until soft so that they can be readily chopped, mashed or crushed with a fork.

Eggs. Many physicians suggest that egg yolk be given the infant when he is from three to five months old. They also suggest that egg white not be given until toward the end of the first year, because infants may be allergic to egg albumen. Egg yolk contains iron and riboflavin as well as protein. It should be hard-cooked, mashed with a fork and fed in small amounts until the infant has become accustomed to it and then gradually increased. It can be given alone or mixed with milk or cereal. When egg white is added to the diet, the egg may be boiled (hard or soft) or poached. Only small amounts of egg white should be given until it is evident that the infant is not allergic to the protein it contains; then the entire egg may be given.

Meat. Many physicians add strained meats to the diet early in the first year. Meat, like eggs and milk, provides protein. Meat especially prepared for infant feeding can be bought in small cans. It can also be prepared by scraping raw meat—liver or beef—with a knife; the scraped meat is then formed into a patty and cooked in a custard cup set in a pan of boiling water. When the meat is thoroughly cooked, the patty will be brown.

At first the infant is given only a teaspoonful of meat prepared in this way, but it is soon increased to 2 tablespoonfuls a day. Liver is especially valuable because of its high content of iron, vitamin A and vitamin B complex. Chicken and lamb are added to the diet later. The infant should not be given fatty meats because fat requires more time for digestion and is therefore less easily utilized. When he is able to chew, his meat may be finely ground rather than scraped.

Fish. Near the end of the first year, fish can be substituted for meat or egg several times a week. The fish should be boiled, baked or steamed, but not fried, because of the increase in the fat content. The fish must be finely divided in order to be certain that it does not contain small particles of bones.

Bread. Dried bread or zwieback may be added to the diet when the infant is about six months old and his teeth are coming through the gums. If he is permitted to hold the bread, he will learn in an easy way to carry food to his mouth. This is the first step in acquiring the ability to feed himself. He will also get exercise for his jaws through chewing the dried bread.

Whole Milk. If the infant is not breast-fed, his formula is discontinued by about six months, and he is given whole homogenized, pasteurized, boiled milk. Some pediatricians are discontinuing formula as early as four months and are not requesting the mother to boil the milk or the water she gives her infant if she lives in a community where the quality of the milk and water supplies are carefully controlled. Since he is receiving carbohydrate in his cereal and other foods, he does not need sugar added to the milk.

Desserts. Desserts are given in the latter part of the first year. Those suited to the infant's needs are fruits, gelatin, milk puddings, junkets and custards.

Home or Commercial Preparation of Infants' Foods

Mothers may prepare the infants' foods at home or buy inexpensive, ready-prepared foods; some may want to can food for his use.* Such foods must be thoroughly cooked without seasoning and strained for feeding the young infant.

Mothers can buy precooked cereal. These powdered cereals can be made into a liquid or paste by the addition of boiled water or the infant's formula. Vegetables, fruits, meats and egg yolk can also be obtained in cans or jars in puréed or chopped form for infant feeding. These containers can be safely refrigerated for two or three days after being opened. It is good practice to remove from the container only one serving at a time. The remainder in the jar or can may be safely covered and refrigerated. The original container was sterilized in processing and is the safest receptacle for the food. The advantages of prepared infant foods are variety, convenience, high retention of nutrients, year-round availability, uniform quality and consistency, and sterility.

Development of Eating Habits

The mother is generally responsible if her child develops poor eating habits. If she makes the feeding period a happy one for him, feeding problems are not likely to develop. It is easier to make a good start in feeding than to correct a bad habit when the infant is older.

By *one month* the infant is able to take food from a spoon if it is offered to him. At *five to six months* the average infant begins to use his fingers in eating (finger-feeding), taking zwieback or dry, thin toast in his hand and learning to carry it to his mouth. At *eight to nine months* he has acquired the skill of holding a spoon and playing with it. At *nine months* the average infant can hold his own bottle and seems to prefer doing so. The *twelve-month-old* child drinks from a cup, although he may want his bottle at bedtime for the comfort of sucking. He should be allowed the bottle at bedtime until he voluntarily gives it up.

During the first year the infant's appetite will be good because of his increasing activity and rapid body growth. At the end of the first year his appetite will decrease because of his slower rate of growth and his corresponding decreased need for food. This is normal and should never be a signal for the mother or nurse to force him to eat or to become anxious lest he starve. Encouraging him to eat too much food at this time often results in feeding problems during the toddler period.

Colic

Colic is most common during the first three or four months of life. By colic is meant paroxysmal intestinal cramps due to accumulation of excessive gas. This causes discomfort and pain. The infant may pass gas from the anus or belch it up from the stomach. In reaction to his pain the infant cries loudly, draws up his arms and legs and becomes red in the face. His abdomen feels hard to the mother's or nurse's hand.

Etiology, Treatment and Prognosis. The causative factors in colic are not known with certainty, but are held to be excessive swallowing of air, too much excitement, excessive intake of carbohydrates which cause fermentation and gas, too rapid feeding or overfeeding, and an anxious, disturbed or easily excited mother or nurse who communicates her tenseness to the infant.

The *treatment* is to bubble the infant gently and frequently, holding him in an upright position to help him get rid of the air in the intestinal tract. Sometimes giving him a drink of warm water will help to expel the gas. He may be turned upon the abdomen, because pressure upon the abdomen tends to aid in the expulsion of gas. To relieve his tenseness he needs loving care, to be held and soothed by his mother or nurse. The physician may recommend a small warm enema or feel that a change in formula is advisable.

Colic is not a serious condition, and infants often gain weight in spite of the periods of pain.

Weaning

Psychologic Background. Weaning from the breast or bottle to drinking from a cup has a psychologic significance apart from pleasure in the new activity and from the mere motor ability to drink rather than to suck. It is the end of an infant's receiving his main pleasure reactions from an object through the use of his mouth and sucking.

An infant usually indicates his readiness for advance in behavior when the old technique is no longer needed and its limitations frustrate him in his desire for new experiences and control of his environment. In his journey toward maturity he must experience a certain amount of frustration at his inability to control his physical and social environment in order to be stimulated to try to achieve this control.

During the second half of the first year the infant both wants and needs more freedom to move about and to acquire increasing control of his body and knowledge of his environment.

---

* Directions for canning fresh foods may be obtained from the United States Department of Agriculture, Washington, D.C., or from a state College of Agriculture.

It is no longer necessary to hold him closely to communicate to him a feeling of love and protection. In fact, he is likely to resist such restraint. He now gains a feeling of trust in others through their smiling faces and through their words spoken in a tone of voice which he has always associated with pleasant experiences. He wants to leave his infant way of taking nourishment — sucking from the breast or bottle — and try to drink from a cup.

In all learning there is an optimum stage of development when a new activity is learned most readily. At this time opportunity for experimentation should be given the infant, under conditions which favor his success. He should not be hurried to drop the old pattern of behavior while he is learning the new. By six months or so he has learned that good things to eat come from dishes and cups and is ready to try milk from a cup when it is presented to him. He shows his readiness to drink from a cup by sitting up and reaching for it. He then looks to the adult for help in the technique of this new way of taking milk. If he fails to take it, the nurse or mother should wait a few weeks and then try again. The old and the new techniques will overlap.

Time for Weaning. The best time for weaning is generally in the second half of the first year. Although some infants learn to drink from a cup at five months, they seldom show pleasure in it and should not be forced to give up sucking pleasure until they are ready to do so.

The infant may be weaned from breast to formula or whole milk feedings, depending on the order of his physician, before six months of age if the mother's milk is diminishing in quantity or if it is necessary that she return to work outside the home. If some breast milk is available, this should also be given to the infant. The feeding should be given by bottle and not by cup, since a little infant needs the comfort of sucking.

Pregnancy and illness are other reasons for weaning before six months. It is a strain on a pregnant woman's physical strength to supply enough of the essential food elements for both the suckling and the fetus and at the same time meet her own physical needs. Chronic illness in the mother, such as cancer and diseases of the kidneys, heart or blood, may necessitate weaning the infant. Severe, long-lasting infections in the mother are also a cause for weaning. Pulmonary tuberculosis in the mother is a contraindication to breast feeding, since the infant would be contaminated from such close contact with his mother.

Methods of Weaning. The infant should be weaned gradually so that he is less likely to be frustrated by the change from sucking to drinking.

As soon as he drinks well from the cup the number of breast or bottle feedings can be slowly reduced. Some breast-fed infants change to taking their milk from a bottle before learning to drink from a cup. It is an individual matter whether to use the bottle feeding as an intermediate step between breast feeding and drinking from a cup. It is a good plan to let the infant learn to like the taste of cow's milk before breast feeding is discontinued completely.

Weaning should never be undertaken when the infant is sick for any but a compelling reason, for he is already under a physical and emotional strain from his illness.

Reaction to Weaning. When the complete process of weaning is too abrupt, the infant may show signs of discomfort (anxiety, sleeplessness and irritability) and may cry a great deal. He is likely to suck his thumb excessively.

If the infant receives extra attention during and after the period of weaning, he will find many other pleasant experiences to compensate for the lost satisfaction of ingesting milk through sucking and will have little or no reaction to the weaning process.

Elimination

As different kinds of food are added to the infant's diet, the color as well as the consistency of the stools will change. For example, if beets are given, the stools will have a reddish tinge. Gradually, as a variety of foods is taken in the daily diet, the stools will be formed, and their predominant color will be brown.

HEALTH PROTECTION: CHILD HEALTH CONFERENCE

The Child Health Conference is part of a continuous program of health supervision which should start in the prenatal period and continue throughout childhood and into adult life. The family is studied in the Child Health Conference so that the personnel can help the family to make the most of their resources in the care of the individual child.

Family Approach

Adjustments of general principles must be made for application to the individual family. It is essential that parents have an easy self-confidence in their ability to fulfill their parental roles. The physician, social worker, counselor or public health nurse must know the socioeconomic status and cultural background of the family when making recommendations, and should make no recommendation which the family will be unable to carry out.

It is difficult for many mothers to measure a child's development in terms of his capacities; they tend to compare growth, development and abilities of one child with those of others. This is a matter in which the Child Health Conference is particularly useful, since it keeps a continuous record of the child's progress.

If the personnel of the Conference work as a team and show an intense interest in the children, the mothers will follow advice and instructions to the best of their ability. Not too much advice should be given at one time, since this might lead to confusion.

Purposes of the Child Health Conference

Overall Purposes. The main purpose of the Child Health Conference is to provide health supervision for infants and young children who would not otherwise receive this service. Some children are not directly under the supervision of any physician, others may be taken to a private physician or to a clinic only when they are sick. The Child Health Conference does not displace the services of the private physician, but supplements them by giving a kind of service which some children would not otherwise receive.

A secondary purpose of the Conference is to educate parents in better ways of caring for children and to give them an understanding of growth and development.

The Conference personnel should strive to meet the mother's needs and to increase her confidence in providing care for her children. Personnel must not be autocratic or judgmental, but rather should be interested and understanding. Many mothers are confused by the conflicting ideas of child rearing gathered from relatives, friends and magazine and newspaper articles. They should be helped to learn the best concepts of child care and feel secure in their ability to adapt these concepts to their particular needs and then put them into practice without doubts and misgivings.

Although direct teaching is one responsibility of the personnel, it is equally important that they accept the mother as she is. If she is suffering from anxiety or is fearful and possibly has feelings of guilt, the personnel should help her to understand the basis for these attitudes, so that the energy wasted in combating her frustration can be used in loving and working for the children.

Specific Purposes. The broad aims of the Conference are implemented through specific aims: (1) to help mothers understand the physical growth and emotional development of their children and to show them how serious problems can be averted if parents know what to expect of a child at various ages; (2) to recognize physical defects or illness through a complete examination and to inform parents of the sources in the community, such as a private physician or a clinic, where these conditions can be treated; (3) to provide protection against certain communicable diseases by immunization procedures; (4) to offer advice about specific nutrition of the child and to give general assistance with budgeting for the whole family diet; (5) to help establish sound child-physician-mother relations and attitudes toward medical treatment; and (6) to provide assistance with behavior problems and to help the family in their total relations with the child.

The physician in some instances may refer a child to a social worker, psychologist or psychiatrist. The nurse will help the mother to understand and accept the need for such service. This is best done by allowing the mother to express her fears and work through the problem with the emotional support of the nurse. The nurse should also help her to extend the constructive relations she has had with the Conference personnel to the new friends in other professions who can provide the service the child needs.

Concomitant Outcomes. Records on the physical and developmental progress of children and on parental reactions to their roles are kept in the Child Health Conference. These records are of potential value in future care of the child. In some cities children are given physical examinations in the Conference, and the completed records of their health histories are sent with them when they go to school.

Mothers and the Child Health Conference

A mother may learn of Child Health Conferences while receiving prenatal care or in the hospital after the birth of her child. Sometimes the public health nurse who delivers the birth certificate may inform the mother if she has not already been told of the availability of the Conference. Any nurse, whether working in a hospital, clinic or public health service, should know of the facilities the community offers for child health supervision and should explain these to the mothers with whom she works. Any infant whose mother does not have a private physician should be taken to such a Conference.

Many mothers come to the Child Health Conference to find out whether they are doing a good job in bringing up a child. They want reassurance that their judgment is sound and that the child is responding normally to their care. Some mothers come because they feel discouraged and inadequate or want to be relieved of a sense of guilt. All come for information and to have their children examined by the physician and given the customary immunizations. Some come because their friends come, and they consider it a pleasant social gathering. Such mothers dress their children to be admired by other mothers and by the clinic personnel. Their attendance should not be discouraged, though obviously they need to take a more serious view of child care.

The Child Health Conference

Personnel. The minimal personnel required to meet the needs of the mother who brings her child to them includes the physician and at least one nurse. If there is a full staff, a social worker, a child guidance worker, a nutritionist and a dental hygienist are available for consultation or treatment. The physician should be a pediatrician or should have had extensive experience with mothers and children. The nurse in charge of the Conference should have had public health experience and have worked successfully with children. In an ideal situation the mother and the child should both see the physician and the nurse at each visit.

Students may be present to have the responsibilities and goals of the Child Health Conference explained to them. Volunteers may have an important part, doing many things to help the nurses.

Administration and Procedures

The Child Health Conference may be a voluntary organization with private support, or it may be a public service supported through public funds. Private physicians in the community are requested to support and to help plan and conduct the Conference.

If possible, the Conference should be held in a place convenient for the parents of the children who will be brought there. In large cities many are located in housing projects or health centers. In rural areas the Conference may travel from community to community; some organization within the community to be visited makes all the necessary arrangements. These Conferences are highly successful and have done much to improve the health of children in rural areas.

The physical setup requires three or four rooms. One room is used as a reception or waiting room and should be large enough to accommodate the mothers and children without crowding.

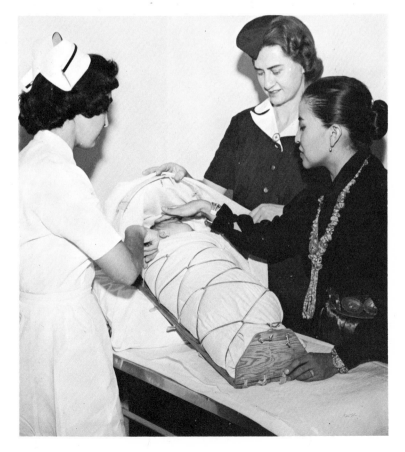

Figure 12–22. A public health nurse of the United States Public Health Service's Division of Indian Health has been instrumental in getting this Navajo mother, in native dress and hair style, to bring her baby for examination to the Indian Hospital at Fort Defiance, Arizona. (Division of Indian Health, United States Public Health Service.)

Posters and exhibits can be placed here. A small room is required for weighing and measuring the children. The physician's consultation room should be equipped for examining the child and should have a comfortable chair for the mother in which she can hold her infant while she talks to the physician. There should also be a separate room in which the mother and the nurse or nutritionist may consult about any problems the mother may have.

If such space is not available, one or two rooms may be divided by screens so that the work of the clinic may be carried on. Ideally, room should be available for taking the child's history, for undressing and examining the child, for comfortable seating of mothers and children while waiting to be seen, and for play among older children. The play area should have small chairs and washable toys for the children. A volunteer worker may be available to supervise the children. The area where immunizations are given should be away from the room where the children and their mothers are waiting, so that they do not hear a child cry when he receives an injection.

Conducting the Conference. The nurse in charge is responsible for the conduct of the clinic. She may have one or more nurses to assist her. The nursing personnel should strive to create an atmosphere of friendliness and dignity. The nurses should thoroughly understand the purposes of the Conference and the recommendations made by the physician for each child so that they may feel secure in conferences with the mothers. Nurses cannot impart a feeling of confidence in the clinic if they themselves are uncertain of the objectives and of the specific recommendations given by the physician for the individual child.

The services offered by the Child Health Conference include the following:

1. Keeping a complete health history of the child
2. Recording the child's height and weight and taking his temperature
3. Giving a complete physical examination
4. Guidance for the regulation of feeding and general care of the child
5. Immunization according to the best medical practice
6. Anticipatory guidance and advice on behavior problems
7. Appraisal of the child's physical and emotional status
8. Nursing interpretation of the physician's advice
9. Referral to private or clinic physicians for illness or correction of physical defects or to a psychiatrist for emotional problems.

HEALTH HISTORY. A careful and complete history is of extreme importance in order to give the clinic personnel a picture of the whole child and to help them establish friendly relations with the mother. The history should not be taken hurriedly. The mother should have time to discuss her problems and those of her child or other family members who are constantly in contact with him. If the nurse takes the history, she should utilize opportunities for health teaching and should explain to the mother the purpose of the Conference. Thereby she prepares the mother for her consultation with the physician.

HEIGHT, WEIGHT AND TEMPERATURE. Recording height and weight and taking temperatures are the nurse's responsibility, though these are often done by a volunteer under her supervision. The undressed child should be observed for rashes or other signs of illness. Demonstrations can be made to the mothers of the procedures of weighing the infant and taking his temperature. As she observes the nurse the mother learns how to utilize safety measures in handling the child.

Procedure for Weighing the Infant. The *purpose* is to determine the exact weight of the infant. The weight provides a way of evaluating the infant's progress or lack of it in his physical status and in growth. Accuracy is therefore essential.

The *equipment* includes infant weighing scales (placed with the head end toward the wall), scale paper, and infant blanket, pencil and paper on which to record the weight, and a paper square with which to handle the scale weight.

The procedure should be done with care for the infant's safety and for the prevention of cross-contamination. The nurse or volunteer should note the infant's weight on the previous visit, undress the infant, wrap him in a blanket and carry him to the scales. To avoid contaminating the scales she should place a piece of scale paper on the scoop and handle the weight of the scale with the paper square. The infant is then placed gently in the center of the scoop with his head to the wall so that he will not fall if he kicks or pushes with his legs. The volunteer or nurse should hold her left hand over the infant while he is weighed to prevent his falling if he tries to sit up. The difficulty in weighing an infant is to keep him still, for if he moves, the weight is not accurate. The mother should stand beside the scale table and speak to him and show him a toy to divert his attention; in this way he will be quiet, and the exact weight can be read. The infant is wrapped in his blanket and given to his mother to hold until the physician is ready to examine him. The scale paper is then removed and disposed of in the receptacle for contaminated paper. The exact weight is then recorded.

Procedure for Measuring Length. The *purpose* is to determine the length of the infant.

The *equipment* includes a metal tape measure or a ruled area on the paper-covered table and a pencil and paper for recording the length.

The nurse or volunteer should place the infant's head against a board or wall at one end of the table. The infant should be stretched lengthwise with his knees flat on the table. A mark may be put at his feet. When the infant is removed, his length can be measured from the board or wall at his head to the mark made at his feet. The length is then recorded.

PHYSICAL EXAMINATION. Physical examination of an infant should be made as often as necessary, but the number of examinations given at various age levels and what is included in the examinations vary in different clinics. In general the schedule is for the infant to be seen by the physician each month during the first year of life, every three months during the second and third years, and every six months during the fourth and fifth years. Such examinations even in infancy should include an evaluation of the infant's abilities to see and hear.

Complete examination at each visit is not necessary. A thorough examination is made when the infant is first brought to the clinic and when he is six and twelve months old. After that once a year is considered sufficient. This is not, of course, a set rule. An infant should be examined whenever the physician thinks it necessary. The need for a complete examination is determined by a limited examination made at each visit or by the mother's report of signs or symptoms of disease, abnormality or lack of normal development.

In general a limited examination is directed toward finding abnormal conditions commonly connected with the stage of development reached by the infant, e.g. conditions of the feet, legs or back when he is learning to walk. The physician's examination, even if limited, consists in noting the mother-child relations, the general growth and development, state of nutrition, general health and evidence of disease or abnormality. A urine test for phenylketone bodies should also be done (see p. 344). The physical examination should precede immunization procedures, which are likely to make the infant cry and be uncooperative.

GUIDANCE FOR FEEDING AND GENERAL CARE. The entire personnel of the Conference give guidance. The physician prescribes the formula and the addition of solid foods to the infant's diet. The nurse should help the mother to understand the recommendations given by the physician, and her own suggestions for his care should be carefully explained. She should be sure that the mother understands in detail *what* is to be done and *how* it is to be done.

The nurse must know enough of the home situation to be sure that the plan of infant care made by the clinic personnel is practical and will fit into the cultural complex of the family. If the plan does not meet these criteria, it should be remade; otherwise the service of the clinic is of little value. If the plan is not suitable, it is not likely to be carried out, or it may cause friction within the family which will adversely influence the mother-child relations.

IMMUNIZATION. Prevention of disease is one of the most important goals in child care. During infancy and early childhood preventive measures can be carried out against certain infectious diseases. Immunization is given at the ages indicated by research and by common practice. Immunization of infants against diphtheria, pertussis, tetanus, smallpox, poliomyelitis and measles should be carried out during the first year of life or shortly thereafter, with booster doses during subsequent years.

Diphtheria, Pertussis and Tetanus. Active immunization against these three diseases can be accomplished at the same time through the administration of 0.5 ml. of combined alum-precipitated or aluminum hydroxide- or aluminum phosphate-adsorbed diphtheria and tetanus toxoids and pertussis vaccine, commonly known as D.P.T. A minimum of three intramuscular injections of this combined toxoid-vaccine mixture should be given at intervals of four weeks, beginning at two months of age.

To reduce the possibility of occasional local or general reactions, the material should be given with a 1-inch needle inserted deeply into the midlateral thigh muscles. In older children it may be given in the deltoid muscles. When primary immunization is being given, inoculation should not be made more than once at a particular injection site. After the injections, reactions of irritability, fever, and swelling and redness at the site of injection may occur. In many Child Health Conferences the nurse may give advice to the mother about the care of the child who has such a reaction to an immunization. If these reactions persist, they should be reported to the physician.

Booster doses of D.P.T. should be given at fifteen to eighteen months and at four to six years. Pertussis vaccine is not necessary for children over this age, since the disease is most severe in infancy. Additional booster doses of diphtheria-tetanus toxoids should be given at twelve to fourteen years and every ten years thereafter.

An acutely ill child should not be given immunization materials. Pertussis vaccine should not be given to any infant or child who has a history of convulsions.

Smallpox. An infant should receive smallpox vaccination by the multiple pressure method by about fifteen to eighteen months of age. The child should be revaccinated between four and six years of age and between twelve and fourteen years. Smallpox vaccination should be repeated every three to ten years thereafter. Smallpox vaccination should not be given to anyone who has eczema or other open skin lesions, nor should it be given if another person in the child's family has eczema and has not been vaccinated. In the latter instance the infant could be vaccinated if he were separated from the other person until

Table 12–3. *Recommended Schedule for Active Immunization and Tuberculin Testing of Normal Infants and Children*

2 months	DTP, trivalent OPV[1, 2]
3 months	DTP[3]
4 months	DTP, trivalent OPV
6 months	Trivalent OPV
12 months	Tuberculin test[4]
	Live measles vaccine[5]
15-18 months	DTP, trivalent OPV, smallpox vaccine[6]
4-6 years	DTP, trivalent OPV, smallpox vaccine
12-14 years	Td, smallpox vaccine, mumps vaccine[8]
Thereafter	Td every 10 years[7]
	Smallpox vaccine every 3-10 years
	Rubella vaccine[9]

Reprinted by permission of American Academy of Pediatrics, from its *Report of the Committee on the Control of Infectious Diseases,* 16 Edition, 1969 (Red Book).

[1]Handling and storage of immunizing agents, dosage, sites and routes of administration and courses should follow product (package) information.

Abbreviations:

DTP is diphtheria and tetanus toxoids combined with pertussis vaccine.

Td is combined diphtheria and tetanus toxoids (adult-type) for those over 6 years of age in contrast to DT, which contains a larger amount of diphtheria antigen.

OPV is trivalent oral poliovaccine.

[2]Trivalent OPV is recommended, but monovalent OPV may be substituted; the order of monovalent virus type fed is type 1 followed by type 3 and then type 2.

[3]If DTP dose is not given to the infant at 3 months, it should be given at 4 and 6 months of age.

[4]Frequency of repeated tuberculin tests depends on the risk of exposure of children under care and the prevalence of tuberculosis in the population group.

[5]Live attenuated measles vaccine (Edmonston strain) with or without gamma immune serum globulin (human) or "further attenuated measles vaccine" (Schwarz strain) without the simultaneous administration of gamma globulin is recommended. Killed measles virus vaccine is not recommended. Measles vaccine should be given to all children with a positive tuberculin reaction after initiation of tuberculosis therapy.

[6]Any licensed smallpox vaccine may be used. The reaction should be read and recorded. Combined administration of smallpox vaccine and OPV may be considered if there is a threat of concomitant exposure or if the patient will be inaccessible for completion of the series.

[7]The 10-year interval for tetanus boosters may be calculated from each dose given for prophylaxis (injury). Prophylactic use for wounds is a matter for clinical judgment. Persons who have had the initial series and booster doses may be expected to have adequate protection for at least 1 year after the last dose without receiving an additional booster dose.

[8]See text of 1969 Red Book.

[9]See text of 1969 Red Book.

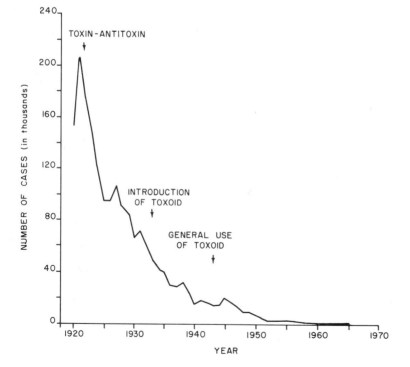

Figure 12–23. Reported diphtheria in the United States, 1920-1965. (National Morbidity Reports.)

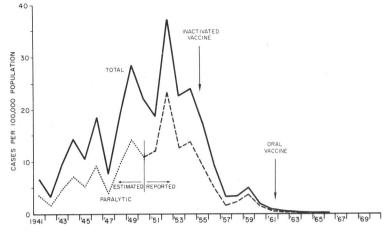

Figure 12–24. Annual polio-myelitis incidence rates, United States, 1941-1966. (Annual Supplement Summary 1966 of the Morbidity and Mortality Weekly Report.)

his vaccination healed. These precautions are necessary to prevent secondary vaccination or generalized vaccinia. Smallpox vaccination should not be given to any child who is acutely ill. Currently research is being done on a small-pox vaccine which can be given as a primary vaccination for infants having eczema.

Poliomyelitis. Two vaccines are now available for the prevention of poliomyelitis: attenuated live oral poliovaccine (Sabin) and form-alin-inactivated poliovaccine (Salk) for parenteral injection.

The Salk vaccine has been effective for many years in producing immunization against poliomyelitis; however, antibody levels fall rapidly in young infants and children after its use. Currently Salk vaccine is generally given only if it was started previously or if the parents request it. The Sabin vaccine against all three types of virus is used more widely now because of its several advantages: it is given orally and stimulates intestinal resistance to reinfection, it stimulates prolonged persistence of antibody, and there is apparently less need for repeated booster vaccinations. Sabin vaccine, however, should not be given within one month of other live vaccines, such as measles and smallpox vaccines.

The trivalent oral poliovaccine is recommended. It should be given at two months, four months, six months, fifteen to eighteen months, and four to six years of age. If monovalent oral poliovaccine is used, type 1 should be given first, followed by type 3 and then type 2.

Measles. If an infant has not had measles, the vaccine should be given at twelve months of age. This is especially important for children who, because of a chronic illness or institutionalization, might possibly suffer serious complications from the disease. Live attenuated measles vaccine is recommended for susceptible normal children. This produces active immunity because it produces a mild, noncommunicable measles

infection. Contraindications to the use of live attenuated measles virus vaccine are, among others, the presence of a severe febrile illness, active tuberculosis, or leukemia (see Table 12-3). Inactivated measles virus vaccine was used in the past; however, since the duration of protection is questionable, it will probably have limited use in the future.

German Measles. Research is currently being done on an experimental vaccine for German measles which would provide immunity against the disease. This would be of great significance especially to young women of childbearing age in the prevention of birth defects (see p. 160).

Mumps. An effective vaccine against mumps

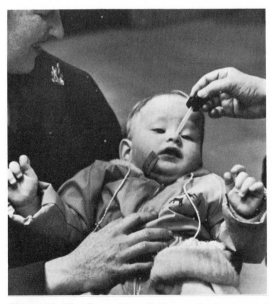

Figure 12–25. For babies, Sabin vaccine is dropped directly into the mouth. (Wyeth Laboratories, Division of American Home Products Corporation, P.O. Box 8299, Philadelphia, Pa. 19101.)

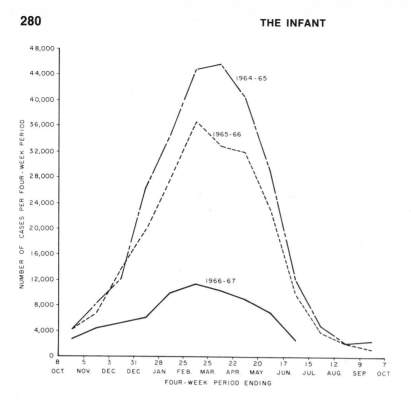

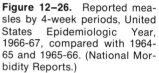

Figure 12–26. Reported measles by 4-week periods, United States Epidemiologic Year, 1966-67, compared with 1964-65 and 1965-66. (National Morbidity Reports.)

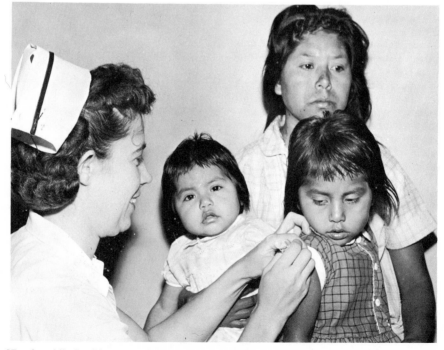

Figure 12–27. A public health nurse of the United States Public Health Service's Division of Indian Health is giving measles immunizations to the children of a Pima Indian family at one of the Division's clinics on the Gila River Reservation in Arizona. (Division of Indian Health, United States Public Health Service.)

made with live but extremely attenuated viruses can be given in one injection. This vaccine is not recommended at present for routine use in infants or young children, pending development of information on the duration of immunity it provides. It is recommended for administration to young boys approaching puberty and for adult males who have not had mumps because of the danger of sterility following the disease. The older killed-virus vaccine against mumps induced immunity for only a short time.

Tuberculin Test. Tuberculin tests should be done on children at twelve months of age. The American Academy of Pediatrics has recommended that all infants one year of age be tested for tuberculosis, preferably before they have been vaccinated against measles or smallpox, depending on the risk of exposure of the child and the prevalence of tuberculosis in the community.

Other Immunizations. If the parents plan to travel to other states or to foreign countries, further information about other immunizations which might be necessary can be obtained from health departments or the Public Health Service, Washington, D.C.

ANTICIPATORY GUIDANCE AND ADVICE ON BEHAVIOR PROBLEMS. These are the responsibility of both the physician and the nurse. The mother can be stimulated to ask questions by mentioning a few of the problems most likely to occur in infants the same age as hers. If the physician is able to spend an adequate amount of time on each mother's problems, it is unnecessary for the nurse to interpret or supplement his recommendations by a thorough nurse-mother conference. But the physician seldom has time to give the mother all the attention she needs, and therefore the nurse-mother conference is commonly held before the mother leaves the clinic. The nurse should be thoroughly familiar with the physician's recommendations so that she does not confuse the mother or alter the physician's plan of care by giving conflicting directions.

APPRAISAL OF THE CHILD'S PHYSICAL AND EMOTIONAL STATUS. Such appraisal is made by both the physician and the nurse of the Child Health Conference, as well as by the public health nurse who visits in the home. In planning care of the infant or child such factors as the history of transmissible defects or diseases, the mother's condition during pregnancy, and the natal and postnatal health history of the infant should be viewed in relation to the socioeconomic background of the family.

All nurses working with children—particularly the public health nurse—should know the norms of infant and child growth and development so that they can recognize and evaluate deviations from the normal. This is true also of students observing or assisting in the Child Health Conference. Experience in the Conference is of little value to them unless they know the general course of growth and development of infants and children.

NURSING INTERPRETATION OF THE PHYSICIAN'S ADVICE. This means more than a nurse interpreting what the physician has said; it means that the mother carries over into her nursing care the *medical advice* given by the physician, including preventive medicine and mental hygiene. Nurses often fail to realize that nursing has something to contribute to the child care program which medicine cannot give. Their recommendations to the mother are based on the physician's orders and on the body of knowledge which belongs to the profession of nursing.

REFERRAL TO PRIVATE OR CLINIC PHYSICIANS. Referral of an infant or child to a private or clinic physician for illness or correction of physical defects, or to a psychiatrist for emotional problems, is certainly a necessary function of the clinic, for it is not prepared to handle such problems. Case finding and referral are two of the main functions of the Conference. The referral is sometimes made by the nurse under the physician's direction, or it can be made by the social worker with his approval.

Functions of the Nurse

In the general management of the Conference the atmosphere should be such as to reduce the strain on the mother and the child and to make them feel at ease. The nurse should greet them pleasantly and introduce them to other mothers. If it is the mother's first visit, the nurse should explain each step of the routine to her. Facilities for privacy should be provided during the mother's conferences with the personnel. The nurse takes the social history of the newly admitted child and talks with the mother before the mother sees the physician. The nurse screens patients and mothers on the basis of their different needs and problems, and it is desirable that the same nurse discuss with the mother the physician's recommendations after her conference with him. The nurse who admits the children to the clinic observes them for signs of illness when they enter in order to isolate any child whose condition may be infectious or to refer him immediately to the appropriate agency or the physician.

The nurse should have adequate time for both individual and group teaching. This will be possible only if a systematic plan of work is in operation and the Conference is running smoothly. The appointment system is essential. Each patient's name should be registered in order of arrival, and all patients should be seen in order of appointment. If a mother brings her child without an appointment, however, it is customary for the physician to see the child if he appears sick or if the mother is anxious about his condition.

The appointment system is a good check on the regularity of the infant's visits to the clinic. Before the mother leaves, the date and time of the next appointment should be given her in writing and should be entered in the appointment book.

Parental Education. Parental education is of little value unless the parents are motivated to receive suggestions from the personnel of the health team. Without motivation they are not likely to put into practice what they are taught. Motivation is increased if teaching has reference to their child and is specific and not general.

Instructions should be simple and should cover the essential information. Excess information is apt to be confusing. Completeness of instruction is measured by the degree in which parents make suggestions and think through their own problems. Self-direction is more effective than direction by others.

Visual aids are valuable in clarifying the application of theory to the child in the home situation. Visual impression is lasting. The parents' understanding of the content covered in parental education should be checked by asking the parents questions. What and how much can be taught parents at any time depends on their social level (i.e. their financial status, living situation) and their intelligence level (how much knowledge they can absorb at one time). Folders or pamphlets should be provided for the parents; they are most effective if given in answer to specific questions and if reviewed with them.

The motivation of the parents is their desire to keep their child well. If they are indifferent to his health, they are not likely to profit from instruction.

The child's daily routine should be planned in sufficient detail to make it of practical value to the mother. Suggestions for guidance of the young child may be given. The feeding of the infant or child is extremely important and is a matter on which there is a great deal of advice from miscellaneous sources.

The purpose and need for regular visits for health checks should be stressed, for parents are likely to feel that these are unnecessary if the child appears well. It is the mother, constantly with the child, who is in a position to observe the early signs of illness. It is imperative that she know these signs and realize the importance of reporting her observations and securing early treatment for the infant or child when he is ill.

Group instruction may be given to mothers on pertinent topics of common interest, such as the kind of clothing suitable to the weather and home conditions, routine immunizations carried out on all children, general principles of feeding and the management of minor behavior problems.

Home Visits. A visit to the home should be made after a child has been brought to the clinic, in order to observe the home environment, to teach the mother and to inspect the child. Ideally, this visit is made by the nurse in charge of the clinic, but if this is not possible, the public health nurse makes the visit and sends a report to the clinic. During the home visit the nurse should observe the socioeconomic status, sanitary conditions, housing, and recreational facilities, which are important to both the infant's and the family's health. In the home the nurse can observe parent-child relations better than in the more or less formal atmosphere of the Child Health Conference.

The Nurse and Volunteer Workers. The work of volunteers is valuable, for they help the nurses to serve as an important means of communication with the public. The nurse should teach the volunteers how to perform nonprofessional duties in the clinic.

Functions performed by volunteer workers in many clinics are as follows:

Check ventilation and light.
Assist in setting up the clinic.
Greet each mother and register the children.
Bring to the attention of the nurse the fact that a child does not appear well.
Begin the admission record.
Take the child's weight and height and record the findings on the chart.
Talk with the mother about educational material and interest her in it.
Supervise the play of the preschool children.
Assist with any additional duties given her.

Need for Expansion

An increasing number of cities and rural areas have organized or are organizing Child Health Conferences. Also some states in this country as well as other countries are establishing, in addition to Child Health Conferences, clinics where nurses are responsible for screening essentially normal children. As the number of these clinics grows they become a factor in reducing the morbidity and mortality rates of children in the area in which they serve. There is, however, still a great need for such facilities in many areas. Nurses must use their influence to secure such services for as many children as possible and encourage attendance at those Conferences which are already in existence. Nurses may exert their influence as a body through their state nurses' associations and through united action in bringing pressure upon the city, county and state legislatures and councils to provide more Child Health Conferences under public auspices. As individuals, nurses can help the public to know the value of such Conferences. Nurses are assuming their professional and civic responsibilities by helping to procure clinic services for all children not fully cared for by private physicians.

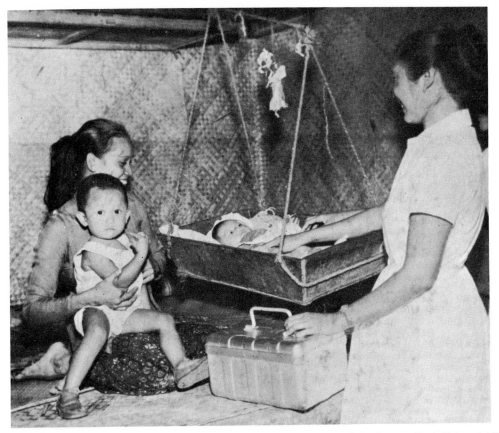

Figure 12–28.   The United Nations Children's Fund introduces modern medicine in a medical clinic established in Indonesia. Instructions on child care are given to a mother by a traveling midwife. (From Free World. USIS, Manila.)

PREPARATION FOR CARE OF INFANTS IN A MAJOR DISASTER

Parents, in addition to learning how to care for their infants and small children under normal circumstances, should also learn how to care for them under mass casualty conditions. Preparation for the care of children in advance of such a disaster might make the difference for them of life or death.

The main problem which would confront parents would be that of feeding the infants. If the infant is breast-fed, further breast feeding should be encouraged. Infants up to six months of age should be provided with 1 quart of fluid per day, such as milk, water, fruit juices or appropriate soft drinks (if nothing else is available). Infants up to one year of age should receive approximately 125 ml. of fluid per kilogram of body weight per day. For a period of thirty days vitamin and mineral supplements should be considered of no importance to a normal child. They should be added to the diet of the child, however, as soon as possible. For an artificially fed infant, bottles and nipples should be boiled before use,

and the formula should be used as soon as it is prepared.

A two-week to two-month supply of uncontaminated water, dried or evaporated milk, sugar, cereal and other foods with which the child is familiar should be stored safely for emergency use for each child under the age of one year. Foods the child likes would be better accepted than those with which he is unfamiliar. Supplies of other necessary items such as diapers, pins, clothing and feeding equipment should also be prestocked for emergency use.

Infants should be immunized according to the usual schedule so that they are protected as much as possible should an emergency occur. Immunization against typhoid and paratyphoid fevers would also be advisable. If diarrhea should occur, food should be withheld and oral electrolytes, if available, or boiled water should be substituted. Injuries to infants or small children should be treated as injuries to adults would be.

At the time of a major disaster infants and children should be kept under the care and supervision of their own parents whenever possible. From their parents they would get the love and security they would need to prevent emotional disturbance during and after such a time of stress.

It has been said that there is nothing new under the sun. This would appear to be true in the case of the cultural beliefs and practices of the family of man. Although we in modern society denounce the primitive practice of allowing weak infants to die for the welfare of the group (see p. 3), this practice is reflected in our present-day concept of disaster nursing. Whether following an atomic or hydrogen bomb explosion or other catastrophic happening, preference in the care of survivors is given to those children and adults most likely to profit from care. The severely traumatized victims, many of them probably infants, who would need extensive therapy would be cared for when time and facilities permitted. In such an emergency would even our civilized society not be selecting those most able to survive in preference to the very young or those least likely to survive? It is obvious that our practices in times when we are not personally threatened change when our own lives are in danger.

TEACHING AIDS AND OTHER INFORMATION*

American Academy of Pediatrics

Child Health Record from Infancy to Adulthood, 1964.
The Health Supervision Program Your Child Should Have.

American Medical Association

A Letter to You, Mother, About Measles and Your Child.
First Aid Manual.
Immunization.
Key Facts About Tetanus.
Measles Vaccine.
Pick Your Shots.
Tetanus—the Second Deadliest Poison.

Child Study Association of America

Auerbach, A. B.: How to Give Your Child a Good Start.
Goller, G.: Permissiveness and the Baby.
Wolf, K. M., and Auerbach, A. B.: As Your Child Grows: The First Eighteen Months. 2nd ed., 1966.

Mental Health Materials Center

Sleeping Habits.
Thumbsucking.

Public Affairs Pamphlets

Carson, R.: Your New Baby.
Riker, A. P.: Breastfeeding.
Saltman, J.: Immunization for All, 1967.

Ross Laboratories

Breast Feeding.
Formula Preparation Instruction Folders.
The Phenomena of Early Development.
Your Child and Sleep Problems.
Your Child's Appetite.

United States Department of Health, Education, and Welfare

A Healthy Personality for Your Child, 1952. Reprinted 1963.
Breast Feeding Your Baby, 1965.
Facts About Pasteurization of Milk, 1967.
Guide for Public Health Nurses Working with Children, 1961.
Healthy Teeth, 1966.
Infant Care, 1963. Reprinted 1967.
Jacobziner, H., Levy, D. M., Suchman, E. A., and O'Neill, G.: Mental Health in the Child Health Conference, 1964.
Jelliffe, D. B., and Bennett, F. J.: Health Education of the Tropical Mother in Feeding Her Young Child, 1964.
Key Nutrients, 1966.
Minimum Sanitary Standards for Community Infant Formula Services, 1967.
Personal and Family Survival, 1966.

---

* Complete addresses are given in the Appendix.

The Care of Your Children's Teeth, 1966.
The Role of the Nurse in National Disaster, 1965.
When It Comes to Fluoridation, 1966.
When Teenagers Take Care of Children, 1964.
Your Baby's First Year, 1962.

REFERENCES

Publications

Ainsworth, M.D., and others: *Deprivation of Maternal Care: A Reassessment of Its Effects.* Geneva, World Organization, 1962. (Columbia University Press, International Documents Service.)

American Academy of Pediatrics: *Report of the Committee on the Control of Infectious Disease.* 14th ed., 1964. Evanston, Ill., American Academy of Pediatrics, 1963.

American Academy of Pediatrics: *Standards of Child Health Care.* Evanston, Ill., American Academy of Pediatrics, 1967.

American Hospital Association: *Procedures and Layout for the Infant Formula Room.* Chicago, American Hospital Association, 1965.

Brackbill, Y., and Thompson, G. G.: *Behavior in Infancy and Early Childhood.* New York, Macmillan Company, 1967.

Close, S.: *The Know-How of Infant Feeding.* Baltimore, Williams & Wilkins Company, 1965.

Décarie, T. G.: *Intelligence and Affectivity in Early Childhood.* New York, International Universities Press, 1966.

Erickson, E. H.: *Childhood and Society.* New York, W. W. Norton and Company, 1964.

Fomon, S. J.: *Infant Nutrition.* Philadelphia, W. B. Saunders Company, 1967.

Foss, B. M. (Ed.): *Determinants of Infant Behavior.* New York, John Wiley and Sons, Inc., 1966, Vol. III.

Frank, L. K.: *On the Importance of Infancy.* New York, Random House, 1966.

Gesell, A., and Amatruda, C. S.: *Developmental Diagnosis.* 2nd ed. New York, Harper and Row, 1964.

Hoopes, J. L.: *An Infant Rating Scale.* New York, Child Welfare League of America, Inc., 1967.

Illingworth, R. S.: *Development of The Infant and Young Child.* 3rd ed. Baltimore, Williams & Wilkins Company, 1966.

Johnson, D. E.: *The Meaning of Maternal Deprivation and Separation Anxiety for Nursing Practice. Nursing in Relation to the Impact of Illness upon the Family.* Monograph 2, 1962 Clinical Sessions. New York, American Nurses' Association, 1962.

Kallins, E. L.: *Textbook of Public Health Nursing Practice.* St. Louis, C. V. Mosby Company, 1967.

Provence, S.: *Guide for the Care of Infants in Groups.* New York, Child Welfare League of America, 1967.

Recommended Dietary Allowances. Washington, D.C., National Academy of Sciences–National Research Council, Revised 1968.

Ribble, M. A.: *The Rights of Infants–Early Psychological Needs and Their Satisfaction.* 2nd ed. New York, Columbia University Press, 1965.

Spitz, R. A., and Cobliner, W.: *The First Year Of Life. (A Psychoanalytic Study of Normal and Deviant Development of Object Relations).* New York, International Universities Press, 1965.

Willis, N. H.: *Basic Infant Nutrition.* Philadelphia, J. B. Lippincott Company, 1964.

Winnicott, D. W.: *The Family and Individual Development.* New York, Basic Books, 1965.

Witmer, H. L., and others: *Maternal Deprivation.* New York, Child Welfare League of America, 1962.

Periodicals

Ben-Or, R.: Perceptual Development in Infancy. *Nursing Science,* 2:453, 1964.

Brody, S.: The Developing Infant. *Children,* 13:158, 1966.

Bruton, O. C.: Diets of Infants and Children in Disaster. *Pediat. Clin. N. Amer.,* 9:1025, 1962.

Calafiore, D. C.: Eradication of Measles in the United States. *Am. J. Nursing,* 67:1871, 1967.

Close, K.: Giving Babies a Healthy Start in Life. *Children,* 12:179, 1965.

Dittmann, L. L.: A Child's Sense of Trust. *Am. J. Nursing,* 66:91, 1966.

Green, S. L.: Hospitalized Infants Need Round-the-Clock Mother Figure. *Psychosomatics,* 5:75, March-April 1964.

Hallstrom, B. J.: Contact Comfort: Its Application to Immunization Injections. *Nursing Research,* 17:130, 1968.

Hymovich, D. P.: ABC'S of Pediatric Safety. *Am. J. Nursing,* 66:1768, 1966.

McCaffery, M. S.: An Approach to Parent Education. *Nursing Forum,* VI:77, November, 1967.

Mumps, Vaccine Proves out in Clinical Trials. *Medical World News,* 8:25, October 27, 1967.

Rakstis, T. J.: How Safe Are Your Child's Toys? *Today's Health,* 45:21, December 1967.

Rubin, R.: Food and Feeding: A Matrix of Relationships. *Nursing Forum,* VI:195, Spring 1967.

Seacat. M., and Schlachter, L.: Expanded Nursing Role in Prenatal and Infant Care. *Am. J. Nursing,* 68:822, 1968.

Wiedenbach, E.: Family Nurse Practitioner for Maternal and Child Care. *Nursing Outlook,* 13:50, December 1965.

13

CONDITIONS OF INFANTS REQUIRING IMMEDIATE OR SHORT-TERM CARE

Hospitalization during infancy is often a new experience for both mother and child. Since the mother is anxious, the infant also becomes anxious. The mother should be encouraged to verbalize her fears about the child's welfare, thereby relieving some of her anxiety.

When an infant becomes ill for even a short time, his well-being both physical and emotional, is threatened. This is especially true if he is hospitalized and deprived of his mother's love while he is in pain, restrained for treatment or not permitted to suck.

RESPIRATORY CONDITIONS

CONTROL OF RESPIRATION. Respiration is controlled by the respiratory center in the brain stem. Changes in carbon dioxide tension affect the respiratory center, which is stimulated by lack of oxygen. Certain drugs (anesthetic agents, opiates, barbiturates), brain injury and hypothermia depress the respiratory center.

MUSCLES OF RESPIRATION. In normal breathing only the inspiratory muscles of respiration are used, mostly the diaphragm. When these muscles relax, expiration occurs. But when breathing is difficult, the intercostal, spinal extensor and neck muscles are brought into use. In forced expiration, as in coughing, the abdominal muscles are used. If these are weak, the child will find it difficult to cough. The nurse can help the older child to cough by exerting manual pressure over the abdomen after he has taken a deep breath.

THE INFANT'S RESPIRATORY TRACT. Naturally the respiratory tract of the infant or little child is very small. This is one reason why any obstruction in the airway is extremely serious. Obstruction may be due to edema, mucus or an aspirated foreign body. If the obstruction is extensive and high in the respiratory tract, the whole lung is affected; if it is in the lower part of the tract, only tissue below the obstruction is involved.

Incidence. Respiratory disturbances as a

group constitute one of the greatest problems in the care of children. The patient's age is important in the kind of disease from which he is likely to suffer and in its clinical picture.

Although respiratory infections are common in young children, it is difficult to identify them as separate clinical entities. The reason for this is that the tissues of the respiratory tract are continuous from the nose, pharynx and larynx to the tracheobronchial tree and also to the paranasal sinuses and the middle ear. Often an infection beginning in the upper respiratory tract will proceed downward to the lower tract.

Epidemiology. Infecting organisms are passed from person to person through the air. As the infant breathes, he draws into his lungs organisms carried on minute droplets of water or particles of dust. These organisms multiply rapidly in the mucous membranes, and the newly infected infant becomes a source of infection to others and of further infection to himself.

These pathogenic organisms die quickly in outdoor air, owing to the action of ultraviolet light from the sun and a temperature unfavorable to their growth. This is the reason why in summer, when infants and children are outdoors and houses are better ventilated, colds are few. In winter, when children are kept indoors, whether at home or at school, cross-contamination is apt to occur, and colds spread through the family, play group or class. Children during the first few years at school are likely to have more upper respiratory tract infections because they are more frequently exposed and have not built up resistance to infection as has the healthy older child. Infected preschool-age and school children thus become a source of infection for smaller siblings at home.

Etiology. Infection is the most common etiologic factor in respiratory conditions occurring after the neonatal period. The infant, however, may aspirate foreign bodies or irritating substances containing oil or zinc stearate.

Acute infection may be caused by viruses mostly or by some bacteria. The influenza virus has been recognized for many years as one of the organisms causing such infections. During recent years several other viruses have also been recognized, such as the adenoviruses, the Coxsackie viruses, the ECHO (enteric cytopathogenic human orphan) viruses and the RS (respiratory syncytial) virus.

Acute Nasopharyngitis (Common Cold)

This is the most common respiratory infection in infants and children. The nasal accessory sinuses and the nasopharynx are involved. The difficulty in caring for children is that the infection spreads quickly, and serious complica-

tions may result. The clinical pattern in infants and small children is different from that in adults.

Etiology. The common cold is caused by a filterable virus or a group of viruses causing an acute catarrhal inflammation of the upper respiratory tract. Bacteria are the cause of the purulent, second stage of the cold; these may be pneumococci, hemolytic streptococci or staphylococci.

CONTRIBUTING FACTORS. Infants and children vary in their susceptibility to colds. Age, nutritional state, fatigue, degree of chilling of the body or emotional disturbance may influence the severity of a cold.

Immunity. Susceptibility to the common cold is universal. Children have little resistance to infection and therefore must be protected from exposure. Serious complications may result, particularly among infants in infants' homes, in a children's hospital or in children's units of a general hospital.

Pathology. The initial lesion is an edema of the submucosa followed by infiltration with leukocytes. There is separation of epithelial cells and destruction of nasal epithelium.

Clinical Manifestations. The child is fretful, irritable and restless. He sneezes and has a nasal discharge which at first is thin and later purulent. The discharge may irritate the edge of the nostril and the upper lip.

Respiration is difficult, owing to congestion of the mucous membrane of the nostrils. The throat is sore, and the cervical lymph nodes are swollen. Gastrointestinal disturbances such as vomiting and diarrhea are common. Fever of 102 to 104°F. is prominent in patients up to two to three years of age. The temperature in older children is not likely to be over 102°F., and the school child and the adult may have little or no fever. Anorexia, cough and general malaise are common. In the small infant obstruction of the nostrils may interfere with sucking, since he cannot breathe and swallow at the same time.

Differential Diagnosis. One of the problems in the diagnosis of the common cold in little children is that its onset resembles that of a number of infectious diseases, e.g. measles, pertussis, poliomyelitis or congenital syphilis. The nasal discharge in allergic rhinitis may appear to be the first sign of nasopharyngitis; it does not progress to a purulent stage, however, as does a cold. Also, in allergy the nasal mucous membranes are pale, whereas in a cold they are inflamed.

Complications. Serious complications such as sinusitis, otitis media, mastoiditis, brain abscess (due to extension of infection from the mastoids), tracheitis, bronchitis, pneumonia, pleurisy or empyema are more common in infancy than in childhood and are caused by extension of the infection from the nose to the sinuses, ears, mastoids, throat, larynx, bronchi and lungs.

Treatment. The treatment is largely symptomatic. In the hospital the child is isolated. It is important to maintain his nutritional state with a suitable diet and adequate vitamins. The fluid intake should be increased. The child should be kept in bed during the febrile stage. Nasal congestion should be alleviated so that the infant may suck properly. Nose drops should be used in an aqueous solution. Neo-Synephrine hydrochloride (0.25 per cent) or ephedrine (0.5 to 1 per cent) are frequently used. Whatever the drug, in general one half to one quarter of the adult strength is used for infants and young children. Oily nose drops should *never* be used because of the danger of lipoid pneumonia. Medication such as aspirin reduces the temperature. The dose is generally figured as 60 mg. (1 grain) of aspirin per year of age up to five years, given two or three times a day; the dose for older children is 0.3 gm. (5 grains) given at the same intervals. Medication should be used only during the first day or two of the cold. Overuse of salicylates may result in salicylate poisoning. Sulfonamides and antibiotics should not be used routinely for the treatment of colds, but are indicated for complications or prolonged infections. Nasal drainage must be carried out, since infants cannot blow their noses.

Nursing Care. REST. Rest is important in the acute stage of this disease. The infant must be spared from many of the ordinary day-to-day noises in the home and from the excitement of family visitors or the activities of siblings.

FLUID INTAKE. Water should be offered frequently, since the infant cannot take large amounts at a time. He has great difficulty in sucking and breathing at the same time and should be allowed to rest frequently while taking his artificial formula, breast feeding or water. The child who is old enough to drink from a cup needs increased amounts of fluid; small amounts may be given frequently. Little glasses, pretty cups with pictures on the bottom and gaily colored straws make the taking of fluids more interesting to the small child. For children of nursery school age a little pitcher from which a cup can be refilled encourages a greater fluid intake. With a group of children of this age or older an achievement chart may be kept where all can see it. Such a chart shows graphically the fluid intake of each child, and they compete in the race to get ahead of the others.

HUMIDITY. The humidity of the room should be 80 to 90 per cent in order to liquefy the secretions in the respiratory tract and reduce the cough. Excellent mechanical devices to increase the humidity of the atmosphere are on the market. If none is available, a long, shallow pan of water may be placed on the radiator. But unless the radiator is very hot, evaporation is slow, and the moisture in the air is not sufficiently increased. The temperature of the room should be about 70°F.

NASAL DRAINAGE. Drainage is facilitated by placing the infant on his abdomen and raising the foot of the bed. A nasal suction apparatus may be used, but with great care, since there is danger of injuring the infant.

NOSE DROPS. Drops should be given only when obstruction is present, not more frequently than every three hours and only for the first two or three days. The therapeutic effect is to shrink the mucous membrane, to relieve the stuffed feeling so characteristic of colds, and to reduce the excessive nasal discharge. The drops are given fifteen to twenty minutes before feedings and at bedtime. The nurse must be certain that the infant's nose is cleared of mucus before feeding and when the infant is put to bed.

Because of the danger of cross-infection, each child should have his own bottle of nose drops and medicine dropper. The dropper is kept in the bottle and serves as a stopper. The dropper has a smooth, bulblike tip or is tipped with rubber tubing so that the infant's nose may not be injured. If one bottle must be used for several children, a separate dropper must be provided for each child and never replaced in the bottle after use. The bottle must at all times be kept out of the infant's reach.

Before instilling the drops, drainage must be secured. To give the drops, the infant is laid on his back, his head over the side of the mattress or his neck extended over a blanket roll. His face is held by the nurse's left hand encircling his chin and cheeks, while she inserts the drops with her right hand. If such restraint is not sufficient and a second nurse is not available to assist in the procedure, it may be necessary to "mummy" him. After the drops have been instilled the infant's head is kept below the level of his shoulders for one or two minutes. The nurse or mother may hold the infant in her lap in any way which is comfortable for him, so long as the head is thrown back.

PREVENTION OF EXCORIATION OF THE LIP. Excoriation of the upper lip with subsequent infection is caused by the irritating nasal discharge. This may be prevented by applying cold cream or petrolatum to the area.

MEDICATIONS. These are difficult to give to little children. Pills and tablets should be crushed into a powder and mixed with water or syrup, or both. They should be given from a spoon.

POSITION. The child's position should be changed frequently. The infant should be propped first on one side and then on the other, with his back supported by a rolled blanket.

CLEANSING THE NASAL PASSAGES. As soon as the child is old enough to understand, he should be taught the therapeutic way of clearing the nasal passages. He should learn to keep his mouth open and blow the secretions from both nostrils at the same time. He should never be told, as many adults do tell children, to "Close the mouth and blow hard."

CARE BY NONINFECTED NURSES. Nurses can contract colds from the children who are too young to cooperate in the prevention of spread of infection. A nurse with a cold carries the risk of infecting the infants even though her technique is good.

MEDICAL ASEPTIC TECHNIQUE. Isolation technique should be maintained as long as a child is infectious. When he is no longer infectious, there is danger of his contracting a secondary infection from organisms carried by nurses or other children. The technique is the same whether we are speaking of the nursing care of an infant having a cold or a contagious disease such as measles or diphtheria which can also be spread by discharges from the respiratory tract (see p. 63).

Medical aseptic technique *in the home* is difficult to carry out. If possible, the isolation unit should include a bathroom. Members of the family other than the mother should not enter the room. She should use the same technique the nurse uses, making any necessary adaptations to the home environment. The person providing care in such a situation is responsible for cleaning the sick room and for concurrent and terminal disinfection.

Prevention. All patients having infections of the respiratory tract should be isolated so that contact between them and well children will be avoided. A child in good nutritional state is not so likely to catch cold. In older children tonsillectomy and adenoidectomy may be indicated. Vaccines are of questionable value in preventing the common cold. Children acquire resistance to infections upon exposure to them by building up protective antibodies. For this reason the older the child, the more likely is he to resist infection.

Otitis Media

Etiology and Incidence. Otitis media is an infection of the middle ear. It is usually secondary to a respiratory infection and for that reason occurs in the colder months of the year. It may also follow measles or scarlet fever.

Organisms causing the condition are generally the pneumococcus, *Hemophilus influenzae* or the hemolytic streptococcus. In older children infected adenoid tissue around the opening of the eustachian tube may be responsible for recurring otitis media. Allergy may also be involved in recurrent otitis media.

Otitis media is most common in infancy because the eustachian tube, lying between the pharynx and the middle ear, is shorter, wider and straighter than in the older child. A contributing factor is that the infant lies flat in bed during the greater part of the day, and infected material is carried more readily through the canal.

Clinical Manifestations, Diagnosis, Course and Complications. The first stage of otitis media is due to swelling of the mucous membrane and consequent closing of the eustachian tube. Congestion, serous exudation and infection of the middle ear follow.

The *symptoms* are nasopharyngitis (inflammation of the nasopharynx) with pain, which is augmented as exudation occurs and fluid pressure increases in the middle ear.

The *diagnosis* is made by examination of the eardrum with the otoscope. The drum appears bulging and lacks its normal luster. Later the bony landmarks and cone of light are obliterated. If the tympanic membrane has ruptured, a culture may be taken from the drainage from the middle ear.

The older child will complain of severe, sharp pain in the ear, but the infant often has no great discomfort and may cry very little. He is likely to rub his ear, however, as if something there annoyed him.

The *course* of the infection is rapid. There is fever, commonly up to 104°F., with possible convulsions in the infant and chills in the older child. The little child is restless and fretful and suffers from gastrointestinal disturbance and anorexia. Fever and pain continue until the inflammation is reduced by adequate treatment, or the eardrum ruptures spontaneously and the exudate is released.

Complications are rare and may result from insufficient therapy. They include chronic otitis media, meningitis, mastoiditis, brain abscess, lateral sinus thrombophlebitis or thrombosis, and septicemia. A chronic condition with a perforated eardrum may lead to impaired hearing or deafness in the affected ear (see p. 440). If mastoiditis occurs, a mastoidectomy may be done.

Treatment. Nose drops are used to shrink the mucous membrane and provide drainage from the blocked eustachian tube. Measures for relief of pain include the application of dry heat to the ear, instillation of warm glycerin or oil into the ear and the giving of aspirin. *Myringotomy,* i.e. a clean elliptical incision of the tympanic membrane, or aspiration of the middle ear may be performed to relieve pressure and prevent the ragged opening made by spontaneous rupture. After a myringotomy, puncture or spontaneous rupture of the drum the physician will probably order irrigations of the ear with hydrogen peroxide. Cultures of the organism will determine the appropriate antibiotic to use.

Nursing Care. Nursing care is based on both the characteristics of little children and the plan of treatment ordered by the physician. The general local treatments will probably include the following.

INSTILLATION OF GLYCERIN OR OIL. The nurse places the infant with his head turned so that he lies upon the unaffected ear, and the ear into which the drops – warmed – are to be instilled in a position for the drops to run down the external canal onto the eardrum. A second nurse may be necessary to hold his head and restrain his hands, or a mummy restraint may be used.

EAR IRRIGATIONS. For these treatments it is necessary to "mummy" the infant unless his mother or another nurse is available to hold him. If the child is under three years of age, the auricle is pulled down and back – if over three years, up and back – in order to facilitate the passage of the fluid onto the drum.

LOCAL HEAT. A hot-water bottle (the water temperature not above 115°F. and the bottle encased in a cotton flannel bag) may be placed under the ear and the child kept upon the affected side.

CLEANLINESS OF THE EAR CANAL. The nurse should wash her hands before touching the ear in order to prevent a mixed infection resulting from her carrying bacteria into the canal. If myringotomy is done or spontaneous rupture of the drum occurs, the physician may request that the purulent material from the external auditory canal be removed by cotton cones or pledgets moistened with physiologic saline solution or hydrogen peroxide. (Some physicians prefer, however, that this not be done.) The area is then wiped dry with sterile cotton.

CARE OF THE SKIN. If the discharge is profuse, the skin around the ear should be covered with cold cream or zinc oxide to prevent impetigo or irritation. If the skin itches, the child's hands should be restrained to prevent scratching and spread of the infection.

USE OF AN EAR WICK. If an ear wick is used, it should be small, inserted loosely and changed frequently. If cotton is packed into the ear too tightly, free drainage cannot occur, and infected material may be forced into the mastoid area. If the infant is placed on the affected side, drainage will be promoted.

OBSERVATION FOR COMPLICATIONS. The nurse should watch for symptoms of complications such as mastoiditis or meningitis or evidence of the less common complications listed above. In some children after the acute infections have been treated, smoldering, low-grade chronic infections of the mastoid bone lead to loss of hearing (see p. 440). Accurate observation is necessary, therefore, to prevent this problem.

Prevention. The most important means of preventing otitis media is by prevention and treatment of the common cold (see p. 288). In older children it may be necessary to remove hypertrophied and infected adenoid tissue.

Serous Otitis Media

Serous otitis media is manifested by an accumulation of uninfected serous or mucoid material in the middle ear. The cause of this type of otitis media is not known, although it is believed that a respiratory allergy may be involved, or the eustachian tube may be blocked. The child has no pain or fever, but may complain of the ear feeling "full." Permanent hearing loss may result.

Treatment includes the use of nasal vasoconstrictors and oral decongestants containing antihistamines. Audiograms should be done periodically to determine the degree of hearing loss.

If deafness becomes a problem, repeated needle aspiration of the middle ear may be necessary, or as a last resort small plastic tubes may be inserted through the tympanic membranes to provide constant palliative drainage. This is a difficult problem which requires the services of the pediatrician and the otolaryngologist.

Acute Bronchiolitis and Interstitial Pneumonitis

These two terms are used interchangeably, especially in speaking of the disease in infants and children. It is difficult to think of a pure bronchiolitis without involvement also of interstitial tissue. In bronchiolitis, expulsion of air from the air sacs is blocked; the result is overdistention of the lung, dyspnea and cyanosis.

Incidence, Epidemiology and Etiology. The majority of infections occur in the first six months of life and are infrequent in children more than two years of age.

The condition occurs most frequently in winter and early spring. Many cases occur sporadically, but there is an increase in the number of infants who contract acute bronchiolitis when there is an epidemic of upper respiratory tract infections among school children and adults. Sex and race do not influence susceptibility to bronchiolitis.

No one organism is always responsible for the disease. A virus would appear to be the causative agent. The respiratory syncytial virus (RS) has been implicated in the illness of infants having bronchiolitis, especially in the winter.

Clinical Manifestations, Diagnosis and Differential Diagnosis. *Symptoms* of bronchiolitis occur several days after an infection of the upper respiratory tract and vary in severity. Respiratory symptoms are more severe than those of toxicity. The infant has a dry, persistent cough with increasing dyspnea. There is widespread inflammation of the bronchial mucous membrane. The mucosa swells, and a thick exudate is produced. Since air can enter the alveoli on inspiration, but is not expelled on expiration, it is trapped in the lungs each time the infant breathes, and the chest becomes overdistended. There is retraction on inspiration, but the chest collapses poorly on expiration.

The temperature is variable, ranging probably between 100 and 101°F. There is no relation between fever and the clinical severity of the disease.

Vomiting and diarrhea are not likely to be severe, but since dyspnea interferes with sucking, feeding may be a problem. The infant is alert, but appears irritable and anxious. The respirations are rapid and shallow and have a characteristic expiratory grunt. The accessory muscles of respiration are used, and there is suprasternal and subcostal indrawing with inspiration. As the lungs become more distended, the alveoli can no longer aerate the blood. Cyanosis may be severe, or the infant may be pale. Rales may not be present or may be scattered and fine, owing to small areas of pneumonia. Chest sounds, termed "wheezing," are common. Dehydration may be severe because of the infant's failure to take fluids and because of loss of water through hyperventilation.

Fluoroscopic and roentgenographic examinations show obstructive emphysema of varying degrees with or without scattered parenchymal infiltration. The white blood cell count is normal. No specific organisms are cultured from the nasopharynx.

The disease has many symptoms which make it difficult to differentiate it from a number of other diseases, among them asthma, cystic fibrosis with pulmonary changes, miliary tuberculosis, pertussis, aspiration of irritating substances and salicylate poisoning.

Prognosis and Complications. The *prognosis* is usually good if the child has received adequate, prompt supportive therapy. The mortality rate is low, but death may occur because of exhaustion and anoxia.

Complications which may follow the acute condition are bacterial bronchopneumonia, otitis media, pulmonary atelectasis with abscess, and cardiac failure.

Treatment. The treatment is aimed primarily at maintaining full oxygenation of the blood. The child requires an atmosphere of high humidity. (Cold vapor is better than hot steam.) This liquefies the secretions and makes it easier to cough up the mucus which fills the air passages. Oxygen therapy should be given to infants with even moderately severe dyspnea before cyanosis appears. Bronchoscopic aspiration may be done if the exudate has accumulated in the tracheobronchial tree. The infant's head and chest should be slightly elevated. In this position respirations are easier because the abdominal organs do not press against the diaphragm. Antimicrobial therapy is used only for infants having a bacterial complication. Large amounts of sedatives or opiates are dangerous, since they tend to depress the cough reflex and respiratory centers. Small amounts of sedatives, however (e.g. phenobarbital), may be given to quiet a child in a Croupette. The fluid intake should be increased. Water-soluble vitamins should be given.

Nursing Care. In planning the nursing care of the acutely ill child his physical and emotional status must be considered. In addition, the emotional reaction of his parents and his nurses cannot be disregarded.

The parents are anxious and fearful and possibly blame themselves for the child's condition. They feel helpless because of their lack of knowledge of the disease, its treatment and nursing care. They may be fearful because of separation from the infant and the financial problem of his hospitalization. They need to have the plan of treatment explained to them and to receive both emotional support and reassurance.

The student nurse may be anxious when caring for a seriously ill infant, and fearful about handling equipment and carrying out procedures which are new to her. By discussing her plan of care and by actually carrying her plan out under the supervision of her instructor, she may overcome some if not all of her feelings of anxiety in such situations.

SPECIFIC CARE. A Croupette is extremely useful in the care of these children (see Fig. 13-1). It provides high humidity and oxygen at a temperature comfortable for the child. The Croupette aids the child's breathing through the higher oxygen content and liquefies secretions in the bronchioles, making coughing less distressing to the child. Air under pressure may be used to provide increased humidity if oxygen is not necessary.

The canopy of the Croupette is made of clear plastic; therefore the nurse can observe the infant easily. Distilled water is used to provide humidity for the child when oxygen or air is passed through it. The bottle containing the water must be thoroughly cleaned each time it is refilled. The container at the back of the Croupette is for the ice which cools the tent. A blanket may be placed over the sheet to absorb the increased moisture from the humidity in the Croupette. An impervious mattress cover is placed under the sheet to prevent the loss of oxygen, which is heavier than air.

The blankets and the child's clothing must be changed when they become damp so that he may not become chilled. This should be done with as little disturbance as possible, and the

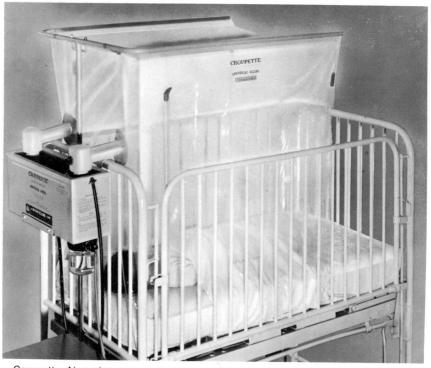

Figure 13–1. Croupette. Air under pressure instead of oxygen may be used to produce water vapor. (Air Shields, Inc., Hatboro, Penna.)

time should be planned to fit into his schedule of feeding and medication.

Complete *charting* of the procedure is important. The date and the time when the child was put into the Croupette and when taken out should be recorded, as well as the amount of oxygen concentration used. It is important to record the infant's response to this therapy as shown by his color, the nature of his respirations and the degree of his restlessness.

If the child is old enough to understand, the procedure of care in a Croupette is explained to him. A favorite toy may be given to keep with him in the Croupette.

Any secretion in the nostrils should be removed. Secretions tend to force the infant to breathe through his mouth. Cotton cones should be used for this procedure.

The fluid intake should be increased through offering water between feedings. If the infant cannot be taken from the Croupette, the nurse should support his head and back with one hand while she holds his bottle with the other. The hole in the nipple should be large enough so that he will not have to suck vigorously to get his feeding, but not so large that there is danger of his aspirating formula coming too rapidly into his mouth.

Water-soluble vitamins, antibiotics and sedatives are given as ordered by the physician.

The nurse should remember that the infant's breathing is labored and should give medications very slowly, raising the infant's head as they are given.

Aspiration of Foreign Bodies

Etiology, Pathology, Clinical Manifestations and X-ray Findings. Small objects which an infant puts into his mouth may be aspirated. Such objects include safety pins, peanuts, beads, and parts of toys, such as the button eyes or squeakers of stuffed animals. Carelessness of mothers and nurses in leaving small objects within an infant's reach or giving him toys unsuited to his stage of development is most often the cause of such accidents.

Some objects are radiopaque, others nonopaque. If they can be located by x-ray study, removal is facilitated.

The lesion resulting from aspiration depends upon the object and upon the degree of obstruction of the air passages it causes. Very small objects may cause little difficulty if they do not obstruct the larynx or a bronchus. Yet an obstructive object may produce atelectasis, bronchiectasis, pulmonary abscess or empyema.

A particle of food may lodge in the bronchus and cause an obstructive inflammatory condition involving eventually the distal respiratory tract. In that case the infant would have a cough, fever and continued dyspnea.

The *clinical findings* may be given meaning by the parents' telling of the infant's playing with a small object which later could not be located.

The immediate symptoms are choking, gagging, coughing and inspiratory stridor. The signs are laryngeal and tracheal in origin. The child may have stridor, dyspnea and hoarseness. If the foreign body is large enough to cause obstruction, cyanosis may occur.

If the foreign body is radiopaque, its location and form can be identified by the shadow it casts on a roentgenogram; the location of a foreign body not radiopaque can be identified by the effects it produces in the trachea or bronchus.

Course. Bronchial obstruction has serious consequences. A foreign body lodged in a bronchus must be removed promptly. If it is allowed to remain more than a few days, it will cause a local purulent infection and a pulmonary abscess. Eventually atelectasis, emphysema and diminished breath sounds will occur. There will be unequal motion of the sides of the chest on respiration.

Treatment. Laryngoscopy or bronchoscopy, if done in time, will permit removal of the foreign body. If the object has lodged in the larynx or trachea, tracheotomy (see p. 406) may be necessary to keep the airway open until further treatment can be given.

A secondary infection should be treated with antimicrobial agents according to the laboratory sensitivity tests done on specimens of the organism involved.

Prognosis. The prognosis is good if there is prompt diagnosis and removal of the object. Nevertheless serious conditions or death may result.

Prophylaxis. Prophylaxis is evident. Keep small objects such as toys with small movable parts, safety pins or nuts out of infants' reach. Older children should not give an infant food which he may put into his mouth in such large quantities that he chokes upon it, or objects which may be aspirated if they cannot be eaten. It is not safe for little children to play with the baby unless the mother is there to supervise them. Adults should not set a bad example by putting pins or other objects in their mouths, for small children tend to imitate people about them and will do likewise.

Lipoid Pneumonia

Incidence, Etiology and Clinical Manifestations. Lipoid pneumonia occurs most frequently in weak and debilitated infants. The condition is caused by aspiration of oils or lipoid material. Vegetable oils are less irritating than animal oils. When oily nose drops are used or when the infant is given such substances as cod liver oil while crying, there is danger of aspiration. A child with defective swallowing ability, e.g. a cleft palate, or a child lying flat in bed without his shoulders and head elevated by a pillow or the nurse's arm is liable to aspirate formula or food while feeding. If this contains lipoid material, lipoid pneumonia may result.

The onset is insidious. There is first an interstitial proliferative inflammation, followed by a chronic proliferative fibrosis. In the last stage there are multiple localized nodules in the lungs.

The *clinical manifestations* are not characteristic of this condition alone. Thus diagnosis is difficult. The infant has a dry and nonproductive cough, his respirations are rapid, and he is dyspneic. Unless there is a superimposed infection, he has no fever or leukocytosis. Bronchopneumonia is a common complication, however.

The roentgenogram shows characteristic features of this condition.

Treatment, Nursing Care, Prognosis and Prevention. There is no specific remedy for lipoid pneumonia, and a mild form of the disease may persist for several months before the child recovers.

Since there is no specific treatment, *nursing care* is all the more important. The child's position should be changed frequently to prevent hypostatic pneumonia. The child should be isolated to prevent his contracting a secondary infection from other children or adults.

The *prognosis* depends on the degree of pulmonary damage and on the severity of any secondary infection.

Prevention is negative rather than positive. Intranasal medication with an oil base is not to be used. The child should receive no vitamins in an oil base, no mineral oil or castor oil.

If the infant is apt to vomit or regurgitate, he should be placed on his side or abdomen after being fed to prevent aspiration of fluid.

GASTROINTESTINAL CONDITIONS

Foreign Bodies in the Gastrointestinal Tract

Etiology. An infant still in the oral phase of development enjoys putting objects into his mouth. As he sucks upon a small object, he may swallow it. Objects which do not stick in the esophagus, but reach the stomach, will generally pass through the intestinal tract. Some objects, however, do not pass through the pylorus and around the bends of the intestine, but become lodged at some point. Sharp objects—needles, bobby pins, hairpins, open safety pins, and the like—may

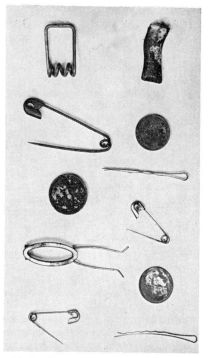

Figure 13-2. Some foreign bodies which failed to pass spontaneously and had to be removed by laparotomy, mostly from the stomach and duodenum. (Gross: *The Surgery of Infancy and Childhood.*)

perforate the intestine. Objects within the stomach can usually be removed gastroscopically.

Treatment. There is no specific treatment if gastroscopic removal of the object is not done. A normal diet is continued; neither a "cotton diet" nor laxatives are used today. Roentgenograms are taken daily. If the object is shown to be moving along in the intestine, perforation is not likely; but if the object is shown to be stationary, operation may be indicated because of the dangers of ulceration and perforation of the bowel. The nurse should watch closely for signs of perforation: nausea, vomiting, blood in the stools, rigidity, or tenderness of the abdomen or evidence of pain. If the physician believes that perforation has occurred, operation is done at once.

Nursing Care. There is no specific nursing care other than close observation of the child for signs of perforation and observation of the stools. The stool should be placed in a fine-meshed sieve and water run with force upon it until the fecal matter disintegrates and an object, if present, is easily seen.

Boric Acid Poisoning

Poisoning by boric acid results from either ingestion of the substance or its use as a powder or ointment on the infant's skin, usually in the diaper area. Symptoms of nausea, vomiting, abdominal pain, diarrhea, and a rash with desquamation of the skin occur. Signs of meningeal irritation, convulsions and coma may follow. The mortality rate in infants is approximately 70 per cent.

Treatment of boric acid poisoning is symptomatic, although exchange transfusion or hemodialysis may be used. Prevention (see p. 418) can be accomplished largely through parental education.

Vomiting and Diarrhea

Vomiting and diarrhea are clinical manifestations of a variety of disorders of infants and young children. These two conditions are together one of the main causes of morbidity among infants and children in many countries where sanitation and hygiene are poor and children are treated with folk remedies rather than with scientific medicine.

Unsanitary and unhygienic conditions have more serious consequences in infancy than in childhood because of the greater susceptibility to, and lesser ability to combat, infection. Vomiting and diarrhea in the infant cause a serious water loss with resulting electrolyte disturbance. Death is most often due to the effects of dehydration and to acid-base imbalance.

Before the student can understand the seriousness of these effects it is important to review certain fundamental concepts of fluid and electrolyte equilibrium and the causes and effect upon the infant of imbalance.

Fluid and Electrolytes. Each body cell is bathed in tissue fluid. The water and electrolyte composition of this fluid has a vital influence on the activity of the cell.

WATER. An adequate and continuous supply of water is a requirement for life in all human beings. Dehydration in the infant is more serious than in the adult, however. About 53 per cent of the body weight of the adult male is made up of water. Infants have an even higher proportion of water, in the newborn being 70 to 83 per cent. But in the first six months of life the proportion of water to body weight declines rapidly. Since fat essentially contains no water, there is a greater proportion of water to body weight in the thin person, whether an adult or an infant.

Water within the body is held in compartments separated by semipermeable membranes. These compartments are of three types, according to the kind of fluid they contain: (1) cellular or *intracellular* fluid (water within the cells), (2) *extracellular* fluid (water within the blood vessels or intravascular water contained in plasma), and (3) *interstitial* fluid (water in the tissues between vascular spaces and cells, which is similar to plasma in composition except that it has a lower protein content). During adult life about one third of the body water is outside the cells; during infancy and early childhood about half of the body water is extracellular.

SOURCE.   The main source of water is through ingestion of fluids and some solid food as vegetables and meats which contain large amounts of water. A second source is through metabolism. When foodstuffs are broken down into simpler elements, water of oxidation is formed.

WATER LOSSES.   Water in the normal healthy person is continually lost through the gastrointestinal tract in stools and saliva; through the skin and lungs, since body heat is removed by the vaporization of water (this volume of water varies greatly, depending on the person's activity, the temperature of the environment and individual make-up); and through the kidneys, whose excretion contains urea and other products of metabolism in combination with water.

In disease these losses may be increased, owing to fever, greater urinary output, diarrhea and vomiting. If, at the same time, a child ingests insufficient water, he will show signs of dehydration such as thick secretions, dryness of the mouth, loss of skin turgor, sunken eyes, loss of weight and concentrated urine.

Besides the difference in the proportion of total body water in cellular and extracellular compartments between infants and adults, there is a further difference. The infant takes in and excretes more water than the adult when these amounts are expressed in milliliters per kilogram of body weight. There are two reasons for these differences: (1) the basal heat production per kilogram is twice as high in infants as in adults. Because of this and because he has a greater body surface area in proportion to his size, the infant loses twice as much water per

kilogram as does the adult. (2) Because of the infant's greater metabolic rate, there is an increase in the products of metabolism and their elimination. Water must be used to eliminate these in greater urinary excretion.

Since the daily turnover of water in the infant is about half of his extracellular fluid volume, any fluid loss or lack of fluid intake depletes his extracellular fluid supply rapidly.

ELECTROLYTES.   It is easier for the student to understand the scientific basis of fluid balance in the body than the electrolyte balance. The following explanation is given as a review to help the student understand the therapy ordered for her patients.

Chemical compounds in solution may either remain intact or may dissociate. Examples of those whose molecules remain intact are dextrose, creatinine and urea. These are nonelectrolytes. Those that dissociate in solution break down into separate particles known as *ions*. Compounds which behave in this manner are known as *electrolytes*. They have gone through the process of ionization and have an important function in maintaining acid-base balance. Each of the dissociated particles, or ions, of an electrolyte carries an electrical charge, either positive or negative.

There are several biologically significant electrolytes. *Cations,* or positively charged ions in body fluid, include sodium (Na^+), potassium (K^+), calcium (Ca^{++}) and magnesium (Mg^{++}). *Anions,* or negatively charged ions in body fluid, include chloride (Cl^-), bicarbonate (HCO_3^-) and phosphate (HPO_4^{--}).

Each water compartment (see p. 294) has its own electrolyte composition which differs from that of the others. *Milliequivalents* (mEq.) indicate the number of ionic charges or electro-

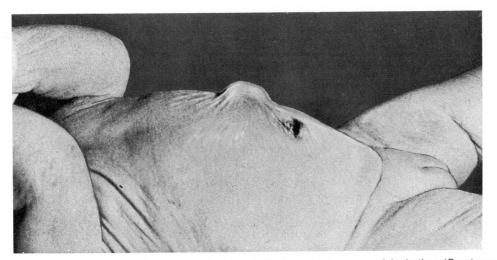

Figure 13–3.   Poor skin turgor. The skin has lost its elasticity, owing to severe dehydration. (Courtesy of Dr. Ralph V. Platou and the American Academy of Pediatrics.)

valent bonds in the ionized solution in each compartment. Although the electrolyte composition of the fluid in each of the compartments is known, in treatment of a particular patient measurement is made of electrolytes within the intravascular compartment, because blood samples are more readily obtainable for analysis. This does not give a true measurement of the electrolytes in the cellular space itself.

Sodium. Most of the sodium in the body is extracellular. The average daily intake of sodium equals the output. The average diet meets normal sodium requirements, but if additional amounts are required in therapy, isotonic sodium chloride in 0.85 to 0.9 per cent solutions and whole blood may be given.

Some sodium is excreted through the kidneys, skin and in perspiration. It is excreted in large amounts when the temperature surrounding the body is relatively high, and during bodily exercise, fever or emotional stress. Loss of sodium through the skin does not regulate sodium excretion; it is simply a by-product of temperature regulation of the body. Normally most of the sodium excretion is through the kidneys, which are the chief regulators of body sodium.

Hormones have a definite effect on sodium excretion. The pituitary antidiuretic hormone influences water resorption from the distal tubules. The adrenal cortical hormones, of which aldosterone is the most important, influence reabsorption of potassium and sodium, thus regulating the concentration of these ions in the blood stream.

Water exchange in the infant into and out of the cell is three to four times more rapid than in the adult. Since the sodium exchange is equally rapid, there are special problems in maintenance of a sodium balance in the infant.

Potassium. The main portion of potassium which is exchangeable is intracellular. The serum potassium ranges between 4.1 and 5.6 mEq. per liter. The daily turnover, intake and output of potassium are balanced, however. The average diet meets the potassium requirements of the body.

Potassium balance may be maintained at a low intake. Renal excretion of potassium, however, is accelerated by ACTH, desoxycorticosterone and cortisone.

The activity of all cells is influenced by the potassium concentration in the fluid around them. A high serum concentration of potassium produces a clinical effect on the heart muscle. A low extracellular potassium level may produce complaints of lassitude and weakness, and a loss of tone of both smooth and striated muscle may occur. Circulatory failure may be seen over a period of time.

Potassium should not be given to a patient until his renal function is adequate; otherwise the serum potassium may be raised to high levels. The main contraindications to potassium therapy are adrenal insufficiency and renal failure not relieved by treatment.

Acid-Base Equilibrium. One of the most important considerations in fluid and electrolyte therapy is the acid-base equilibrium or balance. Whether a solution is acid or alkaline depends on the concentration of hydrogen ions (H^+). If the concentration of hydrogen ions is increased, the solution becomes more acid; if the concentration is decreased, it becomes more alkaline. The amount of ionized hydrogen in solution is indicated by the concept of pH. A solution having a pH of 7 is neutral, since at that concentration the number of hydrogen ions is balanced by the number of OH^- ions present. As the hydrogen ion concentration falls, the pH value rises. In other words, an acid solution has a pH value under 7, and an alkaline solution a pH value greater than 7.

The extracellular fluid normally is slightly alkaline, having a pH from 7.35 to 7.45. If the pH rises higher than this, a state of *alkalosis* exists; if the pH drops below, a state of *acidosis* exists. In acidosis the body fluid may still be considered alkaline, although less alkaline than normal. If the pH of body fluid rises above 7.7 or falls below 7.0, the patient's life is in danger.

Normal function of the kidneys and lungs is important in maintenance of the acid-base equilibrium. The kidneys tend to excrete surplus ions and other substances so that acid products of metabolism are lost from the body. The lungs may vary the rate at which carbon dioxide is lost. If the plasma is too alkaline, the respiratory rate will decrease; if the plasma is too acid, the lungs will eliminate carbon dioxide, which is slightly acid, by increasing the depth or rate of respiration.

Another important concept is that of *buffer solutions.* A buffer solution is one which tends to soak up surplus hydrogen ions or to release them as necessary. They are therefore important in regulating the acid-base equilibrium in the body fluid.

There are several buffer systems in the body. Probably the most important one in the extracellular fluid is the carbonic acid⇌sodium bicarbonate system. A disturbance of acid-base equilibrium can be considered to be the result of imbalance in the carbonic acid⇌sodium (or some other base) bicarbonate system. These bicarbonates are found in the extracellular fluid in a ratio of one part of carbonic acid to twenty parts of base bicarbonate. The acid-base equilibrium and the normal pH of the body fluid are changed when this ratio is disturbed.

In a clinical situation a measurement of the blood concentration of bicarbonate will indicate the severity of the acid-base imbalance. The values of the carbon dioxide content or carbon dioxide-combining power are therefore determined. The normal carbon dioxide content of whole venous blood for an infant or child is approximately 18 to 27 mM. per liter. The normal carbon dioxide-combining power of whole venous blood for an infant or child is approximately 40 to 60 volumes per 100 ml. The equivalent values in *serum* from venous blood may be found in Table 3–2, p. 39. Acidosis is present when these values are below the levels given; alkalosis when the values are above these levels. In certain cases of acid-base disturbance these relations may be reversed.

Purposes of Fluid and Electrolyte Therapy. The physician may order fluid and electrolyte therapy for one or more of the following reasons: to provide for the basic nutrition of the patient, to provide a medium for medication, or to correct an electrolyte imbalance.

Fluid and electrolyte therapy is extremely important in the treatment of vomiting and diarrhea. When a child has either or both of these conditions, a replacement solution is given having an electrolyte content similar to that of the fluid being lost. Many such solutions to meet specific needs are available commercially.

ROUTE OF ADMINISTRATION OF FLUIDS. Size must always be considered when giving fluids to infants and children. If insufficient fluids are given, dehydration may continue. If too much fluid is administered by any route, the circulatory system may be overburdened and collapse may occur. In such a situation the child's heart may not pump fluid at the normal rate, and fluid will ooze from the vascular system to produce edema of the subcutaneous tissues or the lungs.

Diarrhea

Incidence. Diarrhea is a symptom of a variety of conditions which together constitute one of the main causes of morbidity and mortality among infants and children throughout the world.

Contaminated infant foods form a favorable medium for bacterial growth. In countries where the standard of living is low the infant death rate from diarrheal disorders is likely to be high. Breast feeding safeguards the infant from the main source of infection — contaminated milk. Although these general causes of diarrhea are known, the specific cause in any case is proved only by laboratory studies.

Etiology. In many cases of diarrhea the cause is difficult to determine. The following are generally recognized causes of diarrhea.

Faulty preparation of the infant's formula or other food or the technique of feeding may cause diarrhea. Among such factors are overfeeding, an unbalanced diet (unsuitable combination of protein, fats and carbohydrates — excessive sugar causes diarrhea) and spoiled food, often because of the lack of refrigeration and unsterile or unclean technique in the preparation of the formula or other foods.

Socioeconomic causes are difficult to determine. The incidence of contaminated milk and other foods as a cause of diarrhea is highest in the lowest socioeconomic group. In the higher socioeconomic groups the cause is more likely to be an infection by direct or indirect contact with someone who has the organism that causes diarrhea in the child. Causative organisms are pathogenic serotypes of *Escherichia coli* and various viruses, some of which cause respiratory illness in older children and adults. *Staphylococcus aureus* also causes diarrheal diseases, though sometimes the diarrhea occurs in connection with infections from this organism elsewhere in the body. Other organisms — the Shigella (Shiga, Flexner, Sonne-Duval and others), typhoid and Salmonella groups of bacteria — may be causative agents. Sometimes diarrhea results from administration of antibiotics; other organisms may overgrow in the intestinal tract because of a change in the normal flora as a result of antibiotic therapy. Such infectious agents include Proteus and Pseudomonas.

Other causes of diarrhea include allergy to certain foods, emotional excitement and fatigue or the unwise use of laxatives in infancy.

Diagnosis, Clinical Manifestations and Treatment. The *diagnosis* is made from the history and clinical evaluation. The causative factor may be learned from bacteriologic culture from rectal swabs taken at eight- to twelve-hour intervals and from bacteriologic cultures of stools. The laboratory studies usually include determining the carbon dioxide or carbon dioxide-combining power, and the hemoglobin, hematocrit, pH, sodium, chloride, potassium and nonprotein nitrogen values of the blood.

The *clinical manifestations* of mild diarrhea are different from those of severe diarrhea. Severe diarrhea is of two types, that with a gradual onset and that with an abrupt onset.

MILD DIARRHEA. The clinical manifestations are a low-grade fever, possibly vomiting, irritability and disturbed sleep. The warning that these symptoms are due to diarrhea is a change in the nature and number of stools (two to ten a day), tending to looseness and even fluid consistency. At this stage acidosis and dehydration are not severe, though 10 per cent of the body weight may be lost. Weight loss exceeding this is an indication of severe dehydration.

Treatment is by a reduction in the formula feedings, especially in fat and carbohydrate, in order to put less strain on the gastrointestinal tract. The fluid offered by mouth is increased. Five per cent glucose in saline solution may be given orally every three to four hours. In some cases the physician orders a brief period of starvation (twelve to twenty-four hours) followed by giving glucose in saline solution and, later, half-strength skimmed milk or skimmed lactic acid milk.

SEVERE DIARRHEA. The clinical manifestations of severe diarrhea with a *gradual onset* are elevation of temperature, with vomiting, anorexia and abdominal cramps. Diarrhea develops, the stools becoming greenish because of unchanged bile content, containing mucus and possibly tinged with blood. The stools become more frequent—two to twenty a day—and are expelled with force. The infant may be stuporous, have periods of irritability and may have convulsions. Because of dehydration the skin becomes dry and loses its turgor, the pulse is rapid and weak, the fontanels and eyes are sunken, the output of urine is decreased, and the weight loss may be as great as 25 per cent of the infant's former weight. These signs of dehydration are due chiefly to loss of interstitial fluid.

In acidosis the carbon dioxide level may be less than 10 volumes per milliliter. When the amount of urine is decreased and renal function is lost, acidosis is increased, since the kidneys fail to excrete acid-producing metabolites. The depth of respirations increases, while the rate may decrease or increase.

In severe diarrhea with *rapid onset* the temperature ranges from 104 to 106°F. The infant is in extreme prostration; he vomits, and toxic symptoms appear. He is irritable and restless and may have convulsions. Respirations are rapid and hyperpneic. The diarrhea is not as severe as that with gradual onset, but acidosis is present. Collapse is due to loss of intracellular water and diminution of plasma volume. Signs of collapse in the infant are pallor and a flaccid state. The death rate in this kind of diarrhea is high.

The objective of *treatment* in severe diarrhea is first to replace the water loss and restore the electrolyte balance. By comparing the child's weight with that before he became ill the approximate amount of water loss is ascertained. Laboratory studies will show electrolyte imbalance and the level of kidney function. Specifically, the objective of this initial therapy is restoration of renal function by means of a hydrating solution, without potassium, provision of fluid maintenance needs and making up for previous fluid loss by giving a balanced solution. During the initial therapy the infant may be starved for a period of possibly up to forty-eight hours.

Continuous intravenous therapy is used with the very sick infant because fluid will not be absorbed from subcutaneous spaces. Although whole blood transfusions are not given until the infant has been hydrated because of the greater concentration of blood during dehydration, plasma may be given.

When the infant is hydrated, fluids may be given subcutaneously. Hypertonic solutions should not be given, since they draw fluid into the area of clysis and may precipitate circulatory collapse. Hypotonic or isotonic solutions may be used, and hyaluronidase may be given into the site to promote absorption.

When the number of stools lessens and vomiting ceases, glucose and electrolyte mixtures may be started by mouth. Gradually, if no more diarrhea occurs, the concentration of fluids taken by mouth may be increased and fat and protein may be included until the dietary intake is normal within six to eight days. Diluted skimmed milk, lactic acid milk or breast milk may be used initially and gradually concentrated as the infant improves.

Specific chemotherapy is given as soon as the organism causing the diarrhea has been determined. If the diarrhea is accompanied by a parenteral infection, this condition must also be treated.

If the child has fever, a tepid sponge bath may be ordered to reduce the temperature and prevent convulsions. No sedatives or cathartics are given, since they may obscure or distort symptoms indicative of the child's condition.

Prevention. Breast feeding is probably the most important preventive of diarrhea, particularly among the lower socioeconomic group where other preventive measures are difficult to maintain. The proper method for making, storing and giving infant formulas should be taught all mothers, and the nurse should help the mother make the necessary adaptations to the equipment in her home. In hot weather the infant should be offered water frequently, but the food intake is temporarily reduced. The infant should be dressed according to the temperature and not the season of the year. In summer he should be kept as cool as possible, but dressed warmly if the weather turns cool.

The child should be kept from all contact with adults or children having infection, particularly of the alimentary tract, and an infant sick with diarrhea should be isolated to prevent the spread of infection.

Public health measures have a great deal to do with the incidence of diarrhea among infants. Safe sewage disposal, pure water and control of insects and pests are all part of good sanitation. The mother should be taught to make the best use of what she has in protecting the infant from health hazards in the environment which she cannot control. For instance, she should boil all water given to the infant, carefully cover his food to prevent contamination from flies, and place a mosquito netting over him during the seasons when flies and other insects are prevalent.

Nursing Care. Needs as a Basis for Care. When an acutely ill infant is admitted to the hospital, the nurse must be aware of the needs of the infant, the family and especially the mother. She should also be aware of her own needs in fulfilling her responsibilities in the care of the patient and his family.

The *needs of the infant* are paramount to all others; they are also more intimately within the nurse-child relationship. The infant must be given the means to satisfy his sucking needs, since feeding by mouth has been discontinued. He may be given a pacifier. If so, he should be bubbled in order to help him expel air which he may have swallowed. He will need to be comforted when his mother is unable to visit him.

He will need comforting also because of restraints necessary during intravenous therapy. An infant just learning to sit up and move about may find restraint very frustrating. Many of the treatments given him will be painful, and he will need the reassurance of his mother's presence. If she is unable to stay with him, one of the nursing personnel should give him the affection and attention he needs.

If nothing is given by mouth, his lips and tongue become very dry, and he will need mouth care. As long as he is dehydrated he will require special skin care to prevent lesions. He will need to have his position changed frequently, and passive exercise should be given, if possible, during periods of restraint.

The *needs of the mother and the family* cannot be listed in the order of their importance—all are important. The mother needs reassurance if she feels that the child's sickness is in some way her fault. She may feel that she has not been as careful as she should have been in preparing the feeding or in keeping the infant away from other children who had some infection. When she comes to visit the child or telephones to ask about his condition, she should be told of his progress. If his condition becomes worse, the physician should tell her this and take time to answer her questions. The mother may be worried over nonessential matters such as shaving the infant's head for intravenous therapy. Such procedures and the need for the treatment should be explained to her.

The mother may be worried about her ability to pay the hospital bill. If so, she may be referred to the social service department or the credit department of the hospital.

The nurse must think of the other children in the home and whether any of them may have the same infection as the infant.

The *needs of the nurse* are also important. She must maintain her own health at the optimum level so that she can adequately meet her responsibilities as a nurse and in her personal life.

The nurse will need factual information about diarrhea and its treatment so that she can give intelligent care when following the physician's orders and when giving care which promotes the aim of therapy, but is not prescribed by the physician.

Assisting with Venipuncture. The nurse will assist with venipuncture to obtain specimens for blood chemistry studies. Since infants do not have large veins in the antecubital fossa, blood must be obtained from the external or internal jugular vein (see p. 68, Fig. 4-11), femoral vein (see p. 68, Fig. 4-12) or, uncommonly, the superior longitudinal sinus. The nurse is responsible for positioning the infant so that blood can be drawn with the least difficulty for the physician and the least discomfort for the child. *Firm pressure should be applied for several minutes to the jugular or femoral vein after the needle has been withdrawn.*

A sterile syringe must be used because of the risk of reinjection of blood into the vein. A no. 20 or 22 needle may be used even though the smaller the bore of the needle, the greater the risk of clotting of the blood. If the specimen must be obtained under oil, sterile mineral oil may be used.

Mummy restraint is used with infants and young children during treatment and examinations involving the head and neck. The equipment needed is a square sheet or an infant blanket, depending upon the size of the child, and two safety pins. For the method of application see Figure 13-4; Figure 13-5 gives an alternate method. The young child will need to be reassured, for the procedure is more or less frightening, particularly if he knows that it is likely to be followed by an unpleasant or painful experience.

Assisting with Intravenous Fluid Therapy. If the infant has been vomiting, is unconscious or has anorexia or electrolyte imbalance, or if the physician wants to rest the gastrointestinal tract, intravenous therapy may be necessary. The fluids used for such therapy must be sterile, and have a neutral or nearly neutral chemical reaction and the same isotonicity as the interstitial fluid.

When fluids are given intravenously, the physician must take great care to calculate both the amount and the rate of flow. If the circulation is overloaded by too rapid administration or by too much fluid, fatal cardiac embarrassment may occur. With continuous intravenous therapy up to 150 cc. per kilogram a day can be given. Great difficulty is encountered if the nurse attempts to slow a regular intravenous drip to 4 or 6 drops per minute. Adapting devices may be obtained which produce a "mini" or "micro" drop of 1/50 to 1/60 ml. This results in the infant's receiving 50 or 60 mini- or micro-drops per cubic centi-

INTRAVENOUS SCHEDULE
7 A.M. to 7 A.M.

PATIENT __Marcia Allen__   DATE __November 21, 1964__

SPECIAL INSTRUCTIONS TO DOCTORS

1. Write fluid orders for 24 hr. period ending at 7 A.M. or portion thereof
2. Write for various solutions in order of their use. Order bottles by number in a consecutive numerical order.
3. Specify both drops per minute and number of cc's per hr. to be absorbed.

TO NURSES

1. Use this record whenever I.V. fluids are ordered.
2. Check I.V. every half hour on patients under 2 years of age. Record every hour on all patients.
3. Do not discontinue I.V. or let it run dry.
4. Notify doctor if unable to maintain schedule for two successive hours.
5. Notify doctor if I.V. infiltrates.
6. Give solutions in same order as written for.
7. Do not run I.V. at greater speed than has been ordered.

Amount to be absorbed by		Bottle #	Solution	Medication in Solution	CC's in bottle	Amount absorbed	gtt's per minute	Checked by
Run at 40 gtts per minute / Rate of Flow per Hour 40	7 A.M. 0	3	5% G/W	1,000,000 U. Aqueous Penicillin	140	(○)	40	C.L.
	8 A.M. 40	"	"	"	100	40	40	C.L.
	9 A.M. 80	"	"	"	60	80	40	C.L.
	10 A.M. 120	"	"	"	20	120	40	C.L.
	11 A.M. 160	4	5% G/½S	1,000,000 U. Aqueous Penicillin / 2 m.Eq. KCl	0/150	140	increased to 40	C.L.
	12 P.M. 200	"	"	"	110	180	40	C.L.
	1 P.M. 240	"	"	"	60	230	40	C.L.
	2 P.M. 280	"	"	"	20	270	40	C.L.
	2³⁰P.M.	5	5% G/¼S	1,000,000 U. Aqueous Penicillin	0/50/130	290	40	C.L.
	3 P.M. 320			1 cc Multivitamin	130	310		

8 Hr. TOTAL __310 c.c.__

Amount to be absorbed by		Bottle #	Solution	Medication in Solution	CC's in bottle	Amount absorbed	gtt's per minute	Checked by
Run at 40 gtts per minute / Rate of Flow per Hour 40	3 P.M. 0	5	5% G/¼S	1,000,000 U. Aqueous Penicillin / 1 cc Multivitamin	130	(○)	40	C.L.
	4 P.M. 40	"	"	"	90	40	40	J.Z.
	5 P.M. 80	"	"	"	50	80	40	J.Z.
	6 P.M. 120	"	"	"	10	120	40	J.Z.
	6¹⁵pm	6	5% G/¼S	1,000,000 U. Aqueous Penicillin / 2 m.Eq. KCl	0/150	130		J.Z.
	7 P.M. 160	"	"		120	160	40	J.Z.
	8 P.M. 200	"	"	"	80	200	40	J.Z.
	9 P.M. 240	"	"	"	40	240	40	J.Z.
	10 P.M. 280	7	5% G/¼S	1,000,000 U. Aqueous Penicillin / 2 m.Eq. KCl	0/150	280	40	J.Z.
	11 P.M. 320	"	"	"	110	320	40	J.Z.

8 Hr. TOTAL __320__

Amount to be absorbed by		Bottle #	Solution	Medication in Solution	CC's in bottle	Amount absorbed	gtt's per minute	Checked by
Run at 40 gtts per minute / Rate of Flow per Hour 40	11 P.M. 0	7	5% G/¼S	1,000,000 U. Aqueous Penicillin / 2 m.Eq. KCl	110	(○)	40	J.Z.
	12 P.M. 40	"	"	"	70	40	40	Σ P
	1 A.M. 80	"	"	"	30	80	40	Σ P
	2 A.M. 120	8	5% G/¼S	1,000,000 U. Aqueous Penicillin / 2 m.Eq. KCl	0/150	110	40	E.P.
	3 A.M. 160	"	"	"	110	150	40	E.P.
	4 A.M. 200	"	"	"	70	190	40	E.P.
	5 A.M. 240	"	"	"	40	220	40	E.P.
	6 A.M. 280	9	5% G/¼S	1,000,000 U. Aqueous Penicillin / 2 m.Eq. KCl	0/150	260	40	E.P.
	7 A.M. 320	"	"	"	110	300	40	E.P.

8 Hr. TOTAL __300__   24 Hr. TOTAL __930__

MF-16 REV

Figure 13–4. Record the nurse should keep on every child receiving intravenous therapy.

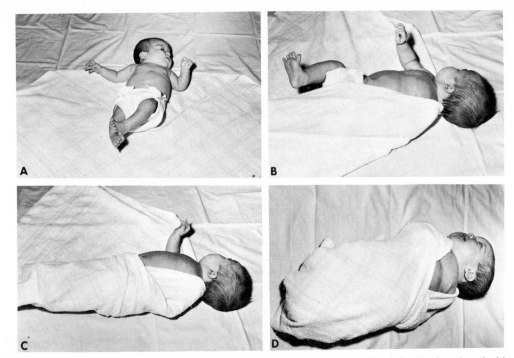

Figure 13–5. Mummy restraint. *A,* One corner of a small blanket is folded over. The infant is placed on the blanket with his neck at the edge of the fold. *B,* One side of the blanket is pulled *firmly* over one shoulder. *C,* The remainder of that side of the blanket is tucked under the opposite side of the infant's body. *D,* The procedure is repeated with the other side of the blanket. The blanket should be pinned in place. (Note: When applying a mummy restraint, be certain that the extremities are not forced into an uncomfortable position.)

meter instead of the 15 drops from the usual intravenous set. Some intravenous sets also have a control chamber which prevents the child from receiving too much fluid too rapidly.

The nurse must still, however, keep an accurate record, at least every hour, of the kind and amount of fluid given, the amount absorbed, the rate of flow or number of drops per minute and the amount remaining in the bottle. She must regulate the number of drops given so that too much is not given too quickly. The regulation of drops should be done when the infant is resting quietly. If it is done when he is crying, the tenseness of his muscles will constrict the blood vessels and cause the fluid to run slowly. Then, when he quiets down, the rate of flow will increase.

The nurse who assists the physician in starting intravenous fluids is responsible for restraining the infant so that the site to be used is immobilized. A mummy restraint can be applied if a scalp vein is to be used; a modified mummy restraint is adequate if another site such as a hand or foot is to be used. Because an infant's veins are very small, it is usual to select one over the temporal region of the skull. In that case the scalp must be shaved over the area. The nurse must hold his head turned to one side as for puncture of the jugular vein. If she presses her fingers against the bony skull and the prominences of the infant's face, she will be more successful than if she puts pressure only on the soft tissue. The head may then be pressed against the pad on the table or bed. Care must be taken to avoid interfering with the infant's breathing while restraining him.

After the physician has inserted the needle it may be supported with folded gauze and taped in place. The infant's head may be mobilized by placing a sandbag on either side; these are held in place by 2-inch strips of adhesive tape. The mummy restraint may be removed and the infant's arms restrained with arm restraints (Fig. 13-7) or clove hitch restraints (see Fig. 10-11).

Other veins in addition to those in the scalp may be used for giving fluids intravenously to infants. Veins in the back of the hands, flexor surfaces of the wrists, (see Fig. 14-1), feet, ankles or the antecubital fossa are used. It may be necessary to expose the veins by surgical dissection. A length of sterile plastic tubing is then inserted into the vein and sutured in place. The plastic tubing is connected with the infusion apparatus (Fig. 13-7).

Recently a needle has been marketed which permits the plastic tubing to be threaded through the needle, which is then withdrawn. With this procedure a cutdown is not necessary.

If the flow of fluid during continuous intravenous therapy is stopped for any reason, another vein will probably have to be used when it is started again. Since this involves repeating the entire procedure, the nurse responsible for

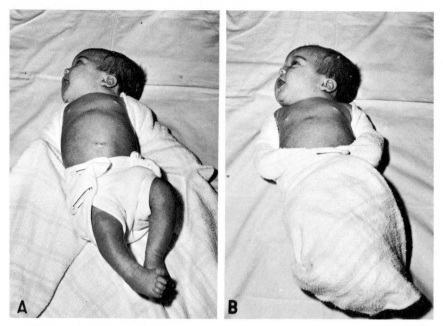

Figure 13–6. Alternate method of applying a mummy restraint so that the infant's chest is exposed. *A,* Pull the blanket firmly over both arms and tuck it under the infant's back. *B,* Wrap the legs in the remainder of blanket on both sides of the body and pin it in place.

checking should report any slowing in the flow to the physician, who may be able to establish a free flow again by flushing the needle.

The nurse is usually responsible for mixing intravenous fluids and adding medications when ordered. Careful aseptic technique must be used, and precise calculation of dosage of medication must be carried out. The nursing student must be supervised in this experience until she has become proficient in the technique. She should know the rules of the institution in which she is gaining experience concerning her responsibility in carrying out this procedure.

Sometimes the physician may order oral feedings to be started while the infant is still receiving fluids intravenously. If the needle is in a scalp vein and the physician does not want the infant removed from his crib, it is important that only clear feedings be given. There is serious danger, since the infant's head cannot be raised, that he might aspirate a little of a milk formula, with the possibility of lipoid pneumonia result-

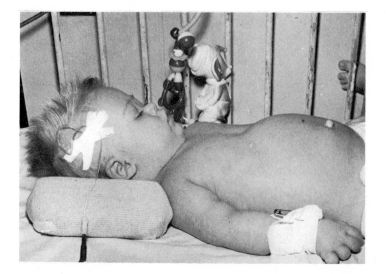

Figure 13–7. Venous cannulation. When the need for fluid administration is urgent and superficial veins are inaccessible, a vein must be cannulated with polyethylene tubing. Sandbags placed on both sides of the infant's head, and extremity restraint used to prevent the child's moving and dislodging the tubing. (R. Kaye, J. D. Bridgers and D. M. Picou: Solutions for and Techniques of Parenteral, Oral and Rectal Administration. *Pediat. Clin. N. Amer.,* Vol. 6.)

ing. If the needle is taped securely to the child's scalp, and with the permission of the physician, the infant can and should be held for his feedings.

SUBCUTANEOUS INFUSION. When ordering fluids to be given by subcutaneous infusion or clysis, the physician orders the total quantity of an isotonic solution on the basis of the child's size and bodily needs. The rate of flow is not ordered specifically as in intravenous therapy, because the flow is determined by the rate of absorption from the subcutaneous tissues. In order to facilitate absorption of such fluids, hyaluronidase may be injected into the area.

Various sites may be used for subcutaneous injection. In the infant the tissues of the pectoral region, the back, the lower part of the abdomen or the thighs are used. If the pectoral region is used, the mummy restraint which exposes the entire chest may be used to immobilize the child (Fig. 13-6). The needles are inserted lateral to and below the nipples. If the subcutaneous tissue of the back is used, the needles are inserted in the upper portion of the back and the fluid is injected from a large syringe. Fluids may be injected into the lower part of the abdomen if the infant is not to have abdominal surgery (such surgery is extremely unlikely in a child with severe diarrhea). The most frequent sites for subcutaneous injection are the anterolateral aspects of the thighs. The infant's arms and legs must be restrained with the clove hitch (Fig. 10-11) or extremity restraint (see Fig. 11-25).

A

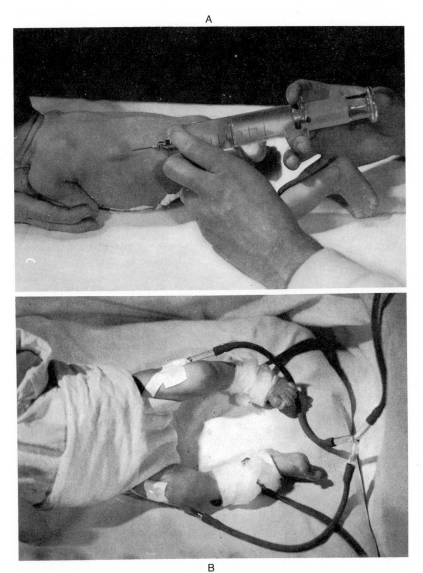

B

Figure 13–8. Hypodermoclysis into (A) tissues of back of a small baby, given with a needle and syringe. B, Common method of giving hypodermoclysis in thighs of babies. The ankles are restrained. Needles are inserted and strapped to each thigh. (Gross: *The Surgery of Infancy and Childhood.*)

Sterile technique must be observed throughout the procedure. Subcutaneous abscesses have sometimes developed after such treatments. The needle point should not be inserted near the femoral or saphenous vessels and should lie between the skin and muscle layers.

Whatever site is used, gentle massage will help to diffuse the fluid into the tissues. If the center of the injected area becomes pale, the position of the needle should be changed.

When an infant is receiving fluids by either the intravenous or subcutaneous route, it is imperative that the nurse recognize his needs for sucking pleasure and for love and attention. A pacifier, unless contraindicated, should be used for the satisfaction of the sucking need. The infant should be bubbled if possible in order to relieve him of swallowed air. This attention, as well as talking to him and playing with him, will relieve his distress so far as is possible during this treatment.

ORAL FLUID THERAPY. If the infant has a mild diarrhea or is recovering from a severe one, fluids may be given orally. The amount of fluid varies with the size and needs of the child. Infants should receive in excess of 125 cc. per kilogram of body weight if their current need and deficit are to be met.

A nurse who is skillful, patient and kind can usually encourage infants to take adequate amounts of fluid if they are physiologically well enough to do so. The nurse should offer at frequent intervals whatever formula or fluid is ordered. An infant who is able to take small amounts frequently will probably retain more than the infant who is encouraged to take too much at a time. Forcing fluids is to be discouraged, because such action too frequently leads to vomiting of all fluid taken.

Before giving the formula the nurse should check the physician's order in case the formula has been changed. After the infant has taken the fluid or formula the nurse should chart the following: type of feeding, amount taken, degree of appetite, occurrence of vomiting.

CHANGE OF POSITION. Change of position and passive exercise are necessary if the infant is restrained for long periods or is too ill to move himself. These measures not only increase his comfort, but also reduce the possibility of intercurrent infection.

SKIN CARE. If vomiting occurs, the skin of the infant's neck and face should be cleansed and carefully dried to prevent excoriation. The skin of the buttocks should be cleansed after changing the diaper to reduce the danger of irritation and a breakdown of the skin. Oil or a bland ointment may be applied after the cleansing. If the skin does become excoriated, the infant should be placed on his abdomen and his buttocks exposed to the air. The nurse must observe a debilitated infant frequently so as to prevent suffocation when he is lying in this position.

Besides exposing the buttocks to the air, a light treatment may be given. All oil should be removed from the skin before the treatment. A 25-watt bulb should be put in a gooseneck lamp clamped to the bed. The lamp should be about 1 foot above the patient, and the buttocks are exposed to the heat for thirty minutes several times a day according to the infant's condition. Care must be taken that the bulb does not touch the bed linen and set fire to it.

BODY TEMPERATURE CONTROL. The infant's temperature should be taken by axilla to prevent undue stimulation of the intestines through irritation of the rectum by a rectal thermometer.

If the infant has a fever, a tepid sponge bath may be necessary. If his temperature is subnormal, additional blankets should be placed over him and tucked about his body. A hot-water bottle (water temperature 115°F.) properly covered may be applied. The hot-water bottle should be examined for leaks before being used. A small infant may be placed in an incubator.

STOOL COLLECTION AND CULTURE. The physician may request that the infant's stools be kept for his inspection. The nurse should wrap the most recently soiled diaper in newspaper or place it in a container for this purpose, discarding the previous specimen. She should always chart the following characteristics of each stool: color, size, consistency, presence of blood or pus, and odor. If a stool culture is ordered, a culture of the freshly passed stool or from the rectal area is taken, depending on the custom of the hospital. In either case a sterile applicator should be used, and the specimen placed in a sterile test tube and sent to the laboratory immediately.

The *frequency of voiding* should also be recorded. Although the amount cannot be measured, it can be estimated.

CARE OF THE LIPS. Since the lips are dry, owing to the dehydration, cold cream should be applied.

ISOLATION TECHNIQUE. Isolation technique, including gown technique, should be followed if the diarrhea is infectious and is spread by fecal contamination. Strict isolation is necessary to protect the other children in the area and the personnel. All persons coming in contact with the patient should wear a gown. All equipment used frequently, such as a thermometer or baby oil, should be isolated with the infant. In the majority of hospitals the laundry is equipped to handle contaminated linen, but if the nurses are to sterilize it, the common procedure is to boil it for ten to fifteen minutes. Feces, urine, vomitus and liquid food waste may be emptied into the sewage in communities with adequate sanitary disposal. In a rural neighborhood or where such facilities are not available contaminated material should be mixed thoroughly with equal volumes of 10 per cent formalin solution or chlorinate of lime, or phenol or cresol in 5 per cent solution, and allowed to stand for at least an hour. Nursing bottles and nipples must be boiled after use. There should be netting over the infant's bed, and screens on doors and windows during the fly season.

If the mother cares for the infant, she must be cautioned to keep her fingernails short so that she will be less likely to carry pathogenic organisms on her hands, and should wash her hands thoroughly after caring for the infant. Nurses should teach the mother the elements of isolation technique so that she can follow the necessary precautions when she visits the infant and avoid carrying infection to the children at home (see p. 63).

PREVENTION OF INFECTION OF THE NURSE. The nurse must remember that she herself may become infected through a break in her technique when caring for the child or his equipment. She must keep her own nails short and clean and wash her hands thoroughly after caring for him.

Vomiting

One of the most common symptoms in infancy and early childhood is vomiting. No attention need be paid to the occasional vomiting of the healthy infant, but an infant who vomits frequently requires medical attention. Persistent vomiting may be serious not only because of its etiologic significance, but also because it results in dehydration and electrolyte imbalance leading to alkalosis. Convulsions and tetany may occur if alkalosis is severe. Alkalosis resulting from severe vomiting is due to a loss of chlorides and potassium. The intracellular fluid has gained sodium ions and lost potassium ions. Potassium ions must be provided in adequate amounts if the normal balance within the cell is to be regained. As soon as renal function and hydration are assured, potassium must be given.

Ultimately, if the infant is not treated and fails to retain any fluid, he may show signs of the ketosis of starvation. Because of the serious consequences of vomiting, every effort should be made to find the cause and to institute immediate treatment.

Vomiting Due to Physical Causes. Faulty feeding technique is the cause of vomiting in healthy, contented infants. Overfeeding leads to gastric distention, which in turn results in regurgitation of the excess formula. *Regurgitation* is the type of vomiting in which the formula comes up in small amounts and drools from the infant's mouth.

The *treatment* for infants who cannot take and retain a large amount of formula is to concentrate the formula so that the stomach will not be overdistended, and yet the infant will ingest the needed calories. If the infant is on a self-demand schedule and takes too much too frequently, reduction of the frequency of feeding tends to reduce vomiting. If he swallows the feeding too rapidly, so that none leaves the stomach before all is taken, overdistention may result. These infants should be fed from a nipple with a smaller hole so that the feeding may pass slowly from the stomach into the intestines while they are nursing. If an infant swallows air in large amounts, the stomach will be overdistended, and vomiting will result. The infant should be bubbled frequently to expel air during the feeding. After he has taken all his formula he should be placed on his abdomen or right side so that formula may pass from the stomach into the intestines and air may more readily escape; thereby the eructed air will be less likely to force milk before it through the esophagus and out of the mouth. Air forced ahead of the milk into the intestines will cause abdominal distention and pain.

Sometimes infants will vomit because of mucus collected in the back of the throat. A preventive measure is aspiration of the nasopharynx before offering the feeding.

Improper feeding leading to irritation of the stomach is a common cause of vomiting. Irritation of the stomach may result from a formula which contains too much carbohydrate or fat. Excessive fat slows emptying of the stomach; fermentation takes place, and this leads to irritation. Prevention and treatment of the condition are by giving the infant a formula better suited to his nutritional needs.

Foods to which the infant is allergic or which are too highly seasoned, new foods or even lumps in the food, if he is unaccustomed to them, may cause him to vomit.

Vomiting associated with infections or conditions outside the intestinal tract is common. Among these are infections of the respiratory tract, ear and pharynx. To these should be added acute communicable diseases; e.g. vomiting often accompanies an attack of coughing in pertussis (whooping cough). When the infectious condition is cured, vomiting ceases. Infections of the gastrointestinal tract which produce diarrhea are likely to be accompanied by vomiting. Such vomiting ceases when the infection is treated successfully.

Conditions other than infections may produce vomiting because of increased intracranial pressure, e.g. hydrocephalus or intracranial hemorrhage. Such vomiting as well as that associated with encephalitis or meningitis is not associated with the feeding time, but is closely related to periods of increased intracranial pressure. The only treatment for this type of vomiting is to reduce the intracranial pressure.

Vomiting may be due to obstruction of the gastrointestinal tract. In the neonatal period vomiting may be due to congenital obstruction (see p. 177) of the intestines or bile ducts. Later, pyloric stenosis (see p. 307), intussusception (see p. 311), volvulus (see p. 177) and strangulated umbilical or inguinal hernia (see pp. 313, 312) may cause intestinal obstruction and vomiting. Treatment of the intestinal obstruction will cause this type of vomiting to cease.

Vomiting Due to Emotional Causes. Some vomiting is voluntary, as in *rumination*. Rumination is the voluntary bringing up of small amounts of food from the stomach within a short time after feeding. The food is brought back into the mouth by manipulating the tongue or putting the fingers far back into the mouth. The food may be reswallowed, but is more likely to drool from the mouth.

The causes of rumination are not known. It may be that the infant dislikes the food or the person feeding him. Rumination may be due to tension in the environment that prevents the feeding process from being satisfying to the infant. This may indicate disturbed parent-infant relations in which the infant lacks affection and probably attention. Whatever the cause, the habit of rumination may lead to death from starvation.

The treatment suggested at present lies in psychotherapy for the mother and increasing the amount of affection shown the infant. Playing quietly with him for some time after his feeding has often proved helpful. Fortunately it is a habit which he will drop if it can be prevented for a few weeks and the conditions which produced it are changed through a general improvement in his care.

Nursing Care. Vomiting is a symptom, and treatment should be directed toward correction of the cause. In addition to correcting the immediate cause of vomiting, parenteral fluid and electrolyte therapy may be indicated to correct dehydration and alkalosis.

In order to determine the degree of renal function and dehydration, the nurse should chart whenever the infant voids, giving the exact time and estimating the amount of urine voided. Only after the amount and frequency of voiding have been ascertained may potassium be given.

If the vomiting is persistent, drugs of the phenothiazine group such as promazine (Sparine) or chlorpromazine (Thorazine) may be given in the form of rectal suppositories. To give a rectal suppository the nurse must lubricate it, insert it gently into the rectum and hold the buttocks together until the tendency to expel it has passed.

The nurse must make friends with the infant so that he feels secure in her care and is relaxed while feeding. Treatments should never be given at feeding time.

The feeding technique should be followed with care. The correct position for feeding resembles the position when feeding at the breast. The infant's head and shoulders should be elevated while his body is cradled in the nurse's arms. Affection is shown by the gentle pressure of his body against hers. If the infant cannot be moved from the crib, his head and shoulders should be raised, if his condition permits, supported by the palm of her hand or her forearm. He should be fed slowly and bubbled frequently if he is in the nurse's lap. If he is fed in bed, he should be bubbled if possible, or allowed frequent intervals of rest. He will probably expel gas before the nipple is again inserted into his mouth. Elevating the head of the bed after feeding mechanically minimizes the tendency to vomit. The infant should be handled as little as possible after feeding, since rest inhibits or lessens the probability of expelling the feeding.

It is important to prevent aspiration of vomitus. The infant's head should be turned to the side so that the vomitus may run from his mouth. If the infant is placed on his right side or on his abdomen after feeding, his head is, of course, turned.

Skin care is important. The face should be cleansed and dried after the infant has vomited. Particular attention should be given to the folds of the neck and the skin behind the ears.

The charting of vomiting must be accurate. The nurse should chart the time in relation to feeding, the amount (estimated), odor, type, color and consistency of the vomitus, whether the infant appeared nauseated before vomiting, and the act of vomiting—whether rumination, regurgitation, vomiting without force or projectile vomiting.

Salmonella Infections

Incidence, Etiology, Pathology, Clinical Manifestations and Diagnosis. Salmonellosis is one of the major public health problems in the United States. The highest age-specific attack rates are for infants and young children.

One of the causes of diarrhea mentioned previously (see p. 297) was the salmonella bacteria. These infections are caused by a number of flagellated organisms related because of their antigenic structure. Specific organisms of the group cause typhoid-like infections in human beings. Infection usually occurs after the eating of contaminated food and may last a long time, especially in infants. Recently it was found that the family's pet turtle may bring the organism causing salmonellosis into the home. For this reason children should be taught to wash their hands thoroughly after handling their turtle.

The water in the turtle's dish should never be disposed of in the kitchen sink.

The chief pathologic changes include acute enteritis and superficial necrosis of the lymphoid tissue in the intestinal tract.

The *clinical manifestations* are headache, nausea and vomiting, abdominal pain, and diarrhea. Elevation of temperature, drowsiness and meningismus may occur. Death results from toxemia, extreme dehydration, and circulatory collapse.

Diagnosis is made on the basis of isolation of the organism and demonstration of a significant agglutinating titer of the patient's serum.

Complications and Prognosis. *Complications* may include osteomyelitis, meningitis, soft tissue abscesses, and bronchitis. The mortality rate depends upon early diagnosis and treatment.

Treatment and Nursing Care. Treatment and nursing care include strict isolation of infected patients, withholding of food by mouth and adequate administration of parenteral fluids. Chloramphenicol appears to be the drug of choice. It is sometimes used with tetracycline for combined antibiotic therapy in salmonellosis. The nursing care is that for a child having diarrhea and vomiting which was discussed previously.

When this diagnosis is made, the public health nurse should visit the home to help the mother prevent a recurrence of this infection and to determine whether any other member of the family has symptoms similar to those of the patient.

Congenital Hypertrophic Pyloric Stenosis

Incidence and Pathology. This is the most common surgical condition of the intestinal tract in infancy. It occurs most frequently in some family strains, in first-born infants and in males. It is uncommon among Negro infants.

Pathologically, there is an increase in the size of the circular musculature of the pylorus. The enlargement is usually about the size and shape of an olive. The musculature is greatly thickened, and the resulting tumor-like mass constricts the lumen of the pyloric canal. This impedes emptying of the stomach. The musculature of the stomach then hypertrophies, owing to the effort required to force the formula through the constricted pylorus.

Clinical Manifestations and X-ray and Laboratory Findings. The symptoms appear in infants two to four weeks old, and only then can the congenital condition be diagnosed. The initial *symptom* is vomiting, which occurs both during and after feedings. The vomiting is at first mild, but it becomes progressively more forceful until it is projectile. The vomitus does not contain bile, but may contain mucus and streaks of blood.

Since little of the feeding is retained, the infant is always hungry. He will take formula immediately after vomiting, only to vomit again. There is either failure to gain or loss of weight. The infant acquires the typical appearance of the starved child—he looks like a little old man. Because little food passes through the pylorus, the bowel movements decrease in frequency and amount. In some cases, however, a starvation type of diarrhea occurs.

The *signs* of pyloric stenosis are dehydration with poor skin turgor, distention of the epigastrium (in badly malnourished infants the outline of the distended stomach and peristaltic waves passing from left to right may be seen during and after feeding) (Fig. 13-9) and an olive-shaped mass, located by palpation, in the right upper quadrant of the abdomen.

Metabolic alkalosis occurs, owing to loss of hydrochloric acid and potassium depletion. There is an increase in the plasma carbon dioxide content and in pH, and a decrease in serum chloride.

If barium is added to the feeding, an *x-ray* film will show the enlargement of the stomach and the narrowing and elongation of the pylorus, increased peristaltic waves and an abnormal retention of the barium in the stomach. A film taken several hours after feeding shows that little food has left the stomach.

Laboratory findings show an alkaline, concentrated urine. Hemoconcentration is shown by elevated hematocrit and hemoglobin values.

Diagnosis and Complications. The *diagnosis* is generally made without difficulty; however, pyloric stenosis may be confused with pylorospasm (see p. 310).

Treatment. Few physicians recommend medical treatment for pyloric stenosis. If it is not successful, the infant's condition worsens and the danger from operation increases. If operation is performed early, however, the prognosis is excellent. But if medical treatment is carried out (it is not usually attempted in breast-fed infants), it is an extension of that for pyloric spasm.

Medical treatment is seldom prolonged unless there is definite evidence of improvement in the infant's condition.

MEDICAL TREATMENT. *Thickened Feedings.* These are mechanically more difficult to vomit than liquid feedings. Cereal or barley flour can be used to thicken the milk formula. A precooked cereal should be used, since the polysaccharides in it are broken down into simpler sugars. The feedings can be made in any desired degree of thickness. When the infant vomits directly after being fed, he should be refed. Some physicians order small-curd feedings such as those made with lactic acid solution added to whole milk.

Lavage. When there is gastric distention, lavage may be ordered to prevent further dis-

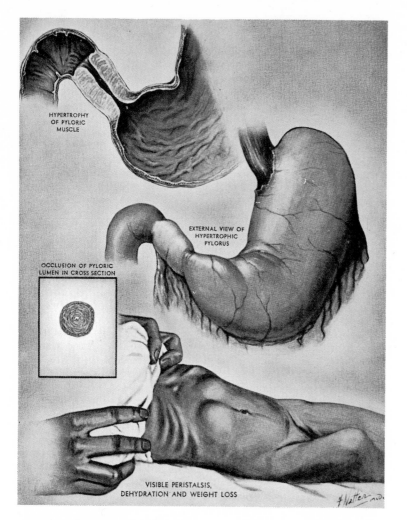

HYPERTROPHY OF PYLORIC MUSCLE

EXTERNAL VIEW OF HYPERTROPHIC PYLORUS

OCCLUSION OF PYLORIC LUMEN IN CROSS SECTION

VISIBLE PERISTALSIS, DEHYDRATION AND WEIGHT LOSS

Figure 13–9. Pyloric stenosis. (Copyright, The Ciba Collection of Medical Illustrations, by Frank H. Netter, M.D.)

tention with subsequent vomiting (see also p. 309).

Drugs. Antispasmodic drugs such as atropine or Eumydrin may be ordered to relax the smooth muscle of the pylorus. These drugs are given fifteen to twenty minutes before feeding. If atropine is ordered, a freshly prepared solution should be given. Most infants have a relatively high tolerance for this drug, though some may show signs of idiosyncrasy. The initial dose should be small and must be carefully measured to avoid overdosage. The dose is gradually increased until vomiting ceases, when it is gradually decreased. If the drug must be temporarily discontinued, a smaller dose is given when it is again administered. If flushing of the face, dilation of the pupils or fever occurs, the physician should be notified. He will probably discontinue the medication or reduce the dose.

Phenobarbital may be ordered for its sedative effect upon hyperactive infants. If heavy sedation or excessive drowsiness occurs, the dose should be decreased.

SURGICAL TREATMENT. Surgery consists in performing the Fredet-Ramstedt operation, or pyloromyotomy. This involves a longitudinal splitting of the hypertrophied circular muscle of the pylorus without incising the mucous membrane. When the lumen has been enlarged by this procedure, food can more readily pass through. If the pyloric mucosa is punctured at operation, there is danger of peritonitis due to the leaking of stomach secretions into the peritoneal cavity.

Preoperative Preparation. The fluid and electrolyte balance must be restored, since a dehydrated infant is a poor surgical risk. If fluid deficiency, electrolyte imbalance and blood losses are not corrected, shock may occur during operation. Replacement of fluid and electrolyte deficits should be made two or three days before operation. After the infant has been hydrated whole blood is given as needed. Vitamins B, C and K are given parenterally.

Just before operation a catheter is passed through the nose and into the stomach. Removal of stomach secretions and swallowed air ensures a deflated stomach during operation and reduces postoperative vomiting.

Nursing Care. PREOPERATIVE EXAMINATION. The nurse assists the physician in examination of the infant to determine the presence of gastric peristaltic waves visible through the abdominal wall. The equipment needed is a bottle of sterile water, a bib and a flashlight.

The procedure is simple. The infant is placed on his back with his face toward his left side. The abdomen is exposed. The bib is placed under his face. While the nurse gives the infant water the physician will hold the flashlight over the infant's abdomen from the left side. He stands on the right side of the infant and observes at the level of the abdomen. If peristaltic waves are present, they will be clearly visible.

PREPARATION AND TYPES OF FORMULAS. *Thickened Feedings.* The formula should be appropriate for the age of the infant. To it should be added varying amounts of pre-cooked cereal. The consistency of the thickened formula may be thin or such that it will not drop from a spoon. The physician will order the precise degree of thickening. A very thick formula may be fed from a teaspoon or may be pressed through a nipple with a large hole, or one from which the tip has been cut, with the bowl of a spoon or a tongue blade.

Fine-Curd Milk. Milk containing a very fine curd is usually prepared by adding acid or, less frequently, by fermentation through bacterial action. In fine-curd milk the casein is so altered that a softer and smaller curd is formed in the stomach. Such a curd is easier to digest and can more readily pass through a constricted pylorus. Lactic acid, U.S.P., may be added to a previously boiled cow's milk formula. The amount of acid ordered varies with the fat content; milk having a higher fat concentration requires more acid. Milk containing 3.5 to 4.0 per cent fat requires 6 cc. (1½ fluid drams) to the quart. Both the ingredients and the equipment must be cold to prevent too rapid curd formation. The acid should be diluted with a small amount of sterile water and added to the milk slowly with constant stirring. Commercial preparations of dried lactic acid milk may be purchased instead of preparing it in this way.

METHOD OF FEEDING. The infant should be fed slowly and bubbled frequently to prevent vomiting. He should also be bubbled before feedings to eliminate gas bubbles in the stomach. After feeding he should be handled as little as possible and moved very gently. He should be placed on his right side or abdomen, and the head of the bed raised slightly. If he vomits after the feeding, he should be refed if the physician so orders.

Charting of the feeding is important. His apparent hunger, whether he vomits—including the type and amount—the presence of peristaltic waves and whether he cries before or after vomiting should all be charted.

LAVAGE. Lavage may be ordered once or twice a day before feeding to cleanse the stomach of formula remaining from previous feedings.

The infant should be placed in a mummy restraint. A basin or pail should be placed on the chair beside the bed. A sterile catheter (size 10 to 12 French) is used, and is connected to a funnel by about 2 feet of rubber tubing. The catheter is lubricated with sterile water and passed rapidly through the infant's mouth into the stomach to a distance of 9 or 10 inches, i.e. from the tip of the nose to the tip of the sternum. If the catheter should pass into the larynx instead of the stomach, the infant would cough, breathing would become irregular and difficult, and cyanosis would occur. In such event the catheter should be withdrawn immediately. The nurse can be certain that the catheter is in the stomach if gastric contents appear in the tube and if the infant breathes normally.

Turn the infant on his left side and siphon off the stomach contents into the basin. Turn the infant on his back and pour an amount of physiologic saline solution or sterile water, a little less than that syphoned off, into the funnel. If the fluid does not flow, owing to air in the tube, "milk" the tube gently. Turn the infant on his left side, invert the funnel over the receptacle, holding it lower than the infant's head, and allow the fluid to drain off. Repeat the procedure until the returning fluid is clear. Usually 500 to 1000 cc. of fluid is used. Upon completion of the procedure, pinch the catheter tightly to prevent fluid from dripping into the pharynx as the catheter is removed.

Lavage is a trying procedure for the infant, and he will need to be held, cuddled and reassured before he is fed.

OTHER PROCEDURES. If drugs are given, the nurse should watch for evidence of overdosage. All symptoms should be carefully charted. If the infant has a fever, the physician should be notified at once.

The nurse may be asked to assist the physician with parenteral fluid therapy (see p. 299).

The infant should be weighed daily at the same time in the day's schedule. Accuracy is essential, for the weight roughly indicates the degree of dehydration and of malnutrition.

The infant must be protected from infection. Unless all other children with infection are isolated in the pediatric unit, the patient should be isolated for his own protection. Nurses and visitors with any infection should not come in contact with him.

The infant's position must be changed frequently to prevent hypostatic pneumonia. The infant must be kept warm, with blankets and hot-water bottles if necessary.

The charting of output is important and includes the color, frequency and estimated amount of voiding and the type and number of stools.

POSTOPERATIVE CARE. Fluids may be given

intravenously for the first few days after operation to meet the daily fluid requirements.

The infant's position is important. The infant should be kept on his right side or on his abdomen; this position aids digestion of fluids or formula because the pylorus is on the right side of the abdomen, and also prevents the infant from aspirating if he vomits. After the immediate danger of vomiting has passed, a fairly upright sitting position tends to prevent vomiting by making it mechanically difficult. The infant's position should be changed frequently, without disturbing him.

The nurse should note the indications of shock: rapid, weak pulse, cool skin, pallor and restlessness. If symptoms of shock appear, the foot of the crib should be elevated and additional warmth provided. It is important to observe the abdomen for distention. Distention might be due to air which the infant has swallowed, but it might also be caused by infection of the peritoneum.

Physicians vary in regard to details of postoperative feeding. Some physicians prefer a modified Down's regimen (Table 13-1), in which feedings are started four to six hours after operation. The infant is given small amounts of 5 per cent glucose and water orally at frequent intervals. This may be increased gradually. A dilute formula of half skimmed milk and water may be substituted for the glucose solution. The formula may be gradually increased in amount and thickened in consistency until the infant is taking the usual quantity for his size and age. If he vomits, a more gradual increase in volume or a temporary reduction in oral intake should be made.

If the infant was breast-fed, the mother's milk should be expressed and given as soon as he can tolerate it. He should be able to feed at the breast three to four days after operation.

The method of feeding is similar to that used preoperatively. A medicine dropper with a rubber tip may be used for the initial feedings, but the bottle or breast should be given as soon as possible in order to satisfy the infant's need for sucking. The bottle-fed infant should be held in the nurse's lap and cuddled before feeding as soon postoperatively as it is safe to handle him. The breast-fed infant should be held as usual, for he derives pleasure from this while satisfying his hunger and his need for sucking.

Prevention of infection of the wound is extremely important if a waterproof collodion dressing has not been used. The diaper should be placed low over the abdomen so as not to come in contact with the incision. If the penis is large enough, it may be taped to the thigh so that contamination of the incision does not occur when the infant voids.

Prognosis. The prognosis is excellent. Complete relief follows successful surgical repair. The mortality rate is low, provided operation is undertaken before the infant has become too dehydrated and malnourished.

Pylorospasm

In *pylorospasm* there is no structural defect of the pylorus. The spasm occurs in hyperactive infants, causing them to vomit frequently and often projectilely as in pyloric stenosis.

The *treatment* of pyloric spasm is by institution of proper feeding technique and administration of antispasmodic drugs such as atropine.

Table 13–1.   *Down's Regimen*

Name		Date	
No. Time of Feeding	Type of Feeding		Remarks
1. at _____	Give 30 minims of glucose water		
2. 30 min. later at _____	Give 1 dram of glucose water		
3. 30 min. later at _____	Give 2 drams of glucose water		
4. 30 min. later at _____	Give 2 drams of glucose water		
5. 30 min. later at _____	Give 2 drams of glucose water and 1 dram of milk*		
6. 1 hr. later at _____	Give 3 drams of glucose water		
7. 1½ hrs. later at _____	Give 2 drams of glucose water and 2 drams of milk		
8. 1½ hrs. later at _____	Give 4 drams of glucose water		
9. 1½ hrs. later at _____	Give 2 drams of glucose water and 3 drams of milk		
10. 1½ hrs. later at _____	Give 5 drams of glucose water		
11. 1½ hrs. later at _____	Give 1 dram of glucose water and 5 drams of milk		
12. 1½ hrs. later at _____	Give 6 drams of glucose water		
13. 1½ hrs. later at _____	Give 1 dram of glucose water and 6 drams of milk		
14. 1½ hrs. later at _____	Give 7 drams of glucose water		
15. 1½ hrs. later at _____	Give 1 dram of glucose water and 7 drams of milk		
16. 1½ hrs. later at _____	Give 1 ounce of glucose water		
17. 1½ hrs. later at _____	Give 1 dram of glucose water and 1 ounce of milk		
18. 1½ hrs. later at _____	Give 9 drams of glucose water		
19. 2 hrs. later at _____	Give 1 dram of glucose water and 9 drams of milk		

Then give 1 ounce of skim milk every 3 hours plus not more than 1 ounce of glucose water between feedings.

*Skimmed milk.

Sedation is helpful, and phenobarbital may be used. Some physicians may order the feedings to be thickened or small-curd feedings to be given (see p. 309).

The most common *complication* of pyloric stenosis is tetanic seizures resulting from metabolic alkalosis and a reduction in the free serum calcium.

Intussusception

Incidence and Etiology. Intussusception is an invagination of one portion of intestine into another. Intussusception and incarcerated inguinal hernia are two of the most frequent acquired types of mechanical intestinal obstruction in infancy. More than half of the children having intussusception are under one year of age. Most of the remaining cases occur in the second year, in male infants who were previously healthy.

The *etiology* is questionable. Often no cause is found. Hyperperistalsis may be responsible. Also the intestinal tract of the infant is freely movable, especially the cecum and ileum, making it easier for one portion to invaginate into another. The immediate cause may be diarrhea, constipation, polyps of the intestinal tract which act as a foreign body, or swelling of intestinal lymphatic tissue. Intussusception may at times occur around a Meckel's diverticulum (see p. 571).

Pathology and Clinical Manifestations. Usually the upper part of the intestine invaginates into the lower. Intussusception is classified according to its location. The majority of cases occur at the ileocecal valve.

The mesentery is carried into the lumen of the intestine, and the blood supply is cut off to the invaginated bowel. Edema results. In some cases reduction is spontaneous, but generally necrosis occurs at the site of intussusception. The strangulated portion may perforate, thereby causing peritonitis and death.

The *clinical manifestations* result from the acute intestinal obstruction. The onset in a healthy infant is sudden. The extent and severity

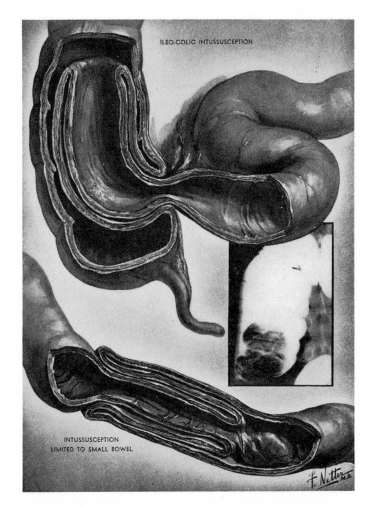

Figure 13–10.   Intussusception. (Copyright, The Ciba Collection of Medical Illustrations, by Frank H. Netter, M.D.)

of abnormal physical findings depend on the duration of the symptoms. There is paroxysmal pain in the abdomen, evidenced by the infant's kicking his legs and drawing them up upon his abdomen. The infant screams. At first, between pains, he may be comfortable. But the pain becomes progressively more severe. Vomiting occurs, first of the contents of the stomach; then it becomes bile-stained. This may be followed by fecal vomitus, depending on the site of intussusception. There are one or two loose stools followed by a discharge of mixed blood and mucus (currant jelly stools) about twelve hours after the onset. No more fecal matter is passed.

The infant is first restless and then prostrated. His temperature may go up to 106 to 108°F. Shock and dehydration occur. A tumor mass may be felt at the site of intussusception; it is usually sausage-shaped. The abdomen is at first soft and then distended or tender. The ring of intestine may be felt on rectal examination if the intussusception is of the ileocecal type. The infant will strain when the intussusception reaches the rectum.

Diagnosis and Treatment. The *diagnosis* is usually easy if there is sudden tenesmus, abdominal pain, vomiting, blood and mucus from the rectum, abdominal tumor and prostration. After a barium enema a roentgenogram may show the intussusception, which is seen as an inverted cap and an obstruction to further progress of the barium.

MEDICAL TREATMENT. Medical reduction is carried out by a surgeon under fluoroscopic observation after a large barium enema has been given the infant. The intussusception is reduced by hydrostatic pressure. The abdomen is not touched during the process. If the intussusception is reduced, the small intestine will fill with barium and the mass will disappear, if not, operation is performed. This procedure is not without risk. The personnel in the operating room should be alerted to the possibility of a surgical procedure if the medical treatment is not successful.

SURGICAL TREATMENT. The infant is prepared for operation by measures to prevent shock and to correct fluid and electrolyte imbalance. Operation is performed as soon as possible. If gangrene or an irreducible mass is present, the involved segment is resected. Usually all that is necessary is reduction of the intussusception. Surgical intervention is preferred because it is certain to reduce the intussusception and allows inspection to seek for a polyp or other cause of difficulty.

Nursing Care. PREOPERATIVE CARE. Good hydration is necessary preoperatively. The nurse assists in giving parenteral fluid and electrolyte therapy, and whole blood if that is needed to combat shock. Deflation of the stomach by constant gastric suction is necessary. The nurse must observe whether drainage is constant and must measure the amount accurately. Antibiotics must be given in proper dosage so that the blood level of the agents will be adequate at operation.

POSTOPERATIVE CARE. Nursing care after a simple reduction is largely symptomatic. Parenteral fluid therapy may be continued until feedings can be resumed. Usually clear fluid feedings are given soon after peristaltic activity has been heard in the abdomen and distention and vomiting have ceased. It is absolutely necessary to keep the operative area clean and dry.

If bowel resection was done, fluids are given parenterally for several days, and gastrointestinal suction is necessary to prevent distention. Accurate measurement of drainage is important, since whatever fluids and electrolytes are lost must be replaced. The nurse must note symptoms of postoperative shock or peritonitis. Changes in vital signs, color, abdominal distention or odor from the incision should all be charted and reported.

Since intussusception may occur during the second half of the first year — when the little child not only misses his mother, but also is afraid of strangers — the importance of his mother's frequent visits must be stressed. These infants are physically uncomfortable and psychologically hesitant to relate to strangers in the hospital situation. Since intussusception is an emergency, the mother will need an opportunity to verbalize her feelings, her shock on learning of the child's condition, and her self-reproach if she did not immediately take him to a physician at the first signs of pain and the change in his stools.

Prognosis. The prognosis is good if operation is performed at once. The chances of recovery are directly related to the duration of illness before operation. After twenty-four hours a high mortality rate is expected. Death in untreated cases results from exhaustion in about three to five days after the onset. Spontaneous reduction may occur in some cases. Recurrences are uncommon after operation.

Inguinal Hernia

Incidence, Etiology and Pathology. Inguinal hernias occur much more frequently in boys than in girls. Such hernias may be present at birth or may occur later. They may be unilateral or bilateral.

As the testis descends retroperitoneally from the genital ridge during embryonic life, a sac of peritoneum precedes it into the scrotum, forming a tube. After descent of the testis the tube normally atrophies. If it does not close completely, intestine or peritoneal fluid may descend into it and produce a hernia. The size of the hernia may vary, depending on whether it extends through the external inguinal ring or into the scrotum.

Although a hernial sac is present at birth, the hernia may not appear until the infant is two or three months old. At this time he has a lusty cry, which increases the intra-abdominal pressure sufficiently to open the sac and force peritoneal fluid or intestine into it. As a result a bulge appears in the inguinal region or the scrotum.

In female infants an ovary may descend into a hernial sac as a result of increased intra-abdominal pressure.

Clinical Manifestations. When the hernial sac is empty, there are no symptoms. When abdominal contents are in the sac, incomplete bowel obstruction occurs. The infant expresses his discomfort and pain in fretfulness. Constipation and anorexia may occur.

If a loop of intestine is incarcerated or caught in the sac, all the symptoms of intestinal obstruction appear. There is danger of strangulation of the bowel with cutting off of the blood supply and ultimately gangrene. Incarceration occurs most frequently in the first six weeks of life. The symptom of an incarcerated hernia is the appearance of a firm, irreducible swelling below the external inguinal ring. The infant may vomit, and he becomes highly irritable. Later there is cessation of bowel movements, abdominal distention, increased vomiting, leukocytosis and fever.

The physician may be able to reduce the incarcerated hernia within twelve hours after it has occurred. If it cannot be reduced, emergency operation must be done. In severe cases bowel resection may be necessary.

If strangulation occurs before operation, the infant has severe pain and symptoms of complete obstruction. Immediate operation is necessary to relieve the condition.

Diagnosis and Treatment. The *diagnosis* is based on the history of intermittent appearance of a mass in the inguinal region and, on physical examination, the finding of a sac which fills when the infant cries or strains, but which can be reduced easily.

Healthy infants are best *treated* by surgical repair as soon as the condition is diagnosed. Operation involves removing the hernial sac and transfixing the neck at the internal ring. Infants tolerate this operation very well. After operation, in the majority of infants, the danger of strangulation and of edema and gangrene is removed.

If incarceration occurs before operation, an ice bag should be applied over the area to reduce the edema. The foot of the bed should be elevated to prevent more abdominal contents from going through the inguinal ring. If manual reduction under sedation is not successful, immediate operation is necessary.

Nursing Care. Preoperatively, as far as possible, the infant should be kept happy and tranquil so that he will not cry. The stools should be regulated, since either a constipated or an irritating loose stool will cause the infant to strain. Both crying and straining tend to raise the intra-abdominal pressure and so produce the hernia.

It is often customary to order "nothing by mouth after midnight" for all patients scheduled for operation the next day. With small children, and especially young infants, such an order may result in dehydration. Since fluid metabolism is rapid in infants, those denied normal intake may become very dehydrated, especially if they have been crying, if they have missed previous feedings, or if they are not to be operated on until later in the day.

POSTOPERATIVE CARE. After an inguinal herniorrhaphy the principal nursing problem is prevention of contamination of the wound unless a waterproof collodion dressing has been used. The area should be kept clean and dry.

Feedings are generally resumed a few hours postoperatively unless a bowel resection was done. The infant should be held for feedings and cuddled while being fed. After a simple hernia repair the older child may be as active as he desires to be.

Umbilical Hernia

Etiology, Incidence and Clinical Manifestations. An umbilical hernia is due to imperfect closure or weakness of the umbilical ring. These hernias occur in all races, but are more common in Negro children.

The *clinical manifestations* are a swelling at the umbilicus which is covered with skin. This protrudes when the infant cries or strains. It can be easily reduced by gentle pressure over the fibrous ring at the umbilicus. The contents of the hernia are small intestine and omentum (Fig. 13-11). The size varies from less than a centimeter to 5 cm. in diameter.

Prognosis, Treatment and Nursing Care. Most small umbilical hernias disappear without treatment, but large ones may require operation. These hernias rarely cause incarceration or strangulation of the bowel.

Physicians differ in their opinions as to the effectiveness of reducing and strapping umbilical hernias. If the physician orders the hernia to be taped, the following procedure may be used.

The area to be taped should be painted with tincture of benzoin to protect the skin and to cause the adhesive to adhere to the skin.

The hernia is first reduced by gently push-

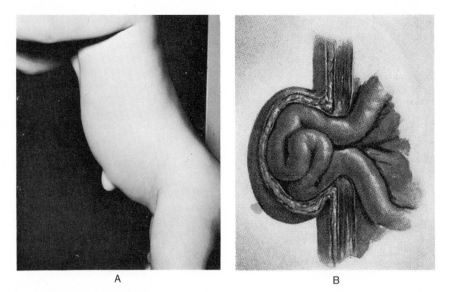

A   B

Figure 13–11. *A,* Side view of infant with an umbilical hernia. *B,* Diagrammatic representation of an umbilical hernia. (Copyright, The Ciba Collection of Medical Illustrations, by Frank H. Netter, M.D.)

ing the abdominal contents back through the umbilical ring. The sides of the adjacent abdominal wall can be brought together in the midline to make a pleat of skin. A 2-inch strip of adhesive can be applied to the abdomen when the tincture of benzoin is dry, from the far bed line, over the pleat of skin, to the near bed line, covering the umbilical hernia. It should be pulled tightly across the pleat.

Usually operation is not done on an umbilical hernia unless it becomes strangulated, enlarges, or persists to school age.

Postoperative *nursing care* requires no special technique. The child may be as active as he desires to be. A normal diet and fluids are given. Pressure dressings, applied at the time of operation, must be kept clean and dry to prevent wound contamination.

GENITOURINARY CONDITIONS

Hydrocele

A hydrocele is an accumulation of fluid around the testis or along the spermatic cord. It may be a congenital condition or may occur during infancy. In diagnosis a hydrocele causing a swelling of the scrotum must be differentiated from an inguinal hernia. A hydrocele appears as a fluctuant, oval, translucent, tense sac. Fluid may gradually absorb during infancy, but if not, surgical correction is necessary.

Pyelonephritis (Pyelitis)

Incidence and Etiology. Pyelitis is an infection of the renal pelvis. Pyelonephritis is an infection of the renal pelvis and renal parenchyma plus, in most cases, inflammation of the ureters and the bladder. Since infections in infants and children are rarely limited to one part of the urinary tract, the term "pyelonephritis" is probably more applicable than "pyelitis."

The condition is relatively common and is the most common renal disease in childhood. The *incidence* is greatest between two months and two years, the period when diapers are worn. The condition occurs more frequently in girls than in boys.

The female urethra is shorter than the male urethra. Infection entering the urinary tract

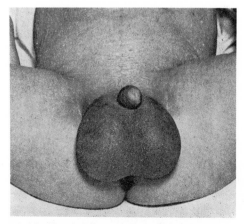

Figure 13–12. A bilateral hydrocele of child. Unilateral hydroceles are common and undergo spontaneous regression, rarely requiring intervention. (Davis and Rubin: *DeLee's Obstetrics for Nurses.* 17th ed.)

from the stool in a soiled diaper contaminates the urethra and may be carried to the bladder, causing cystitis. Infection may enter the urinary tract not only through the urethra, but also by way of the blood stream or the lymphatics. Congenital anomalies causing obstruction of urine are predisposing factors because urinary stasis is associated with chronic urinary tract infections.

Organisms most commonly causing acute infection are the colon bacilli. Staphylococci, hemolytic streptococci and *Streptococcus faecalis* may also cause such an infection. Chronic infections are often caused by multiple types of bacteria. Proteus and Pyocyaneus may also be causative organisms.

Pathology, Clinical Manifestations and Laboratory Findings. There are inflammatory changes in the renal pelvis and throughout the kidney. In the majority of children there are changes also in the ureters and the bladder. The kidney may be large and swollen. Clumps of bacteria may be present. In chronic pyelonephritis there is loss of function because of scarring of the kidney parenchyma. Eventually the kidney becomes small; kidney tissue is destroyed, and renal function fails.

The *clinical findings* are variable. Symptoms related to the urinary tract may or may not be present. The onset may be gradual or abrupt. Fever may be moderate or as high as 104.5°F. (40.3°C.). Prostration, pallor and anorexia appear. Vomiting and diarrhea occur; dehydration may result. Urinary urgency and frequency with dysuria are distressing symptoms. The child is irritable, and convulsions may occur.

It is possible that the infant may show none of the symptoms of localizing of the infection to the urinary tract.

Pain and tenderness in the kidney are signs of the condition. If the infection is chronic, it may continue for months or years, causing anemia and failure of growth and development. Eventually renal failure and hypertension result.

Laboratory findings include pyuria, pathologic organisms in the urine, and leukocytosis. Slight or moderate hematuria may occur, and casts may be present.

Diagnosis and Treatment. The *diagnosis* is made on the basis of pus and bacteria in the urine. A catheterized specimen must be obtained. If there is recurring or persistent pyuria, intravenous or retrograde urography should be resorted to. There may be neurologic or structural abnormalities which cause stasis and continued infection. The cystogram is useful for examining the child for ureteral dilatation.

General *treatment* during the febrile period includes rest; analgesic drugs are given if needed.

Specific chemotherapy or antibiotic therapy is given to shorten the course of the illness and to avoid progressive renal damage. Sulfonamides are most widely used against urinary tract infections. Mandelic acid is effective as a urinary antiseptic only if an acid urine can be maintained. Methionine may be used to acidify the urine sufficiently. Nitrofurantoin (Furadantin) is a bacteriostatic and bactericidal agent against most of the urinary tract pathogens.

During the acute stage the child should be encouraged to take more than normal amounts of fluid to dilute the concentration of urine. Transfusions may be indicated for anemia. If there are obstructive lesions, surgical correction may be attempted. Surgical removal is not always possible, however.

Nursing Care. Clean specimens of urine should be obtained (for collection of specimens, see p. 67). The genitalia must be thoroughly cleansed before the specimen is collected. Zephiran 1:1000 and hexachlorophene solution may be used for this purpose before the specimen is collected. The area is rinsed with sterile water. If a little girl is old enough to use a bedpan, it should be sterilized before use. If a little boy can control himself during urination, a midstream specimen may be obtained; i.e. he voids a small amount, stops, and then voids into a sterile receptacle for the specimen. Laboratory examination of a clean specimen of urine gives a rough estimate of the number of bacteria present.

For bacterial culture only a catheterized specimen should be used. The equipment for catheterization is the same as for the procedure in the adult, with the exception of the size of the catheter. For children size 8 or 10 French is used. Two catheters should be in readiness, since the first to be used may be accidentally contaminated. Various solutions are used for cleansing the genitalia.

The procedure for catheterization of the older child is the same as that for the adult and should be explained to the child. He should be given an opportunity to handle the equipment and should be completely relaxed if catheterization is to be done successfully. The nurse may ask him to breathe deeply through the mouth in order to promote relaxation while the catheter is being inserted into the bladder. For the younger child two nurses are necessary, one to assist him in cooperating and the other to carry out the procedure.

The following points are stressed:

1. The genitalia are cleansed thoroughly with cotton balls dipped in the cleansing solution. *One ball is used for each stroke.* Strokes should be from above downward toward the anus, to prevent organisms from the anus from being carried up over the urethral meatus.

2. The tip of the sterile catheter should be

lubricated with sterile saline solution before insertion into the urethral meatus.

3. The bladder in the infant lies more anteriorly and higher over the symphysis than in the adult, and the urethra lies under and around the symphysis. The meatus in the young child may be exceedingly difficult to locate because of its small size. Because of these anatomic differences it is essential that the light be good so that the meatus can be seen by inspection without causing the infant unnecessary discomfort by probing with the tip of the catheter. Such probing also contaminates the catheter and necessitates use of the second catheter. The catheter is introduced gently, directed downward and inserted along the rounded path to the bladder, lying above the symphysis.

The fluid intake is important. If fluids are ordered in quantity greater than normal, they should be offered between feedings or between meals. The nurse will find it a challenge to discover which fluids the infant likes and his favored way of taking them.

Cryptorchidism (Undescended Testis)

Pathogenesis, Treatment and Prognosis. Cryptorchidism is absence of one or both testes from the scrotum. Early in fetal life the testes develop in the abdomen below the kidneys. During the last two months of intrauterine life they descend into the scrotum. If they have not descended by birth, they may descend at any time until puberty. The missing testis or testes may be in the abdominal cavity or inguinal canal.

At puberty, testes normally increase in size and develop increased androgenic and spermatogenic activity. Since an undescended testis is at a higher temperature within the abdomen than in the normal location—the scrotum—the sperm-forming cells degenerate. If both testes are undescended, sterility results.

Normal secondary sex characteristics develop even though both testes are undescended. If the testis is in the inguinal canal, it may be injured more easily than if it were in the scrotum. Emotional disturbances may occur, especially during the school age, when the young boy finds that he is different from his peers.

Preservation of fertility is the most important factor to be considered in the *treatment.* Either medical or surgical treatment may be used. Some physicians believe that endocrine therapy should be tried during the preschool period. Such therapy is thought to be successful when no hernia is present (hernias are found in more than half of the cases). Gonadotropic hormone is used. If excessive amounts of this hormone are given, precocious puberty may result.

Many physicians believe that *orchidopexy* should be done in all cases of mechanical interference and prefer to operate on children during infancy because of the problem of preservation of fertility and also because of increased fears during the preschool period. Other surgeons prefer to delay operation until the school age.

When the child returns from the operating room, there will be a traction suture in the lower portion of the scrotum fastened to a rubber band attached to the upper inside aspect of the thigh by a piece of adhesive. This anchors the testis to the scrotum. After about a week this attachment is removed. The nurse should not disturb this tension mechanism in caring for the child and must prevent contamination of the suture line. Antibiotics may be given to prevent infection.

If one testis is absent or if a testis must be removed, plastic surgery can be carried out so that the boy will resemble normal boys; thereby no psychologic problem will be induced. This procedure is usually done prior to school age.

The *prognosis* is good if the testis is successfully placed in the scrotum and if no changes occurred in the testis before treatment.

VIRAL INFECTION
Roseola Infantum (Exanthem Subitum)

Etiology and Incidence. Roseola infantum appears to be caused by a filterable virus, although no one organism has been identified as the causative agent. The mode of spread of this infection is also unknown. This condition occurs equally in both sexes, usually between six and eighteen months of age, but it may occur in children three years of age or even older. The incidence of this disease is sporadic in a community; no epidemics have been reported.

Clinical Manifestations, Diagnosis, Treatment and Complications. The onset is acute with an elevation of temperature up to 103 to 105°F. Convulsions may occur. The infant may be irritable, drowsy and anorexic, but he does not usually appear as ill with such a fever as one might expect. The temperature falls by crisis in two to four days, and a macular or maculopapular rash appears. The rash is found principally on the trunk, neck and behind the ears, and less often on the face and extremities. Within a few hours the rash begins to fade and within two to three days has usually disappeared. The occipital and postauricular lymph nodes may be enlarged.* *Treatment* is symptomatic, and *com-*

---

* This disease may be confused with measles and rubella. In roseola infantum there are no catarrhal symptoms or Koplik spots such as are present in measles, and the temperature is too high for rubella to be present.

plications such as residual encephalopathy are rare.

Nursing Care. Isolation of the infant is not necessary. By the time the rash appears and the diagnosis is made, the child is probably no longer infectious, if indeed he ever was.

SUDDEN UNEXPLAINED INFANT DEATH SYNDROME (SUID; CRIB DEATH)

Incidence, Theories of Etiology, Pathology and Prevention. Increasing numbers of infants are discovered dead in their cribs each year for unexplained reasons. These infants usually appear well developed and nourished and are generally between two and four months of age. These deaths occur more frequently during the colder months of the year. They occur more frequently among the nonwhite population than among Caucasians, and in infants of lower-income families living in areas where housing and sanitation are poor. At autopsy only negligible pathologic changes are found.

Suffocation, accidental aspiration of gastric contents causing laryngospasm, bacteremia, hypogammaglobulinemia, acute spinal injury, and allergy to milk or some other substance have been advanced as possibile causes. More physicians are beginning to believe, however, that these tragic deaths are almost always due to a sudden and very acute viral infection of the respiratory tract. Prevention can be aimed only at close medical supervision of infants in the age group affected.

Death is upsetting to any family (see p. 77), but when an apparently healthy infant is found dead in bed, his parents can be deeply crushed and feel very guilty. Siblings who may have become aware of the newly arrived competitor may quickly have to cope with distorted accusations from those outside their families, with their own possible guilt feelings, and with sudden overprotection from their parents. Parents who have lost infants in this way have organized into groups throughout the country in order to support each other during their time of bereavement and to educate the public as to the problem of sudden unexplained infant deaths. Each parent who has lost an infant in this way needs also the emotional support and compassion of the members of the health team.

TEACHING AIDS AND OTHER INFORMATION*

Abbott Laboratories
Fluids and Electrolytes.

Public Affairs Pamphlets
Irwin, M. H. K.: Viruses, Colds, and Flu.

United States Department of Health, Education, and Welfare
Mortality of White and Nonwhite Infants in Major U.S. Cities, 1966.
Sudden Death in Infants: Proceedings of the Conference on Causes of Sudden Death in Infants, September, 1963, Seattle, Washington, 1966.

REFERENCES

Publications
Barness, L. A.: *Manual of Pediatric Physical Diagnosis.* 3rd ed. Chicago, Year Book Medical Publishers, Inc., 1966.
Dutcher, I. E., and Fielo, S. B.: *Water and Electrolytes: Implications for Nursing Practice.* New York, Macmillan Company, 1967.
Gellis, S. S., and Kagan, B. M.: *Current Pediatric Therapy.* 3rd ed. Philadelphia, W. B. Saunders Company, 1968.
Guyton, A. C.: *Textbook of Medical Physiology.* 3rd ed. Philadelphia, W. B. Saunders Company, 1966.
Hughes, J. G.: *Synopsis of Pediatrics.* 2nd ed. St. Louis, C. V. Mosby Company, 1967.
Hughes, W. T.: *Pediatric Procedures.* Philadelphia, W. B. Saunders Company, 1964.
Hutchison, J. H.: *Practical Paediatric Problems.* 2nd ed. Chicago, Year Book Medical Publishers, Inc., 1967.
Kendig, E. L. (Ed.): *Diseases of the Respiratory Tract in Children.* Philadelphia, W. B. Saunders Company, 1966.

* Complete addresses are given in the Appendix.

Metheny, N. M., and Snively, W. D.: *Nurses' Handbook of Fluid Balance.* Philadelphia, J. B. Lippincott Company, 1967.

Nelson, W. E. (Ed.): *Textbook of Pediatrics.* 8th ed. Philadelphia, W. B. Saunders Company, 1964.

Robertson, J.: *Young Children in Hospitals.* New York, Basic Books, Inc., 1958.

Routh, J. I.: *Fundamentals of Inorganic, Organic, and Biological Chemistry.* 5th ed. Philadelphia, W. B. Saunders Company, 1965.

Shirkey, H. C. (Ed.): *Pediatric Therapy.* 2nd ed. St. Louis, C. V. Mosby Company, 1966.

Silver, H. K., Kempe, C. H., and Bruyn, H. B.: *Handbook of Pediatrics.* 7th ed. Los Altos, California, Lange Medical Publications, 1967.

Periodicals

Barness, L. A.: Fluid and Electrolyte Problems. *Pediat. Clin. N. Amer.,* 11:789, 1964.

Berenberg, W.: Roseola Infantum (Exanthem Subitum). *Postgrad. Med.,* 34:234, September 1963.

Berman, D. C.: Pediatric Nurses as Mothers See Them. *Am. J. Nursing,* 66:2429, 1966.

Burgess, R. E.: Fluids and Electrolytes. *Am. J. Nursing,* 65:90, October 1965.

DeFoe, E. C.: Fluid and Electrolyte Therapy in the Nonhospitalized Child. *GP,* 36:125, December 1967.

Donaldson, J. A.: Myringotomy—When and How. *GP,* 29:98, March 1964.

Geis, D. P., and Lambertz, S. E.: Acute Respiratory Infections in Young Children. *Am. J. Nursing,* 68:294, 1968.

Heifetz, C. J.: Let Us Leave Umbilical Hernias Alone. (Editorial.) *J. Pediat.,* 64:303, 1964.

Kraus, A. S., Steele, R., and Langworth, J. T.: Sudden Unexpected Death in Infancy in Ontario. Findings Regarding Season, Clustering of Deaths on Specific Days and Weather. *Canad. J. Pub. Health,* 58:364, August 1967.

Moffet, H. L., Shulenberger, H. K., and Burkholder, E. R.: Epidemiology and Etiology of Severe Infantile Diarrhea. *J. Pediat.,* 72:1, 1968.

Polk, L. D.: Nursing Responsibilities in a Salmonella Outbreak. *Nursing Outlook,* 13:56, December 1965.

Riley, H. D.: Pyelonephritis in Infancy and Childhood. *Pediat. Clin. N. Amer.,* 11:731, 1964.

Rosenstein, B. J.: Salmonellosis in Infants and Children. *J. Pediat.,* 70:1, 1967.

Sanitation Puts Brake on Diarrhea. *Medical World News,* 8:80, October 6, 1967.

Valdés-Dapena, M. A.: Sudden and Unexpected Death in Infants: The Scope of Our Ignorance. *Pediat. Clin. N. Amer.,* 10:693, 1963.

14

CONDITIONS OF INFANTS REQUIRING LONG-TERM CARE

Infancy covers only a short time. An illness of even a few months may retard an infant in accomplishing his developmental tasks. One of the most important of these tasks is to learn to trust people. It is essential that the hospitalized infant keep his trust in his mother's loving protection and learn that others give him physical care and affection. The mother should be encouraged to spend as much time with her child as she can.

The mother's reaction to her child's long-term illness depends, naturally, on the seriousness of his condition. If the illness is severe and the prognosis doubtful, the mother is under a prolonged emotional strain. Her reaction may be to overprotect her baby. The infant may respond with a lack of normal attempts to try out new muscular activities by way of self-help and self-amusement. Even an infant is likely to compensate for a lack of control over his environment by a control over adults who will give him what he wants and do for him what he has not yet learned he can do for himself.

The nurse should understand clearly what activity the physician allows and within that range give the infant opportunity for habilita-

tion. This applies not only to physical activity, but also to psychologic and emotional growth.

The mother should be allowed to verbalize her feelings and thereby relieve to some extent the emotional strain under which she labors. This is not only for her sake, but also because of her influence upon the infant. Unlimited visiting hours in the pediatric unit will give her an opportunity to observe the nurses giving care to her child and to discuss with them the technique of his habilation, whether it is letting him attempt new physical activities or playing by himself without expecting constant attention.

The mother may become overdependent upon the nurse for emotional support. But as she sees the nurse's care of the infant and his response, she will join the health team and cease to cast her responsibilities upon the other members of the team. When she herself is a member of the team, she loses her sense of frustration at others being able to give the child more and better care than she can, and will understand that they excel in professional service, but that she excels in meeting the child's need for affection and security in the love of one person.

NUTRITIONAL DISORDERS (DEFICIENCY DISEASES)

The diets of infants and young children may be deficient in nutriment, i.e. protein, fat or carbohydrate, or in essential vitamins or minerals. Although several factors may contribute to the production of deficiency diseases, the basic problem is usually a lack of intake, though sometimes there may be poor absorption of one or more components of food after ingestion.

Deficiency diseases are especially harmful during infancy because this is the period when growth is most rapid, and the human organism needs adequate supplies of all essential food elements. The deficiency may be of a single food element or of several elements.

Malnutrition (Athrepsia, Marasmus)

Incidence, Etiology and Diagnosis. Malnutrition is less prevalent in the United States and Europe than it was a generation ago. But in India and China and in underdeveloped countries malnutrition of children is one of the problems in which the World Health Organization is vitally interested.

Malnutrition should be considered secondary to the condition causing it. It is a general term indicating undernutrition. Specific vitamin deficiencies are likely in malnourished infants.

The fundamental cause is that the infant does not receive an adequate diet or is unable to as-

similate sufficient nutriment for the metabolic needs of his body, with the result that reserve food elements in the tissues are used. The specific cause may be an inadequate intake or a badly balanced diet; poor feeding habits due to improper training; a physical defect such as cleft lip or cleft palate, or cardiac abnormalities which prevent the infant's taking an adequate diet; diseases which interfere with the assimilation of food (these are generally chronic diseases such as cystic fibrosis); infections which produce anorexia and decrease the infant's ability to digest his food, and yet at the same time increase his need for food; loss of food through vomiting and diarrhea; or emotional problems such as disturbed mother-child relations.

The *diagnosis* of malnutrition may be determined by the obvious symptoms found on physical examination, by failure of growth or by measurement of the blood constituents. Dietary surveys establish the probability of malnutrition in children of any group.

Clinical Manifestations and Laboratory Studies. Failure to gain weight followed by loss of weight is one manifestation of deficiency diseases. Growth of the skeleton and of the brain continues, with the result that the body is long and the head large in proportion to the weight. To maintain metabolism, the body uses its own fat and protein. The subcutaneous fat disappears, but the sucking pads of the cheeks remain, giving the face a factitious roundness. The eyes are sunken. The features have a drawn appearance, and when at last the fat pads have been absorbed, the face takes on an aged look. Tissue turgor

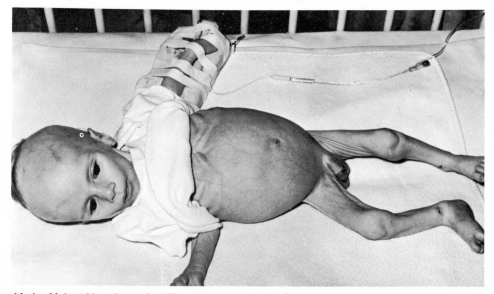

Figure 14–1. Malnutrition due to inability to assimilate food. Subcutaneous fat has disappeared. The infant's skin is wrinkled, especially in the groins. The bones are prominent. Note the arm restrained for intravenous therapy.

is lost, and the skin lies in loose folds on the body. The fat of the abdominal wall and of the buttocks decreases. The skin over the buttocks becomes wrinkled and sags. The skin over the remainder of the body appears loose. The bones are prominent. The infant is no longer active, his muscles are flabby and relaxed, and his cry is weak and shrill.

As his blood volume diminishes and he becomes anemic, his color becomes ashen gray. His temperature is subnormal, the pulse is slow, and the basal metabolism tends to be reduced. His digestive capacity decreases, and his appetite is poor. He may have constipation or starvation diarrhea, in which the stools contain mucus and bile. He is subject to infections and has poor resistance. There may be evidence of a specific deficiency disease such as rickets, scurvy, tetany or nutritional anemia. Nutritional edema may also be present.

The *laboratory findings* show severe hypochromic anemia. The plasma protein level is usually lowered unless hemoconcentration is present. In that case the serum level may be within the normal range.

Complications. Intercurrent infections are frequent. The most common infections are oral thrush (gastrointestinal tract), pyelonephritis (genitourinary tract) and bronchitis or upper respiratory tract infections (respiratory tract). Skin infections such as furunculosis occur, as well as infected bedsores over the bony prominences, e.g. the occiput, heels and knees. Nutritional anemia due to a low iron intake may develop. Nutritional edema results when the body, lacking sufficient protein obtained from food, has burnt its own tissues and destroyed the protein in the plasma, so that the level of plasma albumin becomes low. Nutritional edema is seen in infants who have been malnourished for several months. When sufficient protein is given and the infant has recovered so that the body is able to absorb the necessary amount of protein, the edema disappears.

Kwashiorkor, a widespread condition seen among the underprivileged in tropical and subtropical countries, is a type of malnutrition due to a deficiency of protein and other nutrients. Prevention of kwashiorkor lies in giving an adequate diet after the infant has been weaned.

Treatment and Prognosis. The basic *treatment* of malnutrition is through diet. The initial feedings should be low in quantity and in calories, because the digestive capacity is poor. If too much feeding is given too quickly, the infant will probably suffer diarrhea and vomiting. The initial feeding should be diluted breast milk or, if that is not available, skimmed lactic acid

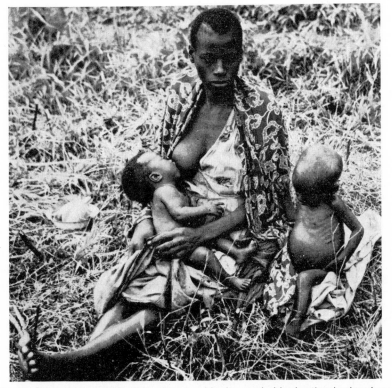

Figure 14–2. The baby is nursing and is doing fine, but his deposed elder brother is already a victim of kwashiorkor. (Jane F. McConnell: The Deposed One. *Am. J. Nursing,* Vol. 61.)

milk. The amount of protein and carbohydrate in the formula is slowly increased. It is necessary to increase the fat content more slowly than the carbohydrate, since fat is more difficult to digest. Evaporated or dried milk may be given within a few days, since the curd is smaller than that of fresh milk. Food requirements for such infants may be as high as 75 to 100 calories per pound a day before they gain weight. They must receive increased protein to build body tissue.

If the infant is dehydrated or shows evidence of electrolyte imbalance, parenteral fluid therapy is given. Depleted reserves of electrolytes must be restored gradually.

Small but frequent blood transfusions may be necessary to correct the anemia and to increase resistance to infection. Medications are aimed at correction of the dietary deficiencies. Intramuscular injections of crude liver extract may be given every two or three days for several weeks, and vitamins A, B, C and D may be given in usual or increased amounts.

Complications such as concurrent infections or skin conditions are treated as they occur.

The *prognosis* depends on the severity of the condition, its length and on whether infection is present. Severely malnourished infants may go into a state of collapse and die suddenly. This is most likely to happen in infants who have continued to lose weight after institution of treatment and have experienced a sudden drop in temperature accompanied with a slow pulse and evidence of a circulatory crisis. Such infants may have acquired a severe, overwhelming infection against which they have no resistance.

Nursing Care. The body temperature must be maintained. If the infant has a subnormal temperature, he should be placed in an incubator or given extra clothing and covered with blankets. Hot-water bottles should be placed on both sides of his body. Since he is subject to infection, his feeding equipment should be sterile to avoid danger of contracting thrush. He should be turned frequently to prevent hypostatic pneumonia, pressure areas on the bony prominences, and skin infections. He requires careful skin care. He should be isolated for his own protection, and nursing personnel who care for him should be free from any kind of infectious condition. Since his resistance is low, he should be kept out of drafts.

The feeding ordered by the physician should be followed carefully and the order checked before each feeding to see whether it has been changed. The infant should be fed slowly and bubbled frequently. During feeding he should be handled gently so that he feels secure in his nurse's care, cuddled and surrounded with emotional as well as physical warmth.

Since collapse is possible, the severely ill infant should be watched at all times for the signs of collapse: temperature drop, slow pulse, cyanosis or gray-white color of the skin, and coldness of the extremities.

The nurse will assist with administration of parenteral fluids or blood (see p. 299). Accurate, detailed charting is necessary and includes the amount of feeding taken, refused or vomited, and whether it was taken eagerly or indifferently. It is important for the physician to know the number and kind of stools and whether abdominal distention is present. The infant should be weighed at the same time daily to determine the exact gain or loss.

Prevention. Prevention of malnutrition is one of the important functions of Child Health Conferences. The amount of the feeding must be adequate. The infant should be fed with good technique so that he may make full use of the feeding ordered by the physician.

Also important in prevention of malnutrition are early treatment of defects, diseases or infections predisposing to malnutrition, and prevention of emotional disturbances.

Malnutrition Due to Disturbed Mother-Child Relations (Failure to Thrive)

Etiology, Diagnosis and Clinical Manifestations. The diagnosis "failure to thrive" is used for infants who have severe malnutrition and faulty physical and emotional development due to a very disturbed mother-child relationship. These infants are usually irritable, apathetic and anorexic, and may have vomiting and diarrhea. They have distortions of social responses (such as refusing eye contact by holding their arms over their eyes) and are physically underdeveloped. Although these infants are not physically separated from their mothers, their symptoms are similar to the syndrome of anaclitic depression (see p. 262).

These infants present a problem in diagnosis and therapeutic management because a physiopathologic state, i.e. congenital anomalies or infections, must be ruled out before the cause can be claimed to be a disturbance in family-infant relations. It is believed that the basic problem of an infant who is normal organically, but who is depressed and fails to thrive, is a mother who cannot claim her infant as her own, who cannot recognize her baby's dependent needs and who has self-doubts about her nurturing ability, and a father who is alienated from both the mother and the child.

Treatment and Nursing Care. The *treatment* of these infants is complex, involving pediatrician, nurse and social worker as a team. The physician must provide a setting in which the family can confide stresses that press upon it. He is responsible for the overall diagnosis based on physiologic studies of the child and background investigation of the parents, and for management of the family as a whole. The social worker together with the physician must furnish noncritical, noncompetitive temporary parent-surrogate figures for the parents themselves. She must help the parents to neutralize stress factors that prevent their assumption of parental roles. The mother especially should have help in finding satisfaction in her motherhood. The nurse must coordinate infant care, teach proper methods of care to the mother, and pass on to the parents what she has observed about their child. She should also share with the public health nurse, if she is to visit the home, her knowledge of ways to help the family. The parents should have ample time to express their feelings to any of the team members. In order for treatment to be successful there must be frank communication between the team and the parents and an accepting attitude on the part of each team member.

Prognosis and Prevention. The prognosis for infants who have failed to thrive is similar to that for those having extreme malnutrition. Much depends on the severity and length of the condition and on whether infection is present. If the pediatrician-nurse-social worker team could function effectively together in establishing positive parent self-images and appropriate parent-child identifications in families in Child Health Conferences, they would promote better mental health and prevent the syndrome of failure to thrive.

Rickets

Etiology and Incidence. Rickets is a deficiency disease of growing children due to a lack of fat-soluble vitamin D (see p. 269).

Since vitamin D increases absorption of calcium and phosphorus from the gastrointestinal tract and decreases renal excretion of phosphate, lack of this vitamin leads to a disturbance of concentration of calcium and phosphorus in the blood and tissue fluids.

Rickets caused by an insufficient intake of vitamin D is now diagnosed relatively infrequently in the United States.

Factors predisposing to rickets are (1) heredity. Dark-skinned people living in temperate zones do not receive an adequate amount of vitamin D from the sun's rays. (2) Age. Rickets may occur at any time from three months to three years. (3) Artificial feeding. A breast-fed infant is not likely to suffer rickets, provided his mother is receiving an adequate amount of sunshine or vitamin D. (4) Prematurity. Prematurity predisposes to rickets because the deposits of calcium and phosphorus at birth are inadequate for the infant's exceptionally rapid growth. (5) Lack of

sunshine. Clouds, fog, dust or smoke in the air or window glass filter out effective ultraviolet rays. (6) Season. The incidence of rickets is greatest in the late winter and early spring.

Pathology and Clinical Manifestations. The manifestations of rickets are most evident in the skeletal system and vary with age and the amount of stress undergone by the affected bone in performing its function in the child's developing body. Deficiency in the structure of the bone is most pronounced in the lack of calcification of the epiphysis. A detectable enlargement occurs in this area. Besides the bones, the muscles are also affected, lacking normal tone.

The *clinical manifestations* are best described under the various parts of the body affected.

In advanced disease the head appears enlarged and square when viewed from above. The anterior fontanel is late in closing, and the cranial bones are soft and make a cracking sound under pressure. This condition is called *craniotabes* and is primarily apparent in the occipital bones.

The thorax shows the rachitic rosary—beading of the costochondral junctions—and Harrison's groove—a bilateral depression at the sites where the diaphragm is attached to the ribs. When the infant is old enough to sit up, a dorsal kyphosis develops. Scoliosis with deformities of the pelvis occurs frequently. If the pelvis of a female infant is deformed, the constricted inlet and outlet will make childbirth difficult later.

The extremities are likely to be deformed. Bowlegs or knock knees accompanied with flat feet are probably the most obvious deformities. There is epiphyseal enlargement of the wrists and ankles.

Later the infant, on sitting, assumes a crouching, froglike position. Because of the poor bone growth and muscle tone the infant is retarded in his motor development and dentition.

The so-called potbelly is caused by relaxed abdominal muscles and may cause the child to be constipated.

The child may have nutritional anemia and a low resistance, especially to respiratory infections.

Diagnosis. Mild and early cases are diagnosed by determining the serum calcium, phosphorus and alkaline phosphatase levels. Advanced cases are easily diagnosed by the gross clinical manifestations and the history of a lack of vitamin D. Radiographically, changes are evident in the bones.

Treatment and Prevention. *Treatment* is by oral administration of large doses of vitamin D, generally 1500 to 5000 International Units a day for about a month. This usually results in cure of the disease. If deformities are present, corrective appliances are used—splints and braces for bowlegs and knock knees. Osteotomy may be necessary.

Both breast-fed and bottle-fed infants should receive supplemental vitamin D in maintenance amounts of 400 International Units per day. This is of greatest importance during the winter months.

Nursing Care. Before the newborn leaves the hospital his mother should receive an accurate explanation of the need for giving him vitamin D. Such instruction is routine for mothers of infants under the supervision of Child Health Conferences. If the infant already has rickets, the mother should have the treatment explained to her. Only a child with severe late rickets or an accompanying concurrent infection requires hospitalization.

Rachitic children should be handled gently and turned frequently. To prevent deformity they should be kept from putting their weight on the spinal column or legs during their illness. In lifting the infant undue pressure should never be put on the bones of the chest. The diaper should be applied loosely lest it bring pressure on the long bones of the legs. Proper positioning lessens the danger of deformity. If the infant lies constantly on his back or on one side, both his head and chest will be flattened by the pressure of his weight on the soft bones. He should lie on a firm mattress.

Administration of vitamin D presents no problem unless it is in a solution containing oil. Then care must be taken that he does not aspirate even a few drops of the substance.

It is important to prevent infection. Frequent changing of his position, required to prevent deformity, will also lessen the danger of lung infection. The physician may order sunbaths for the infant (see p. 266).

Prognosis. Rickets is not a direct cause of death. Minor deformities in general disappear during the preschool period. Severe deformities must be corrected later.

Infantile Nutritional Tetany*
(Tetany of Vitamin D Deficiency)

Incidence and Clinical Manifestations. Infantile nutritional tetany is caused by a deficiency in the intake and absorption of vitamin D. The condition is invariably associated with rickets, but not all rachitic children have tetany. Acquired tetany in a child receiving vitamin D for a rachitic condition is probably due to the rapid deposition of serum calcium in rachitic osteoid tissue and depletion of serum calcium in the blood. It may also result from a decrease in parathyroid activity.

This type of tetany has the same seasonal *incidence* as rickets and occurs in the same age group.

---
* For other forms of tetany, see page 351.

Clinical Manifestations are due to increased neuromuscular irritability. There are two stages in tetany—latent and manifest.

In *latent tetany* the child has a low serum calcium level—less than 7 to 7.5 mg. per 100 ml. —but no obvious symptoms other than "jitteriness" or muscular irritability.

There are four main mechanical or electrical means of producing clinical manifestations of tetany which are used in diagnosis.

1. *Chvostek's Sign.* When the skin in front of the auditory meatus, where the facial nerve is close to the surface, is tapped, unilateral contraction of the facial muscles around the nose, eye and mouth results.

2. *Trousseau's Sign.* If carpal spasm results when the upper arm is constricted for two to three minutes *after the hand has blanched,* the Trousseau sign is positive, showing the presence of tetany.

3. *Erb's Sign.* This test is based on the fact that a patient with tetany has greater muscular irritability than a normal child has. A measured galvanic current is applied, usually over the peroneal nerve just below the head of the fibula. A positive response consists in dorsiflexion and abduction of the foot.

4. *Peroneal Sign.* This sign is positive when tapping the fibular side of the leg over the peroneal nerve causes abduction and dorsiflexion of the foot.

In *manifest tetany* the serum calcium level is often well under 7 mg. per 100 ml. Muscular twitchings and carpopedal spasm occur spontaneously. In *carpal spasm* the thumb is drawn into the cupped palm. The hands are abducted, the wrists flexed. In *pedal spasm* the foot is extended as in talipes equinus or equinovarus. The toes are flexed, and the sole of the foot is cupped. The arms and legs may be adducted and flexed.

There may be spasm of the larynx—*laryngospasm*—indicated by a high-pitched crowing sound on inspiration, due to spasm of the adductor muscles of the larynx which pull the vocal cords together. If the spasm is severe, respirations may cease and cyanosis may occur. Convulsions—generalized seizures including carpopedal spasm—may occur.

Diagnosis and Treatment. The *diagnosis* is made on the basis of the laboratory data and the clinical manifestations. The laboratory tests show a low calcium level, low, normal or elevated serum phosphorus level, and increased serum phosphatase.

The objective of *treatment* in hypocalcemic tetany is to raise the serum calcium level above that causing tetany. Calcium may be given in the form of calcium chloride or calcium gluconate. Calcium chloride is given in a 10 per cent solution orally. Calcium gluconate in a 10 per cent solution may be given intravenously if the child cannot take oral medication. Calcium gluconate should not be given intramuscularly or subcutaneously because of the danger of necrosis at the site of injection.

Convulsions may be controlled by oxygen therapy and intravenous administration of calcium gluconate. If these procedures do not give relief, sodium phenobarbital may be administered intramuscularly. Emergency intubation may be necessary if laryngospasm is prolonged and cannot be relieved with sedatives and calcium salt.

After the acute clinical manifestations of tetany have been controlled calcium therapy should be continued orally; in addition, large amounts of vitamin D should be given daily.

Nursing Care.   Nursing care is of the utmost importance. The nurse will give the medications as ordered.

The nurse should have padded tongue blades to prevent the child from biting his tongue during a convulsion, and oxygen ready in case of convulsions and laryngospasm. She must be trained to give artificial respiration (see p. 182). Intubation equipment should be in readiness.

Prognosis and Prevention.   The *prognosis* is good if treatment is given early. Death may occur from laryngospasm or cardiac failure.

Before the infant is sent home the mother, in her conferences with the physician and the nurse, should be told the importance of vitamin D therapy for all growing children.

The *preventive measures* for infantile nutritional tetany are the same as those for rickets.

Scurvy

Incidence and Etiology.   Scurvy is due to a lack of the water-soluble vitamin C (ascorbic acid) (see p. 268). The vitamin is unstable and is destroyed by heat, and also by alkaline solutions or by oxidation when in aqueous solutions. Ascorbic acid withstands heat fairly well in an acid solution and in the absence of oxygen. Vitamin C is generally given to infants in the form of orange juice, which should never be boiled.

The newborn has an adequate amount of vitamin C if his mother had a sufficient amount in her diet. Since vitamin C, unlike vitamin D, cannot be synthesized by human beings, the total supply must come from the diet.

Scurvy may occur at any age, but is more frequent in infants from six months to two years of age. Scurvy is not seen as often as it formerly was in this country.

Pathology, Diagnosis and Clinical Manifestations.   Pathologically, there is a defect in the formation and maintenance of intercellular substances in supporting tissues, dentin, bone, cartilage and vascular endothelium. Clinical manifestations, including a tendency to hemorrhage, can therefore be seen in the teeth and bones. The tendency to hemorrhage may be the specific result of lack of a maintenance amount of cement substance in the walls of the blood vessels or of collagen around the vessels.

The *diagnosis* is usually based on the history, roentgenographic examination and the symptoms.

X-ray examination shows changes in the distal ends of the long bones. Initially there appears to be atrophy of the bone. In the shaft the bone presents a ground-glass appearance. Subperiosteal hemorrhages of the long bones do not show on the x-ray film *during active scurvy,* but are apparent during the healing process.

It is sometimes difficult to distinguish scurvy from arthritis, osteomyelitis or poliomyelitis because of the tenderness of the limbs and the pain produced on movement. It may also be difficult to distinguish it from dysentery, hemorrhagic nephritis or blood dyscrasias when the tendency to hemorrhage is the most important clinical manifestation.

The *clinical manifestations* appear slowly after the body has been deprived of an adequate amount of ascorbic acid. The infant becomes fretful, irritable and apprehensive. He fears to be touched because of the pain when he is moved, as in changing his diaper. He may have anorexia.

Subperiosteal hemorrhage causes great pain, chiefly in the legs. The pain causes a pseudoparalysis. The child assumes a frog position; i.e. the hips and knees are semiflexed with the feet rotated outward.

There may be bluish-purple, swollen, bleeding gums and blood in the vomitus and stools. Hemorrhages may be seen in the soft tissue around the eyes, and petechiae may appear in the skin.

The infant may have the so-called rosary at the costochondral junction. These scorbutic beads are sharper than those of rickets. In rickets they are due to widening of the softened epiphyses; in scurvy they are due to subluxation (partial or complete dislocation) of the sternal plate at the union of the ribs and the sternum.

The infant's temperature may rise to 102°F. Anemia develops, owing to anorexia and hemorrhage. The infant then becomes very pale. The rate of growth, which is rapid in normal infants, is slowed in those with this condition.

Treatment.   The specific treatment for scurvy is large doses of vitamin C. Orange juice, 90 to 120 cc. daily, or ascorbic acid, 100 to 200 mg. daily, is given orally or parenterally. After several days of such treatment the normal requirement is all that is needed. An adequate diet is given as a supportive measure. Transfusions may be necessary for severe anemia.

Nursing Care. Nursing care centers about the diet and medications and prevention of pain and infection. During the acute stage the child should be fed in whatever position appears to be most comfortable for him.

The pseudoparalysis of scurvy is the chief problem in nursing. Great gentleness in handling is necessary. Since the infant fears that he will be moved when a nurse approaches him, it is well not to come too close to the bed unless necessary care must be given. In diapering the infant the buttocks may be elevated and the diaper slid under from the side. The buttocks should never be lifted by elevating the legs as is customary with a well child. A bed cradle may be used to prevent painful pressure of the bed clothes upon the child's body.

Nursing care, medication and treatments should be given at the same time so that the infant may rest without movement between the times when it is necessary to arouse him.

Prevention of infection is of the utmost importance. The infant's position should be changed frequently, and his mouth should be cleansed with water after each feeding.

Prognosis and Prevention. The *prognosis* is excellent if the treatment is adequate. Pain ceases in a few days, and body growth is resumed.

Prevention lies in giving the infant an adequate diet containing an ample supply of vitamin C. An adequate amount of vitamin C is required throughout childhood; older children need 40 mg. of ascorbic acid a day, and adolescents 45 to 60 mg. a day.

GASTROINTESTINAL DISORDERS

Celiac Syndrome

The celiac syndrome is a state in which the patient has chronic nutritional failure. The clinical manifestations are stunting of growth, wasting of the extremities and buttocks accompanied by abdominal distention, pale, foul-smelling, large stools, anorexia, nervous symptoms, and evidence of mineral and vitamin deficiency.

Two relatively common diseases included in the celiac syndrome are true or idiopathic celiac disease and cystic fibrosis.

Celiac Disease
(Gluten-Induced Enteropathy)

Incidence and Etiology. Celiac disease is characterized by chronic intestinal malabsorption resulting in malnutrition and deficiency diseases. The disease may begin during infancy or the toddler period. It occurs in both sexes and has its highest *incidence* in the white race.

Celiac disease in children seems to be related to nontropical sprue in adults and may occur among different members of the same family. The cause is believed to be an inborn error of metabolism with or without an accompanying allergic reaction. The child cannot ingest the gluten or protein portions of wheat or rye flour. Parenteral infections and emotional disturbances may lead to exacerbations.

Pathology and Clinical Manifestations. The *pathology* is evident in severe malnutrition and secondary deficiency diseases, of which rickets is the most common, but scurvy or hypoproteinemia may also occur.

Typical *clinical manifestations* appear as early as six months and may last to the fifth year of life. Episodes of diarrhea occur. Anorexia, if it occurs, results in failure of growth. Severe abdominal distention may be caused by collections of gas and by relaxed abdominal musculature. There are fluctuations in weight. Loss in weight is most noticeable in the limbs, buttocks and groin. The skin over the flattened buttocks may be wrinkled and hang in folds. The face usually remains plump, and the rounded cheeks may be

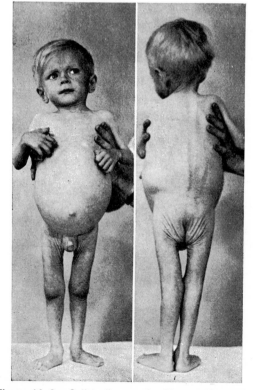

Figure 14–3. Celiac disease. Age 2 years 10 months. (From Murray Davidson in L. E. Holt, R. McIntosh and H. L. Barnett: *Pediatrics.* 13th ed. New York, Appleton-Century-Crofts, 1962.)

flushed. Tooth eruption is often delayed. The child may show increasing irritability and other changes in behavior.

A *celiac crisis* may be precipitated by a mild respiratory infection. The child has dehydration and acidosis caused by vomiting and large, watery stools. His sleep is restless; sweating is excessive, and his extremities are cold. This condition may result in death if the child is not promptly and adequately treated.

The nature of the stools varies with the diet and the severity of the disease. The typical celiac stools are bulky, heavy and of more than normal frequency (particularly during a crisis), mushy, foul-smelling, pale and frothy. The amount of fat (soaps and fatty acids) in the stool is moderately increased in gluten-induced enteropathy. With improvement in the child's condition the stools become formed and normal in color.

There is a mild hypoproteinemia or protein deficiency. A total serum protein level of less than 5 gm. per 100 ml. indicates that the child is seriously ill. Minerals—calcium and iron—are lost in the stools in amounts depending on the severity of the disease.

Treatment. The treatment consists in controlling the diet. Wheat and rye gluten must be excluded entirely, and the amount of fat must be limited. Approximately 6 to 8 gm. of protein per kilogram of body weight should be given daily. If the child is very ill, he is given skimmed or protein milk sweetened with glucose, sucrose or banana powder. Gradually other foods are added, one at a time, at intervals of two or more days. Foods which can be added are eggs, cottage cheese, meat, fruits and vegetables.

The diet must meet the child's caloric needs. Monosaccharides and disaccharides may be given, but not polysaccharides (starches). The parents should be given a list of food products which contain the forbidden wheat or rye gluten, such as gravies, meat loaf, puddings and processed meats, and should be told why these foods are contraindicated for the child.

Treatment during a celiac crisis involves fluid and electrolyte replacement and maintenance therapy. If symptoms of tetany occur, calcium is given until the serum calcium level returns to normal. Liver extract may be given intramuscularly, and large amounts of water-miscible preparations of vitamins A and D should be given to prevent deficiencies. Antibiotics are given if infections develop. Adrenal steroid therapy produces remissions in celiac disease, but a relapse occurs as soon as the medication is discontinued.

Nursing Care. Nursing care involves helping the parents to accept not only the child's physical condition, but also his behavior problems. Typically, the child is irritable and difficult to manage. The nurse must have a sympathetic understanding of their problem. Parents may feel guilty or ambivalent toward the child. They may overprotect him or communicate to him their great concern about his stools.

During hospitalization for diagnosis and treatment the child may need emotional support from the nurses. He is confused and unhappy because of the initial food deprivation. His parents should visit him frequently or, if possible, stay with him. When he is hungry, he becomes frustrated and angry and may have temper tantrums or be withdrawn. The hungry child should feel free to complain either by crying or with words. The understanding nurse will help him to express his feelings in words and will show her sympathy if he cries.

Feeding the child is a problem. Although hunger may be the fundamental cause of his irritability, his appetite is capricious. He should be fed slowly and given small amounts at a time. He should not be forced to eat; when he feels better, he will eat more. New foods should be introduced gradually, one at a time, and may be masked in foods he likes. If he will not take a particular food, this fact should be reported to the physician, and the food should be eliminated from the diet and tried again at some future time. Problems with food may occur when the child is at home if he sees the food other children in the family are eating. He may want their food instead of his own.

Recording of the food intake is important. The nurse should observe and chart the kind and amount of food taken, the child's appetite and his reaction to different foods. With each new addition to the diet she should note the nature of the stools, the child's behavior and the degree of abdominal distention.

It is imperative to prevent infection. Good hygiene must be maintained, since the child is anemic and malnourished. He perspires freely and must be kept dry. If he is confined to bed and tends to lie in one position, he should be turned frequently.

As the child recovers, every effort should be made to provide him with special treats when he cannot have the food which other children in the pediatric unit are enjoying or, after his return home, which the family members are eating.

Children with celiac disease are often withdrawn and do not enter into play with other children. Their play is likely to be passive, since they find active play exhausting. The toddler may retain infantile habits of self-comfort such as sucking his thumb, or he may carry his favorite toy or object wherever he goes to give him a feeling of security. The nurse must be patient and try to provide security for the child in companionship with other children and the unit personnel. As his physical condition improves, his emotional behavior will also change; he will give up infantile habits and seek the companionship of others.

Instructions to the Mother. The parents should learn the underlying concepts of the child's illness and his treatment so that they can give him adequate care after his discharge. In her conferences with the mother the nurse stresses (1) the necessity of preventing infection and emotional disturbances from any cause, (2) the importance of strict adherence to the dietary regimen, and (3) the need for follow-up supervision. This instruction should be given slowly without frightening the mother, for if she becomes too anxious, she will overprotect the child and restrict his activities beyond the limits set by the physician. Overprotection is harmful to positive mental health, particularly in the infant or toddler, who has no relations with a teacher or other professional workers to counteract his mother's attentions.

Prognosis. The mortality rate from celiac disease is low, owing to better understanding and more common use of parenteral fluid therapy, dietary management and control of infection by antibiotics. Recovery takes several months. The course is an intermittent process of exacerbations and remissions. Since celiac disease is a constitutional defect, actual cure does not occur, but clinical manifestations decrease in later life.

Cystic Fibrosis (Mucoviscidosis)

Incidence and Etiology. Cystic fibrosis is a congenital disease inherited as a mendelian recessive trait. For an infant to have this disease, both parents must be carriers. According to the Mendelian Law, the condition may appear in one fourth of all children of such unions. Carriers may with further research be identified by analysis of their sweat.

Cystic fibrosis is a chronic disease, the most serious lung problem affecting children in this country today. The *incidence* in the general population is from 1:1000 to 1:2000 live births, with equal frequency in either sex. The incidence is greatest among Caucasians and rare in Negro infants.

Pathology and Clinical Manifestations. There is a widespread change in the mucus-secreting glands of the body, i.e. in the pancreas, lungs and salivary and sweat glands. The *clinical manifestations* are therefore respiratory difficulties with problems in the maintenance of an adequate nutritional status.

The pancreatic changes are due to obstruction by inspissated secretion, beginning in the acini and extending to the ducts. Eventually acinar tissue dilates and atrophies and is replaced by connective tissue, resulting in fibrosis of the entire gland. The islands of Langerhans, which produce insulin, remain normal.

The air passages in the lungs are obstructed by a thick, mucoid secretion which may produce emphysema or atelectasis and may contain pathogenic organisms causing infection. Later bronchiolectatic abscesses and areas of bronchopneumonia are found. Eventually pulmonary fibrosis and interstitial pneumonia occur. The acini and ducts of the salivary glands are distended. The saliva contains increased amounts of sodium and chloride. The sweat contains a high concentration of sodium, potassium and chloride.

The clinical manifestations may be present at birth if the infant has meconium ileus (see p. 178). Most newborns, however, who have cystic fibrosis may not have meconium ileus because the deficiency of the pancreatic enzymes is seldom complete.

If the infant is normal at birth, between the fourth week and the sixth month there may be a failure to gain weight, indicating the onset of the condition. In the early stage the stools are usually loose, but not fatty or frequent. When the infant receives cereals or fish liver oil, the stools become foul-smelling and frothy. Later the stools are light in color and fatty.

There is failure to absorb sufficient food; therefore the child does not gain weight as he should. At last the fat disappears from the main sites of deposit. There is abdominal distention and emaciation.

During the early part of the first year the child may have persistent severe respiratory infections, usually caused by *Staphylococcus aureus*. The infant may have a spasmodic cough which produces vomiting. He may become dyspneic, may wheeze and become cyanotic. Clubbing of fingers and toes may be seen. Because of persistent obstructive lung disease, the right ventricle of the heart becomes strained and hypertrophied.

Behavior disorders result. The child is irritable and easily fatigued. In spite of these symptoms there may be a good appetite. There is a change in the physical appearance, growth is stunted, the skin appears loose, the buttocks and thighs are atrophied, and the abdomen is protuberant.

Diagnosis. The diagnosis is made on the basis of the history, physical examination, laboratory tests and roentgenologic studies.

Laboratory examinations show a deficiency of pancreatic enzymes (trypsin, lipase, amylase and carboxypeptidase). These enzymes are reduced in or absent from the duodenal fluid. Tests for the presence of these enzymes are done on duodenal juices obtained by intubation and aspiration. Usually only a trypsin test is made, because absence of this enzyme is indicative of

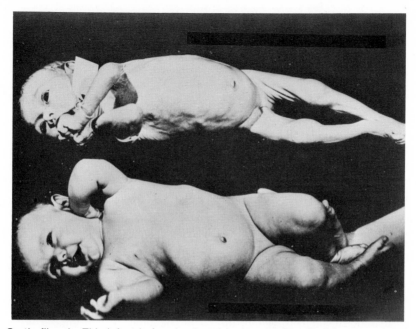

Figure 14–4. Cystic fibrosis. This infant before treatment had a protuberant abdomen and emaciated extremities. After treatment her appearance is that of a normal infant. (Courtesy of Pfizer Laboratories.)

cystic fibrosis. The test for tryptic activity can be done on a stool specimen.

The sweat is tested for chloride content, which is higher than normal in patients with cystic fibrosis (note, however, that this abnormality may also occur in siblings and other relatives who have no clinical manifestations of the disease). In a screening technique the child's hand is placed on agar impregnated with silver nitrate. If the sweat chloride level is high, the hand print is seen on the agar.

Diagnosing cystic fibrosis has been simplified by the Cystic Fibrosis Analyzer. A sample of the child's sweat is obtained by iontophoresis. This analyzer features a new plastic sweat-generating electrode that eliminates the risk of skin irritation. The generation of sweat takes approximately thirty minutes, while the analysis of its electrolyte content takes one to two minutes.

Children who have cystic fibrosis have sodium concentrations in their hair and nails about four times greater than normal children do. A biochemical analysis of infants' fingernails and hair has proved accurate in confirming this diagnosis.

It is possible to test for deficient absorption of fat in the intestines. Microscopic examination of the dilute stool will show excretion of fat in the feces. A low blood cholesterol level may be due in part to poor absorption of fats from the intestines. Since fats are not absorbed, vitamin A given in oily preparations is not absorbed, and some other source of this vitamin must be provided.

Roentgen studies show changes in the intestinal tract and the lungs. A generalized obstructive emphysema, atelectasis, bronchopneumonia, bronchiectasis and bronchiolectatic abscesses may be apparent. Right ventricular hypertrophy of the heart may be seen in advanced cases.

Treatment. Treatment must be planned on a long-term basis, and follow-up care after treatment has been discontinued is extremely important. Good nutrition is essential. The patient should receive a balanced diet which includes a large amount of protein (4 gm. per kilogram of body weight) and a normal amount of fat. If the child cannot tolerate this, the diet should be limited in order to control the bulk and fat content of the stools. In infancy a protein milk formula to which skimmed powdered milk has been added is good. Banana powder and glucose may also be added to the formula. Other foods which are easily digested and are high in protein or low in fat and starches, such as cottage cheese, lean meats, fruits (especially bananas) and vegetables, may also be given.

The caloric intake should be high, from 125 to 200 calories per kilogram of body weight per day, since the child cannot utilize food completely (he loses 50 per cent of the caloric value of his food in the stools). Liberal amounts of salt should be given with the food; in summer and hot weather extra amounts should be provided.

The specific medication in cystic fibrosis is

pancreatic extract. The dose varies with the child's age and his need for the extract. One gram of a patent pancreatin preparation may be given for each 6 to 8 ounces of formula. Two or 3 gm. may be given before each meal to replace the pancreatic enzymes which the child's body cannot produce and which are needed in the digestion of foods. In this way the condition of the stools is improved. If the child does not eat, he should not be given the pancreatic enzyme. Vitamins in water-miscible preparations should be given in large amounts.

Prevention of infection, especially respiratory infection, is of the utmost importance. The child should be isolated from other patients and hospital personnel who have respiratory infections. Because of the danger of cross-infection, hospitalization should be as short as possible. This necessitates teaching the mother to care for the child at home.

Antibiotics may be given prophylactically to minimize the danger from a respiratory infection. If, however, the child contracts an infection, appropriate antibiotics should be given in full dosage.

Digitalis is given if there is evidence of cardiac failure. Oxygen is used for cyanosis due to bronchial secretions or cardiac failure.

Treatments aimed at assisting the child to remove thick mucoid secretions from his lungs include postural drainage, clapping and vibrating.

The specific purpose of postural drainage is to bring the various branches of the bronchial tree into such a position that draining the bronchial branch and the segment of lung it supplies is facilitated. The child is placed in an upside-down position in order that the force of gravity will move secretions to the main bronchi and the trachea so that they can be more easily coughed up. A small child may either be placed on his abdomen on the nurse's lap with his head hanging down or may be placed in the same position over pillows in his crib (see Fig. 14-5). More effective drainage is obtained if the child's position is changed slightly while clapping and vibrating techniques are used over specific areas of the lungs.

The clapping technique is also called cupping or tapping. The nurse's hand must be in a cupped position, and the wrist is alternately flexed and extended as she claps the child's chest gently. This percussion dislodges plugs of mucus from the lung. Air can then get behind the mucus and help move it to the trachea.

Vibrating is another technique which is done only during exhalation of air from the lungs. The nurse places one hand on top of the other or one hand on either side of the child's rib cage and makes gentle, fine vibratory movements. A thumping-vibrating machine can now be obtained and used instead of manual percussion. It can be operated in the home by the parent or by the afflicted child himself. After both cupping and vibrating the child is encouraged to cough.

A physical therapist can instruct and demonstrate the proper procedure for postural drainage, cupping and vibrating to nurses and parents caring for children in the hospital or in the home. The therapist may also need to make suggestions for improving facilities in the home for this purpose. The therapist must stress the fact that *gentleness* is necessary in these procedures. Shaking or jarring the child roughly may only result in the child's refusal to have further therapy.

The child may be placed in a humidity chamber in order to dilute the secretions in the lungs and thus make it easier for him to expectorate them.

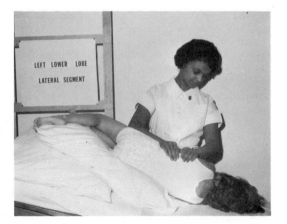

Figure 14–5. There are many positions for postural drainage, and the bed itself may be tilted. Here, a tilt bed and pillows are employed in combination to achieve the desired angle. (Courtesy of The National Cystic Fibrosis Research Foundation.)

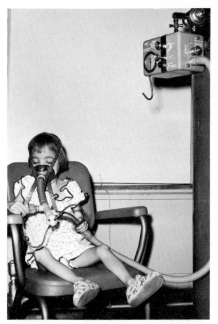

Figure 14-6. The Bird machine provides nebulization under intermittent positive pressure. It has proved effective when used on children having cystic fibrosis.

Aerosol therapy may be given by mask or tent to help remove heavy secretions from the bronchi and to relieve dyspnea. The vapor is given as a fine mist or microparticles at least four times a day. Antibiotic, decongestant, mucolytic and bronchodilator agents, either alone or in combination, may be added to the aerosol solution. Nebulization under intermittent positive pressure may be used. Since the lungs are inflated by positive pressure during inspiration, the aerosols can be administered to every area where ventilation takes place, with the result that bronchial drainage and pulmonary function are improved. Several types of machines may be used for this purpose (Fig. 14-6). It is possible to give this treatment to infants if intubation has been done, but it has proved most successful with children eighteen months to two years of age when a mask is used. The treatment is usually given every few hours and continued until the amount of aerosol medication is exhausted. In severe cases aerosol therapy may be given continuously, with pressure maintained on both inspiration and expiration.

Complications. Rectal prolapse due to emaciation of the buttocks and weak musculature in the rectal area is a possible complication. It occurs most frequently between six months and three years of age.

Heat prostration may result from a high environmental temperature because the child loses electrolytes in perspiration. Osteoporosis may occur because the child cannot utilize fat-soluble vitamin D and therefore cannot make use of calcium in bone growth as the normal child does. Clinical rickets is not often seen, since rickets is a disease of growing children, and these children do not grow. There is vitamin A deficiency due to the child's inability to absorb fats from which the vitamin is obtained. The heart is strained by the exertion required to pump blood through the fibrotic lung. Cor pulmonale, in which the right side of the heart becomes enlarged and dilated, is a frequent cause of death.

Nursing Care. The child's nutritional state is important. The nurse must be patient with

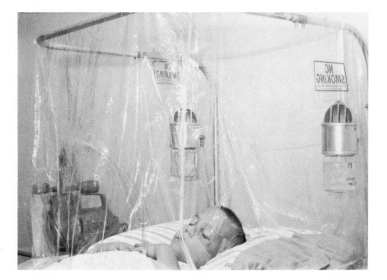

Figure 14-7. Home jet-type "mist tent" nebulization therapy with 2 Mist O$_2$ Gen nebulizers and a 1/12-horsepower compressor for patients with cystic fibrosis. The fog must be so dense that the patient is not visible when the tent is in operation. (From M. Green and R. J. Haggerty [Eds.]: *Ambulatory Pediatrics*.)

the child at mealtimes or when giving the infant his bottle. The patient is apt to be irritable, coughs and vomits easily and often has difficulty in breathing. Small amounts of food should be offered slowly but frequently so that he is not tired by his effort to take food. The infant should be bubbled frequently so that abdominal distention is not increased. The diet should be as varied as possible, with consideration for the child's age and ability to digest various foods. The nurse should carefully chart the child's reaction to new foods and the kind of stools which result from additions to the diet.

It is imperative that the nurse accept the personality changes which take place in the child as his illness extends over months. She should give him love and kindness to promote his feeling of security even during the discomfort of his illness.

Skin care is required. The buttocks must be carefully cleansed after each stool, and ointment applied to protect the skin from contact with further stools. If the skin becomes irritated, the buttocks should be exposed to the air or to the warmth of an electric light bulb (see p. 304).

Scrupulous cleanliness of the diaper area will help to reduce the offensive odor from the stools. Soiled diapers should be taken from the unit as soon as they are removed from the infant. An air deodorant is useful, but should never be made a substitute for cleanliness.

Because of malnutrition the skin may break down over the bony prominences. The patient should therefore be turned frequently, and the entire body must be kept clean to prevent decubiti. More importantly, changing position lessens the danger of pneumonia. Even if the child is old enough to turn himself, he may be too weak to do so; this is the responsibility of his nurse.

The child should not be dressed too warmly, but it is essential that he should not become chilled. If he perspires, his clothes should be changed immediately.

The nurse will carry out the procedures of postural drainage, clapping and vibrating as ordered. She will also assist in intermittent positive-pressure and aerosol treatments. She must explain to the child, if he is old enough to understand, that he is to take a deep breath under regulated gentle pressure and that a fine mist of medication will reach all areas of his lungs. The child should be positioned correctly and helped to sit up straight. This position allows room for movement of the diaphragm and therefore permits deeper respiration. The child should be encouraged to breathe slowly and deeply at first and to relax during the treatment. Demonstration by the nurse with her own breathing may help him to understand what is wanted of him.

If the child is afraid of the procedures, he should be urged to express his fear. The nurse is then able to give support and encouragement. Eventually most children will cooperate. When medication is used in the mist, the infant or young child should be attended by the nurse throughout the procedure of intermittent positive pressure. The nurse must use her judgment in permitting the older child to use the apparatus alone. The machine must be cleaned thoroughly between treatments because of the danger of respiratory cross-infection between children using the apparatus.

Because of the wasted muscles, the usual site for intramuscular injections presents more problems than in the normal child. Injection sites should be examined carefully for hardened areas, and no further medication should be given in any area unless it is normally soft and shows no evidence of trauma. Sites should be rotated whenever injections are given frequently. Massage may help in absorption of the medication and tends to prevent hardness from developing.

Recording of observations should be complete so that the physician may have a clear picture of the child's condition. The stools should be described in detail as to color, odor, consistency and size. The kind and amount of foods taken, as well as those refused, should be charted. Whether the child eats eagerly or indifferently should also be noted. Gain or loss of weight is recorded or shown graphically. The color of the skin has diagnostic value. The nurse should watch for signs of rectal prolapse and report all symptoms of this condition. If the child coughs, the physician wants to know the nature and frequency of the cough. Little children cry readily for many reasons, but crying is also a sign of discomfort or pain. The time, kind and frequency of crying are important both in diagnosis and in judging the effect of treatments and therefore should be recorded in detail. A description of the cry is helpful in appraising not only his physical condition, but also the personality changes which interact with the physical ones.

Heat prostration may be prevented if the nurse observes and reports to the physician the first symptoms.

Prevention of infection must be a constant aim.

Equally important is education of the parents. Conferences with the parents should provide for continuation of the care the child received in the hospital. The mother should be told of the dietary regimen, and time must be taken to be sure that she understands what the diet consists of and also the best ways of making it acceptable to the child. She will also need to know, and emotionally accept, the physician's plan of treatment, including medical follow-up, hygienic measures, prevention of infection, meeting the child's need for adequate rest and the administration of medication. The nurse should not only teach the mother the necessary procedures, but also should explain to her the purpose of each and the expected results. She should also explain the necessity for medication which the physician has ordered and the best way to give it to the child.

The loving mother willingly undertakes the time-consuming and difficult task of caring for her child at home. The nurse will help her to use her affection wisely and set limits to his behavior, even though the prognosis is poor. It is difficult for her to accept the probable regression in his condition during even mild respiratory infections, and even more difficult if she blames herself for some oversight in his care which she believes caused the infection.

The nurse should help both parents to realize their responsibility in caring for the child and the help they must give him in adjusting to his limitations. The danger lies in overprotection by his parents and therefore deprivation of opportunities for normal development. He should be helped to make the best possible adjustment to his handicap. The diagnosis of cystic fibrosis in a child causes emotional and financial problems for a family. The affected child should not be permitted to dominate the family. This is unfair to the other family members. Any guilt which the parents may have should be alleviated. The family should be informed of community facilities available to assist them. They should certainly be informed about the National Cystic Fibrosis Research Foundation and the help it is prepared to give to parents.

Prognosis. The prognosis is unpredictable, but in severe disease is usually poor. Death may occur in the first year from severe malnutrition or overwhelming respiratory infection. The nurse may be of great support to parents at this time, even though they have known the genetic cause of the disease and the prognosis. Spiritual guidance of such parents may be of great value (see p. 75).

Prolapse and Procidentia of the Rectum and Sigmoid

Incidence and Etiology. Prolapse of the rectum is an abnormal descent of the mucous membrane of the rectum. The membrane may or not protrude through the anus. *Procidentia* is an abnormal descent of all the layers of the rectum or sigmoid, or both, which likewise may or not protrude through the anus.

The *incidence* is greatest during infancy, although the condition occurs in children up to three years of age.

Prolapse is precipitated when the intra-abdominal pressure is suddenly increased. Infants and young children who are malnourished, have diarrhea or are constipated are prone to these conditions. Prolapse or procidentia may occur repeatedly with straining at defecation if the sphincter is relaxed and the muscles of the pelvic floor are weak.

Clinical Manifestations. The first manifestation is only protrusion of part of the rectum and sigmoid, which recede spontaneously. Later, manual replacement may be necessary. The protruding mass is bright red to dark purple, depending on the length of time it has been prolapsed and the degree to which circulation has been cut off. The protrusion may be up to 5 to 6 inches in length. The mass may be a flattened, corrugated tumor or just a fold of mucous membrane protruding from the anus.

Treatment, Nursing Care and Prognosis. Treatment is aimed at the underlying problem, i.e. to correct the child's weight by an adequate diet if he is malnourished, to correct constipation by giving a mild medication (e.g. mineral oil) and instituting proper toilet training, and to correct diarrhea if that is the cause of the difficulty.

During defecation the buttocks should be held together manually or with adhesive tape. If the child is able to indicate when he is about to have a stool, manual pressure is preferable, since it can be adjusted to passage of the stool. The buttocks may be taped together after each bowel movement to prevent repeated prolapse.

For reduction of the protrusion the infant should be placed with his head lower than his body. The protrusion may be replaced manually. Toilet paper is put over a gloved finger used to insert the bowel and pressed into the opening of the mass as it is pushed back into the rectum. The finger is then quickly withdrawn, leaving the toilet paper in the rectum. The paper will become soft and be expelled later.

Operation may be necessary if other treatment is not successful.

The *prognosis* is usually good with proper treatment.

Biliary Atresia

Etiology, Pathology, Clinical Manifestations and Prognosis. The cause of biliary atresia is a congenital faulty development of the bile ducts. Bile accumulates in the liver instead of entering the intestinal tract. Bile pigments enter the blood and cause increasing jaundice.

The *pathologic picture* includes jaundice, ascites from portal obstruction, enlarged liver sometimes extending below the umbilicus, absent or deformed gallbladder, and enlarged spleen due to portal obstruction secondary to biliary cirrhosis.

The *clinical manifestation* of jaundice may not be evident until the infant is two to three weeks

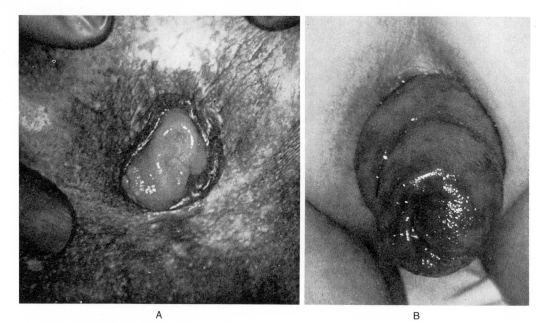

A   B

Figure 14–8. Rectal prolapse. *A,* Partial prolapse; only rectal mucosa involved. *B,* Complete prolapse of rectum (procidentia); entire thickness of rectal wall involved. (From P. Hanley and M. O. Hines, in Ochsner and DeBakey: *Christopher's Minor Surgery.* 8th ed.)

old. Eventually the skin becomes olive-green. The van den Bergh reaction is direct. The urine is stained with bile, and the stools are white or clay-colored and putty-like because of their high fat content and lack of pigment. Infection seems to cause unusual toxemia. The bleeding and clotting times may be prolonged. The prothrombin level is low. Hemorrhage may occur. Absorption of fat, fat-soluble vitamins A, D and K, and calcium is poor.

If operation cannot be done to relieve the obstruction, the *prognosis* is hopeless, although some children live for years.

Treatment and Nursing Care. The diet is high in protein and low in fat. Fat-soluble vitamins A and D are given in water-soluble form. Vitamin K is given to prevent hemorrhage. The child should be carefully protected from infection. Antibiotics are given when infection occurs.

Surgical reconstructive procedures should be done if possible on these children by the age of one to two months. Postoperatively, the child should be observed for symptoms of shock. The vital signs should be taken as ordered. The child's position should be changed frequently and carefully to prevent trauma to the wound. Because healing is impaired the wound should be inspected for bleeding. The abdomen should be observed for distention due to an accumulation of peritoneal fluid or paralytic ileus. Gastric suction may be used until peristaltic movements are heard; therefore elbow restraints should be used to prevent the infant from interfering with the tube. The surgeon may order irrigations of

the tube with warm saline solution in order to keep it open. A rectal tube may be needed to further relieve distention.

The child is fed parenterally until he can take feedings by mouth. If surgery has been successful, the stools will appear more normal when oral feedings are begun. The appearance of the stools should be described accurately and completely.

Research is currently being done on the procedure of transplanting a complete liver into a child who has biliary atresia. No conclusive results concerning this procedure are yet known.

Congenital Aganglionic Megacolon (Hirschsprung's Disease)

Etiology, Incidence and Pathology. In Hirschsprung's disease there is a congenital absence of parasympathetic ganglion ,nerve cells from the intramural plexus of a part of the intestinal tract, usually in the distal end of the descending colon.

The condition is more common in males than in females. The symptoms may be present at birth or may appear during infancy.

The involved portion of the intestine has a narrow lumen and lacks peristaltic activity. The portion of the colon above this area is greatly dilated and hypertrophied, and feces and gas accumulate in it. The muscular coat of the dilated colon, at first hypertrophied, may become thin; in infants the mucosa may become ulcerated.

Clinical Manifestations. A newborn infant

with Hirschsprung's disease may not pass meconium. Vomiting, abdominal distention, an overflow type of diarrhea or constipation may appear in the first few weeks of life.

The subsequent course shows increasingly obstinate constipation with abdominal distention due to the mass of feces and to gas. Abdominal distention may be so great that respiration is embarrassed. Fecal matter may be expelled in pellet- or ribbon-like form or may be fluid. As the disease progresses spontaneous bowel movements are infrequent. Eventually the abdominal wall becomes thin, and the superficial veins are prominent. The fecal mass may be palpated through the abdominal wall. The more severely affected children may appear malnourished and even stunted in growth. Infants and young children may have periodic attacks of intestinal obstruction due to fecal impaction. As a result there is abdominal pain, vomiting and fever.

Diagnosis. The diagnosis is based on the clinical manifestations. If diarrhea is one of the symptoms, as is often the case in infancy,

it is difficult to differentiate this condition from cystic fibrosis. The determining factors are absence of findings positive for cystic fibrosis in the sweat test and the examination of duodenal secretion for trypsin. Roentgen examination after a barium enema in children over six months of age shows the narrowed section of the rectosigmoid. After examination the barium must be removed immediately by colonic irrigation.

Rectal examination shows no fecal matter in the colon lower than the obstruction, in spite of pressure in the bowel above.

Treatment. Frequent or daily enemas are given to remove fecal matter as it accumulates. Retention enemas of mineral or olive oil may be used, followed by colonic irrigations. Some of the solution given by enema may be retained; therefore only isotonic solution should be used. If tap water were used and absorbed in large quantities, water intoxication might result.

When the child is in good condition for operation, the narrowed segment of the bowel in the rectosigmoid area is resected. The normal sig-

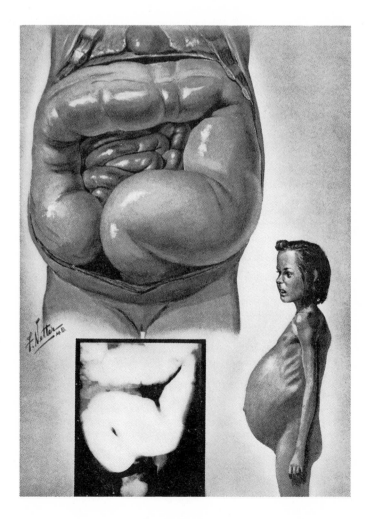

Figure 14–9. Megacolon. (Copyright, The Ciba Collection of Medical Illustrations, by Frank H. Netter, M.D.)

moid section is pulled through and sutured to the anal opening to reconstruct continuity of the bowel lumen.

A more recent type of operation is the Duhamel procedure. This entails preservation of the rectum and its utilization by means of a long, side-to-side anastomosis (by means of a clamp) between it and the normal ganglion-containing proximal colon. This procedure preserves the sensation of the urge to defecate and normal bowel control.

If the child is not in good condition for operation, a temporary colostomy may be done in preparation for further operation. The colostomy is made in the distal portion of the colon where normal ganglia are found.

Nursing Care.   Good general hygiene is important, since these infants are poorly nourished, apathetic and uncomfortable with distention and nausea. Frequent, small oral feedings are better than three large meals a day. A low residue diet is given to keep the stools soft so that they can be easily evacuated. Mineral oil or mild laxatives may be ordered for the same purpose.

Because respiration is embarrassed by the abdominal distention, the infant is more comfortable in an upright position. He can be placed in a sitting position and supported with sandbags and pillows. Enemas or colonic irrigations are given as ordered.

The nurse should record the child's appetite and the frequency and nature of the stools.

If the child is to be operated upon, *preoperative care* consists in emptying the bowel by repeated enemas and colonic irrigations with physiologic saline solution. The physician may order chemotherapeutic agents to reduce the bacterial flora.

The procedure for giving an enema is similar to that for the adult, with some alterations necessitated by the anatomy and physiology of the child.

1. A no. 10 to 12 French catheter is used. It should be inserted only 2 to 4 inches into the rectum.

2. The temperature of the solution should be 105°F.

3. Physiologic saline solution (never tap water) is used, and is made by dissolving 1 dram of salt in a pint of water.

4. Not more than 300 ml. of solution should be given to an infant unless the physician orders a larger amount.

5. The child is positioned by placing pillows under his head and back. The buttocks are placed upon the pan, which has been covered with a folded diaper to serve as a soft pad under the lower lumbar area. Another diaper is used to restrain the legs in position over the side edges of the bedpan (Fig. 14-10).

6. The enema can should not be more than 18 inches above the level of the child's hips so that the solution will run slowly by gravity and without pressure into the bowel.

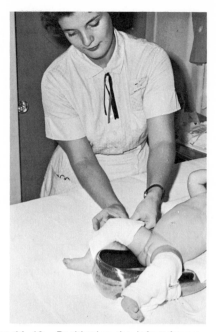

Figure 14–10.   Positioning the infant for an enema. A pillow is under the infant's head and back. The buttocks are placed upon the bedpan, which has been covered with a folded diaper to protect the infant's back. The legs are restrained in position with a diaper brought under the bedpan and pinned over the legs.

7. The results of the enema should be fully and carefully charted.

This is one of the procedures which the mother must be taught in order to give the child adequate care when he is discharged from the hospital. (Commercial enemas may be ordered for children having other diagnoses. If they are ordered, the mother should be instructed in their proper use.)

For an oil retention enema a funnel or syringe may be used. From 75 to 150 ml. of oil is usually given at 100°F. Pressure over the anus is necessary after a retention enema so that it will not be expelled. A cleansing enema should be given thirty to forty-five minutes after the oil retention enema.

In *postoperative care* the nurse will probably be asked to assist in the giving of chemotherapeutic agents to reduce the danger of infection.

The infant's temperature after operation is taken by axilla rather than by rectum until healing is complete.

There should be careful recording of intake and output of fluids and description of the stools. The perianal area should be kept clean and dry at all times, but especially after a corrective surgical procedure. If a colostomy was performed, the infant must be kept clean and dry to prevent excoriation of the surrounding area. The dressing should be changed frequently. If the area around the colostomy becomes irritated, the abdomen should be exposed to the air and the skin protected with soothing ointment.

Complications. The complications to be feared are ulcers in the mucous membrane of the intestine which will cause diarrhea, perforation and peritonitis (unusual but possible), and malnutrition.

Course and Prognosis. The child may outgrow the milder forms of megacolon and improve as his body grows. He may have difficulty in controlling flatus. During his early years this creates no serious difficulty, but during school years it may cause him great embarrassment.

Surgical correction has given excellent results.

Psychogenic Megacolon

Psychogenic megacolon may be difficult to distinguish from a true aganglionic megacolon. The cause of this so-called fear-of-the-pot syndrome is a deep antagonism between mother and child. *Treatment* consists of enemas, laxatives, fecal softeners, increased fluids, and proper elimination or toilet training (see p. 367). This condition usually occurs in the preschool period, but is mentioned here since the presenting symptoms may be similar to those of the more serious disease of infancy. The total attitude of the family and child toward bowel training should be understood if treatment is to be successful.

BLOOD DISORDERS

Blood Formation

Blood cells begin to form in the fetus in the yolk sac about the fourth week of gestation. They form successively in the liver, spleen, thymus and lymphatic tissues and last in the bone marrow. Although the liver produces the majority of blood cells during the first six months of fetal life, blood formation at term is largely carried on in the bone marrow. During the period of growth nearly all the bone marrow produces blood cells, but after growth has been completed hematopoiesis (blood cell production) is limited to the ends of the long bones, vertebrae and certain flat bones of the body. If, however, in childhood all the marrow is hematopoietic and more demand is made for blood, other organs (liver, spleen) and lymph nodes produce additional cells. At times these organs may enlarge because of the need for extramedullary hematopoiesis in certain diseases.

Although erythrocytes, granulocytes and platelets are formed in bone marrow and lymphocytic cells mostly in lymphatic tissue, an examination of peripheral blood may not be adequate for complete understanding of a condition. It is therefore necessary to study by direct or indirect means the states of hematopoietic tissue and the spleen, which is largely an organ of blood destruction.

RED BLOOD CELLS (ERYTHROCYTES). The red blood cells carry hemoglobin, which takes oxygen to the tissues and removes carbon dioxide to be excreted by the lungs. Hemoglobin also acts as a buffer in regulation of the pH of the blood. Production of red cells is stimulated by a reduced oxygen content of the blood as a result of hemorrhage, hemolysis or pulmonary or cardiac disease.

Hemoglobin formation takes place in the reticuloendothelial cells of bone marrow. The red cells are taken from circulation by the reticuloendothelial cells, especially in the spleen. The iron in the hemoglobin is mostly reused; the cell pigment changes into bile pigment and is excreted. When blood is destroyed more rapidly than normal, the liver may not be able to excrete the increased load of bilirubin. Bilirubin accumulates in the plasma, thereby producing clinical jaundice, and may be excreted as urobilinogen in the stools and urine. The spleen and perhaps the liver may enlarge because of increased activity of their reticuloendothelial elements. Rapid formation of new blood cells to replace the old takes place in bone marrow and other tissues.

A mature red cell has no nucleus, but a nucleus is present during the early stage of cell formation. Nucleated red cells are common in fetal blood and may be found in the early days of life, especially in premature infants. Since red cells are constantly being destroyed and created, the presence of some immature cells containing reticulum is to be expected. About 1 to 2 per cent of red blood cells normally are reticulocytes, containing reticulum.

Later in infancy and during childhood the presence of nucleated red cells means that the body is producing them at an abnormally rapid rate in order to meet a demand for them.

The mean number of red blood cells per cubic millimeter of blood is dependent upon the subject's age. In fetal blood the number is 5 to 7 million cells per cubic millimeter. The infant born at term normally has 4.5 to 5.5 million cells. During the first seven to ten days of life the number of red cells decreases rapidly. Because of the immaturity of the liver in early infancy, physiologic jaundice may result (see p. 105).

The destruction of red blood cells then slows down until the lowest point—3.5 to 4.5 million cells—is reached at eight to twelve weeks of life. By six months the infant's blood contains 4 to 5 million red cells per cubic millimeter. The number then gradually increases to 5 million cells and remains at that level.

At birth the amount of hemoglobin is approximately 17 to 20 gm. per 100 ml. of blood. By three months of age the hemoglobin level has dropped to 10.5 to 12 gm. From this level the value rises during childhood to the adult level.

The useful life of a normal red blood cell is about 120 days. Factors such as exposure to hemagglutinins or hemolysins (as in erythroblastosis fetalis or transfusion reactions) or anomalies of structure and shape (sickle cell disease or thalassemia) may shorten the life of a cell to as little as a few days.

The Anemias of Infancy and Childhood

Etiology, Clinical Manifestations and Prognosis. Anemia, a deficit of erythrocytes or hemoglobin, is the most frequent disorder of the blood during childhood. It represents a disturbance in the balance between the production and destruction of these substances.

There are many kinds of anemia, but only the fairly common types will be considered here. The principal types are due to (1) inadequate production of hemoglobin or red blood cells and (2) excessive loss of blood cells. Causes of underproduction of red blood cells or hemoglobin are (1) lack in the bone marrow of some substance or substances necessary in the formation of cells, (2) depressed functioning of the bone marrow, and (3) specific nutritional deficits in the marrow.

Excessive loss of red blood cells may be due to hemorrhage, e.g. acute hemorrhage in the newborn (see p. 167), chronic ulcerative colitis (see p. 500) or hemolysis of the blood. The most common causes of hemolysis are (1) a congenital anomaly of the erythrocytes or hemoglobin (e.g. thalassemia – p. 340 – and sickle cell anemia – p. 341) and (2) acquired anomalies of the erythrocyte or its environment (e.g. toxic hemolytic anemias due to poisons – p. 415 – or drugs, and the hemolytic anemias due to burns – p. 419 – and immune reactions such as erythroblastosis fetalis – p. 165).

Although the causative factors in anemia are varied, the *clinical manifestations* are similar. In the early stage the child is easily fatigued, weak and listless; later symptoms are pallor, cardiac palpitation and rapid pulse rate, or tachycardia. Eventually there is mental slowness and physical sluggishness, cardiac enlargement and inability to carry out the usual activities of childhood.

The *prognosis* varies with the type. When anemia is fatal, it is usually because of weakness of the heart and its inability to maintain the normal circulation of the blood.

Treatment and Nursing Care. The treatment and nursing care depend upon the severity of the condition, its cause and the age of the child.

Transfusions improve the child's condition, his appetite and his disposition. He becomes more active and like other children. Transfusion is lifesaving when anemia has reached the point at which it interferes with cardiac function. The procedure is like that for intravenous therapy (see p. 299). The nurse should note any evidence of discomfort, such as generalized uneasiness, restlessness, crying or chills, which may indicate the onset of a transfusion reaction. There may also be elevation of temperature and changes in the respiratory and pulse rates and in the color of the skin. The child should be observed closely also for changes in the appearance of his urine, the quantity of his urinary output, and for any hemorrhagic phenomena. Whenever the nurse notes such symptoms, she should stop the transfusion and notify the physician immediately.

One problem with transfusions in small children is blocking of the narrow lumen of the needle by the vein wall. To prevent this the blood may be slowly pumped into a small vein by using a syringe. The physician must have assistance to do this procedure. When this technique is used, the blood is given very slowly, with care taken to prevent pumping air bubbles through the needle and also to prevent contamination of the plunger of the syringe.

Medication commonly given includes iron, vitamin C and liver extract. Iron is given if the cause of the anemia is an insufficient intake of iron or loss of iron supply through hemorrhage. Iron may be given by mouth in the form of ferrous sulfate, which is absorbed more efficiently than the ferric salt. The child's mother should be told that iron medication causes the stools to become dark green or black. Iron medication should be given between meals when the stomach is empty of milk products and cereals, because these inhibit absorption of the iron. If the need for it warrants, iron may also be given intravenously or intramuscularly.

Vitamin C is valuable in correction of the anemia caused by scurvy (see p. 325). Liver extract and vitamin B complex may be used in treatment of anemias caused by a megaloblastic bone marrow.

Splenectomy may be performed because of its palliative value or for removal of the pressure of an enlarged spleen upon abdominal viscera.

Preparation of the parents for continued care of the young child having anemia is exceedingly important. In the conference with the mother the physician or nurse will take up the whole problem of the general hygiene of the child. Good hygiene includes an adequate diet, rest, sunshine and fresh air, and will help to build up the child's resistance to infections. The child should be dressed according to the weather and kept from other children and from adults who have colds, sore throats or other infections.

As the child grows older — out of the age group considered in this chapter — he should be as self-reliant and as independent of help from his mother as his age and physical condition permit. The mother must further his desire for independence, but keep it within realistic bounds. For instance, when the child is old enough to feed himself, his mother may give him a spoon while she feeds him with another, letting him take turns with her in bringing the food to his mouth. In the hospital the nurse may do the same thing and so accustom him to the procedure before he goes home. Free play activity should be alternated with periods of controlled, quiet play to allow the child to rest. He should never be allowed to exhaust his strength and should be taught gradually as he matures to protect himself against overexertion and emotional strain.

Prolonged hospitalization should be avoided unless it is necessary because of home conditions detrimental to the child's care or because his condition is such that he cannot be cared for at home. Until recently children who had chronic anemia, such as thalassemia or sickle cell disease, were admitted to the hospital for long periods for blood transfusions. These periods of absence from home and their parents and later from school were detrimental to their normal emotional development. The children often developed a fear of the hospital which made each hospitalization more difficult than the last. They felt insecure as to both their health and the normal pleasures of childhood. Much of this was realistic, but they also developed a chronic anxiety which included fears that were completely illogical and unfounded. In the end their whole lives and indeed those of their parents and siblings revolved around their disease. Hospitalization, if paid for at all, was a great drain on income, often requiring some sacrifice from every member of the family.

Today children are brought to the hospital for diagnostic examination and initial transfusions. They are then admitted to the hospital on a scheduled basis for a one-day stay for further therapy. Children learn quickly about their diseases and feel less threatened by a brief stay in the hospital, during which laboratory studies and transfusions are done, than by prolonged hospitalization. In the pediatric department they are free to talk and play with other children both before the transfusion and afterwards while they are observed for a transfusion reaction. They understand the relation between receiving blood and their feeling of well-being following the transfusion. Children cooperate best when they are familiar with the equipment, the pro-

cedure and the people who carry it out. They should be permitted to handle the equipment initially and to cleanse the area for injection before the transfusion is given.

If a child must be admitted to the hospital for a longer period for examination, laboratory tests or treatment, the nursing personnel should realize the long-term problem involved and do everything possible to make his stay as pleasant as it can be. Nursing personnel might even keep notes as to his likes and dislikes in food, toys and bed location. Often such children, on a return admission to the hospital unit, greet the nurses warmly as old friends instead of threats to their security.

The education of the anemic child should be as like that of his peers as his condition permits. If he is not able to attend school, he should be taught at home. In many cities and towns the school board sends visiting school teachers to homes or hospitals to teach children who are unable to go to school.

Hypochromic Anemia Due to Iron Deficiency

Etiology, Incidence and Pathology. If hemoglobin is not synthesized, pallor of the erythrocytes results. This hypochromia is accompanied by a decrease in size of the cell — microcytosis. If evidence of anemia is also present, as shown by the red cell count, hemoglobin level and hematocrit value below the normal range for the child's age, a hypochromic anemia can be diagnosed.

The cause is almost always a lack of iron in the diet or the child's inability to use the iron he ingests. The young child can produce hemoglobin only if his diet provides a supply of readily available iron. The minimum daily adult requirement of iron is 15 mg. The infant having iron deficiency anemia may need 100 mg. of elemental iron each day.

Iron deficiency is most apt to occur at periods of rapid growth. The premature infant at three to four months of age grows rapidly and is prone to hypochromic anemia. Infants born at term have a greater reserve of iron than has the premature infant, and the results of a diet low in iron, such as one of milk, potatoes and cereals, are not likely to be severe until the term infant is six months to two years old. At two years the growth rate is slowing down, and children are customarily receiving a varied diet adapted from that prepared for the family.

Behind the poor diet which produces anemia may be social and economic conditions — the low income of the parents or their ignorance of or indifference to dietary needs. They may not know what is an adequate diet or, since the infant will take milk, they do not persist in their efforts at feeding iron-containing foods. This may be because they do not know the technique or lack the time or simply will not take the trouble to accustom the infant to taking into his mouth and swallowing any nourishment which is not in a fluid state.

Only in rare cases is anemia due to abnormal difficulty in swallowing or to prolonged vomiting. Even though an infant ingests an adequate liberal diet suited to his age, there may be insufficient absorption or he may suffer from a chronic disease which diminishes the supply of nourishment, such as celiac disease or a chronic diarrhea.

Clinical Manifestations. The onset of hypochromic anemia is insidious and may occur as a complication of an infection, or the anemia may itself be complicated by an infection. Infants having hypochromic anemia due to iron deficiency are especially susceptible to infections.

Clinical manifestations of severe anemia include poor muscle tone, slow motor development, weakness and waxy pallor. The heart may be enlarged, and a loud, systolic precordial murmur may be heard. The spleen may be palpable. The hemoglobin level is often below 5 gm. The red blood cell count may be below 2,500,000, and stained red cells are pale and microcytic.

Treatment. Treatment is aimed at correction of the underlying cause of the condition. An adequate diet includes vegetables and meat. Vitamin supplements are necessary. Vitamin C (ascorbic acid) appears to enhance the absorption of iron. Iron, especially in inorganic form, should be given. Ferrous sulfate is cheap and easily available and has a high iron content. It should not be given in too large amounts, since its absorption is limited and it may produce vomiting. Although other iron preparations may be given, many have a smaller iron content, and therefore a larger dose must be given. Iron may be given parenterally, but this method is seldom used if the child can tolerate oral therapy. Some types of parenteral iron produce irritation at the site of the intramuscular injection and may cause systemic disturbances.

Blood transfusions are given if the child's condition is serious, especially if the infant has myocardial insufficiency. Repeated small transfusions of concentrated red blood cells are valuable.

Nursing Care. Infants suffering from iron deficiency are usually irritable. Feedings must be given slowly. As the anemia improves, the infant's appetite for food other than milk will increase. The infant should receive no more than 1 quart of milk daily. Semisolid and solid foods should be introduced into the diet in the same manner as for younger children (see p. 270).

The infant must be protected from infection, particularly from nursing personnel who have respiratory infections, and clean technique must be used in his care.

Conferences with the mother are important, since prevention of further difficulties lies in her long-term care of the infant. She should be told that his stools will become dark or black because of iron medication. Parents may become anxious at the color of the stools if they do not know the cause.

Some solutions containing iron should be well diluted and given to older children with a drinking tube or straw to prevent discoloration of the teeth by deposits of iron. The older child should rinse his mouth or brush his teeth after administration of the medication. The solution should be well diluted and for infants given with a medicine dropper. Iron in pill form or some newer liquid iron preparations may be given without a straw because they have no effect on the teeth.

Prognosis. Generally the prognosis is good when iron, vitamins and an improved diet are given. Recovery usually takes place in four to six weeks, but treatment is continued for eight to twelve weeks longer. The prognosis is variable if the infant has a concurrent infection.

Thalassemia (Mediterranean Anemia, Cooley's Anemia)

Incidence, Pathology and Types. Thalassemia is a chronic, congenital hemolytic anemia in which the chief defect seems to be an inability to produce cells capable of normal incorporation of hemoglobin. This condition occurs mainly in children whose parents or ancestors came from countries along the northern shore of the Mediterranean Sea, especially Italy, Sicily or Greece. Cases occur, however, among Negroes, Orientals, Europeans and Jews and their descendants.

The *pathology* is that of chronic microcytic, hypochromic anemia. The specific defect is production of cells of abnormal shape which are deficient in hemoglobin and are destroyed more quickly than normal cells would be. They are not capable of normal incorporation of hemoglobin. The hematopoietic tissue attempts to compensate for this defect by producing more fetal hemoglobin than is normal, but does not produce enough for the effective transportation of oxygen. Large numbers of immature and defective erythrocytes are rapidly destroyed.

There are two types of thalassemia, minor and major. Both are familial conditions.

Thalassemia minor occurs when the gene responsible for the defect is a heterozygous trait (see p. 157). The child with the minor form will show mild anemia, moderate hypochromia, and both anisocytosis and poikilocytosis (a condition in which cells are of unequal size and irregular in shape). Sometimes the spleen is enlarged.

These children have no incapacitating symptoms, however, and are able to lead normal lives. Their condition is not likely to be recognized unless blood studies are carried out as part of a family survey.

Thalassemia major is transmitted when both parents have thalassemia minor. On the average, one quarter of their children may be homozygous for the trait of thalassemia major. Such children will have progressive, severe anemia not compatible with long life. This type of anemia responds only temporarily to transfusion therapy. The condition is easily recognized in early infancy because of the onset of a progressive, severe anemia.

Clinical Manifestations. THALASSEMIA MAJOR. Since anemia is not present at birth, the newborn never shows signs of the disease. Severe anemia may develop, however, in the first few months of life. The clinical manifestations are, in general, those of any severe anemia, but certain symptoms peculiar to the condition should be noted.

The infant has a decided pallor, especially of the mucous membranes, and mild jaundice which later becomes a muddy, bronze color. The enlarged spleen of the young infant increases to an enormous size during childhood. This, with an enlarged liver, causes disabling abdominal distention which may lead to cardiorespiratory distress and cardiac enlargement with the danger of cardiac failure. Lymphadenopathy occurs, and skeletal changes are noticeable. Not only the physician but also the mother observes the child's retarded physical development, poor posture, abdominal distention and such skeletal changes as the mongoloid facies—due to the thickened membranous bones of the face and skull, often accompanied with protrusion of the teeth caused by overgrowth of the maxilla—and broad, heavy-appearing hands.

Diagnosis, Treatment, Course and Prognosis. The *diagnosis* is made on roentgen examination. By the time the infant is one year old there is widening of the medullary spaces, thinning of the cortices and decrease in the size of the bony trabeculae (connective tissue beams which extend from a capsule into the enclosed substances). In older children roentgenograms of the skull show radiating bony trabeculae traversing the widened space, resulting in a hair-on-end appearance.

The laboratory findings show microcytic anemia in both forms of the condition. In thalassemia major there is a severe anemia, a low erythrocyte count and a low hemoglobin level. There is a rapid turnover of erythrocytes, with an elevated reticulocyte count and an increase in nucleated red blood cell precursors. Even in laboratory examination it is sometimes difficult to distinguish thalassemia from anemia of iron deficiency, other hemolytic anemias of infancy or sickle cell

disease. The finding of thalassemia minor in the parents aids in establishing the diagnosis.

There is no *treatment* for thalassemia minor. For thalassemia major frequent transfusions must be given to maintain the hemoglobin level above 40 per cent of normal (6 gm. per 100 ml.). The addition of sedimented cells will increase the efficiency of a transfusion and lessen the danger of cardiac embarrassment due to too much parenteral fluid. These children can live with a relatively low hemoglobin level.

One problem associated with repeated blood transfusions is that of transfusion hemosiderosis (hemochromatosis), or excessive deposition of iron in various tissues. Cardiac failure which may be secondary to myocardial siderosis is a serious problem and may be refractory to the usual treatment for this condition. Experimental attempts are being made to eliminate excessive stored iron through increased excretion through the kidneys by the use of chelating agents.

Aspirin with antihistaminic drugs may be effective as prophylaxis against transfusion reactions. If a severe reaction occurs, cortisone may be of some value. Splenectomy may be helpful, since it lessens the discomfort from the enormous spleen; it may also help to prolong the intervals between transfusions and produces more normal growth.

The parents must be encouraged to accept the child's condition with its poor prognosis, and shown how to give the child as normal a life as possible. As with all children with severe anemias, blood transfusions on a brief inpatient or an outpatient basis are preferable to repeated, prolonged hospitalization.

Thalassemia minor is a benign condition which does not interfere with normal growth and activity. The *prognosis* is therefore good. Since the trait is genetically transmitted, young people with this condition should be made aware of the danger involved if they marry a person with the same trait.

In thalassemia major the earlier the onset and the more severe the symptoms, the more rapidly is the outcome fatal. From early infancy these children must depend upon transfusion therapy. As they grow older the need for transfusions becomes even greater. Growth is stunted, and activity is limited. There is constant danger of cardiac failure. Today more patients survive to adolescence than did in the past. If they do survive, there may be some lessening of the severity of the disease. Death may be due to the severe anemia, to progressive hepatic or cardiac involvement or to intercurrent infection.

Sickle Cell Disease

Incidence, Types and Pathology. Sickle cell disease is associated with an inherited defect in the synthesis of hemoglobin. It is confined almost exclusively to the Negro race and is seldom seen in the Caucasian race.

There are two types of the disease—the severe type and an asymptomatic condition. In the *severe* type there is a persistent hemolytic anemia with periodic episodes of painful crises. This severe condition occurs when the abnormality appears in homozygous form (inherited from both parents) (see p. 158). When the defect is heterozygous (inherited from only one parent), an *asymptomatic* condition is present—the *sickle cell trait* (see below). This is much more frequent among Negroes in the United States than is the true disease. If both parents are heterozygous, one of their children will have sickle cell disease, on the average, two will have the trait, and one will be hematologically normal.

Pathologically, the hemoglobin in both forms is abnormal (hemoglobin S). Under reduced oxygen tension this hemoglobin is responsible for forming red blood cells into a sickled shape. In sickle cell disease these malformed cells clump together and obstruct capillaries, thereby causing what is known as a crisis in the disease. Capillary obstruction leads to anoxic changes which cause further sickling and thus still further obstruction in the blood vessels. Pain in the area results. Infarcts occur most often in the spleen, but may also occur in bones, kidneys, lungs, gastrointestinal tract, brain and heart. The spleen may be so badly affected through removing blood cells from circulation and by these infarcts that it may become fibrotic and may atrophy and finally disappear.

Clinical Manifestations. In children with the sickle cell trait there are no clinical symptoms. In sickle cell disease the onset may be as early as the second or third month of life, when normal fetal hemoglobin is replaced by the abnormal hemoglobin which causes sickling. Approximately half of all children affected by this condition have symptoms by one year of age.

The first clinical manifestation the infant may have is sickle cell *crisis*. This is an acute disturbance in which the infant has severe pain in the abdomen and legs. The abdominal wall may have a boardlike rigidity. The child may also have extreme pallor, fever, vomiting and severe flank pain with hematuria, convulsions, stiff neck, coma or paralysis. Two to three days after the crisis, jaundice may appear. Between crises the manifestations are pallor and anemia. Icterus may be persistent.

Growth of a child with sickle cell disease is not stunted, but he may have long, thin extremities, a short trunk, barrel-shaped chest and protruding abdomen. If he is under nine years of age, the spleen may be palpable. There is cardiac enlargement, and murmurs are common.

Laboratory Findings and Diagnosis. Labora-

tory examination shows the sickle-shaped cells which are produced under low oxygen tension. This characteristic may be shown on smears of peripheral blood. If it is not seen on a smear, a drop of blood may be placed under a cover slip and sealed off from oxygen by petroleum jelly; if it is kept for one to twenty-four hours at room temperature, sickled forms of blood cells will appear.

Children having a sickle cell trait can be distinguished from those having the disease. In sickle cell trait the red cell count and hemoglobin level are normal. In sickle cell disease the hemoglobin level ranges from 6 to 9 gm. per 100 ml.; in times of crisis it may fall lower. Each child stabilizes at his own level, and any increase in the level as a result of transfusion therapy is only temporary. The reticulocyte count is elevated to 5 or even 25 per cent, and is usually highest up to a week after a crisis as a result of new cell formation. The leukocyte count is elevated, but the platelets are usually normal in times of crisis.

Roentgenograms of the long bones, skull, feet and hands show widened medullary spaces and thinning of the cortices.

The *diagnosis* of sickle cell disease is at times difficult to make, since other diseases may appear similar to it. This is especially true during crises when vascular occlusion occurs. Conditions which might be confused with sickle cell disease are thalassemia, syphilis, tuberculosis, osteomyelitis, rheumatic fever and acute conditions of the abdomen.

Treatment, Course and Prognosis. *Treatment* consists of supportive measures such as blood transfusions when necessary, and protection against infections. Treatment during crises includes codeine and aspirin for relief of pain, and maintenance of hydration. Antibiotic therapy may be necessary if a bacterial infection is present. Transfusion of erythrocytes may be required. Oxygen is given if the hemoglobin level falls rapidly to as low as 4 gm. per 100 ml. and the child has symptoms of hypoxia. Splenectomy usually has no value in sickle cell disease. In older children autosplenectomy may occur as a result of repeated thromboses.

The *course* depends upon the severity of the sickling tendency, the frequency of crises and the age of the child. As the child grows older crises occur less frequently. In temperate regions crises occur more commonly in autumn and spring.

The *prognosis* depends on the severity of the disease. The condition may interfere to some extent with the child's growth, nutrition and activity. The life expectancy of the small child is probably less than the average because of the physiologic handicap, but many of these children grow up to adult life and are able to earn a living. Death is usually the result of severe anemia or intercurrent infection.

ENDOCRINE DISORDERS

Cretinism (Congenital Hypothyroidism)

Etiology, Incidence and Onset. Cretinism is caused by a congenital insufficiency of the secretion of the thyroid gland due to an embryonic defect in which the gland is absent or rudimentary and unable to produce thyroid hormone. The condition occurs sporadically in the United States. The infant appears normal at birth, but clinical manifestations may appear in the first few weeks or months of life. Cretinism is not to be confused with mongolism, which can be recognized at birth (see p. 220).

Clinical Manifestations and Diagnosis. Early signs of the condition are prolonged physiologic jaundice and feeding difficulties. The infant is pale because of anemia. He is constipated, and an umbilical hernia develops, owing to hypotonic abdominal musculature. There is little perspiration, and the skin is dry and scaly. The child is lethargic, cries little, sleeps most of the time and has little appetite. His temperature is subnormal, his pulse slow. The facial appearance is peculiar, for the eyes are far apart, the bridge

of the broad nose is flat, the eyelids are swollen, and the tongue protrudes from the open mouth. The anterior fontanel is widely open because of poor bone development. Dentition is delayed, and the teeth decay rapidly.

The general appearance is abnormal: the arms and legs are short, the relatively large head is supported on a short, thick neck, and the hands are broad and the fingers short. The hair is coarse, brittle and scanty. The hairline reaches down on the forehead. These infants have an early developmental lag. Bone development is retarded, and physical and motor development is slow. Mental development also is delayed. These children appear lethargic and are late in sitting, standing and walking. They do not learn to talk at the usual time, and sexual maturation is slower than that of the normal child.

They are dull, placid, good-natured babies. Ignorant mothers are often proud of their crying so little and being no trouble. When routine follow-up of newborn infants is neglected, these children are often not given a diagnosis until much valuable time for early treatment has passed.

Early *diagnosis* may be difficult, for the symptoms appear gradually as the child grows older. Roentgenograms show the retarded bone age in untreated cases; multiple foci of ossification appear in the epiphyses. The basal metabolic rate is decreased. The serum cholesterol level fluctuates, but in general is increased. The nor-

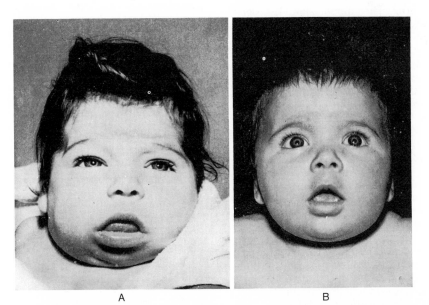

A   B

Figure 14–11. Congenitally hypothyroid infant at 6 months of age. Infant fed poorly in neonatal period and was constipated. Had persistent nasal discharge and large tongue. Very lethargic, no social smile and no head control. *A,* Note puffy face, dull expression, hirsute forehead. Serum cholesterol 172 mg. per 100 ml., alkaline phosphatase 4.8 Bodansky units, negligible uptake of radio-iodine. Osseous development that of newborn. *B,* Four months after treatment with U.S.P. thyroid. Note decreased puffiness of face, decreased hirsutism of forehead and alert appearance. (A. M. DiGeorge in Nelson: *Textbook of Pediatrics.* 8th ed.)

mal cholesterol level is 100 to 300 mg. per 100 ml. of serum; in the cretin it is from 250 to 600 mg. The serum phosphatase level is decreased, and the carotene level is many times increased.

A reliable measurement of thyroid function is the protein-bound iodine level of the serum. The values with cretinism are usually under 2 gammas per 100 ml. Another test of thyroid function is the uptake of radioactive iodine by the thyroid gland. In patients with cretinism a normal concentration in the thyroid is not obtained.

Treatment. If treatment is delayed, the infant may become more and more retarded in growth and mental development. The treatment (substitution therapy) is by oral administration of desiccated thyroid. The dose is usually small when the medication is started and is gradually increased to the maximum amount which can be given without producing symptoms of overdosage. This medication must be taken throughout life. The dose may have to be increased at puberty and during the reproductive period.

In addition, the infant should receive a complete diet with adequate amounts of vitamin D. Since thyroid stimulates bone growth, the child will outgrow his supply of vitamin D if additional amounts are not provided.

The anemia is a problem, since it does not respond readily to hematinics. Constipation, another troublesome symptom, is not easily relieved.

Nursing Care. The nurse should observe children being treated with desiccated thyroid for symptoms of overdosage, e.g. rapid pulse, loss in weight, vomiting, cramps, diarrhea, elevation of temperature, and personality changes such as increased excitability and irritability.

Because of the tendency for decay of the teeth, good dental care should be provided early to preserve the temporary teeth. As soon as the child is able, he should be taught to brush his teeth.

Since one of the main problems in these children is their slowness of mental development, neither the child's parents nor his nurses should attempt to push the child beyond his capacity or compare his general development with that of normal children.

Prognosis. The prognosis in untreated cases is likely to be poor. Death may result early from an intercurrent infection, or the child may become a mentally retarded dwarf. If treatment is begun early and continued through life, the child may be normal physically, but probably somewhat mentally retarded (see p. 526). The earlier and more effective the treatment, the better the prognosis. Even with the best therapy, however, mental development may never be normal.

INBORN ERRORS OF METABOLISM

Phenylketonuria

Incidence, Etiology and Clinical Manifestations. Phenylketonuria is not a common condition; it occurs in about one in every 10,000 births. The condition is equally common in males and females; the majority of affected infants are blue-eyed blonds.

The condition is due to a congenital defect in phenylalanine metabolism. Phenylalanine is an essential amino acid present in all natural protein foods. As the newborn takes in food the phenylalanine accumulates in the blood, and phenylketone bodies are excreted in the urine. The abnormal accumulation of phenylalanine apparently prevents normal brain development.

Phenylketonuria is transmitted by an autosomal recessive gene (see p. 158). The majority of affected infants are offspring of two heterozygous carriers of the gene. With each pregnancy the chance is one in four that the infant will be normal, two in four that he will be a carrier of the defect, and one in four that he will have phenylketonuria. But in some families more than this proportion of children or all the children may be born with this condition.

The *clinical manifestations* begin by about four months of age, when the mother may notice that the infant has a peculiar odor and is not developing normally. Brain development is arrested, and mental retardation of varying degrees may result; hence the condition is sometimes called *phenylpyruvic oligophrenia.* Neurologic symptoms appear; the child may exhibit schizoid-like, disagreeable personality traits. Eczema or convulsions, or both, occur in about one fourth of these children.

Diagnosis. The diagnosis is made by a simple urine test for phenylketone bodies and by blood tests for phenylalanine. When the blood phenylalanine level is above approximately 15 mg. per 100 ml. of plasma, phenylketone bodies usually appear in the urine. The tests are not usually made until the first or second week of life, but are especially necessary on infants born into families with a known history of phenylketonuria or on infants who show signs of mental dullness. The same tests are used for diagnosis and for checking with dietary management. Mandatory laws concerning the testing of infants for phenylketonuria have been enacted in many states.

The *urine test* is made with ferric chloride. One cubic centimeter of urine is placed in a test tube, and 3 drops of a 5 or 10 per cent ferric chloride solution are added. If a green color appears, phenylketone bodies are present. (Phenistix can also be used to test urine.) Normal urine, used in the same combination with ferric chloride, remains yellow.

The *diaper test* is done in many Child Health Con-

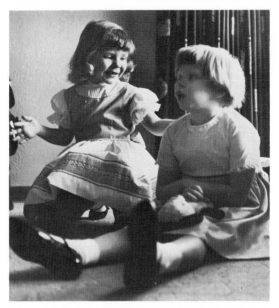

Figure 14–12. A comparison of a child having phenylketonuria (*right*) with her sister who has achieved dietary control of the same condition (*left*). (Courtesy of National Association for Retarded Children.)

ferences (see p. 277), hospitals and pediatricians' offices for early detection of the condition. A drop of 5 to 10 per cent ferric chloride solution on a recently wet diaper will turn it green if phenylketone bodies are present (a positive result is also obtained with histidinemia). If the urine is normal, it remains yellow. The diaper test should be repeated at intervals, since some children with phenylketonuria do not always give positive results.

For many years the diaper test has been the universal method of detecting this disease; however, the screening procedure most prominent at present is the Guthrie test. This test, a simple screening test done on heel blood, can be used to screen newborns for phenylketonuria the day they are discharged from the nursery. Since the blood phenylalanine concentration rises after birth when the infant is given milk feedings, a second test for phenylketonuria should be performed at four to six weeks of age. The earlier the diagnosis can be made, the sooner treatment can be started and the better the prognosis will be. If these tests are not done until after signs of the condition make the physician suspicious, the child will already have been damaged. Recently physicians have advocated screening programs for pregnant women who may have high phenylalanine levels which could lead to mental retardation in their newborns.

Treatment and Nursing Care. Since the clinical manifestations of phenylketonuria are due to accumulation of unmetabolized phenylalanine,

the condition can be controlled by preventing phenylalanine intake from early infancy. Because all natural protein foods contain phenylalanine, Lofenalac (Mead Johnson), a synthetic food providing sufficient protein for growth and repair, yet containing very little phenylalanine, may be substituted. Other foods which are permitted in the diet include 1 per cent protein fruits and vegetables, tapioca and cornstarch as cereals, sugar and butter. Foods which must be omitted include breads, meat, fish, poultry, all types of flour, cheese, milk, nuts and products made with nuts, eggs and legumes. A table of phenylalanine equivalents is available from the Mead Johnson & Company, Evansville, Indiana. Management must be individualized on the basis of response to the therapy, as judged by urine and blood levels of phenylalanine, the level of physical and mental development and the relief of physical symptoms.

The nurse must be aware of the cost of the formula and of the meaning that food has to various cultural groups if she is to understand the reaction that parents may have to this drastic restriction of diet for their child.

The nutritional status and hemoglobin level should be determined frequently, since the infant is on a limited diet. Intelligence tests and other estimates of mental ability are important for infants who have been treated early, to determine the rate of mental growth.

These infants should be observed for evidence of the onset of dermatologic or neurologic symptoms. Nurses should stress in conferences with parents the importance of health checkups of the newborn so that the condition, if it exists, can be treated in the earliest stages. Continued therapy is expensive for the child's family, but they can obtain financial help through federal or state funds or through local health and welfare departments.

Prognosis. The prognosis is at best doubtful, but is far more favorable if a diet with a low phenylalanine content is begun in the early months of infancy. Once brain development has been retarded, the process cannot be reversed; it can only be arrested. If treatment is not given until the child is three years old, he may show improvement in personality and behavior, but not in mental status. Many physicians believe that if the child remains on this diet until he is four to six years old, most of the damage to the brain will be prevented. Termination of the dietary restrictions frequently improves the emotional climate of the family.

Galactosemia

Incidence, Etiology, Clinical Manifestations and Diagnosis. Galactosemia represents an inborn error in the metabolism of galactose.

It is not a common condition. The defect is transmitted as an autosomal recessive trait (see p. 158). The enzyme that changes galactose to glucose in the liver is missing. Galactose is not found in free form in foods; however, intestinal hydrolysis of lactose from milk products yields glucose and galactose. When the amount of galactose in the blood exceeds the ability of the renal tubules to reabsorb it, galactosuria results. These infants appear normal at birth, but galactosuria occurs one or two weeks later when the infant is taking his milk feeding.

Clinical manifestations at first include feeding difficulties, vomiting and weight loss. Later, enlargement of the liver and spleen, cirrhosis of the liver, mental retardation and cataracts are evident. Finally lethargy and emaciation increase, and death occurs from infection or hepatic failure. *Diagnosis* is made on the basis of finding galactose in the blood and urine of these infants.

Treatment and Nursing Care. This defect must be found early and the infant taken off a diet containing milk before irreversible damage has been done to the brain and the liver. A galactose-free diet of milk substitutes containing casein hydrolysates does not raise the blood galactose level. Milk, milk products and lactose-containing tablets must be eliminated from the child's diet for at least the first three years of life. Cataracts, if present, require surgical treatment.

Hypoglycemia

Incidence, Etiology, Clinical Manifestations, Treatment, and Prognosis. In recent years not only infants of diabetic mothers have been diagnosed as having hypoglycemia, but infants of nondiabetic mothers have also been diagnosed as having this condition. This condition is seen mostly in male infants of low birth weight whose mothers had had toxemia.

The *cause* of this type of hypoglycemia is thought to be due to the infant's having inadequate stores of glycogen in the liver before birth, and a very sensitive insulin release mechanism after birth. This may be due to a rare inborn error of enzyme synthesis, but the real cause is not known.

Clinical manifestations may be seen soon after birth and during infancy. These include tremors, convulsions, listlessness, periods of respiratory distress and cyanosis, abnormal cry, and feeding difficulties.

Treatment includes the giving of glucose solution intravenously until the blood glucose level has been stabilized. ACTH may also be given in an attempt to maintain the blood glucose level within normal range. This condition may recur during infancy.

The *prognosis* for life is good; however, these infants may be impaired intellectually as a result of this condition, because the brain, except under unusual conditions, is able to utilize only glucose.

Agammaglobulinemia (Bruton's Disease)

Incidence, Etiology, Clinical Manifestations and Diagnosis. Congenital agammaglobulinemia is a rare condition in which the child is unable to form gamma globulin. This disorder is transmitted by a sex-linked gene (see p. 158); therefore it affects usually only boys, although the mother carries the abnormal gene and can transmit it to half of her daughters, who are not affected clinically.

Children having agammaglobulinemia cannot form antibodies against many bacterial antigens or to antigenic substances such as typhoid vaccine and diphtheria toxoid. They therefore have recurrent pyogenic infections, especially with staphylococci, streptococci, pneumococci and meningococci. Their response to viral infections, however, is normal. Newborn infants acquire gamma globulin from their mothers late in gestation; therefore infections may not occur until the child is approximately six months of age. The diagnosis is made on the basis of a history of repeated infections, a persistently positive Schick test or a negative Widal test result after usual immunization procedures have been done, a lack of lymphoid tissue, especially the adenoids, and a lack of gamma globulin in the blood.

Acquired agammaglobulinemia may appear later in life, but this condition is seen in both males and females.

Treatment and Nursing Care. The *treatment* of agammaglobulinemia consists in prevention of infection and immediate treatment of infections when they occur. The patient should receive monthly intramuscular injections of gamma globulin for the remainder of his life. Acute infections respond to antimicrobial chemotherapy.

A mother, in an attempt to prevent her child from acquiring infections, may overprotect him. The nurse must help such a mother gain a more positive attitude toward her child's illness.

Tay-Sachs Disease (Amaurotic Family Idiocy)

Incidence and Etiology. Tay-Sachs disease is one of a group of cerebromacular degenerative disorders. It occurs most frequently among Jewish people originating in eastern Europe. This condition is one that shows autosomal recessive inheritance (see p. 158).

The cause is thought to be a biochemical abnormality in lipid metabolism.

Pathology, Clinical Manifestations and Diagnosis. The brain becomes atrophic and firm. Stores of lipid are found in the neurons.

The infant is apparently normal at birth. Usually about six months of age, the infant becomes listless, regresses in motor ability, has muscular weakness and is unable to fix his eyes upon an object. By one year he is flaccid and fat. He has hyperactive reflexes, startles easily at the slightest stimulation and is *blind*. This degenerative disease continues with muscular degeneration, spasticity, seizures, malnutrition, decerebrate posturing, dementia and death.

The *diagnosis* is made when macular cherry-red spots surrounded by a gray-white edematous retina are seen in the fundi of the eyes. Optic atrophy is also noted. Blood and cerebrospinal fluid values usually remain normal.

Treatment, Nursing Care and Prognosis. No treatment is known. The family must be informed of the likely clinical course. They should be informed of facilities available in their community for assistance with the child. Genetic counseling about future children should be made available to them.

The aim of *nursing care* is to give the child as much comfort as possible. Stimuli should be reduced to a minimum, for the child startles easily. Nutrition should be maintained by whatever means are possible, including gavage eventually.

The child's emaciated condition necessitates good skin care. He must be turned frequently to prevent breakdown of the skin and to lessen the danger of pneumonia. Since the child is blind, the nurse should speak before touching him so as not to startle him.

The gradual deterioration of the child's condition is hard for the parents to bear. They need much sympathy, particularly since they know that his condition is hereditary. Since it is due to a recessive trait, both parents share the feeling of responsibility for the disease. The rabbi will be a source of comfort and emotional support, but the parents will turn to the physician and the nurse to express their grief at the continued degeneration of the child's condition.

The *prognosis* is hopeless. Death usually occurs before the third birthday.

SKIN CONDITIONS

Infantile Eczema
(Atopic Dermatitis)

Incidence. Many different unrelated inflammatory dermatoses may be grouped under the term of "eczema." Here, however, eczema is considered to be an atopic manifestation of a specific allergen, whether ingested or in contact with the skin. Eczema is a common inflammatory skin condition of infants. It is the most frequent evidence of an allergic state seen in infancy. Seborrhea or diaper rash may be frequently associated with infantile eczema.

Eczema is most frequent in the first two years of life. It is uncommon in breast-fed infants, but not in infants two or three months old, whether bottle-fed or breast-fed, who get some additional solid food. Eczema is relatively uncommon after the second year.

An infant, even a well cared for infant, may receive antigens through contact or by inhalation.

Eczema occurs in both sexes, in any race and at any time of the year. It is most likely, however, to appear in the winter months and to clear up in the summer. It is most frequent in well nourished, fat infants whose general health is excellent.

Etiology. Several factors may be responsible for the condition. There is a decided familial tendency. Anatomically and chemically, the skin of an infant differs from that of an adult. The infant is likely to show greater response to scratching and to other irritants. His skin has a higher water and sodium chloride content that that of the adult. These attributes are exaggerated in the skin of an infant with eczema. His skin may be abnormally sensitive to irritation from clothes, wool garments, soaps, cold, strong sunlight or mild skin infections. Some physicians believe that overfeeding, especially of carbohydrates or fat, may have an adverse effect on infants prone to eczema. It is difficult to prove this, although eczema in obese infants has improved when they lost weight as a result of dietary restriction of fat and carbohydrate.

Although there is general agreement that infantile eczema is due largely to allergy, it is difficult to show specific causes for the sensitivity. The most common allergies are due to various foods, e.g. egg white, cow's milk, wheat cereal and oranges.

Some investigators believe that there is a disturbance in the mother-child relations among infants and children who have eczema. Such children are smothered with love by their parents.

Pathology, Clinical Manifestations and Diagnosis. *Pathologically,* the capillaries of the skin dilate, thereby producing erythema and edema. Fluid escapes from the capillaries into the tissues. Papules and then vesicles form. These rupture and exude yellow, sticky material which dries and forms crusts on the skin (see Plate 1, Fig. 3). The infant scratches, and excoriation of the skin results. Mild and severe lesions may exist at the same time on different parts of the body. The skin becomes thickened, and fissures form. Itching is usually intense, and secondary infection results from scratching the lesions. The regional lymph nodes swell in the area. The cervical lymph nodes may swell if there is an infection of the scalp.

The eczema has periods of exacerbation and remission which are discouraging to the mother, who hopes for steady improvement. Eczema most commonly occurs on the cheeks, forehead and scalp, and less frequently behind the ears, on the neck and on the flexor surfaces of the arms and legs. There may be lesions on the trunk, abdomen and back, but these are usually drier and more scaly than elsewhere. The palms of the hands and the soles of the feet are not involved, though the rest of the body may be.

Because of the constant and intense itching the infant may not be able to sleep and may be highly irritable. If the lesions become infected, he may have a low-grade fever. Although most infants with eczema are overweight, malnutrition may be present if an infant has anorexia, dietary restrictions, a chronic infection or diarrhea.

Eczematous lesions may flare up after prophylactic immunizations. These infants should not be given smallpox vaccination because of the possible development of generalized vaccinia (see p. 277). This condition might also occur if the infant were to come in contact with a sibling or another child who was recently vaccinated. Such contacts should be carefully avoided.

The *diagnosis* is made on the characteristics and distribution of the eruption, the family history, symptoms of severe itching, demonstration of protein sensitivity and a tendency to improve in summer.

Treatment and Nursing Care.   Even the most intensive *treatment* may not produce a cure, but most infants can be helped by therapy.

The mother should be instructed as to the course to be expected, the treatment and the nursing care. She should understand that these infants are prone to infections of the skin and the respiratory tract and that they should be treated at home if at all possible because of the danger of infection in the hospital. Hospitalization may be necessary if the infant already has a secondary infection or if he requires more intensive care and local treatment than the mother can provide. Sometimes there is less external irritation in the hospital environment, and the infant can be kept on a stricter dietary regimen. If the mother is exhausted because of caring for the infant, he should be hospitalized for her sake as well as his own.

If hospitalization is necessary, the infant should be isolated for his own protection, not only from recently vaccinated children, but also from all persons with herpesvirus or pneumococcal or streptococcal infections. These infants are uncomfortable and need mothering. If possible, the mothers should visit frequently, and the nurses should give these infants extra attention.

In local treatment, restraints are important, though they should be applied only when necessary to prevent scratching. These infants scratch their irritated skin instead of crying when they are angry or frustrated. The nurse should help the infant to express his feelings outwardly by encouraging active play or physical movement. Restraints are necessary, of course, when the mother or nurse cannot be with him constantly.

There are many types of restraints, and their use depends on the specific type needed. The following are self-explanatory: elbow cuff, abdominal, jacket, face mask, and ankle and wrist restraints.* Any needed combination of restraints may be used, but they must be checked frequently to determine whether they are constricting the circulation. Cotton socks may be put over the hands and feet after the fingernails and toenails have been cut as short as possible to prevent the infant from digging his skin.

Care must be taken to apply the restraints securely but gently. The restraints should be removed every few hours to allow free movement. If the infant is extremely uncomfortable because of itching, restraints should be removed from only one extremity at a time so that the nurse or mother can easily prevent him from scratching uncontrollably. If he has a paroxysm of scratching, the improvement of several weeks may be undone, and the skin may be opened to infection.

The infant should be picked up frequently and his position changed as often as possible to prevent respiratory infections, especially pneumonia. He should have supervised periods of play out of his crib to minimize his anger at being restrained and to give him opportunity to learn about his surroundings if he is old enough to walk.

To prevent irritation of the skin from rubbing against the sheet, heavy plastic or cellophane sheeting should be placed over the cotton sheet so that the infant can be turned from side to side and lie upon his back without increasing the severity of the lesions. This will also prevent absorption of ointment by the bedclothes. If the parents cannot afford new plastic sheeting, an old pliable plastic table cover can be used. In the hospital large pieces of exposed and washed x-ray film—the sharp edges covered with ad-

---

* An effective elbow-cuff restraint for an infant may be made with tongue blades inserted into a stitched muslin restraint. This restraint may be secured in place by turning the end of a long-sleeved shirt back over the restraint and pinning it securely (see Fig 11-5).

hesive tape—may be used beneath the infant's head.

The infant may be bathed in water if it does not irritate his skin. In general it is better not to use soap; a substitute containing hexachlorophene may be used. Oil baths may be ordered if both soap and this substitute are irritating to the skin. Oil should be applied with a piece of cotton and patted rather than rubbed on. The crusted areas may be soaked with mild antiseptic solution compresses. Saline soaks kept continuously wet for one or two days may be helpful in removing crusts. If large areas are covered with papulovesicles, a soluble starch and sodium bicarbonate bath may be ordered. The water for the bath should have a temperature of 95°F., and the soak should be continued for fifteen to twenty minutes. Floating toys may be used to divert the infant's attention. During the bath only one extremity should be removed from restraint at a time. Although the bath is comforting to the irritated skin, the infant may attempt to scratch his body; if both his arms were free, his nurse or mother would be unable to control him.

It is not advisable to take the infant outdoors if the weather is cold or if there is a strong wind. His clothing indoors should be such that he is sufficiently warm, but not overheated. He should be dressed in as little clothing as possible to avoid overheating and skin irritation. No woolen garments should be used, since he may be sensitive to wool. The diapers should be changed promptly to avoid irritation of the buttocks.

The infant should be held for his feedings in the same way that healthy infants are held. He needs love for his emotional growth. Holding him will tend to change his position and prevent respiratory difficulties. Allowing him to suck on a nipple or pacifier provides relaxation and reduces tension during the first year of life.

Local medication applied to the irritated skin is important. Since different types of lesions may be present on different areas of the body at the same time, different kinds of medication and treatments may be ordered for the various areas. Ointments are not used for weeping areas. On indurated areas the ointment should be thoroughly rubbed into the skin. Whatever ointment or lotion the physician has ordered should be kept on the skin constantly and applied with long, soothing strokes.

Many kinds of ointments and lotions have been used in the treatment of eczema. It is difficult to apply ointment to the skin of the face so as to be effective, because crusts are usually present, and it is difficult to keep ointment on this area. Crusts may be removed by wiping with gauze soaked with liquid petrolatum or by applying saline compresses constantly for one or two days. If an ointment is to be applied to the face,

a mask made of gauze or stockinet may be used to keep the medication in close contact with the skin.

To make a face mask, holes are cut in the material to correspond in shape and location to the eyes, nose and mouth. The holes are stitched so that the edges cannot fray. The mask is secured in place on the infant's head by draw strings. In applying it care must be taken to avoid binding or friction which would irritate the lesions.

If infection has occurred, various lotions or ointments may be used which contain bacitracin, bacitracin with neomycin or other antibiotics.

If the skin surface is dry, red and papular, an ointment containing crude coal tar may be ordered. The ointment should be applied as often as necessary to keep the area covered. Before its application a small area should be treated with it to determine the infant's sensitivity to it. All areas treated with tar ointment should be constantly bandaged, and uncovered only when new ointment is to be applied. Every day all the ointment should be removed with liquid petrolatum, and fresh ointment should be applied. A starch bath may be used to remove ointment from large areas of the body covered with papulovesicles.

In teaching a mother to use tar ointments the nurse should emphasize that the ointment must be kept in tightly covered jars to prevent evaporation of volatile ingredients. Stains on linen can be removed by rubbing both sides of the soiled area with lard and washing with soap and water. The mother should also be told not to expose the infant to sunlight, since tar ointment contains a photosensitizing fraction that will produce further skin irritation. After the papules and the intense itching have disappeared the tar ointment is often discontinued, and a milder

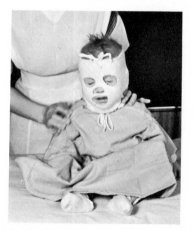

Figure 14–13. Face mask which can be used on a child with eczema to keep medication in close contact with the skin.

medication such as petrolatum or zinc oxide is used.

Many infants improve under these local applications, but if there is no improvement, further measures must be taken. Treatment involves a search for the specific allergens which cause the condition. Whether these are foods, wool or inhalants such as dust, they should be removed.

Wool should be removed from the child's environment. Neither his clothing nor his blankets should be of wool, and adults caring for him should not wear wool. The area about the crib should be kept free from dust. Carpets and drapes harbor dust and should not be used in his room.

A careful history or an elimination diet can be used to determine allergenic foods. If the infant is on an elimination diet, his mother should be given a list of foods he may have rather than a list of foods to be avoided. She should adhere strictly to the diet ordered. Synthetic vitamins may be given to supplement the diet. The diet should be increased so as to be as complete as possible. When a new food is added, the mother or nurse should watch for an allergic reaction to it. Such foods and reactions should be noted for the physician's consideration.

Skin testing as a means of finding allergenic substances is not very helpful in young infants or in children who have eczematous lesions covering their bodies. It is used with older children.

Many infants with eczema are allergic to cow's milk. Substitutes for cow's milk must therefore be provided in their formulas. Some infants can tolerate cow's milk if it has been exposed to a high temperature, thereby altering its protein so that it is less allergenic. For this reason evaporated or dried milk is of great value in the treatment of such children.

Infants sensitive to cow's milk in any form may be given goat's milk, vegetable protein substitutes, formulas made from meat or products made from hydrolyzed casein. Vegetable protein substitutes, largely made of soybeans, are available commercially in liquid or powdered form. With any substitute formula vitamins C and D, as well as other essentials, must be included in the diet.

Various nonspecific treatments may be ordered. Measures which produce mild dehydration are helpful in the treatment of eczema. If a lowered sodium intake is ordered, water retention may be decreased.

Corticosteroids may be given systemically as well as locally to produce relief in severe cases, and are useful in controlling inflammatory skin reactions. Antibiotic therapy by oral or parenteral administration is essential if infection of the skin or other parts of the body is present. Mild sedation may be necessary if the infant is unable to sleep.

Charting is important and should include the condition of the skin (changes in the appearance and location of the rash and the general appearance of the infected areas), reaction to food (both the articles added to the diet and the formula), treatments given, additional allergic manifestations such as asthma and rhinitis, the amount of discomfort caused by itching of the skin, and alteration in personality characteristics.

The psychologic aspect of nursing is as important as the physical aspect. These infants should receive as much attention and affection as normal infants, if not more. Although their appearance may not encourage the nurse to handle, fondle and play with them, they need loving care to prevent emotional deprivation. A gown or a coverall apron may be worn over the clothing of the nurse or the mother in order to protect it from contact with ointment on the child's skin.

Toys suited to the child's age should be provided. The toys must be washable, safe and soft (if possible) and have a smooth surface. Stuffed toys which contain substances such as wool, feathers or kapok, to which children may be allergic should not be used.

The nurse should understand the needs of the parents. Some mothers feel that they have failed to fulfill their maternal role, some are overprotective toward the infant, and others are afraid that their infants have a chronic condition which will result in disfiguring scars and retarded development. The nurse should help the mother to verbalize her feelings about the infant and the care he will need. Helping the mother to overcome her fears about her child while he is in the hospital will ensure better care for him at home.

The nurse must instruct the parents in the methods of local therapy and the diet to be given the infant. She must demonstrate to the mother the ways of applying restraints and providing exercise and diversion for the child. The nurse must help the mother find ways of giving adequate compensation for the kissing and skin-to-skin contact which other infants enjoy and of providing a happy environment in which the infant can lead as normal a life as is compatible with the necessary restraint of his hands and with local applications of ointments. The child should be permitted to move around his crib, playpen or room and feel that he is part of the family group. Normal activity and satisfactions are necessary so that he will not feel frustrated by the discomfort of his itching skin. The mother should have an opportunity to care for him in the hospital with the help of the nurses. This will reduce her fears about caring for him after his discharge.

Prognosis. The prognosis is good, but the course is long-drawn out, with remissions and exacerbations. Parents are likely to become discouraged, especially if they have tried their best to care for the child. The nurse must help them to see the situation realistically and without unwarranted anxiety over the child's evident discomfort. Infantile eczema usually clears up spontaneously toward the end of the second year of life. The condition can be controlled earlier if the causative allergens are eliminated. After two years the child may exhibit other allergic manifestations such as asthma and hay fever.

If infection develops during hospitalization of the infant, the prognosis may be poor, but will depend upon the severity of the condition. To prevent this danger these infants should spend as little time as possible in the hospital.

DISORDERS OF THE NERVOUS SYSTEM

Tetany

Tetany is extreme irritability of the neuromuscular system. It may be caused by any one of a number of conditions. These may be divided into groups: those characterized by a decrease in serum calcium (hypocalcemic tetany) and those in which a state of alkalosis exists (tetany of alkalosis).

Symptoms of *hypocalcemic tetany* occur when the total serum calcium concentration falls below 7 to 7.5 mg. per 100 ml. (normal serum calcium is from 10 to 12 mg.). In tetany of the newborn, i.e. in the first week of life, there is hypocalcemia due to hypofunction of the parathyroid glands. Hypocalcemia also occurs in vitamin D deficiency associated with rickets and is termed infantile nutritional tetany (see p. 324). In celiac disease tetany results because of deficient absorption of vitamin D and calcium (see p. 326).

Tetany of alkalosis occurs when the acid-base balance is shifted to an alkaline level. It is not associated with changes in the serum level of calcium and phosphorus. It occurs with hyperventilation (excessive breathing) and in gastric tetany due to excessive vomiting and the concomitant loss of chloride. It may be observed in pyloric stenosis or in high intestinal obstruction which causes vomiting.

Convulsions

Incidence and Etiology. A convulsion may be termed a symptom of a disease rather than a disease entity. Convulsive disorders are far more common during infancy and the second year of life than in any other age period.

Convulsions during early childhood are due to a variety of conditions, any of which may affect the nervous system.

In the newborn, birth injury, a congenital defect of the brain, and the effects of anoxia and intracranial hemorrhage are the most frequent causes of convulsions. During later infancy and early childhood acute infections of the central nervous system or other parts of the body, with accompanying elevation of temperature, are the most common causes. Less frequent causes are tetany (see p. 324), pertussis immunization (see p. 277), hypoglycemia (see p. 346), poisoning by a convulsive drug or by lead (see p. 416), asphyxia, fluid and electrolyte imbalance, progressive degenerative diseases, neoplasms and postnatal intracranial trauma (see p. 352).

Nursing Care. Though children rarely die in convulsions, few other conditions frighten parents to the same extent. The nurse must be understanding of their fear and help them to a realistic attitude toward the child's condition. They should be told that though seven infants in every hundred have a convulsion, few of them suffer permanent damage. In the other cases the condition is indicative of some deep-seated pathologic state.

The nurse should place the child who has had a convulsion or in whom a convulsion may occur where continuous observation is possible. She should observe the child frequently so that, if he has a convulsion, she will be able to give him care and to report accurately to the physician.

A young child may show changes in behavior indicating the onset of a convulsion, such as irritability, restlessness or the reverse, listlessness. Such changes should be charted with the report of the convulsion. The nurse should note the types of movement and whether they are clonic (i.e twitching, jerking movements) or tonic convulsions (those in which the child becomes stiff and the muscles are in a state of constant contraction), the time the convulsion begins and ends, the areas of the body involved, the amount of perspiration, movements of the eyes and change in size of the pupils, incontinence (this will be influenced not only by the severity of the seizure, but also by the distention of the bladder at the time of the convulsion), the rate of respiration, color, bodily posture, foaming at the mouth or vomiting, the apparent degree of consciousness during the seizure, and the infant's behavior after his return to consciousness.

SEIZURE PRECAUTIONS. The patient must be protected from injury. All hard toys should be removed from the bed, since he might be injured if he fell upon them. A padded tongue depressor should be kept on the bedside stand or taped to the bed to put between the teeth to prevent his biting his tongue. Care should be taken when inserting the tongue depressor to prevent injuring the child's mouth. The sides of the crib should be padded if he has had a convulsion recently or is likely to have one. If the child has repeated convulsions, there should be in readiness an aspirating machine with which to remove accumulated secretions from the nasopharynx, and an emergency oxygen setup in case he has sudden respiratory difficulty.

If the child's temperature is elevated, tepid sponge baths may be ordered. The procedure is as follows.

The water should be tepid. Alcohol is added only if it is ordered. Long, soothing strokes with a washcloth should follow the course of the large blood vessels of the trunk and extremities. In sponging the extremities the stroke is from the neck to the axilla and down to the palms of the hands, and from the groin to the feet. Gentle friction is used to bring the blood to the surface. Moist cloths should be placed over the superficial blood vessels in the axillae and the groins. A warm water bottle should be put to the feet to prevent a feeling of chilliness. This may not be practical with an active infant, but is generally used with an older child. An ice bag is applied to the head for greater comfort.

A sponge bath for an elevation of temperature can be more disturbing to the child than the illness itself. Substitutes for this procedure could be the use of a cold water mattress, or a tepid bath while gradually cooling the water.

If the small child is conscious and refuses to lie down, the nurse may cover herself with a plastic apron and sponge the child in her lap. If he is old enough, he may participate in sponging himself.

Febrile Convulsions

Incidence and Diagnosis. About 7 per cent of all infants and children have febrile convulsions between six months and two or three years of age. After seven years of age convulsions due to elevation of temperature are usually rare. Males are more affected than females, and there appears to be an increased incidence of febrile convulsions in some families.

Diagnosis of febrile convulsions involves diagnosis of the disease of which fever is a symptom. Most convulsions occurring between six and twelve months of age and in early childhood are initial symptoms of an acute febrile disease. A convulsion in this situation is equivalent to a chill experienced by an adult under the same conditions. Any young child who has a febrile convulsion, however, should be examined to eliminate the possibility of other causative factors.

In order to rule out other factors and to be certain of the cause a careful history of previous convulsive episodes and illnesses and a complete physical examination, including a neurologic appraisal, should be obtained. Laboratory examination for calcium, inorganic phosphorus and electrolytes in the blood serum and for sugar and urea nitrogen in the whole blood will aid in the diagnosis. If the convulsion is due to fever, the physician will determine whether the infection is intracranial or extracranial and what the specific problem is.

Treatment, Prognosis and Nursing Care. *Treatment* is aimed at direct control of the seizures by sedatives such as phenobarbital sodium, the dose depending on the age and size of the patient, and control of the systemic conditions causing the convulsion. Therapy includes antipyretic drugs and measures to reduce the body temperature, such as aspirin and tepid sponge baths; anti-infectious therapy. depending on the organism responsible for the illness; aspiration if the nasopharyngeal secretions are excessive; and oxygen inhalation if the patient is cyanotic.

The *prognosis* depends upon the cause of the convulsion. A single febrile seizure is not indicative of a later chronic epilepsy, but repeated febrile convulsions increase the probability of subsequent nonfebrile convulsions (see p. 523).

The *nursing care* is the same as that for convulsions in general (see p. 351).

Subdural Hematoma

Etiology and Incidence. A subdural hematoma is a collection of blood and fluid within the potential subdural space between the tough dura mater, which lines the inner surface of the skull, and the arachnoid. It may be acute, subacute or chronic. The chronic form is generally seen during infancy. The cause is trauma to the head, either extensive molding at birth or injury after birth. The condition is most frequent in infants who have not received adequate care or have been more often exposed to trauma; it may also be seen in infants who have bleeding tendencies as in purpuric states. If the infant has scurvy, the possibility of subdural hematoma following injury is increased. Meningitis may also cause subdural collections.

Subdural hematomas are not rare. They are more common in males than in females and generally appear between the second and fourth months. The *incidence* decreases thereafter to fourteen to sixteen months, after which the condition is less common. In about 80 per cent of cases it occurs bilaterally.

Pathology Clinical Manifestations and Diagnosis. At the time of the injury the delicate subdural veins are torn, and small hemorrhages occur in the subdural space. Fluid collects, and a sac forms in the subdural space between the dura and the arachnoid layers of the meninges. The sac enlarges with further accumulation of fluid and contains a mixture of old and fresh blood and xanthochromic fluid. The brain beneath the sac becomes compressed, and brain

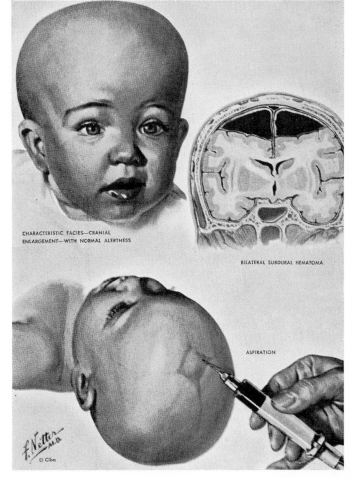

CHARACTERISTIC FACIES—CRANIAL
ENLARGEMENT—WITH NORMAL ALERTNESS

BILATERAL SUBDURAL HEMATOMA

ASPIRATION

Figure 14–14. Subdural hematoma. (Copyright, The Ciba Collection of Medical Illustrations, by Frank H. Netter, M.D.)

atrophy and clinical signs develop. In the long-standing subdural hematoma the fluid may disappear, leaving a constricting membrane that prevents normal brain growth.

Clinical manifestations are varied. In the *acute* subdural hematoma, usually following trauma, there may be a rapid onset of signs of increased intracranial pressure previously described. In the *chronic* form clinical manifestations may have an insidious onset. The mother states that the child had anorexia, irritability, restlessness, vomiting or convulsions. The child who fails to thrive and attain normal developmental milestones may also have a chronic subdural hematoma.

Other signs such as recurrent fever, changes in reflexes, bulging and tense fontanels, enlarged head and possibly abnormal eyegrounds may be present when the mother is interviewed. The degree to which these signs are present is important. The sutures may be separated. The infant may have anemia due to loss of blood. The cerebrospinal fluid pressure is increased,

and the fluid may contain increased numbers of blood cells and an increased amount of protein. On subdural puncture a greater than normal amount of fluid can be obtained.

The *diagnosis* is frequently difficult because of the insidious onset of the signs and symptoms and is best made by bilateral subdural taps. In infants this procedure is easily done by inserting the needle in the lateral corner of the fontanel or farther out through the suture line. In older children burr holes must be made through the skull before the needle can be inserted.

Treatment and Prognosis. Subdural hematoma is usually treated by a neurosurgeon The aim of *treatment* is to remove abnormal fluid and the membrane which forms the sac. Subdural fluid is removed before a craniotomy is done. Frequent aspirations of fluid are performed. Sometimes all the fluid can be removed in this way. Trephine holes may be made to determine whether a membrane is present, and also the estimated degree of cortical atrophy. After confirmation of the membrane a craniotomy is performed to remove as much of the adherent membrane and clot as possible. If the hematoma is bilateral, craniotomies are performed at intervals of several days. In some instances aspiration of fluid must be continued or a shunting procedure may be necessary even after craniotomy.

Transfusions are given to correct the anemia. If scurvy is the cause of the condition, vitamin C is administered. Infection is treated with appropriate antibiotics.

The *prognosis* may be determined by the appearance of the brain at craniotomy. If the brain is severely atrophied, the prognosis is poor. After removal there is often a remarkable clinical improvement. The mortality rate varies because of underlying brain damage.

Nursing Care. One of the most important nursing responsibilities is that of early recognition and prompt treatment of the young child suffering from subdural hematoma, so that the brain will be able to grow normally. If the infant does not receive treatment early, the brain will be damaged, and mental retardation will result.

The infant should be placed on a sponge rubber mattress and turned frequently to prevent pressure areas on the skin. The physician or the nurse who assists him in withdrawal of subdural fluid should shave the anterior portion of the child's scalp and cleanse it thoroughly. She should hold the infant securely to avoid injury caused by a sudden movement.

After the procedure she should observe the dressings for drainage. If drainage seeps through, the dressing should be reinforced to prevent organisms from gaining entrance to the wound, and the physician should be notified at once. The nurse should differentiate between serous drainage and frank hemorrhage. She should also observe the infant for signs of increased intracranial pressure.

Someone must stay with the infant to prevent his attempting to pull the head dressings off, or else his hands must be restrained with elbow cuffs (see Fig. 11-5) or the clove hitch restraint (see Fig. 10-11). Before applying restraints, every effort should be made to quiet him, since restraints make him more restless and increase intracranial pressure. For more detailed care of the postoperative patient see page 593.

Neuroblastoma

Etiology and Incidence. Neuroblastoma is an embryonal malignant tumor arising from the immature cells of the sympathetic nervous system. The adrenal gland is the most common site of the tumor. Neuroblastomas are probably next to brain tumors the most common of all solid tumors in children.

Pathology, Symptoms, Treatment and Prognosis. Pathologically, neuroblastomas are hard, nodular, nonencapsulated tumors which invade adjacent tissues. This condition is often diagnosed late because the symptoms are general. *Symptoms* such as weight loss or lack of gain, abdominal pain, and feeding problems may be due to many causes. Other indications of this condition may be exophthalmos or swelling of the abdomen. The diagnosis is made on the basis of the history, physical examination and possibly a skeletal survey.

Because of its invasion of other tissues and because it disseminates through blood vascular channels to the liver, skin and bones, complete surgical removal is difficult and local recurrences are common, as are distant metastases. These tumors may, however, spontaneously regress after therapy by surgery, radiation or chemotherapy. Chemotherapeutic drugs include, among others, cyclophosphamide (Cytoxan) and vincristine.

In general, children having neuroblastoma have a poorer *prognosis* than those with Wilms's tumor (see p. 223), although they may have spontaneous remissions or spontaneous maturation for unknown reasons.

Nursing Care. The role of the public health nurse visiting in the home is largely one of case finding and referral. The nursing care of these children in the hospital is supportive in nature. The nurse, of course, assists with diagnostic tests and gives preoperative and postoperative nursing care. Since the prognosis of many of these children is poor, the student may find it helpful to review her role in the support of parents whose young children are facing death (see p. 73).

SKELETAL DEFECTS

Craniosynostosis

Etiology and Pathology. In the normal newborn infant the bones of the skull are separated. The sutures, which can be located soon after birth, are separated by a layer of fibrous tissue. The bones of the skull grow in this fibrous strip.

In craniosynostosis one or more of the sutures are closed before or shortly after birth. Growth of adjoining bones is stopped, and there is a reduction in the diameter of the skull in this direction. Where open sutures remain, a compensatory growth or enlargement is found. The result is various deformities of the skull, depending on which sutures are closed. Since other defects of the skeleton may be found with craniosynostosis, it is thought that the skeleton is adversely affected early in embryonic life.

Clinical Manifestations. Since most of the brain growth is completed in early childhood, any pressure which interferes with normal expansion may cause brain damage and mental retardation.

In *scaphocephaly* the sagittal suture is closed prematurely. The head develops in a long, narrow shape. Symptoms of intracranial pressure may be evident.

Oxycephaly is a condition in which the coronal suture closes prematurely, either completely or partially.

Other sutures may also close and various deformities result. Complications arise since the brain may be severely compressed, with resultant headache, loss of vision, and convulsions. Exophthalmos may occur. Examination is likely to reveal strabismus, nystagmus and papilledema. Mental retardation is common. Syndactylism may be associated with this deformity.

Roentgenograms reveal the abnormal shape of the skull and absence of one or more sutures.

Diagnosis and Treatment. Craniosynostosis must be differentiated from microcephaly, which results in a small head because the brain fails to grow. Increased intracranial pressure does not occur in microcephaly.

Surgical intervention may prevent mental and visual defects if it is done before compression of the brain occurs. Early repair of the skull also produces a better cosmetic effect. Operation is therefore done as soon as a definite diagnosis is made during infancy. The surgical procedure includes linear craniotomy along the prematurely closed suture with removal of a portion of bone and lining of the edge of the suture with polyethylene film to slow its reunion.

Nursing Care. The nurse has an important role in early finding of these cases. Often the public health nurse who visits in the home may be the first person to observe the condition in a supposedly normal infant. Although she cannot diagnose this condition, she should refer such a child to a physician.

The nursing care of a patient after operation is similar to that after a craniotomy for brain tumor (see p. 593).

Prognosis. The prognosis is excellent if treatment is instituted before permanent brain damage occurs. Because of rapid bone growth resulting in closure of the sutures, revision of the craniotomy may be necessary.

EMOTIONAL DISTURBANCES

Causes of Anxiety in Infancy. Every infant experiences inevitable frustrations because, basically, "he wants what he wants when he wants it." He may desire to suckle when he is supposed to eat solid foods; he may want his mother to carry him around instead of learning to walk.

These frustrations bring him pain, discomfort and anxiety. Gradually he learns that he can rid himself of these uncomfortable states by adopting new methods of behavior, e.g. by learning to eat solid foods and to walk. Infants learn new skills, therefore, because initially they were frustrated and uncomfortable as a result of depending only upon old skills. Learning new skills eventually brings new pleasures and fewer frustrations.

An infant will desire to learn new skills only if he has an optimum period of satisfaction with the old mode of behavior before the period of frustration begins. Infants should be allowed to experience the inevitable frustrations of life slowly and in small doses. Sudden, overwhelming frustrations, such as weaning within a few days, have an adverse effect on the immature personality.

Behavior of the Infant Who Is Anxious. The anxious infant may react in one of three ways: he may resent or fight against the cause of his discomfort; he may turn away or move from it, without fighting; or he may remain immobile and do nothing.

ANXIETY DUE TO FRUSTRATION IN FEEDING. Young infants frustrated in the feeding process will react in the only way they know, by kicking, crying and by constant bodily movement. If the breast-fed infant cannot get adequate amounts of milk because of inverted nipples, he may regurgitate what he has already taken, he may turn away and refuse to suck, or he may fall asleep. Likewise the infant weaned too abruptly may show the same problem behavior.

The infant may react similarly to complementary foods if the food is too hot, if it contains lumps or if it requires excessive chewing. In such a situation he may vomit repeatedly, may turn his head away from his mother or may become immobile and refuse to participate in the feeding process.

Any of these reactions affects the eating process directly. If the infant blames, as it were, his mother for the discomfort in feeding, he may turn away from her when she approaches him, refuse to eat, cry when she touches him or, when he is a little older, do exactly the opposite of what she requests.

ANXIETY DUE TO FRUSTRATION OF SUCKING. If the desire to suck is frustrated, the infant will suck on non-nutritive objects such as fingers, the blanket or toys for long periods of time and will continue this activity past the second or third year, when such activity is usually given up.

If the parents permit such sucking on non-nutritive objects, the infant will gain his needed satisfaction. But if the parents disapprove, the infant may reject food or will stop the sucking activity completely and learn to find pleasure in frustration.

ANXIETY DUE TO LACK OF PARENTAL LOVE AND OVERWHELMING FRUSTRATION WHICH THE INFANT CANNOT HANDLE. Degrees of anxiety resulting from frustration in feeding or sucking can be observed in many infants at some time during the first year. The response of infants who have overwhelming anxiety due to a lack of parental love and overwhelming frustration has been discussed earlier in this chapter. Infants who fail to thrive even when they have parents or those who have no parents to care for them may ultimately appear to wish death through starvation.

A brief case history may illustrate such a situation.

Timmy, a two-year-old boy, was admitted to the children's unit. He weighed 7 pounds 5 ounces. He had multiple skin infections and suffered from malnutrition and dehydration.

His birth weight was not known. He was the child of an unmarried fifteen-year-old girl. Shortly after his birth his mother left him with a sister and disappeared. His aunt subsequently married and gave him to a neighbor. During the two years of his life he had about eight substitute mothers, neighbors who passed him around at their convenience. Eventually he was given to a woman who really cared for him, but by that time he was so physically retarded and emotionally underdeveloped that her efforts were in vain. He would not suck on a nipple or respond to anyone. She brought him to the hospital, but in spite of gavage feedings, intravenous therapy, antibiotics and the best of nursing care, Timmy died.

The infant equates food with love. Timmy, who received rejection and no love, refused his food and died of starvation.

Symptoms. *Anxiety symptoms* include excessive crying, inability to sleep, restlessness or rhythmic rocking movements and possibly vomiting. In overwhelming anxiety the infant may experience depression with weeping, screaming when strangers approach, withdrawal, and arrest of physical and emotional development.

Feeding disorders, ranging from refusal of food to air swallowing and repeated vomiting, are common. Eventually marasmus may develop, and the infant may die of starvation.

Antagonistic behavior consists in a lack of enjoyment in the companionship of his parents, in a refusal to enjoy interaction with them or in doing the opposite of what they request of him.

Treatment and Nursing Care. Prevention of emotional disturbance is much to be preferred to treatment of the disturbed infant. Many mothers want to be loving and warm to their infants and yet seemingly reject them in some degree because of disapproval by their husbands, relatives or neighbors of a truly maternal attitude toward the infant. Other mothers want to provide warm loving care for their babies, but are separated from them because of their own illness or that of other members of the family.

Such mothers could be helped to a great degree by education in the emotional needs of infants. Such education, given during the prenatal period, could make them more sure of their own judgment and less sensitive to disapproval by others. Although intellectual understanding is not a cure-all for such problems, the support of an outside authority is reassuring. The physician or nurse can help such women to trust their own maternal feelings as guides in their behavior. Those women discussed earlier who desire to do only things that give them pleasure cannot be good mothers regardless of the guidance they receive. Their immature wish for pleasure causes them to be unaware of the infant's need for love and so are unable to give love.

In treating an infant for an emotional disturbance, the cause must first be found. The need which is being frustrated must be clearly understood. It is important for both the mother and the physician to treat the child as though he were a little younger than he was when the traumatic experience occurred. For example, if the infant reacts violently to supplementary solid foods, his mother should cease offering them for a while. Then the foods should be introduced gradually *without force* or even undue urging.

Sometimes the feeding difficulty, vomiting or refusal to eat may become so severe that the infant may need to be removed from his mother for a time. He may be cared for at home by a warm, loving person or may be placed in a hospital. Often such infants may begin to eat well after a brief period of adjustment to the new situation. During the separation the parents should receive guidance so that they may create a more loving environment for the infant when he returns to them.

If the infant is hospitalized, it is the nurse's responsibility to provide the love and tender care he needs. She must hold him closely and show the warmth of her affection, cuddle him and be kind and patient in her feeding methods. Often the nurse can demonstrate to the mother how to hold the infant close to her body to feed him and to give him the loving care he needs.

ABUSED OR
BATTERED-CHILD SYNDROME

Incidence, Etiology, Clinical Findings, Diagnosis and Prognosis. The *incidence* of abused children is not really known, but it appears to be on the increase in our society, especially in large metropolitan areas.

An abused child (usually an infant or toddler under three years of age) is one against whom bodily injury and therefore emotional harm also is done by an adult to such a degree that it comes to the attention of a physician or another member of a helping profession.

The *clinical findings* are the result of injuries which may be due to burning, throwing or knocking the child around or twisting his extremities. They include largely bruises, scratches, burns, hematomas and fractures of long bones, ribs or skull. *Neglect,* which is frequently seen in these children, is the chronic failure of adults to protect the child from obvious physical danger or to provide for him the care he needs. Poor skin hygiene and some degree of malnutrition are usually also evident in battered children.

In *diagnosis* the distinguishing feature of this condition includes variations in stages of healing of several bone lesions as shown on x-ray films. Such bone lesions were incurred at different times prior to examination and hospitalization.

The principal basis for identifying this problem is the judgment of a professional person, since usually the child is too young to complain and the parents will not admit to abusive practices. The *etiologic factor* consists of parents or caretakers who have a defect in character structure which allows aggressive impulses to be expressed too freely when they are under tension. The parents themselves may have been subjected to similar abuse when they were children. In some instances the parent tends to release his rage on one particular child only because he may serve as a symbol of something or someone who once caused the parent unhappiness. A child who was born out of wedlock is many times the target child. Such parents do not volunteer information about the child, they contradict themselves when they describe the injury, become irritated when questioned about the child, are angry with him for his injury and give no indications of feeling guilty about their lack of care of him. They often disappear shortly after the child has been admitted to the hospital, tend not to visit him after admission, and do not involve themselves in his care. These parents are concerned chiefly about themselves, are frequently dependent people who criticize the child and show no indication of having any perception of how the child might feel. These parents demonstrate role reversal, in which they turn to their infants and small children for nurturing and protection as they would to their own parents.

The typical forms of behavior which a neglected and battered child shows are crying in a hopeless manner or very little crying even when uncomfortable, lack of expectation of assurance or comfort from parents, and apprehension when contacted physically. They seem to seek safety in sizing up a situation, finding out what will happen next, rather than from contact with their parents. Children who are loved and cared for turn to their parents for safety in life; battered children endure life as though they were alone with no real hope of safety in a harmful world.

The *prognosis* is variable. The incidence of death is high among these children, but damaged physical health or mental retardation is even greater among those who survive.

Treatment, Nursing Care and Prevention. In any infant with evidence of multiple bone lesions, a subdural tap and x-ray film of the skull must be considered. Fractures of long bones must be reduced and immobilized. The nursing care therefore depends on the specific trauma such a child has. These children need good physical care and love.

Prevention of recurrence involves the cooperation of physicians, police department, social service agencies, humane societies, prosecuting attorneys and nurses. The nurse must be fully aware of the existence of this syndrome because it is she, whether in the hospital, Child Health Conference or public health agency, who may first see a child with evidence of trauma. The nurse may also recognize clues which parents and children give, as listed above. More specifically, when a child is seen in the emergency room of a hospital or in a Child Health Conference who has severe bruises or other wounds on his body and the nurse suspects that he has been abused, she should do the following. She should chart her observations of his physical condition as she would on any other patient, but she should *not* chart her judgment that he had been beaten. If, however, the adult who accompanied the child made a statement about his having been beaten, the nurse may chart these and other statements in quotation marks along with the speaker's identity. The nurse should report her observations to the physician verbally and show him the child's chart. Charting from this time on should include observations of the child's condition and the physician's orders which have been carried out. It is generally the responsibility of the physician or a team of physicians to report violence against children; however, the supervising nurse should be aware of the policy of the agency and the law of the state in which she is working.

The role of the nurse therefore consists in casefinding and reporting to the physician any indications of abuse which she may see, establishing rapport with such families so that she can gain insight into their problems, and caring for the child once he is admitted to the hospital. In working with parents of neglected and abused children a noncritical, nonpunitive approach is necessary in order to prevent them from further acting out their frustrations on their children.

This sort of approach may be difficult for the nurse to achieve because of her own possible feelings of anger or disgust with their behavior.

The nurse must work with other personnel in community services in a coordinated manner. These services include after prompt reporting, rapid and thorough investigation of each family and maintenance of a central registry, since parents of abused children frequently take them to different physicians or hospitals to avoid identification with previous attacks. Prevention in the long run depends on preventing transmission of the kind of social deprivation which results in the neglect and abuse of children, and contributes through those who survive such treatment to the next generation of parents who will not be able to nurture their children either.

The Children's Bureau has issued suggested legislative language which states could use to draft laws making the reporting of child abuse cases mandatory for the physician. The child who is abused could thus get the protection he needs from the appropriate agencies in his community. Most states have within recent years passed such child abuse reporting laws.

CLINICAL SITUATIONS

Michael O'Brien, a four-month-old infant, was brought to the Child Health Conference by his mother. He appeared to be well nourished and well developed for his age, although he had had no previous medical supervision. During Mrs. O'Brien's conference with the nurse the mother asked several questions.

1. "Michael has been breast-fed since birth, but I have been thinking about weaning him to a cup. When should I do this?"
a. "As soon as you can after he is five months old, because continued sucking may cause his teeth to protrude."
b. "As soon as Michael shows a desire to give up sucking and to drink from a cup."
c. "Before summer comes regardless of his age, because it is difficult to wean an infant in warm weather."
d. "Before he is a year old, because he will have several teeth and will not be able to suck properly."

2. "The doctor said that Michael should eat solid food, but he refuses it after he is breast-fed. What should I do?"
a. "Force him to eat, because he will lose weight and develop anemia if he continues to take only milk."
b. "Give him only breast milk as long as he refuses solid food."
c. "Mix the puréed food with some cow's milk and feed it through a large-holed nipple."
d. "Offer small amounts of puréed food before each breast feeding when he is hungry."

3. Michael at four months of age has the following abilities. Select the one that is *not* typical for a child of his age.

a. Enjoys sitting alone.
b. Lifts his head and shoulders at a 90-degree angle when on his abdomen and looks around.
c. Attempts to roll over.
d. Moves his arms rapidly at the sight of a toy.

4. The nurse understands that Michael should be immunized against certain diseases during infancy. These diseases include
a. Measles, pertussis, scarlet fever, chickenpox, diphtheria and possibly tetanus.
b. Pertussis, diphtheria, poliomyelitis, tetanus, and measles.
c. Chickenpox, poliomyelitis, measles, diphtheria, typhoid fever and possibly tetanus.
d. Smallpox, tetanus, diphtheria, pertussis, measles and possibly chickenpox.

5. The important point about Michael's *immediate* safety to stress to Mrs. O'Brien at this time would be
a. "Do not give Michael dry toast to chew, because he may aspirate it."
b. "Do not permit Michael to chew paint from the window ledge, because he might absorb too much lead."
c. "When Michael learns to roll over, you must supervise him whenever he is on a surface from which he might fall."
d. "Lock the crib sides securely because he may stand and lean against them and fall out of bed."

Mrs. O'Brien brought Michael back to the Child Health Conference when he was six months old and said that he had been ill for about three days. The physician observed that Michael's anterior fontanel was sunken, his skin turgor was poor, and his skin was warm. Mrs. O'Brien said that he had had about six stools which were watery and foul-smelling each day and that he had vomited all his feedings. He was referred to the local hospital and was admitted promptly with a diagnosis of diarrhea and vomiting.

6. On admission a blood specimen was drawn from his jugular vein. The nurse restrained the infant by using a
a. Clovehitch restraint.
b. Mummy restraint.
c. Abdominal restraint.
d. Elbow restraint.

7. Intravenous therapy was started promptly. The most important responsibility of the nurse when caring for such an infant is to
a. Check frequently the number of drops of solution running into the vein and regulate the flow of solution as ordered.
b. Remove the needle as soon as the fluid which has been ordered has run into the vein.
c. Change the bed linen promptly if it becomes moistened from the intravenous solution.
d. Add a new bottle of solution when the present one is empty, with or without a physician's order.

Mrs. Smith brought her first infant, a five-week-old son, Bruce, to the pediatric clinic because he had been "spitting up" since he was three weeks of age. Bruce had been breast-fed for the first four weeks of his life, and then had been put on a formula.

8. The physician made a diagnosis of pyloric stenosis on the basis of the infant's history and clinical manifestations, which included
a. Projectile vomiting beginning abruptly, normal stools, and malnutrition.
b. Rumination of feedings, normal stools and a sausage-like abdominal mass.
c. Constant abdominal pain with crying, frequent liquid stools and an olive-shaped abdominal mass.
d. Gradual increase in vomiting, finally becoming projectile in nature, constipation and weight loss.

9. The vomitus of an infant having pyloric stenosis is the color of his formula and does not contain bile because
a. The obstruction is above the opening of the common bile duct.
b. The liver does not secrete bile, since its functioning is impaired.
c. The obstruction at the cardiac sphincter prevents the flow of bile to the stomach.
d. The stenosis of the common bile duct prevents bile from flowing properly.

10. A Fredet-Ramstedt operation was done. Mrs. Smith asks how Bruce will be fed after the operation. In order to answer her question you should know that the feeding regimen after a pyloromyotomy is based on the principle that
a. Thickened feedings aid mechanically in helping food pass through the pylorus because its weight stretches the hypertrophied muscle.
b. Clear liquids are tolerated well because they contain no curds which would have difficulty passing through the pylorus.
c. Easily assimilated fluids are given in increasing amounts so that the newly incised muscle can accommodate gradually.
d. Easily digested fluids are given in large amounts in order to combat dehydration.

When Bruce was seven months old, he was readmitted to the hospital with a diagnosis of eczema. He was irritable and restless, and scratched his skin whenever he could. The skin on his face and scalp was secondarily infected. Mrs. Smith said that Bruce had received a wide variety of foods in his diet and that his appetite had been excellent.

11. Eczema is a skin condition caused by
a. Bacterial invasion primarily by the streptococcus.
b. Excessive secretion of the sebaceous glands.
c. Inflammation around the sweat glands due to excessive heat.
d. Allergy to internal or external irritants.

12. When dressing Bruce after his bath, it is important to dress him.
a. In as few cotton clothes as possible according to the temperature of his environment.
b. In warm woolen clothing, because these infants frequently contract respiratory infections.
c. In only a diaper, because clothing increases the infant's discomfort.
d. In cotton clothing, but wrap him in a woolen blanket for warmth.

13. When using restraints, they must be

a. Kept on constantly to prevent Bruce from scratching.
b. Removed once a day to allow active motion of his extremities under supervision.
c. Kept securely in position so that Bruce remains on his back at all times.
d. Checked frequently to determine whether the restraints are constricting his circulation.

14. Even though Bruce has not yet received his smallpox immunization, it will not be given until he is completely recovered because of the danger of development of
a. Acrodynia.
b. Aganglionic megacolon.
c. Generalized vaccinia.
d. Hypocalcemic tetany.

15. Bruce was hospitalized for several weeks. Mrs. Smith was not able to visit him more frequently than twice a month. In order to prevent emotional deprivation during this time, the most important measure the head nurse could take would be to
a. Place him each day in a playpen near another seven-month-old infant so they could interact with each other.
b. Place his crib near the entrance to the unit so that he would not become lonely.
c. Give him many toys to keep him occupied.
d. Assign the same staff nurse to provide care for him each day.

Mr. and Mrs. Jones had had three children. The first child died at one week of age after an operation for intestinal obstruction due to meconium ileus. The second child is normal. June, their third child, seemed normal at birth and had a good appetite, but she gained weight slowly. At five months bronchopneumonia developed, which responded well to chemotherapy. At eight months she again had bronchopneumonia and continued to have a chronic cough after discharge from the hospital. Upon readmission to the hospital at eleven months because of weight loss, a diagnosis of cystic fibrosis was made.

16. During an evacuation June's rectum prolapsed. After it had been replaced by the physician the nurse prevented the recurrence of the prolapse by
a. Giving a daily colonic irrigation to prevent constipation.
b. Giving a mild laxative each night to prevent constipation.
c. Restraining the child in bed with her head lower than her body.
d. Taping the buttocks together after each defecation.

GUIDES FOR FURTHER STUDY

1. During your experience at the Child Health Conference observe several infants under one year of age with their mothers. Note the apparent differences of maternal attitudes toward the infants when their mothers feed them, comfort them or give them physical care. What immediate effects do these various attitudes have on their individual infants?
2. A mother of an apparently normal two-month-

old infant at the Child Health Conference has complained to you that in spite of all her efforts to teach him to sit alone, he shows no progress toward accomplishing this ability. What would your response be on the basis of your knowledge of the principles of motor development and your understanding of the interrelatedness of maturation and learning?

3. The women's group of a local church has offered to donate toys for the infants hospitalized at Christmas. List the specific toys you would request for infants of various ages and give the reasons for your choices.

4. Visit a foundling home in or near your community. Observe the infants to determine whether their behavior shows any evidence of maternal deprivation. In terms of your knowledge of the care the infants receive, evaluate your findings and make suggestions in seminar as to how the emotional needs of the infants could be met more adequately.

5. Trace the steps in motor development through which an infant must go before he is finally able to stand alone.

6. During your experience at the Child Health Conference or the pediatric clinic list several questions asked by mothers of infants of various ages. Discuss your answers to these questions in seminar. Evaluate your own progress in being able to establish rapport with these mothers and in being able to answer their questions to their satisfaction.

7. Plan a daily menu for infants of three months, six months and one year. Check each of these diets with the recommended dietary allowances given for infants on page 269.

8. What are the most recent statistics in your state on infant mortality? What are the most frequent causes of death? After investigating provisions made for the health supervision and care of infants, give suggestions as to how the infant mortality rate in your state could be reduced.

TEACHING AIDS AND OTHER INFORMATION*

National Cystic Fibrosis Research Foundation

Cystic Fibrosis: For Nurses.
Cystic Fibrosis: For Physical Therapists.
Cystic Fibrosis: Medical Information.
Your Child and Cystic Fibrosis.

United States Department of Health, Education, and Welfare

Children Who Need Protection, 1966.
Phenylketonuria and Allied Metabolic Diseases, 1967.
Recommended Guidelines for PKU Programs, 1966.
Sickle Cell Anemia, 1965.
State Laws Pertaining to Phenylketonuria as of November 1966, 1967.
The Abused Child, 1963.
The Child Abuse Reporting Laws, 1967.
The Clinical Team Looks at Phenylketonuria, 1964.

REFERENCES

Publications

Ainsworth, M. D., and others: *Deprivation of Maternal Care: A Reassessment of Its Effects.* Geneva, World Health Organization, 1962. (Columbia University Press, International Documents Service.)

Barbero, J., Morris, M., and Reford, M.: *Malidentification of Mother-Baby-Father Relationships Expressed in Infant Failure to Thrive. The Neglected/Battered Child Syndrome: Role Reversal in Parents.* New York, Child Welfare League of America, 1963.

Belmonte, M. M.: *Cystic Fibrosis. A Handbook for Parents.* Quebec, Cystic Fibrosis Association of Quebec, 1966.

Cooke, R. E., and Levin, S. (Eds.): *The Biologic Basis of Pediatric Practice.* New York, Blakiston Division, McGraw-Hill Book Company, Inc., 1968.

Cornblath, M., and Schwartz, R.: *Disorders of Carbohydrate Metabolism in Infancy.* Philadelphia, W. B. Saunders Company, 1966.

Elmer, E.: *Children in Jeopardy. A Study of Abused Minors and Their Families.* Pittsburgh, University of Pittsburgh Press, 1967.

Fontana, V. J.: *The Maltreated Child: The Maltreatment Syndrome in Children.* Springfield, Ill., Charles C Thomas, 1964.

---

* Complete addresses are given in the Appendix.

Gellis, S. S., and Kagan, B. M. (Eds.): *Current Pediatric Therapy*. 3rd ed. Philadelphia, W. B. Saunders Company, 1968.

Hsia, D. Y.: *Inborn Errors of Metabolism*. 2nd ed. Chicago, Year Book Medical Publishers, Inc., 1966.

Lewis, G. M., and Wheeler, C. E.: *Practical Dermatology for Medical Students and General Practitioners*. 3rd ed. Philadelphia, W. B. Saunders Company, 1967.

Millichap, J. G.: *Febrile Convulsions*. New York, Macmillan Company, 1967.

Robertson, J.: *Young Children in Hospitals*. New York, Basic Books, Inc., 1958.

Sarner, H.: *The Nurse and the Law*. Philadelphia, W. B. Saunders Company, 1968.

Smith, C. H.: *Blood Diseases of Infancy and Childhood*. 2nd ed. St. Louis, C. V. Mosby Company, 1966.

Stowens, D.: *Pediatric Pathology*. 2nd ed. Baltimore, Williams & Wilkins Company, 1966.

Weatherall, D. J.: *The Thalassaemia Syndromes*. Philadelphia, F. A. Davis Company, 1965.

Young, L.: *Wednesday's Children: A Study of Child Neglect and Abuse*. New York, McGraw-Hill Book Company, Inc., 1964.

Periodicals

Barbero, G., and Shaheen, E.: Environmental Failure to Thrive. A Clinical View. *J. Pediat.,* 71:639, 1967.

Bessken, P., and Miller, W. L.: A Family Copes with Cystic Fibrosis. *Am. J. Nursing,* 67:341, 1967.

Cheney, K. B.: Safeguarding Legal Rights in Providing Protective Services. *Children,* 13:86, 1966.

Clark, J. H., and Sawyer, J. A.: I Solemnly Swear . . . A Nurse Testifies to Child Neglect. *Nursing Outlook,* 16:35, April 1968.

Elmer, E., and Gregg, G. S.: Developmental Characteristics of Abused Children. *Pediatrics,* 40:596, 1967.

Golub, S.: The Battered Child: What the Nurse Can Do. *RN,* 31:42, December 1968.

Haar, D. J.: Improved Phenylketonuric Diet Control Through Group Education of Mothers. *Nurs. Clin. N. America,* 1:715, 1966.

Ingles, T.: Maria—The Hungry Baby. *Nursing Forum,* V:36, No. 2, 1966.

Ireland, W. H.: A Registry on Child Abuse. *Children,* 13:113, 1966.

Johnson, B., and Morse, H. A.: Injured Children and Their Parents. *Children,* 15:147, 1968.

Keleske, L., Solomons, G., and Opitz, E.: Parental Reactions to Phenylketonuria in the Family. *J. Pediat.,* 70:793, 1967.

Krieger, I., and Sargent, D. A.: A Postural Sign in the Sensory Deprivation Syndrome in Infants. *J. Pediat.,* 70:332, 1967.

Kurihara, M.: Postural Drainage, Clapping, and Vibrating. *Am. J. Nursing,* 65:76, November 1965.

Leonard, M. F., Rhymes, J. P., and Solrit, A. J.: Failure to Thrive in Infants. A Family Problem. *Am. J. Dis. Child,* 111:600, 1966.

McConnell, J. F.: The Deposed One. *Am. J. Nursing,* 61:78, August 1961.

O'Flynn, M. E.: Diet Therapy in Phenylketonuria. *Am. J. Nursing,* 67:1658, 1967.

Paulsen, M. G.: Legal Protections Against Child Abuse. *Children,* 13:42, 1966.

Rhymes, J. P.: Working with Mothers and Babies Who Fail to Thrive. *Am. J. Nursing,* 66:1972, 1966.

Schlesinger, B.: Battered Children and Damaged Parents. *Canada's Health and Welfare,* 19:3, November 1964.

Silver, H. K., and Finkelstein, M.: Deprivation Dwarfism. *J. Pediat.,* 70:317, 1967.

Sussman, S. J.: Skin Manifestations of the Battered-Child Syndrome. *J. Pediat.,* 72:99, 1968.

Swenson, O.: Congenital Megacolon. *Pediat. Clin. N. Amer.,* 14:187, 1967.

Wasserman, S.: The Abused Parent of the Abused Child. *Children,* 14:175, 1967.

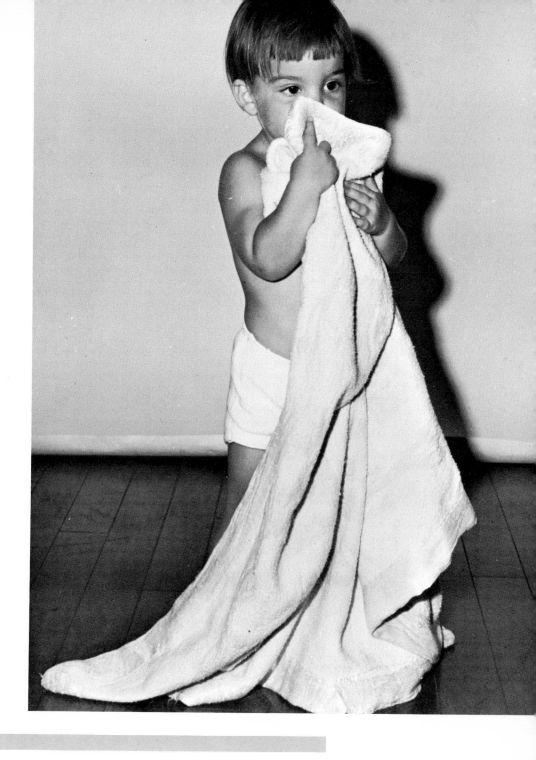

UNIT FOUR

THE TODDLER

15

THE NORMAL TODDLER: HIS GROWTH, DEVELOPMENT AND CARE

The infant by his first birthday has learned to *trust* or *distrust* the adults who care for him. This attitude is modified by experiences throughout childhood and adolescence, but its direct influence on the way he perceives experience during the toddler stage is evident to all who know him.

As the child moves from passive dependency to active interaction with those about him, society or that small section of it which he knows—his family—guides him in conformity with social norms. The most important demand made upon him during the toddler period is that of toilet training.

During the toddler period parents must learn to accept the changes that occur as the child grows and develops. The child becomes more mobile and begins to assert his own independence. Sometimes parents, especially the mother, who enjoyed the total dependency of the infant have difficulty accepting the child's new wish for freedom to explore and to become a person in his own right.

OVERVIEW OF THE TODDLER'S EMOTIONAL DEVELOPMENT

Sense of Autonomy

As the child passes from infancy into the toddler stage (one to three years) he uses his increasing ability to help himself and to develop his *sense of autonomy*. He makes his wants known to those about him to get what he wants. He shows that he has a mind and a will of his own. If he has learned to trust others, he accepts their gentle, considerate guidance in learning new skills. But when they deny him what he wants, he is angry and hates the very people whom he has learned to love—mother, father, siblings and nurse. Their response to his anger is important in forming his personality. If they show him love while refusing him what he wants, he quickly returns to the loving relations which he has learned bring pleasure. He has learned that an angry attitude does not get him what he wants, but that a pleasant response, even when he is denied what he wants, brings him happiness.

Understanding love for the child of this age is shown by giving him all the freedom he can safely use, by giving him all the love and help he needs to keep him safe in an environment which he is unable to control and in which he is dependent upon others for the satisfaction of bodily drives, and by giving him guidance in avoiding hazards in the changing social situations in which he feels himself to be the focal point.

If he has learned by the end of the toddler period to accept and utilize guidance, he has gained a new level of self-control without losing his self-esteem. If he has not learned to be self-helpful, within the limits of his ability and in

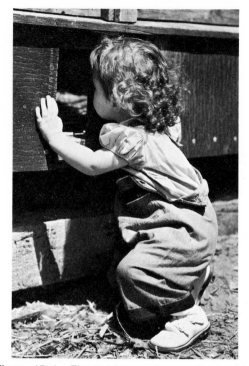

Figure 15–1. The toddler needs security, but she also needs a degree of independence so that she can explore her world. (H. Armstrong Roberts.)

the way that those about him want, and, equally important, to accept adult direction in situations in which he cannot carry on alone, he is likely to feel insecure in his ability to meet the physical and social problems in his environment. He appears withdrawn and may have a *sense of doubt* about himself and others and a sense of what an adult would feel as shame. He avoids new experiences and thus has fewer opportunities to acquire new skills than has the child with an outgoing personality.

Needs of the Toddler

The basic needs of the toddler are the same as those of the infant. The toddler needs security and love, but he also needs graded independence.

Love and Security

Love enables the toddler to grow up and reach out for more mature goals because he feels secure in his parents' affectionate care of him. Since he feels secure, he can endure the frustrations which come to every child in the process of maturation.

Both boys and girls give their first love to their mothers because mothers give them tender,

loving care. As the needs of children become more diversified — less for physical care and more for social pleasures — their attachment to a loving father increases. In a family in which the father gives the infant the same care the mother does the infant generally feels as secure with one parent as with the other. But many infants hardly know their fathers until they reach the toddler stage. Then the father plays with them and takes them about with him. These toddlers, however, still turn to their mothers when they want physical care or feel sick.

During the toddler or perhaps even the early preschool period the child may select in addition to his parents an object which has unusual importance and which seems to provide security for him. This *security or transitional object,* such as a blanket, diaper or toy, is affectionately cuddled and loved, but in the process many times becomes dirty and mutilated. The child may become distressed if the object is cleaned or changed in any way.

Graded Independence

Independence is learned gradually and is given the child only in situations in which he can guard himself from physical and emotional trauma. Independence must be denied him while he is too young to use it successfully, for a painful experience might make him afraid to try out new skills.

FULFILLMENT OF NEEDS

The toddler whose parents give him graded independence which brings pleasurable results develops a sense of self-reliance and adequacy, of autonomy. He finds that he is an individual who may make choices under the guidance of his parents. He may decide to play on the floor or on the chair, to eat the food offered him or reject it, to welcome a visitor or cling to his mother's skirt. Sooner or later he learns that there are many things he would like to do, but *can* not or *may* not. He easily learns that he cannot touch all the objects he wants because some are out of his reach. It will take him a little longer to learn that there are some things he *can* do without being hurt, but *may* not do because his parents say "No."

The child wants to do many things he is not physically able to do. Climbing up stairs is an example of his persistence. If he is constantly with a sibling only a few years older than he, he will attempt many activities which he is unable to do successfully.

As his muscular system matures he develops simple muscular skills, but finds that he cannot coordinate these diverse patterns into a purposeful activity such as he sees older children do so easily. Although he has learned to walk, to hold on and let go, to grasp and manipulate objects in various ways, he is often frustrated in his efforts to make his hands and feet do what he wants them to do. The toddler age is a frustrating age.

Regulating the toddler's activities is an important part of his training and is a challenge to the most mature and resourceful adult. The toddler cannot realize the consequences of what he does. Even if there is no danger of his being hurt, he may make himself ridiculous so that people laugh at him. This hurts his self-esteem if he cannot also join in the laughter.

A gradually expanding area of growth in a safe environment must be provided for him. Since one reason for adult control is that failure may injure his self-esteem, it is evident that an adult should never use shame or ridicule as a means of punishment or of prevention of forbidden activities. Shaming makes the toddler feel even smaller than he is; if it is used to excess, the child may comply when he is watched, but do as he pleases when he is not observed. This has been the cause of many serious accidents.

A certain amount of defiance is normal and may be more apparent than real. "No, no" does not always mean that he will not do what he is asked to do. It may mean, "Don't look so cross, Mama," or "I don't know what you mean." "No" is an easy sound to make, and he may use it for personal pleasure rather than for expression of a negative feeling. Even with the two- or three-year-old it may not mean refusal, but rather a bewildered response to injunctions he does not understand. Too often, however, it means that he will not do what the adult asks of him. His defiance is likely to be increased by anger on the part of the adult. This is because the child is likely to become confused and because he follows the adult's lead with expressions of anger. He lacks words to convey his meaning and strikes the adult, has a temper tantrum, cries or becomes sullen.

Although a certain amount of defiance is part of his growing independence, excessive defiance becomes a habit and, unless wisely corrected, may be a factor in poor adjustment. The repercussion upon himself of the irritation he arouses in others is likely to make him withdraw into himself or become more defiant. If his defiant attitude is not corrected before adolescence, he may find others like himself who are defiant of adult restraint. If he can get along with them, he may become one of the gang whose delinquent acts fill our newspapers. If he cannot fit into the gang because he will not accept the restraint the gang exercises over its members, he may become a solitary delinquent. He may learn to dislike the real world, in which he is disliked, and turn to daydreaming. Outwardly he may appear to be a quiet, obedient child in whom defiance is not suspected. This child is likely to have poorer mental hygiene than the delinquent has.

Parents or their substitutes should have a deep sense of the value of preserving their own dignity as the child sees it, as well as the child's self-respect.

By building on the sense of trust in others which he developed during his first year of life the child normally gains a sense of autonomy during the toddler stage. He must be respected as an individual and helped to internalize the social norms of his group so that he *wants* to do what is *right* and, conversely, hurts his image of himself if he does what is *wrong*.

This developmental task takes two full years to make even a good beginning on which further guidance can be given as the child grows older.

Three specific areas in which the toddler must be given guidance are (1) elimination control, or control of bodily functions of urination and defecation, (2) learning to talk, and (3) learning social norms.

Control of Bodily Functions

Control of the bodily functions of defecation and urination is important, for it is the most personal phase of the young child's learning, closely related to his sensations. The child would like to continue emptying his bladder and bowels whenever he is conscious of discomfort from tension in these organs. Society does not sanction such behavior, and so gradually the toddler must learn to face the frustration of retention, and gain control of defecation and urination with the help of those he loves. Toilet training, or learning elimination control, is at best difficult for the young child, especially if his family places an extreme value on cleanliness. If cleanliness has for his mother a moral aspect (if he dirties himself he is naughty, and if he keeps clean he is good), the child who is not able to keep clean and dry begins to develop feelings of guilt and anxiety because he cannot live up to the expectations of adults who care for him.

The infant, who for the first year received all care, love and attention, is now asked to assume the responsibility of giving up his comfort and to contribute to the comfort of others. He must learn to excrete urine and feces only at the appropriate time and place, although he cannot understand the necessity for this. He is motivated to try only because he wants to please his mother.

In more technical terms, the infant lives according to the *pleasure principle* (wanting what he wants when he wants it). The toddler must begin to accept the *reality principle* (giving up an immediate pleasure in order to gain another pleasure later). In this instance the toddler must give up the pleasure of excreting where and when he wishes in order to gain his mother's approval. If he does not have a trusting relationship with his mother, he will not be strongly motivated to succeed in toilet training.

Other factors, of course, influence him. If he sees an older brother or sister using the toilet, he may want to do the same. As he becomes more active his wet clothing is more uncomfortable. If other children point at the puddles he makes and laugh at him, he may laugh too, but he does begin to connect keeping himself dry with part of the life pattern of the older child whom he imitates.

Learning a new skill is difficult before the stage of maturation at which the child is motivated to learn and is physically able without too great an effort. If he is urged to learn before this stage, unfavorable attitudes may develop. To wait beyond the optimum stage when he is ready to learn a new skill is a mistake, because the happiness of using this skill is kept from him. Then, too, skills normal for his age evoke a favorable response from other people, and his self-image, taken from their attitude toward him, is more satisfying.

Age for Beginning Toilet Training.
Toilet training should be started about the end of the first year when the child is psychologically and physiologically ready. By that age he is usually able to stand alone; this indicates that the tracts of the spinal cord are myelinated down to the anal level. It is useless and too frustrating to the child to attempt toilet training before the neurologic pathways are formed which enable him to control the anal sphincter and the urethra under tension and to excrete when his mother tells him to do so.

Most pediatricians advocate that toilet training may be attempted at the end of the first year, but if the child does not understand what is wanted of him, it should be postponed until later. If training is started before the child is a year old, it is probable that the child is neither controlling nor expelling excreta at will, but rather that his mother has put him upon the toilet chair at the time when tension causes release of the anal or urethral sphincter, or both. As long as the child's diet and fluid intake are about the same each day this procedure may be successful, but any change in routine is likely to change the time of excretion, and he will soil his diaper or training pants. The mother is then apt to feel that the child has retrogressed and may show her disapproval by a scowling face or severe tone of voice.

Bowel training should be started before bladder training, since the number of stools in a day is less than the number of times the child urinates. Bladder training may be started one or more months after bowel control has been fairly well established. Extraneous factors such as moving to a new house or the birth of a sibling may make the process of toilet training more difficult than it would usually be.

Method of Toilet Training.
The first step is to observe the child's usual time of defecation. A little before this time he should be placed on a comfortable infant toilet seat or training chair on which he feels secure. There should be a rest for his arms and feet. He should not be given food or toys at this time, for these distract his attention from the purpose for which he is put on the chair. The mother or nurse should indicate to him by gestures and tone of voice that he is expected to pass his eliminations in this place and at this time. A specific word indicating the act should be selected, a word easily understood by everyone. This is important, for many a child at nursery school or visiting with friendly adults has not been able to tell the adults that he wants to relieve himself, because he does not understand the words they use and they do not know what he is saying. The word used by the child's mother and taught to him often reflects the social class of the parents. Nurses should never show disgust at any word a child may use, though he can be taught a more appropriate one.

Much patience is required of the mother, for the child learns only as the result of repeated attempts. Training should not be made a tense issue for either the mother or the child. The mother will find it easier for herself as well as better for the child if she assumes a casual, matter-of-fact attitude. Toilet training generally covers one or two years, so that there is no need

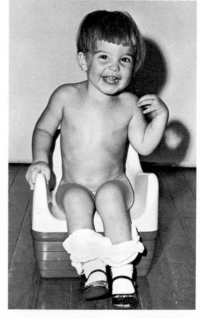

Figure 15–2. The toddler should feel secure when placed on the training chair. She should be able to touch the floor with her feet and should be supported adequately by the back and arms of the chair.

to hurry the process. When the child defecates or urinates in the toilet or training chair, he should be praised and cuddled. But when he fails to do so, the mother should never show disappointment or disapproval, for the child of this age has difficulty in releasing the contents of the bowel or bladder at will.

When the child is old enough to go to the toilet by himself, he should have clothing which he can manage without help so that he can develop increasing independence. His pants should be such that he can slip them down or open them with a zipper. A girl's training pants should have elastic at the waist so that they may be easily pushed down below the knees. Steps which the toddler can climb to reach the adult toilet (with or without the child's toilet seat) are helpful. Boys learn to stand for urination by watching older boys urinate. A step may be necessary for him to urinate into the toilet bowl without wetting the floor.

Enemas, cathartics or suppositories should not be used unless ordered by the physician. The mother should understand that not all children have a daily bowel movement.

Age at Which Toilet Training Is Accomplished.
The average healthy, intelligent child usually accomplishes bowel control by the end of the eighteenth month. Daytime bladder control may be fairly well established by two years of age, and night control by three years. Night control should not be hurried. It is not good to wake the child and take him to the toilet, for he may stay awake for a long time after he has been put to bed again. Withholding fluids in the late afternoon and evening may be tried, but if the child is not physiologically ready, this will not help him to retain urine during the night. Also, he may be thirsty and cry for water during the night.

Training During Illness.
If the child is not trained when he enters the pediatric unit, he should not be taught to use a bedpan or urinal or little toilet chair while he is hospitalized. He would not be motivated to learn because there would be no one person whom he loves and attempts to please by doing what she asks of him. Then, too, a sick child should not be subjected to the strain of breaking old habits and acquiring new ones.

If the mother on admission of the child says that he is toilet-trained, this should be noted in the habit history on the admission chart. The technique used by the mother and the words the child associates with the acts of elimination should be recorded. If the child is old enough to understand, he should be shown the hospital equipment, such as the bedpan, urinal and training chair, if the physician permits him to be out of bed. The nurse should try to keep him on the same schedule as that used at home, but should not be worried if he wets or soils himself and

certainly should not show disapproval. The nurse should explain to the mother so that she will not be disturbed by his behavior that the sick child in a strange environment generally regresses to infantile toilet habits. When he is well again, his mother can help him to resume his former habits of elimination.

Meaning of Toilet Training to the Child.
The child is now asked to do what his mother wants him to do, whereas when he was a baby, she gave him loving care without asking any other response from him than his loving dependence upon her. Instead of being irresponsible, he is now asked to assume some responsibility for himself.

FECAL SMEARING. The child has not yet acquired the adult's distaste for bodily excretions. He likes to manipulate fecal material and smear it upon the floor, wall or furniture. Such behavior occurs between the ages of fifteen and twenty-one months. The toddler thinks of his feces as coming from him and in this sense regards it as a gift. He does not understand why fecal material is thrown away after he has been urged to expel it into the toilet chair. (This is one advantage of a toilet. He can help pull the handle and see the feces disappear with the swirling water. This is to him a satisfying accomplishment.) The parent or nurse should accept the child's feeling about his excretion and never express strong disapproval of his smearing it upon himself or any object. His desire to smear should be gratified in a socially acceptable way by giving him clay, damp sand or mud to manipulate. Later he may enjoy smearing in finger painting, using bright, light, cheerful colors on large sheets of paper.

Smearing with feces can be reduced if the child is cleaned immediately after a bowel movement. Diapers should be applied securely, using four pins, so that he cannot put his hands upon the excrement. After he has learned to use the training chair or toilet, smearing is no longer a great problem.

Influence of Toilet Training on the Child's Personality.
Ambivalence toward his mother is common during the training period. He loves her, but now she asks him to give up the comfort of relieving himself when and where he feels the desire to do so. He therefore feels antagonistic toward her. *His ambivalent attitude is composed of love and hate at the same time.* He may strike at her and pull away and a moment later turn to her for comfort. If she maintains an attitude of friendliness and understanding, love will predominate over hostility in him. It is important to minimize his antagonism so that he does not grow out of the training period with feelings of hostility, rebellion and resentment.

Summary.
If a mother loves her child, he is normally conditioned to please her and will respond to toilet training without too much difficulty. She will not be discouraged if she has con-

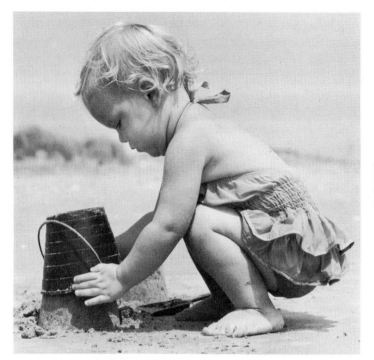

Figure 15–3. Toddlers enjoy playing in sand. This is a more socially acceptable activity than smearing feces. (H. Armstrong Roberts.)

fidence in his intelligence and his desire to do what she asks, and she will give him a reasonable length of time in which to learn.

On the other hand, if the mother shows disgust about the whole process of excretion, the child will feel ashamed of his body. He may feel that he is not lovable. He may even feel that he is a naughty child if he fails in toilet training. Eventually he may acquire the attitude that all physical functions should be brought under rigid control. He may extend this feeling to all his activities and be constantly afraid of doing something which will displease his mother or other adults. In his mind he equates overcleanliness with being good. Unfortunately his desire to keep clean usually inhibits normal active play. Such a child lacks spontaneity and creativity. He is apt to be a child afraid to soil his hands or dirty his clothes when playing. When other children make mud pies, he stands back. Such a child may develop a persistent attitude of anxiously trying to please anyone in authority over him for fear he will lose their approval.

Not only must he be perfect himself, but also he expects his friends to be likewise. He becomes rigid and inflexible and bound by compulsive rituals which to his mind will minimize the danger of his displeasing someone and thus will lessen his anxiety.

Learning Language

Learning to talk takes a long time. From the newborn's cry to the first spoken word is the change from a reflex utterance to something which has a meaning for both the child and others. The infant uses motions, particularly movement of the hands, to indicate his wants. Motions are his substitute for speech.

Between the ages of one and three years the child is increasingly able to understand others and to express his feelings and ideas in words. Infants and little children may continue to use gestures, however, such as holding out their arms and smiling when they want to be picked up, even when they are able to say what they want.

Long before a child can use words in sentences he understands the meaning of many words. The mother's facial expression, gestures and tone of voice help the child to understand the meaning of her words. She may teach him a new word by pointing to an object while she says the word. Or when he is interested in an object, such as a doll, he may say the word as she gives it to him.

Incentives to Speech. In order to speak a child must have satisfying relations with his mother. Unless he feels that she will respond to his words, he is not motivated to speak. He must find it rewarding to talk or he will not be interested in trying. He speaks to express his needs. When he says, "Ma-ma," he is expressing a need for all the pleasant things she does for him. If he says, "Ma-ma," and points to something, he means, "Please give me that." When he learns the names for objects, he will use the names, e.g. cup, dog. If all his needs are supplied without his asking, he is poorly motivated to speak until he feels the need for words to express attitudes, ideas and emotions.

Normally a child's first speech is an expression of his wants. This is followed by words or phrases which indicate ideas or what he thinks the function of objects to be. His idea of animals is expressed in terms of what they do; e.g. a dog barks. He early learns the value of speech in pleasant social relations. He takes great pleasure in talking and talks to anyone, his toys, pets or himself. Even when he can say only a few words, he uses these words to obtain information about himself, other people and things. "Go bye-bye" is not only a request; he is also asking whether he is going outdoors. When he says, "Dog," he may be asking where the household pet is.

Methods of Learning. A young child must have a good model or he will not learn to speak correctly. He will imitate poor speech as readily as correct speech, perhaps more easily because it is often more simple and direct and apt to be accompanied with gestures. If an adult uses baby talk in speaking to him, the child has no model for learning the correct words for objects, experiences and attitudes. He needs not only a model talking *to him,* but also the opportunity to use the word immediately in his answer. Talking to toys, to animals and to himself gives him practice in using words, but since he hears only himself, he may be confirmed in his baby mispronunciation and misuse of words.

There is a plateau stage in learning to talk at which a child makes little progress. The plateau occurs when the child has learned to walk and is so interested in walking that he pays little attention to acquiring new words. Nevertheless he appears to be increasing the number of words he understands.

The child with his limited vocabulary may cry because he is frustrated in his efforts to express his wants or feelings and because he does not get what he wants. He still hits out when he is angry and cries when he is hurt. He has not yet acquired the ability, physically or psychologically, to control his actions and to use words to express antagonism and unhappiness. Later on, instead of hitting his mother or a playmate, he may express his feeling by saying, "I hate you!" or, "I wish you'd go away," and instead of crying because he may not go out and play he may say, "Why does it rain? I want to play," or simply wail, "I want to go out and play." In either case he is asking for the comfort which crying brought him when he was a baby. Even when he is able to speak, if his emotions are too great for him to control, putting them into words is not a sufficient outlet, and he resorts to the immature outlets of anger and disappointment. Whenever he speaks or cries, the child needs acceptance of himself and his feelings, however unreasonable they appear from the adult's point of view. Crying is a distress signal with him as with an infant.

Examples of this sort of situation are often

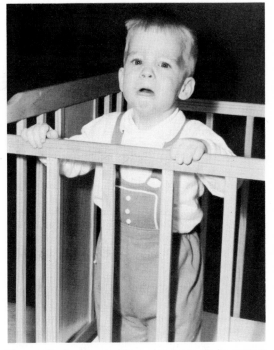

Figure 15–4. The toddler cries because he cannot express his needs in words.

found in the hospital. When a child thinks that he will be hurt because he will get a needle and is reassured by what we say to him, we see the value of his understanding verbal communication and of his ability to put his fear into words. He needs a simple explanation as a preparation for the procedure and both verbal and physical demonstrations of affection so that he does not feel that these strange adults want to hurt him (technically speaking, that he is being attacked). The nurse in such a situation must not say, "Don't cry." To do so would indicate a lack of understanding of how the child perceives the situation. He is still too young not to be afraid of pain. The nurse or mother should explain the need for his being hurt and what is to be done, so far as he can understand the reason or the procedure. If possible, his mother should be there to hold him; if not, one of the nurses whom he knows or at least has made friends with should take her place. The nurse should tell him that she knows he is frightened, saying, "All children feel that way. It will be over soon."

Vocabulary Building. The child builds a vocabulary in the following ways. The first words he learns are nouns of one syllable, nouns like the sounds he has babbled ("Ma-ma, da-da"). He attempts more difficult words until eventually he can give the names of objects and people in his daily environment. He next learns verbs that mean some form of action which he sees about him and whose meaning he understands (e.g. give, take, run). Adjectives he learns from eighteen months on. The first adjectives he learns are usually "good" and "bad," because he hears them frequently. The first adverbs he uses are usually "here" and "where." These are words used by his mother in speaking to him. Last he learns the meaning of pronouns. These are confusing to him because they vary with the person using the word. Johnny is "me" and "I" to himself, but "you" to his mother when she speaks to him, and "he" when she tells his father about him. The same confusion exists with other pronouns.

The size of a child's vocabulary depends on whether he has been helped to learn new words, on whether he has had an incentive to learn and on his intelligence. At nine months he can say "Ma-ma" and "Da-da," and at one year two or three more words. From eighteen months to three or four years his vocabulary increases rapidly. At two years he can say approximately 300 words, and at three years approximately 900. During school age his general vocabulary increases rapidly as the result of being taught new words and of his pleasure in reading.

Sentence Formation. The child's first attempt at making sentences consists in combining two or more words into a phrase and supplementing these with gestures. Early sentences contain nouns, verbs and, at times, adjectives and adverbs, e.g. "Baby go bye-bye."

Delayed Speech. The normal child will begin to speak by about fifteen months of age. If he does not speak by the time he is two years old, the cause for delayed speech should be investigated. Some of the common causes are as follows.

INTELLIGENCE. Speech is delayed in children of low intelligence. The size of the vocabulary depends to a great extent upon the child's intelligence.

SOCIAL AND CULTURAL ENVIRONMENT. Children of poorer social environments are delayed in speech development because they often have poor models to imitate. Children in an orphanage or a similar institution may have extreme language retardation because adults seldom speak to them individually, and when they do, the subject is likely to be merely what the child is to do or not to do.

ILLNESS. Children who are ill in an institution for a long time have slower speech development than well children because they have fewer contacts with other children and also because their needs are answered before they have to ask for what they want. A child who receives much adult attention at home when he is sick may increase his vocabulary rapidly. It is the hospitalized child who is likely to be retarded.

POOR MODELS. If the child has a poor model to imitate in speaking, his speech will be incorrect or retarded.

NEGATIVISM. The child may decide not to talk because he was forced to talk when he had not matured to the point at which he wanted to imitate his mother's words. He may have been laughed at for his babyish pronunciation and had his self-image lowered.

DEAFNESS. If the child cannot hear what others say, he cannot imitate them and therefore will not speak unless he has had special training. Even then he will have a smaller vocabulary, poor pronunciation and a peculiar, flat tone of voice.

SEX. Boys are usually slower than girls in learning to talk. They also have a smaller vocabulary than girls have and make more grammatical errors.

Learning two languages at the same time for the child under five years of age is likely to delay his learning to speak and also causes confusion in both vocabulary and grammatical forms.

Cultural Development

The toddler must learn many other patterns of behavior besides toilet training and language. He learns how to make the simple basic movements in washing and bathing himself and brushing his teeth. He understands what his mother means when she wants him to keep clean, to put his toys away when he has finished playing with them, and to keep his play space neat.

The child is attempting an overall mastery of his world. When he learns to do something by himself, he has a real sense of mastery, independence, and adequacy in meeting his needs. His parents should help him to learn and should approve his success. If parents do not show their approval in ways he can understand, the child experiences a conflict between enjoying what he can do himself (even if this is to get an ashtray and empty it on the floor) and the disapproval of his parents. Since he knows that they will disapprove, he must make a choice between the pleasure of doing what he wants and the pleasure of having his parents' approval. Through such decisions the child eventually learns how to make appropriate judgments, choosing what is considered right in the culture of the group to which he belongs. His basic motivation is love for his parents, a love acquired in infancy and strengthened during early childhood.

Personality Traits of the Toddler

Negativism

In his desire for independence or autonomy the child wants to do many things he should not do. From infancy through the toddler period he has heard his mother say "No" to his many efforts at self-assertion. Gradually he learns to use the words "No, no" to mean "Don't" and a rather stubborn "I won't." In this way he is substantiating his power as an individual in controlling those who love him. The developmental task of this period is to curb his negative responses and to adjust his conduct to the social norms of those in authority.

Each child goes through this period of negativism during his development toward maturity. Two years is said to be the "No, no" age and has been called "the terrible twos." He wants to act as an individual and appears to want power—to have his own way—more than the pleasure of the forbidden activity. Yet when he is frustrated in achieving what he wants independently of the help of others, or when their reaction toward him leads him to believe that they do not love him, he is likely to turn to the adults against whom his aggression was aimed, for comfort in the unpleasant situation he has created for himself.

Sometimes he seems to want to be dependent and independent at the same time. For example, when he is offered ice cream, he may say, "No," and yet eat it quickly in spite of his answer.

A child acts in a negative fashion because he cannot tolerate the frustration of a desire. He cannot accept parental restrictions and at the same time cannot find an acceptable way to gain the results he wants. When he says, "No," he feels as strong as his parents.

Sometimes a child appears to be negativistic when he really is not. He may not object to doing what his parents want, but he does not want to stop what he is doing, e.g. if he is playing happily and is asked to put away his toys and go to bed.

The period of negativism is usually a short one if the child's needs are understood. He needs the support of his parents' love in order to learn how to satisfy his new powers of independence in socially acceptable ways.

Handling Negativistic Behavior. An adult should not use opposition to overcome opposition in a child. Opposition increases the child's desire to show his independence.

An adult should not give the toddler too many commands or interrupt his activities too frequently.

The adult should help the child to participate in what is expected of him by giving physical help, e.g. by putting the toys away when it is bedtime. This allows the toddler to feel that he and the adult are working toward a common goal and not that he is forced to do what the adult wishes. When the mother places food in front of a two-year-old, she may feed him a few spoonfuls, speaking gently to him as she does so. The child may then take the spoon in his hand and feed himself.

The mother must recognize indications of independence in the child. Such recognition increases the child's self-esteem and makes him want to cooperate even more. It helps him to feel self-important. All children learn to know themselves through the attitude of *significant persons* in their environment (particularly members of their own families) toward them. If the mother has a wholesome concept of the child, he has a wholesome concept of himself. If he accepts himself at this age, he can later accept others.

Ritualistic Behavior

The toddler engages in much ritualistic behavior. He makes rituals of simple tasks because he knows that he can master himself in this way. Ritualistic behavior is most common between the ages of two and four years; it reaches its height at approximately $2\frac{1}{2}$ years. As the child leaves the toddler period he has less and less need of a strict routine because he is more sure of himself and can adapt to changes better than he could when he was younger. Adults should recognize these rituals in such phases as bathing (hanging the washcloth in a certain way), eating (having his bib on always in the same way) and sleeping (always taking his favorite blanket to bed with him). The adult saves time and energy by doing so and also gives the child a feeling of security and mastery of himself.

Slowness in Carrying Out Requests

The toddler is gradually learning the difference between right and wrong. He cannot decide which of two actions to take. He is therefore likely to carry out both actions. For example, when his mother calls him from play to use the training chair, he is likely to finish his play activity first and urinate on the way to the training chair, partly because of his nervousness and haste to do what his mother has asked. When the child learns through experience which action he should take, he will be able to make decisions more wisely and more quickly.

Temper Tantrums

Temper tantrums occur when the child cannot integrate his own internal impulses and the demands of reality. He is frustrated and reacts in the only way he knows—by violent bodily activity and crying. When no substitute solution is available, temper tantrums result. Such situations are most common during the toddler and early preschool periods. If the tantrums are abnormally frequent or continue into school age, the child should be taken to a child guidance center for professional help with his problems or with a deep-seated emotional maladjustment.

In the hospital children may have tantrums

because they fear the unknown and are away from those they love. They need help in understanding their environment and care. They also need the security resulting from their mothers' frequent visiting.

In a temper tantrum the child is completely oblivious of the reality of the situation. He does not hear or react to what is said to him unless it shocks him so severely that it penetrates his consciousness.

His release of emotion through muscular activity is either aimless or is directed against himself. He is likely to bang his head against the floor or otherwise inflict pain upon himself. Only rarely does he attack the adult who provoked the tantrum.

Handling the Child. The child should not be given extra attention, but should be observed and restrained from self-injury or from something in the physical environment which may be a source of injury to himself. Restraint increases the severity of a temper tantrum because it prevents the one outlet which the child knows for his anger. If he hurts another child or an adult or breaks a cherished possession, he may feel guilty when the tantrum is over.

The child's tension will be reduced if he can be removed from the immediate cause of the tantrum and be with one adult who he knows loves him. This adult, usually his mother, should be calm and patient with him, but should not force attention upon him until he indicates that he is ready for the comfort of knowing that he is loved and that his unhappiness can be changed to happiness.

Care After Tantrums. It is advisable to make as few comments as possible upon the child's behavior during a tantrum. He should not be punished in any way. If he will cooperate, it is soothing to wash his face and hands. He may be given a toy to divert his attention from the experience he has undergone. He has been so emotionally upset that he needs to quiet down before he is given food.

Prevention. The mother, knowing the child, may see that a tantrum is imminent. She should try to show him better ways of solving his problem and provide more socially acceptable outlets for his anger and frustration. Also a child often fears his own aggression and the disagreeable state into which it throws him. He should be helped to release his tension in a socially approved way, such as through physical exercise.

The sick child may hammer rubber balls through holes in a board or toss bean bags into a can placed on the floor. In the home there is a wide range of activities which can be used as an outlet for his tension. If he may go outdoors, digging in the garden and helping rake the leaves or shoveling snow are tension-releasing activities. In the house he may use a hammer and pegs or build a block tower which he can then knock down.

If the tantrum is caused by an adult's refusal to grant a request, the adult should be firm and not yield to the child. Only by consistency in adult behavior can a child learn to adjust his own behavior to his expectation of the adult's reaction to what he intends to do. Unfortunately, the child does not and never will live in a world of perfect people, and his own imperfections are less likely to arouse guilt feelings in him if he sees imperfections in those nearest him. One value of a large family is that the children talk over imperfections in their parents—whether real or imaginary—and develop a healthy, realistic love of others even while recognizing their faults. It is a comfort to a two-year-old to know that the four-year-old thinks that mother is sometimes mean. The modern mother knows that she is sometimes mean and that the child knows it, but loves her, just as she loves him with all his naughtiness.

Sometimes when a child feels anger and tensions rising, he isolates himself. This is all right as a temporary measure, but if he always withdraws, he will need help in learning to face problems more directly.

Discipline

Discipline has as its goal *self-control*. It is not merely a way of forcing the child's obedience to adult authority. To be most effective, discipline must be carried out through guidance, helping the child to learn how to live comfortably with others. Discipline, if it is to be constructive, must help the child to direct unacceptable, unrealistic and often futile ways of reaching the goal toward which his impulses are directed into socially approved channels that are effective. This socialization process, begun by the parents, should function without demanding too great sacrifice of the child's individuality and creativity.

As the child learns to control himself in his relations with others, he feels more secure and less anxious. To achieve self-control he needs the help of adults in accepting his feelings and handling them in a constructive way. He needs a positive rather than a forbidding, negativistic parent-child relationship.

Discipline is a broad term which includes much of the interaction between the mother or some other adult and the child. A parent uses discipline to establish limits, grant permission, help the child to understand social standards and guide him to direct his impulses into socially acceptable ways of behaving. Much of this is not recognized as discipline by either the parent or the child. It is part of family life or the expres-

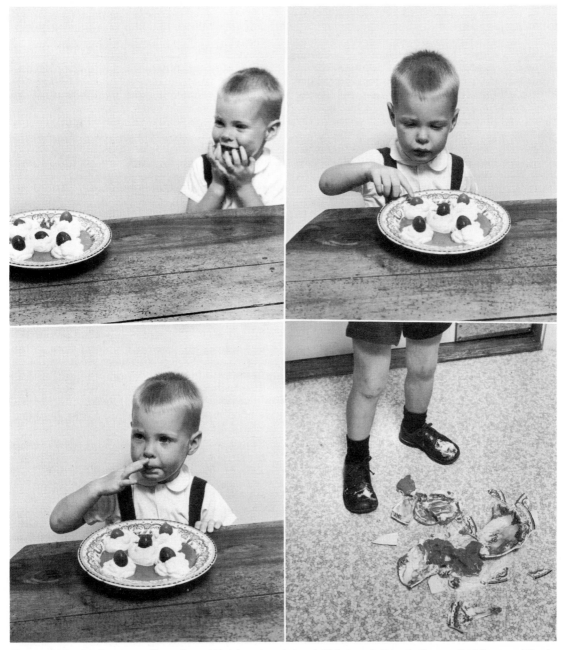

Figure 15–5. Mothers sometimes thoughtlessly put such irresistible temptations in the way that they unwittingly lead their children into mischief! (Courtesy of Lew Merrim and *Baby Talk* Magazine.)

sion of happy parent-child relations. The way in which a parent approaches the problem of discipline is perhaps the best indication of his feelings toward the child.

Setting of Limits. Limits must be set to the child's behavior if he is to feel secure; otherwise he will constantly suffer the consequences of his mistakes in situations in which he is not old enough to function without guidance. Small children do not know the difference between right and wrong; they must learn the difference from their parents. When limits are imposed, the child will probably be angry momentarily, but he is likely to feel more secure because he knows that his parents can create happier situations for him than he can. This is an extension of the sense of trust in adults the infant learned in the first year of life.

It is essential for a child's happiness in relations with other people that he form habits of behavior limited by social approval. Parents who establish habits of behavior which win the toddler friends and give him an acceptable self-image reflected from what others think of him are fulfilling an important part of their function in the training of their child.

The way in which a toddler accepts discipline from his parents or other adults depends upon his love relationship with those adults. Parents who won the trust of their child during his infancy established a relationship in which he was passively cooperative. Passive cooperation lays the foundation for active cooperation.

Constructive Discipline. Parents should be reasonable in their requests and tolerate some delay in the child's response. They should not be overanxious about small details of the child's behavior or say "No" too often. They should never expect from the toddler behavior which is beyond his ability.

The child who has learned the pleasure of cooperating with his parents will carry over the same attitude toward other adults. He will reap the reward of being liked and included in many pleasant situations in which he strengthens his habit of accepting discipline and lays the foundation for self-discipline. Such a child is free to grow, but is given the help he needs with his problems. He is given graded independence, but is not forced to accept more than he can utilize constructively. The adult should do things *with* the child, whenever possible, and not *to* or *for* him, thereby making desirable behavior easy and satisfying to the child.

The child should be shielded from unnecessary fear, but should learn to meet fearful situations courageously. "Courageously" means retaining the ability to think clearly and maintaining full use of all the resources of his body to meet the emergency. This is just what the child loses when he is paralyzed with fear.

If the mother is not *consistent* in her discipline or if the adults about the child do not make consistent demands upon him, he becomes confused and cannot use his developing power of reasoning to determine what will happen if he responds in this way or that. Even if he is motivated to do what the adult says because he loves the adult, he will often disobey because the other parent, whom he also loves, has asked just the opposite of him.

Punishment. Some form of punishment should be given the child who breaks rules which he understands and which are enforced by all adults responsible for his discipline. The child should be allowed to maintain his self-respect when punished, and never be made to feel that his parents do not love him because he has done wrong.

Love should not be used to buy good behavior. Love should call forth love, and the central element in love is furtherance of the welfare, the happiness, of the one loved. Such love is not developed in the child under two years.

Some parents make the mistake of blaming themselves if they feel antagonistic to or angry with (hostile toward) their child. Nurses also may have similar feelings. They never punish a child, because they believe that punishment is an expression of anger. This is a mistake. Punishment is a useful tool in discipline if it is used with discretion. It often clears the atmosphere for further interaction. The child will not resent it if he feels that he "had it coming to him." He should be punished knowing that the adult still loves him. Punishment should never appear to him as an angry retaliation by the adult. Fear of punishment should be reduced to the minimum which serves to reinforce in the child the habits established during infancy of accepting adult decisions to please the adult. Then the child learns the necessity of obedience as he matures and has decisions to make as to what he will and will not do.

If possible, the child should be shown that punishment is the logical consequence of his wrong decision. When a child burns his hand because he disobeys his mother and touches a hot stove, he sees the result of his disobedience, but he also knows that his mother did not inflict the pain. He remembers not to touch the stove again, for he sees the connection between the pain and his act. The connection is not clear to him when his mother punishes him for disobedience. Only if he has learned to trust his parents' judgment and knows that they do not punish him without good reason does he accept the connection between punishment and what he has done in the same spirit with which he accepted the burnt finger when he touched the stove.

It is even harder for him to learn what is morally right and wrong. Burning his finger had no moral implications (unless his mother had told him not to go near the stove); it was a matter of poor judgment on his part. By being hurt he learned about the physical environment in a painful way. If he has learned that "mother knows best," he believes her when she says that he might get hurt or sick, lose his penny, break his toy or tear his new shirt. But when she forbids behavior which interferes with the rights of other members of the family or of the people he meets when she takes him out with her, the reason for her decision is not clear to him. Nevertheless a child who loves his parents does accept their decisions about what is morally right and wrong as he accepts their decisions on the physical results of behavior. He learns to accept punishment as just when it follows his wrong actions. He learns to fear his own extreme impulses which are followed by unpleasant results in his relations with other people and tries to do right.

If a child feels guilty over something he did which his mother did not find out and for which he was not punished, he may purposely do something naughty in order to be punished and so reduce his feeling of guilt over the first offense. Some children who are ignored and rejected by their parents may actually seek to be punished so as to gain some response from their parents. Although this is not a loving response, it is better than being ignored.

Before condemning what a child does, his reasoning, motive and experience must be considered. The child should never be made to feel that the adult condemns him. He must be helped to understand that it is what he has done that is condemned and that he is still loved as before. Punishment should relate to the wrong act and follow directly upon the act so that wrong doing and punishment are brought together in the child's mind. Punishment should not be cruel, and corporal punishment should not be used if it can be avoided and never given so as to embarrass the child before others.

Nurses caring for children in the hospital should set limits on their behavior just as mothers do at home. Too often nursing students have difficulty in doing this in a hospital setting.

Summary of Emotional Development

The problems of this period center mostly around the child's need to develop a *sense of autonomy*. He needs to learn to hold on and let go, as in toilet training. He needs help with the conflict between carrying out his new-found abilities and his continuing need for security and parental love. His accomplishments should be praised and his success in self-control noticed.

Parents should remember that the child has many years in which to complete the developmental tasks begun in the toddler period. They should not try to force him too rapidly into more mature behavior. If they do, the child, instead of submitting, may rebel and defeat the parents' attempts to use compulsion. He may become negativistic.

Two kinds of parents fail in guiding a child during this period. The first is the overdemanding parent, the second is the parent whose policy is *laissez-faire*. With such parents the child has no help in his striving for maturity.

The adult must define reality for the child. If adults do not set limits to his behavior, he cannot learn to live satisfactorily in his society.

OVERVIEW OF PHYSICAL GROWTH AND DEVELOPMENT

Physical growth and motor development are slower between one and three years than during infancy. The toddler period is marked primarily by increasing strength and skill in performance. By the end of the second year the principal types of muscular activities have appeared. Skilled performance in new areas is simply a utilization of old skills in new ways. Old skills become more and more perfected. The result is fewer errors and more speed with smoother, graceful movements. After the basic motor skills have been acquired the repertoire of added skills varies widely, depending upon the child's interest in new activities, his environment and his ability to learn.

Significance of Delayed Motor Development. Although most children progress through the stages of infantile development at approximately the ages given in Chapter 12, some do not. These are not only late in reaching the stage of independent action characteristic of the toddler period, but also are prevented from interacting with other children and from achieving normal social development. The young child whose motor development is retarded cannot join in play with children who can run and climb. He refrains or is excluded from their play and may develop feelings of inferiority which later are the bases for antisocial behavior.

Schedule of Growth and Development. The developmental schedules for toddlers (Table 15-1) are only averages which are in the ranges of ages during which normal children achieve certain levels of development. They are not typical of any one child. There are individual differences. The ages given are *approximate* for the various activities and learnings listed. These developmental schedules provide only a general outline of the growth of a child between one and three years.

PLAY

Purposes. The main function of play during infancy is physical development and early association. As the child grows older the importance of play increases. (1) *Physical development* continues through play. Muscles are developed, and exercise is given to all parts of the body. Surplus energy can be worked off during active play. (2) *Social development* occurs when the toddler participates in activity with other children. Although at this age social interaction is limited, he enjoys *parallel play* (playing *beside* another child, but not *with* him). (3) The *therapeutic value* of play is psychological as well as physical, for it sublimates drives so that they are released in an approved way, and helps the child

(Text continued on page 384.)

Table 15–1. *Developmental Schedules, 15 Months to 2½ Years*

---

15 MONTHS

Motor Control (see also Fig. 15–6)

At this age the toddler has reached a plateau of motor development

Walks alone at 14 months, but with a wide-based gait to steady himself. After he has learned to walk it is to him a form of play

Creeps upstairs

Builds a tower of 2 blocks

Throws objects repeatedly and picks them up again. Throwing is evidence of his new ability to release an object in his grasp

Opens boxes

Pokes finger in holes

Holds a cup with fingers grasped about it. He is apt to tip it too quickly and spill the contents

Grasps a spoon and inserts it into a dish. He cannot fill the spoon well. If he brings the spoon to his mouth, it is likely to be turned upside down, and the contents spilled into his lap

Vocalization and Socialization

Uses jargon

Names familiar pictures or objects

Responds to familiar comments

Vocalizes his wants and points to the desired object

Pats pictures in a book and turns pages

Indicates when his diaper is wet

---

18 MONTHS

Physical Development

Anterior fontanel is usually closed (may be closed as early as 12 months)

Abdomen protrudes

Motor Control (see Fig. 15–7)

Walks and runs with a somewhat wide stance, but increasingly more like the adult gait. He seldom falls

Pulls a toy behind him

Pushes light pieces of furniture around the room

Can walk sideways and backward (16.7 months)

Climbs stairs or upon furniture

Seats himself on a small chair

Throws ball into a box, puts block in a hole

Scribbles vigorously. Attempts straight lines. Differentiates between straight and circular strokes

May build tower of 3 blocks

Holds cup to lips and drinks well with little spilling. Hands cup to his mother or drops it on the floor

Can fill his spoon, but has difficulty inserting spoon into his mouth. Is apt to turn the spoon in his mouth. Spills frequently

Vocalization and Socialization

Knows 10 words

Uses phrases composed of adjectives and nouns

Shifts attention rapidly from one thing to another. Moves quickly from place to place. Explores drawers and closets. Gets into everything

Has a new awareness of strangers

Begins to have temper tantrums if things go wrong

May resist sleep for some time after he has been put to bed. Calls for his mother

May control bowel movements

May smear stool

Thumb-sucking may reach a peak. It usually occurs just before sleep or goes on all night

Enjoys solitary play or watching others' activities

Hugs his teddy bear or doll

Begins to select a favorite toy or object such as a blanket

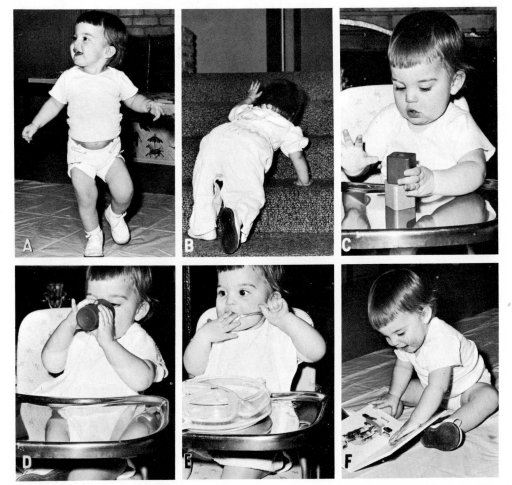

Figure 15–6.   The 15-month-old (*A*) walks alone, (*B*) creeps upstairs, (*C*) builds a tower of 2 blocks, (*D*) holds a cup with fingers around it, (*E*) grasps spoon, but spills contents, (*F*) pats picture in book.

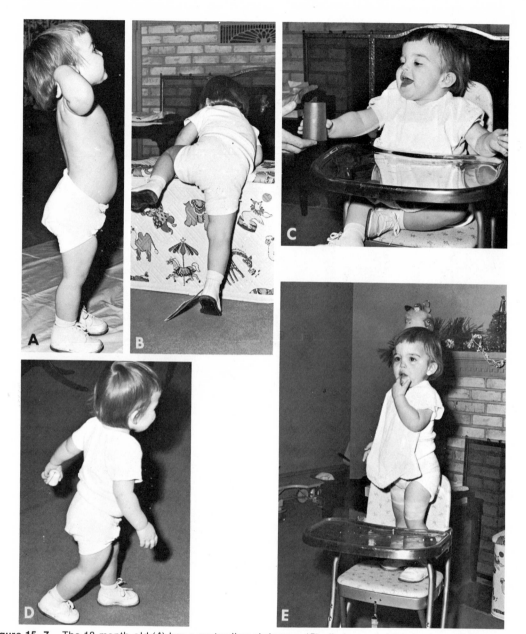

Figure 15–7.   The 18-month-old (*A*) has a protruding abdomen, (*B*) climbs upon high toy box, (*C*) hands cup to mother, (*D*) moves rapidly from place to place and enjoys pulling toy behind her, (*E*) begins to have temper tantrums. This toddler shows increasing frustration because she wants to get out of her high chair. A temper tantrum occurred shortly after this picture had been taken.

Table 15–1. *Developmental Schedules, 15 Months to 2½ Years (Continued)*

---

2 YEARS

Physical Development
  Weight: 26–28 pounds
  Height: approximately 32–33 inches (gain of 3–4 inches in second year)
  Pulse: 90–120 per minute
  Respirations: 20–35 per minute
  Teeth: approximately 16 temporary teeth
  Abdomen protrudes less than at 18 months
Motor Control (see Fig. 15–8)
  More grown up, steady gait
  Can run in more controlled way, has fewer falls and may run away
  Can jump crudely. In initial attempts he usually falls, since his body is propelled forward
  Walks up and down stairs, both feet on one step at a time, and holding onto a railing or the wall
  Builds a tower of 5 or more blocks. Can make cubes into a train
  Can open doors by turning door knob
  Scribbles in more controlled way than at 18 months. Imitates vertical stroke
  Drinks well from a small glass held in one hand
  Can put a spoon in his mouth without turning it
Vocalization and Socialization
  Has a vocabulary of approximately 300 words. Can use pronouns and names familiar objects. Can tell about his experiences. No longer uses jargon
  Makes short sentences of 3 or 4 words
  Shifts attention less rapidly than child of 18 months
  Behaves as though other children were physical objects. He may hug them or push them out of the way. Would like to make friends, but does not know how
  Does not readily ask for help
  Obeys simple commands
  Helps to undress himself. Can pull on simple garments
  Is toilet-trained in daytime. Verbalizes toilet needs
  May still smear with stool
  Thumb-sucking decreased
  Does not know right from wrong
  Number of relatively violent temper tantrums is decreasing
  Is proud of accomplishment of motor skills
  May fear parents' leaving
  Shows increasing signs of sense of individuality
  Enjoys parallel play—no interaction with other children even though their activity is the same. Interaction that does occur may consist in snatching toys from one another, kicking or pulling hair
  Manipulates play materials. Dawdles frequently
  Enjoys playing with dolls, placing beads in box and dumping them out, pulling blocks piled in wagon
  Cannot share possessions. Has great sense of "mine," little of "yours"
  Learns to replace toys in their proper place
  Enjoys hearing stories illustrated with pictures
  Begins play which mimics activities of parents
  Takes favorite toy to bed with him, which helps to quiet him. Has many demands before going to bed

---

30 MONTHS (2½ YEARS)

Physical Development
  Has full set of 20 temporary (deciduous) teeth
Motor Control (see Fig. 15–9)
  Walks on tiptoe
  Rides a kiddie car
  Stands on one foot alone
  Can throw a large ball 4 to 5 feet
  Piles 7 or 8 blocks one on top of the other
  Copies horizontal or vertical line
Vocalization and Socialization
  Temper tantrums may continue
  During the whole toddler period the child has begun to develop a self-concept from reflected appraisal of significant people—his parents and other adults who care for him. He is beginning to know himself as a separate person, and to have a conscience when he can control some areas of his behavior to conform to social demands

---

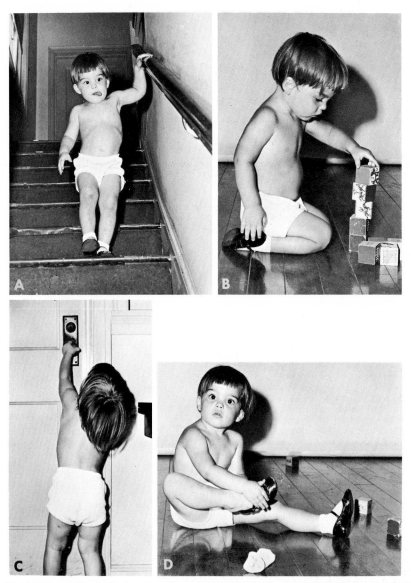

Figure 15–8.   The 2-year-old (*A*) walks up and down steps, both feet on one step at a time, and holding onto the rail; (*B*) can build a tower of 5 or more blocks; (*C*) can open a door by turning the door knob; (*D*) helps to undress herself.

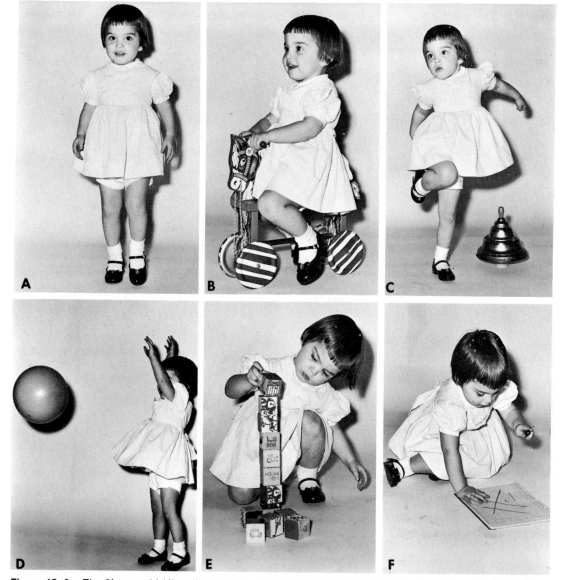

Figure 15–9.   The 2½-year-old (A) walks on tiptoe, (B) rides a kiddie car, (C) stands on one foot alone, (D) throws a large ball 4 to 5 feet, (E) piles 7 or 8 blocks one on top of another, (F) copies horizontal or verticle line.

to release emotional tensions. For instance, an angry child may find relief by pounding boards, or tossing bean bags. (4) Play is a means of *education*. The toddler who plays with toys of all sorts learns to know colors, shapes, sizes and textures of play materials. (5) Play develops a beginning understanding of *moral values*. The toddler begins to learn right from wrong. He begins to learn not to hurt other children by rough play.

The toddler has strong feelings about his toys, clutching at them and saying, "Mine, mine." But he slowly learns the importance of sharing even though it may be difficult for him to do so. He should not be forced to give up his toys until he is older and can understand that play with others involves giving up some pleasures on his part in order to have the greater satisfaction of participation in common projects in which he receives as well as gives pleasure.

Characteristics of Play. Each age group enjoys its own kind of play. Play during childhood follows a pattern of development based on the maturity of the group. Certain play activities are popular at each age no matter what the socioeconomic status, the environment or the ethnic culture in which the child is brought up. In general, play with toys is popular until the eighth year. After this children enjoy games which encourage large muscular activity such as running. After this stage, games or sports for which there are strict rules become all-important.

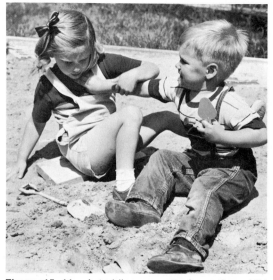

Figure 15–11. A toddler may attack another child because he does not know how to play cooperatively with her. (H. Armstrong Roberts.)

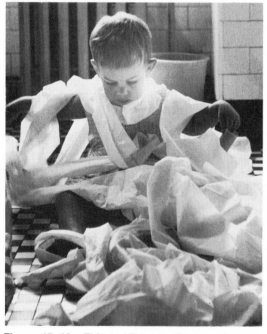

Figure 15–10. This toddler has discovered a new kind of play. (Courtesy of Mrs. Erika Stone and *Baby Talk* Magazine.)

During the toddler period, play is active and is based on the motor and emotional development of the child. Walking in the early toddler period is a delightful game. He has acquired greater skill in the use of his arms. The fifteen-month-old toddler enjoys throwing objects and picking them up again, putting them into receptacles and taking them out again.

At eighteen months the toddler is exceedingly active. Since his attention span is short, he moves freely from place to place and gets into everything. It is difficult to keep him out of drawers. By this age his balance has improved so that he can pull toys behind him or carry a doll or stuffed animal about with him. He enjoys playing alone or watching other children play, but has not learned to play with them in any game requiring group consensus. He notices the activities of his parents and may imitate them.

The two-year-old has less rapid shifts in attention than the younger child. He may dawdle in his play activities. He enjoys manipulating play materials, pounding, patting and feeling mud, sand or clay in his hands. He plays with dolls, strings large beads and puts his blocks into his wagon.

In *parallel play* the toddler plays beside another child in such activities as making mud pies. He wants to be friendly with other children, but does not know how. He may attack another child in his attempt. For this reason adult supervision of toddlers' play is necessary.

The 2½-year-old toddler has developed finer use of his muscles than the two-year-old. He enjoys handling smaller blocks and balls in a sensory way, but he still needs larger blocks and balls for play. He also has enough coordination to ride a kiddie car fairly well.

Play in the early toddler period is mostly free and *spontaneous*. There are no rules and regulations to follow. The child explores as he desires and stops when he pleases. Since he has poor motor coordination, he is apt to be destructive. His toys must be carefully examined to determine whether he might injure himself on broken parts. He does not intentionally break his toys, but his exploration of them—shaking, pushing, rattling—is sometimes more than the toys can stand.

By the end of the second year most children begin to impersonate adults whom they are with and who do what the child considers interesting, e.g. setting the dinner table. If they play with older children, make-believe use of materials leads to make-believe situations such as playing house. Usually when toddlers play house with preschool children, the toddlers are the children in the family.

Even in the early toddler period *constructive* play is seen, such as making mud pies, making holes in sand and playing with clay. Toddlers also enjoy crayons and use them in drawing and scribbling on paper. The product usually has no practical use, but its educational value is great. Toddlers enjoy moving their arms in time to music and singing simple songs, but they are unable to coordinate complex movements of their bodies with the music.

Toddlers, because of their short attention span, require a variety of activities and playthings to keep them busy. They spend most of their waking time in play. Since the span of attention of a two-year-old child is so short, they may leave an activity to do something else, but return later to their original play.

Play is informal. The toddler plays when and where he wishes. He needs no special clothes, toys or play space.

Selection of Play Materials. The toddler's likes and dislikes should be remembered when selecting his toys. He is active and curious. He explores his environment, using his large muscles rather than small ones. He likes to pull and push toys and enjoys pedal-propelled toys, a kiddie car (tip-proof) and low rocking horses. He enjoys toys that open and close. Since he is imaginative, he likes to play with dolls and stuffed animals. His constructive and manipulative activities include playing with sand box toys, water toys, clay, finger paints, blocks, peg boards (large), pounding sets and thick, large crayons. He enjoys being read to while he looks at the pictures in his book.

Safety Factors in Selection of Toys. The toddler needs toys which are safe for him to play with. He should not be given toys that are sharp, have rough edges or small removable parts, nor should he have flammable toys, or beads, marbles and coins that he can put in his mouth to swallow or aspirate. Toys painted with lead paint are dangerous, since he ingests a little of the paint if he sucks them.

CARE OF THE TODDLER

The mother or nurse should adjust adult procedures to the difference in size between the adult and the child. For instance, *when talking to him, the nurse should squat down so that she is on his eye level*. If she merely bends over, her image will still be overpowering for the small child. The toddler lacks the adult's resistance to force and loud sounds; he responds best to a light touch and quiet voice.

Procedures should also be adapted to his level of understanding and endurance of frustration. Although he should be allowed to make decisions on the level of his understanding, he responds best to simple statements or to directions indicating what his mother or nurse wants him to do. Too many choices confuse him, since he does not understand the implications of each choice. He may not ask for what will give him the most pleasure.

The toddler who has learned to trust others

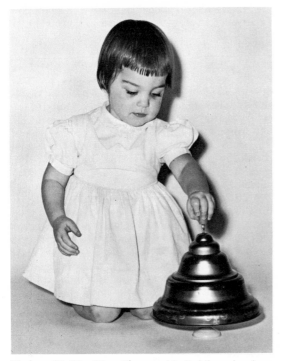

Figure 15–12. The 2½-year-old toddler develops further control of the smaller muscles of the body and is proud of this accomplishment.

knows that the limits they set to his behavior are for his safety and happiness.

Adults often forget that during his daily care the toddler is developing his concept of self and that his self-image is formed from the attitude of others toward him and his behavior. Toddlers are susceptible to the facial expressions of those about them, reading into them their responses to him, to what he does and to his efforts at verbal communication. Because of his ambivalent attitude of love for and aversion to the adults about him, he has difficulty in building his self-image from their behavior toward him. At one time he wants to accept their image of him, at another time to repudiate it. It is during the daily routine contacts with him that loving adults help him build his ego and *conscience* or super-ego. He internalizes the wishes and demands of others, particularly of those he loves the most. The beginning of a conscience is seen when even to a slight extent he is able to control his behavior in those areas in which he is most mature in order to conform to social norms.

Bathing

The toddler's bath need not be as detailed a procedure as that of the infant. It should be given as part of a consistent schedule which fits in with that of his mother and the rest of the family. Many mothers believe that bathing the child before the evening meal is relaxing and induces a quiet mood for the hour before bedtime. He may be bathed in the adult tub, but care should be taken to clean and dry it thoroughly before the water is run for his bath. His face and hands should be washed before meals.

Care of the Teeth

Prevention of decay in the deciduous dentition is important. Proper mouth hygiene and an adequate diet are essential for the prevention of decay.

Brushing the teeth should commence as soon as the temporary or deciduous teeth have erupted. By about two years a child should be taught to use a small toothbrush, brushing from the gum line to the edge of the teeth. Toothbrushing, in addition to cleaning the teeth, also stimulates the gums. He should have a place to keep his toothbrush and be taught how to take care of it. The child of three or four should be taught to brush his teeth after eating and especially before bedtime. Doing it himself establishes interest in keeping his teeth clean and helps to establish a routine which is useful as he grows into later childhood. At first he will not be able to use the brush with perfect technique, but he will improve with practice. His mother should supervise his efforts as long as necessary.

Clothing

Clothing should be light or bright in color, because children like bright colors. Bright colors also have value in accident prevention in that the child is easily seen and is therefore less likely to be injured by vehicles.

Clothing should have large, easily managed buttons and snaps placed where the child can reach them. Girls should wear panties which can be readily slipped down, and boys may have zippered flies which they can manage themselves. All clothing should be easy to put on and remove so that the child can help himself in dressing and undressing.

The average toddler is learning control of urination and defecation and, when two or three years old, may go to the toilet alone. When the mother has decided that he is old enough to be trained, training panties should be used instead of diapers. A change of panties whenever they are even slightly wet will accustom him to being dry. He feels more grown up and like his siblings when he no longer wears diapers and can be changed while standing. If possible, after he has become accustomed to panties, diapers should not be put on him except at night and at nap time. Children find attractive panties a great incentive to keeping dry.

Outdoor clothing should be warm, but not bulky, since the toddler enjoys active play and is irritated when his movements are restricted. He should have rubber boots for rain and snow and some sort of waterproof coat and hood or cap.

Shoes

When the toddler begins to walk, his shoes should be selected with reference to the free development of his feet and his posture. Shoes should have firm soles and should conform to the shape of the foot, i.e. straight along the inside, with broad toes and relatively narrow heels. The soles should not have even a low heel and should be rough to prevent the child from slipping; they should be $\frac{1}{2}$ inch longer and $\frac{1}{4}$ inch wider than the foot. The heels should fit snugly.

A little child outgrows his shoes rapidly. It is well to buy inexpensive ones to last until they are too small and are replaced with the next larger size. If expensive shoes are bought, the mother is tempted to have them used until they are worn out. In so doing she is likely to force the child's feet into shoes too small for him. He is then not only uncomfortable, but also in danger of having the shape of his feet distorted by the pressure of tight shoes.

Fresh Air, Sunshine and Exercise

Toddlers are active, curious and fond of outdoor play. Although the child of eighteen months to two years may be suspicious of strangers, as long as he is with his mother he likes to watch other children play. He enjoys parallel play, but is not yet ready for cooperative play. As he approaches his third birthday he has matured to the stage at which he makes motions of friendliness to other toddlers and some attempt to join in cooperative play. He welcomes a sunshiny day when he may play outdoors, making mud pies, digging in the sand pile or, on a hot day, splashing in water. In winter he likes to play in the snow for a while, but cannot manipulate it as he can mud and sand.

Toddlers need freedom to play where they can wander without danger of being harmed. An adult should be near, however, for it is impossible to foresee what a child is likely to do. Although he wants to run about freely and does not want anyone to be constantly saying "No, no," he feels more secure when he knows that an adult is with him.

Sleep

The amount of sleep the toddler needs depends upon his age, health, emotional tension, activity during the day and depth of sleep. From one to three years the amount of sleep needed gradually decreases. The child may resist sleep for some time after being put to bed, crying for his mother or demanding a drink of water or some other form of attention—anything so that he may have company.

At two years the toddler is likely to have a set ritual which he insists on following when he goes to bed. From $1\frac{1}{2}$ to three or four years he likes to take a favorite toy to bed with him. Since this helps him to relax, he should be allowed to have the toy. As he grows older he will voluntarily give up the habit. Other methods to relieve his tension before going to sleep are headrolling, singing or talking to himself. He should not be restrained or told to be still, for that only increases his tension and delays his going to sleep. The typical child will outgrow these habits by the time he is three years old or shortly after, but may resume them when he is under a strain and anxious, as when he is in the hospital.

Toddlers sleep, on the average, twelve to fourteen hours out of the twenty-four, including a daytime nap of one to two hours. Naps may become a source of rebellion in the two-year-old. Few mothers escape the naptime battles, and mothers should not place too much importance on a child's refusal to go to sleep. His outer clothing should be removed, he should be given a drink of water and taken to the toilet, and then he should be placed comfortably in bed. The shades should be drawn and the room door closed. He may have one toy in bed with him, but a variety of toys tends to keep him awake, for he handles first one and then another. A cuddly toy is the best kind to take to bed. The mother should be firm in keeping to the daily scheduled time for his nap even if he does not sleep.

Dreams and nightmares or night terrors are common, beginning in a mild form at two to three years of age.

Safety Measures

Importance of Accident Prevention. Prevention of accidents is an important aspect of the care of children of all ages. Accidents are the principal cause of death among toddlers and account for many permanent handicaps and disfiguring scars. The majority of accidents occur in or near the home. In approximate order of frequency are deaths due to motor vehicles, burns, drowning, miscellaneous causes, falls and poisons.

Although there has been some advance in the prevention of accidents in early childhood, their incidence has not been reduced as rapidly as has that of serious illnesses which formerly were the main causes of death or permanent disability.

The interests of boys and girls of any age lead them into hazardous situations. When we know the hazards, we are better able to protect the children. Children should be taught what is safe and unsafe for them to do and, until they are old enough to use good judgment, should be under adult supervision.

Nurses as well as physicians must help parents to understand this approach to accident prevention. Then the parents will be able to judge more accurately how much freedom each child should be allowed as he gradually takes over more and more responsibility for his own safety. This applies to the kind of toys given him and to his experimentation in climbing, opening and shutting doors—including slamming the door of the family car—and running ahead of his mother or lingering behind her on the street. If he hurts himself, while sympathizing with him she should point out in terms he can understand the reason why he hurt himself—give him his first lesson in cause and effect of activities which are dangerous for him and cause him pain. In this way his knowledge of what he can safely do will be increased.

Nurses must assume the responsibility of teaching parents and children the importance of accident prevention whenever they meet them, such as in the Child Health Conference and in the hospital unit or clinic. The most effective way for children to learn is through carefully safeguarded, graded experiences in self-protection. There should be a reciprocal relation between protection of the child and the education appropriate to his stage of maturation.

Specific Hazards of Toddler Years. Toddlers naturally fall frequently. In general they sit down suddenly or fall flat without hurting themselves, but if they fall down steps or from some height, they may injure themselves severely. They also tug at the end of table covers and pull objects such as cups of hot coffee over on themselves because they cannot see the top of the table. The modern formica-topped table for the family meals is far safer and more convenient to use than the polished wooden dining table covered with a table cloth.

To satisfy a child's curiosity about what is on top of a table and what mother is doing there, he may be lifted up or placed beside her in his high chair. The average child of two years is tall enough to see over the table edge if he stands on tiptoes, holding on to the table, but this is an uncomfortable position and does not give a complete view of what is there. Also he is so unsteady that if he reaches for something, he is likely to sit down suddenly. This is frustrating and may produce a temper tantrum or tears.

The two-year-old's curiosity leads him into danger. When exploring objects, children poke and probe with their fingers, which may be hurt in one way or another. They may be involved in motor vehicle accidents, may be burned or drowned, may fall from a height, may ingest poison, or may be trapped in an empty refrigerator.

Specific Safety Measures: Shared Parent-Nurse Learning. Safety measures should be designed to prevent accidents which are likely to occur in the daily life of the child. The nurse should help the mother with her individual problems of accident prevention. Both the mother and the nurse will find it helpful to keep in mind the common sources of accidents among toddlers and the preventive measures which can be taken for their safety.

MOTOR VEHICLE ACCIDENTS. Little children are taught to cross the street holding an adult's hand. Their attention is directed to the custom of crossing at the corner rather than in the middle of the block. If there are traffic lights, they are taught that green means "Go" and red means "Stop." They are too immature to gauge the speed of an oncoming automobile with reference to the time it takes them to cross the street, but they will slowly learn while crossing with adults who do not hurry them while a light is changing.

Toddlers should be supervised to some extent at all times, but especially when playing outdoors on a kiddie car, tricycle or sled to prevent their darting into the street between parked cars or coasting down a driveway into street traffic. Parents should be careful when backing a car into or out of the garage, for it is difficult to see a small child directly behind the car.

The incidence of children injured while riding with their parents is increasing as more family cars are on the road. Children share the adult's danger from collision or overturning of the car. A seat belt should be installed for the toddler so that he is not thrown from the seat if the car stops suddenly or is involved in an accident (see

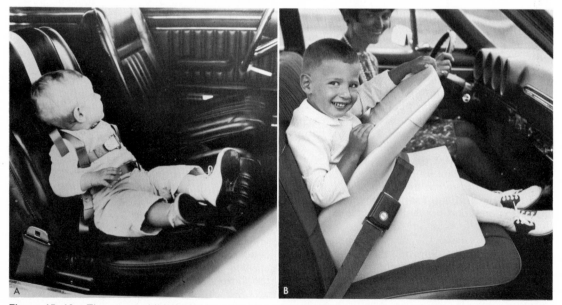

Figure 15–13.   The young child should be protected when riding in a car. *A,* The "safety seat belt" should fit properly around his shoulders and abdomen. (Courtesy of Creative Playthings, Inc., Princeton, New Jersey.) *B,* Tot Guard, a removable shield which helps protect children in collision impacts from any direction. The shield surrounds the child's body and legs without actually restraining him. (Public Relations, Ford Motor Company.)

Fig. 15-13). When a child stands upon the seat beside the driver, a sudden stop is likely to throw him forward. Modern door catches prevent falls from an open door of a moving car.

BURNS. Matches should be kept away from young children, even though few of them in this age group can strike a safety match. Little children should be watched closely in the kitchen so that they do not touch or fall against a hot stove or investigate the top with its fascinating open flames and pots and pans. Pans with handles extending from side to side or toward the back of the stove are less likely to attract the toddler's attention and are harder for him to reach than pans with handles extending to the front of the stove. Hot radiators are a source of minor burns, particularly if the child falls against one. Modern recessed radiators protected by a built-in screen eliminate this danger. Toddlers are interested in electrical outlets and are likely to poke a pin or other bit of metal into them (see Fig. 15-14, *A*). Safety plugs may be used to prevent this.

DROWNING. Children like to play in water, but if they fall they may be unable to get out of even a shallow pool; if they fall into a swimming pool, they are completely helpless (see Fig. 15-14, *B*). There is also danger of their drowning in the home. Children should not be left alone in the bathroom after the water for the bath has been drawn. The bathtub is slippery, and in climbing over the side the child may fall into the water. Should he hit his head or fall into very hot water, he might collapse and drown before his mother returns to bathe him. The old-fashioned washtub is seldom used except in rural areas. Serious accidents have occurred when such a tub was filled with hot water and the child's mother went for a pail of cold water. The child investigated the tub in her absence. If he fell in, he was burned even if he was rescued before drowning. Pails of hot water used for mopping floors are also a danger to small children.

FALLS. Children like to climb (see Fig. 15-14, *C*). Until their muscular coordination and judgment have developed to the stage at which they can climb with safety, special equipment should be provided (e.g. small wooden crates), and all climbing should be under adult supervision.

Children like to look out of windows, but are so short that they often climb on a chair to see what is going on outside. While standing on a chair or a sill they are likely to lose their balance and fall head foremost. Hence all windows should have screens.

Falls on stairs are dangerous. In institutions for children, gates should be placed at the top and bottom of stairways. The modern ranch type of house or one-floor home has obviated the hazard of falls on stairs. If the house has a basement, the door leading to the stairs should be locked.

A child who fell down the basement stairs and was too stunned to cry might lie at the bottom for some time before being discovered.

Falls from open porches were formerly a common source of injury to small children. In modern buildings, however, especially in urban housing developments, porches are likely to be screened and so present no danger.

The side gate of a crib should be kept up at all times and fastened securely so that it will not go down if the child leans against its top.

POISONING. The incidence of poisoning in children is greatest between the ages of one and four years. Children are curious about the taste of substances and often ingest poisonous liquids, powders and even solids which they find in the house. The main source of danger to the little child is the household supply of washing powders and detergents, charcoal lighter fluids and similar products, and substances for cleaning sinks, toilets, and the like (see Fig. 15-14, *D*).

Medicines beneficial in small amounts are often poisonous when taken in larger quantities. If a medicine has little or no taste or if the unpleasant flavor has been camouflaged with some sweet syrup or sugar coating, the child may finish the bottle. All harmful substances should be kept out of the toddler's reach, and common household poisons and medicines should be kept in locked storage places or on high shelves inaccessible to children. Harmful substances should never be kept in containers intended for food (see Fig. 15-14, *E*).

Mothers should be taught what to do if a child does take any of these harmful substances. She should telephone the physician or clinic at once or, if she lives close to a hospital, take the child to the receiving ward. If she cannot get medical attention for the child and she lives in a city having a Poison Control Center, she should telephone there for advice. If she knows what substance the child took and the approximate amount, she should give this information clearly and concisely. If the child has taken the contents of a bottle or can whose ingredients are listed, she should give this information. The Center will tell her the emergency treatment and may furnish emergency transportation for the child to the hospital. In most cities the police car is always available. The container from which the poison was taken should be given to the physician who treats the child. If the child vomits spontaneously or after being given an emergency emetic, the vomitus should be examined chemically. This is particularly important if the mother does not know what the child has taken or the ingredients of some commercial product which she knows the child has swallowed.

In some cities the public health nurse is responsible for visiting the home after the child's

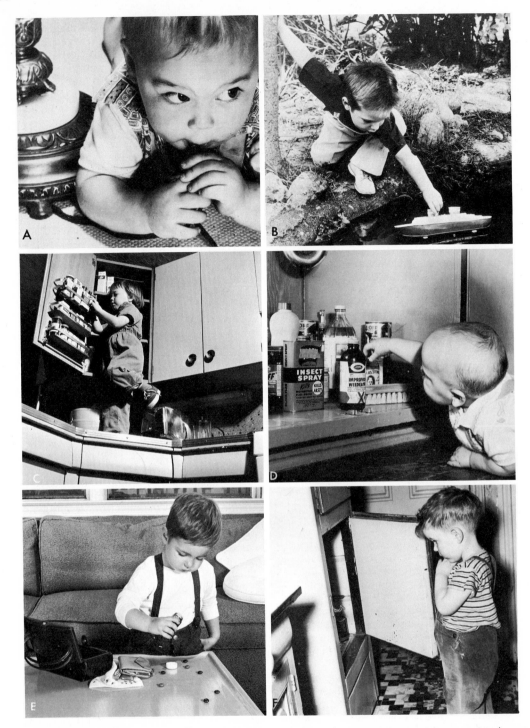

Figure 15–14. The toddler's curiosity may lead him into danger. *A,* Electrical outlets and worn extension cords can be as deadly as the electric chair itself. Plug outlets and keep cords repaired. (Courtesy of the Prudential Insurance Company of America and O. E. Byrd: *Health,* 4th edition.) *B,* A fence around his yard will keep the child from wandering near a pool or fish pond. Teach children to swim early. (Courtesy of the Prudential Insurance Company of America and O. E. Byrd: *Health,* 4th edition.) *C,* The toddler may climb to high places and possibly fall. (H. Armstrong Roberts.) *D,* He may taste or swallow anything he finds in this cabinet containing cleaning products and insecticides. (Photograph by Peter Knowlden, Stanford Medical Center; from O. E. Byrd: *Health,* 4th edition.) *E,* Medications must be kept out of the child's reach. (Courtesy of the Metropolitan Life Insurance Company.) *F,* Doors should be removed from refrigerators when not in use so that small children cannot lock themselves inside. (H. Armstrong Roberts.)

return from the hospital. She helps the parents to correct the situation which led to the accident and gives them a better understanding of the child's level of growth and development so that further accidents may be prevented.

Refrigerator Entrapment

A refrigerator which stands empty and has a door which closes tightly is a menace to any child in the vicinity (see Fig. 15-14, *F*). A refrigerator unit is meant to be airtight to prevent spoilage of food. If a toddler crawls into a refrigerator and the door closes, he may suffocate before he is released. Measures to prevent this accident include completely removing the doors, having the refrigerator destroyed, placing the unit so that the door stands against a wall, or locking the door with a padlock or by other means.

Health Supervision

Visits to the physician or the Child Health Conference, at intervals suggested by the physician, are important during the toddler period. During the second year these visits may be scheduled every two to four months and thereafter twice a year for continued health supervision. During these years, defects may be determined in an early stage. If they yield readily to treatment, they may be prevented from developing into serious handicaps. The physician also records growth progress and gives advice about safety measures, nutrition, the establishment of desirable habits and the prevention or correction of objectionable habits in the child. He will give immunizations to continue the program against the diseases discussed in Chapter 12 (see p. 278).

The toddler period is one in which the physician can establish and develop a rapport with the child that will be valuable when the child is sick, particularly if he must be hospitalized.

Dental care and supervision of daily mouth hygiene are important after the child has his full set of temporary teeth, i.e. by about two to $2\frac{1}{2}$ years. Visits to the dentist should be made about every four to six months. The modern dentist, like the physician, builds up a rapport with the child which is valuable later on when painful dental work must be done. Cleaning the child's teeth, applying a fluoride preparation (see p. 270) and work on superficial cavities in the temporary teeth are seldom painful. The dentist should have a kindly approach to children, explain procedures to them and allow them to handle his instruments.

NUTRITION

Nutrition is important in the maintenance of the toddler's health and normal growth and development. Diets for young children should include the essential nutrients in the amounts necessary for maintenance, replacement and increase of tissue and for energy.

Food should be offered in three well spaced meals. The child may also have nutritious snacks between meals if he is very active. He will be ready to eat the well balanced, varied, yet simple diet offered him at meals if he is not too irritable from intense hunger.

Influence of Growth and Development on Eating Behavior. During his second year of life the child needs less food than during infancy, because he is no longer growing so rapidly. He also has greater interest in the social and physical environment. Many children at this age have anorexia. The mother should remember that the child needs less food per unit of body weight and that this is the primary reason for his anorexia (*physiologic anorexia*). He may have developed food preferences through imitation of his parents or siblings. He may even refuse food for a short time. Food should not be forced upon him. Unless he has some organic disease, serious feeding problems will develop only because adults have tried to impose upon him their

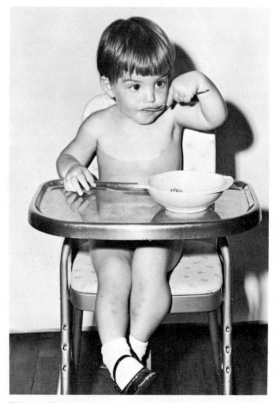

Figure 15–15. A 2-year-old child can put a spoon into her mouth without spilling its contents. She can feed herself most foods fairly well, provided she has had earlier experience in doing this.

ideas of what and how much he must eat. If food is forced upon him when he refuses his meals, he is likely to rebel, and a feeding problem will develop.

Children should be allowed a reasonable freedom in both the amount and the kind of food they wish to eat. Strong likes and dislikes should be respected. The child who dislikes essential food substances should be gradually taught to eat them, or they may be included in the diet in some disguised form, e.g. putting mashed carrots in mashed potatoes. The child may take additional milk if it is used in custards.

At times the toddler may be demanding not only in what he wants to eat, but also in the dishes he uses and the way his food is served. His behavior may be bizarre. He enjoys feeding himself even though he may be slow and clumsy. The mother should be flexible and humor him when the matter is not too essential, since this makes him feel important and reinforces good mother-child relations.

Many children are negativistic at this age, especially in eating. A toddler may test his parents to see how far they will let him have his way. Limits to his behavior must be set. He feels uncomfortable and often fearful if he is allowed to attempt anything his fancy suggests. A child may refuse his food only to be hungry soon after the meal is over. He may feel sick after eating too much or too rapidly. What an affectionate mother asks her child to do is likely to be what makes him feel good physically and emotionally.

Activity influences a child's appetite. A reasonable amount of running about increases his appetite, but if his curious searching of the environment is continued too long, he becomes overfatigued. A rest period before meals serves to lessen fatigue and his resistance to adult suggestion. Furthermore, mealtime may appear to him as an interruption of his play, and so, even though he is hungry, he may resist being called to the table. His mother must determine what is best for him by experimenting with a schedule of meals, snacks, naps and indoor and outdoor play.

The toddler has such a short attention span that he appears to be even more restless than his biologic need for activity demands. He may wander away from the table before he has finished eating. Forcing him to remain in his place may precipitate a temper tantrum. Often his newly discovered interests may be used to bring him back to the table. If he has gone to get his teddy bear, his mother may say, "Here, let's make a place for Teddy at the table."

The toddler is ritualistic in his eating habits; he may have strong preferences for certain utensils and dishes. He may insist on eating foods in certain sequences. Adults should not impose their own eating habits upon the child, whose ritualistic behavior is a normal part of development at this age. His ritual will tend to coincide with family habits if he is made to feel that he is one of the group and not a baby set apart from the group. There are many reasons why a toddler in his third year should eat with his parents and siblings; he is much less likely to acquire eating whims and fancies if they have none than if he eats alone.

Handedness becomes evident during this period. The child should be permitted to use either hand in feeding himself. The spoon should be placed in front of him so that he can pick it up with the favored hand.

It is well to give a variety of foods so that the child learns to like various tastes. It may be difficult during the toddler period to add new foods because the child is likely to have become discriminating in his tastes and detects and appraises new consistencies and flavors in the foods offered him.

Development of Eating Skills. Children differ in their ability and willingness to feed themselves, but the following represents the typical advances in skill.

12–15 months—Drinks from a cup which he himself holds
15–18 months—Holds his own spoon. The mother should spread newspaper on the floor, and he should wear a coverall bib. Help should not be forced upon him, but should be offered if he needs it. The dishes should be unbreakable
24 months—Feeds himself fairly well, provided he has had the requisite early experience in helping his mother feed him. The mother should not make the mistake of feeding him in order that he may not spill his food

Dietary Allowances. Table 15-2 gives the recommended daily dietary allowances for children between one and three years of age.

Specific Suggestions for Feeding. By the time the child is eighteen months to two years old he should be eating table food and three meals a day. Nurses and mothers should remember the following helpful points.

1. Serve food in small portions. The child likes plain food and eats one food at a time.
2. Chop or cut the food into small pieces.
3. The diet for each day should include the following (the particular diet may depend upon the cultural preferences of the family):
   a. Meat or fish, one serving; one egg daily, or cheese
   b. Liver, one or more servings a week
   c. Green and yellow vegetables, two or more servings a day
   d. Citrus fruit, raw or cooked fruit, two or more servings a day (one could be in citrus or tomato juice)
   e. Cereal and bread, enough to meet his caloric needs

Table 15–2. *Recommended Daily Dietary Allowances for Children
1 to 3 Years of Age*

	1–2 YEARS WT. – 12 KG. (26 POUNDS) HT. –81 CM. (32 INCHES)	2–3 YEARS WT. –14 KG. (31 POUNDS) HT. –91 CM. (36 INCHES)
K calories	1,100	1,250
Protein	25 gm.	25 gm.
Fat-soluble vitamins		
Vitamin A activity	2,000 I.U.	2,000 I.U.
Vitamin D	400 I.U.	400 I.U.
Vitamin E activity	10 I.U.	10 I.U.
Water-soluble vitamins		
Ascorbic Acid	40 mg.	40 mg.
Folacin[a]	0.1 mg.	0.2 mg.
Niacin equivalents[b]	8 mg.	8 mg.
Riboflavin	0.6 mg.	0.7 mg.
Thiamine	0.6 mg.	0.6 mg.
Vitamin B_6	0.5 mg.	0.6 mg.
Vitamin B_{12}	2.0 μg	2.5 μg
Minerals		
Calcium	0.7 gm.	0.8 gm.
Phosphorus	0.7 gm.	0.8 gm.
Iodine	55 μg	60 μg
Iron	15 mg.	15 mg.
Magnesium	100 mg.	150 mg.

[a] The folacin allowances refer to dietary sources as determined by *Lactobacillus casei* assay. Pure forms of folacin may be effective in doses less than ¼ of the RDA.

[b] Niacin equivalents include dietary sources of the vitamin itself plus 1 mg. equivalent for each 60 mg. of dietary tryptophan.

From the Food and Nutrition Board, National Academy of Sciences–National Research Council: Recommended Daily Dietary Allowances (1968).

   f. Butter or margarine
   g. Milk – maximum of 1 quart, part of which may be used in cooking or on cereals
4. Satisfy the child's appetite with nutritious foods and avoid offering him candy, cake, ice cream, and the like. Nutritious snacks may be given between meals.
5. Give vitamins as suggested by the physician.
6. Since the child is growing less rapidly, he may eat less than he did at the end of the first year. Do not force him to eat.

Foods to Avoid. The small child does not miss what he has never had and does not need. Foods to be avoided include chocolate, sugar, large amounts of fat (this is difficult to digest), nuts and seeds (there is danger of inadequate chewing and also of aspiration into the lungs), foods which are highly seasoned and stimulants such as tea and coffee.

Importance of Good Eating Habits. During the toddler and preschool years eating habits and attitudes toward foods are developed which tend to persist through life. Meals should be served at regular intervals and in a physical and social situation in which the child feels secure. He should have three or four simple meals a day. Some children with small appetites may need a midmorning, midafternoon or evening snack. Snacks should not be given at a time or in an amount which will interfere with normal appetite at mealtime.

Toward the end of the toddler period most children eat with the family. If his siblings and parents have good or poor eating habits, a toddler will imitate them. Parents who have not already experienced this difficulty with the older children must be told of this problem. They should be advised how to handle problems which may arise and be reminded that the basic factor in forming good eating habits is that eating time be made a happy time. Toddlers are too young to learn good table manners. Eating is an enjoyable experience. Mealtime is a family gathering to share this important and pleasurable activity.

SEPARATION

Meaning of Separation to the Toddler. The toddler, although his security depends upon both parents, is much closer to his mother than to any other adult or to his siblings. He knows his mother as a very special person. His need for her love is as great as his need for food. His attachment to her is possessive and selfish. She can, he believes, protect him from all harm. His parents, especially his mother, make the toddler's world secure and stable.

By the end of his first year the child realizes that it is his mother who gives him love, protects him from harm and provides pleasurable experiences for him. He believes that he cannot survive without her. Because of this feeling he

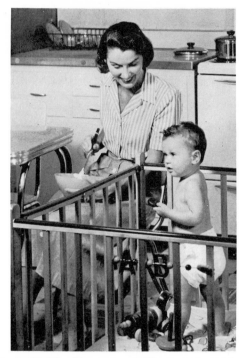

Figure 15–16. The young toddler is protected from harm while mother cooks. (Courtesy of the Metropolitan Life Insurance Company.)

is fearful when she is out of his sight. The infantile game of peek-a-boo is one way by which the child can master his fear of separation from his mother. Since he can bring her back easily, he finds that he can master his separation anxiety more easily. He discovers later, in the game of hide-and-seek, that his mother will search to find him. In these ways he gradually learns that he can bring his mother back to him through his own activity.

We know from his behavior that a child needs his mother, almost an ever-present companion, until about his third birthday. During the toddler period he gains increasing mastery over his fear of separation, and he learns to share his mother with others.

Reasons for Separation. The young child cannot understand why he should ever be separated from his mother. As he matures, however, he becomes increasingly aware that there are others (siblings) whom his mother also loves. He may become resentful of them, and yet his mother expects them to love him and him to love them. At this stage the toddler must be helped to accept his siblings, but he must be shown that he is loved even if he has hostile feelings toward them. He must have all his needs fulfilled, because this means love. Since his mother expects the toddler, who is secure in her love for him, to be like his siblings, he learns one of the first lessons in socialization: to like to be with other people. In this way he gradually matures socially as well as physically. He wins his mother's approval and strengthens her love for him.

As he matures, his mother may work away from home, may continue her studies, and may not be with him constantly. She may become ill or go to a hospital for delivery of another child. The toddler himself may become sick or be injured and be placed in the children's unit of a hospital. His specific response to hospitalization will be discussed in the next chapter.

TEACHING AIDS AND OTHER INFORMATION*

American Academy of Pediatrics

Obedience Means Safety for Your Child.
Seat Belts in the Prevention of Automobile Injuries.

Child Study Association of America

Auerbach, A. B.: How to Give Your Child a Good Start.
Auerbach, A. B.: The Why and How of Discipline.
Auerbach, A. B.: Understanding Children's Fears.

Public Affairs Pamphlets

Baruch, D.: How to Discipline Your Children. Reprinted 1966.
Hymes, J. L.: Enjoy Your Child—Ages 1, 2, 3. Reprinted 1966.

Ross Laboratories

Developing Self-esteem.
Developing Toilet Habits.
The Phenomena of Early Development.
Your Child Becomes a Toddler.

* Complete addresses are given in the Appendix.

Your Child and Sleep Problems.
Your Children and Discipline.
Your Child's Appetite.
Your Child's Fears.

The Children's Hospital Medical Center, Boston, Mass.

Preparing a Young Child for the Doctor.

United States Department of Health, Education, and Welfare

A Healthy Personality for Your Child, 1952. (Reprinted 1963.)
Borlick, M. M.: Guide for Public Health Nurses Working with Children.
Dittmann, L.: Your Child from One to Six, 1962. (Reprinted 1966.)
Feeding Young Children, 1966.
Jelliffe, D. B., and Bennett, F. J.: Health Education of the Tropical Mother in Feeding Her Young
    Child, 1964.
Preventing Child Entrapment in Household Refrigerators, 1965.
Selecting Automobile Safety Restraints for Small Children, 1968.
Su Hijo De 1 A 3 (Your Child from 1 to 3), 1968.
The Care of Your Children's Teeth, 1966.
When It Comes to Fluoridation, 1966.
Your Child from 1 to 3, 1965.

REFERENCES

Publications

American Public Health Association: *Health Supervision of Young Children.* New York, American
    Public Health Association, 1960.
Breckenridge, M. E., and Murphy, M. N.: *Growth and Development of the Young Child.* 8th ed. Phila-
    delphia, W. B. Saunders Company, 1969.
Brauer, J. C., and others: *Dentistry for Children.* 5th ed. New York, McGraw-Hill Book Company,
    Inc., 1964.
Carbonara, N. T.: *Techniques for Observing Normal Child Behavior.* Pittsburgh, University of Pitts-
    burgh Press, 1961.
Chess, S., and others: *Your Child Is a Person: A Psychological Approach to Parenthood Without
    Guilt.* New York, Viking Press, 1965.
Erikson, E. H.: *Childhood and Society.* New York, W. W. Norton and Company, 1964.
Gehman, B. H.: *Twins: Twice the Trouble, Twice the Fun.* Philadelphia, J. B. Lippincott Company,
    1965.
Gesell, A., and others: *The First Five Years of Life.* New York, Harper and Brothers, 1940.
Hurlock, E. B.: *Child Development.* 4th ed. New York, McGraw-Hill Book Company, Inc., 1964.
Hymes, J. L., Jr.: *The Child Under Six.* Englewood Cliffs, N. J., Prentice-Hall, Inc., 1966.
Janis, M. G.: *A Two-Year-Old Goes to Nursery School.* New York, National Association for the Edu-
    cation of Young Children, 1965.
Kastein, S., and Trace, B.: *The Birth of Language: The Case History of a Non-Verbal Child.* Spring-
    field, Ill., Charles C Thomas, 1966.
Landreth, C.: *Early Childhood; Behavior and Learning.* 2nd ed. New York, Alfred A. Knopf, 1967.
Levy, D. M.: *Maternal Overprotection.* New York, W. W. Norton Company, 1966.
Morley, M. E.: *The Development and Disorders of Speech in Childhood.* 2nd ed. Baltimore, Williams
    & Wilkins Company, 1965.
Recommended Dietary Allowances. Revised 1968. Washington, D.C., National Academy of Sciences–
    National Research Council.
Shuey, R., Woods, E., and Young, E.: *Learning About Children.* Philadelphia, J. B. Lippincott Com-
    pany, 1964.
Watson, E. H., and Lowrey, G. H.: *Growth and Development of Children.* 5th ed. Chicago, Yearbook
    Medical Publishers, Inc., 1967.
Watson, R. I.: *Psychology of the Child.* 2nd ed. New York, John Wiley and Sons, Inc., 1965.
Winnicott, D. W.: *The Maturational Processes and the Facilitating Environment: Studies in the
    Theory of Emotional Development.* New York, International Universities Press, 1965.
Witmer, H. L., and Kotinsky, R.: *Personality in the Making; The Fact-Finding-Report of the Mid-
    century White House Conference on Children and Youth.* New York, Harper and Brothers,
    1952.

Periodicals

Baumrind, D.: Parental Control and Parental Love. *Children,* 12:230, 1965.
Berman, D. C.: Pediatric Nurses as Mothers See Them. *Am. J. Nursing,* 66:2429, 1966.

Dark, H., and Dark, P.: Is Your Car Child-Safe? *Today's Health,* 41:14, July 1963.

Hymovich, D. P.: ABC's of Pediatric Safety. *Am. J. Nursing,* 66:1768, 1966.

Kohler, W. C., and others: Sleep Patterns in 2-Year-Old Children. *J. Pediat.,* 72:228, February 1968.

Lamar, L.: A Two-Year-Old. *Am. J. Nursing,* 66:1807, 1966.

Leavitt, S. R., Gofman, H., and Harvin, D.: A Guide to Normal Development in the Child. *Nursing Outlook,* 13:56, September 1965.

McCaffery, M. S.: An Approach to Parent Education. *Nursing Forum,* VI:77, November 1967.

Rakstis, T. J.: How Safe Are Your Child's Toys? *Today's Health,* 45:21, December 1967.

16

CONDITIONS OF TODDLERS REQUIRING IMMEDIATE OR SHORT-TERM CARE

HOSPITALIZATION OF THE TODDLER

In the mind of the toddler his parents are necessary to his very existence. When his parents take him to the hospital and leave him, therefore, he may have a distorted interpretation of the reason for the separation. He may view it as punishment for something he has done or as a complete loss of their love. The child is thus confused about what is expected of him in this strange situation, he is fearful of being hurt physically, and he may become acutely anxious if he thinks that he will not see his parents again. As a result he may revert to infantile behavior, becoming more demanding and self-centered.

The nurse must recognize the child's need to *regress*. She must help him to trust her and to accept his dependence on her while he is ill. Illness may cause the toddler, however, to mistrust adults, the negative counterpart of a sense of trust. The nurse should be aware that the child needs help if he is to trust others once again. The nurse should recognize the ways by which he learned to trust as an infant and provide loving support as he needs it to achieve again this developmental goal.

Specific Responses of the Toddler

On being hospitalized the toddler experiences basic fears: loss of love, fear of the unknown and fear of punishment. He is too young to be reasoned with; he knows only that his mother or his daddy, for whom he calls, does not respond. His distress is potentially harmful to his developing personality and may be dangerous to his physical condition. He may manifest behavior difficulties, sleep poorly, regress in toilet habits and exhibit excessive anger and grief. He may not be able to play as he did at home because of his anxiety. Such reactions have the highest incidence when the child is two or three years of age.

Adjustment to Hospitalization Without His Mother

The stages in the child's apparent adjustment to the hospital are generally as follows:

1. The child is grief-stricken. He calls for his mother almost constantly. He may reject the nurse when she gives him attention.

2. The child sinks into apparent depression.

397

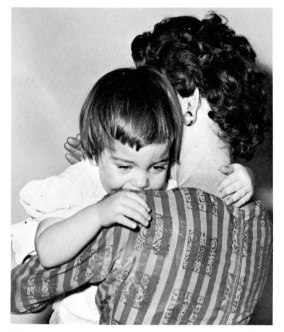

Figure 16–1. The toddler is extremely disturbed when mother says that she must leave her.

He is quieter, withdrawn and apathetic. He mourns deeply for his mother. At this point he may be greatly upset when his mother visits him, because a short visit does not satisfy his need for her.

3. If the child stays in the hospital long enough, he will eventually reach the stage in which he is no longer depressed. He takes greater interest in his surroundings and seems to be happy. At this stage he can no longer tolerate the poignancy of his distress and may repress all feeling for his mother. When she visits him, he barely notices her and does not cry when she leaves.

On discharge he may not want to go home and clings to the nurse to whom he is accustomed. At home it may be some time before the mother-child tie becomes re-established, however strong it was before his hospitalization.

If the child's stay in the hospital is prolonged, he may eventually settle down to hospital life and apparently require neither his mother nor mothering from the nurses. Such maternal deprivation may not result in severe and lasting emotional disturbances; however, some children may be severely emotionally disturbed with no deep attachment for anyone.

The toddler is likely to become a pet of the entire staff. Yet no one has the time or sufficient interest in him to form the loving relation which is needed to stimulate him to learn self-control in order to please his love-object. He is not guided in the development of habits of self-control and obedience through tutelage and discipline. He is not motivated by love for anyone to do what he does not want to do at the moment.

Hospitalization of the Toddler Without the Mother

Some reasons why not all toddlers have their mothers remain with them in the hospital are as follows: (1) arrangements cannot be made for the care of other children at home; (2) some emotionally disturbed children seem to be more upset when mother is present than when they are left alone; (3) some mothers are too anxious and bewildered and are unable to provide care for their sick children; and (4) the physical setup of many pediatric units is not adequate for a visiting parent.

Visiting by the Mother. The toddler separated from his mother has great difficulty in mastering his fear of the loss of her presence. He cannot understand why the separation is necessary, nor can he understand that it is a hospital rule that his mother is not permitted to visit him at all times. Consequently he feels that his mother does not want to be with him. He becomes angry, lonely and frightened. These feelings of anger, fright or hopeless loneliness are psychologically devastating and, through the psychosomatic interaction, physiologically harmful.

When his mother does visit the child, he will express strong emotion. This is good, because then his feelings will not be suppressed, to be expressed later. If his mother understands the reasons for his strong reaction, she will not feel that it would be better if she did not come to visit him. His emotional reaction to her presence may occur on first seeing her, during the visit or when she is ready to leave. If, in spite of his anger, he clings to her and cries, she may be so distressed that she may dread visiting again. Yet at the same time she may be gratified by his evident dependency upon her. The nurse must understand and interpret to the mother the meaning of the child's behavior and, when possible, encourage her to stay with her child longer.

Unrestricted Visiting. An increasing number of hospitals are permitting unrestricted visiting. Although this arrangement is not as comforting to the child as having his mother with him continually, it is far better than restricted visiting. If unrestricted visiting is permitted, the child is able to vent his feelings of distress and anger frequently instead of suppressing them until he has returned home. Parents, in spite of the tears of their children, are often less anxious than they would be if they could see their children only at restricted intervals.

Hospital personnel often feel that unrestricted visiting hours produce confusion on the unit because of the number of parents present. This does not usually happen if parents are shown how to care for their children and if the unit routine is changed to include their services. In general, unrestricted visiting hours, including encouraging the fathers to visit in the morning before going to work, have improved relations between parents and hospital personnel.

If the mother cannot visit her child frequently, the nurse must exhibit a sympathetic understanding of his loneliness and anxiety. She must tell him that she knows that he wants his mother and wants to go home with her. She should not try to make him forget his mother. Instead she should help him to understand that the close tie with his mother is not broken, even though she is not with him. The nurse, of course, will make life in the hospital as pleasant as possible for him.

Measures to help the child feel secure in the intervals between visiting hours include permission to have a favorite toy or blanket with him, allowing him to keep a hankerchief, glove or other object belonging to his mother, and providing cards for him to send to his mother and having her send him cards, which the nurse can read to him. If it is practical, he may speak with his mother over the telephone.

When she must leave, the mother should try to be firm and truthful in telling the child that she must leave and when she will return. She should never sneak out of the unit because she is afraid that he will cry if she tells him the truth. The nurse should stay with him after visiting hours until his initial grief at her departure has passed.

If the mother cannot stay with the child or visit him frequently, he should be assigned to a small group of children whom one nurse regularly attends. She should be relieved during her time off by a nurse who is familiar with the children.

Problems in the Care of the Toddler When the Mother Is Not Present

Rotation of Personnel. Many different nurses offer the child daily care, with the result that no single one loves and cherishes him. He interests himself in material satisfactions and in superficial relations with any adult who notices him. In a situation in which various nurses must care for a toddler, it is especially important for them all to follow the nursing care plan made for him. By doing so, each nurse will know among other items of information, for instance, his favorite foods and toys, how he prefers to take his medicine, and the best approach to be used in giving him injections. Some semblance of consistency in the care of the child can thus be achieved.

Encouraging Adequate Intake. A sick toddler many times will not take the amount of fluids or food he should take to speed his recovery. Some nurses become disturbed when a toddler refuses to eat because this hurts their concepts of themselves as nurturing persons. They must remember that all behavior is caused and that if they can do something about the cause, the behavior can many times be changed. In other words, forcing the child to eat is not the solution to the problem.

A toddler may not eat or drink as much as the nurse believes he should for any of the following reasons: he is not growing as rapidly as he did during infancy and so does not need as much food; he is normally negativistic, in acute conflict between accepting dependency on others and being an independent person with a will of his own; he is reacting to the trauma of separation from his mother and of hospitalization; he may not like the kind of food served in the hospital, or he has anorexia caused by his physical illness. If the nurse is aware of these various reasons for his behavior, she can plan a possible solution to the problem. She could encourage his mother to visit more frequently, especially during mealtimes. She could relax when encouraging the child to eat. She could plan to spend more time with him to gain his trust and permit him the independence of which he is capable or let him be dependent if he wishes. She could ask the mother for a list of the child's food likes and dislikes and attempt to serve him the foods he likes. Once the child gains control of himself, his appetite usually improves. The nurse must realize that a happy, healthy child will eat with little help, but an unhappy, ill child will not eat unless assisted by understanding adults.

Elimination Control or Toilet Training. The child who is separated from his mother will be hindered in the process of achieving control of both his bodily and his socially acquired actions. He may regress in his ability to maintain sphincter control and wet and soil himself. After his return home he will again feel pride in pleasing his mother by keeping himself clean and dry.

The nurse should know and record on the admission sheet the child's stage of development before his admission to the hospital. She should learn from his mother what methods of training (the equipment, words, and the frequency with which he was placed on the toilet seat or potty) were used at home so that as far as is possible the same methods can be continued in the hospital. The nurse must not be too rigid and demanding, since the child is under an emotional strain due to his feeling of abandonment by his mother. The nurse should sympathetically accept the child's inability to cooperate. He needs to learn about the bedpan and the urinal in his mother's presence. Her approval will motivate him to use the new equipment.

If a young toddler has not started toilet training, the nurse should not feel it necessary to initiate training immediately. If he has a prolonged convalescence, training may be begun when he feels stronger. In order for it to succeed, his mother and one nurse for whom the child feels affection should carry out the training process.

The nurse herself may have feelings of repugnancy toward soiling by urine and feces on the diaper and the child's clothing (possibly also a soiled bed). She should understand her feelings and gain control over them. She also needs to understand the toddler's instinctual pleasure and his feelings about his own excretory products.

The nurse should be prepared to forgive "accidents," which are bound to happen. Young children who have achieved control of urination and defecation tend to be upset when an accident occurs. The child needs acceptance. If he knows that the nurse understands and is willing to help, he will more readily cooperate as far as he is able.

Some children use soiling themselves as a means of gaining attention or getting even with the parents who left them in the hospital or as a retaliative measure against the nurses who manifest a lack of understanding of children's needs. They may refuse to ask for a bedpan or urinal and then have an "accident" before or even after it is brought to them. If the nurse censures the child because of an "accident," he may repeat the performance to gain her attention or annoy her.

The nurse must endeavor to find the reason for his soiling and should plan ways to help him to cooperate. The child who resorts to such techniques is in a state of emotional turmoil. The nurse, on whom he depends for guidance, must meet his needs and also help him to work out his problem in a more satisfactory way. She must accept his behavior and yet help him to gain love and attention in a more appropriate fashion.

Hospitalization of the Toddler with the Mother

It is a truism that the most effective way to prevent trauma to a child from hospitalization is to care for him at home when he is ill so that there will be no need for removal to the hospital. But if it is essential that he receive hospital care, every effort should be made to have his mother remain with him. This is not always possible, however, and then ways must be devised to reduce the problem of maternal deprivation.

The child and his mother are first taken to his crib. The nurse should exhibit an unhurried, friendly, sympathetic attitude. The mother should be provided with a chair and helped to relax. Although the nurse shows an affectionate interest in the child, she must not assume the role of the mother-substitute.

The admission procedure (see Chap. 4) should be carefully explained to the mother. The nurse should accept the verbalization of the mother's anxiety and provide emotional support. She should then explain how the mother can help the child in the hospital milieu.

Since the child gains many of his attitudes from his mother, she should be as calm as possible and in every way provide emotional support for him. By her cooperative attitude toward the nurse she can increase the child's faith in his nurse. The mother can explain to the child the hospital procedures and the use of equipment which is new to him. If he is not to use the potty, but rather the bedpan and the urinal, she can explain this in terms he understands. She can undress him and put on his hospital garments.

The nurse should ask the mother about her methods of dealing with the child at home so that the hospital personnel may follow them as closely as possible. If the child's condition permits, the nurse should introduce the mother and her child to other parents and children. She should further orient the mother to the physical facilities of the hospital unit so that the mother can participate conveniently in the child's care. The mother should explain to the child that she will remain with him so that he need not fear abandonment when he sees other children who have been left alone.

A collapsible bed or one of the newer chair-beds can be placed in the unit for the mother. She can then be with her child day and night and provide not only the comfort of being with his mother, but also physical care under the supervision of the nurse.

Hospital personnel do not always realize the advantages of having the mother stay with the child. They fear that she will be difficult to work with. They are mistaken. The more her maternal feelings are satisfied through providing care for the child (feeding and bathing him), the less anxious she will be. She will help her child to stay on a diet if she understands that one is necessary instead of feeding him candy to compensate for lack of mothering. If his physical condition permits, the mother may continue his toilet training during the hospital stay.

The nurse in a unit where mothers give care to their children must determine how much each mother can be trusted to do for her child and how much guidance she will require. Mothers are generally able to give routine care, but the nurse should instruct them in new skills or in any adaptation of methods which the child's condition makes necessary. A mother should never be urged to attempt procedures she does not feel equal to, for she, like the child, is under a heavy strain which may make her less capable than she is at home. Most mothers will help their children through these difficult experiences if they feel that they themselves have the support of the physicians and nurses. There are times, however, when it would be unwise to permit the mother to be with the child, for if she is unable to control herself, the effect upon the child would be disastrous. Whether she stays or not depends upon the situation and upon her reaction and that of the physician and the nurse.

When the mother stays with the toddler, her place at home will have to be filled by the father or the older children in the family. Friends and relatives may help keep the home functioning smoothly. If the child is hospitalized for a prolonged period, however, the mother should be encouraged to leave the child's room periodically for meals and to spend some time at home with other members of her family. She needs some time for herself in order to gain the strength needed to face her child's illness.

Summary of the Nurse's Role in the Care of the Toddler

Although the role of the nurse in the care of the ill child was discussed in general in Chapter 4, significant points in relation to the support of the mother and the toddler will be reviewed here.

The experience of hospitalization does not have to retard the progress of the toddler toward emotional maturity if the nurse helps the child integrate the experience of illness and thus increase his ability to adapt to new situations and strengthen the bond between mother and child. The nurse should be a friend who provides emotional support to the patient and his parents. Emotional support will not be accepted if the nurse is not liked, respected and significant to the family members.

Emotional support refers to those aspects of nursing care which help the person's ego to function in an increasingly effective manner. One of the important functions of the ego is to select and carry out a sequence of behavior which will solve a problem faced by the individual so that he will be able to adapt to the situation. In order for the nurse to provide emotional support to both parent and child she must be aware of their feelings and be ready to respond to them. She must recognize the fact that illness creates stress to which the body reacts in an effort to regain homeostatic balance. She must help to reduce this stress and anxiety by sharing their concerns, showing interest in their problems, and assisting them to adapt to the situation. The nurse must accept the anxiety of the parents and child as appropriate, even though it may cause behavior which seems inappropriate. Any behavior is understood if it is viewed as helping the individual maintain a state of equilibrium.

The manner in which a nurse provides support to the parents has been discussed previously. The way in which she can best provide support to a child is to relieve in a loving way any physical pain or emotional distress he may have. It is not enough for her only to say that she will care for him. She must give the toddler physical care as she did to the infant, but she must also assist the child to become familiar with his surroundings in the hospital, help him adjust to the routines of the unit and make them flexible if necessary to meet his needs, and prepare him for any discomfort he must face. Through her words and actions she must convey to the toddler that he will not be punished for manifestations of regression or anger which he may show, but that he will be accepted as an individual who is loved and respected.

Preparation for Hospitalization

Preparation for hospitalization is minimal, because children of this age cannot grasp the idea that their mothers will really leave them. Emphasis should be placed on how the mother and her child can be kept together.

ACUTE CONDITIONS IN THE TODDLER

Retropharyngeal Abscess

Etiology and Incidence. A retropharyngeal abscess is a suppurative lesion involving one or several of the retropharyngeal lymph nodes. It is generally secondary to a nasopharyngeal infection caused by bacteria or may rarely be due to a penetrating foreign body, e.g. a sliver of a chicken bone. It is most common in the first three years of life and is rare after that because of the normal atrophy of these nodes (the nodes are present in the normal newborn). The incidence even in the toddler period has decreased in recent years, owing to better medical supervision of children and more effective therapy.

Clinical Manifestations, Diagnosis and Differential Diagnosis. Abscess formation is rapid after an acute respiratory infection. The abscess makes it difficult and painful for the child to swallow, and therefore drooling of saliva is prominent. To relieve the pain and facilitate swallowing he tends to keep his mouth open. His head is retracted, and he cries when it is moved. If the lesion is in the upper portion of the pharynx, a bulging of the posterior pharyngeal wall may be visible. Respirations are noisy and are accompanied with a gurgling sound. If the swelling is excessive, obstruction to breathing may occur with stridor and possibly dyspnea. The child's temperature is variable, but tends to be high. Prostration is often severe.

The *diagnosis* is made by inspection if the abscess is in the upper part of the pharynx. Palpation generally discloses a soft midline mass. When the mass is low in the throat, it may be seen in a lateral roentgenogram. The physician may use a laryngoscope through which he can inspect the abscess.

Differential diagnosis must consider tuberculosis of the cervical vertebrae (cold abscess).

Treatment. If antibiotic therapy is started immediately, regression of the infection often occurs without abscess formation. Local heat in the form of hot compresses to the neck should be used if the child is able to cooperate. When the abscess is ready for incision, this is done by puncture; the opening is then spread apart with a hemostat. Frequent aspiration of the pharynx is performed to remove draining material. If hemorrhage occurs, owing to erosion of one of the branches of the carotid artery, ligation of the vessel may be necessary despite the danger of cerebral sequelae.

A general anesthesia is not given, for these reasons: (1) it would abolish the cough reflex, and the child might aspirate the purulent discharge; (2) it would prevent the use of the accessory muscles of respiration; and (3) the child might not be able to breathe after relaxation induced by the anesthetic and before relief of the respiratory obstruction by drainage and decompression of the abscess.

Nursing Care. Nursing care includes assisting the physician in his examination of the throat and incising the abscess, and in postoperative care. When the physician examines the throat, the child should be restrained with a mummy restraint (see p. 301). The nurse holds the child's head still with one hand on each side of his head. The child must be securely restrained so that the examination may be done gently and quickly without damage to the wall of the pharynx and with a minimum of pain and fright to the child.

During incision of the abscess the child is restrained as for examination of the throat. The nurse holds the child's head lower than his body to prevent aspiration of purulent material into the larynx.

After the incision has been made, a position suitable for drainage from the mouth must be maintained. The foot of the bed is elevated, and the child is placed on his abdomen. A pillow may be placed under his chest and abdomen so that the discharge from the abscess will drain through the mouth rather than down the throat. Restraints may be necessary if the child is restless and attempts to move from this position.

The child should be encouraged to take fluids as soon as he can swallow. He must be closely observed for symptoms of respiratory distress and hemorrhage. Frequent swallowing may be an indication of bleeding and should be reported promptly.

Prognosis. The prognosis is good if the abscess is incised as soon as the mass is fluctuant and if proper antibacterial therapy is instituted. An untreated abscess may rupture spontaneously.

Death may occur in untreated cases or in cases in which the child is not brought to a physician until death from anoxia is imminent. Death may occur suddenly because of edema of the glottis, pressure upon the larynx, rupture of the abscess into the larynx or erosion of blood vessels with severe hemorrhage. Less immediate and less frequent causes of death are pneumonia and pulmonary abscess caused by infection carried to the lungs from the draining abscess.

Acute Infections of the Larynx

Acute infection of the larynx is more frequent in toddlers than among older children and is more serious because the airway is smaller and therefore more readily obstructed.

Usually other parts of the respiratory tract besides the larynx are involved. Laryngeal obstruction produces clinical manifestations which are the same even though produced by various types of organisms. The clinical manifestations are aphonia, hoarseness, inspiratory dyspnea, stridor, and retraction of various respiratory muscle groups (intercostal, substernal, subcostal, suprasternal) on inspiration.

Diagnosis can be made by laryngoscopic and bacteriologic examinations.

Croup (Acute Spasmodic Laryngitis)

Etiology and Incidence. Croup is a mild inflammation of the larynx. The predominating clinical manifestation is a reactive spasm of the muscles of the larynx which produces a partial respiratory obstruction.

Spasmodic croup is relatively common between the ages of two and four years, but may occur in any child under five. There appears to be a familial and individual predisposition to the condition. The hyperactive and nervous child seems to be affected more often than the quiet one. Susceptible children are likely to have more than one attack, and the attacks invariably occur at night.

Cold air may precipitate an attack in susceptible children, particularly if an upper respiratory tract infection is present. Even moving the child from a warm room where he has spent the day to the cooler bedroom for the night may induce an attack of croup.

Croup has a low order of communicability,

and mothers should be told this. If they have other children close to the same age, they are likely to fear that these siblings will acquire the condition. Although children seldom, if ever, die of uncomplicated croup, because the child appears to be strangling, croup frightens parents as do few other conditions of like severity.

Clinical Manifestations and Diagnosis. *Clinical manifestations* may appear in a child who has shown no symptoms of an upper respiratory tract infection or other illness. The onset is dramatic, all the more so since it often occurs during sleep.

In a typical attack early in the night the child wakens with dyspnea and coughing. The cough is tight, the sound barking and metallic. Respirations are noisy. The cough wakes the parents, who find the child sitting up in bed, extremely frightened and struggling for breath. He may grasp at his throat because of his feeling of suffocation. With each inspiration a high-pitched rasp, or a sharp stridor, occurs. The child's face is red, and his lips and nails may be cyanotic. The alae nasi may flare with each inspiration. There may be substernal, suprasternal and supraclavicular retractions. The voice is harsh, the pulse rapid, and the child perspires freely. His temperature is seldom over 101°F. After one to three hours the severity of the spasm diminishes, and all clinical manifestations abate. Sometimes more than one attack will occur in a night, or attacks may occur on subsequent nights. The morning after an attack the child may have a loose cough. In a mild attack he may have a croupy cough, but only moderate laryngospasm and dyspnea.

The *diagnosis* is made on the basis of the history, the respiratory difficulty and lack of other clinical manifestations. The physician must differentiate croup from diphtheritic laryngitis, the laryngospasm of tetany (see p. 324) and acute streptococcal laryngitis.

Treatment. Treatment is directed toward reduction of the spasm of the laryngeal muscles. The child should be placed in an atmosphere of high humidity, for this tends to liquefy the secretions in the throat and also reduces the spasm. The physician may order an emetic such as syrup of ipecac to induce vomiting. Vomiting tends to reduce the laryngeal spasm. The dose of the emetic may be repeated once or twice if necessary. A sedative such as phenobarbital may be given after the child has vomited. Chemotherapy may be ordered if the infection is severe, but as a rule is not necessary. Only in rare cases is intubation or tracheotomy needed.

Nursing Care. The nurse carries out the treatment outlined by the physician. The provision of moist air is a primary consideration. The equipment to be used should be shown to the child, and the procedure, if he is old enough to understand, should be explained to him. The water vapor serves to liquefy secretions, and the warmth, if ordered, tends to reduce the spasm of the muscles and to relieve the inflammation of the mucous membrane of the throat. A drug such as benzoin may be added to the water, but actually it is steam vapor that is therapeutic. The child is put in a croup tent to concentrate the warm moist air about him.

THE CROUP TENT. The tent is made in the following way.

Over the upper half or two thirds of the crib (top and sides) are draped a blanket, a piece of plastic or rubber

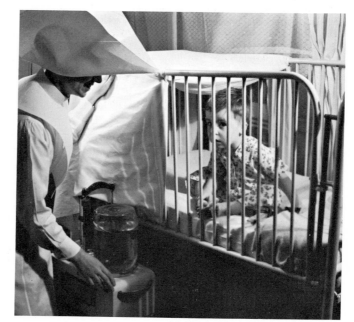

Figure 16–2. Warm moist air can be provided for the child when a vaporizer and a croup tent are used. (William M. Rittase.)

sheeting and a sheet (the blanket forms the inside layer and absorbs moisture). The sheeting is placed between the blanket and the sheet. The sheet and the blanket should be pinned neatly and firmly in place. An electric vaporizer is used to provide steam and should be large enough for an adequate and continuous flow for several hours. The spout of the vaporizer should be pointed forward inside the top of the tent. To prevent burning the child, a piece of wood or protective wire should be placed or tied to the crib rails between the spout and the child. A thermometer should be fastened to the roof of the tent on the crib rail so that the temperature within the tent can be ascertained. Unless the nurse or the mother can stay with the child, a restraining jacket may have to be applied to keep him in the tent. If the child fights the restraining jacket and thereby causes himself further respiratory embarassment, the jacket should be removed. During acute respiratory distress the mother or nurse should stay with him to comfort him and support him in a sitting position if he finds that position most comfortable.

Since the tent is not closed, most children are not frightened by it, but a toddler who is afraid may be told that it is his own little house or tent.

Points in the Use of the Croup Tent. 1. The child must be protected from burning any part of his body by a protective device (a piece of wood or wire netting) placed in front of the outlet nozzle. The nurse must check frequently to make sure that it has not slipped out of position.

2. If it is necessary to remove the child from the tent for some time, as when he is given a bedpan, urinal or the potty, or his bath or morning care, or when his condition improves and he may leave the tent, a warm blanket should be thrown around him so that he is not chilled by exposure to air at room temperature.

3. The child must be kept dry. Steam condenses on the clothing and bed covers. These should be changed when damp.

4. The covers forming the tent must be securely fastened in place so that they do not fall upon the child. Such an accident would frighten him and would impede his respiration until they were removed. They should be pinned on the outside so that he cannot reach the pins.

5. Leaving the lower half or third of the crib uncovered is important, for it permits free circulation of air and also enables the nurse or mother to watch the child without constantly sitting beside him.

6. The temperature within the tent should be checked frequently and kept below 90°F. If the temperature goes much above this, the child's body temperature will also rise.

7. The child should be kept as contented as possible. He should have his favorite toy with him. An adult should be with him as much as is practical.

The physician may order that the child be given cool moist air, rather than steam, to liquefy the secretions in the larynx. This therapy can be given in the home by the use of a cold steam vaporizer. In the hospital cool mist can be provided through the use of a Croupette, using the pressure of oxygen or, if the child does not need oxygen, compressed air. (For setting up the Croupette, see p. 291.) One reason why cool moist air is ordered rather than hot steam is that cool air may lower the child's body temperature, while the warmth of the steam-heated croup tent may raise it. Some hospitals use devices which mechanically vaporize water and fill the crib, cubicle or room with mist.

Home Modification of the Hospital Procedure. The quickest and easiest way to provide warm moist air for the child with an attack of croup is to run hot water in the bath tub or shower, take the child into the bathroom and close the door. This arrangement cannot be continued for long, however, for the steam might damage the paper or plaster on the walls, and the supply of hot water might give out. It does give emergency relief, however, while a croup tent is being prepared.

The crib may be covered as in the hospital. A plastic table cover may be substituted for the plastic sheeting. If the mother does not have a vaporizer, a kettle of hot water may be used. A gas or electric plate can be used to heat the water. Every precaution must be taken to prevent burning the child.

If the child does not sleep in a crib, a sheet or blanket may be draped over a baby carriage, or a card table or a large straight-back chair—tilted—may be placed on an adult's bed, and the child laid under the table or chair. An umbrella may be used instead of the chair, but it does not give a firm support for the tent.

OTHER POINTS IN NURSING CARE. Since syrup of ipecac causes vomiting, the nurse or mother should stay near the child until after he has vomited. He is already anxious because of his respiratory distress, and vomiting increases his anxiety. Soiling his clothing and bed with vomitus may frighten him even if he knows that he will not be blamed for the accident. After he has vomited, a sedative, usually phenobarbital, may be ordered by the physician.

When the child is resting quietly, the nurse should help the mother relieve her anxiety by expressing it in words and provide sympathetic emotional support. The nurse can explain to the mother the child's condition, why treatments and medications are given and the progress of his illness. The mother will then be less frightened if a second attack occurs on the following night.

The nurse is responsible for the administration of any chemotherapeutic agents the physician may order.

In order that the physician may have information essential to the diagnosis and treatment of the condition, the nurse must observe and record all signs and symptoms, both objective and subjective, so far as the child is able to communicate. She should also try to teach the mother the importance and meaning of these observations.

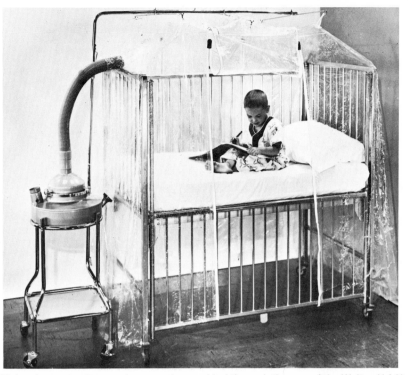

Figure 16–3.   Moist air at room temperature may be provided through the use of the Walton H A Hospital Humidifier. Since the canopy covers the crib, the child has complete freedom of movement. (Walton Lab.)

The most important symptoms to be observed during the attack are the color of the child, the rate and nature of the respirations, the degree of restlessness, the level of anxiety, the presence of cyanosis and the degree of prostration.

If the child's respiratory embarrassment increases, intubation or tracheotomy (p. 406) may be necessary. The nurse must promptly report to the physician such a change.

Prognosis and Prevention.   The *prognosis* is invariably good, although both parents and child are thoroughly frightened.

There are no specific *preventive measures,* but conditions which increase the probability of an attack of spasmodic croup in children known to be susceptible should be avoided. If there is evidence of an impending attack, such as coughing or hoarseness, particularly on the night after an attack, general preventive measures which may be taken include keeping the bedroom warm (temperature approximately 70°F.), humidifying the air of the room and giving the child subemetic doses of ipecac, and phenobarbital for sedation.

Laryngotracheobronchitis

Incidence   and   Etiology.   Laryngotracheobronchitis is an acute inflammation of the larynx, trachea and bronchi. The *incidence* is greatest during the first three or four years of life.

Several viral and bacterial agents may cause the infection. The bacteria usually responsible include *Hemophilus influenzae,* hemolytic streptococci, pneumococci and staphylococci.

Pathology, Clinical Manifestations and Diagnosis.   The *pathology* is manifested in the inflammation and edema of the mucosa and submucosa of the larynx, trachea and bronchi. A purulent exudate which produces crusts may be present. If these accumulate, they may obstruct the air passages.

Clinical manifestations may follow an acute respiratory infection, or the onset may be sudden and accompanied by prostration, elevation of temperature and severe dyspnea. During the onset respiratory difficulty is usually in the inspiratory phase, since the larynx is involved. Later there may also be expiratory difficulty because of involvement of the bronchi and bronchioles.

The child may become restless, owing to lack of oxygen. Hoarseness or aphonia may be present. The chest shows both substernal and suprasternal retractions. His color may eventually become ashen gray or cyanotic. His temperature may be as high as 104 to 105°F., and febrile convulsions (see p. 352) may occur as the result of the fever. His cough is likely to be persistent. If there is an exudate, the cough is loose, croupy and noisy, but if the exudate is too thick to move, the child may not cough at all. When obstruction due to exudate is nearly complete, breath sounds may be barely audible, and dyspnea may be severe.

The *diagnosis* is confirmed and the causative organism is found by laboratory examination of a culture of exudate. Sensitivity tests are performed to determine which antibiotic agent is most effective. The material for laboratory examination should include a direct smear and culture to rule out diphtheria. Blood cultures should also be obtained. Fluoroscopic and bronchoscopic examinations may be done to rule out the possibility of an aspirated foreign body.

Treatment. The basis of treatment of laryngotracheobronchitis is the provision of (*a*) sufficient oxygen, given whenever the accessory muscles of respiration are used for breathing, and (*b*) sufficient humidity to liquefy secretions and so to prevent crusts from forming. Either hot steam (if the child's temperature is not markedly elevated) or cool vapor may be used for this purpose. (*c*) Drugs to control the infection. Broad-spectrum antibiotics may be given; if the infection is of bacterial origin, they are effective, but if it is caused by a virus, no striking response will be observed.

During the treatment a patent airway must be maintained. When there is severe obstruction, relief must be provided by an emergency tracheotomy. *Tracheotomy* consists of an incision into the trachea. It is made in order to open up a passage for air to enter the trachea proximal to the site of laryngeal obstruction.

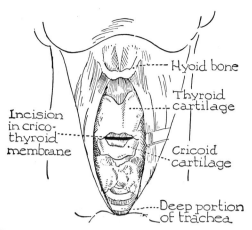

Figure 16–5. Diagram showing landmarks and horizontal incision for emergency tracheotomy. (M. G. Lynch, in Ochsner and DeBakey: *Christopher's Minor Surgery.* 8th ed.)

The incision also aids in the draining of secretions. Indications for a tracheotomy with insertion of a tracheostomy tube are restricted expansion of the lungs (this shows that only a minimal amount of air can enter the lungs), signs of cardiac failure and prostration with severe pallor or cyanosis. The incision is made just below the first tracheal ring (Fig. 16-5).

Drugs such as atropine and opiates are contraindicated because atropine tends to dry up secretions in the respiratory tract, and opiates dull the cough reflex. Digitalization is necessary if clinical signs of cardiac failure (see p. 208) appear.

Parenteral fluid therapy may be required to maintain the proper state of hydration.

Nursing Care. The nurse must observe the child who has laryngotracheobronchitis very carefully for any indication of increasing fatigue or respiratory distress. She should report the occurrence of increased restlessness, pulse rate, temperature, dyspnea or retractions to the physician immediately. She is responsible for recognizing and reporting indications of increased respiratory distress before cyanosis appears.

While the nurse is observing his physical condition she should try to make friends with the toddler so that he will accept her care more easily in case a tracheotomy becomes necessary. She should help to allay the anxiety of both parents and child caused by the distressing symptoms.

After a tracheotomy, maintenance of this artificial airway is of fundamental importance. It is also the outlet for pulmonary drainage. Accidents arise in maintenance of this airway which endanger the child's life. Most of them can be prevented by intelligent nursing care and observa-

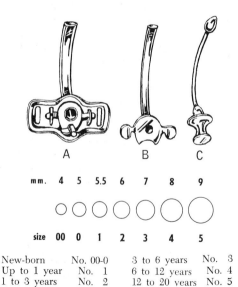

mm.	4	5	5.5	6	7	8	9

size	00	0	1	2	3	4	5

New-born	No. 00-0	3 to 6 years	No. 3
Up to 1 year	No. 1	6 to 12 years	No. 4
1 to 3 years	No. 2	12 to 20 years	No. 5

Figure 16–4. Tracheotomy set. *A,* Outer cannula. *B,* Inner cannula. *C,* Obturator. Diagram below shows sizes of tubes (with the diameters in millimeters) usually used for children of various ages.

tion of the child's condition. The nurse must be prepared to care for emergencies as they arise. Sometimes she will be able to handle the situation herself. If the physician is needed and she puts in a call for him, she will have to give emergency care until he arrives.

Since the situation is frightening, the nurse must use all possible means to reduce anxiety. Confidence in her own ability to give the child optimum nursing care is essential to inspiring confidence in him and his parents.

After a tracheotomy the nurse must provide constant care and observe and report indications of respiratory difficulty and the child's reaction to treatment. She must observe such danger signals as restlessness, extreme fatigue, dyspnea, cyanosis or pallor, fever, rapid pulse, retractions and noisy respirations. She must also watch for bleeding or indications of infection around the incision.

Control of the environment is important in preventing emergency situations from arising. Since inspired air is normally filtered, warmed and moistened in the upper respiratory tract, the environment must be such that the air the child breathes is to some extent moistened and not too cool before it enters the tracheostomy tube. The room should be warm, the temperature of the air he breathes about 80°F. (this temperature will also keep the child warm and prevent his being chilled). To moisten the air, a humidifier or croup tent is used. Oxygen may also be necessary. If continuous oxygen is not necessary, an emergency setup should be kept in readiness.

An aspirating machine with good negative pressure must be kept at the bedside.

A tray should also be kept at the bedside on which is sterile equipment for the routine care of the tracheostomy and for emergency use.

Such equipment includes duplicate tracheostomy tubes with tapes attached, two curved clamps, scissors, obturator, pipe cleaners or tonsil wire, gauze bandage, gauze dressings, a medicine dropper or syringe and needle, applicators, tongue depressors, an extra catheter (no. 8 to 10 French which has additional holes near the tip to facilitate the process of aspiration of the nasopharynx) and an open-tip catheter, preferably of the whistle tip type (this is used in tracheal aspiration, i.e. clearing the tracheal tube of secretions). In addition, there should also be a covered jar of hydrogen peroxide or other solution to cleanse the tracheostomy tube, a covered jar of physiologic saline solution and a covered jar of sterile petrolatum or petrolatum gauze. The jars should be labeled on both sides and on the lids so that the nurse cannot confuse their contents.

A few drops of sterile physiologic saline solution are inserted into the tube to incite a cough which might dislodge crusts in the lower respiratory passages and to liquefy secretions in the lower respiratory tract and so facilitate aspira-

tion of mucus. The sterile petrolatum may be used to lubricate the end of the tracheostomy tube when the physician changes it, and also to coat the area around the tube. The petrolatum may be applied with a tongue depressor.

Care of the Tracheostomy Tube and Incision   The nurse should wash her hands thoroughly before touching the tracheostomy tube and equipment. She *removes the inner cannula* and cleans it by soaking it in hydrogen peroxide or other solution and then passing the pipe cleaners or tonsil wire and gauze through the tube. She aspirates the outer cannula and tracheobronchial tree (the depth to which the nurse is permitted to aspirate the tracheobronchial tree depends on the policy adopted by the medical personnel). If the obstruction persists or if the physician has ordered it with each aspiration, a few drops of sterile saline solution may be instilled into the cannula before aspiration. To do this she uses the medicine dropper or syringe.

The aspirating catheter should be pinched so that the lumen is closed while it is inserted into the opening of the outer tube. (A glass Y tube may be used so that the vacuum can be released by fingertip control instead of by pinching the aspirating catheter.) The catheter should be slowly and gently inserted. After withdrawal for rinsing with sterile physiologic saline solution the catheter should be rotated 180 degrees between the fingers so that its normal curve will carry it down to another bronchus when aspiration is repeated. The catheter should be reinserted and aspiration continued until all drainage has been removed. The inner cannula, thoroughly cleansed, is reinserted and locked in place after the aspiration procedure has been completed.

If the nurse is unable to aspirate the tracheobronchial tree successfully, and if respiratory difficulty or noises on respiration persist, the physician should be notified so that the lower airway can be investigated.

The frequency of aspiration depends upon the need of the child. Immediately after tracheotomy, aspiration is usually performed every fifteen minutes, later every thirty minutes or every hour. The need gradually decreases with improvement in the child's condition.

If the nurse is to change the dressing around the tracheostomy tube, she cleanses the area around the tube with hydrogen peroxide and then coats the area with sterile petrolatum, using a tongue depressor. A gauze square cut to the center should be slid behind the tube and under the tapes to hold it in position.

The prevention of accidents is important in the nursing care of these children. The toddler is too young to understand the necessity of leaving the tube in place, and so his hands must be restrained. For this purpose, elbow restraints may be used. The older child who is restless and has nothing to occupy his mind may attempt to put bits of food or debris into the tube. The nurse should explain the importance of the tube to such a child. She must be certain that the inner

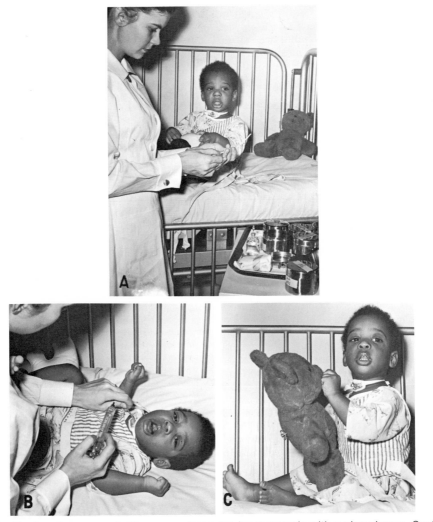

Figure 16–6. Tracheostomy care. *A,* The nurse cleans the inner cannula with a pipe cleaner. Containers are labeled on their tops and sides to prevent accidental interchange of lids. Note the favorite toy of this little boy in the corner of his crib. *B,* Aspiration is done after sterile saline solution from the syringe has been instilled into the tracheostomy tube. *C,* The toddler with his tracheostomy tube in place. After his own aspiration he enjoys aspirating his teddy bear.

cannula is securely fastened in place so that it will not fall out, and that the tapes are applied to the tube properly and securely tied so that the tube is held firmly in the correct position and that the child cannot dislodge it.

If by accident the outer cannula is removed from the trachea, the physician should insert the extra tracheostomy tube. The incision in the trachea must be held open with a hemostat by the nurse while another nurse summons the physician.

If the child stops breathing, because of some obstruction of the airway, the inner tube should be withdrawn and the outer tube thoroughly aspirated. The child should be given oxygen through the tracheal tube. If the outer tube has become dislodged, oxygen should be given through the incision. Artificial respiration may be given; the method is that ordinarily given children (see p. 182), with the fundamental difference that the nurse places her mouth to the opening in the neck rather than over the child's mouth. Other methods of artificial respiration may also be used. When the physician arrives, he will attempt to relieve the obstruction by bronchoscopic examination, if need be.

When the child no longer needs the tracheostomy tube the lumen is partially obstructed by a cork. This compels the child to breathe through his nose, but still permits entrance of supplementary air through the tube. When he can tolerate complete occlusion of the tube, a cork filling the entire opening is placed in position. If this does not cause him distress, the tube can be removed, and a sterile dressing can be placed over the incision. In *decannulation,* since the child may not be able to cough up secretions completely, there is danger of their puddling in the lungs with a subsequent rise in temperature and with restlessness. The child should be under close observation for several days.

There are few conditions in which the nurse's record of observations and the care given the child are more important than in the nursing of a child with a tracheostomy. Whenever the tube is aspirated, the time should be charted, as well as the amount, consistency and nature of the return (whether it contains blood, mucus or crusts), and whether the child breathed more easily after the aspiration. The time when the tracheostomy tube is changed should be charted, together with the child's reaction to the procedure.

Psychologic care is extremely important. The child needs his nurse constantly after a tracheotomy has been done because he is in physical danger without her, and he also needs her emotional support. He has a physical basis for his fear of being alone, and his respiration is further embarrassed when he becomes anxious and excited. In his condition he cannot cry or call for his nurse, and is in danger of respiratory obstruction. He must learn to get used to breathing through the tube, which is at first difficult. He needs the love and reassurance of both his mother and his nurse in order to maintain his sense of trust in himself and others. He is afraid, and the nurse increases his fear when she aspirates the tube, so that he feels insecure and unhappy when she is near him. When he becomes accustomed to aspiration of the tube and finds that it makes him more comfortable, he will learn to depend upon his nurse for relief as he does upon his mother for love. He may even play at aspirating his favorite toy (see Fig. 16-6, *C*). The importance of the tube can be explained to an older child, but the toddler is too young to comprehend its function until he learns from experience that he feels better after it has been cleared.

Until the toddler becomes accustomed to the tracheostomy tube, he is afraid to try to swallow. By placing small quantities of fluid or food in his mouth he will learn that swallowing will cause him little or no pain.

Excitement should be avoided, but the child should be amused with toys, or with stories if his hands are restrained and he is unable to play with toys by himself.

OTHER POINTS IN CARE OF THE CHILD. The vital signs should be taken as ordered by the physician or more frequently as indicated by the nurse's observations of the child. If the child cannot change his position, the nurse should move him frequently to prevent puddling of secretions. A semi-Fowler's position may be most comfortable for the child. It may be necessary to give mouth care if the child is not taking an adequate amount of fluid to keep his mouth moist. He should be helped to get as much rest as possible. It is desirable to give enough fluids—preferably warm fluids—orally to prevent dehydration. If he will not take the required amount, fluids should be given parenterally. His oral intake may be increased by offering small amounts of any fluid he likes at frequent intervals.

Drugs and antibiotics will be given as ordered by the physician.

The physician may discharge the child before the tracheostomy tube has been removed. In that case the mother must be taught the care of the child gradually before he leaves the hospital. He will probably be referred to a public health nurse if he is not under the care of a private physician, and his mother will be instructed to take him for periodic return visits to the outpatient department of the hospital. Not all mothers are sufficiently intelligent and resourceful to undertake the responsibility of such care, but if his mother can be taught to care for him, he is better off at home than in the hospital after he has learned to live with the tube in place and to cooperate in the care it necessitates. The mother should be taught not only the procedures she must carry out, but also what observations she should make of his condition, and what she should report to the physician. She should also be told where she can obtain the required equipment and oxygen for emergency use.

The mother must take great care when bathing the child or when he is near a wading pool with other children that he is not momentarily submerged in the water, for liquid will be drawn through the tracheostomy tube directly into his lungs, and he will drown.

Prognosis. The prognosis depends upon the age of the child, the severity of the infection, the length of illness before treatment was instituted and the kind of treatment the child receives. Death may occur from the primary infection, from a secondary pneumonia or from respiratory obstruction. Septicemia may cause death, but is an uncommon cause.

Pneumonia

Pneumonias may be classified in several ways on the following bases: anatomic distribution, causative organism, pathologic changes in tissue, and response to antimicrobial therapy. None of these methods of classification is completely satisfactory.

In any type of pneumonia the portions of the lung which are affected are not aerated because the alveoli or air spaces are filled with inflammatory exudate. Because of this fact and also because the child breathes in a shallow manner, often owing to pain on breathing, the oxygen saturation of the blood is invariably reduced.

Since there are many varieties of pneumonia and since some kinds occur principally in one or more age groups, only selected types are discussed in this text. Pneumonia of the newborn and aspiration pneumonia were discussed in Chapter 10, and interstitial pneumonitis or bronchiolitis and lipoid pneumonia in Chapter 13. Pneumonias caused by pneumococci and staphylococci are discussed here, since the nursing care of any other type is essentially the same in the toddler period.

Pneumococcal Pneumonia

Etiology, Incidence and Predisposing Factors. Pneumococcal pneumonia is a disease causing more or less consolidation of the affected areas of the lungs. It is caused by the pneumococcus organism, of which there are about eighty types. Certain types are more prevalent among different age groups.

In the past the pneumococcus was the chief cause of pneumonia in infants and young children. Recently the incidence of this type of pneumonia has decreased because of the response of most pneumococcal infections to antibiotic or sulfonamide medications, which are usually given early in the infection. Pneumococcal pneumonia is generally a primary infection. Lobar pneumonia, in which one or more lobes of the lung may be affected, is more common after the period of infancy. The disseminated type, such as bronchiolitis (see p. 290), is seen more often in infancy.

The peak *incidence* is in the late winter and early spring months. In the temperate zone, pneumonia is endemic in the general population. Although pneumonia may occur in more than one member of a family, this is seldom the case. Family members, however, may be carriers of infection. As a result of constant exposure to the infection, most persons have antibodies in their blood against many types of pneumococci.

Predisposing factors are age (the incidence of the disease is highest during the second year of life, the toddler period), and lowered resistance due to malnutrition or severe chilling of the body.

Pathology and Clinical Manifestations. Pneumococci reach the lungs by way of the respiratory passages. The first stage in the attack is termed *engorgement.* During a period of only a few hours the lung becomes dark, bluish-red and heavy. In the next stage, that of *red hepa-*

tization, the infected lobe becomes solid with red cells and fibrin, and air is displaced. In the third stage, *gray hepatization,* the pleural surface lacks luster and is dull in color. The alveoli are filled with leukocytes and fibrin. In contrast to the two previous stages, the third stage is prolonged. In the final stage, that of *resolution,* a creamy purulent material forms and is evacuated via sputum or resorption.

The typical *clinical manifestations* differ with age and are more variable in children than in adults. The onset is abrupt, although it may be preceded by a mild upper respiratory tract infection. In older children the onset is characteristically preceded by a chill, but in younger children the first symptom may be a convulsion. Symptoms referable to the nervous system are more common in children than in adults.

In the early stages the cough is dry and may cause pain. In the stage of resolution the cough is loose and productive. Fever is a characteristic of the early stage as well as of the course of the disease. The temperature rapidly reaches 103 to 104°F. and may or may not show extreme daily fluctuation. Among untreated older children the temperature drops abruptly, usually on the sixth or seventh day. This marks the crisis of the disease.

The respiratory and pulse rates are characteristic of pneumonia. The rate of respiration may be increased to 40 to 80 per minute in infants and to 30 to 50 per minute in older children. Respirations tend to be increased out of proportion to the increase in the pulse rate. They are shallow in order to reduce the pleural pain. The accessory muscles of respiration may be used, with resulting retractions. In children the alae nasi usually expand and contract with respiration.

The pulse rate is increased. The strength and rate of the pulse beat are indicative of the prognosis of the disease. If the pulse becomes weak and the rate extremely rapid or slow, the prognosis is guarded. Chest pain due to pleural involvement is felt especially on coughing or respiratory movement. The pain may be referred to the abdomen.

Gastrointestinal symptoms are common in the toddler. At the onset of the disease he may vomit or have diarrhea. Anorexia is common during the course of the disease. The older child may complain of a headache. Rigidity of the neck may be present.

Diagnosis, Differential Diagnosis and Complications. Examination of the chest is paramount in the *diagnosis* of pneumonia. The physician determines the number and extent of the pneumonic areas by the presence of rales, nature of breath sounds and evidence of consolidation. A roentgenogram is taken to corroborate the foci of consolidation found on examination and the presence of any complications such as atelectasis or empyema.

Laboratory tests may show a slight reduction in the red blood cell count and hemoglobin level and an increase in the white blood cell count—commonly from 16,000 to 40,000 per cubic millimeter. The urine has a high specific gravity, is dark amber in color and scanty in amount. There is usually an acetonuria and a mild to moderate albuminuria. The pneumococcus can usually be isolated from the nasopharyngeal and pharyngeal cultures. Bacteria may or may not be seen in the blood cultures.

Lobar pneumonia must be differentiated from atelectasis and pleural effusion and, if there is severe abdominal pain, from gastroenteritis and appendicitis. If nervous symptoms predominate, meningitis may be suspected.

A common *complication* of pneumonia is plastic pleurisy. It exists to some degree in nearly all cases. The incidence of other complications has been reduced since sulfonamides and antibiotics have been used in the treatment of pneumonia. Abdominal distention or tympanites is a serious complication; if it persists, it may be a reflection of toxic paralytic ileus. Other complications such as empyema or meningitis are extremely rare.

Treatment and Nursing Care. The child can be cared for at home if the physical environment is satisfactory and the mother or another adult in the family can nurse him. This imposes on the physician or nurse the responsibility of teaching the mother how to nurse the child.

Treatment with sulfonamide or antibiotic therapy, or both, is successful and easily carried out by the mother. When these drugs are given early in the course of the disease, administration of oxygen (difficult and dangerous for the mother to give in the home) is seldom needed. If severe complications arise, the child is hospitalized.

Much of the *nursing care* is symptomatic and geared to the needs of the individual child. He should have adequate rest, both physical and psychological. He should be disturbed as little as possible.

At the first indication of pneumonia the physician orders administration of a sulfonamide or an antibiotic, or both. Penicillin in full dosage seems to be the drug of choice. Drug therapy is important throughout the course of the disease. The antibacterial agent should be given for four or five days after the temperature has returned to normal.

An increased fluid intake is necessary to supply the body's increased demand for fluid due to the infection. Fluids should be given in sufficient quantities to maintain the normal specific gravity of the urine. This is important for excretion of toxic products and for avoidance of kidney complications when sulfonamides are given.

If the child vomits, fluids must be administered parenterally. As the child feels better, anorexia becomes less of a nursing problem. He should not be encouraged to eat more than he desires, however.

The child tends to lie on the affected side to lessen the pain. His position should be changed frequently. Although changing position causes pain at the time, it ultimately reduces his discomfort and facilitates drainage from the tracheobronchial tree.

For fever, aspirin is given, and cooling sponges (see p. 352) may be ordered. Oxygen is administered for restlessness or severe dyspnea, even though the child is not cyanotic. A Croupette or an oxygen tent may be used. If oxygen is given early, the need for analgesics and sedatives will be reduced. In severe cases aspirin and phenobarbital may be given.

Drug therapy prevents many of the complications which formerly occurred. Abdominal distention is a serious complication which still occurs in some affected children. Prophylaxis includes early antibacterial treatment of the infection, oxygen therapy before the appearance of cyanosis, and the avoidance of constipation. If distention occurs, an enema may be given and the rectal tube left in place. Prostigmin is the most effective treatment and should be given for even mild distention and repeated if the distention is not relieved.

An adequate convalescent period is essential even though the child seems well after antibacterial therapy. Before the child is permitted to return to his daily activities he should have gained the weight lost during his illness and not be fatigued by normal exercise. Complete recovery usually takes two weeks.

Prognosis and Prevention. Sulfonamides and antibiotics have dramatically changed the course of pneumococcal pneumonia and reduced the mortality from it. After therapy has been begun the temperature usually returns to normal in twenty-four hours, the child's clinical condition improves, and complications are extremely rare. With early treatment the mortality rate is usually less than 1 per cent in both infants and children.

Prevention consists in isolating the child from contact with patients with pneumonia. This is important in the children's unit of a hospital and in the home if any member of the family has pneumonia.

Staphylococcal Pneumonia

Etiology, Incidence, Clinical Manifestations, Pathology and Diagnosis. The causative organism is *Staphylococcus aureus.* Recently staphylococcal pneumonia has become the most important type of pneumonia in childhood. This is due to the emergence of a virulent strain of staphylococci resistant to the common antibiotics.

Staphylococcal infection may be acquired in the newborn nursery, in the hospital unit, in the home or in the community. It may begin as a skin infection, and the child may then become a carrier of virulent staphylococci in his nasopharynx. Later either he or another member of his family may suffer from staphylococcal pneumonia.

The onset of the disease is rapid. Multiple lesions occur in the lungs, pulmonary tissue is destroyed, and abscesses are formed. Lesions on the periphery of the lungs may erode into the pleural space and cause tension pneumothorax or empyema. Other *clinical manifestations* are similar to those of pneumococcal pneumonia.

Roentgenograms of the chest often show multiple lesions and confirm the *diagnosis*. Nasopharyngeal and sputum cultures are positive for the organism. Blood cultures are taken and may also prove positive.

Treatment and Nursing Care. Two essential points in the *treatment* of staphylococcal pneumonia are strict isolation and constant nursing care. An antibiotic effective against the strains of staphylococci found in hospitals should be given, such as methicillin, oxacillin and nafcillin among others. The antibiotic patterns of resistance and sensitivity of staphylococci vary in different areas. Sensitivity tests should be done for the particular organism involved, and drugs should be chosen accordingly.

Oxygen therapy and maintenance of the fluid and electrolyte balance are important. The nurse must observe the child for any symptom suggesting the development of tension pneumothorax, such as the abrupt onset of pain, dyspnea or cyanosis.

Prognosis. The prognosis depends on early diagnosis, the use of an appropriate antibiotic, and the lack of complications.

Intestinal Parasites

Children who have intestinal parasites have few if any symptoms. Such symptoms as picking the nose and restlessness in sleep formerly attributed to such infestations, are more likely to be due to emotional disturbances.

Several varieties of intestinal parasites infest human beings, and frequently infest toddlers. The two most common in the United States are pinworms and roundworms.

Oxyuriasis (Enterobiasis; Pinworm, Threadworm or Seatworm Infection)

Etiology. Oxyuriasis is a parasitic infection produced by the pinworm, *Enterobius vermic-*

ularis, which invades the cecum and the appendix. The worm is white and threadlike in appearance. The adult male is 2 to 5 mm. in length, the female 8 to 13 mm.

Epidemiology and Pathology. Oxyuriasis is the most common variety of parasitic infestation. It is spread by person-to-person contact. Children are especially susceptible. The condition is frequent where large groups of children are in close contact, as in an institution. The child reinfects himself by contaminating his hands when he scratches the itching skin around the anus where the eggs are lodged, or by handling soiled bedclothes, sleeping garments or contaminated objects. He then puts his fingers in his mouth, and the eggs repeat the life cycle upon maturing in the intestinal canal. The child may also become infective by breathing airborne ova. Fertile eggs stay infective for about nine days in the average environment.

In short, the route by which reinfestation is accomplished is anus to fingers to mouth or anus to clothing to fingers to mouth.

Pathologically, eggs which are swallowed hatch in the duodenum and migrate directly to the cecum and the appendix. Adult worms develop from eggs in forty-five days or less. The worms attach themselves to the mucous membrane of the cecum and the appendix by means of their "lips." Usually at night, gravid worms become detached, migrate down the bowel and crawl out onto the perianal and perineal skin, where they lay thousands of eggs and provoke itching. A few hours after deposition the eggs become infective. Gravid worms entering the vagina may cause vaginitis or a salpingitis and encapsulate in the tubules or migrate to the peritoneal cavity and encapsulate there. The worms cause a severe pruritus, and secondary infection and scarification may occur from scratching the anal area.

Infestation usually cannot go on without reintroduction of the eggs by mouth.

Clinical Manifestations. Clinical manifestations are variable. Sometimes there are no symptoms other than itching about the anus at night which causes the child to be irritable and restless. There may, however, be symptoms of acute or subacute appendicitis from appendiceal lesions caused by the worms at their sites of attachment. Bacterial infection of the skin may develop from the pruritus ani, which produces weeping, eczematous areas. Vaginitis often occurs, and little girls are frequently irritable, have a poor appetite, lose weight and suffer insomnia. These difficulties may cause a chronic emotional disturbance. Eosinophilia is present in some affected children.

Diagnosis. A conclusive diagnosis can be made if, on examination, worms are seen to emerge from the anus. The most practical and effective method of diagnosing the condition is by placing a tongue blade covered with cellophane tape, sticky side out, against the anal or perineal area, where it picks up the eggs. The sticky side of the tape is then placed downward on a slide, which can be microscopically examined at any time by allowing a drop of toluene to filter between the tape and the slide. A tape made especially for this purpose may be used instead of cellophane tape. Anal swabbing is best done in the early morning before arising or just before dressing, bathing or defecation. Eggs are not found readily in the stool.

Treatment. The aims of treatment are to destroy the ova and the worms in the intestine and to prevent reinfection from other persons.

Gentian violet until recently was the drug of choice. Two new medications are now being used more extensively. A harmless and effective drug is piperazine citrate (Antepar), a pleasant-tasting fruit-flavored syrup. It produces no side effects when taken as directed. Pyrvinium pamoate (Povan) is an effective single-dose, nontoxic oxyuricide. It will color the stools or vomitus bright red. Since an occasional child may vomit the medication, this possibility should be mentioned to parents. Enemas may also be prescribed.

All infected persons in the household or group must be treated together. After eradication of parasites from the family or group new parasites can be acquired only from outside contacts.

Nursing Care. The nurse has an important part in the cure of children with oxyuriasis. Mothers should be warned of the danger of overdosage of anthelmintic drugs. Some mothers are so anxious to rid the child of parasites that they may give more of the medication than is ordered. The mother should learn how to give the medi-

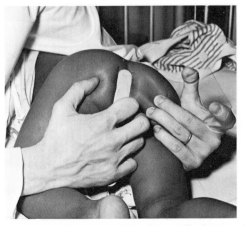

Figure 16–7. Scotch tape test is usually done early in the morning for the purpose of locating the eggs of the pinworm.

cation and to carry out any procedures ordered by the physician. If the mother does not know how to give the child an enema, she should be shown the procedure (see p. 336).

The mother needs to know how to prevent reinfestation. The child should wear mitts or socks over his hands so that he cannot pick up the eggs under his fingernails when he scratches about the anus. His nails should be cut as short as possible. Hand hygiene should be carried out carefully, especially before meals and in the morning. The child should wear a tight diaper or panties so that he will be unable to reach the infested area. The anus should be cleansed carefully with soap and water after each defecation, and a soothing ointment should be applied to allay the itching. The toilet seat should be scrubbed daily. Underclothing, bed linen, night clothing, and towels used to dry the child should be boiled to destroy the eggs which are likely to be on the cloth. In the hospital the child should be prevented from coming in contact with others. His bedpan should be cleansed and sterilized after use.

The worms may be removed from the bowel by enema, cathartics or other drugs prescribed by the physician. This phase of therapy is not often necessary.

The nurse should discuss with the mother the fact that these parasites are not necessarily a sign of uncleanliness so that the mother need not feel guilty about her child's infection.

Prognosis and Prevention. The *prognosis* is generally good.

Prevention lies in scrupulous personal and group hygiene.

Ascariasis (Roundworm Infection)

Etiology and Epidemiology. This condition is a parasitic infestation by the giant roundworm, *Ascaris lumbricoides,* found most commonly in the lumen of the small intestine. The mature worm is similar in both shape and size to a white or pink earthworm and is 6 to 15 inches in length. The circumference of the mature female worm is that of a common pencil; it is slightly less in the male.

These parasites are found in warm climates and in the temperature zones up to latitude 40 degrees north or south. The fertile egg is capable of withstanding almost all external conditions except heat. The egg is contained within the feces of an infected person. Where toilets are not used, eggs may be deposited upon the ground, in cracks between stones or on the flooring. The egg embryonates and contains a motile first-stage larva in nine days in a warm environment. A week later the larva moults, and the egg becomes infective, but does not hatch in the soil. It hatches only after having been swallowed by the infected person.

Even if toilet facilities are available, little children may defecate where they are playing rather than take the time to go to the toilet. They spread the eggs where other children are likely to be contaminated. The eggs develop in the top soil, and the children take them into their mouths on toys, contaminated fingers or food, or by eating dirt. Many children from ages one through ten years have ascariasis where these unsanitary conditions prevail. They are the main source of infestation of older children and adults.

Pathology, Clinical Manifestations and Diagnosis. In the infective stage the Ascaris is swallowed and enters the duodenum, where it hatches. The larvae penetrate the intestinal wall, mesenteric lymphatics or venules, commonly migrate to the liver and then proceed to the lungs through the right side of the heart.

The larvae invade the air sacs of the lungs by way of the pulmonary capillaries and cause the discharge of minute pools of blood at the sites. This results in an acute cellular infiltration which blocks passage of the larvae into the respiratory tree. The larvae moult a second time while in the lungs, ascend to the glottis and are swallowed, becoming established in the small intestine.

If the worms become irritated with their environment, they may proceed down the intestinal tract and be excreted, or they may migrate into the stomach and be vomited or be regurgitated through the nares. Worms may block the appendiceal lumen, perforate the intestinal wall, enter the pleural cavity, block the common bile duct or migrate to the liver and into its parenchyma.

The *clinical manifestations* are those which would be assumed from the pathology. An atypical pneumonia may occur when many larvae are in the lungs. Migrating larvae may cause an allergy; manifestations include asthma, urticaria and eosinophilia. Intestinal symptoms may not be present or may include nausea and vomiting, anorexia and loss of weight. Other symptoms are insomnia, mild fever, nervousness, irritability and physical and mental lethargy. The most frequent symptom in small children is intestinal colic. Large masses of clumped worms may cause intestinal obstruction, perforation of the intestinal wall, intussusception or paralytic ileus.

The *diagnosis* is usually made by recovery of eggs in microscopic fecal films. Occasionally the diagnosis is made by examination of the worms which have been passed in the stools, or have been vomited or have emerged from the nares.

Treatment, Prognosis and Prevention. The drug of choice is piperazine citrate (diethylene diamine), which comes in a pleasant-tasting fruit-flavored syrup (Antepar). It requires none of the auxiliary preparation which other anthelmintics require and has no side effects when given in the recommended dosages.

The *prognosis* is excellent when an appropriate anthelmintic is administered. It is good to fair when secondary complications arise, such as lobar pneumonia, intestinal obstruction or intestinal perforation.

Preventive measures are essential where the condition is common. Reinfestation occurs every three months in endemic areas. Children and adults must be provided with comfortable, clean toilets and must be taught to use them for every defecation. The infested top soil, 2 inches down, should be turned under. All infected persons must receive treatment; otherwise preventive measures are not likely to be successful.

Accidents

Although not all varieties of accidents can be discussed here, the care of children who have suffered some of the more common ones can be considered. These include the insertion of foreign objects into the nose or ears, poisoning, burns, and fracture of the femur.

Foreign Bodies in the Nose

Incidence and Types. This kind of accident usually occurs in early childhood. The infant does not appear interested in so small an orifice as his nostril, and the older child knows that he should not put anything in it. A toddler puts small objects in his nose, such as beads, pebbles, cherry stones, peas and watermelon seeds. He is likely to insert any small object if he happens to get hold of it.

Clinical Manifestations and Diagnosis. The child rarely pushes the object far into the nostril because it hurts him to do so. Inexpert attempts to remove it may push it farther in, however. If the mother does not know that the child has put something up his nose, the first symptom which calls her attention to the accident is his complaint of pain when his nose is touched, obvious obstruction to respiration, and possibly wheezing. If the object is capable of absorbing fluid, it will swell and cause discomfort soon after insertion. If the object is hard and smooth and is not capable of absorbing fluid, it may not produce symptoms for weeks or months. On the other hand, it may irritate the mucous membrane and cause swelling and obstruction. If the object has been lodged in the nostril for some time, a unilateral bloody, purulent discharge may result.

The *diagnosis* is made by examination with a speculum or nasoscope.

Treatment. Sometimes forcible blowing of the nose with the other nostril compressed may dislodge the object. If the foreign body is not easily removed, the physician should spray the nasal cavity with a local anesthetic and attempt removal under direct vision.

Foreign Bodies in the Ear

Incidence, Types and Treatment. This kind of accident usually occurs only in early childhood. The child may put any small object, hard or soft, into his ear.

If the object is visible and within easy reach and the child cooperates, it can be gently removed; otherwise it should be removed under general anesthesia.

Ear irrigation should not be done if the foreign material is organic such as a bean or pea, since the object will swell from absorption of water. A postauricular incision may have to be made in some rare cases.

A small mass of tightly packed cerumen, which is technically not a foreign body, may be removed by careful extraction with a curet or hook. If the mass is large, it should be softened with oil or detergent soap solution and removed by irrigation with warm water.

Poisoning

Poisoning is a morbid condition caused by the ingestion of a toxic substance. A multitude of toxic substances is accessible to the inquisitive, untutored or inexperienced child.

This discussion will be limited to those poisons which children take into their mouths. A child may spit a distasteful poison out, but is also likely to swallow minute particles. He may even swallow repeated mouthfuls. For our purpose we speak of poisons as any substances which, when ingested, even in relatively small amounts, by their chemical action are capable of damaging tissues and disturbing bodily functions.

Poisons may include (1) those which a child is likely to find in the medicine cabinet, such as aspirin, or oral contraceptives, sleeping pills or tranquilizers, or kitchen cabinet, such as carelessly stored insecticides or potent exterminators for insects, mice and rats; (2) those which have an immediate corrosive effect, such as lye or phenol; and (3) others in which the growth of bacteria produces toxins, as in various foodstuffs.

Food poisoning due to bacterial toxins requires the same kind of nursing care as digestive disturbances (see p. 299) and is spoken of here only in connection with teaching mothers the importance of discarding all spoiled food promptly. Bacterial poisoning from spoiled food is far more common in the low-income groups of large cities than in other social classes or in rural areas. Custards and salads do not keep well without good refrigeration and are a common source of food poisoning.

For our purpose poisons must also be divided into those which have an effect within a short time, as an overdose of sleeping pills or rat poison, and those which have a slow but cumulative effect, as chronic ingestion of small quantities of paint which contains lead.

The student should keep these divisions in mind, since each cannot be discussed separately.

Incidence, Diagnosis, Clinical Manifestations and Treatment: General Principles. In the United States poisoning accounts for many cases of accidents, and accidents are the leading cause of death among children over one year of age. Poisoning in children is always an accident due to lack of supervision of the child or to carelessness in leaving poisonous substances within his reach. Approximately 500 children under five years of age succumb annually in the United States from the ingestion of poisonous substances commonly found in the medicine chest or kitchen cabinet. Many more have permanent disabilities such as hepatic damage, esophageal stricture or damaged glomeruli. There are a few cases on record of children being given poison accidentally by mothers or nurses, but these accidents are so unusual that they need no discussion here.

More than 500 toxic substances are used in the home. These include cleaning agents, detergents, bleaches, insecticides, heavy metals, paint solvents, polishing agents, kerosene, cosmetic preparations and drugs such as aspirin, oral contraceptives, hypnotics, sedatives and tranquilizers. The Federal Food and Drug Administration requires that poisonous substances be so labeled. Some commercial preparations have the chemical composition stated on the label, but not always.

Poisoning is more frequent in boys than in girls in the age group under five years. This is probably because boys are more active and venturesome than girls. The poison which children are likely to take varies with the part of the country and with rural or urban status. There is also a class differential. In tenement areas rat and roach poisons are a leading cause of quick poisoning among toddlers. In old sections of many cities poisoning from outmoded lead paint used generations ago on walls and window frames is frequent (see p. 433).

In all cases of ingestion of rapidly acting poisons the *diagnosis* must be made promptly so that the antidote can be administered before the poison is absorbed. For this reason the mother or nurse should endeavor to give the physician a complete history of what has happened. Often, however, she does not know what the child has taken or whether, in fact, he has taken any poison at all. She may think that he has suddenly become sick and take him to the physician for treatment some time after ingestion of the poison. It is essential to know the first indications of poisoning and not make the mistake of believing the child's symptoms to be due to sickness and thereby delay treatment.

Mothers and nurses cannot know the sources, actions and therapy of all known poisons. It is important, however, to know the general principles of management, for in many cases treatment must be instituted before the child can be seen by the physician.

The first step is to identify the poison if this can be done quickly. If it is not known, immediate measures described later should be taken. The mother may see the container from which the child took the poison, or others may give the information. The physician needs this information when he institutes treatment. If the child vomits spontaneously or if the mother has made him vomit causing him to gag (see below), the vomitus should be saved for the physician's inspection. If the child voids, the urine should also be kept for examination. The physician, nurse or the mother may be able to identify the poison by its characteristic odor on the child's breath.

If time and facilities are available, laboratory studies should be made. Unfortunately the immediate treatment (induction of emesis or administration of gastric lavage by the physician or nurse) does not always remove all traces of poison from the stomach before a certain amount has been absorbed into the system. It is advisable to give a specific antidote if one is available. Spectroscopic examination of the blood will show the presence or absence of methemoglobin, sulfhemoglobin and carboxyhemoglobin. The photoelectric colorimeter is used to reveal traces of lead, thymol and many other toxic substances. Later, x-ray studies of the bones can be made to show evidence of lead and bismuth poisoning.

The clinical manifestations and treatment of the different poisons may be found in handbooks on the subject or obtained from the Poison Control Center.

Common clinical *symptoms* of poisoning include (1) gastrointestinal disturbances: (a) abdominal pain, (b) vomiting, (c) anorexia, (d) diarrhea; (2) respiratory and circulatory symptoms: (a) shock, (b) collapse, (c) unexplained cyanosis; (3) central nervous system manifestations: (a) sudden loss of consciousness, (b) convulsions.

These clinical manifestations in a little child are not specific and may indicate acute illness rather than poisoning. The physician must keep in mind the possibility of poisoning; this is essential because he cannot wait for time-consuming laboratory tests to confirm a diagnosis. In most cases of poisoning the effectiveness of the antidote depends upon the time elapsed between ingestion of the poison and administration of the antidote. If the physician does not know the exact nature of the poison or whether the child has actually taken poison, but wishes to rule out that possibility, he may consult the Poison Control Center.

If the poison which the child is believed to have taken is a patent preparation, the ingredients are commonly marked on the container, but if the mother has carelessly put the poison in an old glass jar, its composition may not be known to the mother or physician. The Poison Control Center can usually establish its identity and advise about treatment if there is a clue.

The general principles of *treatment* for ingested poisons may be summed up as follows:

1. Excessive manipulation of the child and overtreatment should be avoided. He should not be treated with large doses of sedatives, stimulants or antidotes. These may cause more damage than the poison itself.

2. In acute poisoning the mother or nurse should remain calm and collected so that she can institute treatment and carry out the physician's orders.

3. Prompt treatment is necessary. Time is of great importance in treatment because the amount of poison absorbed depends on the interval between ingestion of the poison and its removal.

The immediate procedure is to induce vomiting. This may be done by giving the child a glass of milk and then, while holding his head downward, placing a finger, tongue blade or handle of a spoon in his mouth, far back upon the base of the tongue, and depressing it until emesis ensues. Vomiting should be induced in all cases except those in which the child is comatose or in which the poison is a petroleum distillate or a corrosive.

After this the child should be taken immediately to a physician in a hospital or clinic. If the mother or nurse knows from what bottle or other container the child got the poison, she should take it with her for the physician's inspection. She should also take any stomach contents which the child has vomited.

If it is not possible to induce vomiting or if there is reason to believe that not all the poison has been vomited, lavage is advisable. Few mothers have the equipment or know how to lavage the child. This is therefore done by the physician or nurse and is often a lifesaving measure.

Apomorphine given subcutaneously usually causes vomiting at once, and the physician may give this instead of lavaging the child, or he may follow up the vomiting with lavage as a precaution against retention of any poison in the stomach. Apomorphine is a respiratory depressant and should not be given if the child is in a coma, if poisoning is due to a respiratory depressant or if the respirations are slow or labored.

The antidote, if one exists, is then given. The label on the container may state the antidote; if not, the Poison Control Center should be called to obtain the information. The antidote is given even if the child's stomach has been emptied by lavage, for some absorption of poison has taken place.

Symptomatic and supportive treatment for shock or metabolic disturbance is given if necessary. The physician may order oxygen therapy and parenteral administration of fluids and electrolytes. Exchange transfusions may be given in certain kinds of poisoning.

UNIVERSAL ANTIDOTE. If the poison is not known, a universal antidote may render the poison inert or prevent its absorption by changing its physical nature. Such an antidote may be made from the following common household ingredients:

Pulverized charcoal (made from burned toast)...2 parts
Magnesium oxide (milk of magnesia)...............1 part
Tannic acid (*strong* tea)................................1 part

This solution should be given as soon after ingestion of the poison as possible. The carbon will absorb phenol and strychnine; magnesium oxide neutralizes acids; and tannic acid precipitates alkaloids, certain glucosides and many metals.

SALICYLATE POISONING. Aspirin is used so commonly in homes that parents do not realize its potential danger to children. When aspirin, especially the type prepared in flavored form, is left where children can reach it, excessive ingestion may occur. Several recommendations have been made for the purpose of reducing the number of accidental poisonings involving aspirin. Recommendations that have been made include those that aspirin tablets be sold commercially in small quantities so that the child could not take a large amount at one time, that they be sold in containers having lids difficult to open, and that they not be flavored or shaped to look like candy so that they would be less appealing for the young child. Poisoning may also occur from therapeutic overdosage. Aspirin is therefore the most common drug that poisons toddlers. Poisoning may also occur from excessive use of salicylic acid powder or ointment in open, weeping skin lesions.

The clinical manifestations include hyperventilation resulting in respiratory alkalosis which leads to confusion and coma. A metabolic acidosis is also found, due to renal compensation leading to loss of base from the body. Ketosis also follows early symptoms of toxicity. Since salicylates inhibit the formation of prothrombin by the liver, purpuric manifestations

may occur. The child may have anorexia, vomiting, sweating and hyperpyrexia which lead to dehydration.

Treatment includes immediate lavage. Fluids containing electrolytes and carbohydrate should be administered intravenously in order to speed excretion of salicylates in the urine. Vitamin K should be given intramuscularly. Peritoneal dialysis, dialysis using an artificial kidney or an exchange transfusion may be used in therapy.

PETROLEUM DISTILLATE (KEROSENE) POISONING. Poisoning from petroleum distillates occurs because toddlers ingest kerosene, benzine, gasoline, naphtha or some other substance left carelessly around the home. These substances are absorbed quickly from the gastrointestinal tract. Immediate treatment is to have the child swallow quickly 1.5 ml. per kilogram of mineral oil, which reduces absorption, and then begin gastric lavage. Lavage is better than removing gastric contents by an emetic because of the danger of aspiration. The head should be lower than the hips as the gastric contents are removed. Care must be taken that aspiration of the swallowed substance does not occur. For this reason some physicians believe that lavage should not be done.

Further treatment consists of stimulants, the use of an antibiotic given prophylactically intramuscularly, oxygen, and transfusion for methemoglobinemia. Pneumonia and kidney complications may occur later.

POISONING FROM CORROSIVE CHEMICALS. If the child has swallowed a corrosive chemical such as lye, tissues with which the chemical comes in contact are destroyed. Lye is one of the most common causes of poisoning in children. Sources of lye are washing powders, paint removers and drainpipe cleansers.

The manifestations of corrosive esophagitis may be seen in the tissue of the alimentary tract from the lips to the stomach. The symptoms are pain, inability to swallow, and prostration. The mucous membranes of the area are white immediately after the accident, but later become brown, ulcerated and edematous. The edema may be sufficient to obstruct respiration, and tracheotomy may be necessary. The pulse is feeble and rapid, and the child may collapse.

If the child survives, acute symptoms subside, and for a time he may appear well. But esophageal obstruction invariably appears within four to eight weeks as a result of contraction of scar tissue. In severe obstruction the child may be unable to swallow either food or fluids.

The immediate treatment is neutralization of the chemical with dilute vinegar or lemon juice. Pain may be relieved with sedatives. Olive oil or milk taken by mouth may also relieve the pain by its demulcent action. Emetics or lavage should not be utilized for fear of traumatic perforation through the necrotic mucosa. Cortisone therapy may be admininstered to decrease fibrosis or stricture formation.

If the child cannot swallow, food and fluids must be given parenterally. To prevent stricture of the esophagus, the physician may pass a rubber eyeless catheter of appropriate size and filled with small shot. The first treatment is given about four days after the accident. Dilatation by bougie is continued for at least a year. The size of the catheter is gradually increased. The child may be fed by gastrostomy if obstruction has been complete until the lumen is adequately dilated.

Nursing Care. The nurse should prevent the anxious parents from overstimulating or handling and caressing the child too much.

When the child is brought to the clinic, the nurse will save all vomitus and urine specimens for laboratory examination. She assists the physician with lavage or carries out his order for the procedure (see p. 309).

The child in a mummy restraint is positioned with his face to one side. A well lubricated, large-bore catheter is passed. Size 28 French may be used; the actual size depends upon the child's age and the stomach contents. An Ewald aspirating bulb is attached. A small amount of the lavage solution (150 to 200 ml.) should be injected into the stomach and aspirated as necessary. The procedure is continued until all traces of the poison are removed. In all, 2 to 4 liters of solution should be used.

For immediate emptying of the stomach, water or weak salt and sodium bicarbonate solution may be used until a more suitable solution can be obtained. Later, activated charcoal, tannic acid, magnesium oxide or other solution may be used, depending on the poison the child has taken.

Routine lavage is used with the following exceptions: If the child has taken a corrosive poison, there is danger of perforating the esophagus. In strychnine poisoning the stimulation of passing a lavage tube may induce a fatal convulsion.

Good general supporting therapy increases the effectiveness of removing the poison and giving a specific antidote. Supportive therapy will depend, of course, upon the action of the particular poison ingested.

The nurse must watch for evidence of stimulation or depression of the nervous system. Stimulation results in convulsions, restlessness and delirium. Depression results in stupor and coma.

There may be symptoms of respiratory depression, pulmonary edema or pneumonia. To relieve pulmonary distress, the patient may be given artificial respiration (see p. 182) or oxygen, or establishment of a patent airway may be necessary.

The nurse must watch for peripheral circulatory collapse or cardiac failure. Intravenous administration of fluids or digitalis may be necessary.

Some poisons cause intense vomiting and diarrhea. Water and electrolyte loss must be replaced by parenteral fluids.

The nurse must observe the frequency of voiding and collect samples of urine as ordered by the physician. The extent of renal damage varies. The most important aspect of therapy in relation to the influence of poison on the kidneys is administration of the correct amounts of electrolytes and fluids.

The child's temperature must be taken at frequent intervals, since the physician should be notified if hypothermia or hyperthermia occurs.

The child who is poisoned is prone to infection. He must be isolated from other children, and no nurse who has even a slight infection should care for him. The nurse will give antibiotic therapy as ordered by the physician.

Both the child and his parents are in need of emotional support from the nurse, particularly if the child is in pain. The mother may feel guilty, blaming herself for the accident. She should be counseled to avoid such sentiments of recrimination. Competent, comprehensive nursing care is essential.

Prevention. Most cases of accidental poisoning in young children are due to the carelessness of the adults responsible for the care of the children. The immediate responsibility lies with the child's parents. It is also the responsibility, however, of all members of the health team who teach parents the hygiene and care of children to stress the danger to these active, curious toddlers of leaving poisonous substances in any receptacle within easy reach.

All dangerous substances should be kept out of the toddler's reach, on a high shelf or, better still, in a locked cupboard. All drugs, household chemicals and poisons should be kept in the containers in which they were sold, for these are plainly marked, and no adult is likely to carelessly leave them in easy reach of the child. If poisonous substances are stored in containers used for food, there is danger that someone will leave them where the child can sample the contents.* Children should also be protected from poisoning by spoiled food, thus preventing bacterial poisoning.

Burns

Incidence and Classification. A burn is any destruction of tissue caused by heat primarily. Heat may be either dry as from a hot radiator or

---

* This same precaution applies to inflammable materials.

stove, from lighted matches, or from the insertion of a live electric wire into the mouth, or wet as from a cup of hot coffee or soup spilled on the child or from the hot tap being turned on while the child is in the bathtub. Other causes of burns are chemical agents, electricity, overexposure to ultraviolet or roentgen rays and radioactive substances. Burns are one of the most frequent accidental injuries of infants and children. Younger children are apt to be burned at home; older ones may be burned at home or school or during play away from home.

Classification of burns is made according to the degree (depth of tissue destroyed) and percentage of body surface involved. A *first-degree* or *superficial burn* involves only the epidermis. There is redness of the skin, with pain and swelling. Regeneration occurs in superficial burns. A *second-degree* or *partial-thickness* burn destroys superficial skin layers and damages deep tissues. The area is red and blistered and extremely painful. Some scarring may result, but the skin is regenerated from the remaining living epithelial cells. A *third-degree* or *total-thickness* burn produces destruction of the epidermis and some of the dermis. The burned area may appear charred. Nerve endings, sweat glands and hair follicles are destroyed.

Any child having a burn of 5 to 12 per cent or more of his body surface should be admitted to the hospital for treatment. Figure 16-8 shows the rule of nines for the infant and older child or adult.

Problems Associated with Burns; Treatment and Nursing Care. The purposes of treatment of a child having burns are to save his life, to protect him from infection, and to preserve or restore his appearance and functioning as near to normal as possible.

Fluid and electrolyte imbalance presents a serious problem. Shortly after a burn has occurred there is a decrease in the circulatory plasma volume. Electrolytes, water and protein leave vessels and go to the interstitial space around the burned area. The rest of the body is dehydrated. There is increased concentration of the red blood cells. Erythrocytes are destroyed by hemolysis and bleeding into the burned area. Large amounts of sodium enter the edema fluid of the burned area, where there is consequent replacement of intracellular potassium with sodium. The patient may be in negative sodium balance. Acidosis often develops. Infection is a problem and may delay reabsorption of edema fluid in the burned area.

Immediate treatment of a first-degree burn consists in cleaning the area and applying a thin layer of an anesthetic ointment and giving analgesics. A bandage may then be applied securely but not too firmly in order to prevent causing pain.

Another method of treatment which can be used immediately after the injury consists in the application of ice water packs or the immersion of the part in ice water. Hexachlorophene may be added to the water. This treatment, which may produce a varying degree of hypothermia, may be used for burns covering an area of up to 20 per cent of body surface. It may be continued until it can be stopped without the return of pain. With the use of this treatment, pain is controlled, and edema, fluid loss and the rate of infection are decreased.

When a child who has been burned more severely is to be admitted to the hospital, he should be placed in a private room which has running water. Sterile technique must be carried out in his care, so that supplies of sterile sheets, towels, cloths, adult isolation gowns, and gloves (sterile disposable gloves may be used) should be obtained. Also, depending on the policy of the hospital, sterile face masks, caps, and shoe covers may be required. Equipment which must be present in the child's room includes an intravenous setup or cutdown tray, intravenous solutions, blood plasma, a catheterization tray with appropriate size Foley catheters, a sterile container to receive the urine, an emergency tracheotomy tray and a tracheostomy tube of appropriate size, a bed cradle if the open technique of therapy is to be used, an aspirating machine with catheters, and a child's size oxygen mask attached to a wall oxygen outlet or tank.

In second- and third-degree burns the first problem is to combat shock. The child should be placed on a sterile sheet and the burned area covered with sterile towels. Morphine, codeine or another pain-relieving drug is given. Plasma and other fluids are administered intravenously as needed to replace electrolytes (see p. 294). The child should be kept warm by raising the temperature of the room to 78 to 80°F. or by the use of a bed cradle if the open technique of therapy is to be used. Excessive heat, however, may cause dilatation of peripheral blood vessels and aggravate the circulatory disturbance. The hematocrit and hemoglobin levels should be determined as a guide to fluid therapy. Blood chemistry values should be determined frequently.

Typing and crossmatching of blood should be done to prepare for transfusion. A urinalysis is also done. If there is to be débridement, adequate anesthesia is essential. Oxygen should be given to combat anoxia. A tracheotomy (see p. 406) may be done as an emergency procedure if respiratory difficulty occurs. The foot of the bed is elevated in case of shock. Tetanus antitoxin is given if the patient has not had tetanus toxoid. A booster dose of tetanus toxoid may be given if the child had previous immunization. Gas gangrene antitoxin may also be given. Antibiotics should be given to control

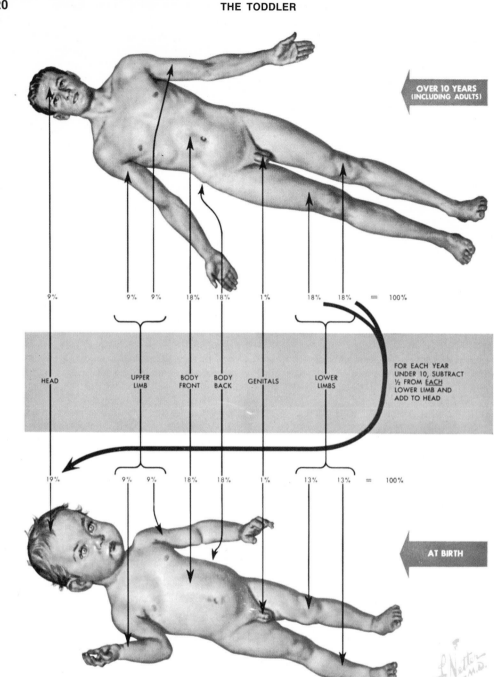

Figure 16–8. The "rule of nines" is helpful in estimating the amount of surface area burned in children of various ages. (Illustrations by Frank H. Netter, M.D., from John W. Chamberlain, M.D., Kenneth Welch, M.D., Thomas S. Morse, M.D. Ciba Clinical Symposia.)

infection. A retention catheter is inserted into the bladder so that an accurate output record is possible.

During the first few days after admission to the hospital the child may have increased thirst due to dehydration. Initially, oral administration of fluids will probably be restricted. Although the child will receive fluids intravenously, he may be permitted small sips of water. If fluids are given too rapidly in large amounts, nausea and vomiting will probably result. Ingestion of fluids and nourishment may become a problem later when a bland high protein and high caloric diet with vitamins, especially vitamin C, and iron for tissue repair is necessary. Since many of these children have decreased appetites due to discomfort and inactivity as well as to their general metabolic and physiologic disturbances, gavage may become necessary. Water to which electrolytes have been added may be offered to the child, but this solution may not be well taken because of its unpleasant taste. The services of a nutritionist may be essential in providing an adequate diet for the child with extensive burns.

There is a difference of opinion among physicians about local treatment, and the nurse naturally follows the orders of the individual physician. In the *open technique* of treatment there is no dressing. The burned area is open to the air, so that an eschar forms. The advantages of open treatment are that the child has less fever and may be ambulatory if the burned area is not extensive, and there is less odor. The open method of treatment is preferred usually for burns of the hands, face, joints and genitalia. The danger in using the open technique is that of infection. One method currently used to prevent

infection includes reverse isolation of the child in a whole-body isolator bed type of plastic tent with portholes through which care may be given. (One such device is termed the "Life Island," which can be obtained from Life Island Hospital Isolation System of the Matthews Research, Inc., Alexandria, Virginia.) The real problem in the use of such a device is that of providing emotional support for the child.

The *closed* or *pressure bandage method* is another method of treatment. In this method the burned area is débrided and gross contamination is removed. A dressing is applied under strict aseptic technique. Pressure is then produced by tightly bandaging the entire dressing. This helps to control plasma loss into the tissues. These bandages should be removed in two or three weeks for grafting, or earlier if the temperature is elevated or there is a foul odor from the dressings indicating infection. Some surgeons apply a light plaster of Paris cast instead of the pressure dressing.

Currently various solutions or ointments are

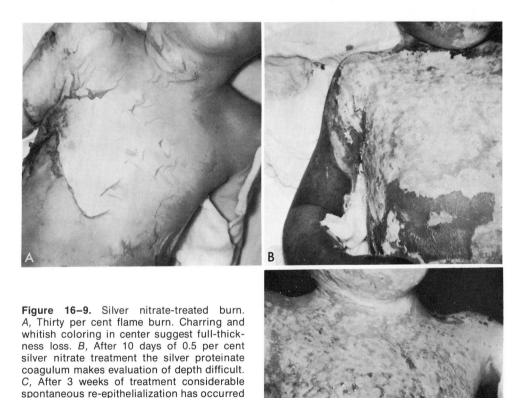

Figure 16–9. Silver nitrate-treated burn. *A,* Thirty per cent flame burn. Charring and whitish coloring in center suggest full-thickness loss. *B,* After 10 days of 0.5 per cent silver nitrate treatment the silver proteinate coagulum makes evaluation of depth difficult. *C,* After 3 weeks of treatment considerable spontaneous re-epithelialization has occurred and multiple islands of granulation tissue are rapidly being covered. Bacterial cultures fail to grow pathogenic bacteria. (From Krizek's article in W. F. Ballinger, R. B. Rutherford and G. D. Zuidema: *The Management of Trauma.*)

used in the treatment of burns. These include 0.5 per cent silver nitrate solution, gentamycin sulfate ointment, Sulfamylon, and silicone solution. The most frequently used of these is a solution of silver nitrate applied locally.

Through the use of 0.5 per cent silver nitrate solution applied after débridement, the dressings are kept continuously wet with the solution. They are changed two or three times a day. The advantages of the use of this method are that it decreases bacteria on the burn wound and results in earlier or less necessary skin grafting and a better cosmetic effect. An important disadvantage is that the solution dilutes the serum electrolytes. Dilution can be prevented by providing electrolytes by mouth or vein. Another disadvantage is that having his dressings changed so frequently is very disturbing and painful for the child. It may also be difficult for the nurse to assist with this procedure when the child is so uncomfortable. If, however, the nurse will keep in mind the advantages of this method of therapy, she will be able to support the child and feel less stress herself during the procedure.

In a civilian disaster the best method of treating burns would be to expose the area to the air, elevate and immobilize a burned limb, and give the patient prophylactic antibacterial drugs.

With severe burns, anemia may appear by the fifth day or earlier. Transfusions and iron therapy may be given.

The *later treatment* of a burned child includes skin grafting and other types of plastic surgery. Skin grafting is successful only if a clean, uninfected, granulating base can be obtained. Eschar formed from open treatment must be softened with sterile wet saline dressings to prepare the wound for a graft. All infection must be cleared before grafting. Necrotic tissue can be soaked off in a tub or by applying wet dressings.

Skin grafts may be of two types: the *homograft,* using skin taken from another person, and the *autograft,* using skin taken from the patient. Skin from a donor is used only to cover extensive burns until the patient is in sufficiently good physical condition to have a graft of his own skin.

There are three types of autografts. For a *pedicle graft* a piece of skin is freed from its attachment on three sides, but left in position on one side. The free end is sutured over the burned area. Later, when the sutured portion is attached, the pedicle is freed at its base. *Patch grafts* are small skin grafts. *Split skin grafts* may also be used. Other types of reconstructive plastic surgery may be done after the area has healed and the child's condition has improved.

The plan of nursing care depends on the location and extent of the burned area, on the needs of the child and on the kind of treatment ordered.

The nurse should observe and record indications of shock (subnormal temperature, low blood pressure, rapid pulse rate, rapid shallow respirations and extreme pallor) and evidence of toxicity. Toxicity commonly appears in one or two days and is accompanied by high fever, prostration, vomiting, cyanosis, rapid pulse rate and decreased urinary output with edema. Unless toxicity is combated, coma and death may result. The child should also be observed for abdominal discomfort or bleeding of the gastrointestinal tract indicating a stress or *Curling's ulcer,* which may occur in burned patients.

The child should be protected from infection and injury to delicate epithelium which grows to replace dead tissue. Sterile gown and mask technique should be used. Thorough handwashing is essential, and sterile gloves may be used. All linen used for the child should be sterilized. Pain is relieved by medication ordered by the physician.

If the open technique is used, a heated cradle covered with a sterile sheet may be placed over the child's body to maintain his body temperature without the need for bed coverings which might stick to the burn sites. If the burned areas on the child's body stick to the sterile cover sheet, spreading the linen with a thin layer of sterile lubricant jelly, with the physician's permission, reduces the sticking and the pain when the child is moved.

A Stryker or Bradford frame (see p. 210) may be used for children having extensive burns to prevent contamination of the burned areas, to facilitate collection of urine specimens if no catheter has been inserted into the bladder, and to keep the body in good alignment.

A retention catheter may be inserted into the bladder so that an accurate intake and output record can be kept. The urinary output should be 25 to 50 ml. per hour. The nurse should report to the physician if it falls below this minimum, since urinary output is an indication of kidney function as well as a valuable guide to the regulation of parenteral fluid therapy.

Body alignment is important to prevent deformity through contractures. If the anterior surface of the neck is burned, a roll placed under the shoulders will prevent contracture. A footboard may be used to prevent foot drop when the child is on his back. When he is on his abdomen, a pillow should be placed beneath each leg to prevent pressure on his toes. The child should be turned every two to four hours, and skin care should be given to prevent pressure areas. The skin around the burned areas should be massaged gently with a soothing lotion approved by the physician. The child should be kept dry to prevent discomfort and contamination of the burned areas. Contracting scars must not be allowed to form during the healing stage.

The child should be given passive exercises to prevent contractures and stiff joints.

Unless his arms and hands are burned, the child should be given toys and equipment for independent play. The nurse should make a sling out of a sheet under the Bradford frame and pin it to the crib sides to support the child's arms and toys. He should be read to, and the pictures in the book shown him. His bed should be placed so that he can see the other children playing. He enjoys a record player, radio or television.

Providing care for a severely burned child may not be easy for his nurses because of his appearance, his possible odor, and his sometimes distressing reaction to having his dressings changed. Nurses must work through their feelings, however, so that they can deal effectively with the child as a person.

Rehabilitation, Response of Parent and Child, Prognosis and Prevention. The goal of *rehabilitation* in the treatment of a burned child is to help him develop and live to his maximum capacity within the limits of his disabilities. This includes helping the child and his parents to accept disfiguring scars and any handicaps he may have. Occupational and physical therapy may be used in the rehabilitation of a child after a burn. He may also be referred to the Social Service Department for an evaluation of his family situation and for aid in providing support to the parents and their child.

The *response of the parent and the child* to his trauma varies in every case. The child may be fearful and anxious because of the fright caused by the accident, his extreme pain and his separation from his parents for a long time. The child may also feel guilty if he was hurt while engaged in some activity which was forbidden by his parents or against which they had warned him. Parents may feel guilty because of lack of supervision of the child – supervision which would have prevented his injury. They may show excessive sympathy for or overprotection of him.

Both the child and his parents need reassurance and understanding. The nurse should discover their fears and give them comfort. If the child must return for plastic surgery, he should have encouragement to face another painful period of hospitalization. He should be encouraged to express his aggression in play if he cannot express it verbally. He should be encouraged to cry if he wishes when painful procedures are done to him. If a nurse whom he knows and trusts is with him at such times to support him, he will be better able to withstand the pain. Such expression of his emotions will facilitate his adjustment to his illness and improve his relations with his parents after his recovery.

In general, the *prognosis* depends on the extent and depth of the burn. Death during the acute phase of the burn results from shock, alterations of blood volume and changes in the electrolyte composition of the blood. Death after the acute phase is the result of toxemia, local or intercurrent infection or debilitation.

The *prevention* of such painful, often fatal, accidents to children is a broad program of education of adults and children in prevention of fire hazards. Not only should they be helped to realize the various ways by which children can be burned, but they should also be helped to understand the importance of teaching their children how to put out their burning clothing should they become ignited and how to escape immediately if a fire occurs in their home. The parents and their children should have frequent fire drills so that they become familiar with the various escape routes.

Fracture of the Femur

Incidence, Etiology, Types and Diagnosis. Many injuries occurring among toddlers are the result of falls. The toddler is learning to climb. He goes up and down stairs and climbs on and off chairs and benches for the sheer joy of it. Although a fracture of the femur is not the only injury he may receive, it is one of the most common serious fractures caused by his many falls. The nurse should stress this danger in her conferences with the mother.

The stairs should have handrails so that the child may hold on to the rail as he goes up or down one step at a time (see Fig. 15-8). Ideally, there should be gates at the top and the bottom of the stairs. The one-story house is safer than the two-story house for the toddler in this respect. Generally there is a door to the cellar steps which can be kept shut.

Fracture of the femur, sometimes accompanied by other serious injuries, also results when the child is struck by a passing car as he chases into the street after a ball or by a car being backed out of a driveway or garage. If the driver is the child's parent, that fact adds to the emotional impact of the accident upon the parents. Climbing over the side of the crib or springing on the bed mattress frequently results in severe falls and skeletal injury.

A *greenstick fracture* is one in which one side of the bone is broken, the other side being bent. This type of fracture is common in children because their bones are soft and not fully mineralized. A severe injury, however, will result in a complete break. In young children, healing may occur with some deformity, though this usually disappears during the process of growth.

The *diagnosis* is made by his history of inability to bear weight, pain on movement and local tenderness. X-ray examination confirms the findings and the position of the broken fragments.

Treatment and Nursing Care. The child's clothes should be removed gently, first from the uninjured side of the body and then from the injured side. The injured limb should be moved as little as possible. It is sometimes necessary to cut off the clothing.

The physician may order cold applications or ice caps for the first twenty-four to thirty-six hours to prevent swelling and edema. Aspirin or a salicylate is effective for relief of pain.

The method of fixation of the legs is by traction. It is developed by a system of weights and pulleys and is applied to both legs by means of skin traction. Traction is applied to reduce the fracture, to maintain the bones in the corrected position and to immobilize both legs. The type of traction apparatus commonly used for children up to approximately two years of age having a fractured femur is *Byrant traction,* and the method is by vertical suspension.

The fundamental principle of the Bryant traction system is a bilateral *Buck's extension* applied to the legs. The procedure is as follows:

1. Shave the legs if any hair is present, and paint the skin with tincture of benzoin so that the adhesive will grasp the skin more firmly. Benzoin also serves as a disinfectant for the skin and allays itching and excoriation beneath the tape.

2. A strip of moleskin should be cut for each leg, long enough to extend above the knee on each side and under the foot. In the center of each strip, at the level of the sole of the foot, place a thin flat board 3 inches long and an inch broader than the widest distance

between the malleoli. There should be a hole in the center of the block through which the traction rope is to be passed. In order to hold the piece of board in place, a second piece of moleskin must be placed on the side facing the child's foot. This piece of moleskin must be as wide as the other and long enough to reach from above the malleoli on one side under the foot to above the malleoli on the other side. This is done to protect the malleoli from pressure from the adhesive. Metal attachments may be used instead of the pieces of wood.

3. Two overhead bars placed longitudinally, or one longitudinal bar with a crossbar, are fastened securely over the crib. One or two pulleys are attached to the bar, in position to apply traction at the desired angle.

4. The moleskin is applied and held in place by gauze, bias-cut stockinet or Ace bandages. A rope is threaded over the pulleys. Sufficient weights are applied *to elevate the child's hips slightly from the bed.* The legs should be at right angles to the body and the buttocks elevated and clear of the bed. A jacket restraint should be used to keep the child flat in bed and unable to turn from side to side. The child may lie upon the mattress of the bed or be placed upon a Bradford frame within the bed. The nurse should never remove the weights once they have been applied, for the traction should be kept constant. In moving the bed the weights should not be supported, but neither should they be permitted to swing against the bed. After traction has been applied to the child's legs it should be checked carefully in order to prevent constriction of circulation or injury to the feet.

CARE OF THE CHILD IN TRACTION. The nurse should observe the traction ropes to see whether the child's body is in correct alignment. She should feel his toes frequently to note any sign of impairment of circulation. The toes should be pink and warm. Any cyanosis, tingling or loss of sensation is an indication that the bandage is

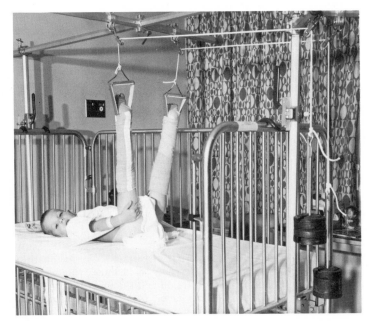

Figure 16–10. Bryant traction is used for the young child who has a fractured femur. Sufficient weights are used to elevate the child's pelvis from the bed. (H. Armstrong Roberts.)

too tight. The nurse should be sure that the weights hang free and that the ropes are in the wheel grooves of the pulleys. Little children in Bryant apparatus are tempted to turn from side to side when they are interested in what is going on about them. This interferes with the even traction exerted by the weights. Movement of the body is an indication that the restraining jacket is not fastened correctly.

Lying constantly supine with the friction which the slight movement of the restraining jacket permits is likely to chafe the child's back. Hence he needs good back care. The nurse should reach under his body and rub his back and buttocks. The bed must be kept dry and free from wrinkles and crumbs or other particles of food.

Lack of exercise often results in the child's becoming constipated. His abdomen may become distended. The physician may order a mild cathartic to relieve the distention. Roughage in the diet and the fluid intake should be increased.

Enemas may be needed, but continued use of cathartics is avoided.

The child in traction may receive overprotection from his nurse, who may believe that he cannot help himself. A child will adapt more easily than an adult to this type of situation and will learn to feed himself, for instance, with minimal help. The nurse, however, should give him greater attention and approval in order to sustain his ego during his enforced bed rest.

These children need their mothers with them also for ego strength. Application of the Bryant traction is frightening to toddlers, and later, when they are accustomed to it, the restraint makes time pass slowly. Unless amusement is provided for them and their mothers visit them daily, they will find hospitalization a traumatic experience.

Prognosis. Femoral shaft fractures in little children heal quickly. There is usually solid union within three to four weeks after the injury.

TEACHING AIDS AND OTHER INFORMATION*

American Academy of Pediatrics

First Aid Treatment of Accidental Poisoning, 1963.
Responsibility Means Safety for Your Child, 1964.

American Medical Association

Buckle Down and Stay Safe.
Danger Lurks.
How Are You Fixed for Poisons?
Protecting Your Home from Unlabeled Poisons.
Seat Belts Save Lives.
Upstairs, Downstairs, All Through the House.

Association for the Aid of Crippled Children

Suchman, E. A., and Scherzer, A. L.: Current Research in Childhood Accidents.

Play Schools Association

Cleverdon, D.: Play in a Hospital, 1964.

The Children's Hospital Medical Center, Boston, Mass.

Accident Handbook: A New Approach to Family Safety.
How to Prevent Childhood Poisoning.

United States Department of Health, Education, and Welfare

Accidents and Children, 1965.
Child Protection Under the Federal Hazardous Substances Act, 1967.
Children . . . and Refrigerator Entrapment, 1965.
Common Intestinal Helminths of Man, Life Cycle Charts, 1965.
Directory, Poison Control Centers, 1967.
Families on Guard Against Accidents, 1967.
Pinworms, 1967.
Safety Tips in, on and Around the Water, 1967.
Shore, M. F. (ed.): Red Is the Color of Hurting, 1967.

---

* Complete addresses are given in the Appendix.

REFERENCES

Publications

Bergmann, T., and Freud, A.: *Children in the Hospital.* New York, International Universities Press, 1966.

Crews, E. R.: *A Practical Manual for the Treatment of Burns.* Springfield, Ill., Charles C Thomas, 1964.

Dimock, H. G.: *The Child in Hospital.* Philadelphia, F. A. Davis Company, 1960.

Dreisbach, R. H.: *Handbook of Poisoning: Diagnosis and Treatment.* 5th ed. Los Altos, California, Lange Medical Publications, 1966.

Ellis, R. W. B., and Mitchell, R. G.: *Disease in Infancy and Childhood.* 5th ed. Baltimore, Williams & Wilkins Company, 1966.

Fagin, C. M.: *Effects of Maternal Attendance During Hospitalization on Post-Hospital Behavior of Young Children.* Philadelphia, F. A. Davis Company, 1966.

Gellis, S. S., and Kagan, B. M.: *Current Pediatric Therapy.* 3rd ed. Philadelphia, W. B. Saunders Company, 1968.

Geist, H.: *A Child Goes to the Hospital: The Psychological Aspects of a Child Going to the Hospital.* Springfield, Ill., Charles C Thomas, 1965.

Green, M. M., and others: *The Concerns of Parents of a Hospitalized Child;* in *Effective Therapeutic Communications in Nursing.* (Convention Clinical Session No. 8.) New York, American Nurses' Association, 1964.

Haller, J. A., Talbert, J. L., and Dombro, R. H. (Eds.): *The Hospitalized Child and His Family.* Baltimore, Johns Hopkins Press, 1967.

Kennedy, R. H. (Ed.): *Emergency Care of the Sick and Injured.* Philadelphia, W. B. Saunders Company, 1966.

Matthew, H., and Lawson, A. A. H.: *Treatment of Common Acute Poisonings.* Baltimore, Williams & Wilkins Company, 1967.

National Safety Council: *Accident Facts.* 1967 Edition. Chicago, National Safety Council, 1967.

Robertson, J.: *Hospitals and Children.* New York, International Universities Press, 1963.

Vernon, D. T. A., and others: *The Psychological Responses of Children to Hospitalization and Illness.* Springfield, Ill., Charles C Thomas, 1965.

Periodicals

Ambler, M. C.: Disciplining Hospitalized Toddlers. *Am. J. Nursing,* 67:572, 1967.

Aufhauser, T. R.: Parent Participation in Hospital Care of Children. *Nursing Outlook*, 15:40, January 1967.

Barrett-Connor, E., and others: Common Parasitic Infections of the Intestinal Tract. *Pediat. Clin. N. Amer.*, 14:235, 1967.

LaDuke, M. M., and others: Germfree Isolators. *Am. J. Nursing*, 67:72, 1967.

Larson, D., and Gaston, R.: Current Trends in the Care of Burned Patients. *Am. J. Nursing*, 67:319, 1967.

Live-In Mothers Aid in Hospital Medical Care. *Medical World News,* 8:58, October 27, 1967.

Mahaffy, P. R.: Admission Interviews with Parents. *Am. J. Nursing*, 66:506, 1966.

Maisel, G., and others: Analysis of Two Surveys Evaluating a Project to Reduce Accidental Poisoning Among Children. *Pub. Health Rep.*, 82:555, 1967.

Markowitz, M., and Gordis, L.: A Family Pediatric Clinic at a Community Hospital. *Children,* 14:25, 1967.

Miller, R. R., and Johnson, S. R.: Poison Control: Now and in the Future. *Am. J. Nursing*, 66:1984, 1966.

Monafo, W. W., and Moyer, C. A.: Effectiveness of Dilute Aqueous Silver Nitrate in the Treatment of Major Burns. *Arch. Surg.*, 91:200, 1965.

Moncrief, J. A.: Early Care of the Burned Patient. *Medical Science*, 18:33, August 1967.

Price, W. R., and Wood, M.: Treatment of the Infected Burn with Dilute Silver Nitrate Solution. *Am. J. Surg.*, 114:641, 1967.

Price, W. R., and Wood, M.: Operating Room Care of Burned Patients Treated with Silver Nitrate. *Am. J. Nursing*, 68:1705, 1968.

Rousseau, O.: Mothers Do Help in Pediatrics. *Am. J. Nursing*, 67:798, 1967.

Roy, Sister M. C.: Role Cues and Mothers of Hospitalized Children. *Nursing Research*, 16:178, 1967.

Rubin, M.: Balm for Burned Children. *Am. J. Nursing*, 66:296, 1966.

Seidl, F. W., and Pillitteri, A.: Development of an Attitude Scale on Parent Participation. *Nursing Research*, 16:71, 1967.

Seidler, F. M.: Adapting Nursing Procedures for Reverse Isolation. *Am. J. Nursing*, 65:108, June 1965.

Skellenger, W. S.: Treatment of Poisoning in Children. *Am. J. Nursing*, 65:108, November 1965.

Webb, C.: Nursing Support for Your Young Patients' Parents. *R.N.*, 30:44, February 1967.

Webb, C.: Tactics to Reduce a Child's Fear of Pain. *Am. J. Nursing*, 66:2698, 1966.

Wu, R.: Explaining Treatments to Young Children. *Am. J. Nursing*, 65:71, July 1965.

17

CONDITIONS OF TODDLERS REQUIRING LONG-TERM CARE

<hr />

LONG-TERM HOSPITALIZATION

Long-term hospitalization of the toddler presents a more serious problem of maternal deprivation than it does in any other age group.

Prevention of Maternal Deprivation. The personnel of the children's hospital or pediatric unit in a general hospital should be educated to understand the toddler's emotional need for his parents so that they appreciate the importance of frequent visiting. If the expense of transportation or loss of time from work is the reason given by parents for not visiting the child, the social service worker may find ways of assisting them. Every effort should be made to keep young children at home, with care given on an outpatient basis. If this is not possible, children should be hospitalized near their homes and, if possible, sent home on weekends and holidays. Arrangements might be made for other young children in the family to go to nursery school so that the mother may be free to visit the sick child. The child's older brothers and sisters should be permitted to visit him.

If the mother is unable or unwilling to visit the sick child frequently, the hospital should compensate for his loss of maternal love by sup-plementing her visits with the long-term care of one of the hospital personnel.

Those who care for toddlers who must stay in the hospital a long time should be permanent members of the staff—graduate nurses, practical nurses, aides or foster mothers. Such nursing intervention helps a toddler to develop autonomy, to establish a relationship that helps him to continue to hope, to retain trust in himself and others, and to learn to handle anger and frustration. Individual care of toddlers prevents much of the emotional trauma seen in hospitalized children who are cared for by a constantly changing series of attendants.

1. The case-assignment system should be used exclusively in long-term care of little children.

2. The same personnel should be assigned to a small group of children throughout their period of hospitalization. This is possible only if nursing care is given by a permanent staff and students are supernumeraries assigned to the care of patients solely for the learning experiences involved.

3. Children needing long-term hospitalization may be placed in hospital units resembling a children's home where medical attention is

provided. The main part of the care should be given by women skilled in meeting the needs of little children; they should be nonprofessional foster-mothers. Each could act as "Mother" to a small group of children. Physicians and nurses could come in only when necessary. In such small family groups a child could form stable relations and lead an emotionally satisfying life.

4. Children confined to the hospital should have as many of the pleasurable activities available to normal children as possible. For instance, they could play with sand and water and do finger painting. In the typical children's hospital unit such play is difficult to provide. In the model hospitals planned solely for the care of children having chronic and orthopedic conditions and in convalescent hospitals a variety of play materials are provided for the children.

LONG-TERM CONDITIONS

Cleft Palate

The incidence, etiology, pathology and clinical manifestations of cleft palate were discussed in Chapter 11 (p. 198). Only the long-term program of care, including surgical correction, will be discussed here.

Total Program of Care or Habilitation. The care and habilitation of the child with cleft palate may require many years of medical, dental, surgical and speech treatment. The personnel involved act as a team, functioning better as a group than if care were given by them individually. The *cleft palate team* includes the pediatrician, plastic surgeon, dentist, prosthetic dentist, orthodontist, otolaryngologist, audiologist, medical social worker, nurse in the hospital, speech pathologist, psychologist or psychiatrist or both, and the public health nurse. The child's physician may act as coordinator of the group so that the mother is not confused by the apparent complexity of the treatment. The mother may need guidance from each of the team members at various times as treatment progresses. Cleft palate teams such as these are usually located in the clinics of the large medical centers.

If the parents cannot afford this care, the child is treated at one of the large medical centers connected with the state program for crippled children or at a children's hospital under private auspices. In either case he is treated without cost to his parents, or for whatever fee they are able to pay.

Dealing with the anxieties of the parents is one of the main functions of the cleft palate team, and specifically of the nurses in the newborn nursery, the public health nurses in the home or clinic, and the nurses in the hospital when the child is admitted for surgery. The parents should be reassured that all possible therapy will be given the child. They must also be told that improvement will take time and will require their full cooperation. The parents must be helped to accept the child with his disfigurement and to help him to adjust to his deformity. The physical defect can be corrected more successfully than can hampering personality traits which may develop if he believes that others turn away from him because of his cleft palate.

Surgical Correction. The child should be placed under the care of the cleft palate team as early as possible so that changes occurring with growth can be observed and plans can be made for long-term needs.

Operation is delayed until the child is between one and five years of age, because the surgeon wants to take advantage of changes in the palate which occur with growth. The time for operation varies because of differences in the size, degree and shape of the deformity. The surgeon tries to correct the defect so that there is optimum union of the cleft in the palate, without injury to the developing maxilla, and so that intelligible speech will be possible.

If operation is postponed until the child is learning to speak—about the third year—a dental speech appliance can be fitted so that the child can speak clearly enough for others to understand him. If the deformity is too severe and surgical repair is not possible, a *prosthetic speech appliance* is used as an important means of speech habilitation. Such appliances must be replaced periodically as the child grows.

Surgical Management and Nursing Care. *Preoperative care* is minimal. Any infection is a contraindication to operation. The nurse must watch the child closely and report any evidence of infection. The clotting and bleeding times should be determined preoperatively. Feedings are given until six to eight hours before operation if the child is in good nutritional condition, with good fluid and electrolyte balance.

Postoperative care is extremely important. Special nursing care is essential immediately after operation to keep the mouth clean and free from irritation. Antibiotics are ordered only if infection is suspected. Directly after the operation the child is placed on his abdomen and may have the foot of his bed slightly elevated to prevent aspiration of drainage material. His head is turned to one side. The nurse should watch closely for signs of an occluded airway and for hemorrhage. If necessary, the child is placed in a position favorable to postural drainage.

The physician may order aspiration of the nasopharynx to reduce the possibility of development of pneumonitis or atelectasis. It must be done very gently. Many physicians, however, prefer that no suction be used.

The nurse should tell the child not to rub the

site with his tongue, in words he can understand, such as, "Don't put your tongue on the part of your mouth which feels sore." Restraint may be necessary to keep the child from putting his fingers or even toys in his mouth. If the child is not old enough to cooperate, his arms must be securely restrained with elbow restraints. The restraints should be placed over the shirt, with the shirt sleeves turned back and pinned in position. The restraints should be removed periodically and passive exercise given.

The nurse may be asked to assist the physician in giving parenteral fluid therapy.

The diet is limited to clear sterile or other fluids as ordered by the physician. Milk is usually not permitted immediately after the operation because of the danger of curds forming along the suture line. The child's mouth should be rinsed or cleansed with sterile water after each feeding.

The diet is fluid or semifluid for ten days to two weeks after operation. For the following two weeks a soft diet is given, and after that a regular diet.

As far as possible all strain on the sutures must be prevented. The first postoperative feeding is given with a rubber-tipped medicine dropper, with the physician's permission, or from a paper cup or the side of a spoon. A straw is not used, for he should not suck.

If possible, crying should be prevented. The child should be kept warm, dry and as comfortable as possible. Quiet diversion such as showing him pictures in his favorite picture book and reading the accompanying story will help to keep him from crying. The physician may order sedatives to be given.

Instructions to the Mother on Discharge of the Child. The mother must be cautioned to prevent injury to the palate. Since the area may be without sensation, the child may show no sign of pain if the healing area is scraped with some hard object such as a spoon. It may be necessary for the child to wear arm cuffs constantly except when he is bathed or when his mother gives him passive exercise and allows him to move his arms freely. At such times she must guard against his putting his hand into his mouth.* Sucking and blowing movements bring a strain upon the wound. If the mother sees that he is amusing himself in this way, she should play with him and divert his attention with a toy.

Upper respiratory tract infection increases his discomfort. He should be kept from infection by isolating him from anyone who has a sore throat or a cold.

Complications. These children may have

---

* The mother can make arm cuffs out of rolled cardboard and tie them in place with string. Care must be taken that the restraints do not rub the skin in the axilla.

recurring attacks of otitis media with resulting loss of hearing. The mother should report any indications of otitis to the physician. Excessive dental decay may accompany cleft palate. The mother should be taught the correct method of brushing the child's teeth so that she can keep them clean when the physician says that it is safe for her to use a brush. Later she will teach the child the correct technique. The mother should also be told of the need for dental supervision of the child. The teeth must receive special attention if an appliance is to be fitted. If displacement of the maxillary arches and malposition of the teeth occur, orthodontic correction may be necessary.

Prognosis. The prognosis is fair, but depends upon the extent of the deformity at birth. A speech defect may still exist after surgical correction of the palatal defect or after insertion of a speech appliance. Speech therapy should be given if the defect persists.

Nephrotic Syndrome (Nephrosis)

Etiology, Types and Incidence. The cause is unknown. It is seldom possible to relate the onset of nephrosis to another condition. Exacerbations of the condition often follow acute infections.

Nephrosis is a disease of childhood, the average age at its onset being $2\frac{1}{2}$ years. It is seldom seen in children under one year of age and for an unknown reason is more common in boys than in girls.

Pathology, Clinical Manifestations and Laboratory Findings. Pathologically, the kidneys are yellowish and enlarged. The cortices are thickened and the tubules dilated.

The *clinical manifestations* may be produced by glomerular lesions which permit excessive loss of plasma protein in the urine with resulting reduction in serum albumin. As a result of this reduction in blood proteins, the colloidal osmotic pressure which tends to hold water in the capillaries is reduced. This increases transudation of fluid from the capillaries into the extracellular space, thus producing edema.

The onset is insidious. Edema is usually the first symptom noted between one and three years of age. At the onset the child rarely appears ill. The edema, apparent around his eyes and at his ankles, becomes severe and later is generalized. As the fluid accumulates, the child gains weight rapidly. In some cases he may double his normal weight. This state may last from several weeks to months. The common sites of collection of fluid are the peritoneal cavity (*ascites*), the thorax (*hydrothorax*) and the scrotum. In some children the swelling is so great that it seems as if the skin would break. Striae may appear

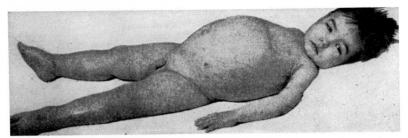

Figure 17–1. Nephrosis in a boy 4 years of age. Edema of insidious origin started several months before admission without any preceding infection and varied from time to time. The urine contained large amounts of albumin and some hyaline casts, but never blood. There was no increase in blood pressure, and no azotemia. (From M. I. Rubin in W. E. Nelson (Ed.): *Textbook of Pediatrics.* 8th ed.)

from overstretching of the skin. The edema in the peripheral tissue shifts with postural change. The urinary output varies inversely with the edema.

Pallor may be out of proportion to the degree of anemia.

Anorexia is a nursing problem. Malnutrition may be severe, but the loss of body tissue is obscured by the edema. Vomiting, diarrhea and abdominal distention may occur. During periods of edema other clinical manifestations sometimes seen include inguinal and umbilical hernias (see pp. 312, 313), respiratory distress, rectal prolapse (see p. 333) and decreased motor activity. The blood pressure usually remains normal, but if the child has advanced renal insufficiency, hypertension is seen. The child is generally afebrile. Behavioral concomitants of his condition are irritability and lassitude.

Nephrotic children are susceptible to infection. It is interesting to note that if the child contracts measles, a remission of the nephrotic condition may result.

A *nephrotic crisis* during the course of the illness may produce such signs and symptoms as fever, abdominal pain and at times erysipeloid skin eruptions. These subside in a few days, and diuresis may occur.

In the final stage of the disease cardiac failure may occur. The child may have hypertension, azotemia and hematuria.

The *laboratory findings* on the urine and blood are important in fitting the treatment to the needs of the child. Typical findings include proteinuria (the presence of protein in the urine). There is heavy loss of albumin in the urine, up to 10 gm. or more of protein daily. Diuresis of large amounts of urine results in disappearance of the edema. Persistent hematuria (red blood cells in the urine) may indicate a serious prognosis. Blood changes involve protein and lipids. Sufficient lowering of the serum albumin level takes place to produce a reversal in the normal albumin-globulin ratio. There is an increase in the blood lipids, especially the cholesterol fraction, with levels of 300 to 1800 mg. per 100

ml. A secondary anemia may be present. The erythrocyte sedimentation rate is rapid.

Complications and Treatment. *Complications* are infrequent, since infections are controlled with antibiotics.

The objectives of *treatment* are control of infections, normal adjustment of the disturbed processes, control of edema and promotion of good nutrition and, of equal importance, good mental hygiene.

Control of infection is achieved through prompt antibacterial therapy if an acute infection develops.

The diet should be well balanced, complete, and high in protein to compensate for the constant loss of protein in the urine. It may be advisable to limit the salt intake for short periods during the course of the disease. Children do not accept salt-poor diets, however, and their nutrition is likely to suffer if such a diet is all that is given them.

Reduction of the edema is induced through diuresis. Hormonal therapy is widely used in the treatment of nephrosis. Short-term therapy stimulates diuresis, but more prolonged therapy is generally used. Corticotropin is given parenterally, and prednisone is commonly given orally. This therapy is started when the condition is first recognized. Steroid is given daily for about four weeks. Then there is a clinical remission with disappearance of the proteinuria. Diuresis usually occurs in seven to fourteen days.

Intermittent hormonal therapy may be given between exacerbations. Smaller doses are ordered than when the child is on intensive therapy during an exacerbation. If the blood pressure is elevated, hormonal therapy is withdrawn. Since hormonal therapy masks the signs of infection, the child should be carefully observed for evidence of infection. Antibiotics are not usually given to prevent infection during steroid therapy.

Attempts to elevate the serum protein levels by giving blood plasma have not been very successful in inducing diuresis. Plasma, concentrated salt-poor albumin or other plasma substitutes may be tried temporarily. Some diuretics are effective in reducing edema. There is a difference of opinion among physicians as to whether nitrogen mustard or another antimetabolite should be used to induce diuresis.

Peritoneal drainage may be necessary if a large ascitic collection of fluid is causing respiratory or cardiac distress. If advanced renal failure is evident, fluid intake should vary with the urine volume and the child's capacity to concentrate urine.

Complete bed rest is necessary only during severe edema and when other symptoms are present. The child is allowed out of bed for supervised activity whenever his condition permits, but he must be protected from infectious contacts.

Reduction of anxiety in parents and child is important. The physician should give the parents support and encouragement during the course of the illness. He should discuss the nature of the disease with them and the therapy he is using. Whenever possible, children should be treated at home and brought to the hospital only for special therapy or expert care.

Nursing Care. Nursing care is the most important element in treatment. The parents should be allowed unlimited or frequent visiting and permitted to help in the care of the child. Thereby the harmful effects of maternal deprivation will be avoided, and the parents may express their love for the child in a way which brings relief from their frustrating feeling of helplessness.

The edematous skin must be protected from injury or infection. The child should be bathed frequently, with special attention to the moist parts of the body. A boy's genitalia should be bathed several times a day and dusted with soothing powder; they may be supported with a soft pad held in place by a T binder. Adhesive should never be used on edematous skin. A pillow should be placed between the knees when the child is lying on his side.

All skin surfaces that are in contact should be separated and cotton placed between them, in order to prevent intertrigo (see p. 121).

The child's eyes may be swollen shut. The edematous area about the eyes and lids requires attention. The eyes should be irrigated with warm saline solution to prevent a collection of exudate. The child's head should be elevated during the day to reduce discomfort from the edema.

In order to prevent respiratory infection the child should be kept warm and dry and turned frequently. He should not be exposed to infection through contact with other children in the unit or with personnel who have a cold, sore throat or other infection.

Nutrition is important, but difficult to maintain, since the child is not hungry during periods of severe edema. The food should be attractively served on colored dishes, with colored straws provided for the taking of liquids. Small amounts of easily digested foods should be offered, and the child may be permitted to help himself to "seconds."

The child should be weighed as ordered by the physician—usually daily or two or three times a week. The gain or loss in weight is evidence of the amount of edema present.

An accurate record of intake and output is always valuable. This is difficult, if not impossible, with little children who are only partially toilet-trained and may have regressed during their sickness. If the urine cannot be measured, the amount voided can be estimated by noting the size of the moist area. The color of the urine should also be charted.

If ascites interferes with respiration, the child may be placed in a semi-upright position until a paracentesis can be done. When abdominal paracentesis is to be performed, the nurse should explain the procedure to the child in order to gain his cooperation. He should void just before paracentesis so that there will be less danger of puncturing the bladder. The equipment and the exact procedure used vary in different hospitals.

In general, the responsibilities of the nurses are as follows:

Nurse No. 1: Sets up the equipment and prepares the area, collects samples of ascitic fluid for culture, and checks the child's color during the procedure.

Nurse No. 2: Explains the procedure step by step to the child. She places him in a sitting position on the edge of the table and supports his back with her body. She clasps the child's hands in hers. No further restraint is necessary if the child cooperates. The nurse should talk to him, have him close his eyes and turn his head away from the site of the puncture.

Ascitic fluid is not permitted to run too quickly or too copiously from the abdomen, because too rapid reduction of intra-abdominal pressure causes the blood to distend the deep abdominal veins and reduce the normal supply to the heart. This may cause shock.

When the procedure is over, an abdominal binder is applied rather snugly, and the child is put to bed. The nurse must observe and carefully chart the amount of drainage and the child's condition.

During the preschool years the little boy who is prone to fantasy may have real concern about his body image. He may believe that his penis, which is inconspicuous because of the extensive edema, has been cut off. The nurse should remain with the child, help him to verbalize his fears, and reassure him that his body is intact.

When his condition permits, the child should be allowed play activities appropriate to his age, interests and state of health. The Play Lady may visit his bed, or he may be taken to the playroom if there is no danger of contracting an infection from the other children.

Instructions to the Mother on Discharge of the Child. The physician explains the nature of the illness and its therapy to the parents. The nurse may further discuss the child's diet, the administration of medications, prevention of infection, skin care and the need for continued medical supervision.

Discipline is a serious problem in any long-term condition in the toddler. Parents should be consistent in discipline of the child and in setting limits to his freedom. A happy home atmosphere is probably the most important factor in discipline. In a happy situation a child is conditioned to cooperate.

Prognosis. The course is variable and is usually characterized by recurrent edema which may be of short duration or may last for some time. Since antibacterial therapy has been successfully used to control intercurrent infections, many children survive until nephrosis spontaneously disappears.

Corticotropin or one of the corticosteroids has had favorable results in many nephrotic children.

If the child does not die from concurrent infection, he has a chance of complete cure, or chronic nephritis or renal failure with a fatal outcome may ensue.

Acrodynia (Pink Disease, Erythredema)

Etiology, Incidence and Diagnosis. The cause is not proved. The disease is believed to be caused by poisoning or unusual sensitivity or idiosyncrasy to mercury. The sources of mercury poisoning include calomel, mercurial ointment and diaper rinses. Children must be protected from accidental ingestion of substances containing mercury. Acrodynia is disappearing from most parts of the United States.

The *diagnosis* is based on the distinctive clinical appearance and the course of the disease.

Clinical Manifestations, Laboratory Findings and Pathology. The *clinical manifestations* are unusual and form a characteristic pattern. The onset is insidious. The child becomes increasingly irritable, restless and at times apathetic. The palms of the hands and soles of the feet are red and slightly swollen. This *pinkness* is accompanied by painful itching. Later the red skin desquamates. The child experiences perverted sensations, such as burning. The body presents a diffuse erythema and profuse perspiration. The cheeks and nose are pink, and the gums are red and swollen. The deciduous teeth, nails

and hair may fall out. The blood pressure is high, the pulse rate elevated. Fever is not usually present unless there is concurrent respiratory infection or pyuria.

The child's personality changes. The hyperesthesia of the skin and muscles results in dislike of and resentment at being handled.

There is a decrease in muscular activity, and the child is hypotonic. He may assume bizarre positions. The knee-chest position is characteristic. Because of photophobia he hides his face.

Anorexia results in malnutrition. Since the child perspires freely, he drinks large quantities of water. He has difficulty in sleeping, owing to severe pain.

The main *laboratory finding* is mercury in the urine.

No characteristic *pathologic changes* have been observed.

Treatment. Dimercaprol (BAL, British antilewisite) is effective against some heavy metal poisons such as mercury. It often causes undesirable side effects such as lacrimation, nausea and vomiting, salivation, headache, burning sensation, pain in the teeth, sweating, a feeling of tightness in the chest, fever, and restlessness.

Opiates are not given except in temporary emergencies for discomfort. Paraldehyde in olive oil may be given rectally to reduce discomfort. Priscoline may also be given for symptomatic relief. If respiratory infection occurs, it should be treated with antibiotics.

The diet should be high in proteins, minerals and vitamins. If anorexia is extreme, gavage feedings may be given. If a child will not drink fluids in sufficient amounts, parenteral fluid therapy may be necessary.

Nursing Care. Nursing care must be adapted to the personality changes in the individual toddler. The nurse must be firm but kind, and react to his behavior with insight into the cause. She must accept the child's reaction, knowing that it is conditioned by his sickness. She must attempt to alleviate his discomfort and anxiety. When he feels more comfortable, his reaction will be more normal.

To keep the child from injuring himself, the sides of the crib should be covered on the inside with soft pads or blankets. When he is placed in his high chair, he must wear a restraining jacket because he is likely to fall. Elbow restraints are required to prevent his chewing his fingers or pulling his hair.

Because of his profuse perspiration and to minimize the chances of a secondary pyogenic infection, the child should have frequent tub baths. The clothing should be light, preferably of cotton.

Gentle mouth care should be given to prevent infection when the gums are inflamed. Because of photophobia, the child should be protected from bright lights.

The child should be offered high vitamin fluids at frequent intervals. He should not be forced to eat, since vomiting may result. If necessary, he may be fed by the nurse or by gavage (see p. 147).

Every precaution should be taken to prevent cross-infection from contact with other children and nurses who have respiratory infections. Sedation may be needed for insomnia and to prevent exhaustion. If BAL is given, the nurse should watch for indications of undesirable effects. The child should be weighed routinely to determine weight loss.

Recreation suited to his condition should be provided. During the acute stage these children are seldom eager to play. But the child will enjoy having his nurse read aloud to him or play his favorite pieces on a record player. Recreation helps the child, and also his parents, to adjust to his condition.

Complications, Course, Prognosis and Prevention. *Complications* which may arise are pneumonia, pyuria, diarrhea and prolapse of the rectum.

The *course* of the disease may extend from several months to a year. Mortality rates are low.

Home is the best place for the acrodyniac toddler. The parents should be made familiar with the nature and the course of the disease. They must be taught how to give adequate care.

Prevention lies in avoidance of medications containing mercury and in keeping the child safe from the accidental ingestion of mercury preparations.

Lead Poisoning

Etiology, Incidence and Clinical Manifestations. Lead poisoning is most common between eighteen months and three years of age. Lead can enter the body through the gastrointestinal tract, skin or lungs. The usual route of entrance in children is through the mouth. Little children suck, or chew when teething, painted or lead toys, crib rails, window sills and furniture. (Paint on repainted wood is apt to come off in flakes.) Toddlers may chew upon painted stair railings, swings or fences, but are more likely to break off and swallow bits of dried paint from wood surfaces.

Lead may be inhaled with the fumes caused by burning storage batteries, motor fuel, or discarded cans containing lead paint, though these are seldom the causes of poisoning in the toddler group.

The *incidence* of lead poisoning appears to be increasing in the tenement areas of large cities. The walls in old buildings are likely to have layer upon layer of paint. Paints used years ago had a higher percentage of lead than paints used today. Paint for outdoor use today has more lead than that for indoor use, which has less than 1 per cent. In old buildings layers of paint come off in thick flakes which the child may put into his mouth, chew and swallow. This increase in incidence may be more apparent than real, however. Today there are fewer missed cases, because children of the lower-income group receive better health supervision than in the past.

The residual effects of lead toxicity on the nervous system may be permanent and progressive.

The *clinical manifestations* and severity depend upon the degree of cerebral irritation. The onset is insidious except in the rare cases of acute poisoning. Progressive poisoning usually occurs as the result of slow absorption or accumulation of lead in the blood and soft tissues. Lead is transferred slowly from the soft tissues to the bone. Lead is excreted in the urine.

Acute lead poisoning occurs most commonly during the summer and only after accidental ingestion of lead salts or inhalation of lead fumes. The child has nausea, vomiting, abdominal pain, convulsions and finally coma. Renal damage is common. Shock may cause death in two or three days. If the child should recover from the acute stage, chronic poisoning may follow.

The clinical manifestations of *chronic lead poisoning* depend on the degree and rate of transport of lead from the intestine or bone (lead is stored in bones) to the blood or soft tissues. In mild cases the child suffers from weakness, loss of weight, irritability and vomiting. He is pale and suffers from headache, abdominal pain, anorexia and insomnia.

Encephalitis occurs after a short period of exposure, owing to the extreme vulnerability of the child's central nervous system. Children suffering from lead poisoning are anemic, and have colic, peripheral neuritis, muscular incoordination, joint pains and a labile pulse rate. Convulsions may occur, followed by stupor and death in coma.

Diagnosis and Treatment. The *diagnosis* is suspected from the history of exposure to lead and the clinical manifestations of poisoning: roentgenographic evidence of increased density at the ends of the long bones, and the presence of radiopaque material in the abdomen indicating the ingestion of foreign substances which may contain lead, basophilic stippling of red blood cells seen on a smear, excessive concentration of lead in the urine, blood or scalp hair, excretion of coproporphyrin in the urine, a mild degree of glycosuria and, when *lead encephalopathy* is present, findings of cerebrospinal fluid under pressure and possibly containing large amounts of protein and a few cells.

The immediate *treatment* of acute lead poisoning is by gastric lavage if poisoning has resulted from the ingestion of lead, followed by catharsis with magnesium sulfate and, if necessary, specific measures to counteract shock. The child should be given milk to form insoluble salts in the intestines. To increase the excretion of lead and thereby decrease its concentration in the blood as rapidly as possible, EDTA (ethylenediamine tetra-acetic acid) may be given. This forms a nonionized chelate with lead which is excreted in the urine. EDTA is usually given by intravenous infusion; it may be administered orally, but its action is delayed when it is given by this route. BAL also causes an increase in the urinary excretion of lead and recently has been used with EDTA in therapy.

Chronic lead poisoning may follow acute poisoning if all traces of lead have not been removed before absorption takes place. For this reason, after emergency care, if there is reason to believe that absorption of lead has taken place, the treatment outlined below is given.

Chronic lead poisoning is commonly the result of taking into the body (with children almost always by ingestion) small amounts of lead over a period of time. When a child is brought to the hospital for chronic lead poisoning, it is not probable that he has ingested lead recently. Lead may be in the intestines, but is not likely to be in the stomach. For this reason lavage is not given routinely. The other measures outlined for the treatment of acute lead poisoning may be ordered. One or more courses of therapy with EDTA may be given to increase the excretion of lead from the body.

The objective of further treatment is to reduce the concentration of lead in the blood and tissues, and to promote its deposition in the bones. To promote and hasten the deposition of lead in the bones, large amounts of calcium, phosphorus and vitamin D are given. Since both electrolyte imbalance (acidosis) and infections inhibit deposition of lead in the bones, such conditions must be corrected. Treatment to prevent absorption from the intestinal tract has been outlined.

Lead colic is treated with antispasmodics such as atropine or opiates. Increased intracranial pressure may be treated medically. When *severe encephalopathy* occurs, the child will show rising blood pressure, papilledema, slow pulse, and unconsciousness. Drugs used to reduce increased intracranial pressure include urea, or mannitol given intravenously. Steroids such as Decadron may also be given. Convulsions due to encephalopathy are controlled with phenobarbital given parenterally and paraldehyde administered rectally. Increased intracranial pressure may also be reduced by repeated lumbar punctures, removing a small amount of fluid at a time to prevent brain-stem herniation. In some children surgical decompression by craniectomy may be necessary. Oxygen may be given for respiratory depression. Parenteral fluids may be administered for fluid and electrolyte imbalance. Urinary retention may be relieved by catheterization.

Treatment to delead the tissues completely takes months, but is essential to prevent recurrence of the symptoms.

Nursing Care. Nursing care is symptomatic. If the child has convulsions, all unnecessary handling should be avoided, since it may stimulate the central nervous system. Nursing care should be planned around periods when medications are to be given. The child who has increased intracranial pressure should be observed carefully for respiratory distress. His head should be elevated to decrease intracranial pressure.

The child in coma is fed by gavage. He must be turned frequently from side to side, and good skin care is essential. For collection of urine specimens the receptacle must be very clean and free from lead, because the amount of lead found in the urine is exceedingly small.

Prognosis and Prevention. The *prognosis* is generally poor. About half of the affected children have manifestations of encephalitis. The mortality rate is about 25 per cent in these cases. Many of the children who recover have permanent mental or neurologic sequelae, such as mental retardation (see p. 526). Close observation is necessary after treatment for a long time in order to prevent further damage to the central nervous system. The incidence of permanent damage to the central nervous system increases with the duration of exposure to lead.

Children who have *pica* or perverted appetite may continue to ingest lead over long periods. All possible sources of lead should be removed from their environment, and they should be closely supervised to keep them from obtaining lead from those sources which it is not feasible to remove.

Prevention is doubly important because treatment is not highly successful. Manufacturers in the United States are required to use lead-free paint on all children's toys and furniture. Amateur painters in the home, however, may repaint furniture with paint containing lead. The public is being educated constantly about the danger involved in the ingestion of paint. The public health nurse also does this in part while visiting in a home where potential sources of lead poisoning exist.

In many areas the incidence of lead poisoning must be reported to the public health department. The public health nurse then makes a visit to the home to guide the parents in removing any source of lead from the environment.

Syndromes of Cerebral Dysfunction

The term "syndrome of cerebral dysfunction" is a relatively new term which includes the diagnoses of cerebral palsy, mental retardation (see p. 526), epilepsy, autism, hyperkinetic behavior disorders and visual and auditory perceptual problems (see pp. 440 and 442). The common bond which brings these conditions together is the fact that in all these disorders intellectual impairment is often present as a reflection of poor integration or organization of the neurologic components involved. These neurologic components include neuromotor, state of consciousness, neurosensory, behavioral and perceptual. Only one of these may be found in a child, or several may be seen in one patient. Usually, since one neurologic component is outstanding for its poor organization, the clinical diagnosis is made on the basis of it.

Cerebral Palsy

Neuromuscular disability, or cerebral palsy, is the term commonly used for difficulty in controlling the voluntary muscles due to damage to some portion of the brain. There is no common cause, pattern of clinical manifestations, treatment or prognosis for such children. The problem ranges from very mild to severe. The damage is fixed, however, and does not become progressively greater. For this reason it is possible to map out a long-term program of development of those capacities which the child possesses.

Diagnosis and treatment are particularly important during the toddler period if parental attitudes are to be properly formed and the child is to have the foundation of experience necessary for normal emotional development in the years to follow. Although for many years children were treated during infancy for the physical manifestations of the condition, only recently have the intellectual and emotional aspects been studied. Proper handling of the child's intellectual and emotional development is as important as his physical care.

Incidence and Etiology. The *incidence* of the condition is from 100 to 600 cases per 100,000 population.

The specific cause is obscure. There are many causes of brain damage which result in this condition; some of these causes are clear, others are not. Damage occurring prenatally, at birth or during infancy has already been discussed. Examples of such causes of cerebral palsy are heredity, prenatal infection or anoxia, developmental malformation of the cerebrum, postnatal anoxia (see p. 181), narcosis at birth, erythroblastosis fetalis (see p. 165) with resulting kernicterus, and intracranial hemorrhage (see p. 178). Damage which may occur in infancy or the toddler period includes lead poisoning (see p. 433), head injury with subdural hematoma (see p. 352), brain damage due to febrile illness, encephalitis (see p. 490), meningitis

(see p. 494) and hydrocephalus (see p. 214). In many children no single causative factor can be established.

Diagnosis, Types and Clinical Manifestations. In some children the *diagnosis* can be made soon after birth. It is based on the following symptoms: asymmetry in motion or contour, difficulty in feeding, i.e. in sucking or swallowing, listlessness or irritability, twitching, stiffening or convulsions, vomiting, excessive or feeble crying, cyanosis or pallor, and failure to follow the normal pattern of motor development (see Chap. 12). In other children the diagnosis is not made until the toddler period, when the question of the child's normal mentality arises.

Two *types* of cerebral palsy account for about 75 per cent of all cases. They are those cases marked by either spasticity or athetosis. *Spasticity* is characterized by tension in certain muscle groups (Fig. 17-2, *A*). The stretch reflex is present in the involved muscles. This is the most common type of cerebral palsy. *Athetosis* is characterized by involuntary or excess motion (fine wandering movements) which interferes with normal precision of movement (Fig. 17-2, *B*). Various degrees of muscle tension are present.

A third type of cerebral palsy is *ataxia*, characterized by a disturbance of the sense of balance and posture. Children with this condition walk as though they were inebriated. A fourth type, marked by *rigidity,* is characterized by resistance in the extensor and flexor muscles. A fifth type is characterized by *tremor,* in which there are

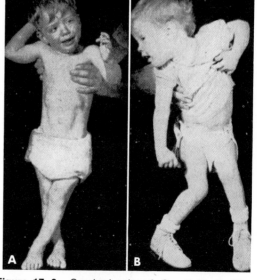

Figure 17–2. Cerebral palsy. *A,* Spasticity. *B,* Athetosis. (From Courville: Cerebral Palsy, San Lucas Press; in Cardwell: *Cerebral Palsy—Advances in Understanding and Care.* New York, Association for the Aid of Crippled Children.)

fine muscular movements with a rhythmic pattern. A sixth type is classified as *atonic*.

The *clinical manifestations* vary with the type or types of cerebral palsy present in the individual child. These children as a group are delayed in their developmental milestones such as learning to sit, walk, talk, or feed themselves. During infancy they tend to have high elevations of temperature in response to even mild infections. They tend to be long, thin infants since their weight gain is usually slow.

Spasticity is the most common evidence of motor disability. The child is unable to control the voluntary muscles, nor can the examiner control them. Certain muscle groups have abnormally strong tonus which keeps portions of the body, mostly the extremities, in characteristic positions. In severely affected children, deformity of position may occur. The child's voluntary efforts to move such muscles result in jerky motions, making walking, eating and other coordinated movements difficult. The parts of the body commonly affected are the legs, which are in a position of *scissoring* (the child crosses his legs and points his toes), the arms (the fist is clenched, the forearm flexed, the upper arm pressed against the wall of the chest) and the trunk (the head is extended and the back arched).

The spasticity varies from very mild to a severe involvement which produces a helpless child. In very severely affected children, swallowing may be difficult because of involvement of the muscles of the face, jaw, tongue and pharynx.

In some cases of spasticity, groups of muscles are weakened. Weakness may be present without spasticity, however.

Topographic designations may be identified as follows: *paraplegia* when only the legs are involved; *hemiplegia* when half the body is involved; and *quadriplegia* when all four extremities are involved. Unusual distributions include *monoplegia* when only one limb is involved or *triplegia* when both legs and one arm are involved.

Disturbances other than these physical problems may be due to brain damage, but they may be caused or accentuated by the parents' reaction to the total problem. Psychologic and emotional problems may be more hampering to the child's development than his motor difficulties. Speech, sight and hearing defects or convulsions may complicate the problem and influence the child's interaction with other members of his family and, later, with his social life in the community. There may be varying degrees of mental retardation, but this is not always an accompaniment of cerebral palsy.

The child with cerebral palsy appears to be emotionally unstable, owing primarily to his physical condition, but also to the psychologic treatment he has received. His basic human needs for acceptance, for love from his parents, his peers and others, for exploration of his environment, for play, for learning as other children do and for the feeling of status which comes through gradually increasing independence are seldom satisfied. He is therefore likely to be chronically emotionally depressed.

If the child has speech problems, he is unable to communicate orally in a normal manner, if at all, with others. If he cannot see well, he is unable to have vicarious experiences through reading or motion pictures—experiences which would enrich the limited use he is able to make of his physical and social environments. If he cannot write, he has further difficulty in establishing satisfactory relations with others. It is in the toddler period that the basis for development of what capacities he has must be laid.

Although the mentality of these children is likely to be affected, many have normal intelligence. With education and special training they may become useful citizens. Even those with intelligence below normal may be trained to earn their living or at least to provide self-care.

Treatment and Nursing Care. The *treatment* of children having cerebral palsy appears to be in a transitional stage. Newer methods of treatment are being proposed. Since there is much discussion and controversy concerning these newer methods of therapy, only the traditional treatment will be explored here.

The aim of *habilitation* is to help the child handicapped since birth to make total use of the abilities he has been able to develop and to help him establish capabilities that the normal child develops automatically. The aim of *rehabilitation* for the child who was once normal, but who because of illness now has a handicap, is to help him relearn or re-establish the abilities he had prior to his illness and to progress in as normal a way as possible. The aim in both habilitation and rehabilitation is to help each person achieve satisfaction in life to the full limit of his capacities.

If children with cerebral palsy are to develop to the fullest extent their capacity to lead normal lives, they should be under the supervision of the cerebral palsy team. This team includes the pediatrician, social worker, surgeon, orthopedist, psychologist or psychiatrist, physiotherapist, speech therapist, teachers, nurses and the child's parents.

It is difficult to identify all children with cerebral palsy during infancy and the toddler period. Such children may be found at school age, since attendance at school is compulsory. The missed children are usually in the low-income group, particularly in families in isolated rural areas. Middle-class parents seek help if they see that their child is not normal; also their children are under the care of a private physician from infancy throughout childhood. Follow-up by public health nurses of newborn infants and continued health supervision through clinics and Child Health Conferences have decreased the number of cases in which professional help has been delayed until school age.

Before treatment can be begun it is necessary to evaluate not only the child's physical condition, but also his intellectual capacity, since treatment will be determined by his needs. It is difficult to evaluate the mental capacity of a child until he is old enough to cooperate on performance tests which use motor abilities. On the best available information realistic short- and long-term programs are planned and re-evaluated as treatment progresses.

No treatment can restore a brain damaged at birth to a normal functioning level. The aim of therapy is *habilitation,* because new habits have to be established rather than lost functions replaced. The goal is to appraise individual assets and potentialities and to capitalize on these in order to create as useful and well adjusted a person as possible. Muscles must be used for new functions, and this training must be made a satisfying, rather than a frustrating, process for the child.

Parents must be helped to accept the child with his assets and liabilities while he is still an infant or as soon as the team is able to evaluate his potentialities. They need help in learning how to care for him and to feel secure in their ability to fulfill the parental role which they have learned to adapt to his needs.

Care includes planning for special problems connected with respiration, feeding, relaxation, play and education.

Problems of respiration in early life are due to cerebral lesions or to mucus in the infant's throat. Mucus can be removed by aspiration. The infant's position should be changed frequently to reduce his discomfort.

Feeding problems may be caused by difficulty in sucking and swallowing. The child may vomit easily. To help him take his feeding, he should be fed slowly. The nurse must be patient when giving him solid food, since often he cannot control the muscles of the throat. Feeding these children requires skill, acquired only by experience, and the student nurse should not be discouraged if at first she is not successful. Helping the child to learn to feed himself is even more difficult. He needs a spoon and a blunt fork (if he is able to control his hand adequately) with special handles so that he can grasp them readily (Fig. 17-3). The plate should be attached to the table so that he does not push it about when he attempts to get food on his spoon or fork.

Problems of relaxation have a special meaning for these children, who are under a constant

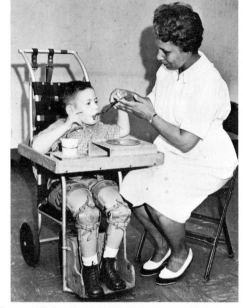

Figure 17–3. An ataxic quadriplegic child learns spoon feeding with the help of a recreationist. Adaptations for this child include a bowl holder, a glass holder and straw, and a built-up spoon handle. (United Cerebral Palsy.)

strain even when attempting to perform the simple acts others carry out unconsciously without giving attention to their movements. Although palsied children tire easily, they find it difficult to relax. They need frequent rest periods in a quiet room with few stimuli of any sort. They should not be excited before rest time or bedtime. The administration of tranquilizers to these children helps to relieve tension and thus promotes relaxation.

These children must be disciplined with understanding. If they feel secure and relaxed, they have far better control over their movements than if they are nervous, angry or afraid. The adult who can be firm, but not rejecting, in her manner and words not only wins their cooperation, but also provides the social environment in which they are physically able to cooperate. The child's success in muscular control reduces his frustration. The palsied child is happier with adults who set limits within which he can function successfully and is thereby less likely to arouse irritation in others. Relaxation is for him a skill which must be learned. After he has learned to relax he can learn purposeful motions which enable him to get the results he desires.

Play problems are many, but can be met successfully. No child leads a normal life if he does not play. But play with these children must be gentle, without excitement, involving only slow changes in stimulation. Mothers and nurses must show creativity and ingenuity in finding toys which will be safe for him and also have educational value, which foster learning, and encourage self-expression or help in social interaction with other children. When he reaches school age, it is important for him to play in groups so that he will make friends and learn to interact successfully with his peers. He should feel that he is their equal, even if he cannot do all that they do and makes uncouth blunders which interfere with play. Some mothers are afraid to permit their handicapped children to play away from them for fear that they will become lost. Proper identification in the form of a pin, chain or bracelet locket or a metal "dog tag" is important for any handicapped child away from his parents.

Education includes training in self-care and social relations as well as formal education. It should begin in nursery school, if not earlier, and must be adjusted to the child's capacity so that he has joy in achieving what is expected of him. When he enters grade school, his work must be adjusted to his mental capacity as well as to his physical limitations. In most cities there are special schools, or special classes in the regular schools, for handicapped children. In these classes or schools, teachers plan the educational programs to meet the needs of small groups of children who have somewhat similar abilities. These schools provide for muscle reeducation and physical therapy and often psychologic help for the child who has emotional problems.

The cerebral palsy team may give other forms of therapy either at the school or in conjunction with the school program. Children whose handicap is not too great may attend the regular school classes, or be in special classes for some subjects and in the regular classes for other subjects in which they can be taught with normal children. When education is adapted to individual potential, the child can gain security from being with normal children. Possibly he may excel in some area of study. Working with other children will help to eliminate feelings of inferiority and self-pity. If the child has difficulty in articulation, speech training will be necessary.

One advantage of the special school or classes is that the furniture is designed so that these children can work in comfort.

HOSPITALIZATION. When a child is admitted to the hospital with the diagnosis of cerebral palsy, the nurses who care for him should learn from his mother the methods of care she has used for him at home. Such information when utilized by the nurse will not only produce a less traumatic transition from care in the home to care in the hospital for the child, but will also provide the nurse with knowledge that she may utilize in the nursing care of other patients.

Parents may need help in meeting the problems connected with hospitalization of the child. Long-term hospitalization is a financial drain upon the income of the average family. When hospitalization is necessary, the parents, even if they carry hospitalization insurance, may be unable to pay the full hospital and medical bills and still maintain the family level of living which is essential for the other children in the family, as well as for the sick child when he returns home. Such parents are referred to the social worker, who will arrange for financial assistance from a state or community agency.

Parents may not understand why the child must be hospitalized, the treatment he will need or how long he must be away from home. They may be unwilling to leave him in the hospital because they think that he, more than a normal child, will suffer from maternal deprivation. The nurse can do a great deal to help the parents view the child's condition realistically.

Life in the pediatric unit of a general hospital or in a children's hospital should be planned for emotional growth as well as physical improvement of the children. Absence from home may be made a maturing experience, particularly if these children have been overprotected at home.

The physical care of children with cerebral palsy includes the prevention of contractures. This is difficult for the parents to understand. They have tried to make the child as comfortable as possible by allowing him to assume any position and maintain it for as long as he wanted. A qualified physiotherapist should teach parents how to carry out passive stretching exercises depending on the specific needs of the child. Corrective splints may be ordered. Usually these are applied only at night, but leg splints may be used during the day to enable the child to stand.

Appliances can be used in the home and the hospital to help these children lead as normal a life as possible. If the child has difficulty in sitting erect or maintaining his balance, he may need a high-backed chair which has arms and a foot platform. If he still cannot maintain his balance, he may require straps to hold him in the chair securely. Such a chair can be converted to a wheelchair by the addition of wheels and handles on the back. Special equipment is available to enable the child to feed himself. Such equipment includes spoons with large straight or bent handles, plates with rims and suction cups on the bottom to prevent slipping, and covered cups with a hole in the lid through which to insert a drinking tube.

Surgical treatment for orthopedic deformities may be necessary. This may involve the severing of nerves leading to the spastic extremities, lengthening of the tendon of Achilles or other procedure to improve the child's muscular control.

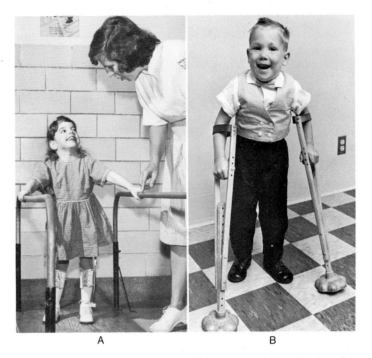

Figure 17–4. Learning to walk. *A,* To educate legs to walk properly, parallel bars and perhaps a small flight of steps are brought into play. The physiotherapist helps this child to achieve the goal of the health team. (Courtesy of the National Society for Crippled Children and Adults, Chicago, Illinois.) *B,* "Kenny sticks" with enlarged crutch tips. (Courtesy of Rehabilitation Institute of The Boston Dispensary, and F. H. Krusen: *Handbook of Physical Medicine and Rehabilitation.*)

A   B

If the child has had a cast applied, the nursing care is that of other patients in casts (see p. 227). If he has not achieved control of bladder and bowel, he may be placed on a Bradford frame (see p. 210). Braces may be used to enable the spastic child to control his motions or to correct his deformity. Medical treatment may include drugs to decrease nervous tension or a tendency to convulsions. Physiotherapy is important to prevent contractures and stimulate control of movement.

Public health nurses and hospital nurses are members of the health team caring for children with cerebral palsy. The team serves the children in their homes, in hospitals, schools and summer camps. Nurses help mothers learn how to give the daily care the child needs and to interpret his needs to other members of the family and to his teachers. As the child grows older his contacts outside the home increase. Even the toddler is admitted to some nursery schools for handicapped children, and older children go to camp in the summer and join play groups planned particularly for them. Nurses contact professional workers and help them to coordinate these special services with the general plan of treatment made by the cerebral palsy team for the individual child.

In large cities there are organizations which offer guidance to the parents of children with cerebral palsy. The nurse works closely with the staff of such an organization. Many of these organizations provide group play for children and vocational training for adolescents. Each year more such groups are supporting research

on the causes and treatment of cerebral palsy and providing funds for the application of research findings to the habilitation and education of these children.

Prognosis. The prognosis depends upon the severity of the physical condition, the child's

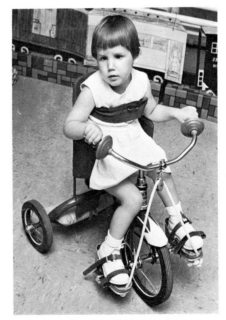

Figure 17–5. Tricycle with back, chest strap, foot plates and pulley system to prevent plantar flexion. (Courtesy of the Minneapolis Curative Workshop, and F. H. Krusen: *Handbook of Physical Medicine and Rehabilitation.*)

mental capacity and the treatment available. Private, state and community programs for these children vary in quality and extent of service, and the prognosis in any case must take into consideration the treatment the child will receive. In general the child with normal intelligence who receives adequate care improves to the extent that he can care for himself and can possibly succeed in a vocation or profession suited to his limitations.

Summary. The role of the nurse includes helping to prevent cerebral palsy, helping to detect it once it has occurred, and helping to provide optimum care for the affected children in cooperation with other members of the cerebral palsy team. The objective in care is that each child develop his potential capacity. In a physically and socially favorable environment many children develop a healthy personality. The foundation is laid during the toddler period. These children must be helped to face reality, to accept themselves objectively, if they are to make a successful adjustment to the problems caused by their handicaps. A child's attitude toward himself and his relations with other people are formed in early childhood, and successful adjustment in adolescence and adulthood is conditioned by his experiences while still a little child. Adults are tempted to make life easy for him rather than helping him face his problems, solve them and go on to the more complex experiences which come with maturation. He needs help with the developmental tasks which come with growing up. Finally he must face the responsibilities of adulthood. If it is possible, he will want to support himself; if he cannot be self-supporting, he must accept support from others. To assume total self-care gives him a feeling of security and of self-respect. He must adjust to his sexual role in life and to the degree of emancipation from his family which is advisable in his condition.

Deafness

Importance of the Problem. Care of the deaf child is a comprehensive problem which requires teamwork for its solution. There are degrees of deafness. Complete bilateral deafness is an extreme handicap. The deaf miss all the pleasure of sound and are without the natural means of communicating with others.

Deafness may not be recognized until the child fails to develop speech or is unable to relate himself to others in the family. If the infant fails to respond to loud noises, the acuity of his hearing should be investigated. A child of twelve months who has ceased to vocalize or one of eighteen months who neither speaks nor recognizes words should be examined for deafness.

Unilateral deafness is different from bilateral deafness and may not be suspected until some accidental occurrence calls the mother's attention to the child's inability to hear in the affected ear. Unilateral deafness, whether partial or complete, should be treated with the same care given in bilateral deafness. The child is, of course, not so seriously hampered in his social relations as is the totally deaf child.

Deafness, whether partial or complete, may cause behavior problems and poor adjustment in group relations. Children who are deaf and have no means of communication may become physically aggressive and unmanageable. They may be alert children with normal or above average intelligence and may be remarkably dextrous.

Etiology and Diagnosis. Deafness may be congenital, owing to anomalies of the ear, or acquired as the result of disease or injury to the auditory nerve or auditory center in the brain. Diseases causing deafness include congenital rubella, congenital syphilis (see p. 185), meningococcal meningitis (see p. 494), encephalitis (see p. 490) and serious chronic otitis media (see p. 289).

Early *diagnosis* is essential. A hearing examination is one of the battery of tests used in institutions participating in the Collaborative Project (see p. 162). Congenital deafness, if complete, is generally recognized in infancy. Unilateral or partial bilateral deafness may not be recognized until the toddler period, when it may be discovered during a routine physical examination (Fig. 17-6). Infants and young children may be tested in a crude manner for their ability to hear. Usually a toy is given to the child. The examiner then stands behind or to the side of the child and produces noise with a buzzer, rattle or other type of noisemaker. A child who hears well will turn toward the sound and forget his play. A deaf child will make no response. In children who are not under health supervision, deafness may not be found until a health examination in nursery or grade school is done. The more refined monoaural tests used at this age level include pure tone and speech audiometric tests. These tests should be done at all frequencies in a sound-proof room. Detection of impaired hearing by routine audiometric tests should be part of the school health examination and repeated every three years. The school nurse or public health nurse may give these tests. When the child has 70 per cent or less of normal hearing, he cannot hear all that the teacher or his classmates say. He needs special help in order to cover the same amount of material as other children.

Treatment. Members of the health team necessary for successful treatment of the deaf or partially deaf child are the physician, otologist, audiologist, speech therapist, possibly psychol-

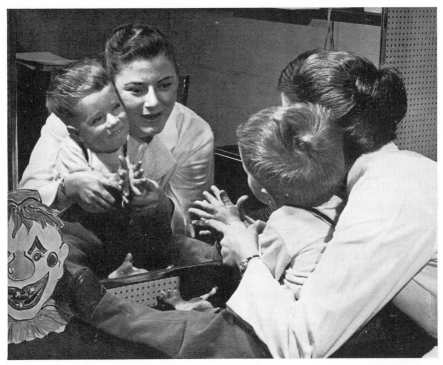

Figure 17–6. The child's speech and hearing are evaluated. Gross hearing tests are followed by audiometric testing if hearing loss is suspected. (From M. Stewart: Role of the Nurse in Pediatric Rehabilitation. *Health News,* Vol. 33.)

ogist or psychiatrist, social worker, nurse, the child's family and the child himself.

Early detection of deafness is necessary for proper speech development and for emotional growth. Training is necessary in understanding the facial expression which goes with words of approval or disapproval, of permission or denial, and in lip reading. Lip reading may start as early as 2½ or three years of age, the period when a child normally learns to talk in sentences. A specialist in lip reading and in speaking seldom begins her work until the child is of nursery school age. The mother should learn to move her lips correctly when speaking in order to supplement the work of the specialist in lip reading. A hearing aid may be provided for the child at a very early age.

Parents are given instruction in the care of their deaf children, and conferences are held in which they can receive help with particular problems.

If deafness is due to recurrent otitis media (see p. 289) or blockage of the eustachian tube, the services of the otologist should be procured.

If there is a serious hearing loss, special education may be necessary. Nursery schools have been organized for deaf children in many communities, and speech training is often given in connection with them. In some communities instruction in lip reading must be postponed

until school age, since there are no facilities for younger children. The sign or finger language may be taught to supplement lip reading. Training to communicate with others lays the founda-

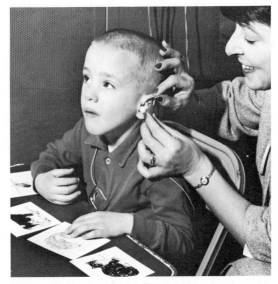

Figure 17–7. A child is fitted with a hearing aid, which will open to him the world of sound. (Irene B. Bayer and the New York League for the Hard of Hearing.)

tion for vocational or professional training or for manual labor, skilled or unskilled, in industry.

Deaf children should be treated as normal children in all respects except their one great handicap; they are normal children who have a hearing loss. Adults who work with them must be patient. Until the child learns to communicate by speech, signs must be used or, if he has learned to write, signs supplemented with written words.

Role of the Nurse. The nurse helps in discovering deafness or impaired hearing in the infants and children brought to the clinic or Child Health Conference. The school nurse often gives the routine tests for impaired hearing. If a child who has been ill appears to have difficulty in understanding what is said in class, the teacher may send him to the nurse for testing. The school nurse routinely sees children who are known to have impaired hearing so that she may supervise the physician's program of treatment. Nurses work closely with the personnel of special classes and special schools for the deaf. In clinics for deaf children and those who are hard of hearing, nurses have direct contact with both the child and his mother.

Prognosis. The prognosis for the improvement or cure of deafness depends on the degree and nature of the pathologic state or structural defect and on whether the child receives optimum treatment. How well a hearing aid and training in lip reading may overcome his physical handicap depends on the availability of such devices and the services of a specialist in teaching deaf children to communicate through speech. If the community does not furnish such help, the child may attend a state school for the deaf or a privately supported institution.

If the prognosis is defined in terms of ability to lead a normal life, then for most deaf children it is excellent. This assumes that deafness is their only handicap. If the child is blind as well as deaf or has low mentality, the prognosis is poorer for social adjustment.

Prevention. The prevention of acquired deafness consists in the prevention of infectious disease which is likely to involve the ear. Respiratory infections are a common example. It is difficult, if not impossible, to prevent all infections, but prompt treatment can be given in all cases of upper respiratory tract infections and otitis media.

Impacted cerumen (wax) impairs hearing and may lead to a lesion of the ear. The wax should be removed by the physician. Sinus infection and infected lymphoid tissue in the nasopharynx should be treated promptly. Drugs which endanger the eighth nerve should not be used indiscriminately.

Relatively few cases of deafness in children are caused by injury. Nevertheless the eardrum can be injured when a child puts something sharp into his ear. Injury to the external ear has little effect on hearing. Injury to the brain can affect the centers of hearing and speech.

Blindness

Etiology and Importance of the Problem. The child may be born blind or may acquire blindness from retrolental fibroplasia (see p. 150), trauma, infection during delivery, ophthalmia neonatorum (see p. 184) or congenital syphilis (see p. 185). Other conditions causing blindness in childhood are numerically of relatively little importance.

Children having visual difficulty may rub their eyes frequently, may squint or frown when trying to see at a distance, or may hold their picture books too close to their eyes when trying to see nearby.

The legal definition of *blindness* is based on a visual acuity of at best 20/200 in the better eye after correction. *Partially* blind children have a visual acuity between 20/70 and 20/200 in the better eye after appropriate correction. Children, like adults, have *myopia* (nearsightedness), *hyperopia* (farsightedness) or *astigmatism* (variation in the refractive power of the various meridians of the eye resulting in a distorted image).

Children who are blind or have extremely poor vision require special education and training for daily life activities. Their condition may be improved by medical or surgical procedures and the use of glasses. They may need help in acquiring the everyday skills needed in self-care. Instruction must be given through the sense of hearing or touch. If the child has normal mentality, he is able to take the same subjects in school as normal children do, although his progress may be slower than theirs. Without the same education that normal children receive, the blind child does not grow up with the interests, attitudes and abilities that the sighted possess.

Treatment. The physical condition is treated, if possible, in order to restore or improve sight or to prevent further impairment of vision.

The totally blind child of school age should be enrolled in a school for the blind or, in a school for normal children, in a special class for children with visual problems. Special classes have been established in public and private schools for children whose vision is so poor that they cannot profit from the regular school system of instruction. These schools emphasize the use of auditory instruction and the development of reading skills through touch perception by the Braille system (Fig. 17-8). For children who are not totally blind books are printed with extra large type so that eye fatigue is minimized. Good lighting and correct posture are emphasized.

Children who have some vision may attend regular classes if a teacher skilled in working

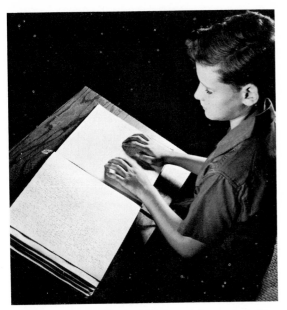

Figure 17–8. A blind child learns to read Braille. (H. Armstrong Roberts.)

with blind children gives them help when it is needed. Such contact tends to develop skill in making friends and joining in the activities of the sighted. Being one of the normal group promotes normal social and emotional development.

Parents must be instructed in the needs of their blind children. Blindness at birth or developing early in childhood prevents the child from knowing what others mean by colors he cannot see and objects he cannot handle (e.g. the sun, a river or a baby robin). The mother should use such words in context so that the child gets some idea of the meaning. Blind children need to handle as much of their environment as is practical and build up concepts which other children acquire by sight. They can handle modeling clay, play-dough, can weave or paint to learn to "feel". They can hear bells, music boxes and record players in order to hear "sound." If these children have been protected from hurting themselves while exploring the world about them, meeting their own needs and doing what gives them pleasure, they acquire a skill in self-help which children blinded later in life seldom acquire.

Parents must be helped to understand the special care required by the blind or partially sighted child. The tendency is to overprotect him. They find it hard to give him the freedom he must have to build up skills and experience which are necessary when he reaches adolescence and must prepare himself for adult life. Vocational training is given the blind, and for those who are capable and desire it a higher education and preparation for the professions which are open to them. Scholarships and main-

tenance are provided from private or public sources if the student is in need of financial assistance.

Role of the Nurse. Early detection of impaired vision or of blindness is essential for the treatment and education of the child. Infants who do not reach for their bottle or toys and do not smile when the mother smiles should be examined for blindness. A toddler who walks into the furniture, has no interest in even large pictures and does not respond to the motions of other people should have his eyesight tested by a physician. Undetected cases of blindness are rare since facilities for health supervision of children in all economic classes have improved, and since physicians and nurses test for vision, using the Snellen E chart for young children as part of the routine physical examinations given in Child Health Conferences and children's clinics, and the Snellen Chart for children who can read in school.

The blind child needs happiness as all children do and is more dependent than normal children upon the moods of the adults about him. The nurse working with blind children knows that they can interpret her moods by the inflection of her voice as other children do by seeing her smile or frown. She should express quiet happiness in her voice. She must let blind children handle all equipment to be used in their examination or treatments, as well as giving verbal explanations.

Community Action. Community action depends upon the attitude of the people in the community toward blindness. Like parents, the community may tend to overprotect the child. Part

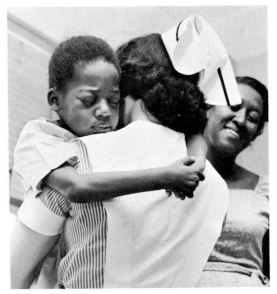

Figure 17–9. A blind child feels secure in her nurse's arms. (Dallas Services for Blind Children.)

of the nurse's responsibility for blind children is to channel the community's sympathy for them into helpful activities.

In some communities play groups for children of preschool age have been organized in which blind children can enjoy play with others like themselves. The playground and the equipment are suited to their needs, and adequate supervision is provided. Such play helps these children to make social adjustments, which serve as a basis for contacts with the sighted and which can be developed into a normal ability to participate in group activities.

Prognosis. The outcome of treatment varies with every child, and no general statements can be made. Great strides are being made in the prevention of blindness from gonorrhea and syphilis, and with improved care of premature infants there are very few cases of blindness due to retrolental fibroplasia.

The prognosis for mental health is good. The child who is born blind can usually make a happier adjustment to his handicap than a child who becomes blind later because of an infection or injury to his eyes. Parent-child relations are more important than any measure which the community can take to help the blind child. But it is the community which provides education and gives the blind person a position in industry or uses his professional services. Children with impaired vision may become self-supporting adults fulfilling all the roles of a normal adult. The totally blind find it more difficult to function in society. Their success depends to a great extent upon their early training.

The Chronically Handicapped Child

Parents of chronically physically or mentally handicapped children should be taught that these children need an environment in which they develop their capacities to the limit, and that the most important element in this environment is the sense of security which loving parents give their children.

Parents may need both financial help and expert counsel in fulfilling their exacting role. It is not easy to be a "perfect parent" to a crippled child. The children also must be helped to grow up normally. Severe personality handicaps interfere with their social adjustment more than their physical condition limits successful social interaction. A child acquires emotional problems as a result of deprivation of emotional satisfactions and lack of opportunity to use, and so to develop, his capacities.

It takes months or years for parents to recover from the shock and frustration of having a child who is not normal. They also fear the additional responsibilities involved in care, and perhaps most of all they fear society's attitude toward them and the child. Anxiety and hostility conflict with their normal love for him.

Such a child disturbs not only parent-child relations, but also all other relations between the members of the family. Parents may manage their feelings in various ways with various reactions on the part of the child. They may deny the existence of his handicap or overprotect him to cover up their negative feelings toward him. Since contact with him causes them anxiety, they may openly reject him and thus not give him the love and security he needs, nor the status of a loved child in the home or that part of the community outside his home where he is learning to adjust to strangers.

Parents may ignore his cues for readiness to learn because they cannot regard him as a person or because they overprotect him. The child therefore does not develop to his potential level. He may even regress.

Help is given to the parents by the whole team of specialists in the crippled children's program: physician, social worker, psychologist or psychiatrist, nurse and others, depending on the child's problem. The nurse must understand normal parent-child relations, the normal developmental process and the needs of the child. She must know how to support parents in accepting problems caused by the child's handicaps, and finally she needs to know the parents well enough to give help when they are ready to accept it. To teach a mother techniques of care before she is ready to learn produces frustration and failure.

The nurse can be a great help to parents when they are discouraged. She must believe in their capacity to care for the child and to give him love and a sense of security. She must communicate to them, not necessarily in words, but by her manner, that she understands their feelings and wants to provide support and assistance.

The nurse must help parents see that their responsibility is to help the child to grow up and to develop his capacity, however little it may be, for self-help in daily living. Other professional workers have the function of educating the child and giving him many of the pleasures which normal children enjoy, e.g. going to camp in summer. But it is the parents who give the child experience in daily life within a family. In order to help the parents in their task the nurse must know the evaluation which the total team makes of the child's potential ability. Without such knowledge she cannot communicate realistic goals toward which the parents and the child can work.

The child's response to the help given him is the final test of its success. If the handicapped child feels that his parents are anxious and frustrated, he will feel unloved and may withdraw into a world of fantasy, never developing to his potential level. Some of these children feel only pity for themselves, some try to hurt others as they have been hurt, and others seek punishment for their own negative feelings.

Children who feel loved and wanted are motivated to overcome the limitations of their handicaps or to compensate through success in activities within their ability. These children are likely to succeed beyond what could be expected of them. The handicapped child does not need pity or sympathy. He needs understanding and a knowledge that others accept his differences and accord him status as an equal.

The nurse must be aware of her own feelings. If she feels repugnance or fear, she should not be ashamed, for most people have the same feelings toward these children. The first step in changing these feelings to a more positive attitude is to know that they exist.

Emotional Disturbances

When a toddler appears anxious, the conflict between his instinctual desires and the demands of his environment is becoming too much for him to endure. Indications of anxiety at his age are refusal to go to bed, "jittery" behavior during the day, restless sleep at night and disturbance of bowel and bladder functioning.

Toilet training is an acute source of anxiety to many children. Children who have achieved bowel and bladder control may have accidents or may play with feces after they have once discontinued this habit. If a child has been too severely trained, he may become afraid of moving his bowels, with the result that he becomes constipated. Constipation may also develop because he is negativistic toward his mother when she has done something he dislikes.

Feeding problems may result from a child's anxiety over toilet training. The child may regress to infantile pleasures in feeding, e.g. sucking.

Stuttering may develop as part of this general pattern of regression. The child adopts the infantile way of breathing; his respirations may become irregular, and he catches his breath. This sort of respiration produces difficulty in speaking clearly, and stuttering may result. This anxiety reaction has its inception in a sudden fright or shock which produces a startle reflex accompanied by catching of the breath.

Some toddlers, instead of regressing, may appear to grow up suddenly. One evidence of this is masturbation rather than the momentary handling of the genitalia seen in infancy. Some toddlers as a result of too severe toilet training become overclean, not wanting to displease mother by soiling themselves in any way.

A toddler who becomes too anxious over the conflicting desires he experiences will not be able to develop satisfying love relations with an adult, nor a sense of autonomy, which is of vital importance. He will, instead, be overcome by shame and by doubt of his own ability. He should be helped to develop a real love for his mother. She should encourage him to take part in activities which he regards as dirty – playing with mud, sand, plasticine and finger paints. She should laughingly praise him for getting dirty when it results from play. If he gets dirty as a means of evincing hostility toward his mother, she should accept this hostility as normal in children of his age, in the same way that she accepts his immature love responses.

Adequate *treatment* of anxiety should be instituted early in life so that the prevailing mood during childhood may be happy and emotional development normal. Untreated, the anxiety of a child is cumulative. It becomes a habitual reaction which may persist into adult life.

Crippled Children's Services in the United States

There are more than 5,500,000 crippled children in the United States known to official agencies. Many others are receiving care elsewhere, and still others are receiving no care. The objective of the *Program of the Crippled Children's Services* of the Children's Bureau is to help each state improve services for locating children having a handicap and for providing them with care. Every state and territory has an official program for their help, generally within the health department. Programs are also developing around medical centers, where personnel needed to help the children are taught by specialists and where research is a principal part of the program. Regional clinics are developed in connection with these centers.

A well run program combines (1) locating crippled children, (2) treatment (correction if possible), (3) management to promote adaptation to their handicaps and to limit the influence of disabilities upon their lives, and (4) prevention of circumstances in which crippling is likely to occur, e.g. safe delivery of the newborn, immunization for poliomyelitis and prevention of accidents. There is also a secondary aim of attempting to prevent the difficulties in physical, mental, social and economic areas of living caused by the condition of the child – difficulties which may involve the entire family and even the community.

Programs for crippled children are broad, covering almost any condition which is a serious handicap in normal living. Each state decides what types of children are to be eligible for assistance under the crippled children's program. Programs often include the following: hearing defects, rheumatic fever, heart disease (congenital or rheumatic), certain eye defects, and epilepsy. The reasons for the extension of coverage are that there are now fewer children having orthopedic problems and conditions requiring plastic surgery, and new forms of management have been found for children for whom treatment was formerly unknown.

The first phase in these programs is locating crippled children. Certainly the public health nurse is assuming more of a responsible role in the case finding and referral of children for care. Necessary treatment follows, either in the agency sponsoring the program or through referral to another agency which can meet the child's needs. The crippled children's team works with the child, and the community is organized to give many forms of assistance. The public not only gives financial aid for crippled children, but also supports, through its vote, the crippled children's program in the state, county and city. The children are provided for in the public school system, and in some localities special teachers may be sent to the home if the child is confined to bed.

The modern type of service may produce heavier case loads, for more emphasis is placed upon coordination of effort with attempts toward more comprehensive patient care. The newer approach brings together all the resources of the community in prevention, treatment and education. Under this program the child lives as normal a life as is possible and is helped to form positive attitudes toward himself and his problem.

CLINICAL SITUATIONS

When Joanne was fifteen months old, Mrs. Wood brought her to the Child Health Conference and complained that her appetite was poor compared with what it had been during infancy. Joanne appeared healthy and was an extremely active child.

1. In discussing Joanne's apparent anorexia with her mother, the nurse would base her comments on the fact that
   a. Since Joanne is not growing as rapidly as she did during infancy, she should not be expected to eat as much.
   b. Probably Joanne's anorexia is due to the fact that Mrs. Wood had stopped giving her vitamins when she was a year old.
   c. Perhaps Joanne should have a complete physical examination by the physician.
   d. Perhaps Mrs. Wood should be more firm in urging her to eat.

2. Joanne must have her basic emotional needs met if she is to develop a healthy personality. During the toddler period she should have
   a. Unlimited opportunity to do whatever she wants and as much independence as she desires.
   b. Recognition as a little child and protection from harm through rigid obedience to parental rules.
   c. Realistic limits set on her behavior by her parents and increasing independence as she is ready for it.
   d. Recognition as a miniature adult who is able to set limits on her own behavior.

3. Joanne's social development is best described by stating that she prefers to play
   a. Alone, but will share her toys and makes friends quickly with strangers.
   b. Alone, but refuses to share her toys and is shy with strangers.
   c. With other children, usually shares her toys and makes friends quickly with strangers.
   d. With other children, refuses to share her toys and is shy with strangers.

4. The accident rate is high during the toddler period because
   a. Parents tend to neglect children at this age.
   b. Their natural curiosity and acitivity lead them into danger.
   c. They do not comprehend their parents' warnings of danger.
   d. They are negativistic about everything and refuse to listen to their parents.

One day while Joanne was climbing up the cellar steps she fell from the top landing to the cellar floor. On her admission to the hospital the physician made a diagnosis of a fractured right femur and multiple bruises.

5. Joanne was placed in Bryant traction. In order to maintain traction, the nurse's most important responsibility was to make certain that
   a. Joanne's hips were resting on the bed and her legs were suspended at right angles to the bed.
   b. Joanne's hips were slightly elevated from the bed and her legs were suspended at right angles to the bed.
   c. Joanne's hips were elevated above the level of her body on a pillow and that her legs were suspended in a position of comfort almost parallel to the bed.
   d. Joanne's hips and legs were flat on the bed with the pull of traction coming from the foot of the bed.

6. In order to prevent Joanne from turning to watch activity on the unit, the nurse would
   a. Apply an abdominal restraint and have other children come to her bed to play with her.
   b. Apply clove hitch restraints to her arms and move her bed so that she could watch television.
   c. Apply a restraint jacket and move her bed so that she could watch other children.
   d. Apply no restraints, but move her bed near the center of the unit so that she could watch the activities of the unit personnel.

Mrs. McIntyre called her pediatrician and explained that Betty Jane, age 2½ years, had had a slight cold for two days, but that within the last few hours she seemed to have increasingly difficult respirations and was extremely restless. After examining the child the physician recommended immediate admission to the hospital. She was admitted with a diagnosis of laryngotracheobronchitis.

7. Betty Jane was placed in a Croupette. Cool moist air is effective treatment of this condition because it

a. Causes dilatation of blood vessels in the bronchi, thus relieving the congestion.

b. Increases the cough reflex, thus making it easier to expectorate mucus.

c. Coagulates the mucus, thus relieving the dyspnea.

d. Relieves the dryness of secretions, making them easier to cough up.

8. Betty Jane became emotionally disturbed when her mother said that she was going home. You as the nurse would suggest that the mother

a. Omit visiting for a few days until Betty Jane adjusted to the hospital routine.

b. Visit only when Betty Jane was sleeping so that she would not disturb the child.

c. Visit as often and as frequently as she could within the hospital visiting policy.

d. Discipline the child because her crying is harmful to her.

Since Betty Jane's respiratory distress became more severe and she showed signs of increasing prostration, an emergency tracheotomy was performed.

9. Immediately after the operation the nurse aspirated Betty Jane's tracheostomy tube

a. As often as secretion appeared at the opening of the tube.

b. Approximately every fifteen minutes.

c. Whenever Betty Jane appeared to have difficulty in breathing.

d. Whenever Betty Jane requested that it be done.

10. Betty Jane was afraid to try to swallow after the tracheotomy had been done. The nurse

a. Offered small amounts of her favorite fruit juice or other liquid at frequent intervals and gave approval when she drank it.

b. Explained to her that she would get a "needle" if she did not take some juice by mouth.

c. Told her that her father would give her a dime for every cup of fluid she drank.

d. Told her she would read a long story to her each time she took a cup of juice.

11. When the nurse aspirated Betty Jane's tracheostomy, she cleaned the inner cannula

a. By running hot tap water through it and aspirating secretions from it with a catheter.

b. By soaking it in an antibiotic solution and cleaning the outside with a detergent.

c. By soaking it in hydrogen peroxide and passing tonsil wire and gauze through it.

d. By running cold tap water through it and wiping it off with petrolatum.

12. The nurse on one occasion found that Betty Jane had torn off the elbow restraints and had succeeded in pulling out the tracheostomy tube. She was cyanotic, and respirations had apparently ceased. The nurse

a. Went immediately to the telephone to call the physician, held open the incision with a hemostat and gave mouth-to-mouth resuscitation.

b. Inserted another tracheostomy tube into the trachea, aspirated the trachea, asked another nurse to call a physician, and gave oxygen through a nasal catheter.

c. Inserted another tracheostomy tube immediately, asked another nurse to call the physician, gave oxygen through a nasal catheter and provided artificial respiration.

d. Asked another nurse to call the physician, held open the incision with a hemostat, aspirated the trachea, provided oxygen through the incision, and gave artificial respiration.

13. When Betty Jane was well enough to play in bed, the nurse would assume, on the basis of her understanding of growth and development, that Betty Jane would enjoy

a. Playing with her favorite toy.

b. Constructing a tower of twenty blocks.

c. Listening to popular songs on the radio.

d. Stringing small beads.

Roosevelt Jones, a two-year-old child, was admitted to the pediatric unit with a diagnosis of chronic lead poisoning. His mother stated that he had eaten paint periodically from his crib and from the window sills over a period of several weeks.

14. Roosevelt should be observed carefully by the nurse for

a. Hemorrhage from the rectum.

b. Convulsions.

c. Edema of the extremities.

d. Respiratory difficulty.

15. Roosevelt responded well to treatment. One day when the nurse was bathing him, he said, "My mommy does it *this* way." His comment indicates that

a. He does not like the way the nurse gives a sponge bath.

b. Routines or rituals learned at home are important to him.

c. His mother gives a bath better than the nurse.

d. He hates his nurse.

16. The nurse found Roosevelt in the bathroom, splashing in the water in the toilet. The nurse should

a. Slap his hands and remove him from the room.

b. Explain that children should not play in such dirty water.

c. Give him a basin of clean water in which to splash.

d. Take him back to his unit and lock the bathroom door.

17. During his nap Roosevelt wet his bed. The nurse would

a. Change his clothes and bedding and make no issue of it.

b. Tell him that he will catch cold if he lies in a wet bed.

c. Promise to give him a piece of candy if he has no further accidents.

d. Explain that only babies wet their beds.

18. Roosevelt had frequent temper tantrums during his hospitalization. The best way to deal with them would be to

a. Punish him by putting him back in his crib for the rest of the day.

b. Reason with him and tell him why he should not become angry.

c. Prevent temper tantrums by pampering him.

d. Protect him during his tantrums and attempt to

prevent them by helping him meet necessary frustrations.

19. The care which Roosevelt should have after a temper tantrum is

a. Ignore him for the rest of the day because he has been a "bad-boy."

b. Wash his face and hands and provide a toy for him.

c. Make fun of him before other children in his group.

d. Make him apologize for his behavior.

20. After a prolonged period of hospitalization Roosevelt became a quiet, withdrawn child who evidenced little interest in his mother when she visited. The nurse should realize that

a. He has accepted his hospitalization well and has matured because of his experience.

b. He has finally been disciplined, and she would expect gratitude from his parents.

c. He had probably become a very disturbed little boy because of his traumatic experience.

d. He was ready to be toilet-trained because he seemed to enjoy playing with his feces.

GUIDES FOR FURTHER STUDY

1. During your experience in the pediatric unit observe the motor development of as many toddlers as you can. Compare the similarities and differences among the children in each age group: fifteen months, eighteen months, two years and 2½ years.

2. Investigate the resources in your community for the dissemination of information about the treatment of children who have taken poison. If your community has a Poison Control Center, familiarize yourself with its functions. If your community does not have such a facility, discuss with your instructor in seminar your role as a citizen and a nurse in meeting this need.

3. Prepare a plan which you could use to teach a mother the home care of a toddler who has had a tracheotomy. In addition to the content and skills she would need to know, investigate the sources and the approximate cost of the equipment she would need to provide this care.

4. Prepare and give a twenty-minute talk on "Accident Prevention" to a small group of mothers of toddlers in your community. Provide pamphlets and a bibliography for them on this subject. Allow time for discussion at the end of your presentation. Make a list of questions which these mothers asked and submit them with your answers to your instructor.

5. What measures are taken to prevent the spread of staphylococcal infections in your hospital?

6. Investigate the programs and services (public and private) offered for crippled children in your state and community. Discuss in seminar the adequacy of these programs in relation to the need for them.

7. List the functions of the health team members who coordinate their efforts in the care and habilitation of a child with cerebral palsy. If possible, interview the parents of a child having this diagnosis to determine their feelings about this condition and their reaction to the child's treatment. Identify the nurse's specific responsibilities in providing education for the parents and care for this child throughout his growth period. Discuss your findings and conclusions in seminar.

TEACHING AIDS AND OTHER INFORMATION*

American Foundation for the Blind, Inc.

Is Your Child Blind?
The Preschool Deaf-Blind Child, 1965.

Association for the Aid of Crippled Children

Richardson, S. A., and Klein, D.: Who Is the Child with a Physical Handicap?
The Child with Brain Damage.

National Society for Crippled Children and Adults, Inc.

McDonald, E. T.: Bright Promise.
Perlstein, M.: Cerebral Palsy.
Spock, B.: On Being a Parent of a Handicapped Child.
Young, W. O., and Mink, J. R.: Dental Care for the Handicapped Child.

National Society for the Prevention of Blindness, Inc.

Gibbons, H., and Cunningham, F.: Finding and Helping the Partially Seeing Child.
Safe Play to Save Sight.
Signs of Eye Trouble in Children.

Public Affairs Pamphlets

Gregg, J. R.: Parents Guide to Children's Vision.
Saltman, J.: Meeting the Challenge of Cerebral Palsy.
Wisnik, S. M.: How to Help Your Handicapped Child.

---

* Complete addresses are given in the Appendix.

United Cerebral Palsy Associations, Inc.

Cerebral Palsy—What You Should Know About It.
Tomorrow Is Today—Planning Ahead for Long-Term Care Legally and Financially.

United States Department of Health, Education, and Welfare

Cerebral Palsy, 1967.
Clements, S. D.: Minimal Brain Dysfunction in Children: Terminology and Identification, 1966.
Educational Programs for Visually Handicapped Children, 1966.
Feeding the Child with a Handicap, 1967.
Haynes, U.: A Developmental Approach to Casefinding, With Special Reference to Cerebral Palsy, Mental Retardation, and Related Disorders, 1967.
Lin-Fu, J. S.: Lead Poisoning in Children, 1967.
Services for Crippled Children, 1968.
Symposium on Environmental Lead Contamination, 1966.
The Child with a Cleft Palate, 1953 (reprinted 1963).
The Child with a Speech Problem, 1964.
The Child with Central Nervous System Deficit, 1965.

REFERENCES

Publications

Ayrault, E. W.: *You Can Raise Your Handicapped Child.* New York, G. P. Putnam's Sons, 1964.
Birch, H. G. (Ed.): *Brain Damage in Children: The Biological and Social Aspects.* Baltimore, Williams & Wilkins Company, 1964.
Cass, M. T.: *Speech Habilitation in Cerebral Palsy.* New York, Hafner Publishing Company, Inc., 1966.
Cruickshank, W. M.: *The Brain Injured Child in Home, School, and Community.* Syracuse, New York, Syracuse University Press, 1967.
Daley, W. T. (Ed.): *Speech and Language Therapy with the Cerebral Palsied Child.* Washington, Catholic University of America Press, 1965.
Drillien, C. M., and others: *The Causes and Natural History of Cleft Lip and Palate.* Baltimore, Williams & Wilkins Company, 1966.
Family Service Association of America: *Casework Services for Parents of Handicapped Children.* New York, Family Service Association of America, 1963.
Ford, F. R.: *Diseases of the Nervous System in Infancy, Childhood and Adolescence.* 5th ed. Springfield, Ill., Charles C Thomas, 1966.
Fraser, G. R., and Friedmann, A. I.: *The Causes of Blindness in Childhood.* Baltimore, Johns Hopkins Press, 1967.
Furth, H. G.: *Thinking Without Language: Psychological Implications of Deafness.* New York, The Free Press, 1966.
Keats, S.: *Cerebral Palsy.* Springfield, Ill., Charles C Thomas, 1965.
Kiernander, B. (Ed.): *Physical Medicine in Paediatrics.* London, Butterworth and Company, 1965.
Levin, A. K.: *Cerebral Palsy.* Baltimore, Williams & Wilkins Company, 1965.
Lowenfeld, B.: *Our Blind Children: Growing and Learning with Them.* 2nd ed. Springfield, Ill., Charles C Thomas, 1964.
Morley, M. E.: *Cleft Palate and Speech,* 6th ed. Baltimore, Williams & Wilkins Company, 1965.
Spock, B., and Lerrigo, M. O.: *Caring for Your Disabled Child.* New York, Macmillan Company, 1965.

Periodicals

Atkinson, H. C.: Care of the Child with Cleft Lip and Palate. *Am. J. Nursing,* 67:1889, 1967.
Banks, H. H., and Panagakos, P.: The Role of the Orthopedic Surgeon in Cerebral Palsy. *Pediat. Clin. N. Amer.,* 14:495, 1967.
Basara, S. C.: The Behavioral Patterns of the Perceptually Handicapped Child. *Nursing Forum,* V:24, No. 4, 1966.
Bledsoe, C. W., and Williams, R. C.: The Vision Needed to Nurse the Blind. *Am. J. Nursing,* 66:2432, 1966.
Chisolm, J. J.: The Use of Chelating Agents in the Treatment of Acute and Chronic Lead Intoxication in Childhood. *J. Pediat.,* 73:1, July 1968.
Cohen, J.: The Effects of Blindness on Children's Development. *Children,* 13:23, 1966.
Downs, M. P.: Hunt to Catch a Handicap. *Today's Health,* 46:46, January 1968.
Gay, M. G.: A Preschool Program for Children with Cerebral Palsy. *Children,* 12:105, 1965.
Griggs, R. C., and others: Environmental Factors in Childhood Lead Poisoning. *J.A.M.A.,* 187:703, 1964.
Healy, H. T.: Variations in Services to Handicapped Children. *Am. J. Nursing,* 68:1725, 1968.
Kapurch, J. A.: Camping Though Handicapped. *Am. J. Nursing,* 66:1794, 1966.

McConnell, F., and Knox, L. L.: Helping Parents to Help Deaf Infants. *Children,* 15:183, 1968.

Marcellus, D., and Hawke, W. A.: Survey of Attitudes of Parents of Children with Cerebral Palsy in Windsor and Essex County, Ontario. *Canad. Med. Ass. J.*: 95:1242, Dec. 10, 1966.

McDermott, M. M.: The Child with Cleft Lip and Palate: On the Pediatric Ward. *Am. J. Nursing,* 65:122, April 1965.

Monroe, J. M., and Komorita, N. I.: Problems with Nephrosis in Adolescence. *Am. J. Nursing,* 67:336, 1967.

Ripley, I. L.: The Child with Cleft Lip and Palate: Through His Years of Growth. *Am. J. Nursing,* 65:124, April 1965.

Ross, J. R., Braen, B. B., and Chaput, R.: Patterns of Change in Disturbed Blind Children in Residential Treatment. *Children,* 14:217, 1967.

Steel, S.: The Preschooler with Nephrosis. *Nursing Outlook,* 12:50, October 1964.

Wolman, B.: Deafness in Children. *Arch. Dis. Childhood,* 38:375, 1963.

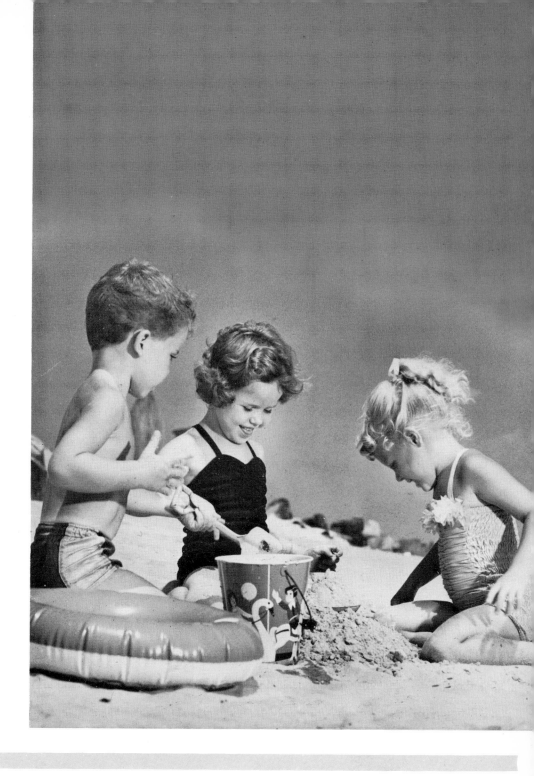

UNIT FIVE

THE PRESCHOOL CHILD

18

THE NORMAL PRESCHOOL CHILD: HIS GROWTH, DEVELOPMENT AND CARE

OVERVIEW OF EMOTIONAL DEVELOPMENT

During the preschool period parents must face the fact that their child is entering increasingly into the activities of the outside world. They then must enter into their own stage of development of learning to separate themselves gradually from their growing child. They must make decisions as to how much free expression and initiative to permit the child, at the same time setting certain limits on his behavior.

The preschool child, having learned to trust others and to know that he is a person in his own right, is ready to find out what he can do. He must learn certain things in order to become the kind of person he wants to be. He watches adults and attempts to imitate their behavior. He longs for the time when he can fully share in their activities.

The preschool child is imaginative and creative. Since he cannot really participate in the adult world, he pretends that he can. The simplest equipment may represent articles used in real life. For instance, a series of wooden boxes or blocks can become a train, or a few small cardboard boxes can furnish a doll's house, the boxes becoming a bed, a chest of drawers, a chair and a table.

The child learns quickly that different materials are suited to specific purposes. He understands language well enough to communicate through speech. This increases his ability to learn from the experiences of others and to understand much that he has not personally experienced. He questions others almost constantly, asking about the world, its people and their activities. He may become loud and persistent in his questioning and at times annoying. He is searching for explanations of the phenomena in his environment, which to him are problems of causation and function which must be solved in order to do what he wants and get what he wants without adult help.

The preschool child is as vigorous in physical activity as in intellectual explorations. He moves freely and violently. He may attack others on purpose or by accident during play. He enjoys gross motor activity, but may also settle

453

down to tasks which develop the finer muscular skills.

The infant and the toddler are guided in their activity largely by the direction of their parents, but the preschool child shows evidence of having a conscience of his own. The "still, small voice" within him guides him or passes judgment on his deeds. Experts state that children may now begin to feel guilty for their errors or wrong doing or even for their thoughts. Their unrestricted thoughts and actions frighten them.

The central problem for the preschool child is to learn about the world and other people. He must also learn to assert his own will in such a way that he will not feel too guilty. If he has the knowledge and the ability to solve this problem, he will develop a *sense of initiative* comfortably controlled by conscience. If he fails to solve this problem, he will emerge from this period feeling overwhelmed and with a *sense of guilt.*

Preschool children may feel guilty because of plans they want to carry out, but may not because of parental disapproval, or because of thoughts or fantasies of which conscience disapproves.

If the child is to develop a sense of initiative and a healthy personality, his parents and other adults in his environment must encourage his plans and the use of his imagination. They must limit punishment to those acts which are dangerous, morally wrong or so socially unacceptable that the result would be unfortunate or harmful to the child or his family.

Preschool children look forward to becoming like their fathers or mothers. They learn adult roles from their parents, who serve as models of behavior. Children enjoy practicing these roles in their play. They begin gradually to learn how to cooperate with their peers and with adults and gain great pleasure from success in their attempts (see p. 472). Parents should encourage the child's efforts to cooperate and let him share in the decisions and responsibilities of family living. If he is denied this opportunity, if his imagination is curbed and he is frustrated too often in his attempts at growing up, he becomes overanxious and spends too much time and energy in purposeless activity. Such children are apt to develop rigid consciences which exercise strong control over their behavior. At the same time they may feel resentment and bitterness toward the adults who restrict their normal behavior.

The child's sense of initiative must be encouraged throughout childhood and youth. If it is not, the good beginning may end in failure.

The Preschool Child and His Family

The Family Romance. During infancy and the toddler period children of both sexes tend to love, and to be more dependent upon, the mother, who cares for them, than on the father, who is not home during the day and may see little of his children except on weekends. Between the ages of three and six a change occurs. The little girl becomes more interested in her father. The little boy, however, remains in love with his mother. This change in the love-object influences the children's behavior toward their parents and the role they assume in play. The girl is "Daddy's little girl" and assumes the role of wife and mother in her play. The boy becomes "Mommie's little boy." He gradually becomes more masculine in his play, taking his role from the pattern set by his father.

During this period the little girl may become possessive of her father and may be in competition with her mother for his love. The little boy may likewise become possessive of his mother and may compete with his father for her love. Children feel some aggression toward the parent of the same sex. Usually they keep their feelings hidden, but at times show their attitude in full force, as when they say to the parent of the same sex. "I hate you, go away!" Such feelings make the child feel guilty and anxious, and he may fear retaliation from the parent. The child feels even more conflict within himself, because at the same time that he hates he really loves the parent, though less than the parent of the opposite sex. This conflict of love and hate is seen in the play of children between three and six years of age. Children love both parents because of the love and attention which parents normally give their children, irrespective of sex.

The parent of the same sex as the child provides a model for the child to imitate as he develops and matures. Parents must give their children much love and understanding during this period of conflict. The child, in order to continue to grow emotionally, must bury his sexual feelings toward the parent of the opposite sex in the unconscious and must identify himself with the parent of the same sex. By the end of this period the boy no longer wants to take his father's place; he simply wants to be like his father. The girl no longer wants to take her mother's place; she wants to grow up to be like mother and to have children of her own one day. The child becomes friends with both parents, not regarding either one as a specific love-object. The *family* then becomes a meaningful love-object. The intensity of response to each member is decreased. The conflict has been resolved.

It is especially important at this stage that the parents be the kind of people that society accepts. If the parents are not acceptable according to society's standards, the child will learn attitudes and feelings which will later be a detriment to his development.

Unfortunately, some children do not make

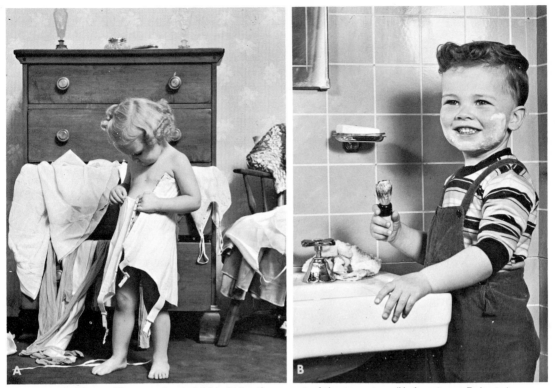

Figure 18–1. The preschool child imitates the parent of the same sex. (H. Armstrong Roberts.)

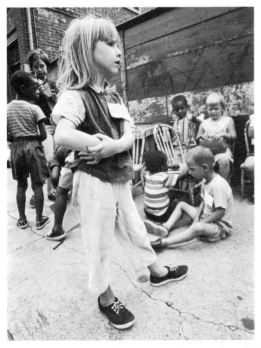

Figure 18–2. Without parental guidance the child will learn feelings and attitudes which may later be detrimental to optimum development. (Courtesy— Photograph by Lawrence V. Kanevsky.)

this shift in emotional attachment. The little boy may continue to love only his mother, and the little girl only her father. These children may not then be able to take the next steps in emotional development because of fixation at this preschool level. Such children may in later years need guidance to change this immature relation with their parents.

The Only Child and the Adopted Child. The only child is the object of all parental relations in the home; attention is concentrated upon him. The only child of young parents is likely to fare better than one of older parents; he is more likely to have young cousins, and parental attention is less likely to be tinged with anxiety. To put it briefly, he is the object of deep affection, but also a source of fun and amusement.

The first child is an only child until the second comes along. Young parents are more likely to be expecting a second child. Expectation of another child has somewhat the same influence as his actual presence would have, and the first child is not wholly treated as an only child. This is different from the attitude of older parents who over a period of years have longed for a child and cannot expect at their age to have other children.

All that has been said about an only child appears to be reinforced through the experience of the death of one or all of the other children.

What has been said of the only child is commonly true of the adopted child. He has in many cases been adopted after the death of a couple's own child or when they find that they are unable to have children. Many child-placing agencies will allow only one child to adoptive parents, since the demand for children to be adopted is greater than the number to be placed. (If twins or siblings are to be placed for adoption, it is customary to give them to parents who desire both children.) The custom of giving adoptive parents only one child works to the detriment of the children, since the life of an only child, lacking contact with brothers and sisters, is not complete.

It is generally considered best to tell the child that he is adopted before this status has any meaning for him. He accepts the parents' attitude that they want him and is satisfied. As he grows older he may feel that he is different from other children and may attribute discipline or punishment to the fact that he is an adopted child whom his parents do not love as they would their own natural child. The increasing number of adoptions during recent years makes the situation more commonplace and less emotionally charged (see p. 463).

Effect of the Birth of a Sibling. *Any environmental change may have a traumatic effect on a child.* Even such a change as moving to a new house should be discussed with him. The birth of a sibling is a change of such magnitude that the child should become accustomed before the baby is born to the idea of no longer being an only child. The birth of another child unavoidably deprives the older child of some parental attention, and a child mistakes this for loss of affection. It is difficult for the toddler or child of nursery school age to accept the situation, for his love is still centered almost exclusively on his parents.

The child feels rejected and may become jealous. Infantile expression of jealousy is of two kinds. It may be shown *directly* in open dislike of the baby, or the child may appear to love the baby more than is normal. In so doing he is laying the foundation of a martyr attitude which may persist throughout life. He usually shows his hostility to the new baby openly and directly. He may make derogatory remarks about the baby. If his parents reprove him, he may feel guilty and may rationalize on the childish level. For instance, he may give as an excuse for hitting the baby the fact that the infant has taken his blanket, though the mother has given the blanket to the infant. Later, when the baby is old enough to take his toy, he grabs it back and says, "It's mine." When his mother intervenes, he sulks or hits the baby or her. Such displacement of his

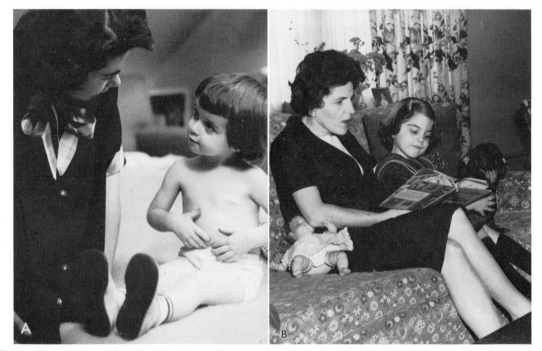

Figure 18–3. A new infant is coming. *A,* "When I get to be a lady, will I have a baby there too?" (Courtesy of George H. Padginton, Hamburg, New York, and *Baby Talk* Magazine, May 1967.) *B,* The child's mother explains to her the coming of the new sister or brother. The use of a book containing pictures of a young infant makes the event seem more real to the child.

anger toward anyone who pets the baby is common.

The child's jealousy may be shown *indirectly* by clumsiness in his contacts with the infant. If his feeling of guilt is great and he is unable to express his jealousy openly, he may drop the baby when given him to hold.

The child handles his hostility toward his mother in different ways. Direct actions against her include physical or verbal attack. On the other hand, he may refuse to have anything to do with her, ignoring her completely because she has brought the new baby home. He may displace his hostility toward her and be hostile to other adults, e.g. his nursery school or Sunday School teacher. He may regress and demand attention similar to that given the baby, refusing to drink from a cup, wanting his milk from a nursing bottle and soiling himself so that his mother must give him the same toilet care she gives "the baby." The mother should accept such temporary regression. If it is too long continued, however, it may be necessary to obtain professional help for the child. The child may repress any outward reaction, without solving his problem. This reaction may interfere with his successful handling of jealousy in later childhood or even throughout life.

Jealousy may begin when the older preschool child learns that the mother is pregnant, possibly during the fourth or fifth month of gestation. It is not wise to tell a young preschool child too early of the pregnancy, since he would have too long a wait before the child's birth. Before the birth of the baby the mother can control the child's jealousy to some extent by giving him as much attention as usual and stressing her pleasure in having him share in loving the coming baby. The baby's coming should be discussed with the child even though he is too young to understand the changes which the arrival of a new infant will make in the family life. Parents should encourage him to talk about his unborn sibling and either to verbalize or express in play his hostility toward the child.

It is a good plan to send the older child to nursery school (see p. 462) in order to develop outside contacts. He may be shown a child's picture book about the arrival of a new baby in the family to help him visualize what his mother means by all the preparations she is making for the coming of the infant.

Jealousy can be handled in a number of ways. A child who shows indications of wanting to hurt the infant should never be left alone with him. A more positive measure is to give the child a pet or a doll so that he has something to care for, just as mother is caring for the baby. He may be encouraged to identify with his parents in lovingly protecting the infant.

All sexual questions should be answered frankly, explanation being adjusted to the child's vocabulary and ability to understand sexual processes. The mother may discuss with him the difference between his needs and those of the infant; this may be done in terms of his being more grown up than the baby. For instance, he can clean his teeth, whereas the baby has no teeth; he can walk, holding mother's hand, or run about and play, but the baby must be carried or go in his carriage; in the car he can be held on the seat between father and mother, while the infant must be in his basket or in mother's arms. The mother should arrange to be alone with the child, or she and his father together with him, while the baby is sleeping in another room. If possible, the child may be with his father when the mother must care for the infant in the evening. Evidences of affection for the infant should be minimized in the presence of the older child.

Needs of the Preschool Child

The preschool child needs security and independence. He needs the security which comes with the knowledge that he has parents who are with him in the home. He needs their love and understanding. Within this circumscribed world of security and love he needs an opportunity to express his hostility and antagonisms. Because of his growing verbal ability he has increasingly less need to use physical expressions of hostility. As he grows he needs opportunities to assume more responsibility and independence. By expressing his hostility and his growing independence he learns what these feelings are like and how he can deal with them.

The child feels love and security when he has two parents with whom he has daily contact. The parents, besides showing love for him, must teach him and guide him toward maturity: (1) From verbal interaction with them he learns how to express himself so that he can communicate with others on a verbal level. (2) In the home he learns to assume more responsibility and be more independent. (3) He gains from them the knowledge he needs to grow up. Two important aspects of knowledge learned in this age period relate to sex and to religion. *More important than the facts he learns are the attitudes he forms toward this knowledge.*

The preschool child turns his interests to the outside world, to the why's and how's of living.

Guidance. There are few, if any, set rules for the guidance of preschool children, but the following suggestions may be helpful. *Limits to the child's behavior must be set and consistently maintained, thereby giving him a basis for prediction of the reactions of other people to what he does and thus making rational behavior possible.*

Limits set by parents give him a feeling of

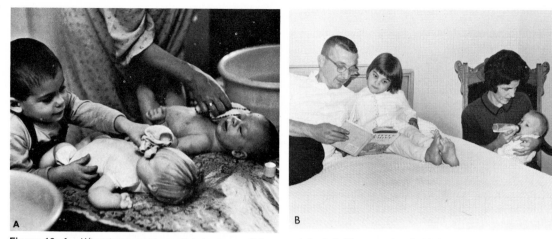

Figure 18–4. Ways to prevent possible jealousy of the new infant. *A*, The preschool child cares for his doll as his mother cares for the new infant. (Photographed by Erika and Bill Stone; courtesy of *Today's Health*, January 1964.) *B*, The father gives the older child attention while the mother feeds the infant.

security which he does not have when he is allowed to decide for himself on matters beyond his ability to decide wisely. Suggestions—not commands—helpful to the child in achieving what he wants at the time, or in forming good relations with other people, should be made in positive form. Commands are seldom necessary, but when given in positive rather than negative form are more effective. The child should not be spoken to in such a way that he feels guilty or fearful. Rather he should be reassured by the sense that his parents are helping him solve problems as they come up in his activities and social relations. A choice of actions should be given him only when he actually may decide which of two or more lines of behavior he may take. A child does not always understand that redirection of his activities is consistent with his own interests. He learns this gradually by experience with the satisfying results which follow parental redirection. He should be encouraged to do as much as possible for himself so that he can grow in independence.

Adults should not make the mistake of playing *for* the child. Instead, he should be helped to enjoy his own activities. For instance, adults should not make art models for him to copy. He should be allowed freely to create his own work. Help should be provided whenever necessary, however; this is an important element in his feeling secure in his parents' protecting love. Children live in the present, and suggestion, to be truly helpful, should be provided and reinforced at appropriate times.

Learning Language. The preschool child learns to communicate his feelings and ideas through language in a more precise form than he did as a toddler. He constantly asks questions and learns about the outside world by seeking the meaning of what he experiences through sensory stimulation. He asks how, why, what, when and where about everything which interests him.

During the preschool period he uses progressively longer and more complex sentences. This is a period of rapid vocabulary growth. Between the ages of two and six years the child learns about 600 words a year, chiefly through the answers given by adults to his questions. He also learns by imitating adults and other children with whom he associates. He may acquire words which his parents do not want him to use, such as ungrammatical terms ("ain't"), slang or so-called bad words. Usually if adults in his environment ignore unacceptable words and do not give him attention when he uses them, he will cease to use them in his conversation.

An analysis of a child's questions shows his need for information, for relief from anxiety and for attention. Answers to his questions should give him increased understanding of his environment and of what is going on about him, as well as a secure feeling that adults can and will help him to learn. Through answers to his questions the child gets not only factual knowledge, but also a concept of adult attitudes and feelings about the topics discussed.

The questions of three-year-olds are rather simple when compared with those of four- and five-year-olds, who want to know how things function. These latter questions require more detailed explanations which adults at times may not be prepared to give. *All adults should remember the guiding principle about answering questions of children and youths: tell the truth to the best of your ability.* If a lie is told, the child will lose his sense of trust in the individual, and his trust in all others may be weakened. *The answer should be in terms of the child's level of understanding.* If an adult does not know the answer, he should tell the child so. Then adult and child are ready to seek the answer together.

Sex Information. The child who learns to trust others and to give as well as receive love has already begun his preparation for a satisfactory marriage and rearing children of his own.

Sex education during the preschool years contributes specific knowledge which the child wants to know and also helps him build desirable attitudes toward this aspect of life. This is especially true when parents love and respect each other and so set a good example for the child to follow. In such a family the child will learn that he or she is a boy or a girl and that each sex has its own role to play in life. The attitudes and feelings which children acquire greatly influence their relations to marital partners and to their own children later. It is essential that the child understands that sex is important to his own personality as well as to that of others.

Although the extent and method of sex education must be fitted to the child's needs, certain general principles are applicable to the sex education of all children. Children are likely to ask simple questions about sex by the time they are three to four years of age, although some may not ask until they are six years old. There are individual differences, of course, depending on factors in the child's environment and degree of maturation. *Information on sex should be given in response to the child's interest in the subject, but never as facts which have no connection with the family life.* In general the child is old enough for correct though simplified answers when he is sufficiently mature to ask questions.

Sex information may be given at home, church or school. The best source of information should be sincere and loving parents who feel comfortable in talking about sex. If for some reason this is impossible, the school or church may give the information. Information acquired from acquaintances unfortunately is likely not only to be incorrect, but also to give the child a distorted attitude to the whole subject of sexual relations. *Parents should answer the child directly and honestly, basing the amount of information given and the phraseology used on the child's physiologic and developmental level. Information should be given promptly when the question is asked.* It is not good to tell more about the subject than is involved in the answer to the question. *The information should be given frankly and unemotionally.* The child will grasp his parents' attitude toward sex more than their answers, and this will free him from worry and preoccupation with sexual problems.

Some of the questions which preschool children ask concern the birth of a child. They commonly ask, "Where do babies come from?" because curiosity is natural to this age group and because conditions pertaining to sex are obvious in the social life about them. After the child has learned that the infant grows within the mother's abdomen, he may ask, "How does it fit inside there?" or, "Can't he move?" The child sees pregnant women, and mass media treat openly of sex. Household pets deliver their young, and rural children learn early of reproduction in farm animals. When the child asks where babies come from and other questions, he should be helped to clarify his fantasies. If his questions are answered frankly and with a positive attitude of acceptance of his interest in the matter, he will receive the information without shame or anxiety. During the preschool period, emphasis should be placed on the physical aspects of sex. The preschool child is too young to understand moral implications, other than the value of doing what his parents ask of him.

In the hospital, children many times will ask nurses questions similar to those they ask their parents at home. The same principles just discussed apply in answering such questions; however, if the mother is present, the nurse can discuss the matter with her and either have her answer the question or answer it herself, knowing that the mother understands what is told to her child.

Many of the problems which beset adolescents arise because they dwell on sex and have fantasies about many aspects of sexuality. If answers had been given during the preschool period and enlarged upon as the child grew older, there would be less danger of such turmoil during adolescence.

Religious Education. Close parent-child relations normally extend through the years during which the child is socialized. The greatest influence in a child's life is his parents' attitude about such basic aspects of life as religion, sex, love of country, economic systems, and education. In answering questions parents must be understanding, objective and kind, particularly in regard to religion, since faith as well as science is involved.

A few general principles pertaining to religious education may be given. *A child cannot be kept spiritually neutral.* Whatever his parents may desire, he hears about religion from other children, and he sees churches and pictures of religious objects.

Whatever the parents tell the child about religion has the same force as does information on other subjects. Yet the child observes what his parents do, and if their actions are not in accord with what they teach him, he is quick to notice it.

A child should be brought up in a genuinely religious home, for a religious attitude toward life is not just an afterthought to living. It is the spiritual atmosphere which pervades the whole of life.

There are two general methods of religious

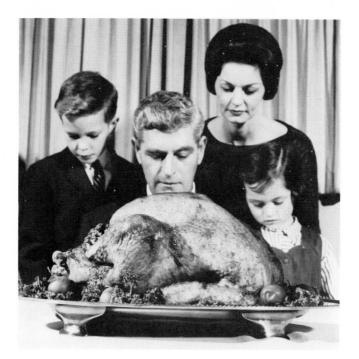

Figure 18-5. In a genuinely religious home the spiritual atmosphere pervades all of living. Children learn more by example than they do from mere verbal explanations. (H. Armstrong Roberts.)

education: that of indoctrination and that of letting the child follow the religion of his choice. Both methods have many adherents. Neither, taken alone, meets the real issue. The preschool child does not follow any religion because he understands it. Rather, he accepts religion because it is expected of him, because someone he loves influences him to do so or because it offers some other concomitant pleasures.

Suggestions for religious training in the home include early training in the faith held by the parents. The preschool child is old enough to go to Sunday School. Religion should be made attractive to him, but should not be forced upon him. He should be taught that God is within our lives, that God loves him. Parents should not give the child the impression that they are condescending to his level when speaking of religion; the discussion should be a shared experience between parents and child. As the child grows up he will learn about religions other than that held by his parents.

Religious training in the hospital is difficult, since the child's questions must be answered only by persons of the same faith as his parents. This avoids confusion of ideas in the child's mind. Furthermore, what the child is told may be a matter of extreme importance to the parents, since the child is not able to think through conflicting statements about religion.

Religious holidays raise many questions in a child's mind. The following explanation of the significance of Christmas and Easter may be given unless the policy of the hospital prohibits discussion of the religious concepts involved. The questions most commonly asked are only indirectly of a religious nature.

There is the old question, "Is there *really* a

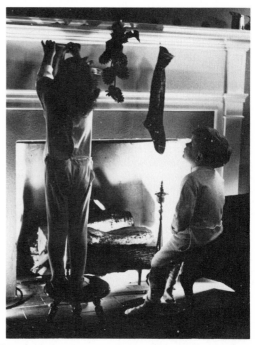

Figure 18-6. A young child truly believes that Santa Claus will come. (H. Armstrong Roberts.)

Santa Claus?" The answer to be given to a very young child is usually, "Yes." He is too young to understand abstract ideas, and Santa stands for the spirit of Christmas. When the child really begins to question this belief, he is already doubting its truth. He should be allowed to discuss his own ideas on the matter. If he actually doubts whether there is a Santa Claus, he is ready for an explanation of what Santa Claus stands for. He may be told that the spirit of Christmas is that of good will. It is a time to make others happy as Santa Claus made him happy on Christmas Day last year and the year before, as far back as he can remember. The origin of Christmas can be told him, and its religious significance, which he probably already knows if his parents are of the Christian faith. Customs which have developed around the celebration of Christmas in different countries will interest him.

The myth of the Easter Bunny can be explained with similar adaptations.

Anxiety in the Preschool Child

Problems which may cause anxiety and tension in the preschool child may come from within or may arise from his environment. They may be due to lack of satisfaction of a need or to an increase in the number and intensity of the child's fears. His response to the problem is to mobilize defenses to deal with the dangers.

Specific Causes. Several causes of anxiety are common during the preschool period. The child may fear being deserted by his parents, that they no longer love him or that he is being punished for misdeeds or for thoughts which he should not have had. He has a great fear of physical injury.

These specific causes are intensified by the peculiar combination of anxiety-producing circumstances which occur during hospitalization. The main causes of anxiety are separation from his parents and fear of pain.

LOSS OF PARENTAL LOVE. To a preschool child parental love is manifested in his daily life with his parents. Separation from his parents means loss of their love. Hospitalization is for most children only a temporary separation from their parents. Long-term or permanent separation must now be considered.

LOSS OF ONE PARENT. A child may be temporarily separated from his father for business or patriotic reasons. He remains with his mother, who builds up in the child a happy expectation of his father's return. If the father is absent for a long time, good parent-child relations may be difficult to establish.

The child who has lost a parent by death or divorce does not live in a complete home. If the parent has died, there is not the same degree of anxiety which is likely to trouble a child of divorced parents. Divorce is generally preceded by a period of unsettled life in which the child may be urged by each parent to love him or her only and to be hostile to the other parent. Generally the court gives the child to the mother, but after the divorce the child may visit his father at times prescribed by the court. The child of divorced parents is confused by the antagonism of each parent toward the other and yet the love of each for him. Of course the child who is loved by only one parent or by neither is deprived of the parental affection which is a child's birthright.

When a boy of preschool age lacks close association with his father, he lacks a male in the home with whom he can identify, against whom he can be aggressive and from whom he can learn about the role of a man in the home, community or country. The boy may become a substitute love-object to his mother for her absent husband. He may develop a feminine outlook on life and never learn the typical masculine technique of competition or aggression.

The effect upon the boy of absence of his mother is generally less serious than that due to his father's absence because there is usually a mother-substitute in the home, e.g. a grandmother, aunt or housekeeper. The boy of preschool age may regress after his mother has left home until he adjusts to her substitute. He may

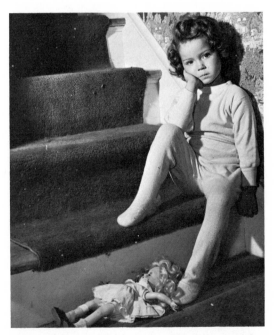

Figure 18–7. A child grieves when her parent has gone away. This overwhelming feeling of loneliness is difficult for her to handle. (H. Armstrong Roberts.)

be deeply hurt by his mother's leaving him when he loves her so dearly and may fear loving a woman who takes her place in the home, lest he be hurt again if she leaves.

The effect upon the girl of absence of the mother is essentially the same as that of absence of the father upon a boy. She will have no one with whom to compete for the father's love, and until a mother-substitute is found she will have no woman with whom she can identify and from whom she can learn the feminine role in life. She may develop a masculine outlook on family and community life.

The effect upon the girl of absence of the father is essentially the same as that of absence of the mother upon the boy. She may become too closely attached to the mother, and also may become afraid of loving a man again and being hurt by his loss. This feeling, if carried over into adolescence, interferes with normal courtship and marriage.

In a situation in which one parent can care for the child, he or she may be assisted by a family member or by the utilization of a homemaker service, or by having the child cared for in a child care center or day nursery or nursery school for part of the day.

Homemaker Service. Homemaker services may be obtained in an increasing number of communities in the United States. Homemakers as individuals must be adaptable, reliable and mature and should be trained in the field of home management skills and child care.

A homemaker can fulfill a very important need in the life of a child who is to continue to live in his own home. Not only can she care for the child who has lost one parent through death or divorce, but she can also provide care for the child who may have two living parents, but whose mother may be ill temporarily or recovering from childbirth, or may be providing care for another seriously ill child. A homemaker could thus help to keep the home together during a period of stress and thus prevent further emotional damage to the child.

Child Care Centers and Day Nurseries. The Social Security Act of 1935 authorized a program to help each state establish or strengthen public child welfare services for the protection of children. The Public Welfare Amendments of 1962 stated that child welfare services were those public services which supplemented or substituted for parental care and included care of children in foster homes, day care centers or other child care facilities.

Child care centers and day nurseries are facilities which provide care for children in the absence of their parents. In these centers or day nurseries children whose mothers must be employed outside the home are provided with food, rest and recreation during the daytime hours.

Since many children needing this type of care come from deprived homes, they may also need intellectual stimulation and cultural enrichment. Thus some type of program is provided to meet these needs.

Nursery Schools. Nursery schools, on the other hand, are for the primary purpose of educating children on the prekindergarten level. They may be operated for a few hours each day because young children cannot profit from a situation the purpose of which is structured learning for a longer period of time. Nevertheless some nursery schools are extending their periods of service for those who need it (see p. 474).

Facilities caring for children are inspected and licensed by state law. Although they must meet certain standards concerning sanitation facilities, area of space and equipment for cleanliness, play and rest, among other requirements, parents should inspect the facility they plan to use in order to determine whether it will be suitable for their particular children. Most parents would also like to meet the adults who will be caring for their children and to determine their ability to provide physical care and guidance for them in their absence.

LOSS OF BOTH PARENTS.   Separation of a child from both parents has all the effects of the loss of a single parent. The trauma to the child is extreme, and he goes through a period of mourning. Since the child is less verbal than the adult, his feelings must be judged from nonverbal behavior. He may show physical symptoms such as vomiting and diarrhea, or a return to more infantile behavior. For instance, although he is toilet-trained, he may soil himself. He may be uncooperative and naughty.

Everyone working with children should know how to help a child who has been separated from one or both parents. No adult should scold or punish a child for his response to parental loss no matter what form it takes. The child should be treated with kindness and helped to express his feelings. He should be encouraged to talk about the parent (or parents) who has gone away. Preschool children may feel that they have caused the death or departure of the parent of the same sex because they wished him or her to leave and be out of the way. The child must be helped to understand that his wish was not the same thing as a deed of violence against the parent.

Substitute parents should be provided as soon as possible for children who have lost both parents, and should make every effort to win the children's love and confidence. Some children may need psychologic help if the trauma has been too great for them to accept.

If by death or divorce of his parents a child is without a home and there is no other relative to care for him, the child will probably be placed by the court in an institution or a foster home, and later, if possible, into an adoptive home.

Institutional Care. The type of foundling home or orphanage (see p. 263) where many children were crowded together permanently in a situation in which they were not likely to thrive no longer exists in the United States. Today shelters are provided temporarily until foster home care or adoption can be arranged for children having no parents, or homemaker service, day care center, or day nursery facilities can be arranged for those having one parent. Unfortunately, however, some of the temporary shelters into which children are placed are overcrowded because of the numbers of children needing such care and the length of time necessary to make appropriate plans for placement. Also, some children are kept in institutions because society is unwilling to terminate parental rights even in those instances in which it is obvious that living parents will never take responsibility for the child. Such parents abandon their children, yet because they retain legal control over them, the children cannot be adopted and thus cannot gain a measure of happiness from living with adoptive parents who would love them.

Institutions for the temporary care of children are usually organized on the basis of small groups, each group being cared for by "substitute parents." These children are dressed like their peers living in the area, and an attempt is made to provide a homelike atmosphere for them. Healthy infants are usually not kept in an institution unless a foster home or an adoptive home cannot be provided.

Foster Home Care. An institution, no matter how well organized, cannot meet the needs of a child as well as good foster parents can. Good foster parents must have a real love for children, must be sensitive to their needs and must have the maturity necessary to let them go from their home when they are to be adopted. Unfortunately, not all foster parents are of this type, and so children may be moved from one foster home to another repeatedly, thus preventing them from developing the sense of security they so desperately need. The social worker of a child-placing agency may be the only adult with whom the child establishes a satisfying and continuing relation throughout a childhood spent in institutions or foster homes.

Foster homes must be inspected and licensed in the state in which they are located. They are inspected for cleanliness, sanitation, and adequacy of space among other requirements.

Adoptions. Many children are available for adoption today; however, the ones most young couples want, the blond, blue-eyed or the dark-haired, brown-eyed, healthy infants may be in short supply. Children who are handicapped either physically or emotionally or are of mixed racial parentage may not be chosen for adoption. These children are indeed the unfortunate victims of circumstances beyond their control.

Nurses who care for infants and children who are to be adopted must remember that, professionally, they are not at liberty to divulge any information either about the biological parents of the child or about the adopting parents, if they are known. If an adoption is handled carefully, an adopted child may have the same love relations with his parents which a child under normal circumstances has with his natural parents.

Children should be adopted through an official adoption agency, rather than independently through a physician or a "friend." These agencies have certain placement practices which deal with the physical, emotional, financial and social status of the adopting parents and the physical and emotional condition of the child, practices which help to assure a successful adoption.

ANXIETY FROM CAUSES OTHER THAN LOSS OF PARENTAL LOVE. *Conscience anxiety,* in which the child feels that he has done something wrong and expects punishment, is prevalent among children of overparticular or strict parents. The bogyman of the modern child is the person who will punish him if he is naughty.

A common and almost unavoidable kind of *anxiety* is that *arising out of inconsistency* in the do's and don't's of parents and parental actions. This difficulty is increased when the parents do not lead the kind of life which they teach the child that he must lead. During wartime, for instance, children are taught to sublimate their destructive feelings and direct them to positive ends, and yet they are given toy weapons with which to play soldier. The children are too immature to understand the difference between personal aggression and that prompted by love of country and group morale. This is a great difficulty in the training of little children during a period of national stress.

Infectious anxiety is acquired from an adult, generally the mother. If the mother is relatively free from overt anxiety under severe circumstances, the child also is apt to be free. But if the mother is overanxious even in commonly accepted situations, the child is also likely to be anxious. This sort of anxiety is often seen in hospitalized children. If the mother is anxious about the child, he will be anxious about himself. This is one reason why the nurse should make the mother comfortable and secure about the hospitalization of the child.

Real or *objective anxiety* or fear is dependent upon the child's ability to understand the nature of the danger which threatens him. Fear of lightning is a needless fear due to the child's not understanding the cause of the lightning. In contrast, a child's fear of needles is gained from experience; he knows that they cause him pain.

Objective fears of preschool children must be managed with consideration of the child's stage of maturation. Many unreal fears may appear real to little children, and most preschool children have one or another of these fears. This is natural, for they have a limited understanding of the world about them. Adults must help a child to handle his fears if they are not to persist, possibly in a compulsive form, in adult life. A real fear of a situation which is dangerous is logical. The remedy is to show the child what may be done in such a situation and how to avoid dangerous situations. Crossing the street is an example. The child should be taught to cross at the corner with, not against, the traffic light.

Ordinary fears include fear of being injured (or seeing people who have been injured or are crippled), being lost or deserted, and being hurt by animals (particularly those which are large or noisy). Some children fear death, but not as adults do. The child may have had a real experience with any one of these fear-producing situations. Children feel most fearful when they are alone or away from their parents among strangers.

Inner anxiety, in contrast to fear, occurs when a child feels unloved. He may have been punished for masturbation, or deprived of his mother's love because of the arrival of a new sibling. To the child who is anxious many things appear to be dangerous, and vague, unknown dangers appear to be ever present. The adult must understand not only the child's fear of external dangers, but also his inner anxiety, in order to help him.

The frightened child needs, more than anything else, to be reassured and to gain a feeling of safety. His mother should hold him and let him feel her protection and strength. After he has calmed down, his attention may be directed from the source of his fear. When he appears sufficiently secure, he may want to talk about his fear and even to have contact with the feared object or situation. Perhaps, before contact, he may want to play out the fearful situation as a game. The adult's role in helping a child to overcome fears is to be supportive and understanding.

Common fears can be prevented to a large extent by imagining how new situations seem to a child and talking to him from his point of view. A puppy which is active and playful, not vicious, to a child may appear to be a monster that cannot be controlled. The adult who protects a child from meeting fearful experiences until he is prepared for them and has sufficient self-confidence will prevent many of the common fears of childhood.

Special Problems of the Preschool Child

The common behavioral manifestations of children's feelings are so important that they must be given detailed consideration in order that the student may learn to give the child comprehensive nursing care. Children of this age group may have such behavioral problems as continued thumb-sucking, enuresis, selfishness, hurting others, destructiveness and masturbation.

Thumb-Sucking

The important danger in continued thumb-sucking is not in the habit itself, but in the response of parents and other adults to it. Parents tend to feel that if a child sucks his thumb in the preschool period, they themselves have failed in training him. They respond to this feeling of failure by becoming inconsiderate of the child in their handling of the problem. They may alternately punish, love and ridicule him because he does not overcome the objectionable habit.

Mothers need not fear that thumb-sucking will injure the thumb or spoil the shape of the child's jaw unless the habit is continued into older childhood and the child exerts maximum pressure when sucking. In any case the shape of the mouth is likely to return to normal after the thumb-sucking has ceased.

Many children who suck their thumbs probably had too little sucking pleasure during infancy. Thumb-sucking may be a sign that the child feels unloved, that he is in danger or is not good enough. It may be an expression of dissatisfaction with life. When parents or other adults exert pressure upon him to give up the activity, his unhappiness is increased.

In order to help the child, parents and other adults responsible for his care must observe the whole child and try to provide a happier childhood experience for him. Adults should note the occasions when a child sucks his thumb and provide more love and security for him at such times. It is essential to find the basis of the problem. Is the child lonely, too excited or bored? Has he too few toys or does he feel neglected? Although children usually outgrow the habit by the age of five or six years, it is important to find and correct the cause in order to prevent the child from acquiring another habit which serves the same function of giving him pleasure and comfort. The matter may be discussed with a child of five or six years who seems to be trying to overcome the habit. He may be encouraged by assurance that he will probably outgrow the habit.

Enuresis

Enuresis, or wetting after control should be established (about three years of age), is both a source of embarrassment and a nuisance to the mother of an enuretic child. Mothers should remember that a child can be toilet-trained only when he is physiologically and psychologically ready for control of urine and stool.

Some of the causes of enuresis are lack of training, too early or too severe training or over-training. If parents would regard toilet training as only a part of the general training of the child, take it in the stride of child training, there would be fewer problems of enuresis. Children who have achieved control of urine and stool may revert to wetting, especially bed wetting, when they meet problems which they cannot solve, such as those connected with the coming of a new baby.

Adults should not make an issue of toilet training. They should not use bribes or punishment or threaten to stop loving a child because he continues this habit. If enuresis is nocturnal only, giving less fluid in the evening may be tried. But the problem is usually more psychologic than physical. Adults should try to be casual and assure the child that he will outgrow this habit. They should help him to achieve a positive attitude toward enuresis – to want to stay dry – and develop confidence in his ability to control elimination. Wetting will not stop at once, but if the child is more relaxed, dryness will be achieved more easily and with less danger to his personality development.

Enuresis may also be due to a physical cause. For this reason children who do not respond to parental training should be examined by a physician. Nocturnal enuresis may be due to environmental factors, such as a dark hall through which the child must walk to the bathroom, or to his reluctance to get out of a warm bed to go to a cold bathroom. Adults should analyze the situation in order to determine his specific problem.

Selfishness

No child is born with the ability to share with others what is his. He can only slowly learn the joy of giving, or even sharing with others, what he wants to keep for himself. He cannot be forced to share. He must first develop a sense of ownership before he can learn to be generous.

Adults can help him to learn to share with others if they let him have possessions which both they and he recognize as his. He should be allowed to decide whether to give or refuse to give his toy to another child. If a squabble occurs over one child's possession of a toy which another child wants, a substitute toy should be provided so that each has what he wants. Many parents make the mistake of taking a toy from its rightful owner and giving it to a smaller child or to a guest or a girl. In order to learn the difficult and often unpleasant lesson of sharing, a child should be helped to enjoy playing with other children. Group play encourages the habit of sharing. He will learn first that using things together is fun and then to share and take turns with his toys and those of other children.

Bad Language

Children learn improper words just as they learn all the other words in their vocabularies. Parents are horrified when their children call names such as "stinker," "louse" or "stupid." They may be shocked when their children say unapproved words in connection with toilet training. They may be hurt when their children say, "I hate you!" or "I'll shoot you."

Bad language generally has more meaning for the adult than for the child, who, as a rule, has little understanding of what such words mean or their connotations. He may use these words on purpose to annoy adults and enjoy the sensation he creates.

In such a situation adults should relax and not be worried or shocked. The child should not be punished, for punishment emphasizes the importance of the words. The adult may say the same word back to the child in an unemotional way and thus make the word seem of little importance, or give the child a more difficult word such as "Mississippi" to say. The adult may say to the preschool child, "I'm tired of hearing that," or he may request the child not to use the word again because it may hurt others. Since no one method will work in all situations, more than one method may have to be tried.

In a nursery school the teacher may try the methods of nonparticipation with the group, suggestion of other words, distraction, or playing with other words or sounds. She should not shame or punish the children for using bad language. The less attention is paid to the use of such language, the sooner will it cease.

Hurting Others

Small children hurt others and are themselves hurt when they play together. If the hurting is accidental, the incident should be overlooked. But if a child persistently tries to hurt others, he needs adult help to control his actions or to prevent him from inflicting some serious injury on another child.

The child who repeatedly wants to hurt others by biting, scratching, pulling hair or hitting is a troubled child. He may be jealous or frustrated, and his behavior may result from his mental state. He must not be allowed to hurt other children. He needs to know that someone who loves him deeply will control him and so prevent the unpleasant consequences of his behavior. He needs to feel secure within limits beyond which he is not allowed to go.

The child should not be punished by having the same injury inflicted on him which he inflicted on another child. He should not be told that he is a bad child. He should not be forced to apologize to the child whom he hurt. Under no circumstances should he be made to feel rejected by the adult who is in charge of the children. The adult should take positive action in situations in which the child is likely to hurt others. If it is evident that a child intends to throw a stone or hit or bite one of his playmates, the adult should restrain him, saying, "Sammy does not want to be hurt." If the harm has already been done, the injured child should be soothed and the offender removed to a less emotional environment in which he is helped to control himself. The attention of the other children should be directed to some activity which they all enjoy in order that happy play may be resumed. As soon as practical, the offending child should rejoin the play group.

Toys and other objects with which a child can hurt others should be removed if a child who is likely to attack others is participating in group play.

The child who wants to hurt others should be helped to identify with the group, accepting them and being accepted by them. He should be given physical outlets in his play through which to work off some of his excess energy and relieve his feeling of frustration. He should be praised for his achievements in group and solitary play and for kindly acts which he does for others.

Destructiveness

All children occasionally break things; such is part of the normal life of a child. Parents must learn to differentiate between accidental and intentional destruction of objects which they may value highly. Much of the child's accidental destructiveness is the result of his boundless energy and endless curiosity. In spite of the damage to property, parents should not too severely limit his outlets for energy and curiosity, for these are valuable qualities which must not be destroyed.

To avoid accidental destruction at home, the parents should remove valuable objects that the child might break or damage. They should provide space for him to play in without danger of his breaking or harming the furnishings of the house.

Toys are apt to be given rough use. Parents should realize that material possessions do not mean as much to a child as to adults. In the course of play children give toys a great deal of wear and tear and may break them by using them in ways for which they were not intended. Adults should set up certain restrictions, however, in the child's use of his toys and of objects belonging to adults. He is then able to learn to value his own possessions and those of others. Progress is slow, however. What he values he will learn to use with care. The child who loves his parents is often intensely sorry if he breaks something which he knows they value, even though he also knows that he will not be punished in any way.

A child who is intentionally destructive is usually an unhappy child unable to control his feelings of jealousy, helplessness, aggression or anger. He may feel unloved, disliked by his peers, or bored by inadequate playthings. Sometimes such children seem to want to be punished, since it is one way of getting attention. The cause of such destructiveness must be found and appropriate treatment given. The parents should avoid scolding or punishing. They should help him direct his energy into appropriate activities.

Masturbation

Parents find it hard to accept masturbation as an almost universal experience in young children. The infant soon discovers that a pleasant sensation accompanies handling of the genitalia, which has no other significance to him and of course is not accompanied by fantasies. In the preschool child, masturbation may be increased and is commonly accompanied by fantasies. Masturbation is utilized in adolescence to fulfill sexual urges which in our culture do not have socially approved release in heterosexual intercourse outside of marriage. It may have a useful part in the ultimate attainment of heterosexual expression of the sex urge.

The child who masturbates excessively for his stage of maturation should not be punished. Rather, he should be helped to work out the problem which is causing him to masturbate more than is normal. The child who has discovered the pleasure derived from masturbation should be given ample opportunity to find other, more socially acceptable pleasures outside his body.

Sex education does not solve the problem of masturbation. It does help the child, however, to understand his pleasure in the practice and to understand that the true function of the sexual organs is reproduction.

Although we should not scold the child for masturbating, the habit, if excessive, may keep him from other pleasures which are necessary for optimum growth and development in childhood. Like any pleasure which is practiced in solitude, it interferes with social interaction. If masturbation is excessive, it may become so fixed a habit that it interferes with the normal desire for heterosexual intercourse within marriage.

Poor handling of the problem of masturbation in the preschool child is likely to result in fixation at the autoerotic level, wherein the child seeks pleasure in himself rather than in relations with others.

Parents should be told that masturbation does not produce nervous diseases or weaken the mind or organs of reproduction, but that parental condemnation of the practice in the child may induce lasting psychologic and emotional harm.

The adolescent who masturbates excessively is failing socially. He is lonely and unhappy. He needs treatment for his social difficulty, not condemnation.

Two important aspects of the problem should be kept in mind. Masturbation focuses feeling in the genital region. This feeling is necessary for the healthy functioning of men and women. Shame and the threats related to this activity can force children to repress sexual feelings. This might eventuate in impotence in the male and frigidity in the female. Both conditions tend to unhappiness in marriage and to increased susceptibility to mental illness.

The important fact to remember about preschool children is that masturbation in excess is a symptom of poor mental hygiene and is not a pathologic process in itself.

There is no one way of helping the child to overcome his tendency to excessive masturbation. He should be assured that he is safe in his parents' affection and that he should not be afraid or ashamed. Threats or punishment would increase his fears. He should be given opportunity for happy relations with playmates and sufficient toys to play with. His parents should be particularly careful to answer all his questions about sex, adapting their answers to his level of understanding.

OVERVIEW OF PHYSICAL, SOCIAL AND MENTAL DEVELOPMENT

Physical Growth and Development

Children grow relatively slowly in the preschool years, but they change from the chubby toddler to the sturdy child. They gain an average of less than 5 pounds a year. The average child of six years of age has doubled his weight at one year of age. During the preschool period the child gains about 2 to 2.5 inches a year. The average height of the six-year-old is 40 inches, or double his birth length. Since the child grows proportionately more than he gains in weight during the preschool years, he appears to be tall and thin by the end of his preschool days.

Children in the years from three to six gain muscular coordination which enables them to explore the physical environment, just as they acquire the ability to explore intellectually through constant questioning of adults and older children or even their playmates.

The child of six years has learned to walk more as adults do. The lordosis of the smaller child has disappeared. During the preschool years the constantly overactive child may suffer from persistent fatigue and may therefore develop poor posture unless preventive measures are taken.

In general, after the second year the child's motor development consists essentially in increase in strength and ease of performance. No distinctly new types of muscle activities are seen after early childhood. New kinds of performance are based on the use of skills already learned. By the time a child is five years old his skill in the use of muscles and his accuracy and speed allow him to be increasingly independent of others.

The pulse rate is normally 90 to 110, the respiratory rate about 20 when the child is at rest. The blood pressure is approximately 85 mm. of mercury systolic, and 60 mm. diastolic.

Social and Mental Development

The child of this age has developed a conscience and has internalized the mores of his group. He has begun to develop for himself such concepts as friendship, acceptance of responsibility, independence (some children show their independence by running away from home), the passage of time, spatial relations, abstract words, and numbers. His attention span has lengthened.

Specifics of Physical, Social and Mental Development

Chronologic age is misleading as a basis for child care. The development of the whole child must be considered; this requires individual consideration. Yet chronologic age is useful for any discussion of classified group characteristics. By using the average of each of the characteristics as the norm for the child of any given age, it is possible to tell how far any child deviates from the norm. No child conforms to the average in all areas of development. He may be far above in one area, behind in another and average in all other areas. For this reason a child's behavior at any time is likely to be that of one age group in certain areas and of another age group in other areas.

Although development does not proceed at a uniform rate in all areas, it follows a logical, precise sequence. The rate at which this sequence occurs is an individual matter. This is the most important point to remember in applying the concept of growth and development to the care of any particular child.

Three Years. The three-year-old child is less negativistic and more easily cared for than the toddler. He has fewer temper tantrums, understands words better and can be given simple reasons and explanations of cause and effect in the phenomena occurring in the world about him. He is interested in new activities; hence this is a period when learning from experience is rapid. Mental activity and verbal expression are increasingly substituted for or reinforce physical activity in the expression of emotions. For instance, a three-year-old is likely to say, "I don't like you," rather than hit someone or throw a stone. Or if he does throw the stone, his emotion is verbalized as he throws.

MOTOR CONTROL. Motor control in the three-year-old is evinced in the following acts:

Rides a tricycle, using the pedals
Walks backward

Walks downstairs alone; walks upstairs, alternating his feet
Can jump from a low step
Can try to dance, but balance may not be adequate
Pours fluid from a pitcher well
Begins to use scissors
Can hit large pegs in a peg board with a hammer
Can string large beads
Builds a tower of 9 or 10 blocks
Tries to draw a picture
Imitates a 3-block bridge
Copies a circle or cross to imitate model
Can undress himself; can unbutton buttons if on front or side of clothing
Helps dress himself
Can go to toilet
Can wash hands
May be able to brush teeth
Can feed himself well
Can help to dry dishes and dust.

VOCALIZATION, SOCIALIZATION AND MENTAL ABILITIES. The three-year-old child feels safe in his world because his mother gave him security in the toddler period. His accomplishments are as follows:

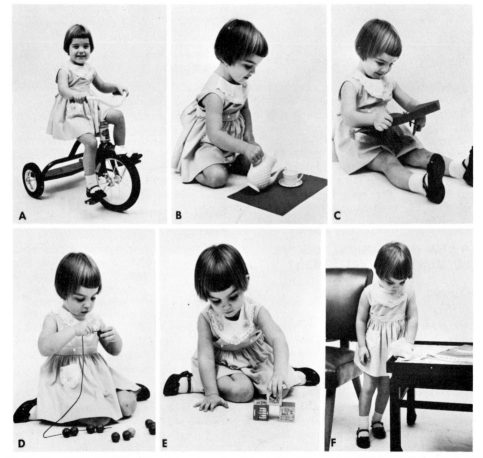

Figure 18–8. The 3-year-old (*A*) rides a tricycle, using the pedals, (*B*) pours fluid from a pitcher well, (*C*) begins to use scissors, (*D*) can string large beads, (*E*) imitates a 3-block bridge, (*F*) can help to dust.

Has a vocabulary of about 900 words

Uses language fluently and with confidence

Talks in sentences about things. Does not appear to care whether others listen or not

Repeats a sentence of 6 syllables. Uses longer sentences than the 2-year-old

Uses plurals in speech

May attempt to sing simple songs

Knows whether he or she is a boy or a girl

Plays simple games with others. Begins to work through the problem of his family relations with other children in play

Begins to understand what it means to take turns

Is toilet-trained at night

Can repeat 3 numbers

Begins to be interested in colors

Knows his family name

Has little understanding of past, present or future

Can name figures in a picture.

The three-year-old may continue to be ritualistic in many of his activities such as arranging toys or going to bed. He is a friendly, laughing child who wants to please others, though he may be jealous of his siblings. He may have fears, usually visual, of the dark or of animals.

Four Years.   The four-year-old is not usually as pleasant a member of the group (family, nursery school or play group) as the three-year-old child. He is more noisy. It is a stormy age. Parents may expect too much of him and clamp down on his manners and the language he uses. *Do's* and *Don't's* become important. His aggression is turned toward his parents. His emotional tone is likely to change suddenly from gay to unhappy.

MOTOR CONTROL.   The four-year-old has the following accomplishments:

Can climb well

Can jump well

Can go up and down stairs without holding the railing, and using his legs alternately like an adult

Throws a ball overhand

Uses scissors successfully to cut out pictures

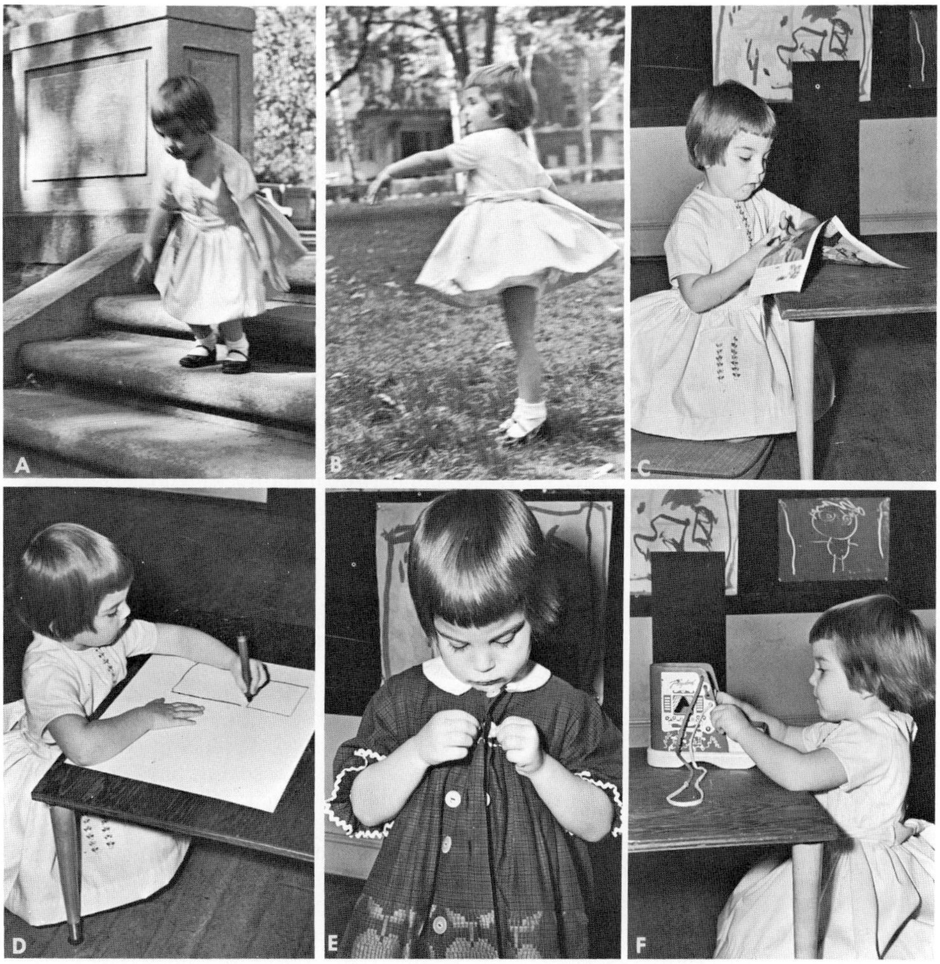

Figure 18–9.   The 4-year-old (*A*) can jump well, (*B*) throws a ball overhand, (*C*) uses scissors successfully to cut out pictures, (*D*) copies a square, (*E*) can button buttons if on front or side of clothing, (*F*) can lace her shoes.

Copies a square
Can build a 5-block gate when model is given
Can button buttons if on front or side of clothing
Can lace his shoes
Can brush his teeth.

VOCALIZATION, SOCIALIZATION AND MENTAL ABILITIES. The four-year-old has the following achievements:

Has a vocabulary of 1500 words or more
Exaggerates, boasts, and tattles on others
Tells family tales outside of home with little restraint
Talks with an imaginary companion, usually of the same age and sex. Projects on this imaginary playmate what is bad in himself. The imaginary playmate is usually forgotten by 6 years of age
May be mildly profane if he associates with older children
Is cooperative in playing imaginative games with several children. Group activities are longer in duration
Can go on errands outside of home
Tends to be selfish and impatient
Takes pride in accomplishments
Aggressive physically as well as verbally
May run away from home
Can name 3 objects he knows in succession
Can count to 3
Can repeat 4 numbers. Is learning number concept
Knows how old he is
Knows which is the longer of 2 lines
Can count 4 coins
Can name one or more colors well
Has poor space perception.

Five Years. This is usually a comfortable age for the child, and for his parents and kindergarten teacher. He has internalized social norms to the extent that he is likely to want to do what is expected of him. He is less rebellious than at four years. With greater strength, improved muscular coordination and ability to reason, he is less frustrated by obstacles in the environment.

The five-year-old is beginning to take more responsibility for his actions. He still needs reassurance and guidance from adults in adjusting to the needs of his group. Kindergarten is important to him; the experience in group membership in an environment which is planned for learning under professional leadership should supplement home training and experience in the play group. The child of this age has developed a personality which gives an indication of what he will be like when he is older.

The outstanding physical change is that the child is beginning to lose his temporary teeth.

MOTOR CONTROL. This includes the following abilities:

Can run skillfully and play games at the same time
Can hop well
Can jump rope
Jumps from 3 or 4 steps

Skips on alternating feet
Can roller-skate on 4 wheels
Can balance on one foot for about 8 seconds
Puts toys neatly away in a box
Can use a hammer and hit a nail on the head
Can form some letters correctly
Can fold paper diagonally
Prints first name and possibly other words
Draws a fairly recognizable picture of a man
Copies a triangle from model
Can wash himself without wetting his clothes
Dresses himself without assistance
May be able to tie shoelaces.

From this age on the child will learn to be more skillful with his hands if he is given assistance and an opportunity to learn. The five-year-old has good poise and excellent motor control.

VOCALIZATION, SOCIALIZATION AND MENTAL ABILITIES. These are as follows:

Has a vocabulary of approximately 2100 words
Repeats a sentence of 10 syllables or more
Talks constantly
Can certainly name 4 colors, usually red, green, yellow and blue. Depending upon his intelligence and his environment, he may learn earlier
Is interested in meaning of relatives—e.g. aunts, uncles, cousins
Asks meaning of words
Asks searching questions
Can determine which of 2 weights is heavier
Can identify penny, nickel, dime
Counts 10 coins
Knows names of days of week and a week as a unit of time
Can put together a rectangular card which has been cut diagonally into 2 pieces
No longer runs away from home.

The five-year-old is serious about himself and is concerned with his ability. He wants to assume responsibility and glories in his achievements.

Summary

At the close of the preschool period the child's basic personality is formed. He has internalized ideals and standards taught him by his parents and teachers. For this reason his conscience influences his actions more than in a younger child. He is less dependent upon the emotional support and reassuring physical presence of his parents, and is content away from them for longer periods of time. Since he has internalized their attitudes and normally has a strong desire to please them, he is controlled by their wishes, even in their absence, far more than the younger child. His socialization, begun in the home, is reinforced by his teachers. He feels guilty if he acts in an asocial way so as to displease the adults whom he loves.

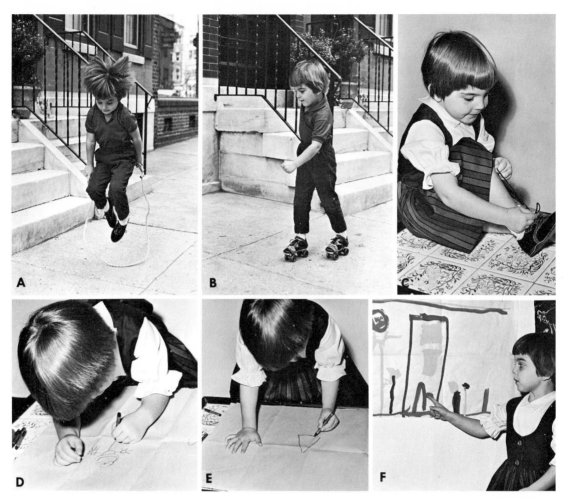

Figure 18–10. The 5-year-old (A) can jump rope, (B) can roller skate on 4 wheels, (C) may be able to tie shoe-laces, (D) draws a recognizable picture of a man, (E) copies a triangle from model, (F) explains the meaning of her picture to the other children in her kindergarten group.

PLAY

Importance of Play. The progress which the preschool child makes in personality development, ability to deal with reality, and control of his feelings can be seen in his play. Through play the child learns to express his feelings, whether of anger of love, less by actions and more by words. Children of this age as they play together are less likely to inflict injury on each other than are toddlers. Through play these children develop concern for their playmates; they are sympathetic with a child who is knocked down or falls.

By observing children at play the adult gains a view into the child's world.

Beginnings of Cooperative Play. The child gradually shifts from solitary and parallel play to a simple form of *cooperative play.* He begins to exchange ideas with other children and gradually to interact with them in play activities. Among children between the ages of three and five years a loosely organized play group emerges. The activity of the group may be continuous, but the membership changes as children join or leave the group at will. These children enjoy social play, but still feel the need of solitary play at intervals; in solitary play they can do what they want in their own way. This loosely organized play goes on despite the bossiness or aggressiveness of some children in the group.

Toward the latter part of the preschool period a more organized type of play emerges. The membership of the group changes less frequently. It is still, however, neither complex nor stable in its organization. Within such groups the typical child takes temporary roles of leader or follower.

Characteristics of Play. *Play is the business of children.* Preschool children play actively.

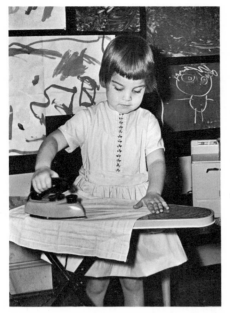

Figure 18–11. The little girl imitates her mother's activities, thus preparing for her own adult role in life.

They climb, run, hammer, and open doors with a bang and slam them shut. Their developing motor skills require practice so that improvement may be progressive.

These children imitate the social life of adults. They play house, enacting the roles of the differ-

ent members of the family, or they may imitate firemen, storekeepers, conductors or their teachers. They change from one role to another as their interest shifts with new experiences.

Preschool play is highly imaginative, but the children are always aware of the difference between the real and their imaginary world. When a child pretends that he is an Indian, he knows that he is not. Yet he plays as if there were no distinction between fact and fancy.

The play of preschool children not only is an imitation of the life about them, but also is repetitive. These characteristics are more notable in some groups than in others. Many play themes stem from a confusion in children's minds about experiences they have had in real life, e.g. the death of a grandparent or the birth of a sibling. The theme may arise from a strong feeling the child has about something in his environment, or from the urge to destroy and demonstrate aggression and power.

THE THREE-YEAR-OLD. Three-year-olds enjoy active games, but they also like to listen to nursery rhymes which they may later dramatize. They are increasingly interested in playing with other children in constantly shifting groups of two or three. Activities shift frequently, but not always with the entrance into the group of a new member or the departure of a child who instituted the activity. These children are beginning to be willing to take turns; this makes cooperative play possible. Such play takes the place of enjoyment in mere physical contact with

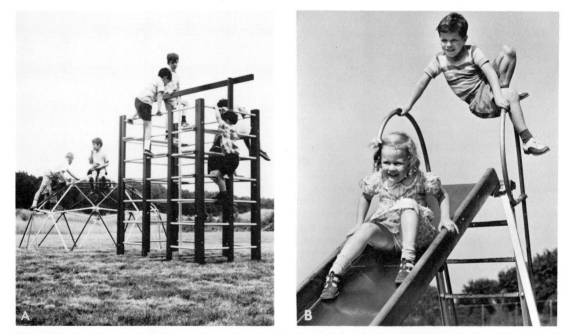

Figure 18–12. Preschool children enjoy active play. *A,* On a dome climber and fireman's gym. (Courtesy of Creative Playthings, Inc., Princeton, N. J.) *B,* On the sliding board. (H. Armstrong Roberts.)

other children. They enjoy activities with sand and water and playing with toys built for dumping and hauling. Quiet activities which they enjoy are cutting, pasting and building with blocks.

Three-year-olds like to combine playthings to make a more lifelike situation. For instance, playing with dolls brings into use the doll's bed, tea set and baby carriage. Imaginative children make substitutes for bought toys; they will use a box for the doll's bed and bits of paper for dishes.

THE FOUR-YEAR-OLD. There is a decided rise in both physical and social activity in the play of four-year-olds. They want to play in groups of two or three and often choose a favorite companion of their own sex. Although they accept the practice of taking turns, they are often bossy in directing others. To be silly in their play, doing things wrongly by intention, is characteristic of this age group.

Four-year-olds have complicated ideas which they are unable to carry out in detail because of lack of skill and of time. They are not able to carry their plan over from day to day as an older child does. They show an increase in the constructive use and manipulation of materials. They are fond of dramatic play and like to dress up. When playing house, the little girl wears her mother's old clothes. Boys as well as girls play house, and each takes the role played by the parent of the same sex. They like not only to play at household activities, but also to help mother with cleaning, wiping dishes, dusting and even ironing and hanging clothes.

Perception of shape in the four-year-old is poor, but he enjoys simple picture puzzles, using the trial and error method of finding the correct place for a piece. He is able to put his toys away, but is not likely to do so unless reminded by his mother or teacher. (In nursery school or kindergarten where all the children replace their toys on the shelf, they remind each other and do not need the teacher's direction.)

THE FIVE-YEAR-OLD. At this age children enjoy varied activities. They like to run and jump. Such expressions as "I can and you can't" are common. Now the child plays in groups of five or six, and friendship with his playmates is both stronger and continued over a longer time. He is definitely interested in finishing what he starts, even though it takes several days to complete it. He plays house and likes to dress in adult's clothing to make his game more realistic. He is fond of cutting out pictures and of working with colored paper or on a specific project with his large blocks, e.g. making a store or boat.

In this last year of the preschool period he becomes cooperative, sympathetic and usually generous with his toys. He is interested in the world outside his immediate environment, likes to go on excursions and listens to stories of things he has never seen. He maintains interest in stories of greater length than does the three- or four-year-old.

Selection of Play Materials. The choice of play materials for the preschool child should be based on the same general principles of pur-

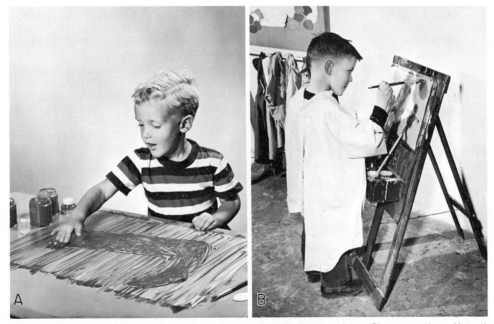

Figure 18–13. Preschool children also enjoy painting with (A) finger paints, (B) water colors. Note the long smock to protect the child's clothing. Newspapers may also be spread on the floor to protect the floor covering. (H. Armstrong Roberts.)

pose, utility and safety as the selection of toys for earlier age groups. Play materials especially enjoyed during this period are housekeeping toys and playground apparatus such as sandboxes, jungle gyms, slides and swings. Toys for active play, such as balls, wagons, tricycles and other transportation toys, and large blocks for building steps and bridges are valuable in muscle development and for learning some basic facts and principles of physics. Manipulative materials, e.g. plastic for molding, water colors or finger paints and musical toys are needed for quiet activities. Children need equipment for cutting and pasting, picture books to color and illustrated books, both prose and rhyme, which adults or older siblings will read to them.

Role of the Adult in Children's Play. Children need help in learning to find pleasure in being with other children and to share and remember that others have rights which they must recognize. They want to please their mothers or nursery school teachers. If a child fears instead of loving an adult, he may cooperate when the adult is present, but when she is not, he knows no limits to his actions.

NURSERY SCHOOL

Children from 2½ or three years to five years are accepted in nursery school. There are several reasons why a child is sent to nursery school: when the child needs the educational experience to supplement what he receives at home, when he needs the socializing experience of contact with other children and total care under the guidance of well qualified people, and when the mother must work outside the home to help support the family. Experience is given in a nursery

school in investigation, experimentation, exercising the imagination, creative activities, problem solving and socializing.

Values. Nursery school promotes growth and development and improves the general health of the child. It increases his capacity for independent action, his self-confidence, and feeling of security in a variety of situations. Since he is in an environment planned to meet his needs and under the supervision of experts in child care, his understanding of himself and of others develops normally, and he is better able to handle his emotions. Nursery school also broadens his appreciation of the avenues of self-expression through art, music and rhythms. As he learns more about the community in which he lives, he is better able to understand the world of which his daily environment is such a small part.

Qualifications. The qualifications for the selection of the school include the qualifications of the teacher, the proportion of teachers to children, health policies, physical setup and educational methods.

Activities. The activities provided at nursery school are first of all those of daily life which the child would perform at home, e.g. eating, toileting, napping, health practices, and play, both indoor and outdoor. The school has equipment for activities appropriate to the child's size and abilities.

Preparation for Nursery School. Even if the child feels secure when separated from his mother for a brief time, she must realize that nursery school, where there are a number of little children, may be a very upsetting experience for him. Unless he is adequately prepared, the child may defend himself against the experience by uncooperative behavior or by

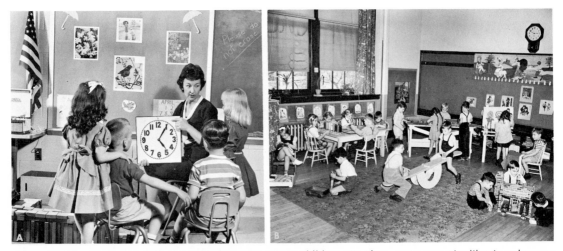

Figure 18–14. At nursery school and kindergarten young children are given many opportunities to solve new problems and to interact with their peers. (H. Armstrong Roberts.)

rejection. Children may adjust in slightly different ways to nursery school, because the school does not present the same situation to all children. Each child has his own past experience and interprets nursery school on the basis of this experience.

Preparation for nursery school generally begins with the mother's own confidence in the school she has selected. If she does not have confidence, it will be almost impossible for her to give the child confidence in the school and make it a pleasant experience for him. She should take him to the building when the school is not in session so that he may become familiar with the physical surroundings before he is left with strange adults and children. He should meet his teacher on these visits and learn to trust her. He may feel more secure if he brings a toy or something else from home to make concrete the continuity of school life with that at home.

After this preparation, decision is made as to whether the child should attend the school. This depends on whether he will be able to profit from the experience, whether he feels at home there, likes his teacher and feels sure that she will take care of him when his mother is not there, enjoys being with other children, knows the routine and is confident that his mother will return and take him home with her. Children must know these things if they are to feel secure when separated from home and mother for more than a short time. If both the mother and the child feel secure about the school experience, future adjustment will probably be advantageous, and the child will enjoy and profit from the experience.

The mother stays with her child on his first day and should continue to come until he feels secure without her. The time he is in the school without her may be gradually lengthened. She should always tell him when she is leaving and assure him that she will return for him at the close of the school day. Some children need to have the experience of mother returning after a short period of being without her, to be certain that her return is part of the nursery school routine. The nurse who supervises the health of children in day care centers, day nurseries (see p. 462) and nursery schools should observe the health of each child so that she can make recommendations for care as necessary.

CARE OF THE PRESCHOOL CHILD

Physical Care

The preschool child is gaining competency in self-care. A feeling of security in his home environment will help him to become independent in self-care. He learns to feed himself without too much spilling, to dress and undress, to wash his face and hands, to brush his teeth and to toilet himself, but he does not take full responsibility for stopping his play and going to the toilet before urgency makes him unable to control elimination.

Even if it is more convenient for the mother to care for the child than to allow him to be independent, she should encourage him to use his abilities so that he may become steadily more independent and that independence may be the goal he desires. Naturally he is slow and often clumsy in his movements. He needs help in his bath, to tie his shoelaces and to manipulate buttons or snappers which are almost out of reach. A little child can seldom brush and comb his hair. The straight, short hair of the boy is more easily arranged than the longer and often waved hair of the girl. The mother should plan the child's day to give him plenty of time for self-care before breakfast and before going off to nursery school or kindergarten, and for the general cleaning up before dinner. The daily schedule of activities should include time for active play, quiet play and, for the younger children in this age group, rest periods, if not naps. Time should be set aside for mother's meeting his need for cuddling and reassurance that she likes to have him home with her. She should hold him on her lap while she reads or sings to him, or as they talk together.

Throughout this carefully planned day his mother protects the child from accidents and from frustrating experiences which retard rather than develop independence.

Sleep

The preschool child is normally so interested in whatever he is doing that he does not know when he needs sleep and rest, and resists going to bed.

The sleep of the three-year-old is frequently disturbed at night. He may have frightening dreams due to his real or imaginary daytime fears. These children may not stay in their beds, but wander around the house or want to sleep with their parents. Sleeping in a room with a brother or sister who is several years older and has outgrown the fears of the preschool period is often reassuring. Children who sleep poorly at night should have naps during the day; otherwise they are restless.

By the time the child is five years old he usually sleeps quietly and peacefully through the night. The child who gets adequate rest at night no longer needs a daytime nap. Most children over four years of age reach a stage at which naptime becomes a battle between mother and child. If the child does not sleep, he cannot be forced to do so, but his mother should insist on a rest period in a darkened room. A sleepy-time record played on his toy record player may be helpful, and he may have his favorite cuddly toy in bed with him. Before kindergarten age even the rest period may be eliminated for the average child, although overactive, excitable children may require rest in the afternoon. Most nursery schools and kindergartens have brief rest periods when the children lie on mats upon the floor or on small cots which can be folded easily and stored away when activity is resumed.

Safety Measures

Since preschool children have more freedom than the toddler has—playing outdoors alone, frequently away from the safe environment of the back yard—more accidents are likely to occur away from home.

Important causes of accidents in this age group are their increased initiative and their desire to imitate the behavior of adults, which leads them into situations hazardous for little children.

Their activities often result in falls, and their interest in new things and investigation of what they can do with them often result in serious accidents. They may play with matches, turn on the hot water faucet, lock themselves in unused or abandoned refrigerators or freezers from which the doors have not been removed, or get an electric shock. Their increased freedom, coupled with their immature understanding of danger, results in their playing around motor vehicles, or garden or swimming pools.

Since preschool children cannot be kept in an accident-free environment, it is important that parents and all adults in charge of children emphasize safety measures to them. They should explain in terms the child can understand the safety measures adults take and why it is not safe for him to attempt all that his parents can do without injury. As he learns what he can do without danger of injury and how to protect himself, the child should be allowed to take greater responsibility for his own safety. Teachers in nursery school and in kindergarten not only provide a safe environment for the children, but also help them to understand the underlying principles of safety measures. The children may play games which teach them the necessary precautions to take in everyday situations such as crossing the street or when riding in an automobile or on a tricycle.

Many children in this age group are accidentally poisoned. The children are less rigidly supervised than they were as toddlers and so are able to investigate all kinds of containers in medicine cabinets, in the kitchen, bathroom or basement. Preschool children are apt to take pills, powders or liquids because they have seen their parents take them. They may take a substance which looks like food because they think that it will taste good.

The care of the preschool child who has taken poison is similar to that of the toddler (see p. 415). The preschool child, however, is more likely to be able to tell from what container he

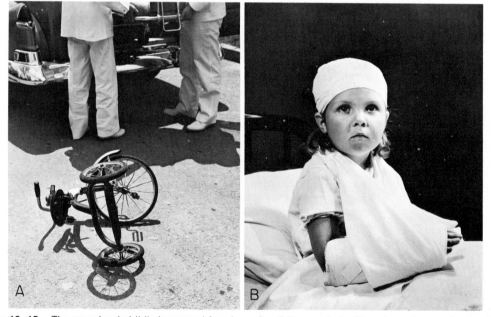

Figure 18–15. The preschool child's increased freedom of activity coupled with an immature understanding of danger may result in accidents. *A,* The child should not have been riding her tricycle in the street. *B,* Immediate hospitalization may result. (H. Armstrong Roberts.)

got the poison and is more cooperative in emergency measures to induce vomiting.

In addition to general sex education, young children should be given information about sex offenders, although this information should not be given at the same time. Preschool children should be taught to protect themselves from child molesters. They should be taught to refuse gifts from strangers, to refuse automobile rides offered by strangers, and to avoid walking alone on lonely streets. Children should learn to know the local policeman to whom they could turn for protection and help should they ever need it in their parents' absence.

Health Supervision

Regular visits to a physician are important, at intervals which he recommends, usually every six months or yearly. The physician gives the child a complete examination, including, when indicated, testing for visual and auditory perception. He records the growth, gives advice about nutrition and any problems which occur in the management of the child, and instructs the mother on essential safety factors. He will give appropriate immunizations against diseases discussed in Chapter 12 (see p. 278).

Dental care is important at this age. Caries of the deciduous teeth commonly begins between the ages of three and six years and tends

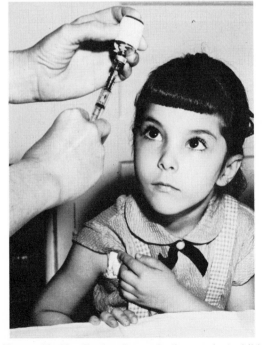

Figure 18–16. Further immunization against childhood diseases is an important part of the health supervision of preschool children. (H. Armstrong Roberts.)

to spread rapidly. Since the deciduous teeth act as pathfinders for the growth of permanent teeth, it is essential that the deciduous teeth be kept in good repair until the permanent teeth erupt. If the deciduous teeth are lost, the permanent teeth may drift or be crowded out of position.

Factors in caries formation include a tendency to decay, position of the teeth, the formation of pits or fissures during dental development, the presence of fermentable carbohydrate or acid-producing bacteria which cause decalcification of the teeth, and the fluoride content of the teeth.

Optimum general health reduces the probability of caries. Dental supervision should be a part of general health supervision, and daily care of the mouth is necessary. The teeth should be brushed after eating, and the child's intake of refined sugar should be limited (see p. 391).

Nutrition

Because of the preschool child's interest in exploring his environment and because of his relatively slow growth, he is less interested in eating than he was during infancy. Attempts to force him to take food he does not want usually result in more strenuous refusal and in persistent eating problems. His appetite will increase as he nears school age. Measures which have proved helpful in increasing his food intake include serving the meal in a quiet environment with few distractions, providing a rest period before meals, using pretty dishes, providing a comfortable chair and table, and giving small servings.

These children like plain food served attractively in separate dishes. Each child has definite likes and dislikes. New food should be added gradually so as to increase the variety of his intake. A small amount, e.g. a teaspoonful, should be served and a second helping given if he likes the food. If he refuses the new food, it should be offered again after he has forgotten its taste.

Children of $3\frac{1}{2}$ years use a spoon, and those of four or five years a fork. They often prefer to eat with their fingers, however. Foods which can be picked up in the fingers should be served at every meal.

By the time the child is five or six years old he can eat a simple adult diet. At this age, however, most children dislike creamed or highly flavored food.

Preschool children are influenced by the example and expectations of their parents in eating as in other activities. In an atmosphere in which everyone is enjoying the meal children are likely to eat more than when the father appears critical of the food and the mother is eating sparingly for fear of gaining weight. Children should not be coaxed, bribed or forced to eat. Distractions should be avoided, and the child should be al-

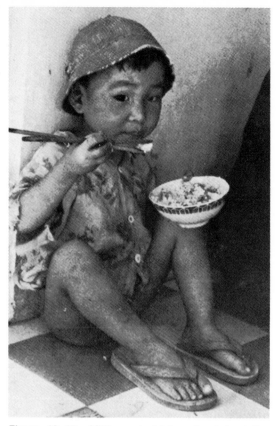

Figure 18–17. Millions of children throughout the world survive on an inadequate diet. (Courtesy of H. E. Devitt, and *Nursing Outlook,* December 1966.)

lowed sufficient time to eat without having attention paid to what he has and has not eaten. He should not be permitted to nibble between meals, although midmorning and afternoon snacks of wholesome food may be given. Children are good imitators and will copy bad eating habits from their parents or siblings just as readily as they follow good habits.

The child identifies with his family. He enjoys eating with them and joining in the conversation. Talk should include the child and not be focused on adult interests alone. It is a good time for parents to answer questions, provided this does not distract the child from eating.

Children of four or five years generally have acceptable manners, but too much emphasis should not be placed on details, and accidents should be accepted without causing the child embarrassment. It is more important that he eat his meal than that he have perfect table manners. The older preschool child wants to help with setting the table and washing the dishes, and should be encouraged to do so. Often helping mother at mealtimes results in the child's taking more interest in food and eating more wholesome food, rather than asking for packaged cookies, cakes, potato chips or pretzels.

If the child refuses to eat sufficient food at mealtimes to keep him healthy, the following factors should be considered: eating too much between meals, an emotional disturbance, overfatigue or imitation of adults who have poor appetites. If the child is ill or has dental caries, he may refuse food because it nauseates him or

Table 18–1. *Recommended Daily Dietary Allowances for the Preschool Child 3 to 6 Years*

	3–4 YEARS WT. – 16 KG. (35 POUNDS) HT. – 100 CM. (39 INCHES)	4–6 YEARS WT. – 19 KG. (42 POUNDS) HT. – 110 CM. (43 INCHES)
Calories	1,400	1,600
Protein	30 gm.	30 gm.
Fat-soluble vitamins		
Vitamin A activity	2,500 I.U.	2,500 I.U.
Vitamin D	400 I.U.	400 I.U.
Vitamin E activity	10 I.U.	10 I.U.
Water-soluble vitamins		
Ascorbic acid	40 gm.	40 gm.
Folacin[a]	0.2 gm.	0.2 gm.
Niacin equivalents[b]	9 mg.	11 mg.
Riboflavin	0.8 mg.	0.9 mg.
Thiamine	0.7 mg.	0.8 mg.
Vitamin B_6	0.7 mg.	0.9 mg.
Vitamin B_{12}	3 μg	4 μg
Minerals		
Calcium	0.8 gm.	0.8 gm.
Phosphorus	0.8 gm.	0.8 gm.
Iodine	70 μg	80 μg
Iron	10 mg.	10 mg.
Magnesium	200 mg.	200 mg.

[a] The folacin allowances refer to dietary sources as determined by *Lactobacillus casei* assay. Pure forms of folacin may be effective in doses less than ¼ of the RDA.

[b] Niacin equivalents include dietary sources of the vitamin itself plus 1 mg. equivalent for each 60 mg. of dietary tryptophan.

From the Food and Nutrition Board, National Academy of Sciences – National Research Council: Recommended Daily Dietary Allowances (1968).

gives him a toothache. Some children use poor eating habits as a means of getting attention or expressing sibling rivalry. These causes are likely to be manifested in other behavior than simply refusal to eat. The cause must be removed to prevent trauma to the child's physical and mental health. He needs reassurance that he is loved.

Table 18–1 lists the food requirements of the preschool child.

EFFECTS OF SEPARATION

The four- or five-year-old child still shows distress when his mother leaves him with strangers, but he has sufficient intellectual maturity to understand her explanation of the separation. He knows enough about the passage of time—the meaning of "soon," "this afternoon" and "tomorrow," or even "the day after tomorrow"—to realize that if he waits, his mother will come back at some fairly definite time.

A child of this age after separation from his mother may cry when he sees her again. This is because seeing her causes his suppressed emotions to be released in tears now that she is there to comfort him. His distress is decreased by crying even if he cries again when she leaves. The child left by his mother in a child care center, nursery school or hospital is reassured by her visit because it shows that she loves him and will come back to take him home.

TEACHING AIDS AND OTHER INFORMATION*

American Academy of Pediatrics

Committee on Accident Prevention: Responsibility Means Safety for Your Child, 1964.
Standards of Child Health Care, 1967.

American Dental Association

I'm Going to the Dentist, 1964.
Pointers for Parents—Your Child's First Visit to the Dentist, 1963.

American Medical Association

Facts Aren't Enough.
Parents' Responsibility.

Child Study Association of America

Auerbach, A. B.: The Why and How of Discipline.
Auerbach, A. B.: Understanding Children's Fears.
Clark, K. B.: How to Protect Children Against Prejudice.
LeShan, E. J., and Rabinow, M.: So You Are Adopted.
Ridenour, N., and Johnson, I.: Some Special Problems of Children; Aged Two to Five Years, 1966.
Weingarten, V.: The Mother Who Works Outside the Home, 1965.
What to Tell Your Children About Sex.

National Society for the Prevention of Blindness, Inc.

Preschool Vision Screening.

Public Affairs Pamphlets

Burgess, H. S.: How to Choose a Nursery School.
Carson, R.: So You Want to Adopt A Child, 1966.
Hymes, J. L.: How to Tell Your Child About Sex.
Hymes, J. L.: Three to Six: Your Child Starts to School.
LeShan, E. J.: The Only Child.
Wolf, A. W. M., and Stein, L.: The One-Parent Family.

United States Department of Health, Education, and Welfare

Better Teeth for Life . . . Fluoridation, 1968.
Children in Day Care, with Focus on Health, 1967.
Chilman, C. S.: Growing up Poor, 1966.
Day Care Services: Why? What? Where? When? How?, 1964.
Homemaker Service—How It Helps Children, 1967.
On Rearing Infants and Young Children in Institutions, 1968.
Rice, E. P.: Homemaker Service in Maternal and Child Health Programs, 1965.
When You Adopt a Child, 1965.

* Complete addresses are given in the Appendix.

Who Are the Working Mothers?, 1967.
Your Child from 1 to 6, Reprinted 1966.
Your Child from 3 to 4, 1967.
Your Preschool Child's Eyes, 1965.

REFERENCES

Publications

Albrecht, M.: *A Complete Guide for the Working Mother*. New York, Doubleday and Company, 1967.
American Academy of Pediatrics: *Adoption of Children*. 2nd ed. Evanston, Ill., American Academy of Pediatrics, 1967.
Brackbill, Y., and Thompson, G. G.: *Behavior in Infancy and Early Childhood*. New York, Free Press, Macmillan Company, 1967.
Brauer, J. C., and others: *Dentistry for Children*. 5th ed. New York, McGraw-Hill Book Company, Inc., 1964.
Carbonara, N. T.: *Techniques for Observing Normal Child Behavior*. Pittsburgh, University of Pittsburgh Press, 1961.
Child Study Association: *What to Tell Your Children About Sex*. New York, Duell, Sloan and Pearce, 1964.
Child Welfare League of America: *Day Care: An Expanding Resource for Children*. New York, Child Welfare League of America, 1965.
de Schweinitz, K.: *Growing up: How We Become Alive, Are Born, and Grow*. 4th ed. New York, Macmillan Company, 1965.
Filas, F. L.: *Sex Education in the Family*. Englewood Cliffs, N.J., Prentice-Hall, Inc., 1966.
Gesell, A., and others: *The First Five Years of Life*. New York, Harper and Brothers, 1940.
Kidd, A. H., and Rivoire, J. L. (Eds.): *Perceptual Development in Children*. New York, International Universities Press, 1966.
National Council for Homemaker Services: *Directory of Homemaker–Home Health Aide Services in the United States and Canada, 1966–67*. New York, National Council for Homemaker Services, 1967.
Piaget, J., and Inhelder, B.: *Early Growth of Logic in the Child*. New York, Harper and Row, 1964.
Prudden, B.: *How to Keep Your Child Fit from Birth to Six*. New York, Harper and Row, 1964.
Rabin, A. I.: *Growing up in the Kibbutz*. New York, Springer Publishing Company, 1965.
Read, K. H.: *The Nursery School. A Human Relationships Laboratory*. 4th ed. Philadelphia, W. B. Saunders Company, 1966.
Recommended Daily Dietary Allowances. Revised 1968. Washington, D.C., National Academy of Sciences – National Research Council.
Stott, L. H., and Ball, R. S.: *Infant and Preschool Mental Tests*. Chicago, University of Chicago Press, 1965.
Thomson, H.: *The Successful Step-Parent*. New York, Harper and Row, 1966.
Winnicott, D. W.: *The Family and Individual Development*. New York, Basic Books, Inc., 1965.

Periodicals

Branan, K.: Day Nurseries: What to Look For. *Today's Health,* 45:49, October 1967.
Brittain, C. V.: Preschool Programs for Culturally Deprived Children. *Children,* 13:130, 1966.
Brooks, P. A.: Masturbation. *Am. J. Nursing,* 67:820, 1967.
Brown, W. E.: The Prevention of Oral Diseases in Preschool Children. *Children,* 13:177, 1966.
Chappelear, E. M., and Fried, J. E.: Helping Adopting Couples Come to Grips with Their New Parental Roles. *Children,* 14:223, 1967.
Colella, R. F. A.: Dental Care. *Pediat. Clin. N. Amer.,* 15:325, 1968.
Eisenstein, F.: A Health Service Program for Children in Day Care. *Children,* 13:237, 1966.
Englund, R. H.: Public Health Nursing in Child Care Homes. *Am. J. Nursing,* 67:114, 1967.
Hargrave, V.: A Statewide Policy for Permanent Foster Care. *Children,* 13:12, 1966.
Hass, R. L.: The Case for Fluoridation. *Am. J. Nursing,* 66:328, 1966.
Jenkins, S.: Filial Deprivation in Parents of Children in Foster Care. *Children,* 14:8, 1967.
Kirkendall, L. A., and Cox, H. M.: Starting a Sex Education Program. *Children,* 14:136, 1967.
Luckey, E. B.: Helping Children Grow up Sexually. How? When? By Whom? *Children,* 14:130, 1967.
Michaela, Mother M. A.: Community-Centered Foster Family Care. *Children,* 13:8, 1966.
Moss, S. Z.: How Children Feel About Being Placed Away from Home. *Children,* 13:153, 1966.
Ostazeski, A. B.: Preparation for Permanent Foster Care. *Children,* 13:9, 1966.
Rakstis, T. J.: How Safe Are Your Child's Toys? *Today's Health,* 45:21, December 1967.
Schreiber, F. R.: What Youngsters' Questions Tell Us. *Today's Health,* 45:34, November 1967.
Sheridan, M. L.: Family Day Care for Children of Migrant Farmworkers. *Children,* 14:13, 1967.
Watson, K. W., and Boverman, H.: Preadolescent Foster Children in Group Discussions. *Children,* 15:65, 1968.

19

CONDITIONS OF THE PRESCHOOL CHILD REQUIRING IMMEDIATE OR SHORT-TERM CARE

HOSPITALIZATION OF THE PRESCHOOL CHILD

The separation anxiety brought about by hospitalization of the preschool child is likely to be less severe than that in the toddler. Children who have made a satisfactory adjustment to nursery school and have become accustomed to their mothers' being away from home for a time generally make a better adjustment to hospitalization than those who have never left their mothers' side for any length of time. Nevertheless preschool children who are ill need the security of mother's presence. The more the mother can be with the child during unrestricted visiting hours or stay night and day with him in his room, the less emotional disturbance will he suffer during and after hospitalization. If she cannot be present, the child may show an excessive desire for affection and even revengeful behavior afterwards.

Preparation for Hospitalization. The preschool child, because of his increased understanding of language, can be prepared for hospitalization in a much better way than can the toddler.

Preparation is most likely to be successful when given by the parents. They should assure the child that they will see him as often as they can and will take him home again as soon as he is well enough to leave the hospital.

The child should be told why he must go to the hospital. A detailed explanation may be beyond his understanding; *what he is told should be the truth expressed as simply as possible.* Young children may feel that they are ill because they have done something their parents had asked them not to do. This may be literally true, as when a child is burned while playing with matches, when he knew that his parents would not permit it. He needs to be reassured that his pain is not a punishment, but the result of dangerous play. Some parents use this childish concept to threaten the child with illness or injury if he is disobedient. For example, a mother may say, "If you do not drink your milk, you will not grow big and strong. You will be sick." When the child is sick, he may believe that he is to blame and that he is being sent to the hospital in punishment, possibly forever. A child should never be threatened in this way, and when hospitalization is necessary, the true reason for it should be given him. Since preschool children are especially aware of defects, mutilations and injuries of other children and are fearful of physical injury to themselves, the child should be encouraged to talk of his fears and fantasies and to ask questions about topics which concern him. Truthful explanations will minimize distortions in his thinking and reduce his anxiety.

The child pictures the hospital as very different from any previous experience he has had. He may have heard adults speak of hospitalization, and always with sympathy for the sick. What he sees on entering the hospital when he is ill may not be alarming in itself, but it stands for a life so different from what he knows at home that he is frightened by ideas of what may happen there.

A few days or even a week before a planned hospitalization the mother should tell her child about the pediatric unit and stress the similarity with his daily life rather than the points of difference. Prior to admission he may even be taken on a tour of the area of the hospital he will see during his hospitalization. Then he will ask questions as they occur to him; e.g. when going to bed, he may ask about nighttime in the hospital and be reassured by his mother's explanation. It is not well to talk too much about the hospital far in advance of his admission, since his attention should not be centered on the experience to the point that anxiety is built up rather than relieved by what he is told.

The mother can tell the child that he will have a bed in the pediatric unit like his crib at home, but of a different color; that meals will be served him, but that he may eat his meals in bed or perhaps at a table with other children. The use of bedpans and urinals often troubles the child just admitted to the unit. This source of anxiety would be relieved if the mother had explained that they are used when children must stay in bed rather than go to the toilet.

The uniforms of nurses and physicians often frighten a child because uniforms make the people about him look different from the adults he knows at home or sees elsewhere. Much of the anxiety over these details of hospital life can be eliminated if a picture book showing the physical and social environment is given the child. Such books can be obtained from a children's library and are often routinely shown to well children by librarians or nursery school teachers. Some parents and some teachers in kindergartens believe it wise not only to discuss a hospital experience with children, but also to visit the hospital while the child is well.

If older siblings have been hospitalized, they often reassure a child because he sees that they really did come back home. They may tell him that he will have ice cream there or that a child care worker or Play Lady will bring toys to him, or that a nurse made a paper cap like the one she wears for a little girl in the bed next to his. Siblings know the details of hospital life which really interest a child.

The parents should prepare the child for unpleasant experiences. If he is going to have an operation, the parents may play through the experience with him, using puppets, or he may play the patient himself, or a sibling who has undergone surgery may enter into the game. A child should be told about going to the operating room and be reassured that his parents will be in his room when he is brought back to it. The parents should know something about the anesthetic to be used. If it is to be given through a mask, this may be enacted. A towel may be used for the mask, and the child should be told to take deep breaths and then pretend to go to sleep. Depending on his age, the concept of deep breathing may be explained by telling him to pant like a dog running, to breathe as though he were blowing up a balloon or as he does when he runs rapidly. The parents may breathe with him to demonstrate how it is done. He should understand that some discomfort will be involved.

It is not advisable to explain all procedures that might be done. The important thing is that he feels that his parents know what will happen to him. After his admission such procedures as injections should be explained to him by his mother or by the nurse immediately before they occur. Then he will be interested in what the nurse is going to do to him and why she is going to do it. He is not interested in the detailed mechanics of the procedure.

The child may enjoy packing his own toothbrush and other articles he will take to the hospital and selecting clean clothes to wear when he goes home. This provides additional assurance that he will be returning home.

If the child has a toy or blanket which he prizes and which provides a feeling of security when he is afraid or tired, it should be taken with him to his bed in the pediatric area. It will be a link with home and will give him comfort in the strange situation. Nursing personnel should recognize the importance of such a possession and protect it from being lost or damaged by other children.

All too often parents are unable to carry out such preparation because of their own anxiety over the child's hospitalization. They may not prepare him at all, or perhaps through ignorance they may give him a misleading impression of what to expect. These parents might be helped if some member of the health team—the pediatrician, head nurse, supervisor, social worker or psychologist—were to explain both the life of the children in the particular area where he would be placed and the treatment necessitated by his condition. Nursing students in some pediatric units visit children in their homes to provide such orientation prior to their hospitalization. A little time spent in this way might save much anxiety on the part of the parents and the child, and also time of the nursing personnel.

Response of the Child to Hospitalization.
The degree to which a preschool child responds to acute illness with anxiety and fear depends on the extent of parental anxiety and on how well he has been prepared by previous experiences for separation. Parents are not able to hide their anxiety completely, and a complete denial of it confuses the child. The parents should master their anxiety by a full understanding and acceptance of the situation. Only then can they build up confidence and courage in the child himself.

Children also feel differently toward their parents because, as the child sees it, the protecting role of the parents has weakened. Parents cannot shield a child from the discomfort or pain caused by his sickness, and he does not understand the reason for this. In the hospital he cannot understand why they let physicians and nurses hurt him. He becomes frightened at his parents' impotence and often angry with them for their failure. The parents must understand his feelings and provide support and comfort through meeting his needs, even if they cannot relieve his pain. The child needs to feel the warmth of parental empathy, not just to hear it expressed in words.

The preschool child's level of understanding has an important bearing on his response to illness. Because of his lack of knowledge of time sequence, he may believe that he will be ill forever. Furthermore, he cannot understand the pain or his feeling of being lost. Because of his physical and emotional state he may have nightmares and lose the ability to evaluate reality as he could when he was well. The very strangeness of his environment arouses fear that new dangers are imminent. These feelings and fears may cause him to become increasingly dependent. He may lose his interest in former activities and center his attention on the part of his body most involved in the pathologic process.

It is important first of all to help the parents handle their own anxiety and then with their aid to assist the child to face reality, understand and accept his illness, and maintain his normal interests in spite of the distraction caused by his condition. The nurse must understand her responsibility in providing emotional support to both the parents and the child. She must realize that an unhappy, anxious child's recovery is retarded by his emotional state, that his progress is not the same as that of a happy child who is neither severely frustrated nor depressed.

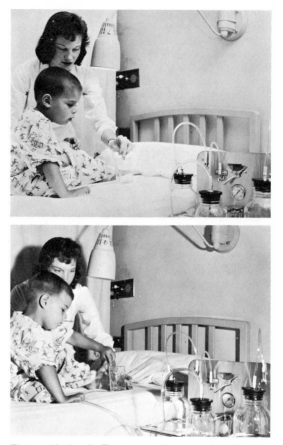

Figure 19–1. *A,* The nurse demonstrates the procedure of suctioning to this preschool child. *B,* The child returns the demonstration, thus becoming familiar with the equipment which will be used in his care later. (Margo Smith, University of California School of Nursing.)

Parental Role During Hospitalization. If the mother is not permitted to participate in giving care to the child, she may feel guilty and think that she has somehow failed as a mother. She may long to have her child back home with her, thinking of all his lovable traits and forgetting a few which are undesirable. When he is discharged from the hospital, he may be anything but lovable at home. His behavior is likely to make her feel even less adequate, especially when she remembers how cooperative he was with the nurses. (If he was not cooperative, she may be subconsciously glad.) She should understand that he is not reacting to her, but to the separation experience as a whole. She must not become irritable and too demanding. Rather, she should give him the love and reassurance he needs, and wait until he has recovered from his hospital experience before expecting the pleasing mother-child relations which existed before his hospitalization.

If the mother is permitted to help with the child's care, little of the reaction just described is likely to occur. If maximum contact is kept between them, she will remain realistic about his illness and the kind of child he is. On discharge from the hospital the child will not find it necessary to unload his feelings of anger on his mother, for these will have been kept to a minimum during hospitalization. Children whose mothers have stayed with them during hospitalization have a low incidence of disturbances afterwards.

Physical Care

Bathing and Dressing. The basic physical care of each child, with the exception of therapeutic procedures, should be similar to what he was accustomed to in his home. It should be based on information obtained from the answers in the questionnaire which was completed at the time of the child's admission (see Fig. 4-9).

On the basis of the questionnaire the nurse can learn to what extent the child can bathe himself and brush his own teeth. If he is physically able, she should let him care for himself as he did at home. If he expresses his dependency needs by wanting the nurse to carry out these procedures, she should do so until he wants to do them himself. The nurse has an excellent opportunity to help him improve his health habits on the basis of what he has learned about such procedures.

If the child is old enough, he should be allowed to choose what daytime clothes he would like to wear. Bright-colored clothing which resembles the kind he wears at home is preferable to the hospital gown that opens down the back. It is disturbing to a preschool child to be dressed inappropriately. The nurse should make certain that such clothing fits so that the little boy does not trip over pant legs that are too long or the little girl be made uncomfortable by a dress or panties that are too tight.

Nutrition. Nutrition may present a challenge to the nurse. While the child is confined to bed it is particularly important that food be made easily available to him and that he be positioned comfortably while eating. If he is permitted to sit up, his back should be supported by a backrest or by a pillow placed against the head of the crib. His tray should be placed before him on a bed table. (These tables are attractively colored and made with collapsible legs.) The nurse should help him if he finds it difficult to feed himself. Any problems about eating which the nurse cannot solve should be referred to the head nurse or to the nutritionist.

The serving of meals for the child who is able to be out of bed should follow the pattern used in child care centers and in nursery schools which provide meals. Regularity is important. A bell may be rung some time before the meal is served. At this warning bell the children stop playing, and preparations for the meal are made. Following the same routine each day makes it habitual, and mealtime is orderly. The meals should be preceded by a quiet period of perhaps fifteen minutes, during which the children relax, stories are told, and they sing or listen to a record player. A positive attitude toward meals stimulates good eating habits. Children in bed should be given bedpans and urinals, and their hands should be washed. Children who are up and about the unit should go to the toilet and then wash their hands with soap under running water. Paper towels are used for drying.

Children whose condition permits should have their meals served at a table. Usually several can be seated at one table. Those with special diets or on limited activities may need individual service.

Chairs should be of suitable height for the table and such that the child's feet touch the floor. Dishes should be attractive and forks and spoons of a size appropriate for the child. All equipment which is not disposable should be sterilized. Brightly colored straws encourage a child to take fluids.

Meals should be well prepared, and a wide variety of wholesome food should be served. In some pediatric units children are permitted to select their diets from menus much as is done on adult units. Small servings are preferable, and the nurse should prepare the food so that the child can eat it. Bread and butter may be served in sandwich form so that the child can handle it more easily. His meat and vegetables should be cut up so that he can take a suitable mouthful on his fork or spoon. If the food is served from a cart set up in cafeteria style which can be brought to the table or bed, he may have a choice of foods and, if able, help himself to what he wants. A meal served in this way is likely to be a happier experience than if a tray is set before him and he has no active participation in deciding upon the foods which will give him a balanced meal. For instance, he may choose between string beans and carrots, ice cream and custard, cookies with pink and those with white icing.

The atmosphere should be happy, the children talking pleasantly with one another. It is a good plan to have an adult eat with the children, to give help to those who need it and to provide a more homelike atmosphere.

Rest

Nap time and bedtime may present problems. The child's needs for sleep and his routine at home must be considered in planning his schedule in the hospital. The room should be darkened and each child prepared for either sleeping or playing quietly in his crib. A child may like to hold one of his toys. If the nurse demands that all children sleep at nap time, one or two may keep all the others awake by their rebellion against such an unreasonable request.

Activity

Children need play activity in the hospital just as they do at home. They need it to fill lonely hours and, by expressing their feelings through it, to reduce the trauma caused by hospitalization. While the child is confined to bed it is important for the nurse or child care worker (Play Lady) to provide toys selected on the basis of his interests and his physical state. When the child is acutely ill and unable to play actively with toys, he may enjoy listening to stories. Telling a story instead of reading it draws children into emotional involvement in it. The story teller can ask questions, insert comments about the individual child and thus make him feel a part of the story itself. If stories about animals or children are told, the child can pretend to be one of the characters and interject his own comments into the narrative. As soon as he is able to be out of bed he should be permitted to play or listen to stories with other children.

Some hospitals have a special nursery school room and an outdoor play area where the chil-dren can play together under the guidance of a nursery school teacher. If no other provision has been made, the children should have a place in the unit such as a sun porch away from the acutely ill children and out of the way of physicians making rounds. One of the unit personnel should be designated to provide the guidance which such a group needs. In the play area children should be free to develop mental, motor and social skills and to express themselves in a variety of art media, such as finger painting or molding with clay or play dough. In some pediatric units facilities for finger painting may not be available because it is a "messy" type of play activity. Even in the hospital, children enjoy playing with household equipment. They also like equipment peculiar to the hospital which will allow them to work out their feelings about hospitalization.

Children frequently select toys such as doctor or nurse dolls, play syringes and stethoscopes with which they can imitate the activities they see around them. Old cloth can be used in such play to restrain a doll, to make a doll's sheet, to make bandages or to improvise a sling for a supposedly broken arm. Much of the equipment which is of value in the play of normal children is also necessary in the hospital play area, particularly simple craft materials, blocks, puzzles, story books and phonograph records. Children enjoy play telephones because they can pretend that they are calling home.

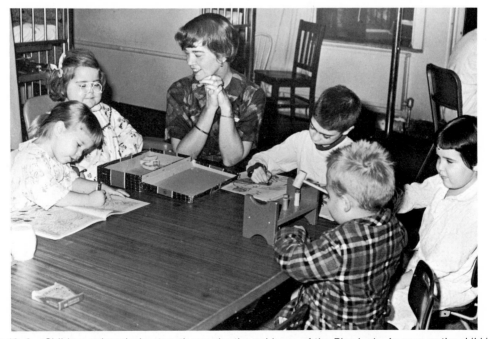

Figure 19–2. Children enjoy playing together under the guidance of the Play Lady. As soon as the child is able to be out of bed, he should be encouraged to play with other children in a group just as if he were at home.

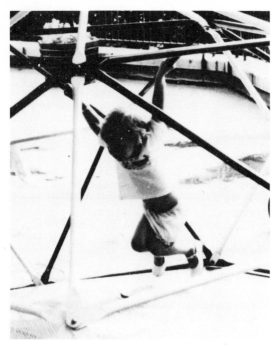

Figure 19–3. An outdoor play area provides a place for the convalescent or less ill child to exercise and to relieve his tension from lack of muscular activity. (Courtesy of Public Relations Department, Children's Hospital of Philadelphia.)

Children's play areas cannot be kept clean and orderly as judged by adult standards. If the nurses are too concerned about the physical appearance of play areas during playtime, the children feel that the unit personnel do not approve of their play and are likely to enter

only half-heartedly into their make-believe, creative work or games.

Children should be taught to take care of their toys which they brought from home or had given them by their parents. They may and indeed should let other children play with them if their social growth is to go forward in the hospital as it normally would in their homes, but a place must be provided where their toys can be safely stored. As a child learns to take care of his own toys he also learns to respect those of other children.

Children also need to have holidays celebrated in the hospital much as they would if they were well and at home.

Nurses should have an opportunity to participate in the play programs for hospitalized children. In this way they not only learn about children and their play, but also have an opportunity to appreciate the contribution of the play supervisor, Play Lady or occupational therapist to the comprehensive care of their patients.

COMMUNICABLE DISEASES

Because of the preschool child's expanding world, his participation in activities with other children in nursery school and play groups, and his exposure to environmental conditions unlike those of his home, he frequently comes in contact with organisms which cause communicable disease. Some of these diseases are preventable, and primary immunizations and booster doses have been given him in infancy (see p. 278), during the toddler period (see p. 278) and during preschool years (see p. 278). Other communicable diseases which are not preventable occur more frequently in this age group than

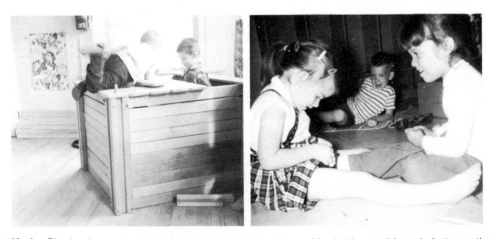

Figure 19–4. Sharing in construction projects and helping others with clothing problems help to continue the preschool child's process of socialization. (Breckenridge and Murphy: Growth and Development of the Young Child, 8th Edition).

in any other. Serious complications common in past years are less frequent today, however, because of early recognition of the disease and prompt treatment.

The morbidity and mortality rates of communicable diseases have declined dramatically during recent decades, but continued research and its application in preventive and curative medicine are still necessary.

The diseases discussed in this chapter are common in young children or those against which immunizations are commonly given.

Definitions. The following definitions are presented as a review of content the student has probably learned in her previous educational experience.

A *communicable disease* is an illness caused by an infectious agent or its toxic products which can be transmitted from one person to another by direct contact with an infected person, by indirect contact with material containing the causative agent or by contact with an intermediate host, vector or inanimate object in the environment. *Sources of infection* may be man, insects, animals or environmental factors such as dust and contaminated water or food. *Causative agents* include bacteria, yeasts, molds, protozoa, viruses and rickettsiae.

Communicable diseases may be endemic, epidemic or pandemic. An *endemic* disease is one that occurs in a proportionately limited number of people in a given area and at a relatively constant rate. *Epidemic* disease is that in which a sharp and sudden rise occurs in its incidence in a given area. A disease is *pandemic* when many cases occur over a large geographic area.

Virulence indicates the ability of the infecting organism to overcome the defenses of the *host,* the body which is involved. The recent habitat of an organism to a large extent influences its virulence. The *incubation period* of a contagious disease is the period between exposure to the disease and the appearance of initial symptoms. The *period of communicability* is the time during which an infected person can transmit the disease directly or indirectly to another person.

A *carrier* is a person or animal harboring an infectious agent without manifesting symptoms, although he or it may infect others. A *contact* is a person or animal exposed to an infection through contact with an infected person or animal.

Immunity is the ability of the body to resist the infecting agent. Protection against specific diseases is due to the presence of antibodies which can weaken or destroy the disease-producing agent or neutralize its toxins. *Natural immunity* is present when immunity exists, although the person has not had the disease or

been given any form of immunization against it. *Acquired immunity* may be either active or passive. *Active immunity* may be acquired by having had the disease or by inoculation with antigens such as dead organisms, weakened organisms or toxins of organisms. The antigens produce immunity by stimulating the production of antibodies which protect the body against the infecting agent. Active immunization against common communicable disease has been discussed in relation to health supervision in the various age groups (see p. 277). *Passive immunity* is relatively short-lived and is acquired by transfer of antibodies from mother to child or by inoculation with serum which contains antibodies from immune persons or animals. Passive immunization is used to modify the disease if a person has been exposed or is already infected. Although various types of serums may be used to produce passive immunization, gamma globulin is the most frequent source of human antibodies.

Skin tests may be done to determine immunity against certain diseases. The most reliable and commonly used tests are the *Dick test,* which determines susceptibility to scarlet fever, and the *Schick test,* which determines susceptibility to diphtheria.

The *treatment* of communicable disease involves helping the body to resist the invading organisms. Recent research on interferon, a protein produced by the body, shows that interferon-treated cells do not support virus growth well. It would follow, then, that interferon is involved in natural recovery from viral diseases. More study is necessary in this area to determine whether interferon can be used in therapy against some of the viruses causing communicable diseases. *Prevention* is dependent on the establishment of immunity and the prevention of contacts with the causative organism. Because of widespread immunization programs the spread of many of the childhood diseases has been checked. *Quarantine* means limitation of freedom of movement of persons or animals exposed to a communicable disease for a period of time equal to the longest usual incubation period of the disease.

Children having a communicable disease are hospitalized only if they require care which necessitates hospitalization. They may be admitted to a *general hospital* if proper facilities for *isolation* are available (see p. 63). All personnel caring for such children must be instructed in isolation technique and conscientiously carry it out as a part of medical or nursing care.

Complications. Children who have had encephalitis following a communicable disease such as rubeola, rubella, mumps, pertussis or meningitis may become mentally retarded (see

p. 526). Many complications of the common communicable diseases can be prevented if adequate care is given to the child when he initially has his illness.

Classification. Communicable disease entities may be classified into one of four groups: *upper respiratory,* such as pneumonia (see pp. 290, 409), measles and diphtheria; *gastrointestinal,* such as dysentery and typhoid fever; *dermal* and *membranous,* such as impetigo (see p. 188) and venereal diseases (see p. 504, Chap. 26); and *parenteral,* such as serum hepatitis and malaria. If these diseases are to be controlled, all personnel in medical nursing, dietary department, laundry, housekeeping and other departments must make combined efforts. Cleanliness is essential in preventing the spread of infection.

The Meaning of Isolation to the Child, His Parents and His Nurse. When a child is isolated, whether for his own protection as when he is burned or for the protection of others as when he has a communicable disease, he is physically separated from other human beings, both children and adults. Not only is he physically separated, but also the process of isolation may psychologically affect the behavior of others toward him. The child may feel forgotten if the nurse does not visit him frequently to care for or to play with him. He may also feel neglected if his parents do not come near him when they visit for fear of carrying infection home to other children in the family.

In addition to the child's feeling of separateness and loneliness, he may also be fearful of the gown and possibly the mask and gloves which physicians and nurses wear when they care for him. He may even be disturbed by the strange gowned appearance of his parents when they visit him.

The nurse must explain to both the parents and the child, if he is old enough to understand, the reason for his isolation. If the parents can understand the reason for isolating their child, they are much more likely to be cooperative in following the isolation procedure, much more understanding of the child's need for physical contact and reassurance, and better able to help the child adjust to his hospitalization. If he can understand, the preschool child who is learning to enjoy the presence of other children will appreciate why other children in the unit cannot come near him or exchange their toys with him.

When the child is well enough, the nurse must provide him with opportunities for social interaction and play activities suitable for his age and level of development. Play materials must be of the type that can be adequately cleaned or disposed of when the child is removed from isolation.

In summary, the nurse must be cognizant of her own feelings toward the isolated child. She should be aware of the possible fears lurking in the minds of his parents. She must be perceptive also of the loneliness and fear of the child who is unable to understand this aspect of his care.

Table 19-1 presents in brief form the common communicable diseases found in the pediatric age group and those against which immunization is given.

ACUTE GLOMERULONEPHRITIS (GLOMERULAR NEPHRITIS)

Incidence, Etiology and Pathology. Acute glomerulonephritis is the most common form of nephritis in children. Approximately 66 per cent of cases of this disease occur in children under the age of seven years. It is seldom seen under three years of age and is more common in boys than in girls. It does not appear to run in families.

Glomerulonephritis is an antigen-antibody reaction following an infection in some part of the body—usually a group A beta hemolytic streptococcal infection of the upper respiratory tract. Nephritis may follow scarlet fever or a streptococcal infection of the skin such as impetigo or infected eczema. Nephritis may occur from one to three weeks after the onset of the infection.

The kidneys become enlarged and pale. On the cortical and cut surfaces there are small, punctate hemorrhages. The glomeruli appear large and relatively avascular. The glomerular capillaries permit blood protein and cells to pass into the glomerular filtrate. The cells of the tubules appear granular and swollen. Capillary damage occurs. (Kidney tissue can be obtained by needle biopsy during life and

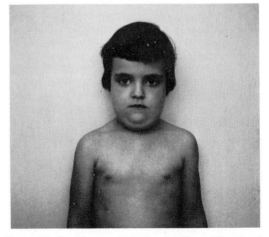

Figure 19–5. Mumps. Note the swelling of the glands bilaterally. This child had extreme difficulty in swallowing.

can provide some information about the pathologic process.) There may be generalized edema with cerebral edema.

Clinical Manifestations and Diagnosis. Glomerulonephritis may vary from a mild illness which may go unnoticed to a severe illness having a sudden onset. *Clinical manifestations* in severe cases may include headache, malaise, high fever, hypertension, oliguria or anuria, and possibly cardiac decompensation leading to death.

In the usual case the child is not critically ill, but has hematuria. The urine may appear grossly bloody or may have a smoky color. There may be mild edema around the eyes; only rarely is there generalized edema unless the child has cardiac decompensation. The temperature at first may be elevated to 104°F., but within a week falls to 100° and continues at this level until the kidneys heal. The child may have a headache, anorexia, vomiting, constipation or diarrhea. Hypertension may occur. The systolic blood pressure may be elevated to 200 mm. of mercury, the diastolic pressure to 120 mm.

Cerebral symptoms may occur when the blood pressure rises, owing to cerebral ischemia as a result of vasospasm. The child complains of headache, may be drowsy, may have diplopia and convulsions and may vomit. The pulse is slow. The cerebral symptoms disappear when the blood pressure is reduced.

The urinary output is usually less than normal. The urine contains albumin, red blood cells, some white blood cells and casts, and has a high specific gravity. The blood urea nitrogen value is elevated. Anemia may be present. The corrected erythrocyte sedimentation rate is rapid.

Clinical improvement can be noted between one and two weeks after the onset. The urine becomes normal between six weeks and several months after the onset of the illness.

Approximately three quarters of all children having glomerulonephritis have cardiac involvement. Cardiac failure may cause death, but if the child recovers, there is complete restoration of cardiac function.

The *diagnosis* is based on the history of previous infection, the presence of hematuria, slight edema and albuminuria. If cardiac failure occurs early in the disease, nephritis may not be the initial diagnosis.

Other diagnoses which must be considered are acute pyelonephritis (see p. 314), scurvy (see p. 325) and blood dyscrasias.

Treatment. The treatment is symptomatic. Bed rest is ordered during the acute stage and until urinary findings are nearly normal. After that, activity does not affect the course of the disease. The urine should be examined at frequent intervals. The child must be protected from chilling, fatigue and contact with others having respiratory infections. The diet during the first few days should consist of milk and sweetened fruit juices. After the acute phase the child may have a soft and then a regular diet. If edema is severe, dietary salt may be limited. During the acute phase, protein may be somewhat restricted.

Penicillin should be given during the acute phase because of streptococci found on pharyngeal cultures. It may also be given orally for two to three months following the acute phase in order to lessen the chances of another upper respiratory tract infection.

If the blood pressure is elevated, indicative of vasospasm, cardiac failure or hypertensive encephalopathy may develop. If the systolic blood pressure is above 140 mm. and the diastolic above 95 mm., a combination of reserpine and hydralazine hydrochloride (Apresoline) is given intramuscularly. These hypotensive drugs reduce the blood pressure rapidly. They may be given orally in divided doses after the initial dose.

Magnesium sulfate may be ordered for intravenous or intramuscular administration as a hypotensive agent. This drug, given to relax the vasospasm, may sometimes produce manifestations of severe respiratory depression and affect the heart muscle. These may be counteracted by giving calcium gluconate or calcium chloride intravenously.

Fluids should be restricted if the child has severe hypertension, unless the urinary output is large.

A child having hypertensive encephalopathy with convulsions may need sedation. A lumbar puncture and oxygen therapy may also be ordered. If he has cardiac failure, sedation with opiates, digitalis and oxygen may be indicated. It is necessary to follow the cardiac status after the symptoms have disappeared.

If the urinary output is decreased, acidosis, edema and uremia may develop. The need is to increase the urinary output and the excretion of waste products of metabolism. Enough water should be taken so that the kidneys can excrete at their maximal capacity. If the child is vomiting, fluids can be given intravenously or subcutaneously to prevent dehydration and acidosis. Solutions containing potassium should not be given when oliguria or anuria is present. Sodium lactate and 10 per cent glucose solution may be given. When nitrogen retention is severe, it may be necessary to eliminate protein from the diet.

Dialysis may be used if anuria persists for five to seven days. Special precautionary measures and modification of the routine use of the artificial kidney for adults may be necessary for the young child. Peritoneal lavage and exchange transfusions may also be used.

Table 19–1. *Communicable Diseases*

DISEASE	INCUBATION PERIOD	COMMUNICABILITY PERIOD	CAUSATIVE AGENT	METHOD OF SPREAD	CLINICAL MANIFESTATIONS
Chickenpox (varicella) (see Plate 2. Fig. 3)	10–20 days	One day before onset to 6 days after first vesicles appear	Virus	Airborne— droplet infection Direct or indirect contact Dry scabs are not infectious	General malaise, slight fever, anorexia, headache. Successive crops of macules, papules, vesicles, crusts. These may all be present at the same time. Itching of skin. Generalized lymphadenopathy
Diphtheria	2–5 days or longer	Several hours before onset of disease, until organisms disappear from respiratory tract	*Corynebacterium diphtheriae* (bacillus)	Droplets from respiratory tract of infected person or carrier	Local and systemic manifestations. Membrane over tissue in nose or throat at site of bacterial invasion. Hoarse brassy cough with stridor. Toxin from organisms produces malaise and fever. Toxin has affinity for renal, nervous and cardiac tissue
Encephalitis	Dependent on type	Dependent on type Types: 1. Virus encephalitis 2. Postinfectious a. Occurs with infectious diseases: measles, German measles, mumps, smallpox and following vaccination; pertussis and following immunization 3. Toxic encephalitis Occurs with acute infections or with lead poisoning		1. Virus is maintained in nature by birds and transmitted from bird to bird by mosquitoes and mites. Transmitted to horses and man by bite of infected mosquito 2. Occurs with infectious disease. Cannot be transmitted to others	Encephalitis is an inflammation of the brain. Several types of virus encephalitides, depending on location in which they were found: (St. Louis, Western [U.S.], Eastern [U.S.] and others). Onset is abrupt with vomiting, fever, stiff neck, convulsions, coma Symptoms may appear early or late. Mild symptoms include headache, stiff neck, fever, delirium. More severe manifestations include convulsions; coma, paralysis. Clinical manifestations may be produced by toxin during the course of illness. Child may be very irritable, have muscle twitching or convulsions and abnormal ocular movements
Epidemic influenza	24–72 hours	Not known— possibly during early and febrile stages	Virus types A and B and subtypes; type C	Airborne droplet infection, direct contact	Manifestations in respiratory tract. Sudden onset with chills, fever, muscle pains, cough. If infection is severe and spreads to lower respiratory tract, air hunger may develop

TREATMENT AND NURSING CARE	COMPLICATIONS	IMMUNITY
Symptomatic. Prevent child from scratching. Keep fingernails short and clean. Sedation may be necessary. Use soothing lotions to allay itching. If secondary infections occur, antibiotics or chemotherapy may be given	Secondary invasion of pathogenic organisms. Erysipelas, abscesses may occur	*Active immunization:* none *Passive immunization:* none *Test:* none
Aims of treatment are to inactivate toxins, to kill the organism and to prevent respiratory obstruction. Antitoxin is given against toxin. A broad-spectrum antibiotic may be given against the diphtheria bacilli in addition to antitoxin. Toxoid is given to immunized contacts. Strict bed rest. Prevent exertion. Cleansing throat gargles may be ordered. Liquid or soft diet. Gavage or parenteral administration of fluids may become necessary. Observe for respiratory obstruction. Equipment for suctioning should be available. Oxygen and emergency tracheotomy may be necessary	Vary with severity of disease— bronchopneumonia, circulatory or cardiac failure. Degenerative changes may occur in kidneys	*Active immunization:* one of suitable antigens may be given as part of diphtheria, pertussis, tetanus immunization *Passive immunization:* (1) newborn obtains it transplacentally from immune mother. (2) Injection of antitoxin *Test:* Shick test—intracutaneous injection of diphtheria toxin. In susceptible persons, discoloration does and vesiculation may occur at site. If immune, no reaction occurs
No specific treatment can be given. Symptomatic care, adequate nutrition and control of convulsions are essential. Nursing care includes providing a quiet environment, aspiration of nasopharyngeal secretions, gavage or intravenous feedings, oxygen, oral hygiene, good skin care, catheterization and enemas. Sedation and broad-spectrum antibiotics are used to prevent secondary infection. Parents must be helped to understand the prolonged convalescence needed for these children	Incidence of behavioral and neurologic disturbances is higher in young children than in adults. Mental deficiency may occur	Immunization is dependent on type of organism involved. Virus encephalitis: some vaccines are available, but not generally used for human patients. Insects such as mosquitoes and mites should be destroyed by insecticides
Symptomatic. Provide bed rest and increased fluid intake. Antibiotics and sulfonamides may prevent secondary infection. Antipyretics, drugs to control cough, and analgesics for pain may be given	In severe cases pulmonary edema and cardiac failure. Secondary invaders may produce bacterial infections of respiratory tract	*Active immunization:* vaccines *Passive immunization:* none *Tests:* none

Table continued on following page.

Table 19–1. *Communicable Diseases (Continued)*

DISEASE	INCUBATION PERIOD	COMMUNICABILITY PERIOD	CAUSATIVE AGENT	METHOD OF SPREAD	CLINICAL MANIFESTATIONS
Infectious hepatitis	14–40 days	Few days before to 1 month or more after onset	Virus	Oral contamination by intestinal excretions; contaminated food, milk or water	Manifestations vary from mild to severe, from mild fever, anorexia, generalized malaise, nausea, vomiting, unpleasant taste in mouth, abdominal discomfort and nonexistent or mild jaundice to severe jaundice, coma and death. Early leukopenia is seen. Bile may be detected in urine; bowel movements are clay-colored. Liver function tests are useful for diagnosis
Measles (rubeola) (see Plate 2, Fig. 1)	7–18 days	From 4 days before to 5 days after rash appears	Virus	Direct contact and airborne by droplets and contaminated dust	Fetus may contract measles *in utero* if mother has the disease. Coryza, conjunctivitis, photophobia are present before rash. Koplik spots in mouth, hacking cough, high fever, rash and enlarged lymph nodes are present. Rash consists of small reddish-brown or pink macules changing to papules; fades on pressure. Rash begins behind ears, on forehead or cheeks, progresses to extremities and lasts about 5 days.
Measles—German (rubella) (see Plate 2, Fig. 2)	14–25 days	During prodromal period and for 4 days at least	Virus	Direct contact or by contaminated dust particles in air. From secretions of nose and throat of infected persons	Slight fever, mild coryza. Rash consists of small pink or pale red macules closely grouped to appear as scarlet blush which fades on pressure. Rash fades in 3 days. Swelling of posterior cervical and occipital lymph nodes. No Koplik spots or photophobia as in measles

TREATMENT AND NURSING CARE	COMPLICATIONS	IMMUNITY
Symptomatic. Bed rest constitutes basic treatment. Diet should be high protein, high caloric, high carbohydrate and low fat. Food should be served in small, attractive, frequent feedings. Chief reasons for hospitalization are persistent vomiting and toxicity. Fluids may be given parenterally. Enteric precautions are necessary: bedpans should be isolated with the child; disposable gloves may be used when carrying the child's fecal wastes from the room, when giving enemas and taking blood samples. Disposable needles and syringes are advisable in drawing blood samples and in parenteral therapy. Protect from respiratory infections. Observation for indications of increasing severity of disease: unusual somnolence, mental confusion and extreme anorexia. Large doses of adrenal steroids may reverse disease process if irreversible hepatic obstruction has not occurred *Prevention:* thorough washing of hands after bowel movements, adequate cleansing of toilets, decontamination of food and water before use	Liver damage, recurrence of symptoms May be a source of chromosomal damage	*Active immunization:* administration of gamma globulin with subclinical level of disease may produce active immunity *Passive immunization:* pooled gamma globulin after known exposure *Test:* none
Symptomatic. Keep child in bed until fever and cough subside. Light in room should be dimmed. Keep hands from eyes. Irrigate eyes with physiologic saline solution to relieve itching. Increase humidity in room to relieve cough. Tepid baths and soothing lotion relieve itching of skin. Encourage fluids during fever. Immune serum or gamma globulin may be given to modify illness and reduce complications. Antibacterial therapy given for complications	Vary with severity of disease: otitis media, pneumonia, tracheobronchitis, nephritis Encephalitis may occur	*Active immunization:* (1) live attenuated vaccine; (2) live attenuated vaccine plus separate gamma globulin; (3) killed vaccine (questionable duration of immunity) *Passive immunization:* pooled adult serum, pooled convalescent serum, placental globulin, and gamma globulin of pooled plasma. Newborn obtains immunity transplacentally from mother *Test:* none
Symptomatic. Bed rest until fever subsides	Chief danger of disease is damaging effect on fetus if mother contracts infection during first trimester of pregnancy Severe complications are rare Encephalitis may occur	*Active immunization:* research is currently being done on a vaccine *Passive immunization:* gamma globulin *Test:* hemagglutination-inhibition test for detection of rubella antibodies

Table continued on following page.

Table 19–1.   *Communicable Diseases (Continued)*

DISEASE	INCUBATION PERIOD	COMMUNICABILITY PERIOD	CAUSATIVE AGENT	METHOD OF SPREAD	CLINICAL MANIFESTATIONS
Meningo-coccal meningitis (cerebro-spinal fever)	2–10 days	Until meningo-cocci are no longer present in mouth and nasal dis-charges	Meningo-coccus or *Neisseria intracell-ularis*	Direct contact	Sudden onset. Fever, head-ache, chills, convulsions, ir-ritability, stiff neck and vom-iting. Petechial and purpuric areas are seen in skin and mucous membranes in men-ingococcal septicemia. Gen-eral muscular rigidity and opisthotonos are seen. Delir-ium, stupor or coma may occur. Spinal fluid is cloudy and purulent
Mumps (infectious parotitis) (see Fig. 19-5)	14–28 days	One to 6 days before first symptoms ap-pear until swell-ing disappears	Virus	Direct or in-direct contact with salivary secretions of infected person	Salivary glands are chiefly af-fected. Parotid glands, sub-lingual and submaxillary glands may be involved. Swelling and pain occur in these glands either unilater-ally or bilaterally. Child may have difficulty in swallowing, headache, fever and malaise
Pertussis (whooping cough)	5–21 days	Four to 6 weeks from onset	*Bordetella pertussis*	Direct con-tact or droplet spread from in-fected person	Coryza, dry cough which is worse at night. Cough occurs in paroxysms of several sharp coughs in one expiration, then a rapid deep inspiration fol-lowed by a whoop. Dyspnea and fever may be present. Vomiting may occur after coughing. Lymphocytosis oc-curs

TREATMENT AND NURSING CARE	COMPLICATIONS	IMMUNITY
Sulfadiazine and penicillin may be used. Sedatives may be needed for restlessness. Intravenous therapy is usually necessary. Symptomatic care includes adequate nutrition (gavage if necessary), frequent turning and good skin care to prevent decubiti, special mouth care to prevent stomatitis, and eye care to prevent drying of conjunctivae. Oxygen administration may be necessary if the child becomes cyanotic. Accurate observation, recording and reporting are necessary if the child has convulsions (see p. 351), drug reactions, urinary retention or constipation. Catheterization or enemas may be required. Cold water mattress may be used to help reduce elevated temperature. Lumbar punctures (see p. 217) are done for diagnosis, intrathecal administration of medication and reduction of intracranial pressure. Suction apparatus and stimulants should be kept at the bedside. Observations must be made of return of function to the extremities, or any change in behavior or symptoms or signs indicating the occurrence of otitis media, pneumonia, obstructive hydrocephalus, subdural collections of fluid, paralysis, spasticity or contractures	Otitis media (see p. 289), ophthalmia or pneumonia may occur. Infection may extend to ventricles and cause obstructive hydrocephalus (see p. 214). Subdural collections of fluids may occur. Headache may persist. Intellectual faculties may be impaired (see p. 526). Child may have paralysis, spasticity, contractures	*Active immunization:* none *Passive immunization:* none *Test:* none
Local application of heat or cold to salivary glands to reduce discomfort Liquids or soft foods are given. Foods containing acid may increase the pain. Bed rest until swelling subsides	Complications are less frequent in children than in adults Meningoencephalitis, inflammation of ovaries or testes, or deafness may occur	*Active immunization:* (1) live attenuated vaccine (not currently used to immunize children); (2) inactivated virus vaccine; (3) placentally transferred immunity is possible for newborns *Passive immunization:* Gamma globulin preferably from serum containing high mumps antibody titers. *Test:* complement fixation test. Skin test with mumps virus antigen
Symptomatic. Pertussis immune antiserum may be given. Protect child from secondary infection. Sulfonamides and antibiotics may be given to prevent secondary infections. Provide mental and physical rest to prevent paroxysms of coughing. Provide warm humid air. Oxygen may be necessary. Avoid chilling. Offer small frequent feedings to maintain nutritional status. Refeed if child vomits. Small amounts of sedatives may be given to quiet the child	Very serious disease during infancy because of complication of bronchopneumonia Otitis media, marasmus, bronchiectasis and atelectasis may occur. Hemorrhage may occur during paroxysms of coughing. Encephalitis	*Active immunization:* vaccine. May be given as part of diphtheria, pertussis, tetanus immunization *Passive immunization:* gamma globulin prepared from hyperimmune human serums *Test:* Agglutinin titer and by complement fixation and mouse protective tests

Table continued on following page

Table 19–1.   *Communicable Diseases (Continued)*

DISEASE	INCUBATION PERIOD	COMMUNICABILITY PERIOD	CAUSATIVE AGENT	METHOD OF SPREAD	CLINICAL MANIFESTATIONS
Poliomyelitis (infantile paralysis)	5–14 days	During period of infection, latter part of incubation period and the first week of acute illness	Virus types 1 (Brunhilde), 2 (Lansing) and 3 (Leon)	Oral contamination by pharyngeal and intestinal excretions	Acute illness. Initial symptoms of upper respiratory tract infection, headache, fever, vomiting. Types of poliomyelitis include abortive, nonparalytic, spinal paralytic and bulbar paralytic forms. Clinical manifestations may vary from mild to very severe after symptomless period following initial symptoms. Later symptoms may include intense headache, nausea, vomiting, muscular soreness, nuchal and spinal rigidity, changes in reflexes, paralysis. Tripod sign is indicative of spinal rigidity. Examination of cerebrospinal fluid shows an increase in protein and in the number of cells, but the fluid is rarely cloudy
Rocky Mountain spotted fever	2–12 days	Not communicable from man to man	*Rickettsia rickettsii*	Spread by wood ticks or dog ticks from animals to man. (If tick is found, it should be removed without crushing it)	Sudden onset of nonspecific symptoms—headache, fever, restlessness, anorexia. One to 5 days after onset, pale, discrete rose-red macules or maculopapules appear
Hemolytic streptococcal infection (streptococcal sore throat and scarlet fever—scarlatina) (see Plate 2, Fig. 4)	2–5 days	Onset to recovery	Beta hemolytic streptococcus, group A strains	Droplet infection or direct and indirect transmission may occur	Initial symptoms of streptococcal sore throat are seen in pharynx. The source of this organism may also be in a burn or wound. Toxin from site of infection is absorbed into bloodstream. The typical symptoms of scarlet fever which may result are headache, fever, rapid pulse, rash, thirst, vomiting, lymphadenitis and delirium. Throat is injected, and cellulitis of throat occurs. White tongue coating desquamates, and red-strawberry tongue results. Schultz-Charlton phenomenon is a blanch reaction occurring after intradermal injection of 0.2 ml. of convalescent serum or diluted antitoxin. Other manifestations may include otitis media, mastoiditis and meningitis

TREATMENT AND NURSING CARE	COMPLICATIONS	IMMUNITY
Both parents and child need support and reassurance, for they are fearful of the term "polio." Treatment and nursing care are symptomatic. Avoid overfatigue. Place child on firm mattress with support for feet. Prevent pressure on the toes when child is on abdomen by pulling mattress away from foot of bed and let feet hang over the edge; when child is on back use a foot board for support of the feet. Change position frequently. Maintain good body alignment. Encourage oral intake of food and fluids appropriate to degree of illness. Physiotherapy may be necessary. Applications of moist heat to alleviate muscular pain. Therapy is required to prevent contracture from muscle shortening and to lessen residual disability. Manipulation of affected extremities within normal range of motion may be done by the nurse with permission of the physician. Antibacterial prophylaxis may be ordered. Catheterization of a distended bladder may be necessary. Since the stools contain the virus, they should be considered infectious. In bulbar poliomyelitis therapy is directed at suctioning of the pharynx and postural drainage to prevent aspiration of secretions, feeding by gavage, parenteral fluids, tracheotomy, use of respirator, oxygen, and prevention of intercurrent infection. Prolonged rehabilitation may be necessary, including braces, splints or surgery.	Emotional disturbances, gastric dilatation, melena, hypertension or transitory paralysis of bladder may occur as complications	*Active immunization* may be acquired from apparent or inapparent infection and from the use of vaccines: (1) attenuated live oral poliovaccine (Sabin) and (2) formalin-inactivated poliovaccine for parenteral injection (Salk) *Passive:* newborn obtains it transplacentally from mother if immune. Pooled adult gamma globulin *Test:* none In epidemic situations children should have limited or no contact with persons outside the family
Early diagnosis and prompt use of chloramphenicol or tetracyclines. Corticosteroid therapy may be given. Supportive therapy, parenteral fluids, oxygen and sedatives may be necessary for seriously ill patients	Central nervous system symptoms, electrolyte disturbances, peripheral circulatory collapse, and pneumonia may occur as complications	*Active immunization:* vaccine *Passive immunization:* none *Test:* none
Penicillin, tetracyclines, immune serum and antitoxin may be given. Adequate fluid intake, bed rest, drugs to relieve pain, and mouth care are important. Diet should be given as the child wishes; liquid, soft or regular. Warm saline throat irrigations may be given to the older child. Increased humidity for severe infection of upper respiratory tract. Cold or hot applications to painful cervical lymph nodes	Complications are caused by toxins, the streptococcus, or secondary infection. Complications of pneumonia, glomerulonephritis or rheumatic fever may occur	*Active immunization:* none *Passive immunization:* none *Test:* Dick test—intradermal injection of streptococcal toxin. In susceptible persons erythema occurs at site of injection. In immune persons no reaction occurs

Table continued on following page.

Table 19–1. *Communicable Diseases (Concluded)*

DISEASE	INCUBATION PERIOD	COMMUNICABILITY PERIOD	CAUSATIVE AGENT	METHOD OF SPREAD	CLINICAL MANIFESTATIONS
Smallpox (variola) (see Plate 2, Figs. 5, 6)	8–12 days	One to 2 days before symptoms until crusts all drop off; usually 3 to 4 weeks	Virus	Direct or indirect contact; possibly airborne. Crusts are infectious	Abrupt onset with vomiting, headache, high fever and generalized aching. Skin eruption occurs a few days after onset, changing from macules to papules, vesicles, then pustules. Umbilication is characteristic of vesicles. Prostration or convulsions may occur. Individual lesions appear in single crop and progress at same rate. Mucous membranes of mouth and eyes become involved. Degree of scarring depends on severity and extent of eruption
Tetanus	3–21 days	Not communicable from man to man	*Clostridium tetani* bacillus	Organisms are found in soil and enter body through a wound. Deep puncture wounds are ideal for growth of this anaerobic organism; burns are ideal because of presence of necrotic tissue	Acute or gradual onset. Bacillus produces a powerful toxin having an affinity for nervous system. Clinical manifestations include muscle rigidity and spasm, hyperirritability, convulsions, headache, fever. *Trismus*, or inability to open the mouth, is present. Spasm of facial muscles results in *risus sardonicus*, or the sardonic grin. *Opisthotonos*, a backward arching of the back, develops, due to the dominance of the extensor muscles of the spine. Clonic tetanospasms may be triggered by slight external stimuli. Consciousness is not lost. Urine may be retained, due to spasm of urethral muscles. Cyanosis and asphyxia may occur, due to muscle spasms of larynx and chest. The rate of metabolism is increased because of the intense muscle hyperirritability. Death may result from aspiration pneumonia or exhaustion

TREATMENT AND NURSING CARE	COMPLICATIONS	IMMUNITY
No treatment except antibiotics and sulfon-amides for secondary infections. Eye care, oral hygiene, and diet as tolerated are given. Severe cases may require sedation and parenteral fluid therapy and gavage. Oxygen, blood transfusions, and digitalis therapy may be indicated	Laryngitis, bronchopneumonia and encephalitis. Infants having eczema may develop generalized vaccinia if vaccinated	*Active immunization:* vaccination, using multiple pressure method *Passive immunization:* vaccinia immune gamma globulin may modify disease *Test:* none
After injury and during illness toxins should be neutralized with antitoxin. Tests for sensitivity to serum must be done before antitoxin is administered. Penicillin is effective against tetanus organisms. Wound should be cleaned thoroughly. Antibiotics should be given to prevent infection of wound. All hospital supplies contaminated with tetanus organism should be adequately sterilized. Good supportive care requires constant attention of the nurse and a physician if possible. Place child in darkened, quiet room. Avoid any stimulation which may cause spasms. A combination of muscle relaxant, sedative and tranquillizing medications will help to control tetanospasms. The child should be relaxed, but not too sedated. Tracheotomy may be necessary if laryngospasm occurs. Parenteral fluid therapy, oxygen, respirator for respiratory failure, suction apparatus, gavage feedings and indwelling catheter may be necessary. After patient recovers, roentgenograms should be taken to detect fractures or avulsion of muscle insertions	Obstruction of larynx, anoxia, atelectasis and pneumonia	*Active immunization:* toxoid is a potent antigen. May be given as part of diphtheria, pertussis, tetanus immunization *Passive immunization:* newborn has placentally transmitted antitoxin, but it is inadequate for protection. Passive immunization results from injection of tetanus immune globulin or antitoxin within a few hours after wound occurs *Test:* none

PLATE 1

1. Thrush (moniliasis of the oral cavity). Erythema, edema and whitish coating of mucous membranes.

2. Mongolian spots. Diffuse, grayish-blue discoloration in sacral region present since birth.

3. Seborrheic dermatitis in an infant. Erythemato-squamous lesions of the face associated with seborrheic cradle cap.

4. Impetigo contagiosa. New lesions covered with heavy, stuck-on, grayish-brown and honey-colored crusts; caused by streptococci. Older healing lesions.

5. Acne vulgaris (comedone acne). Numerous dark follicular comedones; no inflammatory lesions.

6. Acne vulgaris. Numerous superficial and deep erythematous pustules and indurated inflamed cystic lesions of the chin and cheeks.

(From Frieboes/Schonfeld's Color Atlas of Dermatology, by J. Kimmig and M. Janner. American Edition translated and revised by H. Goldschmidt. Georg Thieme Verlag. Stuttgart, 1966.)

PLATE 1

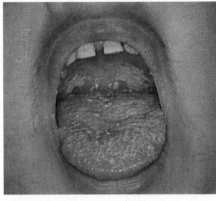

1

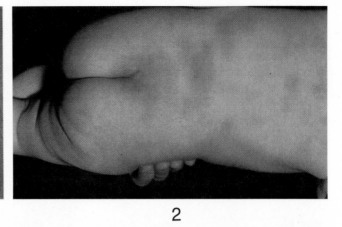

2

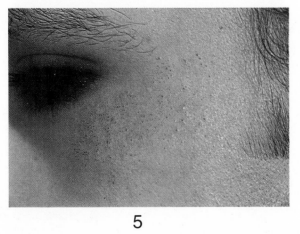

3

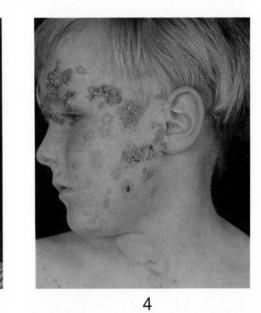

4

5

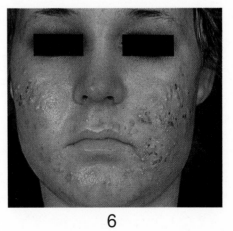

6

PLATE 2

1. Measles (rubeola). Small, round or oval, reddish-brown, partially coalescing macules disseminated over the entire body surface. Photophobia.

2. German measles (rubella). Small, round or oval, pink, non-coalescing maculopapular lesions of varying size. Individual lesions are usually larger than in scarlet fever, and smaller than in measles. Occipital, cervical and post-auricular lymphadenopathy.

3. Varicella in an adult patient. Exanthematous lesions in different stages of development (macules, papules, vesicles, pustules and crusted lesions present simultaneously). Exanthema of oral mucosa with vesicular lesions of the hard palate.

4. Scarlet fever (scarlatina). Diffuse pink-red flush of the skin with punctate (goose-flesh) papular lesions. The rash is best seen in intertriginous areas.

5. Variola vera (smallpox). Generalized eruption with typical umbilicated pustules on an erythematous base associated with severe systemic symptoms. In contrast to varicella, all lesions are in same stage of development.

6. Smallpox vaccination. Between the seventh and ninth days after vaccination the initial vesicle develops into a large necrotic pustule. The surrounding area assumes an erysipeloid appearance, and the regional lymph nodes become enlarged.

(From Frieboes/Schonfeld's Color Atlas of Dermatology, by J. Kimmig and M. Janner. American Edition translated and revised by H. Goldschmidt. Georg Thieme Verlag, Stuttgart, 1966.)

PLATE 2

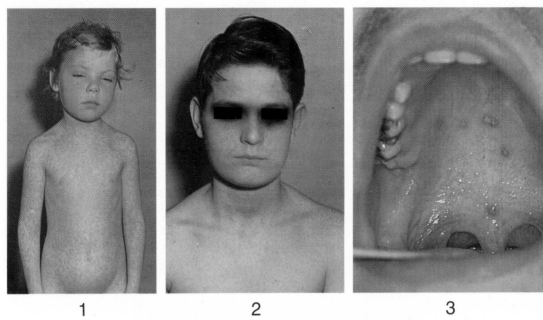

1

2

3

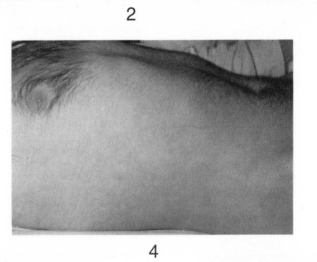

4

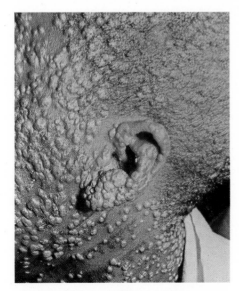

5

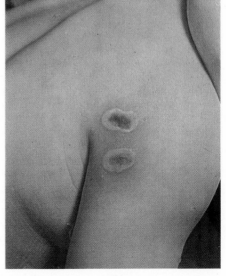

6

Tonsillectomy and adenoidectomy should not be done for several months after the acute phase, and administration of penicillin should precede and follow the operation to prevent bacterial spread.

Nursing Care. Bed rest is essential during the acute phase of glomerulonephritis and until the urine is relatively free from blood cells. The nurse should prevent chilling of the child by dressing him warmly and, when he is in bed, covering him with light but warm blankets. He should be kept in a well ventilated, warm room away from children with infections. When he is allowed up, he should avoid fatigue. He should have sufficient play activities to keep him quiet and contented.

Vital signs should be noted as ordered; the blood pressure should be taken frequently because sudden changes may occur. Any rise should be reported at once. The nurse should observe indications of cerebral manifestations due to hypertension. When these occur, the child should be placed in his crib with the gates raised. If he is in a bed, side bars should be applied to prevent him from falling. When the blood pressure is elevated, the nurse should have equipment on hand to give the medications which the physician may order.

The skin should be kept clean and dry. The diet and fluid intake should be as ordered by the physician, and any limitation of salt, fluids or protein followed exactly. If the fluid intake is restricted, the amount allowed in twenty-four hours should be divided throughout the day. Small amounts of fluid served attractively should be offered at planned intervals. Most of the fluid should be given during the day so that the child can sleep as much as possible during the night. The fluid intake and output should be measured. The child should be weighed at the same time daily to determine progress.

To prevent these children from becoming disciplinary problems when they feel better, all the nurses caring for them should establish limits to behavior and be consistent in their care. They should allow the child as much independence within limits as he is able to assume. If he is sent home for convalescence, the nurse should help the mother plan ways to keep him happy while on prolonged bed rest. The nurse must stress the need for continued medical supervision and continuation of antibiotic therapy if this is ordered.

Prognosis. Glomerulonephritis is usually benign in childhood, and the prognosis is good, but it is unpredictable for the individual child. Second attacks are uncommon, but if healing is not complete, the child may again have symptoms if he has another upper respiratory tract infection or a tonsillectomy. The course of glomerulonephritis may last from ten days to a year.

Chronic nephritis may develop in a small number of children, or they may die as a result of their illness.

VULVOVAGINITIS

Vulvovaginitis occurs with some frequency after the toddler period. There are two types: nongonorrheal vaginitis and gonorrheal vaginitis. Nongonorrheal vaginitis is common, whereas gonorrheal vaginitis is decreasing in frequency.

Prepubescent girls tend to acquire vaginal infections more readily than do adolescents or adult females, because the mucosa of the immature vagina is covered with a very thin epithelium, and the vaginal secretions are neutral instead of acid as in the adult. Since a thick vaginal epithelium and an acid medium are protective devices against infections, the child is relatively open to infection in this area.

Nongonorrheal Vulvovaginitis

Etiology, Clinical Manifestations, Treatment and Prognosis. Practically any pathogenic organism such as a bacterium, virus, parasite or fungus can cause nongonorrheal vaginitis.

If the child is not kept clean, if she masturbates, inserts a foreign object into the vagina or has pinworms, vulvovaginitis may result. If the vaginitis does not respond to therapy, the physician should look for a foreign object causing irritation with subsequent infection.

The *clinical manifestations* are red and swollen genitalia and a vaginal discharge. In some cases a foul odor is present.

The *treatment* is both systemic and local. The child's general health should be improved and the underlying cause of the infection found. The genitalia must be kept clean. If the causative agent is that which produces thrush, Mycostatin or 1 per cent aqueous solution of gentian violet may be applied locally. Mycostatin may also be given systemically. Antibiotic therapy should be given as needed for specific infections. Any foreign body present should be removed. Pinworm infestation should be treated. Douches may be ordered, but usually are unnecessary. Removal of the cause and appropriate treatment assure recovery in most cases.

Gonorrheal Vaginitis

Etiology, Clinical Manifestations and Diagnosis. The *Neisseria gonorrhoeae* causing gonorrhea may gain entrance into the child's vagina during the birth process, from the contaminated hands of the attendants or, later, the hands of the mother. Infection may be transmitted by a rectal thermometer or by contact with contaminated articles such as bathtubs or, with older children, the toilet seat.

The discharge may vary from a thin, watery type to a thick, yellow, purulent type, depending on the severity of the infection. There is redness of the vulva and vagina. Although in some cases there is little or no discomfort, there may be dysuria, fever, and excoriation of the skin of the thighs.

The *diagnosis* is made by laboratory analysis of a sample of the discharge obtained from the vagina or the cervix uteri. Bacterial studies, including culture and a direct smear, should be made.

Complications and Treatment. *Complications* are much less frequent in children than in adults.

The *treatment* generally consists in extreme cleanliness. Penicillin is the drug most frequently used. The child should be examined bacteriologically two weeks after completion of therapy.

Nursing Care. While bathing a child the nurse should examine the genitalia for evidence of a discharge. She should report any discharge to the physician. Individual bedpans and thermometers should be provided. U-shaped toilet seats with paper protectors should be used for each child. Showers or spray baths are preferable to tub baths.

The child should be isolated until cured, and the nurse should be careful in carrying out isolation technique so that she does not transmit infection to other children or to herself. The child should not return to kindergarten or nursery school until the infection is completely cured, because of the danger of spreading gonorrhea among the other children.

Prognosis. The prognosis is good with adequate treatment; without treatment, infection continues for a long time, possibly until puberty.

STRABISMUS (SQUINT, CROSS-EYE)

Significance and Etiology. Strabismus is a condition in which the extraocular muscles do not balance; therefore the eyes cannot function in unison. The child seems to be looking in two directions at once. The normal infant many times appears to have a squint at birth, and this may continue until approximately the age of six months, when his eyes become normal. Other infants appear to have strabismus when they have epicanthal folds and a broad nose. This latter condition is termed *spurious squint,* and no treatment is necessary.

The importance of strabismus in the pediatric age group is that (1) one eye is generally not used as much as the other, and therefore poor vision in that eye results from disuse (*amblyopia ex anopsia*); (2) there is absence of fusion of vision resulting in double images (*diplopia*); and (3) emotional problems occur when the child is taunted by other children about his deformity.

There are several causes for strabismus, and one or more may be found in any case. In some cases it is difficult to ascertain the cause. Strabismus may be congenital or familial, or it may be caused by an acute illness such as encephalitis or diphtheria. It may be due to paralysis of certain muscles or may occur because the muscles do not function together.

Clinical Manifestations and Treatment. The child with strabismus may be able to fuse when he looks in certain directions, but not in others. He may not be able to describe to his mother what he sees. He may tilt his head to bring the images together or close one eye to block out an undesired image. He may appear clumsy and may stumble, or be unable to pick up objects with accuracy. There are various types of strabismus, each producing slightly different effects on the eyes.

The first step in *correction* of strabismus is to prevent double vision and to hide the defect by placing a patch over the good or fixating eye. The patch should be kept on all day and cover the eye completely. The patch may be necessary for weeks or months while the child is forced to develop the deviating eye. The patch covering the good eye may prove to be traumatic to the child, since he has difficulty seeing adequately. He may resist wearing it, and parents need help to devise means of having the child keep it on. Children as young as fourteen months may wear corrective glasses. Orthoptic treatment or muscle exercises may also be effective in developing fusion.

Surgical treatment is carried out on children who do not benefit from exercises or glasses. Operation must be done by the age of three or four years if parallelism of the eyes and binocular vision are to be achieved. Surgery consists in lengthening or shortening extraocular structures.

Strabismus should be corrected before the child goes to school, because other children will laugh at his defect, and he will suffer emotional trauma.

Nursing Care. The nurse should help both the mother and the child to understand the importance of eye exercises and of wearing glasses prescribed by the ophthalmologist. The child who wears glasses must be taught how to protect them when he plays and how to keep them clean. Safety glass should be used in the lenses. A broken lens should be replaced immediately. The child should have his glasses with him when he is hospitalized and keep them in their case, in the bedside table, when he is not wearing them.

A child who is scheduled for operation should

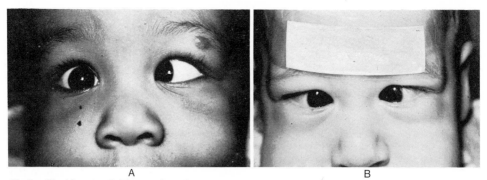

Figure 19-6. Strabismus. *A,* The squint of congenital nonaccommodative esotropia of the left eye. There is also a hemangioma of the left upper eyelid. *B,* The internal strabismus is bilateral and symmetrical. At operation both internal rectus muscles were found to be short, fibrous and ropelike in consistency. (From the collection of Dr. Arnall Patz of Baltimore.) (Schaffer: *Diseases of the Newborn.*)

be hospitalized a few days beforehand. He should be prepared by his mother not only for hospitalization, but also before surgery for the postoperative period when his eyes will be covered and his arms restrained. He should also experience having his eyes covered and his arms restrained by his mother or nurse so that he will not be frightened after his return from the operating room. He should know that as soon as possible the eye dressings and restraints will be removed. His mother should be encouraged to remain with him postoperatively to provide the sense of security he needs. His mother or nurse should read or tell stories to him, play phonograph records or turn on the radio, and play simple games with him so that the hours of blindness pass more quickly. The mother or nurse should speak before touching him so that he is not startled.

A regular diet may be given postoperatively as soon as the child is no longer nauseated. These children enjoy being told about their food while the mother or nurse feeds them. Postoperatively, the nurse can help the mother understand the exercises recommended by the ophthalmologist. She can also notify the nursery school or school nurse so that the same exercises may be continued regularly.

Prognosis. Usually, the earlier treatment is given, the better are the results and personality disorders are prevented. If visual acuity has been affected, permanent reduction of sight may be expected.

TONSILLECTOMY AND ADENOIDECTOMY

Not all children need to have their tonsils and adenoids removed. These tissues act as a defense against occurrence and spread of respiratory infections. The physician considers the necessity for removal in the individual case, and a conservative approach to this problem is becoming widespread. Antibiotic treatment for respiratory infections has obviated the need for tonsillectomy and adenoidectomy in many children.

Indications. The usual indication is recurrent or persistent sore throat. The child may have chronic infection with hypertrophy of the tonsils and adenoids. In considering hypertrophy, it must be remembered that tonsils are normally relatively larger during early childhood than in later years. In some children, however, the tonsils may be small and embedded behind the faucial pillars.

Obstruction to breathing or swallowing is more often due to enlarged adenoids than to tonsils. The adenoid structure, especially on the posterior wall or roof of the nasopharynx, may become hypertrophied and interfere with the passage of air through the nose and obstruct the eustachian tube.

Clinical manifestations of the condition include mouth-breathing, rhinitis and sometimes a dull facial expression. The voice may be muffled and nasal in quality. A persistent cough may be present. Chronic otitis media (see p. 289) may occur, and the child may become permanently deaf unless the obstruction to the eustachian tube is removed.

Infection near the tonsils may be an indication for tonsillectomy, such as retrotonsillar and peritonsillar abscesses and suppurative cervical adenitis.

The decision for performing tonsillectomy and adenoidectomy must be based on problems connected with these tissues. Usually the tonsils and adenoids are removed at the same time, though the child's condition may indicate that separate removal is advisable.

If removal of the tonsils and adenoidal tissue is indicated, but operation is contraindicated, as when a child has hemophilia, the physician may recommend radiologic treatment which results in shrinkage of the tissue.

Age for Operation. Tonsillectomy and adenoidectomy are seldom necessary in infancy or the toddler period, but may be necessary during the preschool period. The operation should be postponed as long as possible for two reasons: (1) the condition may correct itself in a year or more as the tissues normally become smaller, and (2) the operation is psychologically more traumatic to a preschool child because of fears prevalent in this age group.

Time for Operation. Tonsillectomy and adenoidectomy may be done at any time of the year, since immunization against poliomyelitis has become a widespread practice. Colds and sore throats are more prevalent in the winter and spring, but antibacterial agents are given to reduce the danger of such a secondary bacterial infection.

Tonsillectomy and adenoidectomy should not be done until about fourteen to twenty-one days after an acute infection has subsided. If the child has a chronic infection and surgical removal of the tonsils and adenoids is necessary, an antibiotic should be given for a few days before and after operation. When an older child has a history of rheumatic fever, penicillin or sulfonamides, or both, should be given.

Preoperative Preparation. The child's parents should be told of the nature of the operation. The child should be prepared for admission to the hospital. He should also be told something about the operation he is to have. He should know that it will be in his throat. The nurse in the clinic or physician's office may help the mother if she does not know how to prepare the child in terms he will understand. If the mother has not prepared the child before he comes to the hospital, she is probably incapable of doing so. The nurse must then explain to the child in a general way what will be done in the operating room, particularly with reference to how he will feel when he comes out of anesthesia.

Since these children are of an age when the first teeth are loosened and fall out, the nurse should look for loose teeth and report them to the physician so that they may be removed before the child is given the anesthetic.

Usually bleeding and clotting times are obtained preoperatively. One of the barbiturates, together with atropine, is used for preoperative sedation. Food and fluids are withheld for several hours before operation.

Postoperative Care. On his return from the operating room the child is placed in a prone position with a pillow under his abdomen and chest to facilitate drainage of secretions and to prevent aspiration of vomitus. Since many anesthesiologists believe that positioning of pillows in this way hampers respiratory efforts, the child may be placed partially on his side and partially on his abdomen with the knee of the uppermost leg flexed to hold him in position. He should be observed constantly until he is awake and frequently thereafter for several hours. His pulse – rate and quality – degree of restlessness, frequency of swallowing and vomiting should be noted, since these are symptoms indicative of hemorrhage. Materials necessary for stopping hemorrhage and equipment for suctioning should be kept nearby in case of emergency.

Bed rest is indicated for the remainder of the day, and rest periods are necessary for several days after.

Chipped ice may be given when the child wakens. Colored iced popsicles may be more appealing to the child than chipped ice and may encourage his taking more fluids. Soft foods may be started as soon as the nausea following anesthesia is over. Milk and synthetic fruit juices are given at first, and later the natural fruit juices. Synthetic juices are less irritating to the throat than most natural juices. All contact with infection should be avoided. Aspirin may be ordered for discomfort and ice bags applied to the throat to relieve pain.

Complications. Possible complications are postoperative hemorrhage, lung abscess, septicemia and pneumonia. Hemorrhage, the most common complication, may be controlled by packing or ligation. If the hemorrhage is severe, anemia, fever and possibly cardiac dilatation may develop. A transfusion may be indicated.

Reaction of Child to Operation. Children who are able to integrate this experience into their personality structure and who have few, if any, emotional ill effects later are those who have been able to transfer positive feelings from the mother to the nurse, to direct their interest away from themselves to other children and to toys and games, and to express themselves freely, either verbally or by crying.

The children most likely to have emotional problems are those who fail to establish positive relations with the nurse, possibly because the mother-child relations are inadequate, who withdraw from the situation or react with panic to it, who are concerned only with their own discomfort and who cannot express their feelings about surgery or hospitalization. Parents and nurses may consider these children good during hospitalization, but they are likely to show trauma on their return home.

Discharge of the Child from the Hospital. Written instructions should be given parents about the care of the child after discharge and about symptoms which would indicate that he should be seen at once by a physician. Such symptoms are transient earache, frequent swallowing or the vomiting of blood. The instructions should include (1) suggestions for his care, such as keeping him quiet for a few days, fluids and foods to be given, and the necessity of protecting him from infection; (2) information about the giving of medications ordered by the physician; and (3) if the child is not under the care of a private physician, the name and telephone number of the physician to be called in case the mother needs his advice or emergency care for the child, and the location of the place where the child should be taken for the follow-up examination.

TEACHING AIDS AND OTHER INFORMATION*

American Medical Association

Immunization.
Key Facts About Tetanus.
Measles Vaccine.
Pick Your Shots.
Tetanus—the Second Deadliest Poison.

National Society for the Prevention of Blindness, Inc.

Crossed Eyes.
Make Sure Your Child Has Two Good Eyes.
Safe Play to Save Sight.
The Case of the Lazy Eye.

Public Affairs Pamphlets

Saltman, J.: Immunization for All, 1967.

Ross Laboratories

Your Child Goes to the Hospital.

United States Department of Health, Education, and Welfare

A Guide for Teaching Poison Prevention in Kindergartens and Primary Grades, 1966.
Amblyopia ex Anopsia Robs Children's Eyesight, 1965.
Chickenpox, 1966.
Hepatitis, 1966.
Infectious Diseases of the Nervous System.
Influenza, 1966.
Measles (Rubeola), 1967.
Red Is the Color of Hurting, 1967.
Smallpox, 1967.

REFERENCES

Publications

American Public Health Association: *Control of Infectious Diseases in General Hospitals.* New York, American Public Health Association, 1967.

Amos, A. W.: Establishing a Trust Relationship with Children. *Exploring Progress in Maternal and Child Health Nursing Practice.* (A.N.A. 1965 Regional Clinical Conferences, No. 3.) New York, American Nurses' Association, 1966.

Brooks, G.: *Problems Confronting a Navajo Family of a Child with Poliomyelitis. Culture, Atmosphere, and Social Organization: Effects on Nursing Care of the Patient.* Monograph 18, 1962 Clinical Sessions. New York, American Nurses' Association, 1962.

Fagin, C. M.: *Effects of Maternal Attendance During Hospitalization on Post-Hospital Behavior of Young Children.* Philadelphia, F. A. Davis Company, 1966.

Geist, H.: *A Child Goes to the Hospital: The Psychological Aspects of a Child Going to the Hospital.* Springfield, Ill., Charles C Thomas, 1965.

Goerke, L. S., and Stebbins, E. L.: *Mustard's Introduction to Public Health.* 5th ed. New York, Macmillan Company, 1968.

Gordon, J. E.: *Control of Communicable Diseases in Man.* 10th ed. New York, American Public Health Association, 1965.

Haller, J. A. (Ed.): *The Hospitalized Child and His Family.* Baltimore, Johns Hopkins Press, 1967.

Hughes, J. G.: *Synopsis of Pediatrics.* 2nd ed. St. Louis, C. V. Mosby Company, 1967.

---

* Complete addresses are given in the Appendix.

Johnson, D. E.: *The Meaning of Maternal Deprivation and Separation Anxiety for Nursing Practice. Nursing in Relation to the Impact of Illness upon the Family.* Monograph 2, 1962 Clinical Sessions. New York, American Nurses' Association, 1962.

Krugman, S., and Ward, R.: *Infectious Diseases of Children.* 4th ed. St. Louis, C. V. Mosby Company, 1968.

Landon, J. F., and Sider, H. T.: *Communicable Diseases.* 8th ed. Philadelphia, F. A. Davis Company, 1964.

Liebman, S. D., and Gellis, S. S. (Eds.): *The Pediatrician's Ophthalmology.* St. Louis, C. V. Mosby Company, 1966.

Paul, J. R.: *Clinical Epidemiology.* 2nd ed. Chicago, University of Chicago Press, 1966.

Rogers, F. B.: *Studies in Epidemiology.* New York, G. P. Putnam's Sons, 1965.

Silver, H. K., Kempe, C. H., and Bruyn, H. B.: *Handbook of Pediatrics.* 7th ed. Los Altos, California, Lange Publishing Company, 1967.

Silverthorne, N., and others: *Principal Infectious Diseases of Childhood.* 2nd ed. Springfield, Ill., Charles C Thomas, 1966.

Turk, D. C., and Porter, I. A.: *A Short Textbook of Microbiology.* Philadelphia, W. B. Saunders Company, 1965.

Vernon, D. T. A., and others: *The Psychological Responses of Children to Hospitalization and Illness.* Springfield, Ill., Charles C Thomas, 1965.

Periodicals

Adams, M. L., and Berman, D. C.: The Hospital Through a Child's Eyes. *Children,* 12:102, 1965.

Ager, E. A.: Current Concepts in Immunization. *Am J. Nursing,* 66:2004, 1966.

Aufhauser, T. R.: Parent Participation in Hospital Care of Children. *Nursing Outlook,* 15:40, January 1967.

Berman, D. C.: Pediatric Nurses as Mothers See Them. *Am J Nursing,* 66:2429, 1966.

Calafiore, D. C.: Eradication of Measles in the United States. *Am J. Nursing,* 67:1871, 1967.

Friedman, R. M.: Interferons and Virus Infections. *Am J Nursing,* 68:542, 1968.

Gregg, M. B.: Communicable Disease Trends in the United States. *Am. J. Nursing,* 68:88, 1968.

Hallstrom, B. J.: Contact Comfort: Its Application to Immunization Injections. *Nursing Research,* 17:130, March-April 1968.

Krugman, S.: Rubella—New Light on an Old Disease. *Am J. Nursing,* 65:126, October 1965.

Mahaffy, P. R.: The Effects of Hospitalization on Children Admitted for Tonsillectomy and Adenoidectomy. *Nursing Research,* 14:12, 1965.

Mumps Vaccine Proves Out in Clinical Trials. *Medical World News,* 8:25, October 27, 1967.

Ogbeide, M. I.: Measles in Nigerian Children. *J. Pediat.,* 71:737, 1967.

Parrott, R. H.: Conference on Vaccines Against Viral and Rickettsial Diseases. *J. Pediat.,* 72:134, 1968.

Plotkin, S. A.: The Future of Vaccines Against Viral Diseases. *Pediat. Clin. N. Amer.,* 15:447, 1968.

Rapid Rubella Test in Compact Kit. *Medical World News,* 8:60, November 24, 1967.

Rousseau, O.: Mothers Do Help in Pediatrics. *Am. J. Nursing,* 67:798, 1967.

Roy, Sister M. C.: Role Cues and Mothers of Hospitalized Children. *Nursing Research,* 16:178, 1967.

Smith, R. M.: Preparing Children for Surgery. *Hospital Medicine,* 3:68, July 1967.

Squint Can Produce Distorted Outlook on Life. *Medical World News,* 8:34, August 4, 1967.

Use of Mumps Vaccine. *Modern Medicine,* 36:59, February 26, 1968.

Webb, C.: Tactics to Reduce a Child's Fear of Pain. *Am. J. Nursing,* 66:2698, 1966.

Wu, R.: Explaining Treatments to Young Children. *Am. J. Nursing,* 65:71, July 1965.

20

CONDITIONS OF THE PRESCHOOL CHILD REQUIRING LONG-TERM CARE

MEANING OF LONG-TERM ILLNESS TO THE PRESCHOOL CHILD AND HIS FAMILY

The acutely ill child usually requires a brief period of bed rest, but the chronically ill child requires either a prolonged period in bed or frequent, briefer periods of complete rest. This is trying to the preschool child, for his need for physical activity and interaction with other children is curtailed. The care of the chronically ill child in the hospital is difficult enough, but in the home it poses a problem which often seems to be too great for the mother to handle.

It is the mother who is hardest hit when a sick child is cared for at home. She must nurse him, carry on with her usual household tasks and also manage the needs of her husband and the other children. Eventually she becomes over-tired and irritable; she is no longer able to provide the love and support her family needs.

The nurse can often offer suggestions to ease her burden. The mother must accept the fact that she needs rest and that it is useless for her to attempt the impossible. Perhaps she can re-arrange the household duties so that her husband has a greater share of the responsibilities and the other children, family members or neighbors can give assistance with household duties.

If the child can spend the day on a living room couch instead of in his room on a higher floor, the mother does not constantly have to go up and down stairs.

The mother cannot be with the child at all times, and it is good for him to amuse himself. If he is able to sit up, a bed table over his bed makes a play area on which he can draw, color in his picture book or play with small toys.

It is difficult for the mother, in the midst of housework, to remember when medicine is due. An alarm clock set for the time of the next dose may help. A medicine table near the child's bed with plenty of clean spoons and a pitcher of water saves needless errands to the kitchen or bathroom.

Chronic illness also creates difficulties for the child and his siblings. The sick child often seems to the others to be favored and to get more attention than they do. This heightens the normal sibling rivalry. The children should be helped to understand that the sick child needs extra attention, but is not loved more than they are.

Siblings as well as the sick child may have fears which parents find difficult to understand. Illness frightens children and makes them fear pain. If they are old enough to associate sickness with death, they may develop a real fear of

510

death, not only for the sick child, but also for themselves. Parents should be truthful with the children about the condition of the sick child, within the limits of what children can understand. If restrictions must be placed upon the sick child's activities, the siblings should be told why this is necessary.

Sibling jealousy may sometimes be so strong that the well children may have passing or relatively fixed wishes that something "bad" would happen to the sick child. Such thoughts make the children feel guilty. If the sick child's condition becomes worse, it seems to them as if their wish were responsible for his plight. Then their feeling of guilt may reach disturbing proportions. They need the help of an understanding mother who accepts such feelings as a natural result of the disturbed emotional relations in a household where the sick child's needs often take precedence over those of his siblings.

As the sick child improves, he may have to make a difficult adjustment. He may look back longingly to the time when his condition secured for him constant attention. He may be demanding and easily upset if he does not get what he wants. His readjustment to healthful living may take weeks. Parents must be patient and understanding and give adequate love, although less attention, while he adjusts to the real tasks of living.

If disability follows a child's illness or if his activity must be curtailed in any way, the family members should understand the reason for this, and teachers and other adults with whom he comes in contact should be told. Then all persons in his environment can exert a consistent influence on the child. He should be encouraged firmly but kindly to derive pleasure from things he can do. Overconcern about the disability must be reduced; the child must be helped to live with his problem. *Emphasis should be put on the assets he still has rather than on his liabilities, even though these are recognized.*

CHRONIC OR LONG-TERM CONDITIONS

Leukemia

Incidence and Etiology. Cancer is outranked only by accidents as a cause of death in childhood, and leukemia is the principal type of cancer in children. More than 50 per cent of cases of leukemia in children occur below five years of age.

Leukemia is a malignant neoplasm involving all blood-forming organs and causing an overproduction of any one of the types of white blood cells. The normal white blood cell count is 5000 to 10,000 per cubic millimeter; in leukemia it may be more than 50,000 per cubic millimeter.

During childhood acute leukemia is the common form. The disease has no relation to racial, geographic or regional factors or to socioeconomic status. The cause is unknown. Research is currently being done on the relation of viruses to the origin of leukemia. The relation of mongolism to leukemia is also being studied.

Types, Pathogenesis and Clinical Manifestations. The type of white blood cell involved offers a basis of classification, but it is sometimes difficult to distinguish which type of leukemia is present in children. The acute undifferentiated or stem-cell type is common, as is acute lymphocytic leukemia. Subacute or chronic forms are rare in childhood; however, the acute form may be changed to a chronic type with the use of suppressive therapeutic agents.

The number of leukemic cells circulating in the blood is not always high, even though there is overproduction of a single cell type. When a high percentage of blast cells is present and the white blood cell count is high, the leukemia is termed "leukemic." When a low percentage of blast cells is present and the white cell count is low, the leukemia is termed "aleukemic." For a diagnosis of aleukemic leukemia a sample of bone marrow, obtained by aspirating marrow fluid, must be examined.

Pathologic changes are related to the increased number of white blood cells and to secondary changes due to disturbed function of the involved organs. Immature white blood cells multiply rapidly, but do not develop into or function as mature cells. The production of normal blood cells is rapidly reduced. The low platelet count is largely responsible for hemorrhagic manifestations. The liver, spleen and all lymph nodes are enlarged. Renal and osseous changes are seen. Areas of ulceration and secondary infection may be found anywhere in the body.

There are certain common *clinical manifestations* regardless of the type of leukemia. The onset may be rapid or gradual. Widespread petechiae appear. The child is pale and has anorexia, vomiting, weight loss, weakness and fatigue. The temperature is elevated. Palpitation of the heart and dyspnea are distressing symptoms. Episodic abdominal pain may occur, owing to the enlarged lymph nodes. Anemia becomes severe as the condition progresses. When the platelet count drops, the child bleeds easily, and a slight bruise results in large ecchymotic areas; necrotic lesions develop which are apt to become secondarily infected. There are also hemorrhagic areas of the mucous membranes and vital organs.

Clinical manifestations depend on which organ or tissue is invaded by leukemic cells. If the kidney is affected, hematuria results. Necrotic ulcerative lesions may occur around the rectal and perirectal areas, and there is ulceration of the gums. The liver and spleen become enlarged, and lymphadenopathy, especially of deep lymph nodes, develops. The child suffers from leg or joint pain caused by extensive osseous involvement. The pain in the bones is due to the rapidity of osteoblastic and osteoclastic activity along with destruction of the bone by leukemic cells. Increased leukemic foci around the central nervous system may result from the failure of antileukemic agents in effective concentration to cross the blood-brain barrier.

Diagnosis and Treatment. The *diagnosis* is made on the basis of the clinical manifestations. A differential blood smear is done if immature cells are present in the peripheral blood. Anemia is present. Examination of aspirated or surgically removed bone marrow is necessary for a diagnosis of leukemia. The bone marrow shows abnormal leukopoietic tissues and few normal hematopoietic elements. Roentgenograms of the long bones show osseous changes.

Treatment begins as soon as the diagnosis is made. The characteristics of the disease and its treatment should be discussed with the parents. No cure is known, and treatment is palliative.

Adrenal cortical hormones, folic acid antagonists, 6-mercaptopurine, cyclophosphamide and vincristine are used in treatment. The administration of corticosteroids, usually prednisone or ACTH, results in rapid relief of signs and symptoms in children who have acute leukemia. The remission may last for a few weeks to months. Side effects such as rounding of the face and fluid retention develop when heavy doses or prolonged therapy is given. Nevertheless when symptoms recur after a remission, further therapy can be given. Antimetabolite drugs, such as folic acid antagonists are given. The most commonly used drug in this group is methotrexate. These drugs interfere with folic acid metabolism (folic acid is essential to the synthesis of nucleoproteins required by rapidly multiplying white cells). These drugs are toxic and may cause depression of bone marrow and gastrointestinal bleeding. Toxic symptoms include oral ulcers, diarrhea and possibly alopecia. 6-Mercaptopurine acts differently from the folic acid antagonists; it is a purine analogue. The chief manifestation of toxicity of 6-mercaptopurine is interference with hematopoiesis. Children treated with methotrexate or 6-mercaptopurine who have remissions are seen by the physician at monthly intervals. The approximate duration of these remissions is from four to seven months. An alkylating agent, cyclophosphamide (Cytoxan), which may be given orally, has been used also to induce remissions in children having acute leukemia. Toxic effects of this drug include depression of bone marrow, alopecia and hemor-

rhagic cystitis. Still another drug used in the treatment of acute leukemia is vincristine (VCR). Sensory and neuromuscular toxicity as well as constipation may occur with the use of this drug. Symptoms of toxicity resemble those of intracranial leukemia. Remissions last approximately two months. These various drugs may be given in cycles to postpone clinical relapses of leukemia.

As the illness progresses, the body becomes gradually resistant to the drugs, and a remission can no longer be obtained.

Antibiotics are given to control intercurrent infection. Blood and blood derivatives such as platelets and white cells are used for transfusions, whether during a brief or long-term hospital admission, to correct severe anemia, to stop bleeding and to combat infection. Sedatives are given whenever needed to make the child comfortable.

Bone marrow aspiration is necessary in the diagnosis and treatment. Marrow is obtained from the sternum or iliac crest. The child should be told the purpose and something of the details of the procedure. He will feel the restraint necessary to hold him in position, the cleaning of the area, the injection of procaine and the pressure of the needle as it enters the tissue. After bone marrow aspiration the patient should be observed for bleeding from the site.

In *chronic leukemia* busulfan (Myleran) may be used.

Nursing Care. The child who has leukemia is usually hospitalized only for diagnosis, for the regulation of therapy, for periods of exacerbation and for terminal care. During the periods of remission he should live at home with his family and lead as normal a life for his age as is possible. Although it may be difficult for them to do, the parents should attempt to provide a happy atmosphere and keep anxiety to a minimum. The child should not be treated too permissively or be overindulged because he is ill.

In some pediatric units children having leukemia are cared for in a strictly sterile environment. This requires reverse isolation, utilizing a whole-body bed isolator type of plastic tent with portholes through which care may be given (see p. 421).

The nursing care is similar to that for anemia (see p. 338). The nurse should handle the child's body *gently,* since the extremities are painful when touched. Oral hygiene is needed and must be done with the utmost care to prevent trauma to the sore and bleeding gums, especially if oral ulcers are present. When these children have sore throats, they may not wish to talk or eat. These children are prone to infection; therefore care should be taken to prevent them from becoming chilled. An adequate fluid intake is important. To prevent nausea, small amounts of fluids which he likes should be offered frequently. The intake and output are routinely charted.

Well balanced meals can be planned from foods which he likes, and should be served when he is awake. He should not be wakened at mealtimes, since he needs his rest.

Accurate charting is important. The nurse should watch for bleeding and report both the site and the amount. It is difficult to get these children to say how they feel, but any complaints should be charted, together with the circumstances bearing upon the complaint.

The child is irritable because he is extremely uncomfortable. While the child is receiving intravenous therapy throughout the day the nurse should expect him to be irritable because of the pain involved and because of his inability to move as he would like. All who care for him should be patient and try to provide a quiet but happy atmosphere in which there are as few frustrations as possible. The mother should be with him as much as possible, both to give him the constant loving care he needs and to learn how to nurse him during his periods at home. Parents have a natural and positive outlet for their affection when they are allowed to help in the nursing care of their child while he is in the hospital.

When alopecia occurs as a result of drug therapy, the child should be prepared for the possible loss of his hair. Parents many times purchase a wig for the child to wear when he feels well enough to do so.

During his illness the child may be nauseated, lonely and easily tired. The company of parents who have accepted his fatal illness and adjusted to it helps him also to accept and adjust to his condition. The child may at times appear to be anxious. This may be partly the result of anxiety which his parents were unable to conceal from him. Since the child may be ill for months, with remissions and exacerbations, the parents will need emotional support from physicians and nurses who they know have cared for such children before.

When the child is cared for at home, he may be brought back to the outpatient department for periodic transfusion therapy. The parents in this situation may contribute to his care by helping to observe and possibly regulate the rate of flow of the blood, platelets or white cells being given. The nurse must remember, however, that there is a difference between mothering and nursing and that it is she, the nurse, who is ultimately responsible for the care of the child.

Terminal nursing care is difficult. Parents may know intellectually that the child will die, but emotionally they continue to hope for a cure. Nurses need to appreciate that parents may be extremely demanding and difficult during their child's illness because of their intense anxiety. The child must be given physical and emotional support, for he is most uncomfortable as long as he is sufficiently conscious to be aware of his sensations. His nose and throat should be kept clean, and his lips and mouth moist. Frequent bathing is necessary to keep the skin clean, and his position should be changed as often as possible without disturbing him, in order to prevent bedsores. Sedatives may be given when necessary.

To minister successfully to the dying child and his parents, the nurse must be able to accept the way in which they express their fear and grief. To do this she must face her own feelings about death. When the critically ill child lapses into unconsciousness, the nurse must remain with the parents at his bedside so that they know that everything possible is being done for his comfort. If the nurse leaves them alone with the dying child, she may thereby indicate to them rejection of their grief. If parents cannot be present, the nurse must remain constantly with the dying child to prevent loneliness and the feeling that there is no one to help him when he is suffering and afraid of the change that is coming over him. The children in the unit sense tension of the nurse and that of the other personnel. They need her emotional support, most especially if they know they have the same illness as the dying child. The question as to whether to tell such children that they too will die is one which must be answered on an individual basis. (See page 73 for further discussion of the dying child and his family.)

Complications and Prognosis. *Complications* arise as a result of lack of normal white blood cells. Intracranial and visceral hemorrhages may occur. Intracranial hemorrhage is the most common immediate cause of death. Death results from the disease itself or from intercurrent infections, or both.

Without treatment the course of acute leukemia is usually that of rapid deterioration, death occuring in about two months. With treatment acute · leukemia may be changed to a chronic form and the child may survive from one to three years or longer. When the child is in the terminal stage of his illness, the question of how long to help him survive by mechanical means is a difficult decision to make.

Tetralogy of Fallot

Preoperative Care and Treatment. Tetralogy of Fallot was described in connection with congenital defects in the newborn infant (see p. 204). Since operation is usually postponed until between three and five years of age, preoperative and postoperative nursing care and a description of the types of operation are included here. The student, after learning the detailed care of children having one type of congenital cardiac anomaly, should be able to transfer this knowledge to the care of children having other kinds of cardiac surgery.

Surgical Correction. One of several types of surgical correction may be done on children having tetralogy of Fallot. In closed-heart surgery (palliative surgery) there are the Blalock-Taussig operation, the Potts operation and the Brock procedure.

CLOSED-HEART (PALLIATIVE) SURGERY. In the *Blalock-Taussig operation* a branch of the aorta is anastomosed to the pulmonary artery. In children under two years the innominate artery is used; in children over two years the subclavian artery is preferred. The result of this operation is that a connection is made between a systemic artery and the pulmonary artery, thus increasing the blood flow to the lungs, improving exercise tolerance and reducing cyanosis.

In the *Potts operation* a direct connection is made between the aorta and the pulmonary artery. The same results are achieved as with the Blalock-Taussig operation.

None of these operations is corrective. The operative risk with anastomotic procedures is low. Although the immediate clinical improvement is good, some incapacity may remain.

The *Brock procedure* is a direct operation for the pulmonary stenosis and is done through a right ventricular approach. This operation increases the flow of blood to the lungs, but does not correct the ventricular septal defect.

OPEN-HEART (CORRECTIVE) SURGERY. Techniques developed to permit open-heart surgery include the following: (1) hypothermia. Hypothermia may be induced by the use of water-cooled mattresses of varied sizes, ice bags, or gastric lavage with iced liquid. The degree of cooling is dependent on the surgeon; however, maximum benefit with minimal danger can be achieved when the child's temperature is reduced to between 86 and 90°F. (30 to 32.2°C.) Some surgeons may request temperatures lower than these. Vigorous shivering must be prevented if this therapy is to be effective. The use of hypothermia is not without danger, and therefore the child so treated must be watched carefully by a team of experts for complications. In hypothermia the body temperature is lowered so that the metabolic rate is reduced. Reduction of the metabolic rate decreases the need for oxygen in the tissues of the body and so lessens the danger of anoxia. (2) Heart-lung machine. The heart-lung machine is interposed in the circulation, allowing blood flow to bypass the heart and lungs. Gaseous exchange occurs within the apparatus. The venous blood passes through two catheters in the venae cavae to the machine, and the oxygenated blood is returned to the large arteries for systemic distribution. Since the machine

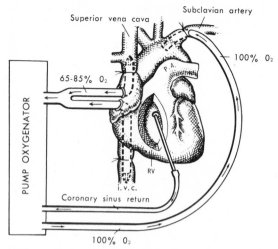

Figure 20–1. Cardiopulmonary bypass. Cannulation of venae cavae for withdrawal of venous blood and of aorta for perfusion with oxygenated blood from apparatus. The sucker for collecting blood from the open chamber of the heart is placed beneath the tricuspid valve, returning this blood to the apparatus. (Courtesy of American Heart Association. Adapted from Ventricular Septal Defects with Pulmonary Hypertension, by James W. DuShane and others: *J.A.M.A.*, Vol. 160.)

carries on the functions of the heart and lungs, the surgeon is able to open the bloodless heart and repair the defective structures. (3) Hyperbaric oxygenation. Hyperbaric oxygenation involves placing the patient in a specially built chamber having the content of oxygen from 21 to 100 per cent under one to five atmospheres of pressure. Because of this the amount of oxygen is greatly increased in body tissues and fluids. Recently research has been done on the use of this technique in surgery in cyanotic congenital heart diseases of children. Problems associated with the use of hyperbaric oxygenation at present include oxygen toxicity, and the hazards of decompression, explosion and fire.

Open-heart surgery would seem to be best for the child having tetralogy of Fallot, since it affords relief of the pulmonary stenosis and closure of the ventricular septal defect. The operative risk is higher than that of the anastomotic procedures. The results are spectacular, however, in successful cases.

During these operations a thoracotomy tube is usually inserted into the pleural space and attached to a gravity suction bottle placed lower than the chest. The pleural space is thus kept free from drainage. If the fluid were permitted to remain in the chest, the lungs would not be able to expand completely, and the fluid might become infected, resulting in empyema. The fluid in the tube oscillates with respiration, indicating that there is an airtight seal at the site where the thoracotomy tube is inserted.

EMOTIONAL PREPARATION FOR SURGERY. Not only should the parents explain the procedure of admission to the hospital to the child, but they should also have explained to him in simple language the nature of his illness and the treatment to be done. If the child has siblings, they should also understand the child's condition so that they do not become jealous of the extra attention which of necessity he must receive.

The child admitted for cardiac surgery is usually somewhat insecure and unstable in spite of the preparation he may have had. He has probably observed the anxiety of his parents over his physical health, and he in turn becomes anxious about his own welfare. Since the majority of parents, realizing that crying by a child who has a cyanotic type of cardiac defect results in frightening cyanosis, they have minimized frustration for him so that he has not been able to learn to stand the usual frustrations of childhood. In addition, he has to minimize his physical activity, not only by not playing actively with other children, but also by becoming overdependent on his parents for meeting the normal physical needs which other preschool children handle themselves. Although some children will revolt in the face of such restrictions and exercise to the limit of their tolerance, most of them submit because of the attention they receive. These children may lack self-confidence, may feel inferior to their peers, and may withdraw from other children, yet may be demanding and aggressive with their parents and other adults.

In order to plan her care for the child the nurse through discussion with the parents should determine how much preparation for his operation the child has actually had, what experiences he has had in the past which would prepare him for this experience, and how he usually relates to adults other than his parents. On the basis of this information the nurse should be able to determine her approach in order to make the child feel more secure in her care.

The parents who bring the child to the hospital usually regard surgery with an ambivalent attitude: of exaggerated fear because of the relative newness of cardiac surgery and of hope for the child's recovery. The parents need someone with whom they can discuss their hopes and fears and from whom they can get easily understood answers to their questions.

Both the child and his parents need emotional preparation for the tests and operation which the child is to undergo. Any diagnostic procedures which may be done, such as the exercise tolerance test, roentgen examination and fluoroscopic examination, oxygen saturation tests, electrocardiography, cardiac catheterization and angiocardiography, should be explained when appropriate. The child and his parents may be taken to the operating suite and to the intensive care unit so that they will become familiar with the physical setting, the brightness of the lights and the increased activities as well as the appearance of the gowned and masked personnel. Details of the operation such as how the anesthetic will be given, where the incision will be, and what types of tubes will be inserted can be discussed in a nonthreatening manner. The purposes of therapy should be discussed. The equipment to be used should be shown *gradually,* such as that used for the administration of parenteral fluids, tracheal suctioning, drainage apparatus, intermittent positive-pressure apparatus, the oxygen tent, and the inevitable injections. The child should be placed temporarily in the oxygen tent in order to accustom him to the experience. He should also be taught how to use the intermittent positive-pressure respirator if this is to be used postoperatively. This machine is frightening to many children because of the gust of air it emits and because the face mask makes them fear that they will suffocate when it is used. Suggestions for gaining the child's cooperation include a demonstration of the use of the mask by the nurse, and making a game of the treatment by pretending that the mask is of the same type as astronauts use. Prior to operation the child should also be oriented to other aspects of the nursing care which he will receive: the taking of vital signs, taking of fluids, necessity for turning, coughing, and deep breathing. If the child understands that he can tell the nurse how he feels about the care he receives, he will be free to express his emotions freely postoperatively. The nurse should stress the fact that the child and his parents may forget some of the aspects of the care she has described. Then when they do forget something postoperatively, they know that the nurse expected this to happen, and they feel confident in asking for assistance.

Throughout this preparatory phase, the nurse should make every effort to assure both parents and child that a nurse will be with the child constantly so that he will not be alone. The nurse, through her accepting manner, can also convey the fact that emotions which either parents or child feel should be expressed to her, whether of fear, anger or dependency, and that they will be accepted. Regression, which is a usual response to stress, should also be recognized and accepted.

The nurse at this time can also help the parents to understand that she will be very busy attending the child after operation and that her increased activity is not an indication that the child's condition has become worse.

PHYSICAL PREPARATION FOR SURGERY. Since many children are not in optimum physical condition preoperatively, adequate diet and fluid intake, rest and controlled exercise are needed. Adequate hydration is especially needed if the child has a compensatory polycythemia (see p. 204). If cardiac failure is present, absolute rest, digitalis, diuretics and oxygen therapy may be needed. Antibiotics are given prophylactically before operation. The child must be protected from patients and personnel having infections. Fluids are given parenterally before and during the operation to prevent dehydration.

The child's skin is shaved and prepared on the evening before operation. A cleansing enema may be ordered. Sedation is given so that he may get as much rest as possible. He is weighed on the same scale that will be used to weigh him after the operation. By comparing the difference in weights it can be determined whether the child received too much or too little parenteral fluids during the operation. The child should be permitted to take his favorite toy or security object with him to the operating room.

The nurse who cares for the child preoperatively should care for him postoperatively so that changes in his condition can be easily noted and the child may feel secure in her presence. During operation the nurse must give the parents support by answering their questions and preparing them for the child's appearance after operation so that their anxiety may be reduced. It may be wise to show the parents a child who has had the same operation their child will have so that they are not overwhelmed by his appearance.

During the operation the nurse should also check on the equipment needed for the child's care, including a cardiac arrest tray, and make certain that it is assembled in readiness for his return. Immediately postoperatively she should become familiar with the operative procedure which was done, the medications and parenteral fluids which he received, and the orders which were written for his postoperative care.

POSTOPERATIVE CARE. On admission to the intensive care unit or recovery room the child is given oxygen immediately. Each catheter in his chest must be carefully checked and attached to the suction machine. The vital signs must be taken, and if there is any indication for the use of a cardioscope, it is attached to the patient. The heart rate and rhythm and the electrocardiogram can thus be observed constantly. The administration of intravenous fluids must be checked and regulated carefully, perhaps using a special regulating pump if one is available. If a tracheotomy has been done, the child should receive the care described on page 406.

When the child reacts from his anesthesia, he should be told that his operation is over. The child may be confused, restless, drowsy and in obvious pain. A narcotic may be given on the physician's order. The child may be unaware of his environment and the medical and nursing personnel around him, and be concerned only with himself and his pain.

The vital signs are taken each hour, or more often if necessary. The nurse must take the temperature rectally, since the cool atmosphere (68 to 72°) in the oxygen tent may affect an oral reading. If fever is present, rectal administration of aspirin, tepid water sponges, ice bags to the groin and axillae, an ice-water mattress or a hypothermia blanket may be ordered. Fever must be reduced, since this increases both the rate of blood flow through the body and the metabolic rate.

The nurse should check the rate and depth of respirations and note whether chest expansion on both sides is equal. If the child has noisy or rapid breathing indicating an accumulation of mucus in his respiratory passages, the nurse should use suction to remove the secretions. She should also note the difference in the rate, quality, rhythm and volume between the radial and pedal pulses. The blood pressure should be taken with the other signs. If the pulse rate becomes irregular and the blood pressure drops, the physician should be notified immediately, because these signs may indicate impending cardiac arrest. If the pulse and respiratory rates rise, if the blood pressure drops, and if the child is very thirsty, the physician should also be notified, because these are signs of hemorrhage. The cardiac monitor in use in many institutions is of great value in the care of these patients. The color of the child's nailbeds and skin and the condition of his skin, whether moist, dry, cool or warm, should also be observed and recorded. If cyanosis and respiratory embarrassment are severe, a tracheotomy may be necessary (see p. 406) if it was not done previously.

Intravenous fluid therapy is given by cutdown in the child's arm or leg. The administration of fluids must be carefully recorded (see p. 299) in order that they are not given too rapidly. It must be remembered that a change in the child's position or a change from a resting to a crying state may change the rate of flow. The nurse must also check on whether the tubing is kinked or obstructed in any way and whether fluids are infiltrating into the tissues.

Fluid intake by mouth is usually limited during the postoperative period in order to prevent added strain on the heart due to overloading the circulation. A Levin tube may be inserted to prevent gastric dilatation. Mouth care and frequent rinsing of the mouth with water will alleviate some of the thirst the child experiences. Since both the parents and the child may be disturbed by this limitation of fluids, the nurse should assure them that thirst is a normal reaction and explain the reasons why unlimited fluids may not be given.

If the child is unable to void within eight to

twelve hours after operation, a Foley catheter may be inserted. The specific gravity, color and the amount of urine should be recorded.

Immediately after operation the one or two chest catheters were connected to underwater suction. These tubes remove fluid which has collected in the pleural cavity. By observation of the drainage, bleeding can be readily detected. If the physician so orders, the tubes are "milked" in the direction of the drainage bottles to assure that they are patent and free of blood clots, and to facilitate drainage. The nurse must check to see that the tubing is not kinked and the connections with glass connectors are tight, that the tubing is long enough to permit the child to move, that there is no rapid increase in the amount of drainage, and that the fluid in the tube fluctuates with each respiration. The nurse must remember that the drainage bottle and the water bottle must remain below the bed level, i.e. below the bottom level of the child's thorax. To ensure that they are not elevated, they should be attached to the floor or placed in a holder which cannot be moved easily. Chest drainage must be observed accurately for color, amount and consistency. The time is marked on the vertical tape on the side of the drainage bottle every hour so that the amount of drainage can be easily seen.

The nurse must realize that if air leaks into the pleural cavity, a pneumothorax may occur with restlessness, apprehension, cyanosis, sudden sharp chest pain around the area of insertion of the catheter, tachycardia and dyspnea. If these signs and symptoms occur, the nurse should clamp the chest catheters as close as possible to the child's chest and immediately call the physician.

Postoperatively chest x-rays are taken so that the lungs can be visualized. Because the oxygen is turned off while the x-ray picture is being taken, the child may become very apprehensive. His vital signs should be taken, and he should be reassured of his progress.

Although the child was oriented preoperatively to the necessity for coughing and deep breathing, he may have difficulty cooperating postoperatively when such activity produces pain. The nurse can help him by supporting his chest, especially over the incision area, with both her hands. The child should be praised for any effort he makes to cooperate. Since coughing is important in order to prevent retention of secretions and atelectasis and to promote lung expansion, the physician should be notified if the child cannot cooperate.

The use of the intermittent positive-pressure respirator may be helpful in encouraging the child to cough. The nurse should observe his color, respiratory and pulse rates and his general response during this treatment. She should remember that coughing is very painful and tiring for the postoperative cardiac patient. Therefore, if a narcotic is ordered, it should be given prior to this therapy. Either hot or cold steam vapor may be used to prevent drying of mucus in the respiratory tract with resulting greater ease in expectoration.

The child's position should be changed every hour to promote good circulation and ventilation of the lungs, and to maintain good range of motion of the extremities. The child's body should be adequately supported with pillows if he cannot maintain his position. As soon as possible the child should be encouraged to help move himself. After moving the child, some increase in drainage from the chest tube may be noted.

The nurse should make the following additional observations: the absence of pedal pulses, or presence of cyanosis or coldness of the legs indicating a possible embolus in an artery, distention of the veins in the neck, nausea, abdominal distention, or bleeding or infection of the incision of the intravenous site. Any twitching of the extremities, signs of congestive heart failure, petechiae or complaints of dizziness, restlessness or headache should be reported. The nurse is responsible also for assisting the physician in the removal of the chest tubes, and, if one was used, the pacemaker wire from the heart muscle.

Rest is of primary importance; therefore the nurse should plan her care so that the patient has as much rest as possible. Narcotics or sedation should be given as prescribed; however, careful nursing care can relieve the child's fear and thus lessen his need for medication. Depending on the severity of the surgical procedure, the child may be permitted out of bed in a wheelchair within a few days after the chest tubes have been removed.

As was mentioned previously, children who have had cardiac surgery may regress to an infantile state. They may cry, become more demanding, or require more physical contact than they did before the operation. The nurse, recognizing their need, provides care as she would to an infant in order to help the child rebuild his sense of trust in others. The nurse must, as the child's condition improves, help him once again gain control of his situation, to regain the autonomy he has temporarily lost. As convalescence progresses the child feels increasingly well and is ready to assume more responsibility for his own care and to play with other children.

Before the child is discharged from the hospital the physician, parents, social worker, public health nurse and the hospital nurse must work out together a plan of care for the child. The child is usually more active, aggressive and independent than he was preoperatively. These changes may frighten the parents because they fear that he will overexert himself. Also the mother may have difficulty in giving up the pleasure she gained from caring for a sick dependent child prior to surgery. The nurse can help them by pointing out his obvious enjoyment of new activities and his new freedom from dyspnea and fatigue. The mother must be helped to find satisfactions to replace those of caring for an ill child.

Complications and Prognosis. The *prognosis* is generally good after operation and depends on the quality of the surgical correction. If complete correction is achieved by the open-heart technique, the prognosis is excellent.

Hemophilia

Incidence. Hemophilia is not a single disease entity, but a syndrome which represents distinct inborn errors of metabolism (see p. 158). There are defects in any one of several factors in blood plasma needed for thromboplastic activity. It would be well for the student to review the mechanism of normal clot formation before she attempts to comprehend the problem in hemophilia.

Hemophilia A is due to deficiency of factor VIII, antihemophilic globulin (AHG); *hemophilia B,* of factor IX (Christmas disease), plasma thromboplastin component (PTC); and *hemophilia C,* of factor XI, plasma thromboplastin antecedent (PTA).

Children may have deficiencies of other factors; however, the two most important types of hemophilia are A and B. Hemophilia A is the true or classic form of the disease. Since the nursing care is approximately the same in all types, the others will not be considered in this text.

Hemophilia A is inherited as a sex-linked recessive trait. Though it appears only in males, it is transmitted by symptom-free females. Male hemophiliacs can transmit a latent form of the disease to female children, however. Spontaneous mutations may have occurred to cause this condition when no other family member has had the disease. It is a congenital defect in the blood-coagulating mechanism leading to severe bleeding.

The disease is seldom diagnosed in early infancy unless the newborn bleeds from the umbilical cord or after circumcision. As children grow older and become more active the condition is apparent, for even a slight injury produces continued bleeding.

Pathogenesis, Clinical Manifestations and Treatment. The disease is characterized by a tendency to prolonged bleeding caused by an extremely delayed clotting time. Normal blood clots in three to six minutes; hemophiliac blood may require an hour or more for clotting.

The prothrombin time and the bleeding time are normal when a test cut is made because the cut is smooth and small; the incised surfaces are approximated, with the result that adequate thromboplastin becomes available from damaged cells. But hemorrhage may be spontaneous or result from a slight injury. In children hemorrhage frequently occurs from the nose or into the knee, where repeated hemorrhage may result in permanent crippling. Hemorrhage into the joints is known as *hemarthrosis.* This is extremely painful, since bleeding occurs in a confined space. Therapy consists in the use of sedatives or narcotics, immobilization with splints, and the application of cold to the part. A bivalve plaster cast may be applied for the purpose of immobilization, with physiotherapy after its removal to prevent the development of contracture of the joint. A bed cradle may be used to keep the weight of blankets off the affected part. Careful handling is necessary to prevent further bleeding. Anemia, moderate elevation in platelets and leukocytosis may occur if hemorrhages have been extensive.

Immediate *treatment* of an open wound consists in cleansing it thoroughly and placing in the laceration fibrin foam or absorbable gelatin foam with thrombin. Bleeding may also be stopped by pressure on the area, cold applications, blood transfusions and administration of concentrated plasma containing the necessary factor. Antihemophilic globulin in stored blood loses its activity rapidly; therefore transfusion of fresh whole blood or plasma is essential for treatment of hemorrhage. Anticoagulant substance may form in the blood of the hemophiliac, and subsequent administration of fresh blood or plasma may be less effective in controlling hemorrhage. Therefore local measures for control should be tried before blood or plasma is used. Sedatives may be required if the child must be kept extremely quiet during treatment. If repeated hemorrhages cause the joints to become involved, orthopedic treatment may be necessary.

Nursing Care. Because of repeated hospitalization for transfusions and treatment, it is necessary for the nurse to understand the attitude of the child and of his family toward the disease and his hospitalization. Careful handling of the child is necessary, and the nurse must be alert to symptoms of pain or pressure, since bleeding may occur anywhere in the body.

Medications should be given orally; however, if injections are necessary, the sites should be carefully chosen and rotated. The medication should be injected slowly, and pressure should be applied for at least five minutes, whether manually or with a pressure dressing.

If the condition is diagnosed in infancy, the child's toys must be soft and the sides of his crib and playpen padded to protect him from injury. When learning to stand and walk, the child must be protected from falling. He may wear sponge rubber pads on his knees and buttocks and a football helmet on his head. As he grows older, both he and his parents must understand the danger of trauma in his more active life. His teachers, the school nurse and his classmates should be informed of his condition and the problems it creates. While adults supervise his activities they must guard against assuming an overprotective attitude and allow the child some activity within the limits of safety.

The nurse must provide continued emotional support. During periods of freedom from bleeding his parents may become less conscious of the necessity for medical follow-up. The nurse should emphasize the necessity of medical supervision. He should also receive optimum dental care and supervision early in order to prevent extraction of teeth. If removal of teeth becomes necessary, the child should be hospitalized for the procedure.

When a child has a chronic illness such as hemophilia, he may be absent from kindergarten or school many days of the year. When he is not in school, a tutor may be obtained or he may be kept in contact with his class by a school-to-home telephone hookup.

Because of the long-term nature of his illness the child and his family may need counseling and financial assistance. Replacing blood or plasma may create a problem for the parents. If the child has had repeated episodes of hemarthrosis, he may become sufficiently crippled so that in order for him to be rehabilitated, surgery or the use or braces, casts, crutches or a wheelchair may become necessary. The National Hemophilia Foundation can provide assistance in the form of information, the location of parent groups, and clinics as well as other types of aid.

Parents, especially the mother, may feel guilt at having given birth to the child and resentment at having to care for him. If they are too anxious, the child will become self-centered and fearful. As a result he may withdraw from other children and become overdependent on adults. He may use his disease to control his parents and purposely do things dangerous for him. The parents must undertake the difficult tasks of preparing him for a satisfying role in adult life by helping him to develop his autonomy, initiative and independence, both for himself and for his community.

Prognosis. The prognosis is uncertain. A cyclic pattern may be noted in which periods of little bleeding and of severe bleeding occur. Death may follow intracranial hemorrhage or exsanguination from a serious hemorrhage elsewhere in the body.

Purpura

Spontaneous hemorrhages are characteristic of the condition known as purpura. These hemorrhages may occur in the skin, mucous membranes or internal organs. Such hemorrhages may develop in any condition in which there is a decreased number of platelets in the blood, defective capillary walls or in which damage is done to normal capillary walls beyond the point at which platelets can stop the bleeding. Petechiae, or minute hemorrhages into the skin, may also occur as an allergic manifestation when a local specific tissue reaction results in capillary stress.

Two specific types of purpura are discussed in this text: idiopathic thrombocytopenic purpura and anaphylactoid purpura.

Idiopathic Thrombocytopenic Purpura

Etiology, Incidence, Clinical Manifestations and Laboratory Findings. Purpura is associated with a deficit in the number of circulating blood platelets. This deficiency is caused by factors outside the platelets themselves.

The disease has its greatest *incidence* in the age group between three and seven years. It is uncommon in Negro children. The most frequent form of the disease during childhood is the acute, self-limited type.

The onset of the acute type is sudden. It may follow a mild respiratory infection or measles. There is fever and prostration. Characteristic, spontaneous small hemorrhages into the skin, mucous membranes or other tissues occur. Large ecchymoses may result from trauma. In the severe form of the disease there may be hemorrhages from the vaginal and nasal mucous membranes and from the urinary and gastrointestinal tracts. Cerebral hemorrhages are to be feared.

In the chronic form, infrequent in children, the onset is gradual. The child may have a history of prolonged bleeding following injury and of ready bruising. Periods of good health alternate with periods of excessive bleeding.

The *laboratory findings* confirm the diagnosis made upon the clinical manifestations. The platelet count is always below 100,000 per cubic millimeter of blood (normal is between 200,000 and 500,000). In the chronic form of the disease, iron deficiency may occur from loss of blood. The bleeding time is usually prolonged. The clotting time is normal, but the clot fails to retract in the usual manner. The bone marrow is studied in order to rule out leukemia.

Treatment, Course and Prognosis. Supportive *therapy* includes transfusions of whole blood to replace blood loss, antibiotic therapy to treat infections, bed rest for moderate or severe bleeding, a well balanced diet and vitamin therapy. If severe bleeding occurs, an infusion of platelet-rich plasma or whole blood is necessary.

ACTH or cortisone can control severe bleeding, but the effect upon the platelet count cannot be predicted. Splenectomy may be performed if the disease continues for six to twelve months or if hemorrhaging is severe. Splenectomy may induce lasting remissions in children with the chronic form of the disease. The operation modifies symptoms in children who are not cured.

The majority of children who have the acute form of purpura recover in about two months under supportive therapy. Intracranial hemorrhage is uncommon, but is responsible for most deaths from purpura. About 10 per cent of the children with purpura have the chronic form with remissions and exacerbations.

Anaphylactoid Purpura (Schoenlein-Henoch Syndrome)

Schoenlein-Henoch syndrome is the term used for anaphylactoid purpura because the illness is a polymorphic systemic disease. Skin and visceral lesions are manifestations.

Incidence and Etiology. The disease is not uncommon; it affects all races. It has its highest *incidence* between the ages of three and seven years, the average being about five years.

The cause is unknown. The onset may occur after contact with a specific substance. In such cases allergy seems to be important. It is possible that this is one type of hypersensitivity response to a variety of antigenic stimuli. The onset may follow an upper respiratory tract infection with beta hemolytic streptococci.

Clinical Manifestations and Laboratory Findings. A series of *clinical manifestations* take place, possibly following an infection. Abdominal pain or arthralgia, or both, may occur. After the initial symptom a skin rash appears on the legs and the buttocks, and spreads to the face, arms and trunk. The rash consists at first of urticarial wheals; then a variety of maculopapular erythematous lesions appear. The lesions may finally become petechial or purpuric, changing from red to purple, to rust, and then fading. Several types of lesions may be present at the same time. Hemorrhage and edema may occur in the gastrointestinal and urinary tracts. There is usually malaise and a low-grade fever.

Other manifestations are acute, colicky abdominal pain, vomiting and melena. In children having renal involvement there may be albuminuria and hematuria. About half of the children with kidney involvement also have hypertension or azotemia. The joints, usually the knees or ankles, may be involved. If so, they are painful and swollen, and motion is limited. These symptoms may be confused with symptoms of rheumatic fever. Cerebral edema and hemorrhage may cause convulsions and coma.

Laboratory findings show no change from the normal in clotting time, platelet count, bleeding time, clot retraction or in the blood and blood-forming organs. Anemia results if the blood loss is great. The erythrocyte sedimentation rate is elevated.

Treatment, Complications, Course and Prognosis. There is no specific *treatment*. If a specific allergen (food substance, bacteria, drug or pollen) is involved, the child should be kept from contact with it. If purpura follows a bacterial infection, antibacterial treatment should be given to eliminate pathogens. During the acute phase bed rest is necessary, and the child should be observed closely for signs of involvement of the kidneys or brain. Corticosteroids may give relief from symptoms and reduce hemorrhage, but they do not shorten the course of the illness. They are usually given on an experimental basis only, since adverse effects may occur. Blood transfusions are given as needed.

Renal *complications* may occur, and renal insufficiency may manifest itself several years after the acute phase of the illness.

The *course* and *prognosis* are extremely variable. The condition may last from about six weeks to one or two years. Usually it is mild and lasts for only a few days. Death, however, may occur from gastrointestinal and kidney changes, from hypertension or intracranial bleeding.

Allergy

Etiology and Predisposing Factors. The term "allergy" denotes an altered tissue reactivity to one or more substances. When an antigen or a foreign substance enters the body, the individual defends himself by creating an antibody to destroy the foreign material or change it into a harmless substance. Histamine is produced in large amounts by these reactions in allergic persons and is responsible for causing unfavorable allergic effects on body tissues. In nearly all cases the antibody is already present because of the body's responses to previous doses of antigen. Such sensitization may result from inhalation, absorption through the skin, ingestion or parenteral injection.

The antigen most frequently responsible for the allergic state is a foreign protein, one from a different animal species than man. Carbohydrates, lipids or chemicals may be protein-linked and may act as antigens in the production of antibodies.

The development of allergic manifestations depends partly on inheritance, in which case the term to be used is *atopy,* partly on the nature of the allergen and partly on the degree and duration of exposure. Although all persons are potentially allergic, susceptibility to allergy varies.

Approximately 75 per cent of allergic children have a positive family history of allergy. The child's allergens and his allergic manifestations need not, however, be exactly the same as those of his parents.

The fetus may be passively sensitized *in utero,* but does not exhibit manifestations of the sensitivity until his first exposure to the allergen. Infants and children who have had severe gastrointestinal disturbances may develop sensitivities due to unchanged protein which enters the bloodstream because of increased permeability of the intestinal wall. Psychologic factors involved in stress are important in the development of allergy.

Clinical Manifestations, Diagnosis and Laboratory Findings. *Clinical manifestations* may differ, depending on the age of the child. An infant who has eczema (see p. 347) may suffer allergic rhinitis or asthma as a child. New sensitivities may appear in children, while old ones may continue or be lost.

Children having allergic manifestations should be skin-tested in order to determine the offending substance. Although they react to test allergens as do adults, reactions must be interpreted in the light of clinical findings. The intensity of the reaction does not necessarily indicate the importance of the particular test substance in causation.

The *diagnosis* of an offending allergen may also be made by giving the child an elimination diet. This is effective in determining the causative agent in an infant whose diet includes only a few foods. The mother should understand that certain foods must be eliminated completely from the diet and that the child's reactions to other foods must be accurately observed.

Except in acute asthma, eosinophilia of the peripheral blood is usually present in allergic persons. Eosinophilia of the mucous membranes of the nose may be present in any kind of allergic manifestation.

Treatment, Prognosis and Prophylaxis. The physician must obtain a detailed history of the child and his family, and the parents must be willing to cooperate in a long-term program of treatment. Three methods of *treatment* may be attempted: the offending allergen may be removed; sensitization to specific known allergens may be decreased; or the response toward the offending allergens may be altered.

Probably the most effective way to manage food allergies is to eliminate the particular food from the diet. Care must be taken that the subsequent diet is adequate for a child of his age.

There is no exact method of determining the dosage necessary for desensitization to a known allergen. Desensitization to inhalants is usually done by injection of extracts of the material in gradually increasing doses. The initial dose is usually the smallest amount which, given subcutaneously, will produce a positive intradermal test. Subsequent doses are given at three- to five-day intervals, and each is larger than the preceding dose. At no time is an amount given which will produce symptoms. Desensitization to foods is accomplished by giving a gradually increasing amount of the substance which causes symptoms.

The third method of treatment is altering the response of the body to the offending allergen. Disturbing emotional factors should be corrected, since the emotional state influences the response of the body. Any endocrine imbalance should be treated. Certain drugs may be beneficial in treatment, including antihistamines, epinephrine and ephedrine. Corticotropin (ACTH) and the cortisones may also be used. Any respiratory infection should be treated, since it may predispose to an allergic state. Dehydration depresses the allergic response. Allergic manifestations may be reduced by provision for adequate rest and improvement in general health.

An allergy to a substance cannot be cured, but it may be kept sufficiently under control so that no symptoms are produced. Partial or complete removal of the allergen from the environment of sensitive persons should be attempted. It is important that children whose parents are known to have allergies avoid contact with substances which may produce allergy.

If one or both parents are allergic, the newborn should not be given cow's milk before he begins breast feeding, since sensitization to cow's milk may occur. Furthermore, during infancy and childhood additions to the diet should be in the form of single, simple foods. If a combination of new foods were given at the same time, and an allergic manifestation developed, it would be difficult to know which food was the cause. Children of allergic parents should not be given foods which commonly cause an allergic response, such as cow's milk, eggs, chocolate, wheat and oranges.

Types of Allergy in Children. The most important clinical manifestations of allergy in children include eczema (see p. 347), asthma, allergic rhinitis (hay fever) and serum sickness. Chronic conditions of the nose, throat and gastrointestinal tract may also be due to allergy.

Asthma

Incidence, Etiology and Pathology. Asthma is a pulmonary disorder caused by an allergy. Infantile eczema is a common forerunner of asthma. The disease is uncommon in infancy; its *incidence* increases in children three years of age and older.

Asthma may be evoked by particular foods, inhalants or infections, particularly those of the respiratory tract. It may also follow vigorous activity, exposure to cold or an emotional upheaval. Asthmatic attacks often occur at night after the child has been put to bed, because of his contact with a feather pillow, a wool blanket, a fuzzy, stuffed toy or even dust in the area.

The smallest bronchioles undergo the greatest change. Initially the bronchiolar musculature goes into spasm, and the mucous membrane becomes pale and edematous. Then thick, tenacious mucus collects, and there is further obstruction of the air passages. During the attack not all the inspired air can be expired, and some collects in the alveoli, thereby causing obstructive emphysema. Wheezing and rales, due to the presence of bronchial secretions, are heard. Atelectasis may develop, caused by obstruction of a bronchus.

The attack may last for a few hours or continue for a few days. The child eventually coughs up the mucus, and the spasm relaxes. If infection is present, further respiratory embarrassment is observed.

Clinical Manifestations and Treatment. Asthma is characterized by paroxysms of an expiratory type of dyspnea with wheezing and generalized obstructive emphysema. The onset may be gradual with sneezing, nasal congestion, a watery discharge, and a slight cough before the attack. In other cases the onset may be sudden, often at night. The child may sit up in bed to breathe more easily. He perspires profusely and appears anxious. The wheezing occurs largely on expiration. He may cough almost continuously. If a bronchus becomes plugged with mucus, atelectasis occurs in that lobe, and the mediastinum then shifts toward the involved area. The neck veins become distended, and cyanosis is common. During the asthmatic attack the child should never be left alone. The parents become extremely anxious, and their anxiety may further alarm the child, who then becomes increasingly emotionally disturbed.

With treatment such an attack may be over quickly. Untreated, it may last several days. If the child has *status asthmaticus* (refractory asthma), the attack may continue for several days, both day and night. Death may occur during status asthmaticus.

The most effective way to treat asthma is to eliminate the offending allergen, whether food or an environmental allergen. If this cannot be done, hyposensitization to the allergens involved may be carried out. The child should avoid fatigue and chilling and should be kept calm and emotionally at ease.

The most effective drug in the *treatment* of asthma is epinephrine given subcutaneously. Epinephrine may also be administered by a pharyngeal spray; it should be sprayed deeply into the larynx as the child inhales.

Other drugs frequently used are ephedrine sulfate or hydrochloride, aminophylline (ethylenediamine), which is a bronchodilator and may be used when epinephrine has lost its effectiveness, and antihistamines. A corticosteroid may provide relief quickly when other medications have failed. Prednisone may be given orally. Potassium iodide is of some value because it liquefies bronchial secretions so that the child can cough them up. Atropine is not used because it tends to dry up secretions.

The asthmatic child should have a generous fluid intake in order to liquefy secretions in the bronchi. Sedation may be needed if he shows indications of becoming exhausted. Sedatives which may be given include phenobarbital, chloral hydrate and paraldehyde. Morphine decreases the cough reflex and makes it difficult for the child to get rid of secretions.

Oxygen may be given to reduce anoxia and cyanosis. Increased humidity in an oxygen tent or in the air of the room tends to liquefy secretions and enables the child to expectorate. If a bronchus becomes plugged and atelectasis results, bronchoscopic aspiration may be necessary to open the airway.

Antibacterial therapy should be given when the child has an infection along with an asthmatic attack. To prevent respiratory infections he may be moved to a warm, dry climate during the winter months. Some physicians recommend giving the child small doses of an antibiotic as prophylaxis against infection during the winter months. Others recommend the use of bacterial vaccines to reduce the incidence of respiratory infections.

In the treatment of an asthmatic child the services of an allergist and a child psychologist or psychiatrist may be necessary.

Nursing Care. The nurse, besides cooperating in the therapy, should also make accurate observations of the child's behavior when he is with other children or hospital personnel, as well as the interaction between the child and his mother during her visits. A continuous record of observations is of great importance to the physician or psychiatrist in determining the emotional factors involved.

It is important that the asthmatic child be kept in good health. He should receive a balanced diet with vitamins. Since he may eat slowly because of his respiratory difficulty, sufficient time should be permitted for meals. Smaller meals at frequent intervals may be less tiring than large meals at longer intervals. The child should have adequate rest. He will probably be more comfortable sitting up than reclining. He should be kept as emotionally calm as possible. Simple amusements and quiet play are necessary to keep him happy.

Although the nurse should be patient with the child, she must set limits for his behavior. Inconsistency tends to create emotional conflicts which increase the respiratory difficulty. These children should be permitted to attend nursery school and later, school, provided the teachers and school nurses understand their problem, so that they can live as normal a life as possible.

Prognosis. The prognosis is most favorable if treatment is begun early. Many children cease to have asthmatic attacks at puberty, though others continue having them into adult life. If the asthmatic attacks cease, the child may exhibit some other allergic manifestation.

Allergic Rhinitis (Hay Fever)

Etiology and Incidence. Hay fever is an allergic manifestation involving the upper respiratory tract. Attacks may be perennial. Allergic rhinitis may be caused by pollen or by exposure to other inhalants. Ragweed and roses cause allergic rhinitis in susceptible persons. The condition is seldom seen in children under three or four years of age.

Clinical Manifestations and Treatment. *Clinical manifestations* include sneezing, which may be paroxysmal, rubbing the nose to relieve itching, and nasal stuffiness. Itching and erythema of the conjunctivae may also occur. The mucous membrane of the nose is pale and swollen. The nasal discharge may at first be clear and profuse, but as secondary infection occurs, it becomes purulent.

Allergic rhinitis is milder than other allergic diseases. The most effective method of *treatment* is elimination of the allergen from the environment if that is at all possible. Air-conditioning and filtering devices may be used. Desensitization may be attempted if the allergen cannot be eliminated.

Antihistamines such as Benadryl or Pyribenzamine are frequently used for seasonal hay fever. Agents to constrict the nasal mucous membranes, such as ephedrine, are helpful. Epinephrine is seldom used unless asthma is also a problem.

Serum Sickness and Anaphylactic Reactions

Incidence and Etiology. All persons may potentially get serum sickness if the amount of injected foreign serum is sufficient. It may occur at any age in both sexes.

The most common cause of serum sickness is the prophylactic injection of horse serum, although other serums may also produce clinical manifestations. Injection of the serum incites the production of antibodies, which unite with the rest of the serum to produce the allergic reaction.

The first injection of minute amounts of serum may sensitize a person for years. Total reactions may resemble anaphylactic shock and may occur in persons sensitized to horse serum.

Causes of anaphylactic reactions seen less commonly in children than adults include the injection of products containing or derived from penicillin, or insect stings.

Clinical Manifestations, Prognosis and Prevention. The *clinical manifestations* vary from mild to severe. The onset is usually about two days after the injection of serum, although it may vary from a few hours to a month. The skin eruption, an urticarial wheal, occurs first at the site of the injection, but spreads over the entire body. In more severe cases purpura and exudative eruptions may occur. Angioneurotic edema involving the eyelids, lips, tongue, hands or feet may occur, and generalized edema may be present. Itching is intense. Generalized lymphadenopathy and enlargement of the spleen may be present. The joints may be swollen and red. Muscular pain, headache, fever and malaise are frequent. In severe cases neurologic and cerebral complications may be seen. If the person has been sensitized previously, clinical manifestations appear early after serum injection.

When the skin test is done for serum sensitivity or when serum is given, epinephrine should be available to control anaphylactic symptoms and urticarial eruption. Ephedrine may also be used, as may antihistaminic drugs and corticosteroids. Cold compresses, starch baths and antipruritic lotions may be used to relieve itching. Sedatives and salicylates may be ordered to make the child more comfortable.

The reaction to serum is self-limited. It usually lasts from one to three days, but may last a week or longer.

Prevention requires sensitivity tests. It is important that the nurse understand the purpose of this procedure, because serum is frequently used in the prevention of disease.

Before any foreign serum is injected the child should be tested for sensitivity. An intradermal injection of horse serum, for instance, is made, especially if the child has a history of allergic eczema, asthma or hay fever. If the child is known to be sensitive, a very weak testing solution should be used at first. If the area becomes red after twenty minutes, the reaction is considered positive. The ophthalmic test may also be used as a guide in determining sensitivity to serum. If the eye becomes red in a few minutes, the reaction is considered positive. An antihistaminic drug may be given prophylactically to prevent serum sickness.

Epilepsy (Chronic or Recurrent Convulsive Disorder)

Convulsions in infancy have already been discussed (see p. 351). Convulsions during the preschool period may indicate that the child has epilepsy.

Epilepsy is characterized by paroxysmal, recurrent attacks of impaired consciousness or of unconsciousness. Tonic or clonic muscular spasms or another type of abnormal behavior occurs. Epilepsy is not a specific disease entity in itself, but rather a general term which includes a variety of recurrent seizure patterns.

People in the community as well as family members sometimes fear those who have epilepsy, or they consider the disease socially disgraceful. Physicians, nurses, social workers and other team members must educate the public to the real meaning of the disease as a chronic illness. A large amount of information should not be given at once, but slowly so that it does not pose too great a threat.

There are two types of epilepsy—idiopathic and organic.

Idiopathic Epilepsy. More than half of the children who have recurrent seizures before puberty have idiopathic epilepsy. The cause of the seizures cannot be found. Heredity may be a factor, but this can seldom be clinically demonstrated. The onset is commonly between four and eight years of age. Treatment to control the seizures is possible in about 85 per cent of these children.

Organic Epilepsy. Organic epilepsy may result from a number of focal or diffuse injuries to the brain which have left residual damage. Such injuries may be caused by direct laceration of brain tissue due to trauma, hemorrhage due to trauma or the hemorrhagic diseases, anoxia (asphyxia neonatorum), infections (e.g. meningitis, encephalitis) or toxic manifestations due to kernicterus or lead poisoning. Degenerative changes may take place in the brain. Congenital problems such as phenylketonuria or hydrocephalus or diseases such as syphilis or toxoplasmosis may result in organic abnormalities in the brain. Organic epilepsy usually shows abnormalities on electroencephalograms.

Clinical Manifestations and Diagnosis. The *clinical manifestations* are used as the basis for the classification of seizures: grand mal, petit mal, psychomotor, focal and infantile myoclonic seizures.

Grand mal seizures in children are not likely to be preceded by an aura such as is common in adults. Older children may have a headache, may be irritable and lethargic or may have digestive upsets before seizures. The seizure is a generalized convulsion; a tonic phase and a clonic phase are usually seen.

A *tonic spasm* is an involuntary, violent, persistent contraction. In the tonic phase the child falls to the ground, the pupils dilate, and the face is distorted. The neck, abdominal and chest muscles are held rigidly. The limbs stiffen. As air is forced out of the lungs a brief cry may be heard. The child may bite his tongue and may

void or defecate as the result of contracture of the abdominal muscles. Since respiratory movements are arrested, cyanosis occurs. This phase usually lasts up to forty seconds.

The *clonic* phase, which consists in alternate contraction and relaxation of muscles, lasts indefinitely. After this the child goes into a deep sleep. When he wakens, he may complain of headache and may appear confused or stuporous. A child may have seizures at night (*nocturnal epilepsy*) and in the morning find his bed wet or discover that he has bitten his tongue.

A child who has grand mal seizures may become egocentric and negativistic, owing to the attitudes of others toward him and his illness.

Petit mal seizures consist of transient loss of consciousness with possibly rolling of the eyes, lip movements or slight movements of the head, limbs or trunk. The child does not fall. He usually stares into space. After the age of three years petit mal occurs more frequently in girls than in boys. These attacks last up to thirty seconds. The child may not realize that he had a seizure. He may have as many as a hundred or more in a day or as few as one a month. He is usually confused after an attack.

There is a third type of seizure—*psychomotor seizures*—which cannot be recognized easily because there seem to be purposeful but repetitive inappropriate muscular acts. Usually no tonic or clonic movements are noted. The child may have a slight aura and may sleep after an attack. He is usually not confused.

Focal seizures (*jacksonian epilepsy*) may be either motor or sensory. The manifestation depends on the location of the focal area in the brain which has the abnormal neuronal discharge. Unilateral jacksonian attacks are usually clonic, indicating that their origin is in the motor cortex. The muscles involved are usually those of the hand, tongue, face and foot. A focal seizure beginning in one area such as the hand spreads to areas of the body on the same side in a fixed pattern. Consciousness may or may not be disturbed.

Infantile myoclonic seizures are seen before the age of two years and involve one group of muscles. The child may lower his head and flex his arms innumerable times a day. He may also flex his legs on his abdomen. This type of convulsion usually disappears by the third year, and grand mal seizures appear. The condition is usually accompanied by mental retardation.

Diagnosis is made on the family history and the child's record of convulsive seizures. Different types of epilepsy show a variety of electroencephalographic abnormalities. For diagnostic purposes, therefore, whenever a convulsive disorder is present, an electroencephalogram is made. Roentgen studies of the skull are also necessary. Other tests such as pneumoencephalography and examination of the cerebrospinal fluid may be done if indicated.

Treatment. During an attack the child should be protected from injury. His clothing should be loosened around the neck, and he must be turned to one side so that he does not aspirate secretions. Oxygen should be given if cyanosis occurs and if the convulsion is prolonged.

A prolonged series of grand mal seizures is termed *status epilepticus.* Oxygen is given, and phenobarbital sodium is administered intramuscularly. The environment should be quiet while the child is recovering from a prolonged convulsion. He and his parents need reassurance.

Prolonged therapy has three purposes: control of the convulsions, education of the child's family and others in his environment to accept him, and help so that he may function to full capacity. The treatment includes anticonvulsant drugs, good care of the whole child, diet therapy and psychotherapy if necessary. The family and the child should have a positive attitude toward his illness. He should lead as normal a life as possible. Anxiety tends to increase the occurrence of seizures. If the child appears anxious, the social worker or child psychiatrist may help the family find the sources of his anxiety. The child should be kept at home rather than institutionalized if his capacities permit home care.

The choice of drugs and the dosage needed to control convulsions depend upon the individual child and the type of seizure. Phenobarbital is often used over a long period for grand mal seizures. If the child has an idiosyncrasy to phenobarbital, a maculopapular skin eruption, drowsiness and fever may be noted. Mebaral (mephobarbital) is also used in some cases of grand mal seizures. Dilantin (diphenylhydantoin sodium) is an effective anticonvulsant, but does not produce excessive drowsiness as barbiturates may. Nonhemorrhagic, painless hypertrophy of the gums may follow administration of Dilantin. No special treatment is required. Drowsiness and ataxia may occur if the child receives too large a dose.

Ethosuximide (Zarontin) is presently the drug of choice in the therapy of petit mal, since it is less toxic than other compounds. Tridione (trimethadione) is also effective in the treatment of petit mal seizures. This drug may increase the occurrence of grand mal attacks if the child also suffers from such seizures. Phenobarbital or Dilantin may also be ordered. Prolonged or excessive use of Tridione may produce drowsiness, nausea, photophobia or skin eruptions. Aplastic anemia may also occur. Mysoline (primidone) is given for grand mal and psychomotor seizures. Side effects include drowsiness and ataxia.

Diet therapy is important. A fasting diet, ketogenic diet and a reduction of fluid intake tend to prevent seizures. Diet therapy may be used with the older child who cooperates with treatment, but is usually more difficult than with the little child. The diet should be varied so that it is palatable, since a ketogenic diet containing large amounts of fat is not appetizing over a long period.

Nursing Care. The nurse must record her observations of a convulsion. This is important because the physician is seldom present when the child has a seizure. Although the child must be closely watched, he should not be made to feel that he can never be left alone. The physical aspects of his care are similar to those of the infant during a convulsion (see p. 351). Prevention of injury to the child is a principal concern.

The nurse should keep the child as free from anxiety as possible. Unnecessary stimulation should be avoided. Diversion appropriate to his age and ability should be provided. His play equipment should be such that it will not cause injury during a seizure.

The nurse assists with the diagnostic tests. All procedures should be explained to the child in a way that he will understand. The nurse must see that he swallows his anticonvulsant medications and must watch for side effects of the drugs.

Parent-child relations should be observed for indications of rejection or overprotection of the child. He should be watched for traits of egocentricity, emotional instability and selfishness, and what is noted should be reported to the physician. These traits develop as a reaction to adult attitudes toward the child and his illness. The parents and the child must understand the need for continued medical care and supervision to control convulsions.

Course and Prognosis. Since the child is better off at home than in the hospital if the mother can give him the care he needs, it is important that she learn how to care for him. The child should have as normal a life as possible. Outdoor activity should be provided. If the convulsions are not too severe and the child is mentally able to profit from the experience, he should go to nursery school and later to school. The attitude of adults and their treatment of him when he has a seizure influence the attitude of other children toward him.

The role of parents of an epileptic child is difficult; the child's role is even more difficult. Parents and child need emotional support, reassurance and praise for their achievements. The seizures can be reduced in frequency so as not to interfere too much with the child's activity. Personality changes can be minimized if parents treat the child as though he were essentially normal. They must prevent him from becoming overdependent on them.

The *prognosis* depends on the mental and

physical handicaps the child has and on the adequacy of medical and environmental management. If the child has adequate treatment and was mentally normal at the beginning of his illness, he can be expected to remain essentially normal throughout his life.

As the child grows to adulthood he may find that because of his diagnosis certain of his activities may be limited. Certain states have laws forbidding the epileptic to drive an automobile, to work in certain occupations or to marry. These laws may be changed as the public develops a better understanding of the disease and its therapy.

Mental Retardation

Incidence and Etiology. Mental retardation is any interference with intelligence that causes a limitation in the way the child is able to adapt to his environment. It is not a disease entity itself, but is a complex of symptoms due to a variety of causes. Between 3 and 4 per cent of all children born in the United States will at some time in their lives be classified as mentally retarded.

Heredity may be the cause; in some cases mental retardation can be traced through generations and an incidence above average among relatives proved. There are so many other factors, however, that it is difficult to single out heredity. Some of these factors may be classified as follows: (1) *prenatal* causes, including metabolic disorders such as phenylketonuria (see p. 344), hypothyroidism (cretinism) (see p. 343), mongolism (Down's syndrome) (see p. 220), cranial malformation (see p. 354), maternal infections such as German measles or syphilis, maternal irradiation, anoxia and isoimmunization (kernicterus) (see p. 166); (2) *neonatal* causes, including intracranial hemorrhage (see p. 178), anoxia (see p. 181) or birth trauma; (3) *postnatal* causes, including intracranial injury or hemorrhage (see p. 352), infections such as meningitis (see p. 352) or encephalitis (see p. 490), poisoning such as with lead (see p. 433), cerebrovascular thrombosis, anoxia, neoplasms (see p. 592) or recurrent convulsions.

Diagnosis. Such factors as epilepsy (see p. 523), cerebral palsy (see p. 435), severe malnutrition (see p. 320), emotional disturbances (see p. 445), blindness (see p. 442), deafness (see p. 440) and speech disorders (see p. 599) may lead to an incorrect diagnosis of mental retardation which may result in the child's being treated as a mental defective and deprived of the opportunity to attain his potential mental development.

A definite diagnosis of mental retardation should be made only after a thorough study of the family and the child. Such a study should be done by a team composed of members selected from among the following: a pediatrician, a psychologist, a psychiatrist, a social worker and public health and hospital nurses. In order to participate with other team members the nurse should have a good knowledge of community and state resources for such children. She may also help to implement and to interpret the recommendations of the team to the parents. Centers have been established, usually in connection with medical schools of large universities, for research and diagnosis and for the development of plans of care for individual retarded children.

Mental retardation of a severe degree may be recognized as early as birth. It is indicated by failure of the infant to learn to suck at the breast or from a bottle. If a three-month-old infant who has lived in an adequate environment fails to develop normally, mental retardation must be considered. Throughout infancy, before the child learns to talk, rough estimates of his mental ability may be made by testing his motor abilities. Does he sit, stand and walk within the usual age limits for a physically and mentally normal child? Mentally retarded toddlers may be slow in trying to help themselves, in speaking, in feeding themselves or in toilet training. Until the child is of preschool age, slowness of development may not be recognized. It becomes a disturbing problem, however, as soon as the child is with normal preschool children living in the same environment. A child who is only mildly mentally retarded may pass through infancy and even the preschool years with no indication of retardation. When he enters school, however, and is expected to understand abstract concepts, his handicap may become apparent.

Causes of delayed development should be sought whenever a child has retarded physical and motor development. The child should have a thorough examination to determine whether there is a physical cause for which therapy can be given.

Intelligence tests and other evaluation devices should be given to provide an estimation of mental capacity. A study of emotional reactions and social adjustment should be made. Personality characteristics of mentally retarded children vary; some children are pleasant and get along well with other children and with adults, but others are restless, irritable and disobedient. These traits interact with mental capacity in social adjustment. Children of low intelligence are usually clumsy in their movements and slow to respond to stimuli.

Classification and Clinical Manifestations. Mentally retarded children may be classified in three groups. (1) Those children who are *mildly retarded but educable* and have an intelligence quotient between 51 and 75 can reach a mental age of eight to twelve years. (2) Those children who are *moderately retarded but trainable* and have an intelligence quotient between 21 and 50 can reach a mental age of three to seven years. (3) Those children who are *severely retarded and are completely dependent on others for their care* and have an intelligence quotient between 0 and 20 can reach a mental age of zero to two years.

Children who are mildly retarded but educable may learn to function fairly well in the home if they are able to care for themselves, and in the community by learning to perform simple manual services or trades. Children who are moderately retarded but trainable may learn to talk fairly well and understand what is said to them. Their ability to concentrate varies, but is not long upon any one task. They may be able to dress themselves, to acquire socially acceptable elimination control and to feed themselves without assistance. Some children who are severely retarded may not be able to speak or walk until five years of age, and others may never learn. They require constant care and supervision. Although they may make some progress slowly, they are usually institutionalized.

Management. Management of the mentally retarded child is the responsibility of the home, school, community and state. The initial step is for the physician to inform the parents of the problem. They should not be told, however, until the diagnosis is definitely established. Although parents may have suspected the diagnosis, they face it with great anxiety and, when it is confirmed, may have a feeling of guilt. They need sympathetic understanding of their problems and acceptance of their attitudes in order to free themselves from their feeling of guilt, or at least responsibility for the child's condition, for lack of normal parental love and the feeling that he is a burden. As soon as possible they should be included with other health team members in making realistic plans for the child's care based on the parents' reaction to the handicap, the degree of the child's retardation and the community facilities in the area in which they live.

If the cause of the retardation can be found and is amenable to treatment, every effort should be made to help the child. Thyroid extract is given for cretinism, operation is performed for subdural hematoma, hydrocephalus or craniosynostosis, and dietary management is provided for phenylketonuria.

Parents should be educated as to a child's potential and should have a realistic concept of his ability. Parents and teachers should not use pressure in an attempt to force a retarded child to learn. Such pressure leads only to frustration, which causes further emotional problems. The retarded child needs from parents and

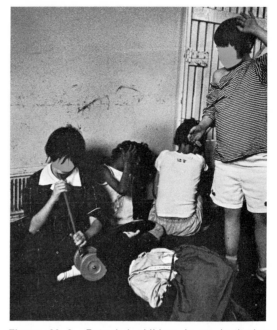

Figure 20–2. Retarded children in an institution where no activity program has been planned for them and they spend the day in a drab, barren room, doing nothing. The result is that they become increasingly retarded in their behavior. (From B. Blatt and F. Kaplan: *Christmas in Purgatory: A Photographic Essay on Mental Retardation.* Boston, Allyn and Bacon, 1966.)

teachers the same kind of love, security and help that a normal child needs, but he needs them longer because his dependence extends beyond the usual age.

The plan of management should include environmental arrangements in which the child can utilize his capacities to the best advantage. For some children institutional care is best. For others special training can be given at home. Mentally retarded children as well as those having emotional problems may benefit from foster home care, day care, or the utilization of foster grandparents in long-term care. Some children may profit from attendance at special nursery and grade schools. They should be taught to care for themselves and should learn a vocation if possible. These important decisions must ultimately be made by the parents; however, the health team can give some guidance based on the child's diagnosis.

Before realistic plans can be made the parents of retarded children must accept the diagnosis. If they do not, they may continue to search for a medical reason for the problem and cure of the condition. Once they have accepted the diagnosis and plan for the child's care, they may gain confidence and emotional support by joining a group of parents whose children have the same problem as theirs.

Siblings of any handicapped child, but especially those of the mentally retarded, may feel neglected because of the amount of time mother devotes to the retarded child. Some children may regress to the level of the retarded child in order to gain the attention they feel they deserve. When the siblings are older, they may hesitate to bring friends to the home, to date, or to marry because of fear that the condition may be inherited. Adequate explanation should be given to the siblings of a retarded child and free communication established so that misconceptions can be eliminated and anxiety reduced.

Nursing Care. The nurse may be the first to detect early signs of mental retardation. She may see the child in the outpatient department, hospital or his home. Often, because of her understanding of normal growth and development, she can observe lack of development which the parents are unaware of. She should report her observations to the physician, who, with the other team members, can determine the degree of retardation and its possible cause.

The nurse should be a member of the team which plans and carries out recommendations for the care of the child at home and for his education and training. *Operant conditioning,* behavior therapy, or behavior modification utilized in the care of mentally retarded and emotionally disturbed children, are conditioning techniques based on the principle of *reinforcement.* Reinforcement simply means that a reward should be given for a certain response so that the probability of recurrence of that same response will be increased. The reward, such as food, candy, praise or encouragement, must be given *immediately* and *consistently* after the approved behavior is done. Behaviors which are not to be strengthened do not lead to reward. This technique makes it possible to teach complex behaviors when these are broken down into small steps which the child can easily achieve. Behavioral changes in the areas of toilet training, feeding, dressing, and the reduction of destructive behavior, among others, are possible with the use of this technique.

In helping the mother to provide care for the child the nurse should make it clear that a child, no matter what his chronological age, will proceed in his development and thus need to be treated according to his mental age. Thus in teaching self-help skills, it is necessary to teach the child at whatever level of mental ability he has at that time. When helping the mother teach the child habit formation, it is essential that the nurse remember the ages at which the average child is ready to perform certain acts successfully, such as elimination control or toilet training, feeding himself, and dressing himself among others. (See the growth and development charts in Chapters 12, 15 and 18.) Also, any physical handicap must be taken into consideration when teaching a skill. If the child has cerebral palsy (see p. 435), for instance, his progress will be slower than that of a child who has adequate muscular control. The child who is mentally retarded lacks the ability to do abstract reasoning; therefore the purpose of teaching is for habit formation with little expectation of his being able to transfer knowledge from one situation to another. When training for habit formation, it is necessary first of all to help the child to relax, then to proceed through the routine, repeating it sufficiently so that he will eventually be able to do it himself.

When the mother wishes to teach the child elimination control, she should first of all keep a record or schedule of when the child routinely urinates and has his bowel movements. The child should then be placed on the toilet approximately every two hours according to his own schedule. Gradually his schedule could be modified to fit into the family routine. Each time the mother takes him to the toilet, he should be taken to the bathroom. The training chair should not be moved about the house to accommodate his activities. The mother should explain simply in words and gestures what he is to do and give him approval if he succeeds. As when teaching an essentially normal child (see p. 367), if he does not succeed in his attempt, he should not be condemned.

The mother who wants to teach the child to dress himself should provide clothing that is easy to put on and take off and place articles of clothing consistently in an order for his use. As clothing having zippers, buttons and ties are purchased, the child should be guided in practicing these skills.

In helping a mentally retarded child to feed himself, the mother should follow the same general principles of teaching as are used for the essentially normal child in addition to the principles of operant conditioning. Special eating equipment may need to be obtained for the child's use (see p. 437).

In disciplining the mentally retarded child, the principles utilized for the average child as well as those of operant conditioning should be followed. These include consistency in action, the use of simple language to explain what he has done wrong, and the establishment of a routine in his daily living, so that the child learns what is expected of him. If punishment is necessary, it should follow the misdeed immediately so that the two events are connected in the child's mind.

The mentally retarded child needs stimulation from his environment if he is to achieve his potential. He needs as many, if not more, objects to look at, sounds to hear, items to handle and manipulate as the mentally normal child does.

When such a child is hospitalized, the nurse's specific functions are provision of physical care as for a normal child and supervision of the child to prevent self-injury. Close restraint is not good for such children. They should be given constructive play activity so that their attention is focused on acceptable behavior.

The nurse may help the parents select toys on the basis of the child's mental, not chronologic, age. She should help them to understand that his attention span is short, and that they should give approval for his successes and provide for him simple responsibilities at home.

Prognosis, Prevention and Planning for the Future. Unless the child is severely retarded, the outlook for length of life is about that of normal children. His adjustment to society will depend on the extent of his retardation and on the extent to which he has learned to use his mental resources.

Great strides are being made in the *prevention* of the causes of and the problems due to mental retardation. Research is being done to find means to reduce its incidence. The *Collaborative Project on Cerebral Palsy, Mental Retardation, and other Neurological and Sensory Disorders of Infancy and Childhood* instituted by the National Institute of Neurological Diseases and Blindness has already been discussed (see p. 162). During recent years there has been a growing commitment of federal funds to the care of the retarded. Many communities are making strides in providing special services for retarded children. Even greater efforts must be made to increase funds available for research, for the preparation of personnel to care for retarded children, for the organization of more parent groups and for comprehensive programs to help these children.

EMOTIONAL PROBLEMS

Two emotional disorders that occur most frequently during the preschool period are phobias, or irrational fears, and temper tantrums.

Phobias

Children usually have many fears of dangers in the real world. They learn fear of such things as fire, sharp knives or a busy street from their parents, who wish to protect them from accidents or harm. But children also fear things which could not possibly cause them harm. They may be afraid of the dark, of the dead, of noises or of ghosts. Boys are more commonly afraid of injury to their bodies, and girls of the dark and of strange noises. The incidence of these fears is greatest during the preschool period.

When an unreasonable fear produces panic in a child, he is said to have a *phobia*. Not even the reassurance of a loving adult can reduce the emotional feeling toward the dreaded object. If the cause of the phobia is close to reality, e.g. fear of a dog which actually is capable of harming a child, the phobia is not too serious. If the cause is not close to reality, the child is emotionally ill. The real problem is not the phobic object, but an insoluble emotional conflict. Most children re-

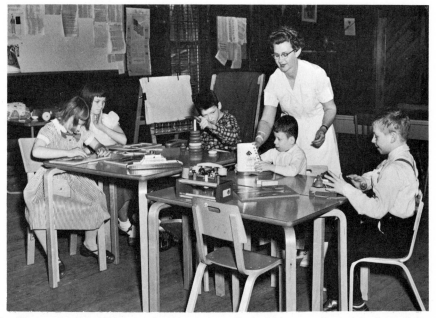

Figure 20–3. These retarded children are learning to coordinate their muscular activity through play. (Charles P. Jubenville, Ed. D., Director, Daytime Care Centers.) (*Nursing Outlook,* July 1960.)

cover from their phobias, but they may need help to do so.

The most effective way to help a child rid himself of a phobia is to help him slowly cope with the situation or object. The adult should gradually give him an opportunity to be near the feared object and have a chance to inspect or ignore it. The adult should also help him actively to participate in the dreaded situation or with the feared object.

Sometimes reassurance and demonstrations that the object is really harmless or that other children do not fear it will help the child to master his own fear. Under no circumstances should his fear be ignored, nor should he be forced to contact the object.

The child should be encouraged to be more self-helpful and to spend more time with other children instead of with his parents. He should be permitted to express his hostility verbally or to engage in active games in order to work out his feelings.

Children whose activity is seriously limited because of a phobia or whose phobic object is not close to reality should have psychiatric treatment.

Temper Tantrums

Temper tantrums are normal during the toddler period, but if they continue into the preschool period and become more severe, the child has not learned how to handle the normal frustrations of growing up.

During a severe temper tantrum the child is unconscious of his surroundings and of reality. He uses a great deal of muscular energy, striking out against his surroundings or himself, rarely against the adult responsible for his frustration. The child's reaction is usually out of all proportion to the apparent cause.

In taking his frustration out on himself the child is, in effect, angry with himself. When he becomes exhausted as a result of so much physical activity, he is remorseful because he allowed himself to act like a baby or toddler.

Temper tantrums occur in every child's life. If they are serious or prolonged or recur too frequently, the child is probably not developing as he should do. Possibly a child having pathologic temper tantrums has been overindulged and has not learned to control his impulses or to react within normal limits to frustrations. Treatment consists in helping such children to gain more control of their infantile desires and to get pleasure from more mature forms of satisfaction. A nurse can help by causing a child to feel more pleasure in pleasing her than in giving way to every impulse.

Pathologic temper tantrums may occur if the child has been forced too early to be independent and to exert too rigid control over his behavior.

He tries hard to behave in a way that will make his parents approve of him. Treatment consists in helping him to lower his own standards of behavior so that he can act in accordance with his age. Under psychiatric care such children learn to control themselves and to function at their age level.

EMOTIONAL ILLNESS

Childhood Schizophrenia

Incidence. The number of preschool children having severe mental illness admitted to pediatric units appears to be increasing. More child care units for these patients are being opened in both general and psychiatric hospitals. With better diagnosis, children with mental retardation and those with a schizophrenic illness are being separated and treated in more appropriate ways. The need for nursing personnel in children's psychiatric units remains urgent.

Clinical Manifestations. These children have an arrest of personality development, usually accompanied by a return to earlier, more primitive thinking, behavior and ways of com-

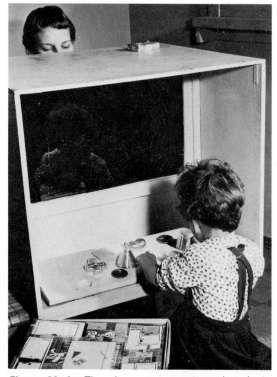

Figure 20–4. The observer can note and evaluate the actions of the child in play through the one-way glass screen. Such observations assist physicians in their evaluation of a child's intellectual and emotional status. (Byrd: *Health.* 4th ed.)

municating with others. The parents believe that these children develop normally until the obvious deviant symptoms appear. The developmental history of these children, however, is atypical in that the smooth, interrelated pattern of emotional, social and intellectual development of normal children is not found.

Withdrawal of these children from contact with people in their environment is generally seen between the third and fifth years, but may be seen as early as the second year. Even though they may have learned to talk, they do not feel the need, nor are they able to communicate in meaningful language.

These children cannot distinguish what is real from what is unreal, and those with severe or very early involvement are unable to differentiate themselves from other persons in the environment. The ability to test what is real develops in the first year of life in a child who receives mature, loving maternal care. In childhood schizophrenics this ability either has not fully developed or has been lost.

Children showing decided withdrawal or *autistic behavior* wander about, hiding in places such as closets where they have little human contact. They enjoy oral activity, mouthing various objects, and must be protected against swallowing harmful substances.

Some of the markedly autistic children cannot be fitted into organized routines. Such efforts result in increased temper tantrums, masturbation, preoccupation and anxiety. When they are permitted to remain by themselves, they enjoy solitary play or bodily preoccupations such as sucking or head-banging. Other children cannot tolerate changes in routines and remain inflexible in their behavior.

Management. The severely psychotic child may benefit from residential care and the use of techniques of operant conditioning. When he is hospitalized, it is the function of the nurse to provide the love, security and acceptance that have not been available to him in a healthy, reciprocal relation with his mother, as well as good physical care. Nurses thus become therapeutic agents who act in close cooperation with the child psychiatrist.

Further treatment includes helping the children to identify their own bodies as separate from those of other people, helping them to integrate their concept of self and to develop relations with other human beings, and protecting them from their own destructive impulses. The nurse must try to see the world as the disturbed child sees it, thereby increasing her ability to understand the child and his behavior. As the autistic child improves, routines can be gradually introduced. Those with rigid or stereotyped patterns of behavior should be encouraged to tolerate some flexibility of routines and some innova-

tions in play. The aim of routines is to provide a cycle of rest and activity and to help the child learn to help himself with such functions as bathing, dressing and eating. Young children having lesser degrees of emotional illness are being helped through attendance at centers where they can interact with essentially normal children or with others who also have problems. Many parents of emotionally disturbed children also receive psychotherapy while their children are under treatment.

Prognosis. The earlier a schizophrenic illness begins, the more guarded is the prognosis because these children present an extremely difficult problem in therapy. These young children have not developed strength of personality with an ability to relate to the mother. The psychiatrist must help them to develop their personalities from the earliest foundation. The older the child when his withdrawal occurs, the better is the prognosis.

Most younger children showing profound autistic behavior are considered extremely mentally ill, and only concentrated therapy and care can provide hope for their recovery.

CLINICAL SITUATIONS

Mrs. Rashofer brought her three-year-old son, Barry, to the pediatric clinic. Although her other four children were well, Barry had recently become pale, had been losing weight and seemed to be tired constantly. On physical examination the physician found that the child had widespread petechiae of his skin and ulcerations of his gums. The tentative diagnosis of acute leukemia was made and was later confirmed when a sample of bone marrow was examined.

1. Methotrexate was ordered for Barry. The nurse should know that this drug is
   a. A folic acid antagonist.
   b. An adrenal cortical hormone.
   c. A salicylate.
   d. A purine analogue.

2. When the nurse cares for Barry, she should observe him especially for
   a. Vomiting and diarrhea.
   b. Tinnitus.
   c. Cyanosis.
   d. Hemorrhage.

3. The physician has told Barry's parents that although he may have periods of remissions, the eventual prognosis of a child having leukemia is extremely poor. During Barry's illness the nurse would encourage Mrs. Rashofer to assist her in giving him care because
   a. No nurse has time on a busy pediatric unit to provide all the detailed care a child having leukemia requires.
   b. Barry cries whenever his nurse cares for him. He would probably be happier if his mother gave him care.
   c. His mother apparently is not satisfied with the

care the child is receiving, since she has several times discussed the possibility of employing private duty nurses for him.

d. His mother needs help in expressing her affection for him and also in learning how to care for him when he is discharged from the hospital.

4. Barry has had a remission of his illness, and the physician has decided to send him home. Just before Barry's discharge from the hospital he and Dickie (three years old also) were playing with blocks in the hospital play area. Barry took one of Dickie's blocks, and Dickie began to cry. The nurse would

a. Encourage Barry to return the block to Dickie.

b. Tell Dickie that he cannot play with the blocks unless he can share them.

c. Take the blocks away from both children.

d. Give Dickie another block similar to the one Barry took.

5. In a few weeks Barry was readmitted with his initial symptoms. Mrs. Rashofer assisted the nurse in giving him care as she had on his previous admission. One afternoon the nurse found her crying in the hall outside the pediatric unit. Mrs. Rashofer explained, "I just cannot satisfy Barry any more. Every time I touch him he cries." The nurse would show her understanding in this situation by saying,

a. "I think Barry probably would stop crying if you bought him a new toy. What do you think he would like?"

b. "Perhaps he misses his father. Could he come to care for him awhile this evening?"

c. "Barry is very uncomfortable now. Perhaps you could help him most by just holding his hand and reading his favorite story to him."

d. "Children sometimes cry when they are feeling better. Why don't you get a cup of coffee? He will be happy to see you later."

6. Barry had lapsed into unconsciousness, and the physician had told the parents the gravity of his condition. Mr. and Mrs. Rashofer sat quietly sobbing beside his crib. To comfort these parents the nurse said,

a. "After Barry dies you'll have to forget him and devote your lives to your other children. They have probably missed you since you have been spending so much time in the hospital."

b. "All of us have done everything possible for Barry. In helping to care for him I have learned to love him too. I believe I can understand to some degree your feelings about your son."

c. "I know you would prefer that I leave you alone with Barry. Please call me if you need me."

d. "I just cannot understand why little children have to suffer. What sin did Barry commit to deserve punishment such as this?"

Martin Schleer, a four-year-old boy, has been admitted to the pediatric unit with a diagnosis of acute glomerulonephritis. Mrs. Schleer said that all three of her children had recently been ill with scarlet fever. Martin's clinical manifestations on admission included slight edema of the face, hematuria and hypertension.

7. When Martin was admitted to the hospital, the head nurse purposely did *not* put him to bed near

a. Barry, who has leukemia.

b. Susan, who is mentally retarded.

c. Wanda, who has a streptococcal tonsillitis.

d. Marsha, who has rheumatic fever.

8. After the nurse had given Martin an intramuscular injection he said, "I hate you. Go away." The nurse should answer

a. "I hate you, too."

b. "You should not say that. You are a naughty boy."

c. "I am sorry you hate me. I like you."

d. "I won't let your mother come to see if you say that again."

9. When the nurse took Martin's blood pressure, she found it to be 150 mm. systolic over 110 mm. diastolic. She reported this finding to the head nurse, who said that the physician would probably want to give the child

a. Ammonium chloride.

b. Apresoline and reserpine.

c. Aminophylline and magnesium sulfate.

d. Diamox.

10. One day during visiting hours Martin's mother told him that he had a new baby cousin, Doris. Martin asked his mother where his baby cousin "came from." His mother should

a. Give him a complete description of the normal birth of a baby.

b. Tell him that he must not ask questions like that.

c. Tell him her mother bought Doris at the hospital.

d. Tell him the baby came from inside her mother's body.

11. Martin was in the hospital during the Christmas season. His mother had told him about Santa Claus. Some time during the next few years Martin will question the truth of this myth because Santa could not possibly fit through their chimney. At that time his mother should

a. Insist that there is a person named Santa Claus.

b. Tell him truthfully about the spirit of Christmas.

c. Tell him that Santa will forget him if he persists in asking questions.

d. Feel ashamed that she had told the child a falsehood.

12. Martin was discharged from the hospital. On his first return visit to the outpatient department his mother told the nurse that he had recently become fearful of dogs. In this situation Mrs. Schleer should

a. Force him to touch a dog so that he would get over his fear.

b. Tell him that dogs will not hurt him, that it is a very unusual dog that will bite children.

c. Encourage him to talk about his fear and to play with a small dog in his mother's presence.

d. Ignore the fear because he will outgrow it in a few years anyway.

Mrs. Rinell thought that Susan was slow in developing motor skills in comparison with her other two older children, but she did not become too concerned about her until she observed her behavior with other five-year-old children in kindergarten. Although her family physician had said that Susan was a healthy child, she consulted a pediatrician who admitted Susan to the hospital for diagnosis.

13. After a thorough study of the family and the child by the health team members Susan was found to have an intelligence quotient of 65. The nurse should know that she is

a. Within the lower limits of the range of normal intelligence.

b. Mildly retarded, but educable.

c. Moderately retarded, but trainable.

d. Severely retarded and will be completely dependent on others for her care.

14. The nurse should realize that one of her principal objectives in the care of this child is to

a. Help the parents gain a realistic concept of Susan's ability.

b. Encourage her parents in their persistent efforts to have Susan learn something new each day.

c. Help her parents to develop a *laissez-faire* attitude toward Susan's training.

d. Encourage her parents to be lenient in their setting of limits on Susan's behavior.

15. Mrs. Rinell, who lives in a community where there is a poliomyelitis epidemic, called the public health nurse and told her that Susan was not feeling well. The nurse's advice to her was to

a. Take Susan and her siblings to her grandmother's home in another town so that she would not be exposed to poliomyelitis in her weakened condition.

b. Take Susan to the isolation unit of the local hospital for treatment.

c. Ignore her symptoms since her complaint seemed indicative of an upper respiratory tract infection.

d. Put Susan to bed and call her pediatrician.

GUIDES TO FURTHER STUDY

1. Compare the development of three children during your observation in nursery school according to the following: motor ability, independence in dressing, toileting and eating, selection of playthings, sociability with adults and children, and ability to rest.

Discuss in seminar the similarities and differences in behavior and abilities of these children.

2. During your observation in nursery school observe the behavior of the same three children as in Question 1 as they part from their parents. Note the age of each child and the length of time they had been attending nursery school. Answer the following questions for each child. Did the child hang his outer garments in the coatroom in the parent's presence? Did the parent wait until the child was inspected? Where did the parent actually leave the child? What words did the parent use when parting? Did the child appear unhappy when the parent left the school? What could have been done to make the parting more happy if it was unhappy?

3. Observe the health inspection in nursery school and plan to discuss the following in seminar: the purpose of the daily health inspection, the time it occurred, the procedure of examination, and the way the nurse gained the children's cooperation. Did the children learn anything from this routine? If the nurse encountered any difficulties in gaining the children's cooperation, discuss each situation as it occurred and make suggestions as to how the problem(s) could have been resolved.

4. As the nurse in The Little Friend's Nursery School it is your responsibility to inform both teachers and children about Rhonda Evans's illness. She has recently been hospitalized with a diagnosis of epilepsy. Discuss what you believe both groups should know about this illness so that positive attitudes can be formed toward this child.

5. Billy Jeffries, three years of age, has been admitted to the hospital for treatment of hemophilia. Describe the role and responsibility of the nurse in relation to both parents and child from the time he is brought to the hospital to the time of his discharge. What guidance should the parents have had by the time of discharge?

6. Preschool children fear bodily injury. During your experience in caring for children collect incidences in which children have shown such fear, expressing it either verbally or nonverbally. How could these manifestations of fear have been prevented? What was your role in reducing these fears?

TEACHING AIDS AND OTHER INFORMATION*

American Heart Association

Heart Disease in Children.
If Your Child Has a Congenital Heart Defect.

American Medical Association

Emergency Medical Identification Card.
Mental Retardation Handbook.

Joseph P. Kennedy, Jr. Foundation

Education for the Mentally Retarded: What You Should Know: What You Can Do.
Recreation for the Mentally Retarded: What You Should Know: What You Can Do.
The Mentally Retarded . . . Their New Hope.

---

* Complete addresses are given in the Appendix.

National Association for Mental Health, Inc.

Directory of Residential and Day Treatment Resources for Mentally Ill Children, 1967.
Organizing Discussion Groups for Parents of Mentally Ill Children.
The Mentally Ill Child: A Guide for Parents.

National Association for Retarded Children, Inc.

A Proposed Program for National Action to Combat Mental Retardation.
Bensberg, G. J.: Teaching the Mentally Retarded.
Boyd, D.: Three Stages in the Growth of a Parent of a Mentally Retarded Child.
Dittmann, L. L.: Home Training for Retarded Children.
Dittmann, L. L.: The Family of a Child in an Institution.
Dittmann, L. L.: The Mentally Retarded Child at Home, a Manual for Parents.
Dybwad, G.: New Horizons in Residential Care of the Mentally Retarded.
Dybwad, G.: Trends and Issues in Mental Retardation.
Feeding Mentally Retarded Children.
Holtgrewe, M. M.: A Guide for Public Health Nurses Working with Mentally Retarded Children.
How to Provide for Their Future.
Jensen, R. A.: The Clinical Management of the Mentally Retarded Child and the Parents.
Mental Retardation—Its Biological Factors.
Murray, M. A.: Needs of Parents with Mentally Retarded Children.
Schild, S.: Counseling with Parents of Retarded Children Living at Home.
Standifer, F. R.: Parents Helping Parents.
Zwerling, I.: Initial Counseling of Parents with Mentally Retarded Children.

Public Affairs Pamphlets

Hart, E.: How Retarded Children Can Be Helped.
Hill, M.: The Retarded Child Gets Ready for School.
McGrady, P.: Leukemia: Key to the Cancer Puzzle?

The Epilepsy Foundation

A National Listing of Medical Facilities for the Treatment and Diagnosis of Epilepsy.
Children with Epilepsy—A Series of Pamphlets.
Epilepsy, A Survey of State Laws.
You, Your Child and Epilepsy.

United States Department of Health, Education, and Welfare

A Modern Plan for Modern Services to the Mentally Retarded, 1967.
Asthma, 1966.
Children's Bureau Activities in Mental Retardation, 1966.
Dittmann, L. L.: The Mentally Retarded Child at Home, reprinted 1964.
El Problema del Retraso Mental, 1967.
Epilepsy, 1967.
Feeding Mentally Retarded Children, reprinted 1965.
Hemophilia, 1966.
Holtgrewe, M. M.: A Guide for Public Health Nurses Working with Mentally Retarded Children, 1964.
Kugel, R. B.: Children of Deprivation: Changing the Course of Familial Retardation, 1967.
Recreation and Mental Retardation, 1966.
Research Relating to Mentally Retarded Children, 1966.
Social Security: What It Means for the Parents of a Mentally Retarded Child, 1966.
The Care of the Retarded Child, 1965.
The Child with Epilepsy, 1966.
The Prevention of Mental Retardation Through Control of Infectious Diseases, 1968.
The Problem of Mental Retardation, 1966.
Wolff, I. S.: Nursing Role in Counseling Parents of Mentally Retarded Children, 1964.

REFERENCES

Publications

Baumgartner, B. B.: *Guiding the Retarded Child*. New York, G. P. Putnam's Sons, 1965.
Bensberg, G. J. (Ed.): *Teaching the Mentally Retarded*. Atlanta, Georgia, Southern Regional Education Board, 1965.
Bergman, T., and Freud, A.: *Children in the Hospital*. New York, International Universities Press, Inc., 1966.

Boggs, E. M.: *Equal Protection for the Unequal. Prevention and Treatment of Mental Retardation: An Interdisciplinary Approach to a Clinical Condition.* New York, Basic Books, Inc., 1966.

Borgatta, E. F., and Fanshel, D.: *Behavioral Characteristics of Children Known to Psychiatric Outpatient Clinics.* New York, Child Welfare League of America, Inc., 1965.

Carter, C. H.: *Medical Aspects of Mental Retardation.* Springfield, Ill., Charles C Thomas, 1965.

Crome, L., and Stern, J.: *The Pathology of Mental Retardation.* Boston, Little, Brown and Company, 1967.

Ehlers, W. H.: *Mothers of Retarded Children: How They Feel; Where They Find Help.* Springfield, Ill., Charles C Thomas, 1966.

French, E. L., and Scott, J. C.: *How You Can Help Your Retarded Child: A Manual for Parents.* Philadelphia, J. B. Lippincott Company, 1967.

Gasul, B. L., and others: *Diagnosis and Treatment of Heart Disease in Children.* Philadelphia, J. B. Lippincott Company, 1966.

Hallas, C. H.: *The Care and Training of the Mentally Subnormal.* 3rd ed. Toronto, Ontario, Macmillan Company of Canada, Ltd., 1967.

Hirshfeld, H.: *Your Allergic Child.* New York, Arco Publishing Company, 1965.

Hughes, J. G.: *Synopsis of Pediatrics.* 2nd ed. St. Louis, C. V. Mosby Company, 1967.

Keith, J. D., and others: *Heart Disease in Infancy and Childhood.* 2nd ed. New York, Macmillan Company, 1967.

Kennedy, The Joseph P., Jr. Foundation: *Mental Retardation.* Springfield, Ill., Charles C Thomas, 1966.

Kessler, J. W.: *Psychopathology of Childhood.* Englewood Cliffs, N. J., Prentice-Hall, Inc., 1966.

King, J. K. (Ed.): *Early Childhood Autism – Clinical, Educational and Social Aspects.* Long Island City, New York, Pergamon Press, Inc., 1966.

Murray, D. G.: *This Is Stevie's Story.* (National Association for Retarded Children). Nashville, Tennessee, Abingdon Press, 1967.

Nagera, H.: *Early Childhood Disturbances, The Infantile Neurosis, and the Adult Disturbances.* New York, International Universities Press, Inc., 1966.

Penny, R.: *Practical Care of the Mentally Retarded and Mentally Ill.* Springfield, Ill., Charles C Thomas, 1966.

Philips, I. (Ed.): *Prevention and Treatment of Mental Retardation.* New York, Basic Books, Inc., 1966.

Robinson, S., Abrams, H. and Kaplan, H.: *Congenital Heart Disease.* 2nd ed. New York, Blakiston Division, McGraw-Hill Book Company, Inc., 1965.

Smith, C. H.: *Blood Diseases of Infancy and Childhood.* 2nd ed. St. Louis, C. V. Mosby Company, 1966.

Thurman, W. G.: *Acute Leukemia and Pediatric Malignancies.* Philadelphia, Lea & Febiger, 1966.

Wing, J. K. (Ed.): *Early Childhood Autism: Clinical, Educational and Social Aspects.* Long Island City, New York, Pergamon Press, 1966.

Periodicals

Adams, M. L.: Care of the Retarded Child in The Home. *Nursing Forum,* VI:403, Fall 1967.

Arnold, I. L., and Goodman, L.: Homemaker Services to Families with Young Retarded Children. *Children,* 13:149, 1966.

Bailey, T. F.: Puppets Teach Young Patients. *Nursing Outlook,* 15:36, August 1967.

Barnard, K.: Teaching the Retarded Child Is a Family Affair. *Am. J. Nursing,* 68:305, 1968.

Bright, F., and France, Sister M. L.: The Nurse and the Terminally Ill Child. *Nursing Outlook,* 15:39, September 1967.

Cassell, S., and Paul, M. H.: The Role of Puppet Therapy on the Emotional Responses of Children Hospitalized for Cardiac Catheterization. *J. Pediat.,* 71:233, 1967.

Christ, A. E., and others: The Role of the Nurse in Child Psychiatry. *Nursing Outlook,* 13:30, January 1965.

Curfman, H. G., and Arnold, C. B.: A Homebound Therapy Program for Severely Retarded Children. *Children,* 14:63, 1967.

Desmond, M. M., and others: Congenital Rubella Encephalitis. *J. Pediat.,* 71:311, 1967.

Dybwad, G.: Who Are the Mentally Retarded? *Children,* 15:43, 1968.

Edward, J.: Extending a Hand to Parents of Disturbed Children. *Children,* 14:238, 1967.

Fackler, E.: The Crisis of Institutionalizing a Retarded Child. *Amer. J. Nursing,* 68:1508, 1968.

Geis, D. P., and Rochon, D.: Home Visits Help Prepare Preschoolers for Hospital Experience. *Hospitals,* 40:83, February 1966.

George, P., and others: A Study of "Total Therapy" of Acute Lymphocytic Leukemia in Children. *J. Pediat.,* 72:399, 1968.

Goodman, J.: A Nurse Is a Heck of a Nice Thing. *Am. J. Nursing,* 67:550, 1967.

Hammer, S. L., and Barnard, K. E.: The Mentally Retarded Adolescent. *Pediatrics,* 38:845, 1966.

James, E. E.: The Nursing Care of The Open Heart Patient. *Nursing Clin. N. Amer.,* 2:543, 1967.

Johnston, R.: Foster Grandparents for Emotionally Disturbed Children. *Children,* 14:46, 1967.

Legeay, C., and Keogh, B.: Impact of Mental Retardation on Family Life. *Am. J. Nursing,* 66:1062, 1966.

Linde, L. M., and others: Growth in Children with Congenital Heart Disease. *J. Pediat.,* 70:413, 1967.

Linde, L. M., Rasof, B., and Dunn, O. J.: Mental Development in Congenital Heart Disease. *J. Pediat.,* 71:198, 1967.

Livingston, S.: What Hope for the Child with Epilepsy? *Children,* 12:9, 1965.

Mandelbaum, A.: The Group Process in Helping Parents of Retarded Children. *Children,* 14:227, 1967.

Mansmann, H. C.: Management of the Child with Bronchial Asthma. *Pediat. Clin. N. Amer.,* 15:357, 1968.

Mental Retardation and the Nurse. *Nursing Forum* VI:178, Spring 1967.

Meredith, D. A.: Speech of Psychotic Children as a Tool in Therapeutic Nursing Care. *Nursing Clin. N. Amer.,* 1:245, 1966.

Miller, R. M.: Prenatal Origins of Mental Retardation: Epidemiological Approach. *J. Pediat.,* 71:455, 1967.

O'Neill, J.: Siblings of the Retarded: Individual Counseling. *Children,* 12:226, 1965.

Pappas, A. M., and others: The Problem of Unrecognized "Mild Hemophilia." *J.A.M.A.,* 187:772, 1964.

Peterson, L. W.: Operant Approach to Observation and Recording. *Nursing Outlook,* 15:28, March 1967.

Pitorak, E. F.: Open-Ended Care for the Open Heart Patient. *Am. J. Nursing,* 67:1452, 1967.

Saunders, E. F., Kauder, E., and Mauer, A. M.: Sequential Therapy of Acute Leukemia in Childhood. *J. Pediat.,* 70:632, 1967.

Segal, A.: Some Observations About Mentally Retarded Adolescents. *Children,* 14:233, 1967.

Spurgeon, R. K.: Nursing the Autistic Child. *Am. J. Nursing* 67:1416, 1967.

Spurgeon, R. K.: Some Problems in Measuring Nonverbal Behavior of Autistic Children. *Nursing Research,* 16:212, 1967.

Vernick, J., and Lunceford, J. L.: Milieu Design for Adolescents with Leukemia. *Am. J. Nursing,* 67:559, 1967.

Whitney, L.: Operant Learning Theory: A Framework Deserving Nursing Investigation. *Nursing Research* 15:229, 1966.

Wood, J. W., and others: Mental Retardation in Children Exposed in Utero to the Atomic Bombs in Hiroshima and Nagasaki. *Am. J. Pub. Health* 57:1381, 1967.

Wright, M. M.: Nursing Services in a Mental Retardation Clinical Research Unit. *Nursing Clin. N. Amer.,* 1:669, 1966.

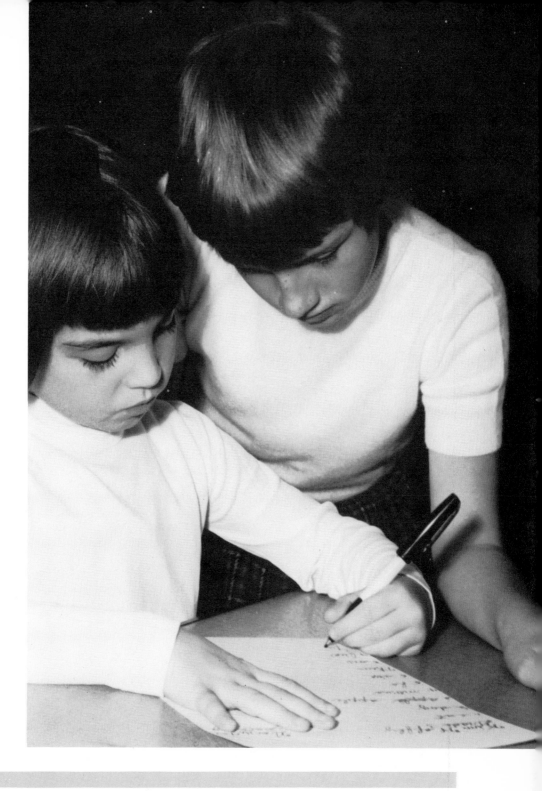

UNIT SIX

THE SCHOOL CHILD

21

THE SCHOOL CHILD: HIS GROWTH, DEVELOPMENT AND CARE

OVERVIEW OF EMOTIONAL DEVELOPMENT

At some time during the school-age period parents must learn to adjust to what appears to be almost total rejection by their child. He may exhibit an overt independence of them and of the standards they have tried to impress upon him. At this time parents may feel hurt, disappointed and angry. Yet, in spite of what appears to be true, the child still needs unobtrusive parental support, given with respect for the child's feelings of independence.

By the time the child reaches his sixth birthday he should have learned to trust others and should have developed a sense of autonomy. He should also have learned the fundamentals of getting along in his particular environment, through experience in living and through questioning his parents and other adults. He should have developed a sense of initiative, but his activities should be controlled to some degree by his conscience.

These stages which the child passes through before he is six years old are probably the most important for healthy personality development. Children whose personality growth has been warped are likely to remain handicapped unless help is given them. There are exceptions to this, of course, for experiences in later childhood and in adolescence influence the trend in emotional development.

Sense of Industry. Between the ages of six and twelve years the child develops a *sense of industry* and a desire to engage in tasks in the real world. He is internally motivated to put forth effort on a purposeful activity which will yield a sense of worth. Even before he is six years old a child may show evidence that he enjoys doing socially useful tasks for others, that he wants to do things and to learn to do them well.

These years are usually a calm period, and few overwhelming upheavals are apt to occur. The child continues in a steady growth toward learning how to attain the goal of becoming a responsible citizen. He acquires knowledge and skills which will help him to make a worthwhile contribution to society. He learns how to cooperate with others, to play fairly and follow the rules of the game, and to conform to social norms so that his life with others will be a positive experience for him and for those with whom he interacts. With all this, however, the school-age period is characterized by alternate conformity and rebellion against adult authority.

Instead of developing a sense of industry,

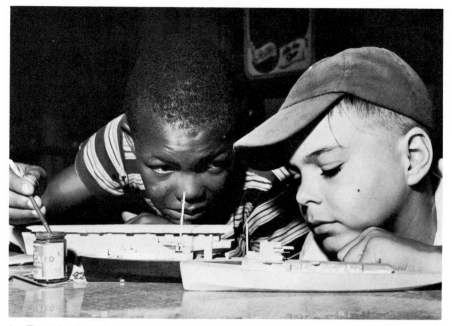

Figure 21–1. The school child wants to learn to do things and to do them well. (H. Armstrong Roberts.)

the child may acquire, or intensify earlier, *feelings of inferiority* and inadequacy. This is more likely to happen if he has not successfully passed through the previous stages of personality development.

The Child and School. At school the child has a task, one that will continue throughout childhood. If he is adequately prepared, if his needs as a growing person are regarded and if he is successful, the school experience will have a positive influence on personality development. If he is not successful in school because he is dull, his self-image is that he is stupid. If he is too maladjusted to make friends among his peer group, he feels that nobody likes him. He may stay in school, passively accepting his inferiority, or leave school as soon as the law permits.

Out of school he may find a job in the attempt to secure a sense of accomplishment. To succeed, he needs the sense of industry which he failed to develop during his school years when it was a major developmental task. If he fails in the job, he may turn to delinquency to gain the status and recognition among his peers which he failed to gain in school and at work. If his delinquency is extreme, he also gains attention from adults which he could not secure by legitimate means.

The importance of adapting the school experience to the needs of the growing child is evident.

School is not the only place where a child may gain a feeling of mastery and acquire a sense of industry. The child may be given useful tasks at home. Parents may delegate to him responsibilities which contribute to the happiness and

well-being of all the family. Such tasks and responsibilities should not be those which adults do not want to do themselves, but rather should be based on a division of labor in which the child's tasks are suited to his abilities. The work should not be so time-consuming that the child has no opportunity to study, to take on status-giving tasks outside the home and to play with siblings and friends.

Community organizations for children stress both recreation and work, e.g. the 4-H Clubs and the Girl Scouts and Boy Scouts of America.

The school child must grow out of the dependence upon his family which was natural for the younger child, and must find satisfaction in the company of his peer group and adults outside the home. He must develop neuromuscular skills so that he can participate in work and games with others. He must acquire sufficient knowledge to interact with adults outside of school and thereby learn from them about the social life of his society. He must gain some understanding of adult concepts, logic and ways of communicating.

More specifically, during the school years the child should develop wholesome attitudes toward himself as a person and should learn his or her appropriate masculine or feminine social role. He should learn how to get along with his age mates, yet should be able to act according to his conscience and his scale of values. He should achieve independence in caring for himself. He should learn the fundamental skills of reading, writing and calculating, and the physical skills necessary for ordinary games.

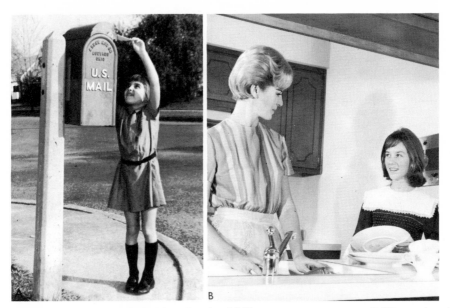

Figure 21–2.   The sense of industry is developed as the child learns to assume responsibilities such as (*A*) mailing letters and (*B*) wiping dishes. (H. Armstrong Roberts.)

By the time he is twelve years old he should have developed positive attitudes toward his own and other social, racial, economic and religious groups, and have learned the concepts necessary for participation in daily living with adults in his environment.

The School Child, His Family and His Friends

Relations with Parents.   The child between six and twelve years should have widened his social horizons beyond the confines of his own home. Although he is still dependent upon his parents' love, companionship with his peers and adults outside the home has become of increasing importance.

The child's relation with the parent of the opposite sex which existed during his preschool years has been resolved. He has come to respect and love that parent, but now identifies with or tries to be like the parent of the same sex. By imitating that parent's role he learns his own social role.

Children gain increasing ideological as well as physical and emotional independence from their parents. They gain new ideas from adults outside the family: teachers, parents of their friends, policemen, television performers, newspaper writers and authors of textbooks and of fiction. Often these ideas and attitudes conflict with those of their parents. This is likely if the parents are immigrants or of a low socioeconomic status. The adults who teach these children must help them to understand this conflict so that they

do not become impatient with their parents and lose respect for them.

Health education is a part of modern general education in the public schools. Health measures such as taking a bath every day, accepted by the children, may seem foolish to their parents, who went to school twenty to thirty years ago. Daily baths may be almost impossible in a crowded tenement flat. There is then a conflict between what the child is taught at school and at home, which places a serious strain on parent-child relations.

The school child learns to think of himself as a person in his own right and may resent rigid limits which parents continue to impose on his behavior. Furthermore, he dislikes a show of affection when he is feeling well and in no danger. He often pulls away from the adult's embrace and turns his face from kisses. The parents may be confused and thrown into emotional conflict by the new concepts which children bring home, by their efforts at independence and by the apparent disinterest in a physical show of parental affection. The parents may be surprised, however, as the well child who refuses to have an adult hovering over him turns to these same adults for affection and protection when he is threatened by illness or injury.

Parents need help in understanding the normal growth and development of their children when such conflicts arise. They may discuss these matters with the child's teacher, alone or during parent-teacher conferences, with their physician, religious advisor or a nurse who visits in the home or cares for the child in the hospital.

There are certain guidelines which would help parents to counsel and discipline their children in an easier manner. First of all, parents should invite the confidence of their child as a parent, not as a buddy or school chum. Parents should leave the door open, so to speak, to discussions, but they should never intrude on the privacy of a child, because privacy is the right of every human being. Parents should set a good example for their child to follow in building character traits such as honesty and loyalty. Parents cannot expect their child to obey the rules of society when they themselves do not. Both parents should set consistent limits on their child's behavior, because even though he may be upset at the time, he will understand ultimately that their interest is evidence of their love for him. Parents should also try to see their child as others see him, not as an idealized extension of themselves. Finally, parents should not compare one child with another in the family. Each child should be accepted because he is *himself* and different from his siblings or cousins.

Relations with Siblings. Whether the school child is an only child or one of a group of siblings has more and more effect upon his personality. If he is an only child, he tends to cling longer to his concept of being the center of the family. When he goes outside the family to make friends in his peer group, he still expects to be the center of the group and becomes frightened when he finds that he is not. He finds it difficult to learn the give and take of social living with other children. An only child who does not succeed in establishing himself as a group member may find that playing by himself is a lonely existence. He may come to resent being an only child and long desperately for siblings such as his friends have. In addition, since he is the recipient of the undiluted force of his parents' attitudes and feelings, he is likely to be limited in his freedom.

Children in a large family find adjusting to children outside the family and sharing with the group easier than does the only child. They learn early that some are given opportunities and restrictions, while others are not. They learn that no one of them, unless it is the youngest child, is singled out as the center of interest, although each in his own way is loved by his parents. Although they may disagree among themselves, each sibling has a deep affection for the other children in the family.

Children in large families have problems, however, which the only child does not have. Sibling jealousy is a problem even in families in which all the members love one another. Although it is more acute in preschool children than among children over six years of age, it still exists. An older child may envy the attention which the younger siblings receive. He may resent the fact that his discarded toys are being broken by a younger child and the fact that, despite his feelings, he is expected to love and often to take care of his siblings.

If the school child is a younger sibling, he may envy the older child his freedom and skills. He may strive to be like the older child and be defeated in his attempts. The school child's jealousy of his siblings, younger and older, may actually increase as he strives to keep ahead of the younger child or to catch up with an older brother or sister. Scholastic ability is a principal cause of sibling jealousy among school children, particularly in a child who is mentally inferior to his siblings.

School children often prefer to be with their friends rather than their siblings. Relations with a friend are less emotional and freer from parental interference. A child chooses his friends; the sibling relationship is one he is born into and cannot be discontinued when he wishes to be free of it. Ideally, experience with siblings should facilitate a child's social adjustment outside the family, but it does not take the place of friendships of his own choice.

Relations with Friends. As the child psychologically moves slowly away from home, his friends become increasingly important to him. He learns to take his place as a member of a group, and his social life begins. In making this adjustment children tend to avoid the company of the opposite sex. During this period boys consider girls sissies, and the girls think boys too rough. Each sex tends to develop its own language and its own activities and behavior.

Children of school age can be exceedingly cruel to each other. They want to control or feel that they are able to control another person. The state of being "picked on" is common during the school period. Some children are excluded from friendship groups and verbally are made to feel uncomfortable. School children can also be cruel to adults whom they dislike.

Gangs or Groups. Since school children have learned that their parents are not omnipotent, that they make mistakes and are sometimes afraid, they tend to confide not in them, but in their friends. They form close friendships and ultimately join a group of other children of their own sex. Such a group may be merely a friendship group or it may be a secret society or an antisocial gang, depending upon the needs of the children who form it. Among themselves the children discuss the problems they face. They discuss their own theories about life, death and sexual matters; they share attitudes, values and beliefs with the peer group.

Much of a boy's hostility and aggression is worked off in his peer group through fighting, either in a supervised, organized game such as baseball or football or while playing "cops" and robbers or cowboys and Indians. Unfor-

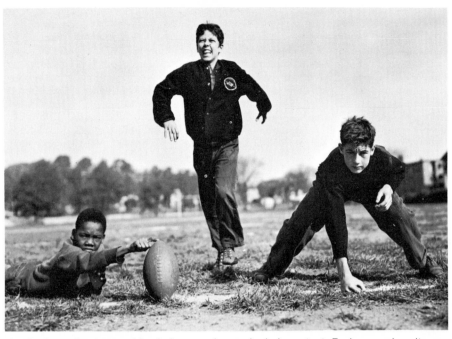

Figure 21–3. During school years friends become increasingly important. Each sex enjoys its own language and its own kinds of activity. (H. Armstrong Roberts.)

tunately some of these juvenile gangs turn their hostility not against their own age group in play, but against other youths or adults in deadly earnest. When this occurs, the pattern is laid for delinquent behavior.

Girls also form their own groups and discuss their own problems. They do not, however, as a rule engage in the aggressive and hostile activities common in the boys' gang.

Toward the end of the school period children have learned to compete and to compromise with others and to cooperate so that they can accomplish something in their group which no one child could do without adult help. They have learned how to get along with their own and other groups and to follow the rules of the larger society. They have developed a sense of responsibility about matters which they know are important.

Parents should be understanding and accepting of the activities of their school children and willing to give independence when it is needed. All too often only the mother is interested, and she seldom understands the boy's interests. The father often appears disinterested in his children's individual or group activities. This is unfortunate because the boy especially needs his father's loving interest at this time.

OVERVIEW OF PHYSICAL, SOCIAL AND MENTAL DEVELOPMENT

Physical Development. During the school years the child shows a progressively slower growth in height, but a rapid gain in weight. He tends to lose the thin, wiry appearance of the earlier years. General growth is slow until the spurt just before puberty. Muscular coordination improves steadily; posture should be good (the earlier lordosis has disappeared). The lymphatic tissue reaches its height of development in the early school period. The frontal sinuses are fairly well developed by six years of age. From this time on all the sinuses are potential foci of infection.

This is the period of eruption and growth of the permanent teeth. The six-year molars are the first to erupt and are the keystone for the

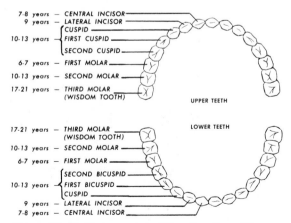

| 7-8 years — CENTRAL INCISOR |
| 9 years — LATERAL INCISOR |
| CUSPID |
| 10-13 years — FIRST CUSPID |
| SECOND CUSPID |
| 6-7 years — FIRST MOLAR |
| 10-13 years — SECOND MOLAR |
| 17-21 years — THIRD MOLAR (WISDOM TOOTH) |

UPPER TEETH

LOWER TEETH

| 17-21 years — THIRD MOLAR (WISDOM TOOTH) |
| 10-13 years — SECOND MOLAR |
| 6-7 years — FIRST MOLAR |
| SECOND BICUSPID |
| 10-13 years — FIRST BICUSPID |
| CUSPID |
| 9 years — LATERAL INCISOR |
| 7-8 years — CENTRAL INCISOR |

Figure 21–4. Permanent dentition. Eruption of these teeth occurs between six and twenty-one years of age.

permanent dental arch. The receding mandible, characteristic of the younger child, has extended forward to allow room for the permanent teeth.

The temperature, pulse and respiration approach the adult norms. The normal temperature is 98.6°F. The average pulse rate is from 85 to 100 per minute, the blood pressure 95 to 108 systolic and 62 to 67 diastolic. The rate of respiration is 18 to 20 per minute.

The physical changes which indicate pubescence may begin to appear toward the end of the school age.

Social and Mental Development. In school the child has an opportunity to widen his social contacts while he develops his mental abilities. The school hours of the six-year-old in many places are shorter than those of older school children. This makes the transition from home to school life and the adjustment to new experiences easier for the child.

SPECIFICS OF PHYSICAL, SOCIAL AND MENTAL DEVELOPMENT

The older a child becomes, the less is it possible to set norms as standards for his behavior or abilities. Such norms illustrate merely the kinds of behavior that often occur at a certain age. The student should recall from Chapter 2 that not all development proceeds on a steady upward curve. It has periods of acceleration, plateaus, and even lags in some areas, while other areas of development proceed normally. Yet all physical growth and mental and emotional development are interrelated in the individual child. Individual differences and the effects of his health status and home, school and community environment become more and more pronounced as the child grows older.

Six Years

The sixth year is a year of transition, of physical and psychologic changes which society has taken as the criterion for readiness to enter school. It is a difficult period for parents, and also for the child because he wants to assume increased responsibility and self-direction and yet lacks the basis for making wise decisions. Typically, he is upset and tense, self-centered and a show-off. He enjoys bossing others, but is easily hurt by the criticism he evokes. He is ready to start anything, but not anxious to finish the task. He may be defiant and rude with adults as a result of his unstable emotional reactions.

Six-year-olds feel tension because they are growing up and are leaving the security of home to go to school. This means that the child is feeling a new wave of separation anxiety which is felt periodically, even in adolescence. They want

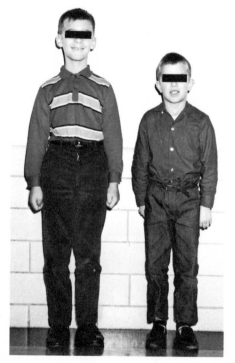

Figure 21–5. The older a child becomes, the less it is possible to set norms of physical development, behavior or abilities. These two boys are six years of age, but show an obvious difference in growth.

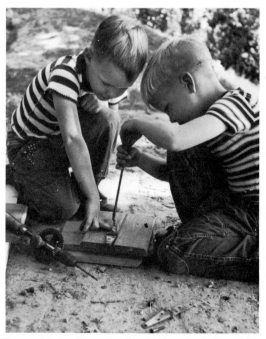

Figure 21–6. Six-year-olds enjoy physical activity, but their movements are not as coordinated as those of older school children. (H. Armstrong Roberts.)

the role of the little child again. Parental love and praise are important to them.

Boys and girls play together. Their play is apt to end in chaos. There are disputes and physical battles in which boys and girls take equal parts. The individual child is still more important than the play group as a whole.

The six-year-old may still be troubled by some of the sex questions he asked in the preschool period. He may indulge in sex play. Although he looks forward to marriage, he pays little attention to the sexual aspect and may invite one of his relatives to be his marital partner. He is likely to want his mother to have a baby even if there is already one in the family.

Physical Development and Motor Control. Physical development and motor control are seen in the changing characteristics and abilities of the six-year-old. The loss of the temporary teeth continues, and the first permanent teeth, the six-year molars, erupt. In school, if he did not go to nursery school or kindergarten, he is exposed to infection more frequently than he was at home, and ear, nose and throat problems are common. He appears to be in constant motion. He enjoys physical activity, but his movements may be clumsy because of his fatigue from overactivity—wrestling, playing tag, tumbling, and jumping with other children. His balance is improving; he climbs, skips, hops and gallops well. Girls jump rope, a single rope, but not double. Both sexes can walk steadily on a chalk mark and learn to skate. Some children can ride a bicycle.

These children can throw and catch a ball. They are aware of their hands as tools, cutting and pasting well. They can hammer, build simple structures, manipulate fasteners on clothing with the aid of sight to guide their hands, and tie shoelaces.

Vocalization, Socialization and Mental Abilities. The six-year-old has command of practically every form of sentence structure. Speech is fixed, and he is no longer experimenting with its use. He asks questions which show thought and uses language as a tool and less for the pleasure of talking as he did during the preschool age. He may use language aggressively, expressing himself in slang and even swearing. He uses language to share in the experience of others and

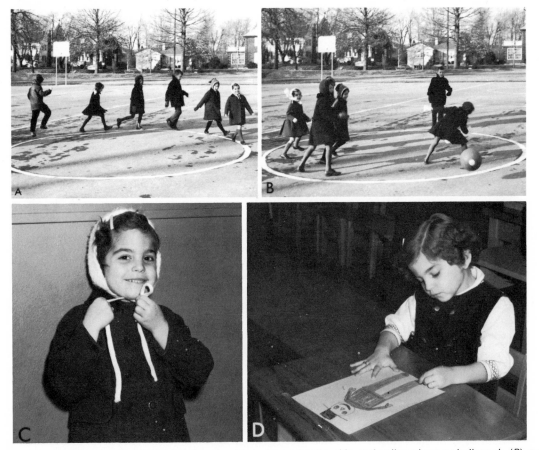

Figure 21–7.   The six-year-old (*A*) has improved balance so he can skip and gallop along a chalk mark, (*B*) can throw and catch a ball well, (*C*) can tie a bow easily, (*D*) can draw a man with hitherto absent features.

is interested in learning more about his relatives and his own and their place in the family tree. He still defines objects in terms of their use: a chair is something to sit on, and a spoon is what he eats with. But he has some concept of abstract words; he knows whether it is morning or afternoon. He knows his right hand from his left, can count to twenty or more, but when printing, he may reverse one or two of the digits or capital letters. Since he can now recognize shapes, he can read, and describe objects seen in pictures. He can draw a man with hitherto absent features such as hands, neck and clothing, and he can distinguish between what he has been taught is attractive and what is ugly when shown a series of faces. He is able to obey three commands given in succession, e.g. "Wipe your hands, put the dishes on the table, and close the door."

Probably his greatest achievement in abstract thought is his beginning interest in the concept of a power greater than himself or his parents—God.

Seven Years

Seven is an assimilative age, a quieting-down period. The child is less of a problem than he was at six years, more often quiet than boisterous. Many teachers find the second-grade group the easiest to teach in elementary school. The child has less intense relations with others; he does not ask for trouble. But he enjoys teasing, and this often gets him into difficulty with children younger than himself and with adults who take their part. He likes to play alone, although he prefers group play. When playing, he is more passive than the six-year-old.

The seven-year-old sets high standards for his family and feels both a personal inferiority and anger over even their minor failures, as he sees them, in living up to their respective roles. His ethical sense is developing; he is conscious of right and wrong in the conduct of others and in what he himself does. He may tattle on other children from a sense of justice. On the whole he is now a cooperative member of the family and wants the approval of his parents. Parents must respect his inner life, his strains of sadness and his uncalled-for periods of shyness. It is during these periods that he is becoming aware of himself and thus of others.

The seven-year-old is more modest about sexual matters and indulges in less sex play. Many seven-year-olds would like to have a baby brother or sister. The seven-year-old may become involved in an elementary love affair with someone of the opposite sex.

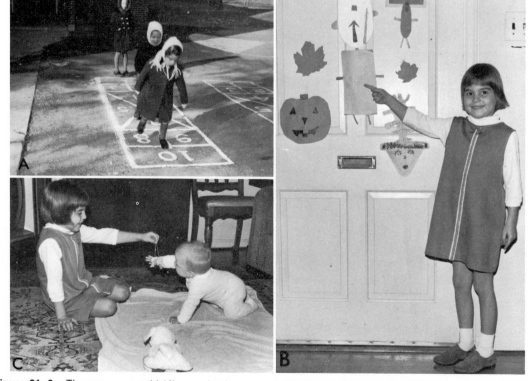

Figure 21-8. The seven-year-old (A) can play hopscotch, (B) knows which month of the year it is, particularly months in which some event such as Halloween occurs, (C) is a cooperative member of the family.

Physical Development and Motor Control.
The general level of activity is lower at seven years than at six, but varies widely in individual children. The child has a trait which annoys his elders, but fascinates him and other children – wiggling a loose tooth.

The books he reads need no longer be printed with type larger than average, for his eyes become fully developed between seven or eight years of age. His posture is now more tense and ready for motion than that of the younger child.

Boys and girls enjoy skating and other active sports. There begins to be a division, however, between boy and girl sports. Girls jump rope and play hopscotch, games which boys are likely to participate in only in a teasing way. Although seven-year-olds are active, they enjoy games in which they can sit down and rest.

Vocalization, Socialization and Mental Abilities. The child is becoming oriented in time as well as space. He knows which month it is and the season of the year, particularly months in which some event in which he is intensely interested takes place – Christmas or his birthday. He begins to read the clock, both the hours and the minutes.

His hands are becoming more steady, and he often prefers a pencil with an eraser to a crayon. He can print several sentences, though the letters become smaller toward the end of the line. Reversal of letters is less common, and he is likely to correct such errors. He can repeat five numbers in succession and three numbers backward, count by two's and five's, grasp the basic idea of addition and subtraction, copy a diamond without confusing it with a square, and tell what parts are missing from an incomplete picture of a man. His attention span is lengthening, and he enjoys repeating activities that afford him satisfaction. He is more self-helpful, needing little assistance in dressing, undressing and going to bed. He is increasingly interested in God's place in the world and wants to know where heaven is and what it is like.

Eight Years

The eight-year-old is at an expansive age and wants to do everything. This is an age of broadening experiences and intellectual exploration. He is more creative and active in his solitary play and work, but he needs other children and their approval, and he actively seeks their company. He is full of enthusiastic energy and wants to be considered important by adults. He wants to assume responsibility and to spread his influence in the culture of his group by putting on dramatic shows and inventing new ways of doing tasks. He tries to understand adult ideas and standards by listening to what is told him. He learns by experience and from others what is necessary for group living. If his mental ability is average or above average, he becomes very much interested in reading, group activities and school, especially in science as he sees it pictured in space ships and machinery. He likes science fiction. Hero worship begins at this age.

He likes to join clubs if they are not too rigidly organized and takes group fads seriously. Eight-year-olds appear to be sex-conscious, choosing playmates of their own sex. Boys are usually secretive about girl friends, especially if *she* is a new girl in the neighborhood. They show less active interest in sex questions which are beyond their comprehension than does the younger child, but they may ask questions at appropriate times. Mothers should suggest to their children that it is better not to discuss the answers to sex questions with siblings or friends.

The eight-year-old behaves best when strangers are present or when he is away from home.

Physical Development and Motor Control.
There are subtle changes in the body of an eight-year-old; the arms are growing longer in proportion to the body, and the hands are also proportionately larger. His movements are becoming smoother, more graceful and perfected. His amusements change as he matures. He now likes hiking, playing ball and such games as follow-the-leader. The boy wants to improve his skill in boxing and wrestling, and the girl in jumping rope, hopscotch and roller skating. Both boys and girls are dramatic in their activities and accompany speech with descriptive gestures.

Vocalization, Socialization and Mental Abilities. In school the child of eight is writing rather than printing, and enjoys his new skill. In mental tests for his age group are found questions such as naming from memory similarities and differences between two objects – e.g. ball and block – and counting backwards from twenty. In school and daily life he has new abilities. He is beginning to understand perspective in drawing. He can repeat the days of the week and has some concept of the number of days which must pass before some pleasant event will take place – a holiday, his birthday or, in the hospital, visiting day and that eventful day when he goes home.

Some children enjoy going to Sunday School and are interested in hearing about heaven as "the place you go to when you die."

Nine Years

The nine-year-old is neither a child nor a youth. He is only beginning to take part in family group discussions. He is not as restless as the eight-year-old and is more interested in family activities. He is impelled to show others that he is an individual and resists or ignores adult authority when it conflicts with ideas or values of

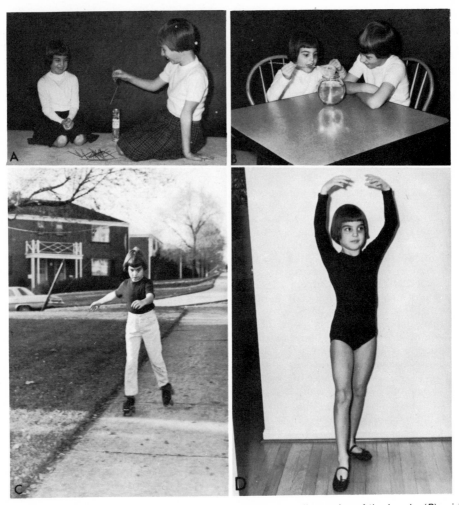

Figure 21–9. The eight-year-old (A) enjoys games of skill using small muscles of the hands, (B) evidences interest in science, (C) can move more smoothly when skating, (D) can balance gracefully.

his peer group. Teachers find the children in fourth grade difficult to teach. In broadening his experiences outside the home he grows toward independence. He is better able to accept blame for his acts and assumes responsibility for care of younger siblings and for keeping his room in some sort of order. He is motivated, as well as more likely, to complete the tasks he begins.

He fluctuates between childhood and youth in his actions and thoughts. Hero worship is becoming pronounced. Girls still prefer to play with girls, and boys with boys. They are usually less concerned with the reproductive aspect of sex than when they were eight. This depends, however, on whether their desire for information about the conception and bearing of children was satisfied when they first asked for it. The nine-year-old is in a state of constant urgency, as though he were in a contest with time.

Physical Development and Motor Control. These children have more variation in skills than they had during their first three years of school. Normally, hand-eye coordination is developed, and the child becomes skillful in manual activities. In general, children of this age can use both hands independently.

The child works and plays hard and enjoys displaying his motor skill and strength; he shows great interest in competitive sports such as baseball.

Vocalization, Socialization and Mental Abilities. New abilities, which show his mental development, include describing common objects in detail not in terms of use as he did when he was six years old, repeating the months of the year in order, knowing the date, telling time correctly, writing (usually with small, even letters), matching the material which he reads with reality, making correct change from a quarter, arranging five weights according to their heaviness, multiplying and dividing (simple division) and repeating four numbers backward (this is one item in a commonly given mental test).

The child can take care of his bodily needs

completely; this is a great step away from early childhood and toward adult self-reliance. He has developed acceptable table manners and shows them without coaching from his parents. Although he has fewer fears than when he was younger, he has become a worrier. His advance toward adult attitudes is shown in his rejection of the Santa Claus myth, and yet he does not intentionally destroy it for a younger sibling. In contrast to the two preceding years, he may show a lack of interest in God and in religion.

Ten Years

The average child of ten years is at the beginning of the preadolescent period. The girl is further advanced than the boy toward puberty. The ten-year-old is even more reasonable than the nine-year-old, for he has acquired greater mastery of himself and his environment. He is courteous and well mannered with adults, and shows more self-direction in his actions. He wants to measure up to a challenge, defined in the social norms of the group. He has broad interests and is beginning to think clearly about social problems and social prejudices. Special talents appear in this age group.

The child adjusts better than before to home routines; he can live by rules and tolerates frustrations. He is entering the age when the need for group activities is at its highest point. To him, attaining a goal for the group is more important than his own ideas or desires. He is capable of great loyalties and intense hero worship; both are qualities making for successful group membership.

The ten-year-old is interested in matters of sex, but is more likely to discuss the subject with his peer group than with his parents. Children of both sexes investigate their sexual organs. Some children are modest, but others present problems of sex play.

Outside the classroom the two sexes rarely mix. Although kissing games may be played in children's entertainments arranged by adults, they are seldom played spontaneously. Children tease each other about friends of the opposite sex.

The ten-year-old wants to be independent. For this reason requests should be made positively and with tact. Negative requests affront his sense of personal worth. The power of suggestion is important at this age and can be used to help the child develop a good character.

Physical Development and Motor Control. As the child's body matures, sex differences are more pronounced. Both boys and girls have perfected most of the basic small motor movements. They desire perfection in their complex abilities. Girls have more poise than boys, partly because of their earlier maturation.

Vocalization, Socialization and Mental Abilities. The child now thinks of situations in terms of cause and effect. He has some insight into the fundamentals of human relations and wants to accomplish great things in life.

His education is more advanced, and he uses what he knows and the skills he has acquired in his daily life. He can write for a relatively long time and maintains good speed. He likes mystery stories, science fiction and practical magic. He can use numbers beyond 100 with understanding and can do simple fractions.

Ten to Twelve Years
(Preadolescence)

The years between ten and twelve are known as the preadolescent period. It is a time of rapid growth and development, when many problems occur. As he approaches adulthood the child may become overcritical of adults, comparing them with the self-image of the man or woman he or she intends to be. The child wavers between dependence and independence and is likely to withdraw when he is frustrated instead of voicing his anger. He may rebel against parental standards of bathing and dressing.

Friends in his peer group are extremely important to him; he shares their attitudes and tells them his thoughts rather than confiding in his parents. He enters with enthusiasm into group community projects such as collecting worn clothing for charity or old newspapers for the Boy Scouts.

He is critical of what he does. He wants to become somewhat financially independent of his parents; he is happy to do small jobs after school or during vacations. He seeks an adult friend of the same sex with whom to identify and to whom he can express criticism of his parents. The composure and control of the ten-year-old gradually vanish at eleven to twelve years. He becomes annoying, sloppy, exhibitionistic and negativistic. He tries hard to master reality in preparation for adolescence. He is interested in how things work and curious about the world in general, but his interest in acquiring academic knowledge may lag.

He needs to gain strength of personality so as to be able to make healthy solutions to the conflicts of adolescence. The adult who is responsible for the preadolescent at home, in the community or at school must accept the fact that the child needs to rebel and depreciate others in order to work through his conflict between dependence and independence. He is still dependent, but he does not wish to be made to feel infantile. He rejects his parents because he does not want to feel dependent on them; he meets his dependency needs by relations with other adults. The adult whom the preadolescent selects to fill this role must handle the child through democratic guidance. He must accept the child, yet provide limits to his behavior as the parents did when the child was younger. The preadolescent needs help to channel his feelings and energy in the proper directions—sports and work suitable to his stage of growth and development. He needs help in accepting himself in his new role of preadolescent. Adults in his environment should help him to build up his self-esteem and strengthen his personality in order to prepare him adequately to meet the problems of adolescence.

Physical Development and Motor Control
Children in this age group are filled with energy and are constantly active. Their muscular control is good, and manipulative skill almost equals that of the adult. They appear to be under tension, which is relieved by foot-tapping on the floor or finger-drumming on table tops.

The twelve-year molars erupt, the last teeth to erupt during childhood. The preadolescent spurt in growth comes earlier in girls than in boys, but girls lag behind boys in endurance and physical strength.

Vocalization, Socialization and Mental Abilities. Before he is twelve years old the average child is able to define some basic abstract terms such as honesty and justice. His development of vocabulary and diction depend upon his intelligence, experience and environmental opportunities. Children in this age group can see the moral of stories. Their interests and intellectual pur-

suits vary. Intellectual growth is seen in their interest in world affairs, both past and present, and their attitude toward social problems, especially those which touch their daily lives.

They are eager to learn about health. They want to know why the mouth should be covered when coughing. They are capable of self-care in ordinary situations, but should still be under some supervision of sympathetic adults. They can assume some responsibility for the care of younger children. Their contact with children and adults goes well beyond the limits of home.

The peer group is very close to the eleven-year-old. This is a period for sharing secrets. Even a secret language may be devised and used strictly with the close peer group. These children still prefer to play with their own sex group, but accept the opposite sex in their activities.

SCHOOL

Attendance at school is an important part of the growing child's life. The school is the institution in society specifically designed as the formal instrument for educating its children. Its purpose is to help each child to develop his potential to the fullest. This includes helping each child develop his *sense of industry.*

The basic tools for achieving this objective are the communication skills and the arithmetic

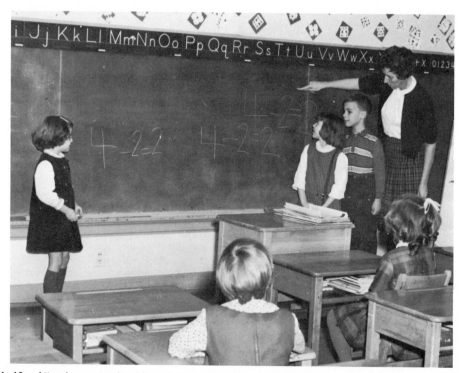

Figure 21–10. Attendance at school is an important part of the child's life. In school, children should be helped to develop their sense of industry.

fundamentals. Mastery of these tools then makes it possible for the child to extend his educational horizons to areas such as history, geography, science, social studies, health education and the creative arts.

From the earliest years the school program provides experience which contributes to the child's social development as a member of a group. It is here that he should be learning to think critically, to make judgments based on reason, to accept criticism, to cooperate with others and to be both a leader and a follower as the occasion warrants.

The extent to which a child acquires a sense of personal worth and a respect for the contribution of others is an important measure of the effectiveness of the school program. Attendance at school is important for all children, irrespective of their socioeconomic group and intelligence level. The course of instruction should be such that every child will be able to get a feeling of successful accomplishment in some area.

All children should feel that they can accomplish something both in school and, later, in community life. This does not mean that all children should be passed along with their group in school whether they do well or not. They do not want to be rewarded when they know that they have failed. They need opportunities for success on their individual level of achievement.

Not every child is capable of excelling intellectually in academic courses, but the school should help each child to realize his potential ability and find real satisfaction in his achievement in other areas of living — areas in which the child who does not do well at school may be more successful than those who excel in class work.

Preparation for School. Not all children are emotionally ready for school at the same chronologic age. If the preschool child has attended and adjusted well to nursery school, he probably will have little difficulty with adjustment to school. He will consider school a normal responsibility of childhood.

As soon as school starts there is an enforced separation of the child from his home. The unprepared child, more than those who are prepared, may be uncertain of the expectations of the teacher, a new adult in charge of part of his life. He may be frightened by leaving his parents and by the demands of a group of children different from those he has known before. In general, however, if he has attended kindergarten in the public school of his neighborhood, he will have friends in the first grade and will be accustomed to the school building. If a younger sibling is entering kindergarten, he is protective and tells him all about it. He will go to and from school with siblings or neighborhood friends.

Preparation for school experience is much like preparation for attendance at nursery school (see p. 474). The child should know his full name and address before entering school. He should know certain safety rules, such as how to cross the street safely. He should also know how to care for himself for the most part in matters of dressing and toileting. He should have a physical examination and must meet school requirements for immunization.

The mother should take the child to school before school starts in order to orient him to the physical environment and to meet his teacher. Parents should talk positively about school experience at all times, but particularly to the child entering school. Older siblings will present school as a matter-of-fact experience for all six-year-olds and as something to brag about to younger children. After school has started, if the child appears afraid of the school experience, the mother may stay with him in the classroom for a while until the teacher has established a positive relation with him. Before parents allow a child to go to school alone they must be certain that he knows the way or, if he must take a bus, which bus to ride. Generally the school either is in easy walking distance or sends a school bus to collect the children who live too far away to walk to school.

A problem may arise after the child has become familiar with school life in that he pays more attention to the job of gaining friends than to gaining knowledge. This is to be expected, especially if none of his old friends from home, nursery school or kindergarten are in his class at school.

Parents should not expect too much from children upon their return from school. Children have put in a day of school work and recreation under supervision, both of which are planned to promote growth and development. Nevertheless the child should gradually assume some home responsibilities, planned so that he has time for play with his siblings and friends and also to be by himself. This last is a need often overlooked even by thoughtful parents.

During the orientation period as well as during all his school life the child's parents should be willing to listen to his tales about his school experiences. This strengthens his ability to use language and also helps him to become more of a person in his own right. Parents' unflagging interest in school and the child's activities does more than anything else to invest education with its real importance.

If the child refuses to attend school, is chronically unhappy there or is not learning at the rate he should, his parents should investigate the situation in conjunction with his teacher or other school personnel.

Role of the Teacher. Teachers play a definite role in helping children develop a sense of industry through their assignments, stimulation of group activities and their suggestion that children accept responsibilities for nonacademic duties in the classroom. In addition, teachers can also deepen their students' sense of trust, autonomy and initiative, or encourage the growth of these traits.

A teacher has a profound influence because, next to the parents, he or she is the most important person in a child's life. This is especially true during the grade-school period when the child needs an older person of his own sex to "worship." This is one reason why it would be beneficial to have more male teachers; the grade-school boy is apt to lack this model. The teacher should be the kind of person whom the child can profitably imitate. Unfortunately some parents want the teacher to take too much responsibility for their children; they want relief from their own duty of rearing them. They want the teacher to solve all the child's problems while he is in school. These parents should be helped to understand the proper function of the school and to recognize their own responsibilities as parents.

Parents may seek guidance from teachers or school counselors individually or collectively. Parent-teacher groups are especially valuable for interpreting the function of the school in the child's life, growth and development at various age levels, and problems such as discipline, sibling rivalry, sex education and special health problems of children. The leader of such a group may not always give advice; she should let the group solve the mutual problems facing its members.

PLAY AND WORK

Play is a child's tool for learning, and his play changes with his developmental needs. The child during the school years adds realistic features to his play, yet he becomes at the same time more imaginative. His fantasy and his concept of reality do not now become mixed as they did during the preschool years. He has his daydreams, but his dreams and fantasies are his secret and are not shared with his parents. Adequate play materials should be provided.

In general, time spent in play and the number of play activities decrease as the child matures. Nevertheless the time spent upon specific activities increases because the attention span becomes longer and the child has a deeper interest in what he is doing. Play during the school years becomes more formal than it was during early childhood, more organized, more competitive and to some degree less physically active. The child begins to have an interest in hobbies or collections of various kinds because in so doing he is actually collecting facts and knowledge about the world in which he lives.

As the child participates in more organized, competitive sports such as football, baseball or running matches he needs the help of adults in learning the rules. Parents should spend more time with their children. The adult should not be the leader, however. Children respond best when they plan their own play experiences. In this way they learn self-government and self-direction of activities.

Another responsibility of the parents during the school years is helping the child learn to work. He should be encouraged to assist with duties in or around the house. Allowing him to help may take more time than doing the work without him, but ultimately the adult's time is saved and the child has developed his sense of industry. If he is not allowed to help when he is young, he may not be interested in helping later in life. The work he is asked to do should definitely contribute to the welfare of the group.

As soon as the child shows interest in earning his spending money — this will be during his later school years — he should be helped to decide the kind of work he would like to do, whether delivering papers, mowing lawns or baby-sitting. The attitudes toward work which he develops in these early years will be important in shaping the kind of workman he is during adult life.

Six to Eight Years

From six to eight years of age the child is interested chiefly in the immediate environment and the immediate present. He needs, in play, an opportunity to express his feelings and find acceptance. Play must be suited to his interests and concentration span. Since he knows more about family life than any other kind of living, he enjoys playing house. A child also takes the role of a member of various occupational groups which he comes in contact with: storekeeper, milkman or trainman. What a child pretends to be gives the adult insight into his personality.

Six Years. The child six years of age plays with spreading scope and movement. Sex differences in play are defining themselves more clearly. Both sexes, however, enjoy many activities in common. For instance, both girls and boys like to paint and color and to cut out and paste. Boys enjoy drawing airplanes, trains and boats; girls are more likely to draw people and houses. Boys enjoy digging more than girls do, though it is a favorite activity of both sexes. Boys are more likely to have bicycles than girls are, but all children of this age want to learn to ride. If they have none of their own, they borrow the bicycles of their older siblings and friends. Both sexes enjoy running games, tag, hide-and-seek, roller skating and swimming. Girls enjoy jumping rope.

Both boys and girls like to pretend, but there is a sex difference. Boys pretend that they are conductors, motormen or soldiers or imitate some other masculine role in which there is plenty of activity. Girls dress up in costumes and play at being mothers or teachers, with younger children or dolls as their children. This is the age when doll play is at its height, and every toy pertaining to the mother role adds to the child's pleasure. Irrespective of sex, these children start collections of miscellaneous items such as bits of fancy paper, pictures or anything that takes their fancy.

Children six to eight years old like to "read stories from memory," look at comic books, play simple table games and listen to radio and television programs.

Boys and girls may play school and house together, but boys do not do so when playing only with boys. Boys particularly enjoy games characterized by getting under cover and shooting the enemy. They are interested in construction and transportation games.

Suitable toys for girls include dolls, doll clothes, wash baskets, doll strollers or baby carriages, swings, stoves, suit cases and make-up equipment. Boys like electric trains, airplanes, boats, trucks and automobiles.

Seven Years. Play at seven is approached more cautiously than at six years, and there are fewer new ventures. The child is more obsessive in his play interests. He enjoys funny books and coloring in books with pictures suited to his age. He likes table games, jigsaw puzzles, magic and tricks. He reads simple books fairly well, and enjoys reading. He is content to play by himself when no companions are about and is better able than the six-year-old to plan what he wants to do next. He listens to the radio and watches television programs in which there is plenty of shooting and wild horseback riding. Boys like to invent and then construct playthings and gifts for mother, using cereal boxes, fruit crates and even packing boxes. Girls enjoy designing dresses for paper dolls.

These children enjoy collecting in quantity, not for quality; they collect stones, bottle caps and almost anything they find which is out of the ordinary.

They demand more realism in their play. They need guns and caps to play cowboys and Indians or "cops" and robbers. All seven-year-old "mothers" want dolls the size of a real baby, which can "suck" from a bottle and wet the diaper. These "mothers," who want a realistic family of "children" whose ages range from newborn to four, also love "older" dolls with hair which can be brushed and combed. They like large "sister" dolls, but find them too big for mothering.

Both sexes enjoy active games. Girls like hopscotch, jumping rope and the quiet game of jackstones. Boys play ball, climb trees, race and play marbles. Both sexes ride bicycles well, and learn to swim under supervision. If they have the opportunity, many learn to ski. Girls enjoy almost all forms of play which boys engage in, but are not likely to be as proficient as the boys in active sports.

Eight Years. Eight years is an active age, in which there is a wide variety of interests. Unsupervised play among eight-year-olds becomes noisy and may end in a quarrel. They do not enjoy playing alone. With an adult they demand his complete attention; with other children they demand full participation. Their drawings are full of action.

Girls like to mix dough for cookies, make jello in fancy molds, frost cakes and experiment with simple cooking. Boys enjoy simple chemistry sets and equipment for making telegraph sets and performing magic tricks. They are fond of dramatics, and of fighting and rushing to fires. Girls also enjoy dramatics, though of a less masculine type, and always want an audience.

Boys and girls of this age make collections, but are now conscious of quality, and they classify and organize the items. Boys collect stones and rocks, marbles, cards of baseball stars or cars. Girls collect paper dolls, valentines and Christmas cards or similar items.

Eight-year-olds begin to form loosely organized, short-lived clubs. They have secret passwords which must be given before permission is granted to enter the club house, hut or hangout.

These children enjoy active games. In spite of their fondness for exuberant activity, they respond well to supervision.

They enjoy various sports in season. They are interested in table games such as checkers and dominoes. They may invent their own rules for an old game, often to such an extent that it is virtually a new game. Rules may be short-lived, but must be adhered to by all participants while they are in effect. Children of this age do not accept losing a game easily, they argue about decisions, and they often walk out of the group if they are beaten.

Most eight-year-olds can read well enough to enjoy childhood classics such as books on travel and geography. Comic books are still prime favorites. These children are at the peak of wanting prizes and objects given with coupons from breakfast cereals plus a small sum of money. They are thrilled to receive mail as adults do. Radio and television are extremely important in their lives. They like stories of adventure and mystery. Science fiction is becoming a favorite.

Nine to Twelve Years

The interest of children in this age group expands to distant places, backward into history and forward into the jet age. They like tales

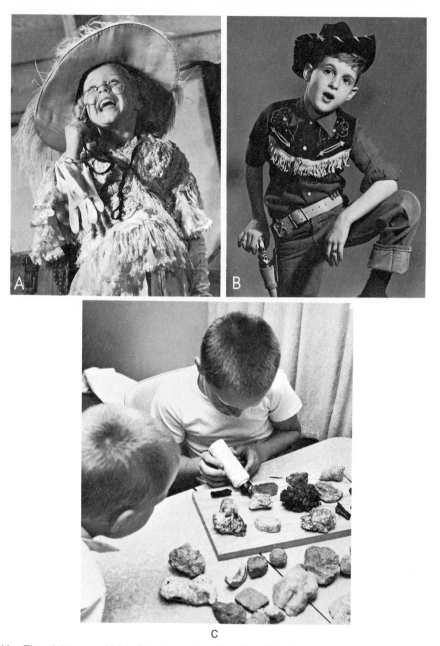

Figure 21–11. The eight-year-old (A, B) enjoys dramatic play, (C) enjoys making collections. (H. Armstrong Roberts.)

which do not point a moral, but give examples of courage, kindness, endurance and adventure. They feel responsible for performing some service as part of their day's activities. They are developing a sense of satisfaction from contributing to group activity, and the beginning of group loyalty which characterizes the gang age of older siblings. They are now able to receive help in understanding the advantage of mature behavior, although they can seldom live up to their ideal of a self-image. They are interested in their future as they say, "What I'm going to be . . ." Parents should be observant of natural inclinations, although vocational decisions may not be made until the child reaches adolescence.

Nine Years. The nine-year-old plays and works hard, often to the point of fatigue. He is busy with his chosen activities; he enjoys reading, listening to the radio and viewing television for prolonged periods. Boys play football or baseball, and girls play with dolls for hours on end.

Both boys and girls enjoy active sports. They

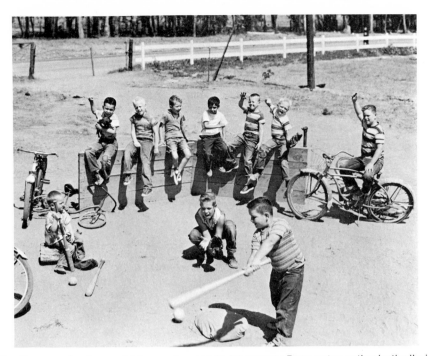

Figure 21-12. Young school-age children enjoy sports in season. Boys enter enthusiastically into sand-lot games of baseball. The youngest boy in this group has been assigned the job of holding the bats. (H. Armstrong Roberts.)

are old enough to want to improve their skills, and there is a purpose in their play which they seldom had when younger. Boys often disturb the peace of the home by roughhousing.

Nine-year-olds are great readers, reading their favorite books over and over again. They often read the junior classics, but comic books and books on adventure, war and slapstick domestic humor still fascinate them.

Many children are interested in music and take music lessons in school or from a private teacher. They often apply themselves well to music study and acquire skill through hours of practice. Talents appear at this age, especially in the creative arts. Children have an opportunity to hear good music on the radio, television and record players at home or school. They still have favorite programs on the television, but are not as rigid about viewing only these as when they were younger. They all want to go to the motion pictures.

Ten Years. Sex differences in play are pronounced among ten-year-olds. Boys and girls are developing the skills which each sex needs in society. At school the boy works with speed and likes the challenge of mental arithmetic.

The ten-year-old is so conscious of needing the support of his peers that he often esteems the opinions and attitudes of his gang or club more than those of his family. He is interested in social welfare and social justice. He is loyal to his group and does not divulge group secrets. He may indulge in hero worship.

On the radio and television the likes of the ten-year-old are much the same as those of the nine-year-old. Boys spurn romance and love stories. The two sexes are well separated.

Girls enjoy dramatizing life situations, and the subjects they choose are likely to deal with engagements and weddings. They still play with dolls, however, taking the role of mother and "bringing up their children." They are becoming much more interested in their appearance.

Eleven Years. The eleven-year-old is full of energy and activity. He experiments with various projects and is intensely interested in the activities of his group. His interest in school may diminish, particularly if he is not a good student. Play is no longer paramount in his life; companionship has become more important than play.

Although these children may seem bungling in motor skill at home, they have acquired new types of agility in play. Everything interests them. This is the gang age, and the gang enjoys meeting in its own hut or tree house. The child's interest in reading and motion pictures has increased; the characters he learns about appear to be alive, people he would like to know or perhaps punish in some way.

Twelve Years. The twelve-year-old is enthusiastic, so much so that he acts without con-

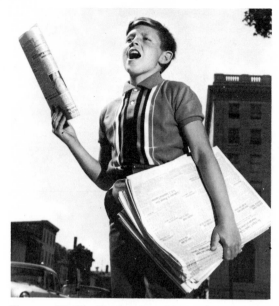

Figure 21–13. Twelve-year-olds enjoy earning money. (H. Armstrong Roberts.)

sideration of consequences. Although he is very much a part of his group, he also likes to be alone. He engages in sports with more team spirit and less wandering of attention to something else in the environment which is of personal interest to him. He has not the same need for praise that he had a year before. His broader interests are seen in his wanting a pen-pal from a foreign land.

Twelve-year-olds are becoming interested in earning money not for running errands or little jobs for their parents, but in some form of organized project, especially a twosome project, in which they are heavily motivated to succeed. They may be interested in publishing a news bulletin, and many boys have paper routes. Boys and girls still tend to stay apart.

CARE

Physical Care

Bathing, Dressing and Toileting. Children between six and twelve years of age are fairly self-sufficient in bathing, dressing and toileting, but they need some help with the niceties of manicuring, neatness and even cleanliness. There are, of course, individual differences; some children resent having their ears kept clean, and others do not like to have their hair combed and brushed. Sex differences are apparent: girls are generally more careful of their appearance than boys are.

The six-year-old needs help, though he does not readily accept it. He dawdles and needs management. In undressing he drops his clothes on the floor or flings them aside. The seven-year-old still dawdles, but tends to complete his tasks. The eight-year-old is more efficient in caring for himself. From nine years to the end of the school age children show increased responsibility in selection of clothes, adapted to the occasion and the weather, hanging them up and disposing of soiled garments. They can take care of toileting and bathing, but may still need reminders to brush their teeth or wash their hands thoroughly, and girls need help with long hair.

Sleep

The sleep of the school child is rarely quiescent. Fears in the form of night terrors or nightmares prevent his sleeping peacefully because for one reason he has reached the point in his mental development at which he has a concept of death (see p. 76). The bedtime hour should be a quiet time when the parents and the child feel greater interdependency. It is a good time for confidences, questions and answers, and discussions. Routine prayers may be said.

The older child may become self-assertive about the time when he wishes to go to bed. Parents must judge the amount of sleep the child needs and see that he is in bed in time for sufficient sleep. The amount needed decreases with age. The six-year-old may need eleven to twelve hours of sleep, while the twelve-year-old generally needs only ten hours.

Safety Measures

With the broadening scope of activity among children during the elementary school years, parents cannot hope to be with them constantly in order to prevent accidents. If parents and nursery school and kindergarten teachers have emphasized safety measures, a child should be ready to build on the foundation of past experience and develop further his ability to meet the accident hazards common to school children.

Between the ages of six and twelve years the most common cause of accidental injury and death is *motor accidents*. Children may cross a street against the light or from between parked cars, or be injured while riding in cars or on bicycles.

The second most frequent cause of accidental death is *drowning*. Children should be taught to swim as early as possible. They should also be taught water-survival techniques.

Accidents resulting in injuries to the eyes are not too uncommon during the school years. Children should be taught to wear protective devices when doing any activity which is potentially dangerous.

Accidents also occur when children are skating, riding the school bus, or playing with other children or with animals.

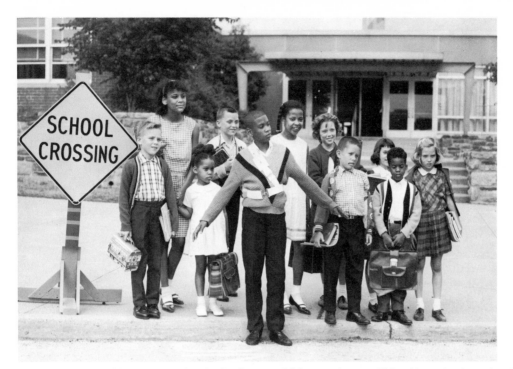

Figure 21–14. Motor accidents cause the death of many children each year. This older school-age boy is a member of the safety patrol. He takes his responsibility of protecting other children very seriously. (H. Armstrong Roberts.)

HEALTH

Responsibility for the child's health rests with the parents. Health of the school child is influenced by the health supervision he receives from the family physician and the dentist, by the health instruction given by his parents and teachers, by the environment of his home and school, by the community public health program and by the direct services he receives in school.

Preschool Health Examination

Every child should have a preschool health examination. His height, weight, posture, hearing and vision should be checked carefully. Beginning problems of school children may be due to faulty hearing and vision. If glasses are necessary to correct a defect in vision, they should be made of safety glass to reduce the possibility of injury to the eyes. A dental examination and correction of defects are essential. If the child is to gain the optimum benefit from school, he needs to be physically well.

The physician will continue the immunization program against communicable diseases discussed in Chapter 12 (see p. 277).

The preschool examination should be done in the spring, before the child enters school, so that treatment for any defects or problems can be given before school opens.

Parents should see that the child receives a thorough physical examination every year. If he is not well, he should be taken to a physician. Dental examinations should be made twice a year or as often as the dentist recommends.

School Health Program

The school health program is an important part of the national health program. The main purpose of the school program is to maintain, improve and promote the health of every school child. Adequate supervision of the physical, mental, emotional and social aspects of school life should be included in the program. The program also includes planning the course content in health education and nutrition, and putting it into effect through instruction and the routine life of the children during school hours. Accident prevention, recreation and physical education should be included.

The school nurse and other personnel in the program should see to it that routine health appraisals are done on all children, with follow-up on those who need care to see that they receive it. Parent education and parent counseling are also necessary. Teamwork by parents, teach-

A

STANDARD HEALTH EXAMINATION RECORD

AMERICAN ACADEMY OF PEDIATRICS, INC. ©1959

(THIS PART TO BE FILLED IN BY PARENT BEFORE PRESENTATION TO PHYSICIAN)

ORGANIZATION OR SCHOOL

NAME_____   PARENT OR GUARDIAN _____ PHONE_____
        LAST   FIRST

ADDRESS_____ BIRTH DATE_____ AGE_____ SEX_____

_____ RELIGION_____

PAST ILLNESSES: (CHECK — GIVING APPROX. DATES)

		DISEASES DATE	SUGGESTIONS FROM PARENTS:
FREQUENT COLDS	STOMACH UPSETS	CHICKEN POX	
FREQUENT SORE THROATS	KIDNEY TROUBLE	MEASLES	
SINUSITIS	HEART TROUBLE	MUMPS	
ABSCESSED EARS	RHEUM. FEVER	SCARLET FEVER	
BRONCHITIS	CONVULSIONS	POLIOMYELITIS	
ASTHMA	TUBERCULOSIS	WHOOPING COUGH	
ALLERGIES	DIABETES		

OPERATIONS OR SERIOUS INJURIES

SERIOUS IVY POISONING

OTHER DISEASES OR DETAILS OF ABOVE

COMMENTS FOR CAMP:

BEHAVIOR_____ SLEEP WALKING_____ BED WETTING_____ NIGHT TERRORS_____

FAINTING_____ MENSTRUATION_____ CONSTIPATION_____ OTHER_____

ANY CONTRA-INDICATION TO SWIMMING?_____ TO DIVING?_____

ANY SPECIFIC ACTIVITIES TO BE ENCOURAGED?_____ ANY RESTRICTED?_____

IS STUDENT UNDER ANY SPECIAL MEDICAL OR DIETARY REGIMEN TO BE CONTINUED?_____

B

IMMUNIZATIONS			PHYSICAL EXAMINATION (BY LICENSED M. D.)
IMMUNIZATIONS	DATE PRIMARY SERIES COMPLETED	DATE OF LAST BOOSTER	DATE OF EXAMINATION
WHOOPING COUGH			HEIGHT_____ WEIGHT_____
DIPHTHERIA			MUSCULOSKELETAL
TETANUS			
POLIOMYELITIS			SKIN
SMALLPOX			SCABIES
OTHER			ATHLETES FOOT
			IMPETIGO
			OTHER
TUBERCULIN TEST	DATE_____	RESULT	

PHYSICIANS COMMENTS AND RECOMMENDATIONS

THIS PERSON IS IN SATISFACTORY CONDITION AND MAY ENGAGE IN ALL USUAL ACTIVITIES EXCEPT AS NOTED.

EYES_____ VISION: R 20/_____ L 20/_____

EARS_____ HEARING_____

NOSE_____

THROAT_____

TEETH_____

HEART_____

LUNGS_____

ABDOMEN_____

GENITALIA_____

_____ M.D.   HERNIA_____

ADDRESS_____

URINALYSIS_____

Figure 21–15. Standard Health Examination Record approved by the American Academy of Pediatrics for use with children of school age. (Courtesy of American Academy of Pediatrics.)

ers, nurses and private and school physicians is essential. Local physicians should understand the school health program and wherein it supplements their service to children. Other personnel who may cooperate include the child's dentist, the school dentist, the principal of the school, the school counselor, the school custodian and engineer, school psychologist, social worker, physical education teacher and special education staff.

Preventive services should be used to control tooth decay, accidents, emotional disorders, poor nutrition, infectious diseases, unhygienic environment and insufficient care after an illness.

Health Problems During School Age

Among the most important health problems of the school child is greater exposure to communicable diseases. Diseases against which he is immunized or which he had in the preschool period present no problem. The mother should be informed of the school regulations about keeping him home from school when he has a fever, cold, rash or other symptoms of communicable disease, to prevent exposing others.

A second health problem which the school has is to meet the needs of the handicapped child on entrance to school. His condition poses a special problem for the school personnel. They should be kept informed of the total rehabilitation program being carried out and their specific part in it.

A third problem is presented by the older children, who should be told something about the physical changes they will experience at puberty. Both sexes should be informed of this. Although parents should talk over these matters with their children in order to maintain good parent-child relations, the school nurse or a teacher may also discuss them individually or in class. Stressing the universality of the experience makes it less personal and more objective. Parents should know what the children are taught in school. Pictorial presentation should be supplemented with discussion. The material should be selected according to the interest, chronologic age and level of understanding of the children. It should be factual and presented unemotionally. The child who is unprepared for the physical changes which accompany puberty may be terrified when they occur.

In our speeded-up society which is overstimulating children of eleven or twelve years to go "steady," many parents are confused about how much restriction to place on their preteen's behavior. Children of this age are not ready emotionally for serious boy-girl involvement and are likely to welcome a firm parental "no" to this sort of behavior.

A fourth problem which has emerged is that of smoking and drug abuse. Since the incidence of smoking and drug abuse is increasing even among children who have not yet reached puberty, many physicians and educators believe that programs on these subjects should begin in elementary school.

NUTRITION

During the school age caloric requirements per unit of body weight continue to decrease, but the nutritional requirements remain relatively greater than in a mature person.

Table 21-1 gives the nutritional requirements for children of school age.

School children usually eat well and have fewer food fads than preschool children. Eating

Table 21-1. *Recommended Daily Dietary Allowances for Children of School Age (6 to 12 Years)*

	6-8 YEARS	8-10 YEARS	10-12 YEARS	
			BOYS	GIRLS
	WT.-23 KG. (51 POUNDS) HT.-121 CM. (48 INCHES)	WT.-28 KG. (62 POUNDS) HT.-131 CM. (52 INCHES)	WT.-35 KG. (77 POUNDS) HT.-140 CM. (55 INCHES)	WT.-35 KG. (77 POUNDS) HT.-142 CM. (56 INCHES)
K calories	2,000	2,200	2,500	2,250
Protein	35 gm.	40 gm.	45 gm.	50 gm.
Fat-soluble Vitamins				
Vitamin A activity	3,500 I.U.	3,500 I.U.	4,500 I.U.	4,500 I.U.
Vitamin D	400 I.U.	400 I.U.	400 I.U.	400 I.U.
Vitamin E activity	15 I.U.	15 I.U.	20 I.U.	20 I.U.
Water-soluble Vitamins				
Ascorbic acid	40 mg.	40 mg.	40 mg.	40 mg.
Folacin[a]	0.2 mg.	0.3 mg.	0.4 mg.	0.4 mg.
Niacin equivalents[b]	13 mg.	15 mg.	17 mg.	15 mg.
Riboflavin	1.1 mg.	1.2 mg.	1.3 mg.	1.3 mg.
Thiamin	1.0 mg.	1.1 mg.	1.3 mg.	1.1 mg.
Vitamin B_6	1.0 mg.	1.2 mg.	1.4 mg.	1.4 mg.
Vitamin B_{12}	4 μg	5 μg	5 μg	5 μg
Minerals				
Calcium	0.9 gm.	1.0 gm.	1.2 gm.	1.2 gm.
Phosphorus	0.9 gm.	1.0 gm.	1.2 gm.	1.2 gm.
Iodine	100 μg	110 μg	125 μg	110 μg
Iron	10 mg.	10 mg.	10 mg.	18 mg.
Magnesium	250 mg.	250 mg.	300 mg.	300 mg.

[a] The folacin allowances refer to dietary sources as determined by *Lactobacillus casei* assay. Pure forms of folacin may be effective in doses less than ¼ of the RDA.

[b] Niacin equivalents include dietary sources of the vitamin itself plus 1 mg. equivalent for each 60 mg. of dietary tryptophan.

From the Food and Nutrition Board, National Academy of Sciences–National Research Council: Recommended Daily Dietary Allowances (1968).

problems relate more to the time of eating, e.g. whether it interferes with television programs or group activities, and the manner of eating than to the content and amount of food consumed. Since a child may be hungry after school, nourishment is necessary. Milk and fruit are preferable to candy and cookies.

Because the child wants to be like his peers, the kind of lunch he wants will depend on whether his friends take a lunch box to school or eat in the cafeteria. If the noon meal is not adequate, breakfast and dinner should make up for the deficiency.

School children can be helpful to their mothers at mealtime. They can help plan menus, set the table, shop for food and wash dishes. Although these activities develop a sense of industry and responsibility, parents should not ask too much of young children, who spend many hours in school and require outdoor play to keep them well.

Eating Habits. Mealtime should be a pleasant, restful period in the day, but many parents do not keep it so because of overemphasis on manners. The child's eating habits will improve as he grows older.

The six-year-old stuffs his mouth, spills food and grabs for it and may be very talkative while eating. He is more interested in eating at the beginning than at the end of the meal. His appetite is good. He may refuse to use a napkin.

The seven-year-old talks less during the meal. He may bolt his food, but he is quieting down. His napkin may not remain in place.

Eight- and nine-year-olds eat more neatly, using napkins as their elders do. They are apt to have better table manners in public than at home.

Ten- to twelve-year-olds eat an adult meal and have table manners similar to those of their parents, whether at home or elsewhere.

Children's eating habits would improve more rapidly if less stress were laid on table manners. A friendly atmosphere and enjoyment of the meal are the best aids to appetite.

EFFECTS OF SEPARATION

If the child has experienced good parent-child relations, he will probably suffer little trauma due to separation from his parents for short periods. The school child has learned to relate to adults and children outside his family and so is not emotionally disturbed when he is left with strange people. He knows the meaning of time gradations and is better able to tolerate separation from his parents. He knows when they will return. Prolonged separation, however, for weeks or months, as during hospitalization, is likely to produce emotional trauma. If his parents do not visit him frequently, particularly if he knows that they are able to come, he feels a sense of rejection which interacts with the physical strain of his illness or injury. The reasons for prolonged separation should be explained to the child in a factual, realistic way by a sympathetic adult, preferably one of his parents. Other evidences of parental love besides visiting should be shown him.

TEACHING AIDS AND OTHER INFORMATION*

American Academy of Pediatrics

Report of the Committee on School Health.

American Medical Association

Suggested School Health Policies.
Your Friend, the Doctor.

American Nurses' Association

Functions and Qualifications for School Nurses, 1966.

Child Study Association of America

Clark, K. B.: How to Protect Children Against Prejudice.
Frank, J.: Television: How to Use It Wisely with Children, 1965.
Redl, F.: Pre-Adolescents: What Makes Them Tick?
The Wonderful Story of How You Were Born.
What to Tell Your Children About Sex.

Mental Health Division, Department of National Health and Welfare, Ottawa, Canada

Promoting Mental Health in the School.

---

* Complete addresses are given in the Appendix.

National Society for the Prevention of Blindness, Inc.

Vision Screening in Schools.

Public Affairs Pamphlets

Carson, R.: Your Child May Be a Gifted Child.
Gruenberg, S. M.: Your Child and Money.
Hunt, J. McV.: What You Should Know About Educational Testing.
Lambert, C.: Understand Your Child—From 6 to 12.
Neisser, E. G.: Your Child's Sense of Responsibility.
Osborne, E.: Democracy Begins in the Home.
Osborne, E.: How to Teach Your Child About Work.
Sunley, R.: How to Help Your Child in School.

United States Department of Health, Education, and Welfare

Health of Children of School Age, 1964.
Moving Into Adolescence: Your Child in His Preteens, 1966.
School Health Program, An Outline for School and Community, 1966.
The Protection and Promotion of Mental Health in Schools, 1965.
Your Child from 6 to 12, 1966.
Youth Physical Fitness, 1967.

REFERENCES

Publications

American Academy of Pediatrics: *Report of the Committee on School Health of the American Academy of Pediatrics.* Evanston, Ill., American Academy of Pediatrics, 1966.
Brauer, J. C., and others: *Dentistry for Children.* 5th ed. New York, McGraw-Hill Book Company, Inc., 1964.
Breckenridge, M. E., and Vincent, E. L.: *Child Development. Physical and Psychologic Growth Through Adolescence.* 5th ed. Philadelphia, W. B. Saunders Company, 1965.
Cromwell, G. E.: *The Nurse in the School Health Program.* Philadelphia, W. B. Saunders Company, 1963.
Davis, C.: *Room to Grow: A Study of Parent-Child Relationships.* Ontario, Canada, University of Toronto Press, 1966.
Erikson, E. H.: *Childhood and Society.* New York, W. W. Norton and Company, 1964.
Filas, F. L.: *Sex Education in the Family.* Englewood Cliffs, N.J., Prentice-Hall, Inc., 1966.
Gesell, A., and Ilg, F. L.: *The Child from Five to Ten.* New York, Harper and Brothers, 1946.
Grout, R. E.: *Health Teaching in Schools.* 5th ed. Philadelphia, W. B. Saunders Company, 1968.
Krause, M. V.: *Food, Nutrition and Diet Therapy.* 4th ed. Philadelphia, W. B. Saunders Company, 1966.
Lerrigo, M. O., and Cassidy, M. A.: *A Doctor Talks to 9- to 12-Year-Olds.* Chicago, Budlong Press, 1964.
Mielach, D. Z., and Mandel, E.: *A Doctor Talks to 5- to 8-Year-Olds.* Chicago, Budlong Press, 1966.
Nemir, A.: *The School Health Program.* 2nd ed. Philadelphia, W. B. Saunders Company, 1965.
Oberteuffer, D., and Beyrer, M. K.: *School Health Education: A Textbook for Teachers, Nurses, and Other Professional Personnel.* 4th ed. New York, Harper and Row, 1966.
Ojemann, R. H. (Ed.): *The School and the Community Treatment Facility in Preventive Psychiatry.* Iowa City, State University of Iowa, 1966.
Piaget, J.: *The Child's Conception of Number.* New York, W. W. Norton Company, 1965.
Recommended Dietary Allowances. Revised 1968. Washington, D.C., National Academy of Sciences–National Research Council.
Strang, R.: *Helping Your Child Develop His Potentialities.* New York, E. P. Dutton and Company, 1965.
Verville, E.: *Behavior Problems of Children.* Philadelphia, W. B. Saunders Company, 1967.
Wallach, M. A., and Kogan, N.: *Modes of Thinking in Young Children.* New York, Holt, Rinehart and Winston, 1965.
Watson, E. H., and Lowrey, G. H.: *Growth and Development of Children.* 5th ed. Chicago, Yearbook Medical Publishers, Inc., 1967.
Watson, R. I.: *Psychology of the Child.* 2nd ed. New York, John Wiley and Sons, Inc., 1965.
Wheatley, G. M., and Hallock, G.: *Health Observation of School Children.* New York, Blakiston Division, McGraw-Hill Book Company, Inc., 1965.
Wilson, C. C. (Ed.): *School Health Services.* 2nd ed. Washington, D.C., National Education Association, and Chicago, American Medical Association, 1964.

Periodicals

Abolishing Childhood. *Today's Health,* 45:57, September 1967.

Abraham, W.: How Important Are Your Child's Friends? *Today's Health,* 42:6, March 1964.

Berlin, I. N.: Working with Children Who Won't Go to School. *Children,* 12:109, 1965.

Brion, H. H., Johnson, M., and Bardin, R.: A Day in the Life of a School Nurse-Teacher. *Nursing Outlook,* 15:58, August 1967.

Brooks, B. R.: Aggression. *Am. J. Nursing,* 67:2519, 1967.

Bruce, S. J.: What Mothers of 6- to 10-Year-Olds Want to Know. *Nursing Outlook,* 12:40, September 1964.

Bugg, R.: Danger Rides the School Bus. *Today's Health,* 45:21, November 1967.

Coakley, J. M., and Parker, J. M.: Education of Nurses for School Nursing. *Am. J. Nursing,* 65:84, November 1965.

Cromwell, G. E.: The Child in the School. *Nursing Outlook,* 13:27, February 1965.

Fredlund, D. J.: The Route to Effective School Nursing. *Nursing Outlook,* 15:24, August 1967.

Gorlick, H. S.: Are School Nurses First-Aiders or Health-Leaders? *RN,* 30:52 October 1967.

Illingworth, R. S.: How to Help a Child to Achieve His Best. *J. Pediat.,* 73:61, July 1968.

King, J. S.: A School Nurse in Bolivia. *Nursing Outlook,* 16:37, November 1968.

Kornblueh, M.: The Cafeteria Food Game. *Nursing Outlook,* 15:47, February 1967.

McGuigan, R. A., and others: Children Under Pressure: Four Doctors' Views. *Today's Health,* 45:62, September 1967.

Medaris, E. B.: Incorporating Health Concepts in School Nursing. *Nursing Outlook,* 15:60, August 1967.

Millner, B. N.: Health Needs of School-Age Children – What Are They? *J. School Health,* 36:277, June 1966.

Rich, L. E.: Volunteers Plan a School Health Exhibit. *Nursing Outlook,* 13:35, February 1965.

Saunders, F. M.: An Ever Present Help. *Nursing Outlook,* 15:41, August 1967.

Schroeder, C. E.: Mental Health Facilities in the School. *Nursing Outlook,* 13:30, February 1965.

Sparrow, A. G., McNeil, H. J., and Grace, K. M.: Prevention Begins at Home. *Nursing Outlook,* 15:52, March 1967.

Stitt, P. G., and Shultz, C. S.: Fivefold Focus on Child Health. *Nursing Outlook,* 15:29, August 1967.

Wayne, D.: The Lonely School Child. *Am. J. Nursing,* 68:774, 1968.

What Does a School Nurse *Do* All Day? *RN,* 29:87, December 1966.

22

CONDITIONS OF THE SCHOOL CHILD REQUIRING IMMEDIATE OR SHORT-TERM CARE

HOSPITALIZATION OF THE SCHOOL CHILD

The school child is usually able to accept his illness and separation from his parents better than does the preschool child. His reaction to hospitalization is related to his previous personality structure and to the nature of the parent-child relation.

Preparation for Hospitalization. Children of school age should have much the same kind of preparation for hospitalization as that given the preschool child (see p. 481). Because of his greater verbal ability the school child usually understands more readily the explanation given him. School children can read booklets about the hospitalization experience. The parents will adapt this material to the needs of the child. He should be told the truth about the experience before him. He should be assured that his parents will visit him as often as possible, and send cards and telephone him so that he knows that they are thinking of him.

Response of the Child to Hospitalization. When a school-age child is admitted to the hospital he is probably outnumbered on the pediatric unit by younger children, and his needs may be overshadowed by those of the infants, toddlers or preschool children. The nurse should therefore understand his needs and respond to them in order to make his hospital experience a positive one, since most school children in spite of the preparation given for this new experience may believe that they caused their own illness, or were to blame for it in some way such as by being "bad."

Children between six and eight years of age conform or rebel alternately against adult authority. If the child rebels, he will have guilt feelings and expect to be punished. When the rebellious act results in hospitalization, the therapy he is given may be viewed as punishment. The young school-age child also experiences renewed separation anxiety when he is away from his mother. He may evidence indications of this anxiety by enuresis, night terrors, insomnia or nail-biting during his hospitalization.

Since the child from eight to ten years of age has a better developed ego, he can respond more appropriately to the limitations and requests of adults responsible for his care. The child has little real knowledge about how his body functions until he is about nine years of age, and even then he may have gross misconceptions mixed with truth. He may believe that he can get diabetes from eating too many desserts, a respiratory infection from not wearing his coat, a nose-bleed from exercising too much, or osteomyelitis simply because he fell. He still has little understanding of the specific cause of illness and may feel that he has been singled out from his peer group for punishment.

The child from ten to twelve years of age has already experienced stress in school and is less likely to be disturbed by the problems of hospitalization. He may, however, be disturbed because of the lack of privacy, especially if he is self-conscious about the bodily changes accompanying puberty. He may also be anxious about his absence from school and his loss of friends, and have fear that permanent harm to his body may occur as a result of his illness or injury.

The hospitalized school-age child may be very angry or anxious, and have various fears and fantasies. Children in general dislike staying in bed because motility is important to them. The child's control of the outside world, his inner impulses and his very self-preservation are achieved to a great degree through his own activity. *Immobilization, then, is probably the most difficult aspect of a child's illness.* When he is restricted in his activity he becomes anxious, and his anxiety leads to a need for greater activity. When he is confined to bed he has little outlet for his deep feelings, and he may become subject to fears and fantasies. He may over-exercise when adults are not around or he may be frozen with his fears. If the child must be completely immobilized, he may become depressed and submit with hopeless resignation to his treatment. The child needs help in understanding his illness and must accept some responsibility for his own therapy.

In summary, the school child may feel guilty, anxious and angry during his hospitalization. Emotions such as these are harmful and may retard his recovery from illness.

The Nurse and the School Child. The school child needs nurses who understand his level of growth and development, his needs and the experiences he should have for continued personality growth while in the hospital. The nurse should be warm, friendly and fair, yet able to set reasonable limits to his behavior. She should try to understand each child as an individual who is having unavoidable frustrations due to his illness or injury. She should try to provide satisfactions which make his situation more endurable.

Problems which the nurse must help the child solve are those of his feelings of guilt, fear of physical harm and anxiety due to immobilization. The child who is very affected by his condition will talk less about it than one not so deeply concerned. The nurse must use every bit of ingenuity she can to break down the emotional barrier between herself and the child.

Since children do not usually discuss such feelings openly with adults, the nurse must help the child understand that illness occurs whether he is "good" or "bad." The nurse should encourage the child to talk of his ideas about the cause of his illness and give him factual information as to the real cause of his condition. The nurse should use various tools to help explain to him the physiologic problem and the necessity for his inactivity. She may use models or pictures of the heart or other organs of the body, plastic models of the visible man and visible woman, and line drawings of the body indicating what is to be done during certain procedures. The nurse must further help the child to overcome his fear by describing what is to be done, by telling him that the treatment will help him to feel better eventually, although it may hurt for a while, by permitting him to handle the equipment used, and by encouraging him to help her with the procedure. Since the child as he grows through school age is curious and eager to learn, the nurse should remember the level of his understanding at various ages and tailor her teaching to his ability to comprehend. The nurse must provide a warm emotional atmosphere so that he feels free to discuss his problems, fears and fantasies of illness or injury with her. Although the six- to twelve-year-old child has better ability to cope with stress than a younger child, he still needs the opportunity to discuss his fears and fantasies of illness or injury with a meaningful adult, his parents or a nurse whom he trusts.

The feeling of anger previously discussed may be shown by the child either verbally or through actions. The child may actually tell the nurse that he hates her even though he knows that she has given him good care, or he may refuse to do what she requests. The understanding nurse accepts the child's emotion, but sets a limit on his further active expression of it. She might say, "I realize that you are very angry, Joey, but I cannot permit you to throw your books on the floor. Could you tell me how you feel?" If the nurse is calm, the child can verbalize his emotion without acting it out further. Sometimes simply by reflecting the emotion a child shows by saying, "You feel angry, Joey," the nurse can make the child feel understood and perhaps open the door to further communication with him.

When school children have many frustrations during the day and are forced to keep strict self-control, they often release their aggression and tension during the hours when the evening nurse is alone on the unit. She may be faced with pillow fights, arguments, toys thrown on the floor or paper wads hurled from bed to bed.

The best way to handle this situation is by prevention. The children should have the opportunity during the day to use their aggression in constructive activities. Ambulatory as well as bed patients can have self-directive physical activity under supervision of the Play Lady or volunteers.

The nurse can also permit the child to help plan his daily schedule, thereby building up his self-confidence. She should visit him frequently. If the physican permits, another child's bed can be brought close enough to his for them to play together. The child may also enjoy making his own rules for keeping himself quiet. If he continues to be agressive, his behavior should be brought to the attention of the physician, who may recommend further psychologic help or treatment.

Children have preconceived notions of what the nurse will be like. If the child perceives qualities of his parents in his nurse, he may react to her as he does to them. For this reason he may not react to his nurse in terms of how she reacts to him, but rather as he is accustomed to react to his mother. Such behavior on his part gives a clue to his past experience and to his needs for guidance.

The school child normally does not like an adult hovering over him and protecting him; but when he is injured or ill, he wants adult protection and support. A boy especially may think of nurses as a threat to his independence, yet when a painful procedure is to be done, even he will seek the nurse for strength and support.

Nurses in the hospital and in the community should learn ways to help convalescent children to be constructively happy. Hospitalized children enjoy continuing the collections they started at home (see p. 553), and starting new collections better adapted to items found in the hospital. They may collect empty antibiotic bottles, paper cups or greeting cards. They may enjoy reading, playing table games, listening to the radio and watching television. The nurse must supervise these activities so that they will not be too exciting for the children.

School children who enjoy assuming responsibility and caring for younger children may help in the hospital unit during convalescence. This will help them gain confidence and recognition and acquire skills. They may cooperate in cleaning up the playroom and the schoolroom in the afternoon. They may help to put away supplies and pass nourishment. Often they can help feed younger children, read to them or play with them. This enables the older children to identify with adults in the unit and gives them a feeling of self-confidence.

Physical Care of the Child. School children who have become fairly independent in caring for themselves become embarrassed when they are ill because they are physically cared for by the nurse. This is especially true of boys ten years of age or older. The nurse should remember that the school-age child can contribute to his own physical care in the areas of bathing, feeding and dressing unless he is too ill or handicapped to do so. If he cannot care for himself, the nurse should help the child to accept the situation and cooperate rather than feel that he is forced to submit because it is the custom in the hospital. The child associates such care with being a baby and feels threatened by his loss of power. It is a good plan to speak casually of the care adult

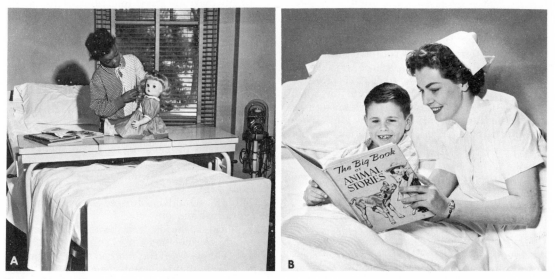

Figure 22-1. The school-age child needs nurses who understand his need for rest and the experiences he should have for continued development while in the hospital. *A*, The nurse may provide toys which the child wants to play with in bed so that she gets the rest she needs. *B*, The nurse may encourage another child to improve his reading skill while he is hospitalized. (H. Armstrong Roberts.)

patients receive, asking a little girl whether she would like to be a nurse when she grows up or telling a boy of nursing in the military service. The child should be encouraged to regain his independence as soon as he is physically able to do so. Normally he is anxious to do all that he can for himself. This, in part, is the reason why children of school age enjoy wearing regular clothing instead of hospital gowns, because this indicates that they are no longer very ill. The nurse should also recognize the fact that the older school child can and should have an opportunity to participate and cooperate with his parents in the efforts of the health and nursing teams.

School children have learned the terminology of their group, especially in connection with urination, defecation and the organs of reproduction. The nurse should understand that the child learned his attitudes and expressions at home and from his friends. To make him feel ashamed of the only terms which sound familiar to him would cause a younger child to feel that he was among strangers who did not love him. He might be afraid to tell the nurse when he again needed to go the toilet. In school he asks to be excused, but that request does not fit the hospital situation. The older child may feel that the nurse rejects him because she comes from a low socioeconomic class. His sense of worth, his self-image, is hurt, and he may withdraw from the situation.

The child from eight to eleven years may have sleep phobias associated with fears of dying, especially when he first realizes the irreversibility of death. These may occur in the hospital when he is physically ill, especially when he is frightened because of impending surgery and possible loss of control of body functions. The nurse should comfort the child and remain with him until he is quiet.

School in the Hospital. Children hospitalized for short-term care may not have the time to become actively involved in school work as do those children requiring long-term hospitalization. Nevertheless the individual child may need the support of a visiting teacher even though he is in the hospital for only a few days. For a more complete discussion of the education of the hospitalized child see Chapter 23 (p. 574).

ACUTE CONDITIONS

Epistaxis (Nasal Hemorrhage, Nosebleed)

Incidence, Etiology, Clinical Manifestations, Treatment and Nursing Care. Epistaxis is common throughout childhood, especially during the school age, but the incidence decreases after puberty. It is caused by external trauma, foreign bodies, forcible blowing of the nose or picking the nose. Rhinitis may also lead to nosebleed.

The strain of emotional excitement or physical exercise may be enough to start nasal bleeding. If there is a circulatory, renal or emotional condition which produces an elevation of blood pressure, nasal hemorrhage may result. It may also result from a blood dyscrasia or an infection. As girls reach puberty, epistaxis may occur as vicarious menstruation.

The onset is sudden. Blood may flow from both nostrils. Bleeding is usually minimal and stops spontaneously, but it may be fatal if the child has a hemorrhagic disease.

The child should be kept in a semi-erect position. His clothing should be loosened around the neck. He should not blow his nose. An ice bag over the bridge of the nose is helpful. Gentle but firm compression of the nasal alae against the septum should be made with the fingers or some type of clamp. A solution of epinephrine may be applied to the nasal mucous membrane with a cotton applicator (epinephrine is a vasoconstrictor). The physician may cauterize the point of bleeding with silver nitrate. In more severe cases packing the nares with thromboplastin or Gelfoam may be necessary. In hemorrhagic disease blood transfusion may be required if much blood is lost.

Respiratory Infections and Communicable Diseases

Incidence and Care. If the child has not had the common communicable diseases in the preschool period, he is likely to get them when he goes to school because of close contact with many children. For the same reason the child is prone to respiratory infections. This is especially true if he comes from a small family in which he is overprotected or has been brought up in a rural area where infections are less common. The greatest *incidence* of infections is in the first grade.

Health teaching should begin in the early grades. The child should be taught to cover his mouth with his handkerchief when coughing and to turn his face toward the floor. This is particularly necessary at the table, where coughing would spread droplets on food. He should not contaminate his hands and then contaminate toys, books, door knobs and other objects which others touch.

Children should be dressed according to the temperature and protected from rain and snow with slickers, hoods and boots. They should be taught to come home to change their clothing if they get wet. (If the mother scolds them for getting wet, they will not come home at once, but will wait, hoping to dry off before she sees them.) Teachers should make provisions for children caught in the rain on the way to school.

Every teacher should tell her class to report

symptoms of a cold, sore throat or other illness. The children should be taught to wash their hands when contaminated and always before eating. It is essential, but difficult, to teach them not to offer each other bits of candy, apples, laps of ice cream cones and sucks of pop from the bottle or common straw, because they think it friendly and generous to share what they have with another child.

Children should be kept away from others who have respiratory infections. The child with an infection should not be sent to school. If he comes and the teacher finds that he is sick, she or the school nurse may send him home, provided there is someone there to care for him, or should telephone for his mother to come for him. If there is no adult at home to receive him, the child may be kept in the infirmary. If the school has no infirmary, and his condition permits, he should be placed in the rear of the classroom away from other children. If someone comes for the child, she should be told how to care for him. Such instruction includes home isolation technique and how to make paper bags to receive the child's paper handkerchiefs. Immunization techniques should be recommended if necessary. If the child is so sick that he will need considerable nursing care, the mother should be helped to schedule her time so that she gets enough rest.

Ringworm (Tinea)

Ringworm is a superficial fungus infection of the skin. Ringworm is classified according to the area of the body affected or the shape of the lesion produced. Since several fungi may cause ringworm, laboratory examination is often necessary before adequate treatment can be carried out. All types of ringworm are contagious.

Ringworm of the Scalp (Tinea Capitis)

Incidence and Etiology. This condition, practically limited to children, is common among neglected children. It is a serious problem in schools of disorganized, low-income urban areas.

In the United States the most common causative agent is *Microsporum audouini*. This infection is transmitted by human beings and is highly infectious. *Microsporum canis* is transmitted to the child from an animal. These conditions tend to disappear spontaneously at puberty.

Infection may begin at the base of a single hair, but it spreads in a circular fashion, forming lesions up to 2 inches in diameter. The spores of the fungus invading the hair at the base cause the hair to break off close to the skin, leaving a bald area. The scalp of this area becomes red, and grayish scales appear. A secondary infection may occur. The child may complain of mild itching.

Diagnosis, Treatment and Prognosis. The *diagnosis* is made by examination of the scalp under a beam of ultraviolet light from a Wood's lamp. Microscopic examination of extracted hairs may also be made.

The response to *treatment* with griseofulvin

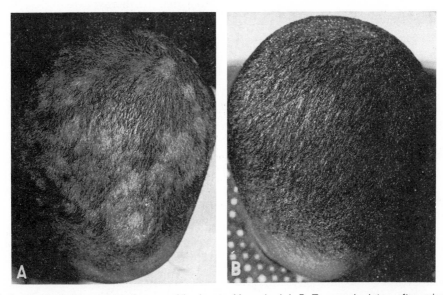

Figure 22–2. *A,* Noninflammatory tinea capitis due to *M. audouini. B,* Ten weeks later, after griseofulvin (1 Gm./day) had been given for one month. A single dose, 3 to 5 Gm., may suffice, in place of prolonged therapy. (From Pillsbury, Shelley and Kligman: *A Manual of Cutaneous Medicine.*)

administered orally is good. The lesions can be cured in seven to ten days. Locally, a strong antifungal ointment such as Whitfield's ointment can be used. The head should be covered with cloth or a stockinet skull cap. This is washed and boiled each day to prevent spread of the infection. The child can be considered cured when a direct microscopic examination and a culture are negative.

The *prognosis* is good.

Ringworm of the Skin (Tinea Corporis; Tinea Cruris)

There are two types of ringworm of the skin — tinea corporis and tinea cruris.

The lesions of *tinea corporis* are on the neck, face, forearms and hands. The lesions begin as rounded or slightly irregular, reddish-pink, pea-sized, slightly raised scaly patches. The centers of the patches clear, and the periphery spreads. The outline takes on the form of a ring. Mild itching is present.

The lesions of *tinea cruris* occur in the groin. Local warmth in the affected area causes inflammation, itching and infection, with small pustule formation.

Treatment and Prognosis. The response to *treatment* with combined griseofulvin and conventional topical antifungal therapy such as an ointment containing sulfur and salicylic acid is good. For edematous, exudative lesions wet dressings of Burow's solution or potassium permanganate are used.

With treatment the *prognosis* is excellent.

Ringworm of the Feet (Tinea Pedis)

Incidence. This condition is common among school children during the summer months. The infection comes from other children and adults. It is acquired at swimming pools and other places where people go barefoot. The infection usually appears between the toes. There is no scale formation, but the superficial epithelium is macerated and desquamates. The raw surface is often fissured. Itching is intense, and pain may follow if the child rubs or scratches the area.

Treatment and Prevention. Ointment such as Desenex or half-strength Whitfield's ointment should be applied. The feet may also be soaked in Burow's solution. Stockings and other foot coverings contaminated by the fungus should be sterilized or discarded. Light, ventilated shoes which reduce sweating are less aggravating to the condition than heavy footwear.

As a preventive measure children should wear shoes when walking where others are going barefoot and contaminating the area. Infected persons should stay away from swimming pools and gymnasium dressing rooms and all such places where they may spread infection.

Pediculosis

Types, Etiology and Incidence. There are three types of pediculosis in children: (1) pediculosis capitis, or infestation with the head louse, which is exceedingly common among neglected children; (2) pediculosis corporis, or infestation with the body louse; and (3) pediculosis pubis, or infestation with the crab louse. Since pediculosis capitis is the most common type in children, only this will be discussed here.

Pediculus capitis, or head louse, is present on the scalp, and the ova (eggs) or nits are attached to the hair. The ova are grayish, translucent, oval bodies which adhere to the shaft of a hair. They hatch in three or four days. The lice are usually seen on the heads of neglected, unclean children. They are easily transferred from child to child in schoolrooms and in tenement areas. They are more common among girls than among boys because of the girls' long hair.

Clinical Manifestations, Treatment and Nursing Care. There is severe itching of the scalp. Scratching leads to excoriation with serous, purulent or sanguineous exudation. Crusts form, and the hair is matted.

The posterior cervical lymph nodes become infected from the scalp lesions. Excoriations may also be present on the face and neck.

Treatment and *nursing care* are effective. The aims of therapy are to kill the pediculi, devitalize nits and bring relief to the child. All inflamed areas must be healed. Clothing should be dry cleaned or laundered and ironed, and hats should be dusted with 10 per cent DDT in talcum powder. Various preparations containing DDT (chlorophenothane) powder, benzyl benzoate-DDT-benzocaine emulsion (Topocide), or Kwell (benzene hexachloride) may be used on the child's head. Treatment may be repeated as often as necessary on the physician's order. Nits may be removed by combing the hair with a fine-tooth comb dipped in hot vinegar. If the hair is heavily infested, it may be advisable to cut it close to the scalp. If pustules are present on the neck and face, an antibiotic may be used. Children should be cautioned not to exchange hats with other children. The remainder of the family should also be examined for infestation. They should be referred to the local public health agency so that the home can be evaluated and so that the nurse can encourage the family to go to the clinic for examination. This should lead into general health teaching of the total family unit.

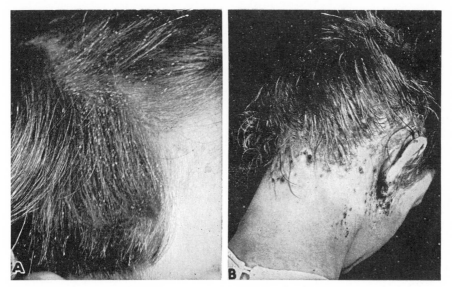

Figure 22-3. Pediculosis capitis. *A,* Numerous nits are visible. *B,* Impetiginous lesions frequently develop secondary to scratching, especially in children. (Lewis: *Practical Dermatology.* 2nd ed.)

Scabies

Etiology and Clinical Manifestations. Scabies is caused by *Acarus scabiei (Sarcoptes scabiei),* or itch mite. The female acarus burrows under the skin to deposit her eggs. The itch mite is easily transmissible from person to person. The body is involved where the skin is moist and thin, between the fingers or toes, on the wrists, in the axillae and around the abdomen and genitalia. The path where the mite burrows under the skin, about ½ inch in length, but superficial, may be seen easily. Secondary infections with papules, vesicles or pustules may occur. Itching is intense.

Treatment and Nursing Care. The objectives of care are to kill the parasite and to relieve the itching. *Treatment* consists of a hot bath followed by three applications of benzyl benzoate-DDT-benzocaine emulsion (Topocide), Kwell or Eurax, one each twelve hours. Twelve hours after the last application another hot bath should be taken. A broad-spectrum antibiotic can be used to treat secondary bacterial infection. Treatment should include all infected persons in the household so that all mites are killed simultaneously. All contaminated clothing and bed linen must be dry cleaned or boiled.

For **impetigo contagiosa** (see Plate 1, Fig. 4) and **furunculosis** see pages 188 and 189.

Osteomyelitis

Incidence, Etiology and Pathogenesis. The *incidence* of osteomyelitis is highest among children five to fourteen years of age and twice

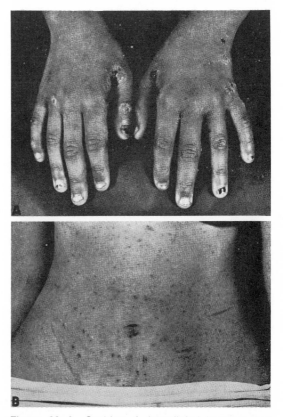

Figure 22-4. Scabies. *A,* Interdigital burrows and excoriations, with some secondary pyoderma. *B,* Excoriations over abdomen and lesions in the umbilicus. (Lewis: *Practical Dermatology.* 2nd ed.)

as frequent among boys as among girls. Acute osteomyelitis is due to deposition in the bone of bacteria from some primary source, usually on the skin, as furunculosis, impetigo or infected burns.

The causative organism commonly is hemolytic *Staphylococcus aureus*. Bacteria enter the bloodstream and are carried to the metaphysis of a bone. Infection spreads laterally along the epiphyseal plate, penetrates the cortex and locates under the periosteum, causing an abscess. The medulla of the bone may become infected. Dead bone forms a sequestrum which may be extruded or absorbed. The periosteum forms new bone and may completely cover the dead shaft with an involucrum.

Clinical Manifestations and Diagnosis. The first *clinical manifestation* is a furuncle or other infection of the skin. One or two weeks later malaise, septicemia, fever, chills and vomiting develop abruptly. The child suffers a sharp, localized pain in the affected bone. Signs of inflammation — swelling and redness — are present over the bone. The child may become very ill with fever and toxic symptoms.

The *diagnosis* is made on a leukocyte count of 15,000 to 25,000 or more cells. A blood culture is usually positive. If so, the causative organism is located. Roentgenograms may be made after changes in the bone have occurred, i.e. in five to ten days after the onset of symptoms.

Treatment and Prognosis. *Treatment* consists in giving antibiotics according to the organism found. Usually antibiotics effective against several strains of *Staphylococcus aureus* are used until the specific organism is proved. A splint is applied to the affected extremity to immobilize it and lessen the pain. Analgesics are given for pain. If an abscess forms, it is drained.

The course and *prognosis* depend on early therapy and its continuance over an adequate time. If the condition is treated early and adequately with antibiotics, the prognosis is excellent. The mortality rate has decreased greatly since specific antibacterial agents have become available.

Supracondylar Fracture of the Humerus

Incidence, Etiology, Pathology and Clinical Manifestations. Supracondylar fractures are common injuries of childhood and are most likely to occur when the child is climbing or engaged in a competitive sport that requires physical skill. Supracondylar fracture of the humerus occurs just above the elbow and is due to direct trauma to the arm.

The distal fragment is displaced posteriorly and presses on the brachial artery, thus interfering with the circulation to the forearm. Swelling and bleeding in the area also hamper the return of venous blood from the forearm. The combination of these two factors can produce serious ischemic paralysis.

Diagnosis, Treatment and Nursing Care. The *diagnosis* is made by roentgenogram. It is essential to reduce the fracture promptly and adequately and re-establish the circulation and drainage to and from the forearm. The surgeon may manipulate into place bones with only slight displacement. A splint is applied to hold the elbow in flexed position. The arm may be placed in an overhead suspension apparatus to reduce edema. X-ray films should be taken to check the position of the fragments. The arm should be immobilized for three to four weeks. After the fracture has healed, the child can re-establish motion with his own muscles without forceful manipulation.

If swelling was great at the time of injury, traction and suspension are used to reduce the fracture. The color of the skin and the quality of the radial pulse must be checked with both kinds of treatment.

Upon admission to the hospital the child is usually apprehensive, unhappy, and perhaps feeling guilty because the injury occurred while he was doing something he should not have done. Since there was no time for preparation for hospitalization, he needs a nurse who is a friend.

The nurse should check the radial pulse and the color of the skin of the arm frequently — usually every thirty minutes. She should continue her observations for the first twenty-four to forty-eight hours after the injury. If the child complains of numbness or if the fingers are discolored or cold or if the radial pulse is weak, the physician should be notified immediately.

Upon admission the child should be placed on a firm mattress. Proper positioning is important and depends on the kind of treatment to be given. Ice bags may be ordered to aid in the control of swelling and to relieve pain. The bags should be well covered and only partially filled with small pieces of ice. They should be placed under, not over, the arm, since their weight should not rest on the injured area.

To prevent a feeling of dependency, the child should be encouraged to do as much as possible for himself. Various kinds of activity appropriate to his physical limitations should be provided.

Appendicitis

Incidence, Etiology, Pathology and Clinical Manifestations. Appendicitis is rare during the first two years of life, but the *incidence* increases throughout the school years and adolescence.

Obstruction, especially with fecal concretions, is the principal factor in the majority of cases. Obstruction may also be caused by infection or allergy. Organisms found in the appendix include streptococci, *Staphylococcus aureus* and coliform bacilli. Pinworms may be an initial cause of inflammation (see p. 412).

The mucosa is inflamed and ulcerated. The lumen becomes distended, thereby impairing the blood supply. Bacteria may escape through the wall and cause diffuse peritonitis or an abscess confined by adjacent intestine and omentum.

The *clinical manifestations* may be variable. The onset may be abrupt or may follow gastroenteritis. The manifestations may include nausea, vomiting, abdominal pain, constipation or diarrhea, localized tenderness, and absence of peristalsis unless diarrhea is present. Abdominal pain in children may not be localized in the lower right quadrant. The child may not be able to report accurately the site of the pain.

Other manifestations are anorexia, mild leukocytosis (12,000 to 15,000 cells), fever of 99 to 102°F., flushed face, increased pulse and respiratory rates, restlessness, irritability and sleeplessness.

Diagnosis, Treatment, Nursing Care, Complications and Prognosis. The *diagnosis* of appendicitis in childhood is difficult, since a number of other conditions produce somewhat similar symptoms. If the child has a respiratory infection, abdominal pain may be due to incipient pneumonia or mesenteric adenitis. Inflammation of a Meckel's diverticulum or gastroenteritis may also cause symptoms suggestive of appendicitis. Irritation of the peritoneum may occur in rheumatic fever and resemble appendicitis. Repeated examinations may be necessary before a definite diagnosis is made.

Appendectomy—surgical removal of the appendix—should be done as soon as possible after the diagnosis has been made and the child is in condition for operation. Preoperative preparation is routine and consists in withholding of food, establishment of hydration by the intravenous route and reduction of temperature below 102°F. (rectally). Administration of antibiotics to prevent or minimize the danger of peritonitis and enemas may be ordered, but cathartics are not given. Operation is done immediately after admission or as soon as possible.

Recovery after appendectomy is rapid, and the child usually returns to school in two weeks. If he had peritonitis or a peritoneal or appendiceal abscess, continuous gastric suction, chemotherapy and parenteral fluids may be ordered. The child may be placed in semi-Fowler's position to assist in localizing the infection. He is ambulated as early as possible even if he still has a gastric suction tube in place. Recovery, naturally, will be slower than in the uncomplicated case.

The *nursing care* of a child undergoing appendectomy is usually simple and similar to that of adults.

Complications include a localized abscess and diffuse secondary peritonitis. The appendix may perforate, thereby causing complications, because the parents gave the child a cathartic (lay treatment for any abdominal pain in childhood) or because the child, interested in play and not wanting a cathartic, did not tell his mother of his discomfort.

The operation is practically without risk if it is performed before perforation occurs. Even after perforation has occurred the risk is relatively slight.

Meckel's Diverticulum

Etiology, Pathology and Clinical Manifestations. When the intestinal remnant of the omphalomesenteric duct from the terminal ileum to the umbilical cord persists and does not close, a Meckel's diverticulum is formed. It arises from the ileum, but usually does not have a connection with the umbilicus. A Meckel's diverticulum may be $\frac{1}{2}$ to 3 inches in length and may be lined with intestinal mucous membrane. In some cases it may also contain gastric mucosa.

The diverticulum usually is not responsible for symptoms. When its gastric mucosa secretes

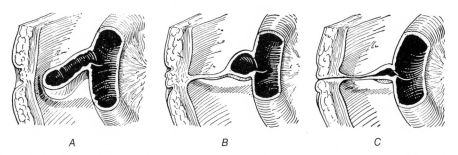

A   *B*   *C*

Figure 22–5. Meckel's diverticulum of the ileum. *A*, Ordinary blind sac. *B*, Diverticulum continued to umbilicus as a cord. *C*, Diverticulum with fistulous opening at umbilicus. (Arey: *Developmental Anatomy.* 6th ed.)

gastric ferments, complications arise. It may produce ulceration in the ileum or in the diverticulum which may lead to massive hemorrhage, perforation and peritonitis. The diverticulum may cause intestinal adhesions, strangulation or intussusception, and this may result in intestinal obstruction.

When hemorrhage occurs, the stools may be black at first, and then bright red. With hemorrhage there will be pallor and an increased pulse rate. If transfusions are not given immediately, collapse and death may occur.

Finding the diverticulum is the only way of confirming the diagnosis.

Treatment and Nursing Care. Transfusions are given for hemorrhage, and surgical excision of the diverticulum is necessary.

Nursing care after removal of a diverticulum is similar to that given after other abdominal surgery.

TEACHING AIDS AND OTHER INFORMATION*

Canadian Mental Health Association
Suddenly It Happens—Your Child Is Ill, 1967.

Mental Health Materials Center
Preparing Your Child for the Hospital.

Play Schools Association
Cleverdon, D.: Play in a Hospital.

The Children's Hospital Medical Center, Boston, Mass.
Johnny Goes to the Hospital.

United States Department of Health, Education, and Welfare
A Guide for Teaching Poison Prevention in Kindergartens and Primary Grades, 1966.
Poison Ivy, Poison Oak, and Poison Sumac, 1967.
Red Is The Color of Hurting, 1967.
Ringworm (Including Athlete's Foot), 1966.

REFERENCES

Publications
Catzel, P., and Cohen, S.: *The Paediatric Prescriber.* 3rd ed. Philadelphia, F. A. Davis Company, 1966.
Dimock, H. G.: *The Child in Hospital.* Philadelphia, F. A. Davis Company, 1960.
Ellis, R. W. B., and Mitchell, R. G.: *Disease in Infancy and Childhood.* 5th ed. Baltimore, Williams & Wilkins Company, 1966.
Geist, H.: *A Child Goes to the Hospital: The Psychological Aspects of a Child Going to the Hospital.* Springfield, Ill., Charles C Thomas, 1965.
Gips, C. D.: *The Interpretation and Misinterpretation . . . by Hospitalized School-Age Children . . . of Being Sick: Implications for Nursing.* Phases in Human Development: Relevance in Nursing. Monograph 15, 1962 Clinical Sessions. New York, American Nurses' Association, 1962.
Haller, J. A., Jr. (Ed.): *The Hospitalized Child and His Family.* Baltimore, Johns Hopkins Press, 1967.
Hutchison, J. H.: *Practical Paediatric Problems.* 2nd ed. Chicago, Year Book Medical Publishers, Inc., 1967.
Larson, C. B., and Gould, M.: *Calderwood's Orthopedic Nursing.* 6th ed. St. Louis, C. V. Mosby Company, 1965.
Paul, J. R.: *Clinical Epidemiology.* 2nd ed. Chicago, University of Chicago Press, 1966.
Powell, M.: *Orthopedic Nursing.* 5th ed. Baltimore, Williams & Wilkins Company, 1966.
Robertson, J.: *Hospitals and Children.* New York, International Universities Press, Inc., 1963.
Shirkey, H. C. (Ed.): *Pediatric Therapy.* 2nd ed. St. Louis, C. V. Mosby Company, 1966.
Vernon, D. T. A., and others: *The Psychological Responses of Children to Hospitalization and Illness.* Springfield, Ill., Charles C Thomas, 1965.
White, R. R. (Ed.): *Atlas of Pediatric Surgery.* New York, Blakiston Division, McGraw-Hill Book Company, Inc., 1965.

* Complete addresses are given in the Appendix.

Periodicals

Cluster, P. F.: A One-Room School for Hospitalized Children. *Nursing Outlook,* 15:56, August 1967.

Coles, R.: Violence in Ghetto Children. *Children,* 14:101, 1967.

Erickson, F.: When 6- to 12-Year-Olds Are Ill. *Nursing Outlook,* 13:48, July 1965.

Howe, J.: Children's Ideas About Injury. *ANA Regional Clinical Conferences,* American Nurses' Association, 1967. New York, Appleton-Century-Crofts, 1968, page 189.

McCaffery, M., and Moss, F.: Nursing Intervention for Bodily Pain. *Am. J. Nursing,* 67:1224, 1967.

Petrillo, M.: Preventing Hospital Trauma in Pediatric Patients. *Am. J. Nursing,* 68:1468, 1968.

Winchester, J. H.: They're Almost Never Too Sick to Study. *Today's Health,* 46:31, August 1968.

23

CONDITIONS OF THE SCHOOL CHILD REQUIRING LONG-TERM CARE

REHABILITATION OF THE SCHOOL CHILD

The process of rehabilitation begins as soon after recognition of the illness as possible and continues throughout illness until the child is rehabilitated to the fullest possible extent. Rehabilitation in our culture is based on the belief that all persons should be helped to maintain or regain their best possible physical or mental health. Whether the child has multiple handicaps or a chronic disease, rehabilitation is geared to averting further preventable damage, and to helping him gain his maximum physical potential while bolstering his psychologic defenses for the future. If the members of the health team and the nursing team do not make a positive effort to rehabilitate their patients, these children may *regress* in their abilities and interpersonal relations. Thus rehabilitation becomes one goal in the comprehensive care of patients. The nurse must work closely with other members of the interdisciplinary health team to achieve this end.

By school age and adolescence the child must assume increasing responsibility for his own rehabilitation after illness. His cooperation must be gained through understanding the necessity for this. The nurse has an important role in interpreting this need to him and in helping him to assume this responsibility.

In order to help the child achieve the goal of rehabilitation, his own goals must be considered. Thus the nurse has the responsibility to investigate these goals through discussions with him. She must relay pertinent information to other members of the health team. In our society it is our privilege and responsibility to help prepare each child, whether normal or handicapped, to take his rightful place in the world of tomorrow.

School in the Hospital. In our culture going to school has become identified with the mainstream of child growth and development. It is of utmost importance that the hospitalized child be assured of a continuing relation with this mainstream. When the child cannot go to school, the school must come to him. School to the older child is his "life work." He is just as serious about it as an adult is about his employment. For this reason many hospitals maintain a school program for hospitalized children. The program may include the acutely ill child; however, the majority of children attending class are the chronically ill and convalescent children.

The purpose of the school program is, first, to keep the child up with his grade group academically; second, to keep the child with his peer group socially; third, to act as a supportive factor in the child's total adjustment to his hospitalization. Attendance at school gives him an opportunity to express himself and to use his time

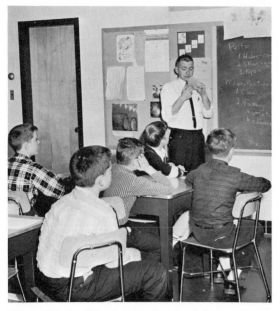

Figure 23–1. Attendance at school is an essential part of the rehabilitation program. (H. Armstrong Roberts.)

in a constructive manner. It brings some of the familiar outside world into the hospital.

Many times the chronically ill child needs individual or remedial help. School in the hospital presents an excellent opportunity for the child to receive such help.

With the liberalization of visiting privileges parents see their children more frequently. This provides a unique opportunity for parent-teacher communication. Parents become the link between the child's home-school and his hospital-school.

Attitudes toward school and school work can be important factors in understanding the child. Sometimes these attitudes have implications for the physicians, nurses and all other personnel who work with the child. They provide clues to his motivation, his potential, the satisfaction he derives from his work and the degree to which he has learned to function effectively. They reflect his self-image as well as the quality of his home and school backgrounds.

In many hospitals the child is taught by a visiting teacher, either at his bedside or in a group of children in a classroom made to accommodate wheelchairs and even beds on rollers. The classroom should have the usual equipment, including blackboard and movable tables and chairs. The hours spent in study are short, and no child is under pressure to learn. His program is suited to his condition.

Hospitalized school children miss not only school, but also many opportunities for learning

which other children have. They should be given what opportunities are available in the hospital setting. They can learn facts about their own bodies and something about preventing disease. Convalescent children may be taken on picnics and sightseeing trips. Those who cannot leave the hospital may have motion pictures and exhibitions brought to them. School children become bored and withdrawn if they are not given an opportunity to learn.

After a child has been discharged from the hospital he may have to convalesce at his home for weeks or months. If he lives in a community which has a school-to-home telephone or closed-circuit television service he may be able to participate in his regular classes. Thus he can continue his education without feeling left out. If such a service is not available, a visiting teacher may come to the home to tutor him so that he will be able to return to his class when he is fully recovered.

LONG-TERM CONDITIONS

Rheumatic Fever

Collagen Diseases. Collagen diseases are a group of diseases characterized by damage to the ground substance of connective tissue, followed by changes in collagen fibrils. The connective tissue of all organ systems is usually affected, and the small blood vessels are frequently involved. The following are collagen diseases (they are heterogeneous from the clinical point of view, but have certain symptoms in common): rheumatic fever, rheumatoid arthritis, periarteritis nodosa, disseminated lupus erythematosus, scleroderma and dermatomyositis. All these diseases respond symptomatically to corticotropin (ACTH) or cortisone during some stage. The basic problem in these conditions is the deposition of fibrinoid material in the tissues. Histopathologically, fibrinoid is extensively deposited in the lumen and walls of blood vessels and in the surrounding connective tissues.

Etiology, Incidence and Pathology. Rheumatic fever is a general systemic disease characterized by frequent recurrences following infection with group A beta hemolytic streptococcus. The etiologic importance of this organism is based on clinical epidemiology, as shown by its association with a sore throat preceding rheumatic fever by one to three weeks, and by immunologic response seen in the antigen-antibody reaction. A streptolysin which causes a clear zone of hemolysis around bacterial colonies on blood agar plates causes an antibody response in the patient's blood which can be measured as the antistreptolysin-O titer (ASO titer). The level of this antibody response reflects the intensity of tissue reaction and is an aid in diagnosis. The common origin of infection is in the throat (possibly followed by scarlet fever) or skin.

The pathologic sequence in rheumatic fever is (1) the initial infection with group A beta hemolytic streptococcus, (2) usually a latent or nonsymptomatic period lasting one to three weeks, and (3) the onset of rheumatic fever.

Rheumatic fever is one of the leading causes of chronic illness and death in children. It has its highest *incidence* between the ages of five and fifteen years; the majority of first attacks occur between six and eight years. It is most prevalent in the temperate zones. Climate is a more important factor than racial susceptibility. The incidence varies with the season and geographic location, but it always follows the curve of incidence of streptococcal infections. It is most common in the spring months in the United States, but in the later months of the year in England. Overcrowded living conditions and general lack of hygiene among the lower socioeconomic groups in large cities are predisposing factors. The disease has a high family incidence; hereditary predisposition is possible.

The characteristic lesions of rheumatic fever are found in the connective tissue of the heart, subcutaneous tissue and in the arteries. Collagenous structures become edematous and may form granulomas or *Aschoff bodies*. These bodies are usually found in the wall of the left ventricle and interventricular septum. Structures resembling Aschoff bodies may also be found as *subcutaneous nodules* under the skin. These lesions may develop exudative manifestations. Such rheumatic effusions are usually absorbed, but adhesions may be found, especially in the pericardium. They are found in the hearts of the majority of children who succumb to acute carditis. Valvular lesions which form scars as they heal may result in thickening of the leaflet and shortening of the chordae tendineae. Such deformities of the valves result from repeated infection.

The heart may be impaired after rheumatic fever, owing to damage to the myocardium, the endocardium (including the valves) or the pericardium. The effects of the contracting scar tissue may not be evident for several years after the initial attack of rheumatic fever. Chronic valvular heart disease results.

Clinical Manifestations. The symptoms and course of the disease are variable. The three principal clinical manifestations, however, are carditis, migratory polyarthritis and Sydenham's chorea. The typical attack may present any one of the clinical manifestations, which tend to recur at varying intervals. The onset may be acute or insidious with symptoms of "growing pains," pallor, nosebleed, malaise, and attacks of abdominal pain. Attacks last from one to three months, and recurrence may follow if the child acquires a streptococcal infection.

Carditis tends to occur in younger children. It is a more serious manifestation than arthritis or chorea, since it may lead to permanent disability or death. The pathologic changes include exudation and proliferation. The pericardium, myocardium and endocardium may be affected with subsequent scarring. The temperature may rise to 104°F. Leukocytosis, anemia and severe pallor may occur. The respirations are rapid, and the cardiac lesion results in tachycardia, especially during sleep, and a pulse of poor quality. In severe cases the following manifestations may be seen: prostration, weakness, orthopnea, cyanosis, precordial pain and cardiac decompensation and dilatation. Cardiac murmurs are present and may change in quality.

Arthritis of a migratory polyarthritic type is usually seen in older children. The larger joints—hips, knees, ankles, shoulders, wrists and elbows—are characteristically involved. The duration of involvement varies, and the pain moves from one joint to another. In older children the affected joint is hot, tender, red and swollen. Permanent deformities do not follow this type of arthritis.

There is moderate leukocytosis, and the erythrocyte sedimentation rate is increased. The child's temperature usually runs from 101 to 102°F. Cardiac involvement may follow polyarthritis. So-called growing pains may be distinguished from migratory polyarthritis because they tend to occur only at night, are not associated with other manifestations of rheumatic fever, and are generally muscular rather than joint pains.

Sydenham's chorea (St. Vitus's dance) is a disorder of the central nervous system. It usually occurs in older children. See page 583 for a discussion of this condition.

There are other clinical manifestations of rheumatic fever (Fig. 23-2): (1) subcutaneous nodules of varying size which may be found on the extensor tendons of the hands and feet, on elbows, scapulae, scalp, patella and vertebrae. The skin moves freely over these nodules; they are not painful, and they disappear gradually. (2) Pericarditis, in which there is pain in the precordial area and a friction rub heard over the precordium. (3) Muscle and joint pains (the so-called growing pains) may indicate rheumatic fever, and the child should be examined to rule out this disease and also orthopedic problems. (4) Epistaxis is a common manifestation of the onset of rheumatic fever. (5) Abdominal pain may be severe and may be mistaken for appendicitis. It is usually located in the epigastrium and may be due to enlargement of the mesenteric lymph nodes or to inflammation of the peritoneum. (6) There may be low-grade fever

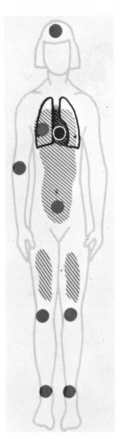

Figure 23-2. Sites of involvement in acute rheumatic fever. (From Disease Panorama on Rheumatic Fever. Courtesy of the Schering Corporation.)

(2) The erythrocyte sedimentation rate is almost always elevated in children who have rheumatic carditis and polyarthritis, thereby indicating the presence of an inflammatory reaction. The sedimentation rate may remain elevated after clinical manifestations have subsided, showing that the rheumatic process is still active.

The rheumatic process should not be considered over until the white blood cell count is below 10,000 per cubic millimeter. Leukocytosis indicates inflammation. As long as anemia persists, the infection is probably still active.

Streptococci may be present in the upper respiratory tract of the child, a member of his family, or others whom he contacts. The organism may not be present if treatment has been given, but certain antibodies formed against streptococcal products may be present. Laboratory examinations may detect antifibrinolysin, antistreptolysin or antihyaluronidase.

Electrocardiograms may provide evidence of carditis. The P-R interval is often prolonged in the presence of carditis.

Treatment. Since treatment of a child having rheumatic fever is a long-term problem, it involves especially the following members of the health team: physicians, nurses in the pediatric unit, public health nurses, social service worker, teacher and Play Lady.

No specific treatment will stop the rheumatic process. Bed rest is essential until the C-reactive protein is negative, the pulse rate normal, the erythrocyte sedimentation rate decreasing, the pain gone and the hemoglobin level normal.

in the afternoon. If the diagnosis is uncertain, the erythrocyte sedimentation rate should be determined. (7) There may be skin manifestations. Various types of erythema may appear, e.g. erythema marginatum (Fig. 23-3) or erythema multiforme. Erythema marginatum is a pink eruption with serpiginous outline, occurring mainly on the trunk. These lesions may appear and disappear for years. (8) Pleurisy and rheumatic pneumonia may be complications. (9) The child tires easily, loses weight, and is pale and anorectic.

Diagnosis. The diagnosis may be difficult because many other conditions show clinical manifestations similar to those of rheumatic fever. Each laboratory test must be interpreted in the light of other test results and of the child's total clinical picture.

Laboratory tests are of value in diagnosing rheumatic fever and in evaluation of the disease. (1) There are several abnormal proteins found in the serum of children having rheumatic fever as in other inflammatory states. C-reactive protein is never present in normal blood. This protein disappears as the child's condition improves.

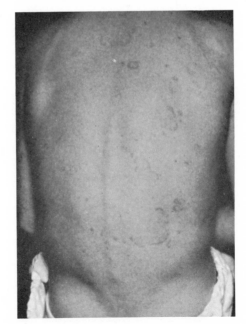

Figure 23-3. Erythema marginatum. (Nadas: *Pediatric Cardiology.* 2nd edition.)

The child should have begun to gain in weight before activity is permitted. If the work of the heart is reduced until the healing process occurs, a minimum of scar tissue in the heart will result.

Penicillin is given only to eradicate group A streptococci from the body. It does not alleviate symptoms. Salicylates quickly relieve fever, joint pains and swelling. Symptoms of toxicity such as tinnitus, hyperpnea, purpuric manifestations, nausea and vomiting should be recorded. Salicylates are usually given orally. Aspirin (acetylsalicylic acid) or sodium salicylate is given. This therapy should be continued until C-reactive protein is negative and the erythrocyte sedimentation rate is decreasing. If the child cannot tolerate salicylates, aminopyrine or phenylbutazone (Butazolidin) may be used.

Therapy with corticoids produces the same effects as salicylates. ACTH, prednisone or cortisone may be used. Prednisone is preferred because it may be given orally and causes less sodium retention than cortisone. Laboratory findings tend to return to normal more quickly than with the use of salicylates. Corticoids are considered by many to be beneficial in the treatment of rheumatic carditis, especially in extremely acute phases of the condition or if life-threatening failure is present. These drugs do not terminate the rheumatic process, but suppress it. There may be a mild recurrence of symptoms when the drug is discontinued.

Steroid therapy masks symptoms; thus it is necessary to watch the child closely for symptoms of infection or complications. These children do not have a fever when they have infections. The blood pressure should be taken daily and the drug discontinued if the diastolic pressure rises to 100 mm. or above. The salt intake should be moderately restricted.

A side effect of steroid therapy is the production of a *Cushing-like syndrome* characterized by acne, moon face, increased pigmentation, hirsutism and abnormal fat distribution. This disappears when therapy is discontinued.

Morphine is given to control precordial pain, and sedatives such as phenobarbital to allay apprehension. Oxygen may be necessary. Digitalis may be indicated if cardiac failure is present.

Nursing Care. ACUTE PHASE. In the acute phase of rheumatic fever, rest is all-important in order to reduce the work of the heart. The need for absolute bed rest should be explained to the child, and he should be reassured that it will be a restriction only as long as necessary. The bed must have a firm mattress, since this promotes good posture and is less uncomfortable than a mattress which sags. If the child is dyspneic, or if the position provides comfort for him, the head of the bed may be elevated. During the period of complete bed rest when the head of the bed is elevated, the child's arms should be supported at his sides with pillows to reduce their weight from the shoulders. If the pillows are of the proper height, the child will find it easier to expand his chest, and his arms will not bring pressure on his abdomen when he folds them across his body. The child's legs should

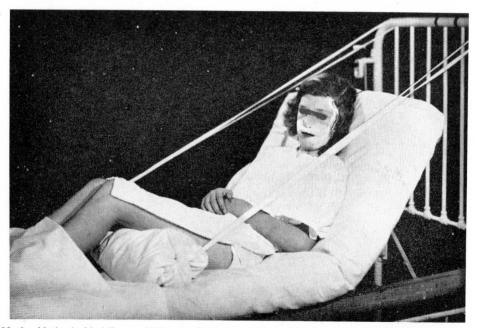

Figure 23–4. Method of holding a child up in Fowler's position with a knee roll. (Gross: *The Surgery of Infancy and Childhood.*)

be in proper alignment, and his feet should be supported with a foot board to prevent foot drop and external rotation of the hips. A bed cradle may be used to prevent pressure from the bed clothes on his toes.

Nursing care should be given at appropriate times so that the child can have long periods of complete rest without being disturbed. Since bodily movement causes pain, he should be moved unnecessarily as little as possible. The nurse's movements must be smooth, sure and unhurried; this helps to inspire confidence of the child in his nurse. If he is hurt by her, he becomes anxious and does not want to be touched. The nurse should explain what she is going to do, e.g. insert the thermometer or lift him. What the child may be permitted to do for himself depends upon the physician's orders. If the child becomes irritable and more restless in bed than he would be out of it, the physician may permit a limited amount of activity in spite of the fact that laboratory findings are not normal.

The nurse is responsible for providing the child not only with physical comfort, but also with emotional rest. His needs must be anticipated and met in order to alleviate his anxiety.

The child with rheumatic fever who is on bed rest should have frequent skin care, especially of the back and buttocks. A rubber ring may be used to prevent pressure on the sacrum and buttocks, since these children may be constantly in a sitting position. His position should be changed frequently in order to prevent breakdown of the skin, to increase expansion of the lungs and to prevent his extremities from becoming stiff. Sore joints should be handled carefully when he is moved. The child's elbows should be massaged with lotion because they may become irritated by rubbing on the sheets. The child should be helped to use the bedpan as necessary.

If the child breathes through his mouth or has a limited fluid intake, good mouth care is essential.

Small, frequent feedings of light, nourishing food are better than meals served at the usual intervals. It may be necessary to cater to the child's appetite; he should not be forced to eat, nor allowed to overeat, since without exercise he might become obese. When food is brought, he should be placed in a comfortable position for eating and, if he is unable to help himself, should be assisted by the nurse.

If oxygen is ordered, it is usually given in a tent (Fig. 23-6). The procedure should be explained to the child. The school child is not likely

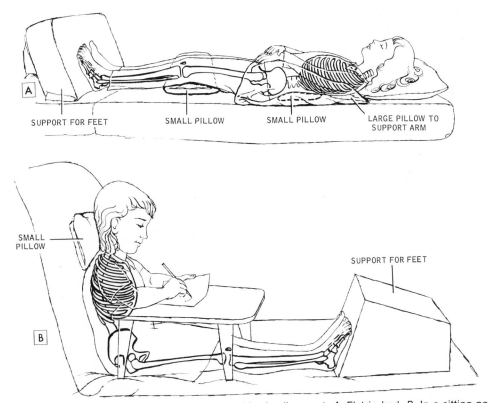

SUPPORT FOR FEET   SMALL PILLOW   SMALL PILLOW   LARGE PILLOW TO SUPPORT ARM

SMALL PILLOW

SUPPORT FOR FEET

Figure 23-5. Methods of positioning a child for good body alignment. *A,* Flat in bed. *B,* In a sitting position.

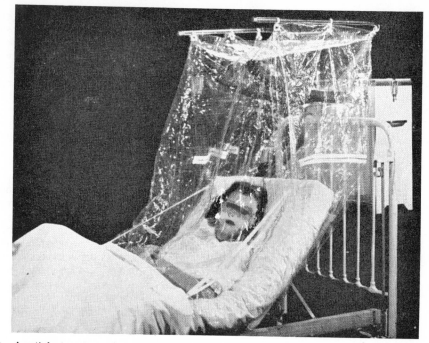

Figure 23–6.   A satisfactory type of oxygen tent for administration of a high concentration (90 per cent) of oxygen. (Gross: *The Surgery of Infancy and Childhood.*)

to be frightened as is the younger child. He should be given a bell so that he can summon his nurse. He should wear adequate clothing so that he does not become chilled.

Nursing records must be full and specific. The rate and nature of the pulse are indicative of the child's progress. If the physician so orders, the pulse should be taken when the child is sleeping as well as when he is awake. The pulse rate should be counted for a full minute, before the thermometer is inserted. The temperature and respiration rate should also be taken as ordered and accurately recorded.

If digitalis is ordered, the nurse should count the pulse rate before the administration of each dose. If the rate has decreased or the quality of the pulse has changed, the dose should be withheld until the physician can examine the child. Criteria by which improvement can be measured include the quality of the pulse rate when the child is resting and its ability to return to its former rate after mild exertion. If heart damage is evident, the child's activity must continue to be limited.

In general, an intake and output record is required. If possible, the child should be allowed to keep his own record. If fluids are limited, he should have a schedule which he may follow. The reason for limiting fluid intake and for keeping the intake and output chart should be explained to him. The amount and kind of food taken should also be charted.

The nurse should also observe and record the emotional state of the child, fatigue, respiratory excursion, orthopnea, venous distention in the neck, dyspnea, cough, pain, color of the skin, lips or nails, skin lesions, and edema.

The personnel caring for the child should understand the parents' attitude toward the child and his illness. The nurse and the physician should begin early in the illness to evaluate the family's attitude toward the child. These attitudes may vary from apparent unconcern to extreme anxiety. Parents must be helped to a more positive approach to the illness if the child is to be successfully rehabilitated.

CONVALESCENT CARE. Probably the first requisite in successful nursing of the convalescing child is to keep him happy and contented. These children become depressed because they see other acutely ill children admitted, recover and be discharged, while they themselves remain in the hospital. The child's activities must be confined to the limits permitted by the physician. There is a gradual increase in the child's ability to care for himself (bathing, feeding, and so on) as he improves.

If schoolwork is permitted, the child has this interest and the satisfaction of feeling that he is keeping up with his class. This helps him to look forward to the time of his discharge from the hospital. Recreational and occupational therapy helps him by teaching him new skills which he is interested in learning and which are related

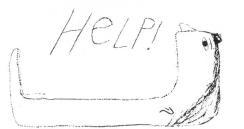

Figure 23-7. This plea for "HELP" was drawn by a long-term hospitalized, seriously ill school child whose deep needs for love and acceptance could not be met. Although he was not able to express his needs verbally, he could put his feelings into one word on paper. (Courtesy of Miss Mary Brooks.)

to the physician's plan for his care while in the hospital. Suitable activities include finger painting, making beads from macaroni and stringing them, or making other kinds of jewelry, making puppets or cuddly toys, soap carving, spatter prints, spool knitting, making model airplanes and boats, leather construction, clay modeling, knitting, and so on. Making collections of items which interest children of his age is also appropriate. These children enjoy guessing games, many of which have educational value. This acceptance of activities within the limits set by the physician helps the child to understand and accept quiet games or a physically inactive role in an active game when he plays with his friends after his discharge.

The play period in the hospital should be short and should be followed by periods of music, story telling or reading, during which the child relaxes.

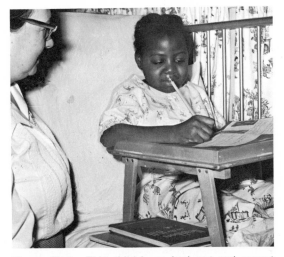

Figure 23-8. This child is on bed rest and cannot be taken to the classroom in the hospital with other children. The school teacher therefore visits her in her room and helps her to gain the satisfaction of keeping up with her class.

The time out of bed is gradually increased. A comfortable chair (not a wheelchair) may be placed by the window, and the child may be given playthings which interest him and ensure quiet activity. A wheelchair is used when the nurse pushes him about to explore his environment. After several weeks or months he is allowed to walk, but must be closely supervised so that he does not overdo it.

Home is the best place for the convalescent child, but if this is not possible because of overcrowding and general lack of facilities, he may be sent to a convalescent hospital where the environment is planned to give him the emotional security he needs, opportunities for play, education, work and group life, as well as continued supervision of his physical health. The public health nurse or home care personnel may make an evaluation of the home as to the adequacy of facilities prior to the child's discharge from the hospital. In some cases the child may be sent to a foster home, but it is extremely difficult to find such a home.

Resumption of normal activities is gradual over a period of several weeks to months.

If the child is sent to a convalescent hospital or a foster home, he should help to make plans, know about total plans and meet his foster parents before he leaves the hospital. His parents should remain in contact with him, since such arrangements are only temporary.

It is necessary to work out a plan with the parents or foster parents for the child's care when he leaves the hospital. Not only his physical but also his psychologic needs must be met. Gradual independence must be given and behavior disorders prevented. All aspects of his care should be discussed. If any item of equipment is needed, e.g. overbed table, back rest or footboard, the parents may be shown how to make these from orange crates and suitcases, or, if they cannot be made at home and the parents cannot afford to buy them, they may be provided through some agencies.

The home atmosphere should be cheerful. The child should have the same kind of quiet recreation which was provided in the hospital. In some cities a visiting school teacher will be sent by the school board, or a telephone connection may be made between his room and the classroom of the school he has attended. This enables him to hear the instruction given his class and their responses.

Not too much attention should be directed toward the child's heart condition. The whole child should be helped to develop confidence. He should learn how to set his own standards for activity. The ultimate aim should be kept in mind: to restore the child to his place in society with the least possible emotional trauma. When he returns to school, the health team, including teacher and school nurse, must know the health plan to be carried out. They should understand his illness and thus help other children to understand and accept the difference in his routine; e.g. he will use the elevator, but they will not; his hours in school may not be as long as theirs.

The parents and the child should be helped to understand the need for visits to the clinic or his private physician for prophylactic medications and dental care. The social service department may be helpful in arranging for transportation for these visits. Parents should understand and accept his daily routine and also be able to recognize respiratory infections and skin infections, possibly caused by streptococci, and to get adequate medical care when these occur.

Caring for the child in the home is difficult for the mother, especially if she has other children who need her attention, if the home is crowded, or if the mother must work outside the home to supplement the family income. Another problem which the mother may have is that of keeping appointments for regular follow-up care for the child when transportation is difficult and when there are small children for whom a baby-sitter must be found. A more subtle problem emerges when the child is well enough so that he requires little professional care. The mother no longer has the support of physicians, nurses and social workers at a time when she needs increasing psychologic support in coping with the child's convalescence. The public health nurse, if she visits in the home, can help the mother find solutions to many of these problems as they emerge.

Prognosis and Prevention. The mortality rate seems to be declining from both initial attacks and recurrences of rheumatic fever. Recurrences are most common during childhood and decline after puberty.

Serious cardiac damage results from repeated, severe rheumatic attacks (Fig. 23-9). The *prognosis* for children who have their first attack before six years of age is graver than for those who have it later, because they usually have carditis with residual cardiac damage. If the child has chronic valvular disease resulting from rheumatic carditis, his heart will become hypertrophied, owing to the increased work load. When his heart is compensated, the only finding may be a cardiac murmur. When the heart is decompensated, the circulation is inadequate, and blood accumulates in the venous system. Edema, ascites, congestion of the lungs and liver, dyspnea and cyanosis result. The treatment of cardiac decompensation in the child is similar to that in the adult and includes reduction of the work of the heart by keeping the child in bed and rested by the use of sedatives. Further treatment includes the administration

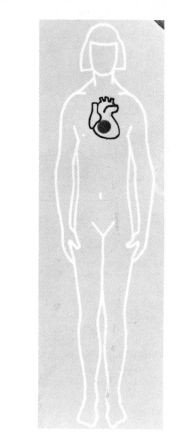

Figure 23–9. The single site of chronic involvement—the heart. (From Disease Panorama on Rheumatic Fever. Courtesy of the Schering Corporation.)

of oxygen to relieve dyspnea, digitalis to slow the heart rate and diuretics to relieve edema. The diet usually ordered is one low in salt. Fluids may or may not be limited. Often the residual heart condition may be so severe that it handicaps the adolescent or adult in his home and community life. (See Figure 23-10.)

The prognosis is good for children who have no evidence of cardiac involvement. Death in childhood is apt to be due to further rheumatic infection rather than mechanical failure of the heart. Operation to place artificial valves like those used in the affected hearts of adults is not usually done in children.

Rheumatic polyarthritis does not result in permanent joint changes, and chorea does not produce permanent changes in the central nervous system.

The *prevention* of rheumatic fever lies in the prevention of infection with group A beta hemolytic streptococci. Prevention of the first attack is through elimination of streptococci from the upper respiratory tract when the child has pharyngitis or scarlet fever. Penicillin is given for ten to fourteen days. This is preferably given

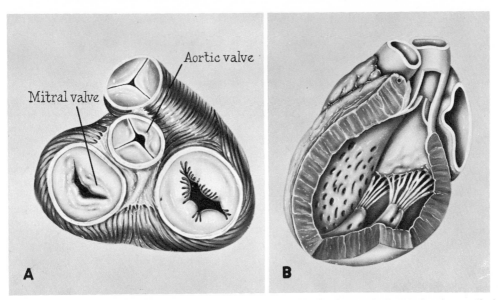

Figure 23–10. Chronic rheumatic heart. *A,* Superior view of chronic rheumatic heart showing aortic insufficiency and mitral stenosis. *B,* Dissection of chronic rheumatic heart showing fibrosis of mitral valve and thickened chordae tendineae. (From Disease Panorama on Rheumatic Fever. Courtesy of the Schering Corporation.)

orally except in those instances in which the certainty of the patient's maintaining his own prophylaxis is questionable.

Recurrence must be prevented, since each attack increases the threat of additional cardiac damage. The child should be kept from persons with upper respiratory tract infections. If he does acquire a respiratory illness, he should have a throat culture taken, possibly by the school nurse. Ideally, he should live in a warm climate and an uncrowded environment. As a prophylactic measure, benzathine penicillin is given monthly by intramuscular injection, or penicillin or sulfadiazine is given by mouth daily indefinitely after the initial attack. It is essential for the nurse to stress the importance of taking this preventive medication to both the parents and the child. These drugs may be obtained either free of charge or at minimal cost, depending on the ability of the parents to pay. The responsibility for the full cost of the drug may be assumed by the health department, the heart association, the welfare department, the crippled children's agency or a combination of these. This eases the financial burden for the parents and facilitates oral prophylaxis.

Currently a highly purified vaccine designed to prevent childhood streptococcal infections which lead to rheumatic fever and glomerulonephritis is being tested. The effectiveness of this vaccine in producing immunity against the streptococcus probably will not be known for some time.

If it is necessary for the child to have a tonsillectomy and adenoidectomy or undergo dental

work, an increased dose of penicillin should be given to prevent bacterial endocarditis.

Public Health Aspects. There is need for a community program of control, case finding and preventive work. There should be long-range programs for the care of these children. Improved living conditions of the lower-income group and better health programs in the schools would do much to prevent this serious disease. In some cities the coordination of team efforts for the benefit of these patients needs to be improved.

Sydenham's Chorea (St. Vitus's Dance)

Incidence, Clinical Manifestations and Diagnosis. Sydenham's chorea is one of the clinical manifestations of the rheumatic process. It is primarily a disorder of the central nervous system. It is most common in girls during later childhood and early adolescence — from seven to fourteen years of age. The highest *incidence* is at eight years. Some authorities believe that the disease occurs in certain families more than in the general population (thus heredity would appear to be important) and that nervous persons are most apt to have the disease. It is seldom seen after puberty.

Sydenham's chorea is characterized by involuntary, purposeless, irregular movements involving any part or all of the voluntary musculature.

The *clinical manifestations* may vary from mild to severe. The onset is gradual. The child becomes increasingly nervous, and his jerking, spasmodic, purposeless, incoordinated, irregular movements cause him great discomfort. These movements are different from, and more severe than, those of tic. The first symptom of the condition may be clumsiness, and the child may be reprimanded for dropping something or spilling food at the table. The movements of the facial muscles produce grimaces which often may appear to the adult as rude and to other children as silly. The child's handwriting shows lack of muscular control and may become almost illegible. The child cannot suppress his spasmodic movements, which become worse with excitement and embarrassment, but cease when he is asleep. Muscular weakness may become so great that he is unable to walk or even sit up. He talks with difficulty, and it is often impossible to understand his speech. He is "jittery," and slovenly in his personal habits, and may be unable to dress himself, having greatest difficulty in buttoning his clothes and tying his shoelaces. He may be unable to feed himself and may have difficulty in swallowing. Some children become incontinent. Emotional instability is shown in giggling, crying, fretfulness and rapid shifting from depression to elation. Usually the child does not have fever. The school teacher is apt to recognize the early signs of chorea: the child's lack of ability to sit still in school, his grimacing and the obvious changes in his handwriting. Teachers should be educated about the early signs of such illnesses as chorea which affect school children.

The *diagnosis* is based on the clinical manifestations, the most important of which are increase of choreiform movements when tense, increased dysfunction of speech and rapid changes of facial expression from a grin to tears. Laboratory tests such as the sedimentation rate, the leukocyte count and the antistreptolysin O titer may be normal and the C-reactive protein negative.

Treatment, Nursing Care and Prognosis. Both *treatment* and *nursing care* are based on the relief of symptoms. Since there is no really effective treatment, nursing care is of central importance.

Drugs are given as ordered. The child should have absolute mental and physical rest. He should have a private room or be with a few carefully chosen children who meet his need for companionship. Prolonged, warm baths may have a sedative effect and tranquilizers and phenobarbital may be given. He must be fed by his nurse. He should be protected from injury by padded sideboards for his bed. Blankets, sheets or pillows may be used for this purpose. His toys should be those with which he will not hurt himself. The nurse must anticipate his needs. Waiting for a bedpan or urinal increases his nervousness.

Gradual exercise, both physical and mental, is given in accordance with the physician's orders as the child's condition improves.

Since these children move constantly, they need adequate nourishment. They should be fed frequently with a light, nourishing diet, high in protein and iron. Vitamin supplements should be provided. The child should be fed with a spoon rather than a fork, because he might injure himself upon the prongs.

Skin care is important. Soothing baths to relieve his nervousness are also part of good skin care. Constant motion is likely to produce abraded surfaces on his elbows and knees. His skin should be massaged with a soothing lotion or ointment, and his pajamas should be of soft material to protect his skin from friction on the bedclothes. If he is incontinent, the bed should be changed as soon as it is soiled or wet, and the skin of the buttocks and the genitalia should be washed and dried thoroughly.

Psychologic care is as important as physical care. The nurse must be patient and understanding because the child's movements constantly interfere with her giving care, and also because he is emotionally unstable and irritable. He should be allowed to help himself as much as the physician permits, since this gives him a feeling of independence. He needs both love and happiness in his contacts with his parents and nurses. The nurse should help the parents to give him these essentials.

Child-parent relations may have been strained by the child's behavior before his condition became so evident that he was taken to a physician. Some parents will feel guilty at having blamed him for clumsiness he could not help, and others will find it difficult to understand that his irritating behavior was and is due to his disease, and not under his control. They doubt whether his recovery will bring a return to good behavior. The nurse's understanding attitude will help them to see the situation objectively and to give the child the emotional support he badly needs.

The convalescent child may be taught at home or in a special school where the hours of study are short and the whole educational plan is adapted to his needs. During his convalescence, play material appropriate to his needs should be provided. At first toys which exercise large muscles should be given, and then those which promote the use of small muscles. In this way the child will learn muscle control again.

The *prognosis* is good. There is spontaneous recovery in eight to ten weeks. Attacks may recur, but recovery is eventually complete. The child's progress may be gauged by observing the improvement in his handwriting. He is therefore asked to write his name daily. The disease is seldom fatal, but death may occur, owing to exhaustion or cardiac disease.

Rheumatoid Arthritis (Still's Disease)

One of the conditions with which rheumatic polyarthritis may be confused is a chronic systemic disease, rheumatoid arthritis. Although this condition may have its onset during the preschool years, it is especially important during the school period because of the possible development of deformities which have a crippling effect on the child and may prevent normal growth and development.

Etiology, Pathology, Clinical Manifestations and Diagnosis. The cause is unknown, although the disease was thought in the past to be a response to infection somewhere in the body. It is unrelated, however, to infection with the group A streptococci as is rheumatic fever. Rheumatoid arthritis appears to occur in response to stress; it occurs in the spring months, in the temperate zone and in girls more often than in boys.

The *pathology* includes joint lesions involving the synovial membranes, joint capsules and ligaments. Fibrous or bony ankylosis, which may occur eventually, and flexion contractures result in deformities. The spleen, liver and lymph nodes may be enlarged. Carditis may occur. The erythrocyte sedimentation rate is increased, and the C-reactive protein is positive. The antistreptolysin O titer is seldom elevated.

The *clinical manifestations* may become apparent during the preschool period. The onset may be acute with fever up to 106°F. and possibly joint enlargement, or the onset may occur gradually. The elbows, shoulders, fingers, wrists, knees and ankles may become affected symmetrically. Local bone growth may be disturbed. The children guard their joints against movement. The fingers become swollen and taper from a thick base to a fine tip (*spindle fingers*). The child may have anorexia, appear quite anxious, and seem to prefer to be left alone. A macular eruption may be seen on the skin. The course of the disease is characterized by recurrent remissions and exacerbations until puberty; however, exacerbations may occur in adult life.

The *diagnosis* of rheumatoid arthritis may be confused with rheumatic fever (see p. 575), osteomyelitis (see p. 569), or leukemia (see p. 511).

Treatment, Nursing Care and Prognosis. The *treatment* must be understood by both parents and child, since the disease may be chronic, and its course is unpredictable. Therapy usually requires the services of many members of the medical team under the leadership of the pediatrician or the family physician. Therapy is aimed at promoting the normal growth and development of the child.

The components of rehabilitation are early diagnosis, alleviation of pain, correction of deformities and prevention of other deformities, and acceptance of the disease by the child and his family.

Anti-inflammatory drugs such as large doses of aspirin may be used. The nurse must watch constantly for toxic symptoms of aspirin if very large doses are given. Prednisone may also be used; however, unfortunately when the drug is discontinued, symptoms reappear. In the acute phase of rheumatoid arthritis the child may need to be fed, bathed and dressed by the nurse because of the severe involvement of his hands. Later the child should be encouraged to be as active as possible since inactivity hastens decalcification of the bones and encourages ankylosis. Physiotherapy is essential in the care of these children. If joints are held in flexion, muscles may become shortened. After inflammation in the joints has been reduced, the joints should be put through the full range of motion at least once a day. The child should lie on a firm mattress and should be encouraged to lie flat rather than curling up on his side, which may be his position of comfort. Half-shell splints applied to the legs at night help to prevent foot drop. Since these children would probably be more active at home than they are in the hospital, they should be discharged from the hospital as soon as possible.

The parents should be helped to learn how best to care for these children. If the children are given hot tub baths in the morning, the stiffness of joints which develops through the night is reduced. Since rheumatoid arthritis is a long-term condition, both the parents and the child need support from the members of the team. The child's anxiety about his condition should be relieved in order to sustain any remission of symptoms he may have. He should be encouraged to attend school and compete in nonstrenuous activities.

The *prognosis* for life and freedom from disability is good; however, there may be some residual deformity. The course of the disease may last for years.

Diabetes Mellitus

Incidence and Pathology. In diabetes mellitus the body is unable to metabolize carbohydrates, owing to insufficient production of insulin, an internal secretion of the pancreas. There is also abnormal metabolism of fat and protein. Approximately 5 per cent of all people with diabetes show the first symptoms in childhood. The disorder is not common among children, but it tends to be more serious than in later life. The disease is inherited as a recessive characteristic.

Diabetes mellitus having its onset before fifteen years of age is called *juvenile diabetes.* This disease must be distinguished from *diabetes insipidus,* which is a disease of the pituitary or the hypothalamus.

Since there is a deficiency of insulin, or since its effect is inhibited in diabetes mellitus, diabetic acidosis, coma and death may result. Hyperglycemia is produced, which, when it exceeds the normal threshold, causes glycosuria. Hyperglycemia initiates diuresis, and as a result excess glucose is excreted. In addition to glucose, electrolytes and water are lost from both the intracellular and extracellular compartments of the body.

Tissue breakdown is due in part to osmotic forces and in part to tissue catabolism because of the body's inability to use glucose for fuel. Protein and fat are oxidized more rapidly than is normal. Because of the increased rate of breakdown of fats, ketonuria results. Ketonuria, dehydration and kidney dysfunction result in acidosis.

In uncontrolled diabetes, hyperglycemia is found; body water, electrolytes and fixed base are lost; the plasma carbon dioxide content is lowered; acidosis develops; and glycogen stored in the muscles and liver is lost.

Nurses must be alert for evidence of diabetes in children, especially if there is a family history of the illness. They should educate the family about potential danger signals, such as a child's unusual thirst and frequent need to void.

Clinical Manifestations, Laboratory Studies and Diagnosis. Diabetes may develop slowly or may first be recognized when the child is in coma. The onset in children is generally more rapid than in adults, and the child is likely to be underweight at the onset. Obesity does not appear to be a factor in juvenile diabetes.

The *symptoms* are increased thirst and appetite, weight loss, polyuria (this may be the cause of bed wetting in children who had achieved night control of urination), possibly weakness and, over a period of time, pruritus, dry skin and excessive hairiness. In the nonacidotic stage the child will have glycosuria, possibly ketonuria, and hyperglycemia.

Nurses and all others responsible for the daily care of children should know the symptoms of *diabetic coma* or *acidosis.* Coma usually follows an infection in untreated diabetics who are not able to burn up carbohydrate and therefore utilize fat for energy. The symptoms are drowsiness, dry skin, cherry red lips and flushed cheeks, hyperpnea, acetone odor to the breath, abdominal pain, nausea and vomiting. The child in coma has Kussmaul breathing or severe hyperpnea, a rigid abdomen, rapid and weak pulse, lowered blood pressure and temperature and soft, sunken eyeballs.

Laboratory studies show a lowered carbon dioxide content of the blood and a shift of pH to the acid side. Albumin and casts may be present in the urine when the child has acidosis.

The *diagnosis* is based on the family history and the history of the child's previous health, and on the clinical manifestations and laboratory studies. A fasting hyperglycemia with glycosuria is diagnostic of diabetes mellitus. Other conditions, however, may have to be ruled out. Whenever glucosuria is found, a blood sugar determination should be made. If the blood sugar level is more than 200 mg. per 100 ml., a diagnosis of diabetes mellitus is tentatively made. A glucose tolerance test may show prolonged, high levels of sugar in the blood, indicating that the body cannot burn carbohydrates. A high white blood cell count may be present with diabetic acidosis.

Treatment. Management of the preadolescent diabetic is usually not too difficult if he and his parents understand the disease and his care. Management of the adolescent diabetic is more difficult because of his desire to rebel against the authority of his parents and the physician. If he is adequately treated, the diabetic should be able to compete with his peers in physical, mental and social development.

Treatment includes a *diet* which supports normal growth and development and satisfies the child's appetite, and the administration of insulin in sufficient amount to maintain glycemic equilibrium. An important aspect of treatment is instruction of the child and his parents so that they can manage the treatment in the home. This requires acceptance by the child and his family of the fact that he is essentially a normal child.

Should *diabetic acidosis* develop, treatment involves close cooperation of the physician, nurse and laboratory personnel. Laboratory examinations are needed to determine the blood sugar level and carbon dioxide-combining power or carbon dioxide content, and urinalysis for sugar and acetone. Intravenous therapy is used. Electrolytes, carbohydrate and water are given with insulin. Vitamins may also be given. If the child is in severe acidosis, with a pH of less than 7.1 and a carbon dioxide measurement of less than 6 mEq. per liter, sodium bicarbonate may be given. Urine should be collected each hour in order to guide modification of the dosage of insulin and carbohydrates as therapy progresses. Warmth and comfort are essential for the child with acidosis. The nurse should watch for changes in color, type of respiration and degree of consciousness. Gastric aspiration may be carried out to relieve distention, to prevent pulmonary aspiration of vomitus and to hasten the time when the child can take fluids by mouth. Sodium bicarbonate solution may be introduced through the tube into the stomach after the stomach has been emptied. Large doses of appropriate antibiotics may be given if infection is present.

Oral feedings may be started when the child regains consciousness, usually after twelve to sixteen hours of parenteral therapy, and then carbohydrate and electrolyte mixtures are given. This dietary stage is followed with an adequate fluid diet. Small doses of insulin are given to cover the oral intake of carbohydrates; the amount is based on the findings of urinalysis for sugar. While taking oral feedings the child should be checked for symptoms of insulin shock or diabetic acidosis. An average diet may be given in a few days if he shows no untoward symptoms.

Management after correction of the acidosis or of the child in whom diabetes was not adequately controlled requires the same teamwork that is necessary in the acute crisis, but nursing care becomes the center of the program. The child must be treated individually; each child needs a satisfactory diet and insulin dosage. The diet should be approximately that of a normal child and similar to the family's diet. The specific requirements of the diet are that it supply caloric intake for activity and growth, sufficient protein intake for growth, and the required vitamins and minerals.

One of two types of diets may be ordered. (1) Quantities of food may be *measured.* Many parents find that children feel more secure when a definite dietary program is ordered and exactly followed. (2) The so-called *unrestricted* or *free diet* is that of a normal child. It is restricted only in that excesses, such as high carbohydrate intake, are avoided. On this diet the child feels as free as a normal child because he may eat practically whatever he wishes. The present trend in therapy appears to be toward the unrestricted diet.

In general, the child is on a stabilized, measured diet only at the beginning of treatment. Upon discharge from the hospital he and his parents should be given a list of foods which are exchangeable in planning his meals for the day. For such a diet gross household measures are adequate. They are not as rigid as in a weighed diet. Occasional deviations are not important. The child on such a diet should receive a satisfactory intake with adequate distribution of caloric intake at various meals. He should learn to manage his diet himself as he grows older.

The child should be stabilized on his diet and the amount of insulin he needs while he is in the hospital. Since the amount of exercise he takes changes his needs, for several days before his discharge he should take about the same amount of exercise as he will when he is at home. The diet should be so planned that his appetite is satisfied and his growth and development are normal when he is leading the same kind of life his friends lead.

Insulin is a specially prepared extract of the pancreas. Injected into the body, it enables the body to burn sugar. All juvenile diabetics need insulin. At present it is necessary to give it by subcutaneous injection. Although adult diabetics have profited from sulfonylureas (orally administered hypoglycemic agents) and the biguanides (Phenformin-DBI), these do not provide a reliable replacement for insulin in the treatment of diabetic children.

Seven types of insulin are used in the treatment of children. *Regular (unmodified insulin)* or *Semi-Lente insulin* affects the blood sugar in thirty minutes after injection, and the effect lasts from six to twelve hours. *Protamine zinc insulin* and *Ultra-Lente insulin* affect the blood sugar in approximately four to eight hours after injection, their influence lasting for twenty-four hours or more. *NPH insulin, globin insulin* and *Lente insulin* produce initial and long-maintained effects; the time in which these preparations are effective is between that of unmodified insulin and protamine zinc insulin. The physician generally orders a combination of unmodified insulin and another type which produces prolonged action. Both Lente insulin and NPH insulin can be given in the same syringe with unmodified insulin, but protamine zinc insulin cannot.

The dose of insulin is estimated on the basis of qualitative tests of the urine for sugar. Urine specimens should be collected at the following hours: before breakfast, at 7 or 8 a.m., before lunch, at 11:30 to 12 noon, before the evening meal, at 5 to 6 p.m., and before bedtime, at 7 to 9 p.m. Actually, another specimen obtained approximately thirty minutes after the initial specimen will be more accurate when tested than the first. Obtaining the second specimen from a young child may be difficult, however; therefore it is probably wise to test the urine each time the child voids. Usually Clinitest tablets are used in preference to other methods. If too large a dose of insulin, too little food or too much exercise is taken, insulin shock may result. With an even balance between the diet and the dosage of insulin the urine should be essentially sugar-free. Some physicians prefer to have recorded a trace of sugar in the urine, since the danger of insulin shock from a constantly negative result would be prevented.

Several factors are important in varying the need for insulin. Adjustment must be made periodically in the relation of *diet* to insulin dosage. All children need *exercise,* but diabetics must take exercise that requires a relatively definite amount of energy expenditure. Exercise produces a lowering of the blood sugar level and may cause shock in children taking insulin. Only when the diet and exercise are standardized is it possible to give the requisite amount of insulin. Changes in diet and in energy output make adjustment of the dose to the child's needs essential. This is difficult because of the differ-

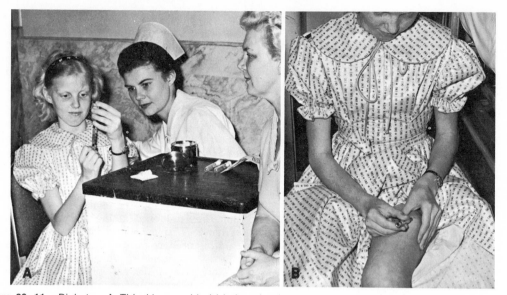

Figure 23–11. Diabetes. *A,* This 11-year-old girl is learning how to prepare her dosage of insulin. Her mother, who has already learned the procedure, is interested in her progress. *B,* Having practiced the procedure, this child is now able to inject the insulin and thus to assume more responsibility for her own care.

ence in the child's activity on school days and on vacation days, and in wet and sunny weather. The child should always carry sugar with him and take if it he feels the symptoms of shock. If unusually strenuous activity is planned, insulin dosage must be reduced proportionally. Some physicians maintain diabetic children on an insulin dosage which permits some spilling of sugar daily so that their margin of safety is a little greater with changes in the amount of exercise they have.

Since *infection* increases the need for insulin, the child may go into acidosis easily if he has an infection. During such periods additional amounts of insulin may be needed to prevent glycosuria. The amount is reduced during convalescence.

Emotional disturbances also increase the child's need for insulin. Diabetic children who are emotionally stable can be regulated more easily than those who are easily upset.

Adjustment in dosage may also need to be made on the basis of *body growth.* Some children require more insulin as they approach puberty and adolescence, but some do not.

Nursing Care. An important part of the nursing care of the diabetic child is helping him and his parents to develop positive attitudes toward his condition. Probably the central problem is to help them accept the fact that the child can be healthy and active if dietary rules are followed and insulin is given in adjustment to his needs. Their initial attitude is likely to be that restriction is necessary only when the child is sick. The parents and the child must learn that constant care is necessary. The nurse should listen to the parents when they express their feelings about the illness and try to reconcile both parents and child to maintaining the prescribed diet and dosage of insulin, together with regular exercise.

As with other illnesses, the child having diabetes should be encouraged to express his feelings about his disease and his treatment. Many children believe that they are being punished because of the dietary restrictions and the use of injections in treatment. The child's questions should be answered, and he should also be encouraged to reduce some of his anxiety through play.

If a free diet is ordered, the child will have little problem in controlling his food intake. If a measured diet is ordered, the nurse must condition the child to self-control and make it easy for him, and instruct the mother in the need for, and the means of, helping the child conform to his regulated life. He should have exercise *after* meals. All tempting but restricted food should be kept out of the way as far as possible. Nevertheless school children must learn to go without, while others eat, the foods they are denied. The diet should be made attractive. Snacks should be permitted and planned for at bedtime and between meals. The child should understand that if he reports breaks in dietary rules, he will not be punished or scolded, but that unreported breaks may cause sudden sickness.

No attempt should be made to hide the fact that the child is a diabetic. He and those about him should know this so as to understand his restriction of diet and need for a regular life. But he should not be permitted to use illness as a defense against accepting the role of a well child. He should be encouraged to assume his share of family responsibilities. He should also participate on an equal basis with his peer group, not looking on his diabetes as a handicap.

Table 23-1 presents material which nurses will find useful in understanding the child's treatment in the hospital and care at home. If this information is given to parents, it supplements, but does not take the place of, individual instruction which the physicians, nurses and dietitians will give the parents and the child. Understanding the care given the child in the hospital not only brings about better cooperation between the child, his parents and the nurses, but also is the basis for the acceptance and following of the program for his care at home. The nurse should be thoroughly familiar with the information the table gives. Student nurses will find it an aid in learning the total care of the diabetic child and in teaching parents and children this care.

The teacher and the school nurse should be aware of the child's illness and the manifestations of shock and coma so that they can help him in such emergencies. The child's parents and the school nurse should keep emergency kits containing glucagon available for use in case the child becomes unconscious from insulin shock. The school personnel, parents and the child must realize that readmission to the hospital will be necessary for evaluation and ad-

justment of the diet and insulin dosage.

The school nurse can also help the child in school to collect and test urine specimens by providing a place for him to do so privately. The child should be taught to record the results of his urine tests on a homemade or commercially available chart. The importance of honesty in keeping this record should be stressed.

Children who have diabetes may learn more about their disease by attending a summer camp for diabetics. Programs vary from camp to camp, but all attempt to develop the child's self-confidence, self-esteem and independence.

As the child approaches preadolescence and the rapid growth spurt his need for food increases. Since at this time his need to be like his peers is great, the child may eat what they eat even though he knows that he should not do so. The preadolescent diabetic then needs support and understanding so that he can keep his disease under control. If the child is threatened or punished for eating food he should not eat, further dietary indiscretions may result. The diet may need to be readjusted in order that the preadolescent gets the food he needs.

The period of adolescence may be a difficult one for the diabetic youth and for his parents. While the young person may wish to become independent and rebel against restraints such as are involved in his own care, his parents may seek to protect him, thus keeping him dependent on them. The social worker with other team

Table 23–1. *Care of the Diabetic Child*

SYMPTOMS OF INSULIN SHOCK AND DIABETIC COMA

Insulin Shock (Due to overdose of insulin, reduction of diet or increase in exercise)		*Diabetic Coma* (Acidosis)
Early manifestations:	Pallor Weakness Dizziness Changes in disposition* Sweating Tremor Sudden hunger Dilated pupils	Changes in mental state (lethargic)* Vomiting Abdominal pain
Severe reactions:	Semiconsciousness Later: convulsions, coma, death Low blood sugar Urine sugar-free Acetone absent	Acetone odor on breath Dehydration Hyperpnea Face flushed Lips cherry red Little perspiration Blood sugar high, low carbon dioxide Sugar and acetone present in urine

*The emotional reaction of the child is characteristic of him. He may cry, be hostile or appear happy.

The child and his parents should recognize the need for immediate assistance if symptoms of shock or acidosis occur. In case of shock the child should be given fruit juice or sugar. The child should carry a lump of sugar with him and, if he recognizes symptoms of shock, take the sugar. If the child becomes unconscious, he should be kept warm. The parents or school nurse should inject glucagon in the amount of 1 mg. When the child regains consciousness, sugar can be given by mouth. If the child does not respond, he should be seen by a physician who will administer glucose intravenously. Recovery after treatment for shock is usually rapid.

Table 23–1. *Care of the Diabetic Child (Continued)*

GENERAL CARE

1. Skin care to prevent infection
   a. Give frequent baths, at least every other day
   b. Provide inexpensive shoes which may be discarded when the child outgrows them
   c. Teach the child to report any break in the skin and treat it promptly

2. Maintenance of resistance to infection
   a. Dress the child appropriately according to the temperature, not the season of the year
   b. Keep the child away from anyone who has an upper respiratory tract or other infection
   c. Report infections promptly to the physician
   d. Immunize the child against common communicable diseases

3. Proper elimination

4. Regulation of exercise
   a. In the hospital keep him as busy as he would be at home
   b. At home encourage him to take moderate exercise regularly each day

5. Accuracy in saving of urine specimens
   a. Save and test a specimen of urine at prescribed hours. Parents and child can be taught to test urine specimens
   b. Be careful that the child does not dilute the urine to cover a break in adhering to his diet

6. Diet
   a. Let the child eat with other diabetics in the hospital, for he is then more likely to accept his diet
   b. Teach the child to keep to the diet ordered by the physician. Give the child the list of allowed exchanges of food if such is ordered
   c. Make adherence to the diet as easy as possible by varying it as much as is permitted
   d. Teach the child to manage his own diet as early as possible

7. Administration of insulin
   a. Parents and child should learn the reason for and the procedure of administration of insulin
   b. Children 7 to 10 years of age can usually be taught to give insulin to themselves (even an intelligent younger child can learn). The earlier the responsibility is given the child, the better it is for him. The public health nurse can provide assistance with this procedure to parents and child at home
      (1) Make the explanation simple. After the nurse has explained the procedure initially, another diabetic child can assist him better than an adult can, perhaps because he has more time to spend on showing how and why each step is done
      (2) Let the child practice frequently under supervision
         (a) Use routine sites of injections: upper right arm, upper left arm, left thigh, right thigh (each extremity may be used for several weeks if injections are given $1/2$ inch apart)
         (b) Check the dose measured by the child until his accuracy is proved
         (c) Pinch the skin, or teach the child to do so, when using a site on the thigh, because this minimizes the pain of injection
         (d) Do not give insulin too near the surface of the skin

8. Records
   a. The child should be taught to keep daily records of the insulin dose, diet, and urine test findings until he learns about his illness and it is under control

9. The child's part in his recovery
   a. Keep the child under supervision as long as necessary, but give him independence as soon as possible
   b. Get his cooperation in
      (1) Voluntary self-control in diet so that other children cannot tempt him
      (2) Taking regular exercise
      (3) Honest reporting if he transgresses against the physician's orders
      (4) Not fooling his parents with faked symptoms of insulin shock
      (5) Avoiding self-pity or exaggerating his handicap
      (6) Carrying on his person at all times an identification card or tag which reads "I HAVE DIABETES" and gives his name, address, telephone number and his physician's name and number where he can be reached
   c. Guide the child to normal adolescence by understanding his aggressiveness, withdrawal or rebellion against restraint. Bring him, through understanding of his problem, to normal adulthood in which he can take his place in society

members can help both parents and child in their struggle so that the adolescent can reach adulthood and take a productive place in society. Psychiatric assistance may be necessary to achieve this goal.

Complications, Course and Prognosis. *Complications* are uncommon except in children who have been inadequately treated or have had the condition for a long time. The following may possibly result from diabetes: lack of development, stunted growth, amenorrhea and lack of development of secondary sex characteristics. Children may also suffer cataracts, gangrene and arteriosclerosis after the disease has been present for years. Infections are common and heal more slowly than is normal in the poorly treated diabetic child. These include infections of the skin, respiratory tract and lower urinary tract. Dental caries is also common.

Complications which may occur as a result of insulin injections include atrophy of the subcutaneous fat and allergy to insulin.

The *course* and *prognosis* depend on the accuracy of control measures. Serious degenerative lesions appear in young adults who have had diabetes mellitus for ten to twenty years. These include arteriosclerosis with hypertension, nephropathy and retinal changes.

Precocious Sexual Development (Precocious Puberty)

Etiology and Treatment. Precocious sexual development can be diagnosed when secondary sexual characteristics appear before the child is eight to ten years of age.

These children may be divided into two groups: those with true precocious puberty, and those with precocious pseudopuberty, in which no sperm or ova are formed.

Most cases of *true precocious puberty*—with menstruation and ovulation in girls and the presence of sperm in the discharge of the organs of reproduction in boys—are due to a constitutional premature maturation of the endocrine control of the genital tissues. Although the appearance of the child may be embarrassing, other children eventually catch up with the preadolescent in development. There is a decided spurt in physical growth resulting in early epiphyseal closure of the long bones. The eventual height of these children therefore tends to be below average on maturity. The physician will explain this condition to the parents and to the child. These children should be guarded against sexual abuses, which, in a girl, may lead to pregnancy. No treatment is necessary for this condition.

A second type of true precocious puberty is due to a central nervous system infection such as encephalitis or a lesion which usually involves the hypothalamus or the floor of the third ventricle. Convulsions or mental retardation may also be present in these children. Treatment should be directed to the cause itself. The prognosis depends upon the cause.

Precocious pseudopuberty, the least common cause for precocious puberty, is due to a tumor of the ovary or the adrenal cortex, or the accidental ingestion of estrogens or androgens. Treatment consists in surgery or the withdrawal of the medication. The prognosis depends upon the cause of the condition.

Head Trauma

Active school children acquire head injuries usually as a result of automobile accidents, falls from bicycles, falls when climbing, or being hit on the head when playing.

Cerebral Concussion

Clinical Manifestations, Treatment and Nursing Care. The *clinical manifestations* of cerebral concussion following a sudden blow on the head include a transient loss of consciousness, headache, pallor, vomiting, apathy and irritability. If the child is unconscious for a prolonged time with varying degrees of amnesia, the diagnosis of *cerebral contusion* or *laceration* should be made. Convulsions may occur.

The *treatment* and *nursing care* for the first twelve to twenty-four hours after a head injury include the following: careful observation at least every two hours of the level of consciousness, recording of the vital signs, and notation of the movement of the eyes and equality of the pupils, including their size and reaction. Any change in these signs or deepening of the level of unconsciousness may indicate intracranial bleeding. If the child is very restless, a sedative such as chloral hydrate may be ordered. The side rails should be padded to prevent injury in case a convulsion occurs. The child's bladder should be examined for overdistention, which may be a cause of continued restlessness.

Skull Fracture

Clinical Manifestations, Diagnosis, Treatment and Nursing Care. The *clinical manifestations* of a basilar fracture include blood in the external auditory canal, a discolored tympanic membrane, periorbital ecchymosis, epistaxis or bleeding from the mouth, subconjunctival hemorrhage or facial weakness. The *diagnosis* of fracture may be made on the basis of roentgenograms of the skull.

The *treatment* of a depressed fracture includes elevation of the depressed area of the skull. Children having linear fractures usually require treatment similar to that for those having cerebral concussion. Repair of the dura must be considered. Antibiotics may be given as necessary.

The *nursing care* of these children includes careful observation for changes of vital signs indicating increased intracranial pressure. If cerebrospinal fluid is leaking from the nostril or ear, the nares of the external auditory canal should not be irrigated or plugged with cotton.

Extradural Hematoma

Clinical Manifestations and Treatment. The *clinical manifestations* of extradural hematoma are usually seen within twenty-four hours after the injury even if the child has no skull fracture. The child may have been unconscious immediately after the injury, become conscious, then lapse into a stupor or coma. He may have signs of increased intracranial pressure, ipsilateral dilatation of the pupil and hemiparesis.

The *treatment* consists in immediate neurosurgery to prevent compression of the brain stem. Post-traumatic epilepsy may follow head injury.

Brain Tumor

Etiology, Incidence, Clinical Manifestations and Types. The majority of brain tumors in children are due to abnormal growth of cells already present in the brain; few are due to metastases from noncerebral neoplasms. Generally these tumors are located beneath the tentorium cerebri. (Most brain tumors in adults are located above it.)

The *incidence* of brain tumors among children is only one sixth that among adults. Tumors increase in incidence up to six years of age and then remain at a uniform level during the school period.

Most of the *symptoms* are due to increased intracranial pressure. Such symptoms include *vomiting,* usually in the morning, at first nonprojectile, but later projectile; *headache, diplopia* and *head enlargement,* if the tumor occurs before the sutures are firmly united; and *changes in mental awareness,* such as lethargy, behavioral changes, drowsiness, stupor, coma and ultimately death. Many times the initial personality changes are first noted by the child's school teacher or school nurse, who may encourage the parent to have the child evaluated medically. Changes in *vital signs* are important in diagnosing increased intracranial pressure. Convulsions are rare in infratentorial tumors, but may occur in some children having these lesions.

Other clinical manifestations depend on the type and location of the tumor.

Five types of tumors may be seen, as follows. *Medulloblastoma* is a fairly common tumor in children. The incidence is greatest during school age and reaches its highest point at five to six years. It is a highly malignant, rapidly developing tumor usually found in the cerebellum. Clinical manifestations are unsteadiness when the child walks, anorexia and vomiting, and headache, usually in the morning. Papilledema and ataxia are present. The child is drowsy, and nystagmus can be observed. Death usually results in less than a year.

Astrocytoma may occur at any age, but the peak incidence is at eight years. The tumor is usually located in the cerebellum. The clinical manifestations differentiate this tumor from others. The onset is insidious, and the course is slow. Signs of focal disturbance or increase in intracranial pressure may occur. The child may have ataxia, hypotonia, diminished reflexes and nystagmus. Papilledema is present. Without operation the prognosis is poor. Total surgical removal with complete cure is possible.

Ependymoma is located in the fourth ventricle or in one of the lateral ventricles of the brain. Increased intracranial pressure and other manifestations are present, depending on the location of the tumor. The child will have vomiting, headache, enlarged head and unsteady gait. Hydrocephalus may occur. The treatment is by incomplete internal compression and roentgen therapy.

Craniopharyngioma occurs in late childhood. The tumor is near the pituitary gland. There is pituitary or hypothalamic dysfunction. The most common hormonal disturbance observed is diabetes insipidus. The child may be stunted in growth and may have myxedema or delayed puberty. The cerebral disturbance results in defects of the visual fields. Later there may be memory or personality disturbances. There is evidence of increased intracranial pressure due to obstruction of the flow of cerebrospinal fluid. Headache and vomiting are noted. A roentgenogram of the skull reveals separated sutures. Surgical removal of the entire tumor is usually impossible. Roentgen therapy may control for years a tumor which was not surgically removed.

Brain stem gliomas have a peak incidence among children about seven years old. The clinical manifestations are multiple cranial nerve palsies, ataxia of the trunk and little sensory loss, without indications of increased intracranial pressure. The course is slow, but the tumor is inoperable. Roentgen therapy may permit the child to survive for a while.

Diagnosis and Treatment. Early *diagnosis* of brain tumor may be impossible because of its insidious beginning. The diagnosis is based on the history of symptoms of increased intracranial pressure or focal cerebral disturbances, and the findings on physical examination. An electroencephalogram assists in locating superficial supratentorial tumors. Pneumoencephalogram may be done, but this procedure is not without danger. A positive *Macewen's sign* is associated with separation of the sutures. Roentgenograms may show splitting of the suture lines or calcification within the tumor. Ventriculograms and arteriograms help to localize the tumor. Lumbar puncture should not be done when increased intracranial pressure is present, because of the possibility of pushing the medulla into the cervical spine. Brain scans performed on children may be useful as diagnostic screening procedures for suspected intracranial neoplasms.

The symptoms listed under the different types of tumors may also be found in children with encephalitis, brain abscess or some degenerative brain disease, and such conditions must be ruled out before a diagnosis of brain tumor is made unqualifiedly.

The *treatment* may be surgical or with deep radiation. In surgery as much of the tumor as possible is excised. Most brain tumors cannot be removed completely. Deep radiation may be of value in some cases. With recent advances in anesthesiology and with improved endocrinologic therapy, especially with the corticosteroids, the results of neurosurgery have been improved. Even when complete cure is not possible, symptoms may be relieved and the child may be able to enjoy life for a variable time.

Nursing Care. EMOTIONAL SUPPORT. Both the parents and the child should become familiar before operation with the nurse who will care for the child postoperatively. The relation should be one of mutual trust. The parents are naturally anxious. They as well as the child should be prepared for neurosurgery, for how the child will look postoperatively and for the treatment and procedures which will be necessary after operation. Conversation that would be anxiety-producing should not be carried on where the child can hear what is said, even though he appears to be unconscious. Parents need continued understanding and support from the nurse during the preoperative and postoperative periods. Maintenance of his general nutrition and of his and his parents' morale and outlook about the condition is important.

PREOPERATIVE CARE AND OBSERVATIONS. Preoperative care consists in placing the child in a bed with crib sides or, if he is too large for a crib, side bars, because of the danger of his being confused or drowsy and falling out of bed.

The child should receive a nourishing diet. If he vomits, he can be refed, because usually he is not nauseated. Enemas are not given because of the danger of increasing the intracranial pressure.

Observations by the nurse in order to help the physician in localizing the tumor and appraising the increasing intracranial pressure are of the utmost importance. She should listen to the complaints or comments of the older child and observe children of all ages. She should chart both complaints and observations fully and with the conditions under which they occurred.

Specifically she should note lowering of the pulse rate and change in its nature, gradual or sudden change in body temperature, decrease in the respiratory rate and change in the nature of respiration, especially irregular respiration, and any change in blood pressure, particularly a rise in the systolic pressure with widening pulse pressure.

The nurse should record vomiting, and indications of headache, lethargy and drowsiness. Any convulsions should be recorded in full. (Seizure precautions should be followed —see page 351.) If possible, the nurse should ascertain whether there is limitation of the visual field or whether the child sees a double image of a single object. She should record the degree and situation of muscular weakness. Fecal and urinary incontinence or retention is routinely recorded. All complaints of pain and discomfort are noted.

The nurse should know where emergency equipment—such as oxygen, aspirator, sterile gloves, ventricular tap tray, emergency drugs and other supplies and equipment—is kept in case they are needed. Whenever the nurse is in doubt, she should call the supervisor or clinical instructor for instructions and explanations of the care the child requires or the procedure to be used for a specific treatment which must be done.

POSTOPERATIVE CARE. Postoperative care is exacting and requires both skill and experience in the nursing care of children undergoing brain surgery. Parenteral fluid therapy is given when the child cannot take fluids by mouth. Any difficulties with the intravenous setup should be reported at once. The rate of absorption of fluid should be noted carefully. Too rapid administration may produce a dangerous increase in intracranial pressure. Mouth care is essential to prevent parotitis and monilia infection.

The child's position immediately postoperatively is lying flat on the unaffected side. After the danger of vomiting has passed and the nasopharynx no longer needs to be aspirated, his position should be changed frequently from side to back in order to prevent pressure areas and hypostatic pneumonia. The surgeon may prefer that the head be slightly elevated. For turning the child who has had surgery in the cerebellar area the nurse's movements should be slow, and his body should be kept in a straight line; the position of the head should not be changed or turned. In moving the child the head, neck and shoulders should be well supported so that no twisting of these parts of the body occurs (Fig. 23-12). Two nurses are needed to move the child of school age. Further measures to prevent the formation of pressure areas on the child's head or body include the use of a sponge rubber pad over the mattress and the use of cotton doughnuts under pressure areas such as the ears or the side of the head.

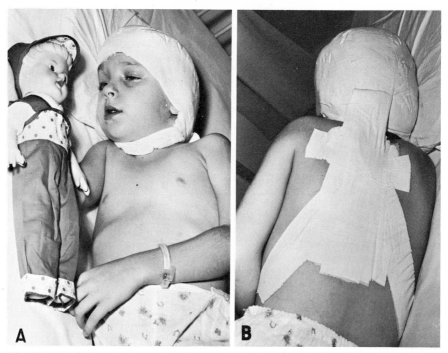

Figure 23–12. Suboccipital craniectomy dressings assist in keeping the head in correct alignment with the child's body even when the child is turned. *A*, Front view; *B*, back view.

The patient should be kept clean and dry at all times. Back care is given frequently, and the area around pressure points is massaged. If paralysis or spasticity of the extremities occurs, pillows or other support should be used. Foot drop must be prevented by adequate support.

The vital signs are taken as ordered by the physician—every fifteen minutes at first and then less frequently as the condition warrants —to determine indications of rising intracranial pressure.

The nasopharynx is aspirated as necessary. The child is encouraged to breathe deeply at regular periods, hourly or as ordered.

If shock occurs, warm blankets are applied. Emergency stimulants, fluids for intravenous therapy and oxygen should be kept on hand for immediate use. The foot of the bed is usually not raised because of the danger of increasing intracranial pressure. The nurse must be alert for, and immediately report, urinary incontinence or retention.

Restraints should not be used unless they are absolutely necessary, because the child may struggle against them and increase intracranial pressure. They should be used if the child pulls at his dressings, tries to dislodge the intravenous or gavage tube or in any way tries to injure himself. Elbow restraints, mitts for the hands or clove hitch restraints (see p. 180) may then be used.

If the head dressing becomes wet with drain-age, the area is circled with gentian violet. If there is rapid enlargement of the stained area or if bright red blood appears on the dressing, the surgeon should be notified immediately. The nurse may reinforce the dressings with sterile pads held in place with a bandage. Meningitis may result from contamination of the surgical area.

Edema of the face, eyelids and brain may result from injury during operation. Because lacrimal secretion cannot circulate over the eyes when edema is present, the conjunctivae may become dry and infected. Warm saline irrigations of the eyes, eye drops or the application of cold compresses to the swollen eyelids may be ordered to prevent this complication. Some physicians recommend that the eyelids be taped closed with small pieces of cellophane or covered with eye shields. Corticosteroids or other hormonal substitutes may be given preoperatively and postoperatively to lower intracranial pressure by reducing edema.

Hyperthermia may be caused by intracranial edema, bleeding, or disturbance of the heat-regulating center. The temperature should be taken at least every half-hour when it is elevated. Methods to reduce fever include undressing the child and covering him with a sheet or only a diaper over the pubic area, reduction of room temperature, tepid sponge bath, cold water mattress, ice water enemas or small retention enemas containing aspirin. The body temperature is usually not brought down to normal, but it may be kept fairly low. If the child cannot swallow, gavage feedings may be given. If they are given, distention should be noted.

As soon as the child has ceased to vomit and shows signs of being able to swallow, small amounts of water may be given. Nourishing liquids and a soft diet are added gradually. Fluids and foods should not be encouraged too much because vomiting, which increases intracranial pressure, may result. Solid foods are given as soon as the child can tolerate them.

As the child recovers from operation he should be helped to gain greater independence in his own care. He should be given opportunities to play alone and with other children. Parents need assurance that he should continue to be given independence after discharge. They should also understand that the child needs continued medical supervision after discharge.

Course and Prognosis. The *course* depends on the type of tumor involved. Illness may last from a few weeks to several years. The *prognosis* for living into adulthood is very poor.

Minimal Cerebral Dysfunction (The Brain-Damaged Child) and School Underachievement

Incidence, Etiology, Clinical Manifestations, Diagnosis and Treatment. The term *minimal cerebral dysfunction* is one applied loosely to an extremely heterogeneous, chronically disabled group of children. It is not a clear-cut entity or specific diagnosis. This condition may be due to actual brain damage, but it may also be due to genetic, cytogenic and morphogenic developmental defects or maturational irregularities of the nervous system. The number of these children appears to be increasing either because of improved diagnostic skill or because more of these children are living because of improved medical science.

Children having minimal cerebral dysfunction may have behavioral and learning disabilities which are observed only after they enter school. These children are characterized by psychologic, behavioral, academic and neurologic deviations from the normal. They may have one or many of the following problems: difficulty in paying attention in class, and problems in the general areas of remembering, language, conceptualization, perception, impulsivity and sensory and motor function such as hyperactivity, underactivity or awkwardness. These children have normal, near-normal or above-normal intelligence, although they may have difficulty in learning; therefore they can be distinguished from the mentally retarded group.

Management of the child having minimal cerebral dysfunction is best accomplished through the efforts of all involved, the parents, pediatrician as leader of the team, specialized physicians, psychologists, school administrator, teachers, social workers, school nurses, and nurses in the hospital when he is admitted for diagnosis or treatment.

Evaluation of the child is made on the basis of behavior, academic performance, psychologic evaluation, a carefully taken medical history, and medical and neurologic examinations, including an electroencephalogram among other tests. Positive therapeutic results require detailed evaluation of the child's status and a plan based upon the assets and liabilities of the individual and his environment. Establishment of a firm, consistent environment with attention to the social problems of the family probably contributes more to therapy than reliance on drugs.

Nursing Care. The nurse's role in the care of the child having minimal cerebral dysfunction includes early case finding and cooperation in the efforts of the team caring for the child. These efforts involve diagnosing and providing counseling for the parents, including the need for appropriate pedagogic techniques and occasional psychotherapy.

Nursing intervention when the child is hospitalized should be directed toward controlling an overstimulating environment and providing a stable structured environment in which he can achieve success. Since the child has difficulty in adjusting to changing conditions, the nurse should provide for continuity of care and avoidance of tension-producing situations, possibly through the consistency of nurses assigned to his care or by the mother's staying with the child. The nurse should tell the child in a simple, direct manner what is expected of him. She should also praise him when he accomplishes desired behaviors. He will respond to understanding guidance and approval. A confident attitude toward his abilities and liabilities will improve his self-image.

If the mother lives in the hospital with the child, the nurse can observe the mother-child relations for emerging emotional problems. The social growth of a child having perceptual disorders is poor if the parents refuse to recognize his problems and consider him just a "bad child." The nurse should also have knowledge of the community agencies to which the family can be referred. The parents should be told what to expect from their child now and in the future and that he will probably improve with maturation and therapy.

Legg-Calvé-Perthes Disease (Perthes's Disease, Coxa Plana)

Etiology and Incidence. Perthes's disease is an aseptic necrosis of the head of the femur.

The cause is unknown. It is a self-limited disease occurring in children between five and ten years of age. The condition affects boys more frequently than girls, possibly as a result of trauma to the hip.

Pathology, Clinical Manifestations, Treatment, Nursing Care and Prognosis. The *pathology* may be divided into three stages, each lasting about nine months to a year. The first stage is an aseptic necrosis. Roentgen films show a relative opacity of the epiphysis. The bone becomes necrotic. The second stage is revascularization. On roentgen study the epiphysis is shown as fragmented and mottled. The third stage is reossification. Roentgen examination shows the head of the femur to be gradually re-forming.

If weight is placed on the leg, the head of the femur tends to become flattened and mushroom-shaped. Later in life degenerative changes occur because of discrepancies in shape between the acetabulum and the head of the femur.

The *clinical manifestations* are those of synovitis, i.e. a limp, and pain in the hip. The pain is often referred to the knee. Muscle spasm is not commonly severe. Motion is usually restricted only in relation to abduction and rotation.

The most important point in *treatment* is avoidance of weight bearing. Some physicians believe that the child should have complete rest and traction on the leg during the course of the disease. Others immobilize the hip by surgery, casts or braces to prevent the deformity resulting from weight bearing.

The *nursing care* includes stressing to both the child and the parents the importance of not bearing weight on the extremity for several months. The child should be kept in bed on a firm mattress and bed board. If the child is in traction, he may be either supine or prone. He should be turned at least every four hours. He must be encouraged to move his joints and to maintain good muscle tone. If a cast is applied, he should be cared for as outlined previously (see p. 227).

One of the most difficult aspects in the care of the very active school child who has Perthes's disease is the necessity of prolonged immobility. If the child is to be confined to bed for a prolonged time, the home should be evaluated and guidance given to the family for implementation of their facilities for his care. The ingenuity of the mother or nurse may be taxed in providing activities which will keep him occupied. The child might possibly be referred to an institution for the care of convalescent children.

The younger the child at the onset of the condition, the more likely is he to retain a spherical than to acquire a deformed, flattened head of the femur. Complete recovery depends on when treatment was given and whether gross deformity of the hip occurred.

Dental Problems

Pedodontia has as its main purposes the maintenance of healthy teeth, the prevention of disease, the treatment of defects and the restoration of function. Common dental problems include dental caries (see p. 477), malocclusion, traumatic injuries and discolored teeth.

Dental caries is the leading dental problem of children. There seems to be a positive correlation between parental dental health education (see p. 391) and the incidence of dental caries in children. Thus it would be expected that children from socioeconomically deprived areas would have more dental caries than those from other groups. Genetic factors, adequate diet, good oral hygiene and the use of fluoride are important in the incidence of this condition. Dental caries in children is treated much as it is in adults.

Malocclusion is a term which is applied to irregular positioning of the teeth and the improper coming together of the teeth when the jaws are closed. The causes of malocclusion may be inherited, such as the size of teeth and jaw, or may be acquired, such as due to harmful habits or early loss of teeth through decay. This condition results in decreased masticatory functioning and possibly a disfigured mouth, facial deformities, faulty speech, nutritional disturbances and emotional problems. The dentist should evaluate a child's occlusion as it develops. An orthodontist, a dentist who is especially trained to diagnose and treat malocclusion, should be consulted if malocclusion is evident. If the deciduous teeth are lost prematurely or if there is congenital absence of teeth, treatment should be begun early in order to prevent malocclusion. Treatment may include either placement of space-maintaining appliances or actual movement of the teeth. Preventive orthodontics may save many children from becoming dental cripples.

Children having *traumatic injuries* to the teeth should be examined immediately after the accident. The kind of treatment given depends on whether it is a deciduous or permanent tooth, the stage of tooth development, the nature of the fracture and the status of the dental pulp.

The normal color of the permanent teeth is usually darker than that of the deciduous teeth; thus parents become anxious lest their child's teeth be permanently *discolored*. They should be told that when all the permanent teeth have erupted, their color will probably be uniform. Teeth may be stained by extrinsic agents. These stains can usually be removed by cleaning and polishing by the dental hygienist.

EMOTIONAL DISTURBANCES

By the time the child is six years of age his personality is fairly well established. He should be free to gain further skill in the use of his body and mind and to develop both stronger inner controls and relations with children and adults outside his family. He needs time to achieve these goals; during the same period he is making a good adjustment at school.

If the child shows behavior problems which are symptoms of emotional disturbances during the school years, his response usually resembles some adult reactions to difficulties. The child may present neurotic symptoms such as nervousness, finger-sucking, nail-biting and fears; school phobia; conduct disorders (the problem child); language disorders such as stuttering; and psychosomatic illnesses such as anorexia, overeating, constipation, colitis, abdominal pain and enuresis.

These disorders, serious in themselves, may also prevent the child from making a good adjustment at school. *Failure in school may thus be due to emotional disturbance as well as to mental retardation.* The child who is overanxious and tense cannot concentrate on learning even if he has the intellectual capacity to achieve.

The teacher and the school nurse should be aware of such problems as they arise. They should be able to work with parents and other team members in order to help the child.

Neurotic Symptoms

Physicians often find it difficult to differentiate between normal behavior and neurotic behavior of children. Some behavior, however, when it is consistent, must be classified as neurotic.

Nervousness

Etiology and Clinical Manifestations. Nervousness is not a separate condition in itself, but represents a group of symptoms. Nervous children are physically and mentally restless, overexcitable, timid and easily fatigued.

The inciting cause of nervousness may be a continued heavy load of anxiety or stress, or severe illness. Some children become nervous because of parental pressure to achieve. Children may also be nervous because they feel inferior to others, are overstimulated at play or acquire anxiety from their parents.

The *manifestations* are easily recognized. The child is tense and restless, the pulse and respiration rates are increased, the movements are jerky, and the child's responses are too rapid.

Treatment and Prognosis. *Treatment* may be given by a physician or a psychiatrist, depending upon the severity of the problem. The child should have adequate nutrition and sleep without excessive excitement, discipline or

stimulation to achieve in either motor ability or school work. The nervous child needs support and a well planned routine. Sometimes he may need to be placed in a new environment away from an anxiety-producing home.

The *prognosis* depends upon the cause and the management of the child and his problems.

Finger-Sucking

The average child gives up thumb- and finger-sucking by the time he is two years old; others relinquish it by five or six years of age. If a child continues past this time and into the school age, investigation should be made into the life of the child and his parents to find out the cause of his neurotic behavior. Punitive measures or those producing physical prevention of the sucking activity, e.g. splints on the arms and bandages on the fingers, or making the practice unpleasant, such as putting bad-tasting lotions on the thumb or fingers, should be avoided.

If a child stopped sucking his fingers at an early age and resumed the habit at seven or eight years, he probably met an unsolvable difficulty in his development and regressed to gain satisfaction. Such difficulties include the birth of a sibling, the mother's leaving home to work, the death of a loved grandparent or moving to a new home. The treatment is to learn and correct the child's attitude toward the traumatic event.

Nail-Biting

Nail-biting is an indication of tension. If the parents resist his attempts to gain satisfaction by nail-biting too traumatically, a parent-child conflict is begun. Severe nail-biting may become an attempt by the child to humiliate and annoy his parents. It is physically painful; thus the child punishes himself for his hostility to his parents. He should be given a manicure set as soon as he is able to use it and praised for his well kept hands. He should be helped to express his hostile feelings so that he no longer needs to bite his nails. His self-confidence should be increased in the home situation.

Imitation may also be important in nail-biting. The child may be simply imitating a parent who has the same habit. The parent may accept the behavior in himself, but not in the child.

Fears

Children must develop certain fears based on dangers that exist in the real world. Such things as bonfires and sharp knives should arouse a degree of fear in children that they will be harmed unless they take necessary precautions.

Fear of the dark, one of childhood's most common fears, is due to the fact that in the dark the child feels alone and deserted. The dark may be peopled for him with dangerous persons of his fantasy. Parents should assure him that they have not deserted him and that they do not fear the dark.

Crippling anxiety replaces fear when there is an unconscious distortion of reality. The distortion occurs because the real situation is equated with an unconscious conflict or an anxiety-charged previous experience. Usually the exact meaning of the previous experience is repressed.

If anxiety persists in spite of the child's experience which should disprove it or of the passage of time which should weaken the fear, some symbolic significance is attached to what is feared, and professional help should be sought.

Children should not be exposed thoughtlessly to situations which generate anxiety. If they are exposed, they can handle the anxiety best if they have secure relations with their parents and can talk about their fears or act out their feelings in relation to the fear.

School Phobia

School phobia is a term which indicates a symptom and not a disease, since many of these children are not phobic (see p. 529). These children may refuse to go to school. They may prefer either to remain at home or to become truant away from home. This latter category will not be included in this discussion. Manifestations of this problem may be the development of somatic complaints, fear of the teacher or children, or some situation at school. This problem may also be an indication of psychosis. Actually, these children are afraid to leave their parents, especially the mother, and their parents do not want their children to leave them. Central to the problem, therefore, is an exaggerated dependency on the parents.

The aim in therapy of children having a school phobia is to have the children return to school immediately, with the use of force if necessary. Failure to have the children returned to school is the responsibility of the parents as much as the children themselves. After these children have returned to school, therapy is aimed at correcting the underlying family relation problems in order to prevent a recurrence. If the child, as indicated by other manifestations, is very emotionally ill or psychotic, he should be referred to a child psychiatrist for therapy.

Conduct Disorders (The Problem Child)

Etiology, Types, Management and Prognosis. The child whom the parents and teachers call a problem child is usually merely trying to solve a problem with his behavior. Such behavior may occur in any socioeconomic group. It usually occurs because the child's basic emotional needs have not been met. The problem generally arises because his methods of expressing his distress are limited. Such children may steal, be truant from school, hurt smaller children, tell dirty stories or engage in sex play. In recent years some of these children have found that glue-sniffing provides a form of intoxication which they enjoy. Under the influence of glue vapors some of them commit misdemeanors. If untreated, these children who have learned to enjoy the experience of becoming intoxicated may turn to alcohol, narcotics or other drugs (see p. 648) during their adolescent years. Behavior may be, but is not always, directed toward those who, the child feels, are responsible for his problems.

In the management of this problem the psychiatrist first of all gains the child's confidence. He does not blame the child for his behavior. He encourages the child to tell his own story. *Treatment* must be extended in every phase of the child's life. It may require a team approach to the whole problem, including parents, physician, teacher, spiritual adviser, scout leader, social worker and nurse. The child also should be a partner in making the therapeutic plan. Treatment is usually directed at the parent-

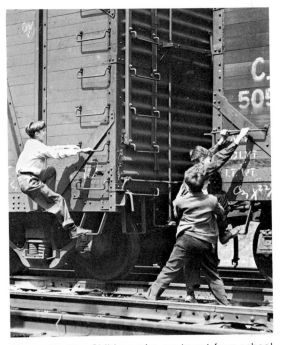

Figure 23–13. Children who are truant from school may engage in extremely dangerous activities. (H. Armstrong Roberts.)

child relations and at the child's feelings of inferiority over a variety of problems.

The outlook is usually good if these children are given the understanding help which they need.

Language Disorders

Etiology and Incidence. The cause of any language disorder is usually complex. The *incidence* of speech defects is greatest between the ages of four and eleven years. Boys are more frequently affected than girls.

Types, Diagnosis and Management. There are three *types* of speech disorders: functional disorders such as stuttering, defects due to anatomic malformations such as cleft palate (see p. 198) and cleft lip, and defects due to central nervous system lesions such as cerebral palsy (see p. 435). The whole child must be considered when the *diagnosis* is made and management is planned. *Management* depends on the basic problem causing the speech disorder.

Stuttering

Stuttering is the most common functional speech disorder. The child is unable to speak freely because of incoordination and spasmodic action of the muscles involved in speech. Although there is some question about the cause, there is increasing evidence that stuttering is a symptom of a profound emotional disturbance. Some experts believe that the emotional disturbance may be due to an enforced change of handedness. Before treatment can be planned the child's physical, intellectual and emotional status must be ascertained.

Management consists in reducing the child's anxiety about his stuttering, and treatment of any other problem found in the evaluation. The child should receive adequate health care and be helped to gain insight into, and understanding of, his disorder. Usually the services of a psychiatrist and a speech therapist are needed.

Psychosomatic Illness

Etiology. Psychosomatic illness is a physical disturbance that has a psychologic origin. There may also be an organic basis for such illness, but the element of emotions enters into the causation. Every child may have emotional reactions which interfere with his bodily functions. The degree of interference and the location of the problem vary with the individual child. In school children several psychosomatic illnesses arise in connection with the gastrointestinal

tract, including anorexia, overeating, constipation, ulcerative colitis and abdominal pain. Enuresis (see p. 600) and asthma (see p. 521) may also be classified as psychosomatic illnesses in children. The diagnosis and treatment of psychosomatic illnesses are the joint responsibilities of the physician and the psychiatrist.

Anorexia Nervosa

The child who has anorexia nervosa seems to have a relentless drive toward self-destruction through starvation. Such a child at first deliberately refuses food, even though he has an excellent appetite. Anorexia nervosa occurs only if the child has some deep emotional problem. There is often an intense conflict between mother and daughter. The girl is likely to have many misconceptions about pregnancy and indulges in sexual fantasies. As the period of starvation is prolonged, real anorexia and self-induced vomiting of food directly after it has been eaten produce rapid weight loss and bodily changes due to food deprivation. The child may gain sympathy from the family because of these symptoms.

Treatment includes correcting any electrolyte imbalance and increasing the diet. The child is usually hospitalized. Psychiatric consultation should be obtained.

Anorexia nervosa is a chronic condition, and the ultimate prognosis is questionable even with adequate medical and psychiatric therapy.

Overeating

Overeating which results in extreme obesity is usually thought to be due to the child's need for love, which he equates with food. It may also be due, however, to his wanting to grow big in size or to other emotional factors. Treatment is generally difficult. Many times the services of both a physician and a psychiatrist are necessary to curb the child's desire for food.

Constipation

Many cases of so-called constipation in children exist only in the minds of the parents. They feel that their child is constipated because he does not have evacuations as often as the parents think he should. Nevertheless children do have true constipation, and on occasion it is due to emotional factors.

There are two main causes of this sort of constipation. One occurs in children who show disgust at any form of dirt, especially excreta. These children, in the toddler and preschool ages, before control of elimination was definitely established, feared that their parents would punish them even if they defecated at socially approved times and places, and hence became afraid of *all* defecation. This early fear conditioned them to feel anxiety about defecation even after control was thoroughly established, with the result that they restrained the normal need to have bowel movements. The usual treatment for this sort of constipation is to add a small amount of bulk to the diet and to praise the child whenever he becomes dirty during play periods. The older child may have the hygienic aspect of regular evacuation explained to him.

The other kind of constipation is due to excessive early toilet training and results in the child's feeling that excreting is a hostile act against his parents. Such a child needs psychiatric help in order to uncover and remove his fear of his own emotional reactions.

Chronic Ulcerative Colitis

Etiology. This is an inflammatory condition whose cause is unknown. Several theories have been advanced about the cause; the most commonly accepted theory is that it is a psychosomatic illness.

Pathology and Clinical Manifestations. Part or all of the colon may be involved, as may be the ileum. The mucosa may be largely denuded, and multiple longitudinal ulcers may form a network over the colon. There may be fibrosis, and the colon may be decreased in size.

The onset may be insidious or acute. The most important symptom is frequent passage of small stools containing mucus, blood and pus. Diarrhea may occur on occasion. There is usually no fever, abdominal pain or vomiting, although these may occur during exacerbations of the condition. Hemorrhage from the bowel or rectal prolapse may be a complication. Emaciation, anemia, nutritional edema and vitamin deficiencies may also be present.

Diagnosis and Treatment. The *diagnosis* is made on the basis of the history, lack of causative organisms in the stools, and finding of ulceration and inflammation on proctoscopic examination. When the condition is prolonged, the colon becomes a smoothly outlined tube.

There is no specific *therapy.* The diet should be soft and bland with a low residue. Additional vitamins and minerals should be given. Blood transfusions may be given for anemia. Temporary relief may be achieved with one of the corticosteroids. Ileostomy or colectomy may be done. The most encouraging plan of therapy is that carried out jointly by the pediatrician, the psychiatrist and the surgeon. Emotional and environmental stresses should be relieved. To this end, the parents as well as the child may require psychotherapy.

Course and Prognosis. The chronic course is interrupted by periods of remission and exacerbations. The disease may continue for years. Death is usually caused by exhaustion.

Abdominal Pain

Recurrent abdominal pain without organic cause is a frequent symptom in older school children. It occurs with little regularity in relation to meals, evacuations or time of day. The intensity of the pain varies from mild discomfort to severe pain. Appendectomy or exploratory laparotomy procedures are of no benefit to the child.

These children generally seem to be older and more pleasant and responsible in their behavior than their peers. Their parents may have a high expectation of themselves and their children or they may fear that the child cannot cope with the usual process of development. The child, not being able to handle the anxiety of his parents, looks for direction and safety and does not then achieve as well as other children his age. This behavior only reinforces the parental anxiety over the child. The services of a physician and a psychiatrist may be necessary in the treatment of such children.

Enuresis

Enuresis is wetting after the age when toilet training should have been completed. Although these children are usually normal, they should have a physical examination to rule out such conditions as diabetes, pyelitis or nocturnal epilepsy.

Enuresis has many causes. One of the most serious is a personality or character maladjustment. These children need psychiatric help for their emotional problem. Other kinds of enuresis may perhaps be due to jealousy of a new sibling, revenge enuresis because of lack of love from parents or a regressive neurosis. Treatment of these types consists in changing the parents' attitude toward the child so that they can give him more love. Treatment by restricting fluids before bedtime, with charts of achievement, or by mechanical devices to waken the child may cure the enuresis, but not the basic problem.

Inadequate bladder capacity has been implicated recently as a cause of nocturnal enuresis. Delayed bladder development makes it physically impossible for some children to store urine throughout the night. Therapy in this situation consists in increasing bladder capacity by having the child retain progressively larger amounts of fluid during the day. Medications may be given to reduce the tone of the muscle wall of the bladder, thus decreasing the amplitude and frequency of contractions and allowing the bladder to dilate.

Additional causes of enuresis in the school child include retardation, lack of toilet training or a situation in which the child's bedroom is too far from the bathroom. Treatment here is easier than for the child with a severe emotional problem who may require psychiatric care.

Therapy

Parents may make mistakes, and the child may not be too much affected. Too many mistakes, however, will affect the child's behavior. Parents are too close to the situation to see what is really happening. They may be bothered by the child's behavior, but may not realize the basic problem involved.

Sometimes a child's behavior is upsetting to parents even though it is only a manifestation of his growth. All that such parents need is an explanation of the normal growth and development of a child. Usually no therapy is required.

Professional help may be needed, however, if the cause of the problem is deep-seated and not understood by the parents. Such help may be required if the child is afraid to leave his level of development and advance toward maturity, is not growing and developing according to the usual pattern of maturation, is oversubmissive, overaggressive or not learning at a rate commensurate with his ability, cannot deal with frustrations or challenges in a way socially acceptable for a child of his age or shows behavior characteristics which are socially unacceptable.

Sources and Types. Outside help may be gained from the family physician, pediatrician, psychiatrist, parent study group, teachers or guidance counselors.

Parents often hesitate to seek help for emotionally disturbed children. They feel that they should know all the answers. A psychiatrist would want a detailed history of the parents' development and problems, as well as a history of the child. He would also want to know the relations between parents and other family members.

The psychiatrist may believe that the problem is typical for a child of this age and will help the parents handle the particular problem; he may believe that it is largely the parents' problem and recommend a change of environment for the child or secure help for the parents; or he may believe that it is largely the child's problem and ask to see him frequently in order to help him gain an understanding of his problem and see other ways to handle his needs.

Prolonged therapy may be necessary. At times during such therapy the child's behavior may seem to become worse in that he may act out impulses that previously were under control. Parents need the help of the psychiatrist to understand what is happening in the parent-child relations and to know how to deal with the child's behavior. The psychiatrist does not divulge the material which the child gives him without the child's permission. This is difficult for the parents to understand, but it is essential that they accept this element in the counseling situation. In addition to therapy for the child, the parents may also be involved in psychotherapy. Group therapy which involves the child and his parents as an educational and therapeutic experience is becoming more widely used.

The emotionally disturbed child may be placed in a foster home, a day school, a boarding school or a structured residential treatment center or psychiatric hospital. These several types of facilities provide children with various degrees of emotional problems a way of receiving therapy outside the setting of their own homes.

Role of the Nurse. The nurse who cares for children having psychosomatic illnesses or emotional disturbances must be able to observe their behavior accurately and record what she hears, feels and sees. Such observations help those who are treating these children, as well as helping the nurses themselves in the care of the children.

Close cooperation with the therapist is essential. The therapist can help nurses to understand the meaning of the behavior they observe and help them provide the kind of nursing care skills these children need. Therapists are interested in the child's relations with his parents, his peers and other adults. They would also like to know his adjustment to the hospital, to school and to play activities.

More nurses who have been educationally prepared as clinical specialists in the area of child psychiatry are needed to improve the care of emotionally disturbed children by working even more closely with the children's therapists.

Group conferences of all team members, including physicians, social workers, school teachers, play therapists, nurses, aides and other auxiliary personnel who have contact with these children, are necessary. They help everyone to understand the care of the child as well as the cause of his illness. Such conferences often also help the nurse to understand her own personality and thus improve her relations with the children under her care.

CLINICAL SITUATIONS

Marsha Dullin, a nine-year-old girl, has been admitted to the pediatric unit with a diagnosis of rheumatic fever. She lives with her parents, three brothers and two sisters in an apartment in a tenement house. Her father is a manual laborer, and the family income is $100.00 a week. On admission Marsha's temperature was elevated, and she complained of joint pains.

1. When Marsha was admitted to the hospital, the nurse found nits in her long blond hair, but she could see no pediculi. The physician ordered applications of DDT powder. The nurse removed the nits by

  a. Washing Marsha's hair daily with soap containing hexachlorophene.

  b. Sliding each nit off its hair shaft after applying DDT powder.

  c. Applying benzyl benzoate lotion and brushing the nits out of the hair.

  d. Combing her hair with a fine-tooth comb dipped in hot vinegar.

2. Marsha had been ill at home only a brief time before her admission to the hospital. She is fortunate that her illness was diagnosed and treated early because

  a. Cardiac damage can be minimized or prevented.

  b. Manifestations of chorea can be prevented.

  c. Spread of this infection to her siblings is minimized.

  d. Large amounts of medications will not be necessary in her treatment.

3. The most important point in providing nursing care for Marsha during the acute phase of her illness is

  a. Maintaining contact with her parents.

  b. Physical and psychologic rest.

  c. A nutritious diet.

  d. Maintaining her interest in school.

4. The physician has ordered sodium salicylate for Marsha. The nurse should be aware that some of the toxic symptoms of this drug are

  a. Tinnitus and nausea.

  b. Dermatitis and blurred vision.

  c. Unconsciousness and acetone odor of the breath.

  d. Chills and an elevation of temperature.

5. Significant instructions which Marsha's mother will receive before the child is discharged will concern

  a. A high protein diet, adequate immunization and avoidance of contact with anyone having an upper respiratory tract infection.

  b. Routine immunizations, limited activity and adequate nutrition.

  c. Adequate nutrition, avoidance of contact with anyone having an upper respiratory tract infection and prophylactic medication.

  d. Limited activity, administration of sodium salicylate and a high vitamin diet.

6. Marsha's one desire before the onset of rheumatic fever was to be a ballet dancer. Now that she may possibly have some cardiac involvement, the team in long-range planning for her rehabilitation would

  a. Avoid all reference to dancing in their discussions with her.

  b. Investigate Marsha's feelings about her future and help her to consider other career interests.

  c. Assure Marsha that a career in dancing would be possible if she promised to take care of herself.

  d. Ignore her questions related to dancing because this problem can be discussed later.

Elaine Watson, an eleven-year-old child, was admitted to the pediatric unit four weeks ago in diabetic coma. Both her parents and her two older sisters have shown a deep interest in her condition. Elaine is in the sixth grade in school. Her teachers are proud of her level of achievement.

7. In the management of juvenile diabetics, which one of the following factors is considered the *least* important?

  a. Taking of regular daily exercise.

  b. Prompt treatment of all infections.

  c. Maintenance of emotional stability.

  d. Treatment of allergies.

8. In evaluating Elaine's ability to care for herself the nurse believes that

  a. Elaine is too young to give herself insulin.

  b. A visiting nurse should teach Elaine to give herself insulin after she is discharged.

  c. Elaine should be taught to give herself insulin while she is in the hospital.

  d. Elaine's mother should assume the responsibility for insulin administration until Elaine is an adolescent.

9. When Elaine returns to school, she should certainly remember to carry with her at all times

  a. A lump of sugar.

  b. A bag of salted nuts.

  c. Her insulin and a syringe.

  d. Sufficient money to telephone her mother in case she feels ill.

10. Mrs. Watson asks the nurse whether she believes that Elaine should join the Girl Scouts of America. Although the mother should make her own decision, the nurse could base her comments on her belief that

  a. If her closest friends are members of the troop, she should join regardless of whether she wants to or not.

  b. The leader will teach her many things a young girl should know.

  c. Elaine will meet many girls her own age who share her interests.

  d. If Elaine joins, she will probably lose interest in her school work.

11. Mrs. Watson is concerned because Elaine's friends have recently begun to use lipstick. Elaine has expressed a desire to use it also. The nurse believes that

  a. Mrs. Watson should forbid the use of lipstick for another year at least.

  b. Mrs. Watson should permit Elaine to use it, but that she should teach her to apply it correctly.

  c. Mrs. Watson should explain to Elaine that the use of lipstick at her age is not refined.

  d. Mrs. Watson should degrade the mothers of Elaine's friends because they have permitted their daughters to use lipstick.

GUIDES TO FURTHER STUDY

1. The children's clinic in your hospital does not have a playroom. Plan the room, including the furniture and the equipment (creative materials, toys, records and books) that would be needed. Indicate the personnel

necessary. In your planning indicate your knowledge of safety factors for children of various ages who will be using the room.

2. Eight-year-old Rebecca Schwartz was recently admitted to the pediatric unit with a diagnosis of diabetes. She is the only child of older parents. Her father has a small grocery business of his own. Rebecca is in the third grade in school and has average scholastic ability. Discuss in seminar the guidance this child and her parents will need. Role-play with another student the process of teaching this child regulation of diet, testing of urine and administration of insulin. Discuss the principles of learning to be considered as well as the content to be presented.

3. Discuss with a school nurse in your community her total program in relation to prevention of disease, treatment of illness, rehabilitation of the handicapped and health education of children. Is her program based on the level of growth and development and understanding of the children in her school? Has she taken into consideration the cultural background and the socioeconomic level of these children and their families? What is the role of this nurse in relation to the children's parents? In your discussion of this question in seminar give specific illustrations to support your answers.

4. During your experience in the pediatric unit you have been caring for a school-age child with a diagnosis of ulcerative colitis. Incorporate in your plan of care the recommendations of his psychiatrist. Did your patient show any change in behavior as a result of your altered approach? Discuss any problems you had in attempting to carry out the recommendations of the therapist.

5. You are providing care for two eight-year-old boys whose oral fluid requirements are greater than normal. On the basis of your understanding of growth and development, suggest ways by which you could help these children to cooperate with you in meeting this particular need.

TEACHING AIDS AND OTHER INFORMATION*

American Dental Association
Your Guide to Oral Health, 1964.

American Diabetes Association, Inc.
Facts About Diabetes, 1966.
The Child with Diabetes.

American Heart Association
Have Fun . . . Get Well!
Home Care of the Child with Rheumatic Fever.
Now You Can Protect Your Child Against Rheumatic Fever.
Prevention of Rheumatic Fever.
What You Should Know About Rheumatic Fever.

Child Study Association of America
Atkin, E. L.: Aggressiveness in Children.

Medic Alert Foundation
Why? Medic Alert.

Mental Health Materials Center
Bed-Wetting: How Can I Correct My Child's Habit?
Destructiveness: What Can Be Done About It?
Stuttering: How Can My Child Overcome It?

National Society for Crippled Children and Adults, Inc.
A Directory of Camps for the Handicapped.
Johnson, W.: Toward Understanding Stuttering.

The National Foundation—March of Dimes
When Your Child Has Rheumatoid Arthritis.

United States Department of Health, Education, and Welfare
Clements, S. D.: Minimal Brain Dysfunction in Children, 1966.
Haynes, U.: A Developmental Approach to Case Finding, 1967.
Heart Disease in Children, 1966.
Learning Disabilities Due to Minimal Brain Dysfunction, 1968.

---

* Complete addresses are given in the Appendix.

REFERENCES

Publications

Aichhorn, A.: *Delinquency and Child Guidance.* New York, International Universities Press, Inc., 1965.

Bakwin, H., and Bakwin, R. M.: *Clinical Management of Behavior Disorders in Children.* 3rd ed. Philadelphia, W. B. Saunders Company, 1966.

Barbara, D. A. (Ed.): *New Directions in Stuttering: Theory and Practice.* Springfield, Ill., Charles C Thomas, 1965.

Chapman, A. H.: *Management of Emotional Problems of Children and Adolescents.* Philadelphia, J. B. Lippincott Company, 1965.

deGutierrez-Mahoney, C. G.: *Neurological and Neurosurgical Nursing.* 4th ed. St. Louis, C. V. Mosby Company, 1965.

Dimock, H. G.: *The Child in Hospital.* Philadelphia, F. A. Davis Company, 1960.

Duncan, G. G., and Duncan, T. G.: *A Modern Pilgrim's Progress for Diabetics.* 2nd ed. Philadelphia, W. B. Saunders Company, 1967.

Farmer, T. W. (Ed.): *Pediatric Neurology.* 2nd printing. New York, Hoeber Medical Division, Harper and Row, 1966.

Fischer, A. E., and Horstmann, D. L.: *Handbook for the Young Diabetic.* 3rd ed. New York, Intercontinental Medical Book Corporation, 1964.

Frank, I., and Powell, M.: *Psychosomatic Ailments in Childhood and Adolescence.* Springfield, Ill., Charles C Thomas, 1967.

Ford, F. R.: *Diseases of the Nervous System in Infancy, Childhood and Adolescence.* 5th ed. Springfield, Ill., Charles C Thomas, 1966.

Luper, H. L., and Mulder, R. L.: *Stuttering: Therapy for Children.* Englewood Cliffs, N.J., Prentice-Hall, Inc., 1964.

Markowitz, M., and Kuttner, A. G.: *Rheumatic Fever. Diagnosis, Management, and Prevention.* Philadelphia, W. B. Saunders Company, 1965.

Morley, M. E.: *The Development and Disorders of Speech in Childhood.* 2nd ed. Baltimore, Williams & Wilkins Company, 1965.

Redl, F.: *When We Deal with Children.* New York, Macmillan Company, 1966.

Redl, F., and Wineman, D.: *Children Who Hate.* New York, Macmillan Company, 1965.

Rexford, E. N.: *A Developmental Approach to Problems of Acting Out. Monographs of the Journal of The American Academy of Child Psychiatry.* New York, International Universities Press, Inc., 1966.

Root, H. F., and others: *Joslin's Treatment of Diabetes Mellitus.* Philadelphia, Lea & Febiger, 1967.

Schulman, J. L.: *Management of Emotional Disorders in Pediatric Practice.* Chicago, Yearbook Medical Publishers, Inc., 1967.

Terry, F. J., and others: *Principles and Technics of Rehabilitation Nursing.* 3rd ed. St. Louis, C. V. Mosby Company, 1966.

Traisman, H. S., and Newcomb, A. L.: *Management of Juvenile Diabetes Mellitus.* St. Louis, C. V. Mosby Company, 1965.

Verville, E.: *Behavior Problems of Children.* Philadelphia, W. B. Saunders Company, 1967.

Wohl, M. G., and Goodhart, R. S.: *Modern Nutrition in Health and Disease Dietotherapy.* 4th ed. Philadelphia, Lea & Febiger, 1968.

Periodicals

Ambinder, W. J., and Falik, L. H.: Keeping Emotionally Disturbed Foster Children in School. *Children,* 13:227, 1966.

Basara, S. C.: The Behavioral Patterns of the Perceptually Handicapped Child. *Nursing Forum,* V: No. 4, 24, 1966.

Brewer, E. J.: Rheumatoid Arthritis in Childhood. *Am. J. Nursing,* 65:66, June 1965.

Brockmeier, M. J.: Nursing in Two Community Health Settings. *Nursing Outlook,* 16:55, April 1968.

Cluster, P. F.: One-Room School for Hospitalized Children. *Nursing Outlook,* 15:56, August 1967.

Conners, C. K.: The Syndrome of Minimal Brain Dysfunction: Psychological Aspects. *Pediat. Clin. N. Amer.,* 14:749, 1967.

Flesch, R.: Counseling Parents of Chronically Ill Children. *Pediat. Clin. N. Amer.,* 10:765, 1963.

Geis, D. P.: Nursing at Camp Needlepoint. *Nursing Outlook,* 15:46, May 1967.

Haynes, U. H.: Nursing Approaches in Cerebral Dysfunction. *Amer. J. Nursing,* 68:2170, 1968.

Leiner, M. S., and Rahmer, A. E.: The Juvenile Diabetic and the Visiting Nurse. *Am. J. Nursing,* 68:106, 1968.

Long, P. J.: The Diabetic Child at Home. *Nursing Outlook,* 12:55, December 1964.

Martin, M. M.: Insulin Reactions. *Am. J. Nursing,* 67:328, 1967.

Medical Notes: The Syndrome of Minimal Brain Dysfunction. *Nursing Clin. N. Amer.,* 3:375, 1968.

Michener, W. M.: Ulcerative Colitis in Children: Problems in Management. *Pediat. Clin. N. Amer.,* 14:159, 1967.

Miesem, M. L., and Wann, F.: Care of Adolescents with Anorexia Nervosa. *Am. J. Nursing,* 67: 2356, 1967.
Moore, M. L.: Diabetes in Children. *Am. J. Nursing,* 67:104, 1967.
Nelson, M. B.: Laramie's Rheumatic Fever Control Program. *Nursing Outlook,* 14:31, August 1966.
Paine, R. S.: Syndrome of Minimal Cerebral Damage. *Pediat. Clin. N. Amer.,* 15:779, 1968.
Pearson, H. A.: Marrow Hypoplasia in Anorexia Nervosa. *J. Pediat.,* 71:211, August 1967.
Starfield, B.: Functional Bladder Capacity in Enuretic and Nonenuretic Children. *J. Pediat.,* 70:777, 1967.
Walike, B. C., Marmor, L., and Upshaw, M. J.: Rheumatoid Arthritis. *Am. J. Nursing,* 67:1420, 1967.
Wayne, D.: The Lonely School Child. *Amer. J. Nursing,* 68:774, 1968.
Westin, G. W.: The Limping Child. *Pediat. Clin. N. Amer.,* 14:601, 1967.

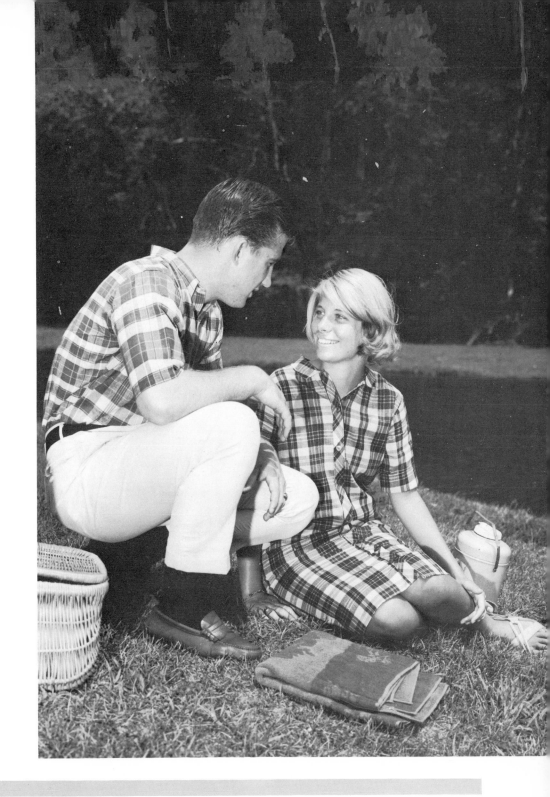

UNIT SEVEN
THE PUBESCENT AND THE ADOLESCENT

24

THE NORMAL PUBESCENT AND THE NORMAL ADOLESCENT: THEIR GROWTH, DEVELOPMENT AND CARE

When their child reaches the pubescent and adolescent years, the parents must take still another step in their own development. Their teenager, in trying to build a *sense of identity* of his own, may tend to separate himself to some degree physically and emotionally from his family. His parents must then learn to build a new life of their own and, standing in the background, watch their adolescent with increasing maturity proceed to shape his own life.

Adolescence is unique to human beings. All other mammals achieve sexual maturity early, but man, with his long period of dependency, achieves sexual maturity much later. Thus the sexual function takes on certain features peculiar to man. This refers to the point that man is a social animal and in his highest state of maturity is able to find a balanced integration between his social part and his animal nature. Adolescence, then, is the period when the young person is struggling to find this balance within himself.

A host of possibilities enter into the success or failure of this struggle: genetic factors, health, family constitution and attitudes, economic level, the culture of the group to which the adolescent belongs and the various educational, recreational and vocational opportunities afforded him by society at local, state and national levels.

In order to differentiate the terms used in this chapter, the following definitions are given. The *prepuberty* or *prepubescent* period refers to the period of rapid physical growth when secondary sex characteristics appear. *Puberty* may be said to have occurred when the girl begins to menstruate and the boy to produce spermatozoa. *Menarche* refers more specifically to the time of the first menstrual period. *Adolescence* begins when the secondary sex characteristics appear and ends when somatic growth is completed and the individual is psychologically mature, capable of taking his place as a contributing member of society. It is a period of conflict, stress and anxiety, as well as one of self-realization and accomplishment.

609

By about ten to twelve years of age the child begins the last period of life before adulthood. Before that time the child should have developed a sense of trust in others, a sense of autonomy in that he is a human being with a mind and a will of his own, a sense of initiative in that he wants to learn to do what he sees others doing, and, during school age, a sense of duty, industry or accomplishment of real tasks which he can carry through to completion. The young person who approaches puberty and adolescence has two additional strides to make in his personality development. These can be termed a *sense of identity* and a *sense of intimacy*. Adolescence ends gradually with the beginning of adult life — about eighteen years in our culture. The termination of adolescence may be prolonged to the mid-twenties or later because of social and economic factors.

Although the chronologic age of ten years may be given as the beginning of prepubescence and the chronologic age of eighteen years as the end of adolescence, few specific times when definite changes occur may be given during this period. As the youth grows older, the span of time in which a specific step in development occurs becomes wider. It is therefore possible to describe only the overall changes in growth and development which occur during prepuberty, puberty and adolescence. Adolescence is basically a time when the individual battles for recognition of his adulthood, and yet at the same time desires unconsciously to remain a child.

Many young people at some time during these years reach a period of emotional crisis or change, with the outcome not easily assured. Such a crisis may lead to backtracking in development or to further growth and maturing. This crisis provides a new chance to resolve emotional problems which were not resolved before and have remained quiescent.

OVERVIEW OF EMOTIONAL AND SOCIAL DEVELOPMENT

Puberty

The pubescent period may be considered a pause of two or three years between childhood and adolescence. It is basically the organic phenomenon of adolescence. It is a period of rapid physical change and personality growth when the individual achieves nearly his adult bodily stature. Girls begin their preadolescent growth spurt by about ten years and boys by about twelve years. Between twelve and fourteen years for girls and one or two years later for boys, they approach the end of puberty. Children who, during school years, resembled each other

in body build now show definite indications of belonging to one or the other sex, of becoming taller, shorter, thinner or more obese than others.

The child during pubescence shows strides in personality development as well as physical growth. He becomes increasingly more adaptable, approaching his peer group and problem situations at home and at school with greater confidence. He enjoys games that involve not only physical skill, but also team cooperation. Although there is a revival of love for the parent of the opposite sex, he argues with his parents frequently. He is able to assume increasing responsibility in what to him is reality. Parents may not have the same values that he holds during this period. The parents may want him to assume greater responsibilities around the home, but he may feel that his responsibility lies in helping his friends with a game or in completing a project he has started.

The pubescent seems able to handle important emotional problems easily. If a parent, grandparent or sibling dies, the child may appear on the surface to adjust very well, turning rapidly to other activities in his environment. Later, however, he may have to face the problem again because it was not worked through satisfactorily; it was only hidden from his own as well as an observer's view.

Parents become aware that during pubescence the hostility which previously existed between boys and girls is gradually disappearing. There is an interest in "dating," in going to mixed parties, especially dances, and in talking about members of the opposite sex. Such activities do not really mean that the children have become emotionally mature. They merely indicate that the youngsters are trying to leave childhood and to assume the pattern of behavior of the adolescent or adult group.

The child realizes that he is inadequate in these initial attempts to be grown up. He knows that he is not mature and that most of his activity still centers around school, friends, play and home. Unfortunately, many parents try to capitalize on this step in development and urge more rapid development of interest in the opposite sex than the child is ready for. There may be reasons for parental pressure in this area, not the least of which is their wish that the child be popular with both sexes, that he be well accepted in his peer group. Severe pressure of this sort usually does not achieve the positive goal that parents might wish.

On the whole, however, puberty is a period of comparative quiet for the child and for the adults in his environment. He seems now to be a relatively independent person. Parents can reason with him and come to some kind of solution for their problems. Both the school and society expect him to understand the mores

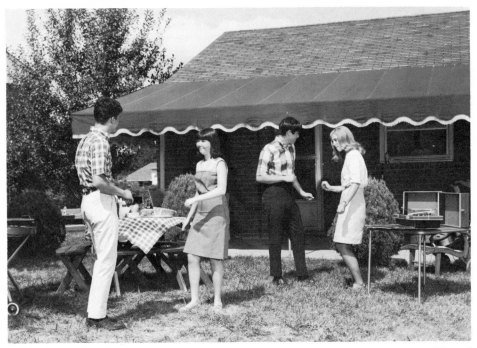

Figure 24–1. Pubescents and adolescents enjoy attending mixed parties, especially dances. These fourteen-year-olds, in addition to learning to dance, are learning how to get along with each other. (H. Armstrong Roberts.)

of his group. Behavior such as lying and stealing, which were not punished too severely in earlier years because of his immaturity, are now unacceptable because he is presumed to know what behavior society expects. Adults expect the child during puberty to make a fairly adequate adjustment to the demands of reality in our society.

Adolescence (the Sense of Identity and the Sense of Intimacy)

The transition from childhood to adulthood is not a smooth one. Adolescence is a period of stress for young people and parents alike. The adolescent must learn who he is and must modify his conscience for his adult role in life. He now questions many of the beliefs that he held as certain and true. Besides this intellectual and emotional upheaval, his rapid body growth causes him anxiety, and the cultural pressures of today's world add further stress to his uncertainty.

Adolescents today are faced with many pressures which the older generation did not have. The rapid rate of social change, the threat or presence of war, increase in the speed of travel and rapid technological progress impose problems unknown in previous generations.

Perhaps more important is the fact that adolescents are faced with a problem of finding employ-ment at a time when they seek independence from home. Child labor laws, which greatly restrict adolescents in terms of employment, have had beneficial effects, but have also made problems. This in turn makes for great problems for schools in that compulsory education laws become exceedingly difficult to administer in view of the increasing number of adolescents who are actually uneducable. This refers not only to mentally retarded children, but also to those having emotional difficulties.

Erikson has called the central problem of the early period of adolescence the establishment of a *sense of identity*. In the words of a modern adolescent girl: "I could never begin to discuss my feelings and conflicts because of their confusing order. My ideas on life and people are always changing because I am going through that process of trying to find myself."

The adolescent wonders how he appears and will appear to others in the future. Does he fit what society expects him to be? This is really a question about the continuity of the individual, from early childhood to adult years.

Adolescents in primitive societies have an easier time defining their role than do those in our culture. They have initiation rites which symbolize to themselves and to others that they are young adults. For instance, in the Navajo religion the ceremonial of the Blessing Way is performed for girls at puberty. In our society confirmation, or acceptance into the Church, is

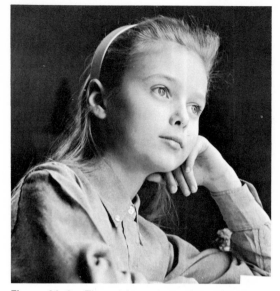

Figure 24–2. The adolescent wonders who she is and what her role in society will be after graduation from high school. (H. Armstrong Roberts.)

do not have the significance that initiation rites have in primitive societies.

Nevertheless, even though the rites in primitive societies do add a measure of security to the individual youth's life, they take away the freedom of choice which children of our culture have.

Since our society does not have rigid rules, mores, customs and taboos which govern the behavior of adolescents, they themselves must organize them. Patterns of dress, behavior or prejudice are set by the group and tend to make the members feel worthwhile. Unfortunately, such limits on behavior tend to form groups from which many young people are excluded. Those who are excluded then have a much more difficult time in gaining a sense of security and of identity.

The young person in our society may be disturbed not only because he is not certain of himself, but also because he is not certain of who he is to become. There are so many choices to be made in growing up, so many opportunities ahead, that instead of being comforting, they are confusing.

The adolescent who is not able to face himself and life squarely, who has a feeling of *self-diffusion,* may become delinquent, neurotic or psychotic. The outcome of the adolescent's struggle to establish his sense of identity is dependent largely on what his personality development was during childhood. The problem is further

a ceremony that has similar meaning to the young person. Graduation from grade school or junior high school and the ceremonies of various youth organizations may mean the same thing to the adolescent who belongs to them. Although these ceremonies are important, they

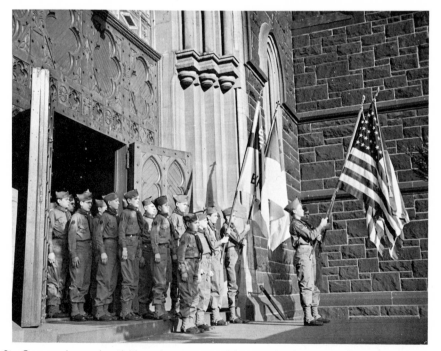

Figure 24–3. Ceremonies and activities of young people's organizations help them to understand their role in our society. (H. Armstrong Roberts.)

complicated in our society for the individual who belongs to a minority group.

The child whose personality development was not adequate may be helped during pubescence and the adolescent years through psychiatric therapy or helpful guidance of teachers and others. Less fortunate is the child whose security during his early years was based on the mores of a minority group. During adolescence he may decide to reject his past and try to become a true American middle-class citizen. This step may be too difficult, and he may falter and become delinquent. Although many professional persons are trying to find an answer for this problem, it has no easy solution.

Although the sense of identity is difficult to achieve, the young person must gain it in order to be saved from emotional turmoil. He must be able to find for himself a meaning to life; he must be able to see clearly that life has continuity for him individually. Probably never before in history has youth faced the difficulty that it faces today in a world of rapidly changing values and ideas, a world facing destruction at the same time that the youth is trying to save himself.

After the youth has developed a sense of identity during early adolescence he should be able to develop a *sense of intimacy* with himself and with persons of both sexes. If the youth is not certain of himself, he will not be able to form close ties of friendship or love with other people.

Although closer relations between boys and girls begin during pubescence, they are not intimate relations and serve only as settings for discussion of what they think and feel. During later adolescence these relations serve another purpose. They help to resolve the individual's preoccupation with the integration of the sexual function. They help one young person to unite with another. If the young person cannot do this because of his lack of a valued personality, he may become an isolate who keeps his relations with others on a cool, rigid, formal basis. If such a person rushes into an early marriage, it will probably fail because, lacking the ability to know himself, he is not able to know and love another.

While the healthy adolescent is establishing his sense of intimacy he has a real struggle with sexual feelings. This new force drives him to his peers. In the healthy adolescent this does not lead to the sexual act, although some physical expressions of affection are common. Such an adolescent does not usually want to proceed with the sexual act, because this involves a feeling of loss of independence. Sexual promiscuity in adolescence is usually an attempt to find an infantile relation rather than a mature form of psychosexual development.

Unfortunately our culture places less emphasis on the young person's developing a sense of intimacy than on his becoming independent and industrious. In our materialistic society the emphasis is often on success, not in interpersonal relations, but in the competitive world of work. For this reason many "successful" young people and adults have not developed the ability to understand the personality of others. They tend to be unhappy even though to the world they appear to be highly successful.

Problems of the Adolescent

The adolescent must face five important problems and find a solution to them if he is to gain a sense of identity and a sense of intimacy and to reach some degree of emotional maturity as an adult: (1) *integration of his personality for future responsibility,* (2) *emancipation from his parents and family,* (3) *creation of satisfactory relations with the opposite sex,* (4) *acceptance of a new body image after the rapid physical changes of this period, and* (5) *a decision about the vocation he will follow as an adult.* If his development to puberty has been satisfactory, these goals will not be too difficult, provided parents and other adults give him the help and guidance he needs. All too frequently, however, much friction and misunderstanding between parents and their adolescent children exists, making the process of growing up more difficult than it might be.

Integration of Personality. By the time the child reaches adolescence he should already have made a beginning toward the integration of his personality. He should have some consistent ways of acting in certain situations. He should have a healthy way of meeting reality, of doing something constructive in problem situations. If he has not reached this point in development, he may enter adolescence shy, anxious and with a desire to retreat and isolate himself when a problem arises. He may avoid social contacts and responsibilities whenever possible. He may, without help, complete adolescence poorly equipped to face life.

In order to achieve integration of personality the adolescent must participate in society as a whole, not only in relation to himself as an individual. He must be able to accept people — friends, and later his wife, children, neighbors and those of cultures other than his own. He should refrain from being too critical of others and should try to see their point of view. He should take part in the life of the larger community. He must have a deep feeling of willingness to help others in order to achieve a feeling of social unity and thus gain social strength. As one adolescent said: "By giving of myself I receive satisfaction and contentment. But by giving I also receive much more. It is a chance to mature and understand myself through others."

The Adolescent and His Family. Parents, teachers and other adults may not be as important to the adolescent as they were previously. He may be hostile to them and resent their authority. He is torn between his need for support and acceptance, to be dependent as a child, and his need for independence. He must defend himself against his unconscious love for the parent of the opposite sex and resolve his ambivalence toward the parent of the same sex. Although parents may consider the adolescent unmanageable and say that they cannot understand him, they should recognize his growing feelings of maturity and also his occasional need for help.

The adolescent, instead of wishing to be like the parent of the same sex, may attempt to be as different as possible. He may even ridicule his parents at home, but still value them highly outside the home. Affection is turned from the parents to adults outside the family. This begins a series of brief "crushes" typical of adolescence. The adolescent loves the adult, desires to please him and identifies with him. The young adolescent thus makes some of the characteristics—a trait, a manner of speaking, a skill—of the adult a part of his own personality. Often the adult, whether a teacher, Scout leader, relative, minister, priest, rabbi, physician or someone in public life, never realizes the effect he has had upon these young people. Many times parents who do not wish their child to grow up resent the fact that another adult is imitated in this way.

On the other hand, such relations may be extremely helpful for the adolescent and his family. A trusted, respected adult outside the family can help the adolescent find himself and his role in life more easily than can the parent, who may be less objective. Such an adult can help the adolescent clarify his thinking, work out his solution and find more mature patterns of behavior. When an adolescent reaches this point, his behavior gradually becomes determined by his own judgment rather than by controls imposed from outside. His parents and friends become less frustrating, and his hostility toward them diminishes.

Some parents need as much help and understanding as their adolescents do. Having had stormy periods of adolescence themselves, they may have acute apprehension over the trials of their own children. If they do not get the help they need, they may be either too strict or too lenient in setting limits to their children's behavior. Neither of these extremes provides the help which youth needs at this crucial time. The adolescent needs acceptance and guidance as a growing individual. Only in this way can he discover his limitations and powers.

The adolescent's relations with his siblings may become exceedingly strained. This is especially true of a boy whose younger sister has already reached puberty and left him behind in growth. Yet both the brother and the sister should feel more confident about approaching the problems of adolescence, especially in adjusting to the opposite sex, because they have learned the acceptable patterns of behavior from each other.

In some families younger siblings may place an adolescent sister or brother in the role of a parent-substitute. This kind of identification is probably not harmful if it does not interfere too much with the adolescent's own development and social activities.

The battle for independence is fought in practically every family. The parents fight to maintain authority and prestige in the eyes of the young person, and the young person fights for liberty. The youth who fights such a battle should probably be less a source of worry than one who causes no conflict over his strivings to become independent. The latter will probably stay emotionally in childhood and not weather the storm of the adolescent period.

Adolescence is the ideal time for children to begin to have their own lives. Unfortunately parents often say that they want their children to mature, but block them at every turn. The greatest harm parents can do is to expect the worst from their children, because they will probably get it. If parents expect the best, children are more apt to live up to this expectation.

Emancipation from the family is difficult because both sides have their own problems. The adolescent is often reluctant to accept responsibility and fears criticism if he does accept it. At the same time that he needs to feel cared for he lacks a desire to cooperate with adults who could give him this feeling of security. Parents also usually unconsciously have their problems. They have great difficulty sharing the adolescent's love with others. They tend to underestimate his strength to function away from them. They may desire to continue dominating the adolescent. They may say that they fear that he will be harmed if he leaves home. The mother often feels these problems more than the father does, since she is left alone while he works.

Any activity of daily living may be the basis of conflict: the time of leaving or coming home, whether the car may be used, whether the adolescent may have a key to the house, the selection of clothes, and the like. The adolescent should gain emancipation slowly. Just as his parents should try to understand his role in this conflict, so he should attempt to understand their problems.

If parents and child build a good foundation during the first six years of life, these battles will not wreck the adolescent's life. Parents must let the youth develop his judgment and skills, tell him the truth and avoid attacking or ridiculing him.

There has been a tendency in recent years to be too permissive with adolescents, perhaps as a reaction to the former trend to handle all young people too rigidly. Some limits are still important. A tolerant parent need not condone everything the adolescent does. One of the most difficult problems parents face is the establishment of a relation that enables them to give their children the freedom they need while assuring their acceptance of guidance.

Eventually the adolescent's anxiety decreases, and his return to the more immature relation with his parents is no longer necessary. He is then able to have a mature, interdependent relation with them and others because his independence is more confidently maintained.

The Adolescent and His Friends. The young adolescent who becomes a group member is fortunate because then the whole group repudiates adult influence and tends to strengthen the individual's concept of his own capabilities. His ideas are dominated by the social and ethical codes in the group. Fads are important, whether they involve clothes or behavior. The adolescent must be accepted by his group to feel secure. He may not express his individuality beyond the limits imposed by the group.

As a result of mutual soul-searching by individual members of the group, standards for basic concepts of living are worked out. Attitudes about morality, ethics, religion and social customs are formulated and adopted by group members. The group thus plans how the individual member should behave and becomes an island of security in what seems to be a confused world.

As soon as an adult leader is introduced, this function of the group is lost. The young people are no longer fully able to develop themselves as individuals or to learn how to get along with their peers.

The child who does not reach puberty at the same time as others may have emotional problems that are difficult for him to solve. He may find himself alienated from his peer group, yet not accepted by a younger or older group. Children who reach puberty late are especially at a disadvantage because feeling weak and less capable physically and physiologically hurts their pride.

Adolescents may develop a strong bond of friendship with just one or possibly two other adolescents of their own sex. This relation is based on similarities in interest, age and personality factors. Such friendships are important to personality development. These friends are devoted to each other and become inseparable. They have a relatively mature understanding and appreciation of each other's needs, reacting without the selfishness evident in earlier periods of development. They share each other's ideas, deepest secrets, and troubles, and thus develop a sense of responsibility and loyalty to others that had not existed before. A great

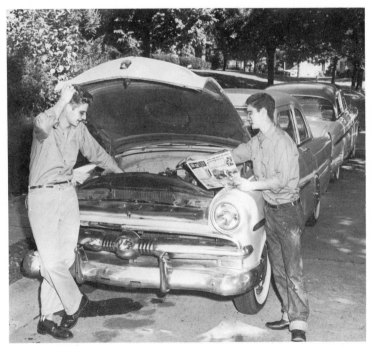

Figure 24–4. Close friendships are formed during adolescence, characterized by a more mature understanding of each other's needs than was possible during earlier periods of development. (H. Armstrong Roberts.)

deal of whispering is evident in these friendships.

These relations help the adolescent girl especially to break away from her attachment to her mother. Boys do not seem to have the intense friendship with other boys that girls have with other girls. Boys work out their feelings in horseplay, teasing and wrestling.

Gradually short-term attachments develop with members of the opposite sex which tend to break up the intense friendships with members of the same sex.

Adjustment to the Opposite Sex. When interest develops in the opposite sex, great secrecy surrounds it at first. When the boy sees a group of girls, he may perform physically in a way to attract their attention. He may say to himself and others that he was "just getting some exercise." The girls may giggle in response to attract the boy's attention.

Later, real interest and romantic love affairs develop, usually between a girl and a boy one or two years older than she because of the difference in physical maturation rates of the two sexes. These attachments are usually short-lived, but they do give those concerned some knowledge of the personality characteristics of the opposite sex which will help later when each is in a better position to fall in love.

To establish heterosexual relations the adolescent must rebel against and free himself from the forbidding infantile conscience. If he reduces his inner standards too rapidly, his anxiety becomes intolerable, and he tries even harder to control himself. Although he resents his parents' authority, the adolescent may at this time seek their control. He may also turn to religion or to the pursuit of intellectual interests to reduce his conflict. Ultimately his fear of his instincts will lessen, he will learn to control himself, and he will be able to enjoy pleasures which are needed for his growth.

Since marriage and parenthood lie just ahead for many adolescents, the two sexes must become accustomed to each other and learn to know each other well. Adolescents get practice in this by participation in dances, picnics, and the like. Physical expressions such as hand holding, kissing and embracing are normal functions of a person preparing for marriage.

In their efforts to develop an understanding of the other sex adolescents are often inhibited by adults. Parents are afraid that if young people are too much interested in the opposite sex, they will marry too soon and be unable to finish their education or support themselves well. They are afraid of pregnancy out of wedlock, disease, and disgrace to the family. The adolescent needs help from parents in accepting a masculine or feminine role and in understanding sex drives. Parents often do not remember

that if good parent-child relations have existed, if the young person has been given adequate sex education and has been taught social responsibility and consideration for others, he will usually abide by his parents' wishes about sex behavior. Young people should have an opportunity to mix with each other without anxiety and shame.

Many parents in the past discouraged young people from "going steady." They were afraid that the adolescents would be hurt when the friendship ended because the relationship seemed to be a demimarriage. More recently adolescents consider themselves to be "going steadily" instead of "going steady." In our socially mobile society many are wary of entangling alliances and are more convinced that a relationship depends on what emotions the couple invest in it, not by what the relationship is called.

If the child has had adequate sex education, if he was taught respect for others in these matters, and if he has had religious training on which he can base his decisions about his conduct, few problems are likely to arise during the adolescent years. Adolescents may need guidance, however, on specific problems that may arise in relation to their assuming an adult role. The adolescent must be helped to understand the moral and social customs that should govern his conduct in the matters of "dating" and sexual intercourse. He should be helped to find socially acceptable outlets for his interests.

Threatening the adolescent does more harm than good and may serve to encourage the very behavior that adults term undesirable. The adolescent can thus rebel against adult authority and standards in a way that may be disastrous to him. Since the conduct of adolescents is controlled not only by what adults say, but also by what the group dictates, it is vitally important that the individual be a member of a group that upholds society's standards of conduct.

Emotional Maturity

No one ever really becomes emotionally mature in all facets of his personality. There is always some development of the past that is incomplete, although the stages of development are the very cornerstones upon which a mature personality is built.

Theoretically, an emotionally and physically mature person is able to face reality, to use good judgment, to select a mate, to provide a home and to rear his children wisely. He should be able to meet responsibilities and get pleasure from activities participated in alone or with others. He should be able to balance responsibility and pleasure in a way that keeps him free from tension. Yet while he is master of himself and of his world, he should be humble, recognizing his own limitations as well as those of reality.

The mature person should be able to accept dependency, both of others and of himself, when necessary. This capacity for mutual dependency is a crucial part of social living.

A mature person believes in himself and in others who love him and whom he loves. He is able to deal wisely with those who dislike him and whom he dislikes.

Toward this goal the adolescent must work. He must formulate his own code of behavior and philosophy of life. These must be based on his individual decisions, but both are greatly influenced by previous family life, by teaching in school and church, by all his contacts in his lifetime and by all the experiences he has lived through.

OVERVIEW OF PHYSICAL DEVELOPMENT

During puberty and adolescence the young person not only makes great strides toward emotional maturity, but also reaches physical maturity. Changes in appearance as a result of physical development may cause disturbances in emotional well-being.

Puberty

Pubescence is associated with reaching sexual maturity. During the year or two preceding puberty rapid changes occur in the rate of growth in weight and height, in body contours and in the physiology of the body as a result of maturation of the gonads and hormonal activity. These changes usually continue to puberty, which occurs by about twelve to fourteen years, with a range of eleven to fifteen years in girls and a year or two later for boys. Girls tend to develop more rapidly than boys and to maintain their lead until they reach adult maturity.

Physical changes in the boy include, in order of appearance, (1) increase in size of the genitalia, (2) swelling of the breasts, (3) growth of pubic, axillary, facial and chest hair, (4) voice changes, and (5) production of spermatozoa. Boys grow rapidly in shoulder breadth from about the age of thirteen years.

Boys can become disturbed by *nocturnal emissions,* the loss of seminal fluid during sleep. If they have not been told that this is normal, they may regard it as a disease, or a punishment because of masturbation or thinking too much about sex. They may also believe that it is devitalizing. Nocturnal emissions are due to the activity of the sexual glands, and occasional release of spermatic fluid during sleep should cause no concern. If boys are not adequately prepared for this phenomenon, they ask either

their father or their friends about it. Boys generally are able to talk more freely among themselves than girls are and therefore usually find a solution to this problem.

Changes in the girl, in order of appearance, include (1) increase in the transverse diameter of the pelvis, (2) development of the breasts, (3) change in the vaginal secretions, and (4) growth of pubic and axillary hair. Menstruation has its onset between the appearance of pubic hair and that of axillary hair. Girls begin to have broad hips from about the age of twelve years on.

Because of lack of adequate information, girls may have ambivalent feelings about menstruation. They may resent the fact that they cannot completely control all their bodily functions, and may therefore consider menstruation a burden.

Many parents do not adequately explain to girls the various changes in body contour indicative of puberty. Before puberty and adolescence the child should be well oriented as to the anatomic and functional differences between the sexes. The girl should have a clear conception of ovulation, fertilization, pregnancy and birth. She should certainly have been told about menstruation before it occurs. Especially in discussing menstruation, adults are likely to pass on to their children the same beliefs and taboos which were told to them. They may say that the girl should rest or not participate in social activities during the menstrual period, thus implying that she is not well.

Menstruation is a normal physiologic phenomenon. There is no reason why women should curb their normal activities at this time. Menstruation is not debilitating. The blood loss is quickly made up. If mothers would only stress that menstruation is a normal phenomenon, young women would have fewer problems.

In discussions about sex, parents should impress upon their children that the realities of sex are far more complex than the image presented by sensation-seeking media which are likely to contain more fiction than fact. Parents should provide guidance to counteract the false information many adolescents obtain from such sources. They should also encourage discussion of sexual matters, allowing sex its proper place as a healthy part of life.

Other physical changes also occur in children of both sexes at adolescence. The sebaceous glands of the face, back and chest become more active. If the pores are too small, sebaceous material cannot escape, so that it collects beneath the skin and produces pimples or acne (see p. 627). Perspiration is increased. Vasomotor instability produces blushing.

Growth in height tends to decrease each year from birth, but with the onset of pubescence there is a rapid increase, and the child becomes tall. Gain in weight is proportionately greater than gain in height during early adolescence; therefore the adolescent appears to be stocky. This obesity has an important effect from both a physical and a psychologic standpoint.

There are differences in the rate of growth of various organ systems. The skeletal system often grows faster than its supporting muscles. This difference in growth rate tends to cause clumsiness and poor posture. Since large muscles may grow faster than small ones, the youth is likely to lack coordination. His extremities, his hands and feet, may grow out of proportion to the rest of his body and cause more problems in coordination.

Since the heart and lungs usually grow more slowly than the rest of the body, the supply of oxygen may be inadequate, and the pubescent may feel constantly tired.

The youth, and sometimes the parents, not realizing that this is just a stage every adolescent must go through, may feel inferior and socially embarrassed by these bodily changes. The youth may try to compensate for his supposed inferiority by ridiculing others, by trying to force his body to behave and to appear better by exercising and dieting, by attracting attention to himself by giggling and fidgetiness or by developing his intellect so that his physical appearance can be tolerated. Other pubescents may withdraw so that they cannot be compared with others. Parents should not scold or ridicule a child at this stage. Further growth will correct many of the problems. Instead, children should get from their parents reassurance and help to face the conflict between the image of themselves as they would like to be and as they are.

At puberty the child is flooded with new sensations and feelings which he cannot understand. This is one of the reasons why the youth may be alert and interested in everything for a time and then shortly after be bored, withdrawn and disinterested. By withdrawing, he is able to assimilate and digest the incoming sensations. This developmental phenomenon may occur about the time he is thirteen years old. He may do poorly in school for about a year at this time. Parents and teachers can help him by being patient and by explaining to him that this is just a period in his growth. He should not be ridiculed.

Motor behavior is influenced by the rapid changes taking place in the body. The young adolescent may appear awkward in his gross body movements because of his difficulty in adapting to these changes and because of his fear of ridicule, although he is actually gaining in strength and skill. As a result of rapid growth, pubescents may not have sufficient energy left for activity; therefore they may tire easily.

Girls do not usually develop the gross motor ability that boys do. This may be partially due to the fact that girls have many interests other than sports.

When rapid physical changes and changes in motor skill occur, the pubescent may become intensely interested in his physical appearance. During preadolescence he had an image of what he would be like as an adult. If what he is becoming is unlike his previous image, he may become uncertain of himself and of his body. Parents should help the young adolescent to make a realistic appraisal of his appearance and to make the most of his outstanding qualities.

Adolescence

After the pubescent years growth slows, and the change in body proportions occurs more gradually. The adolescent must continue to live with organ systems and functional capacities of widely varying levels of maturity. Usually by fifteen to sixteen years the secondary sex characteristics have developed fully, and adolescents are capable of reproduction. During the first year or longer of menstruation, periods are frequently missed or are irregular. Conception is unlikely until a year after periods have begun and usually does not occur until around the sixteenth year.

By this age the adolescent's motor abilities are similar to those of adults; thus adolescents can perform tasks which require muscular control and skill. Parents must guard against the adolescent's trying to live up to that part of his development which is most advanced, such as stature. They must try to help him set limits to his behavior as a result of understanding the problems involved.

At the end of adolescence the young person appears physically like an adult. His head is approximately one eighth of his body length. When his wisdom teeth erupt, between seventeen and twenty-one years of age, he has his full set of thirty-two permanent teeth (See Fig. 21-4).

SPECIFICS OF PHYSICAL, EMOTIONAL, SOCIAL AND MENTAL DEVELOPMENT

Pubescence and adolescence are best understood if they are considered a period of accelerated maturation and not a span of a certain number of years with specific steps in development to be accomplished each year. To subdivide this span of years is artificial, since development proceeds at varied rates. The rate of growth and development depends on all the factors mentioned throughout this text: heredity and con-

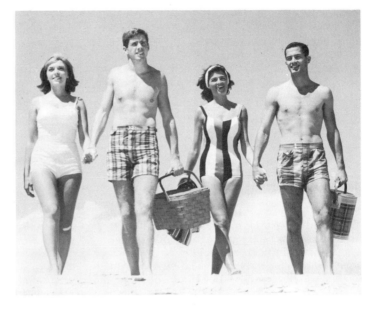

Figure 24-5. After the pubescent years the rate of growth slows, and changes in body proportions occur more gradually. These young people have nearly achieved their adult size. (H. Armstrong Roberts.)

stitutional make-up, racial and national characteristics, sex, environment — including prenatal environment — socioeconomic status of the family, nutrition, climate, illness and injury, exercise, position in the family, intelligence, hormonal balance, and emotions.

School

Adolescents as a group can do much more abstract thinking than they did when they were in the lower school grades. As their school subjects become more complex, there is a period of rapid increase in vocabulary and language development. Unfortunately, mental growth is not exactly correlated with increase in size. Parents and teachers should therefore not expect more mentally from a young person simply because of his rapid increase in physical size.

Adolescents have some difficulties in adjustment to school. They may spend more time in extracurricular activities than in academic work. They may be so disturbed by the problems inherent in adolescence that they may not be able to concentrate long enough to study. The school, recognizing that such problems exist, should offer activities that will help them find answers to their problems and satisfy their social needs.

There is great variation in academic ability and interest. A few adolescents excel in all areas, more excel in a few areas, and some excel in no areas. Often the degree of interest in school is based on the ultimate goal the adolescent has set for himself. If he needs further academic preparation leading to a professional role, he will apply himself to his studies. If his goal is to be an unskilled laborer requiring no additional

preparation, he may not see the necessity of achieving excellence in his high school work.

Besides academic preparation for adult life, high school offers the adolescent opportunities in extracurricular activities for satisfying his needs for security, recognition and success for himself and his group. Adolescents should have

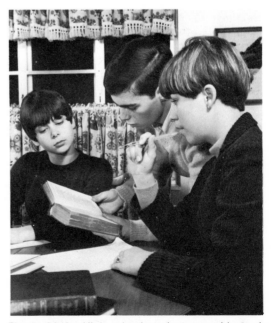

Figure 24-6. High school students are able to do more abstract thinking than they could when in elementary school. They involve themselves deeply in subjects that interest them. (H. Armstrong Roberts.)

opportunities to develop intellectual and physical skills and to satisfy their interests in areas such as crafts, music and art.

School programs should take into consideration the stage in development each child is going through. This is especially essential since the children in any one class may be prepubescent, pubescent or early adolescent, depending on their rate of growth.

Parents should continue to take an interest in the school life of the adolescent. They should also invite him to some of the social activities of adults in the community. It has been said that high school activities such as sports events, dances and parties are too expensive and that this is one reason why some children develop feelings of inferiority in their group and a desire to leave school before graduation. Adults in the community can help such children by providing opportunities for them to make their own money for these purposes.

Adults may also assist adolescents in their selection of a vocation by being willing to talk to groups about their own vocational choices.

Play and Work

During pubescence and adolescence sex makes more of a difference than ever in play and work interests.

Girls develop interests in social functions such as parties and dances, romance, housekeeping and child-rearing responsibilities. They enjoy romantic motion pictures and television programs. They may spend hours making themselves more attractive, experimenting with hair styles, cosmetics and new clothes. They learn to cook, clean and sew. Their interests widen in such fields as art, poetry and music. They, as well as boys, may spend a long time talking on the telephone to someone they have just seen a short time before the conversation began.

Boys are usually interested in competing and excelling in sports. They develop team loyalty and spirit. They are interested in mechanical or electrical devices ås hobbies. Their acceptance in the group depends not so much on personal appearance as on manliness, physical abilities and ability to complete a job.

Adolescents enjoy part-time work by which they can earn spending money for themselves. They may serve newspapers, mow lawns, shovel snow or care for young children. Although these activities have little relation in most cases to their ultimate work in life, the way they carry out their responsibilities gives some indication of their level of industry in whatever work they perform as adults. The adolescent thus learns to work with others, to cooperate even with those to whom he has no real personal attachment. He should find satisfaction in knowing that he has done a job well and that he can contribute in some way to society.

Adolescents gain great satisfaction from working for a worthwhile cause. Feelings of altruism are well developed at this age, and the individual and the group can make valuable contributions to a worthwhile effort.

Choice of Vocation

Three types of vocation face the young person: the vocation of citizenship, the vocation which will make a living for himself and his

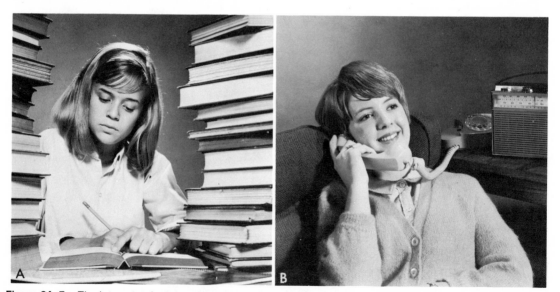

Figure 24–7.   The interests of adolescents vary. *A,* Some enjoy earnest study. *B,* Some enjoy seemingly endless telephone conversations. (H. Armstrong Roberts.)

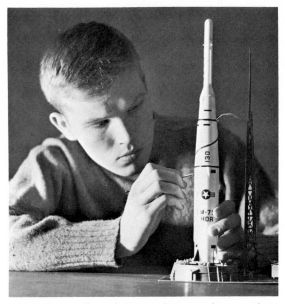

Figure 24-8. The adolescent boy may have an interest in mechanical or electrical devices. Such an interest may influence his choice of vocation. (H. Armstrong Roberts.)

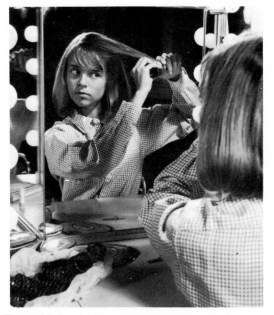

Figure 24-9. Adolescents become very much aware of their appearance. (H. Armstrong Roberts.)

family, and the vocation of parenthood. Parents should be honest with their children and tell them the problems involved in each type.

Probably the vocation which the adolescent believes is most immediately important is a career. The attitude among some groups that everyone will be taken care of, that adolescents need not worry about working, is an unhealthy one. The adolescent girl should probably prepare for both a career and marriage.

The adolescent should be guided in vocational preparation with consideration for his limitations and capacities. Simply that the father wanted to be a physician all his life is no reason why the son should be encouraged to study medicine. The young person can make his best contribution to society by doing something he is sincerely interested in. It is unfortunate if an adolescent's desires about his future must be changed because of his socioeconomic status or level of intelligence. Guidance in vocational choice is essential if the young person is to avoid such a disappointment or is to make plans so that he can achieve his goal.

CARE

The adolescent, after his attention has been turned to the opposite sex, becomes very much aware of how he appears to others. Parents are usually amazed at the change in the young person's behavior at this time. He becomes unusually clean, neat in dress and careful of grooming. Appearance is of the utmost importance socially. After this time parents need have little concern about the daily care of the adolescent, other than to see to it that he gets adequate rest and a balanced diet. Adolescents require about eight to nine hours of sleep a day. They require a higher caloric intake than ever before because of their rapid growth.

Safety Education

Although much effort in the home, schools and youth organizations has gone into safety education for young people, the accident rate among adolescents continues to be distressingly high. In the teen-age group the greatest cause of accidents is motor vehicles. In an effort to reduce mortality and morbidity from this cause, many schools offer driver-training and safety programs for older children. Adolescents must learn to discipline themselves in order to become safe and courteous drivers, to save their own lives as well as those of others.

Adolescents are especially susceptible to injury when riding on motorcycles, a sport which is increasing in popularity. Girls who ride behind the driver of a motorcycle may burn their legs on the exhaust pipe. Boys may be thrown from the motorcycle for many reasons. Since most motorcycle deaths are caused by head injuries, any person who drives a motorcycle, motor scooter or motorbike should wear a safety helmet for protection in case of accident.

Other causes of accidental death during the adolescent years are drowning and firearms. Such accidents are largely preventable. Young people should learn to swim and should be taught to use firearms safely, if they are interested in using them at all. They should be cautioned against playing with a loaded weapon, especially against playing the game Russian roulette.

To a degree adolescents must be safeguarded to prevent physical trauma when they want to do something beyond their physical endurance.

As soon as interest in personal appearance develops, girls especially may resent the fact that they seem to be gaining too much weight. They may go on a diet which may endanger their health. Parents should supervise the diet without being obvious about it. The adolescent may have practice in planning meals, in marketing and in balancing a day's meals and thereby learn the essentials of an adequate diet. This is especially important so that the young woman may be in a state of adequate nutrition when she is married and begins her childbearing period.

Both parents and school personnel should educate young people in the essentials of a good diet, because often adolescents tend to drink too many carbonated beverages and to eat too many pizzas and French fries. Since group consciousness is strong, at times a whole group must be helped toward an understanding of better eating habits. They should learn that only by eating a diet that includes meat and other protein foods, vegetables, fruits, whole grain cereals and milk will they achieve the health status in adulthood that is desired. The teenager's interest in his own health and appearance can be used to encourage wholesome food practices. Boys many times eat properly because of their interest in being in good physical condition for competitive sports.

NUTRITION

Adolescents must receive adequate nutrition, especially at the time of their greatest growth. Appetite usually poses no problem at this time. Adolescents are known for their propensity to raid the refrigerator.

Because of rapid growth the girl may need 2400 calories daily and the boy 3000 calories. Table 24-1 gives the nutritional requirements of adolescent boys and girls at different ages. The difference in requirements between the sexes is due largely to the difference in ultimate size and the fact that boys in general are more interested in physical activity than are girls.

Table 24–1. *Recommended Daily Dietary Allowances for Pubescents and Adolescents (12 to 18 Years)*

	BOYS		GIRLS		
	12–14 YEARS	14–18 YEARS	12–14 YEARS	14–16 YEARS	16–18 YEARS
WEIGHT	43 KG. (95 POUNDS)	59 KG. (130 POUNDS)	44 KG. (97 POUNDS)	52 KG. (114 POUNDS)	54 KG. (119 POUNDS)
HEIGHT	151 CM. (59 INCHES)	170 CM. (67 INCHES)	154 CM. (61 INCHES)	157 CM. (62 INCHES)	160 CM. (63 INCHES)
K calories	2,700	3,000	2,300	2,400	2,300
Protein	50 gm.	60 gm.	50 gm.	55 gm.	55 gm.
Fat-soluble vitamins					
Vitamin A activity	5,000 I.U.	5,000 I.U.	5,000 I.U.	5,000 I.U.	5,000 I.U.
Vitamin D	400 I.U.	400 I.U.	400 I.U.	400 I.U.	400 I.U.
Vitamin E activity	20 I.U.	25 I.U.	20 I.U.	25 I.U.	25 I.U.
Water-soluble vitamins					
Ascorbic acid	45 mg.	55 mg.	45 mg.	50 mg.	50 mg.
Falacin[a]	0.4 mg.	0.4 mg.	0.4 mg.	0.4 mg.	0.4 mg.
Niacin equivalents[b]	18 mg.	20 mg.	15 mg.	16 mg.	15 mg.
Riboflavin	1.4 mg.	1.5 mg.	1.4 mg.	1.4 mg.	1.5 mg.
Thiamin	1.4 mg.	1.5 mg.	1.2 mg.	1.2 mg.	1.2 mg.
Vitamin B$_6$	1.6 mg.	1.8 mg.	1.6 mg.	1.8 mg.	2.0 mg.
Vitamin B$_{12}$	5 μg.	5 μg.	5 μg.	5 μg.	5 μg.
Minerals					
Calcium	1.4 gm.	1.4 gm.	1.3 gm.	1.3 gm.	1.3 gm.
Phosphorus	1.4 gm.	1.4 gm.	1.3 gm.	1.3 gm.	1.3 gm.
Iodine	135 μg.	150 μg.	115 μg.	120 μg.	115 μg.
Iron	18 mg.	18 mg.	18 mg.	18 mg.	18 mg.
Magnesium	350 mg.	400 mg.	350 mg.	350 mg.	350 mg.

[a] The folacin allowances refer to dietary sources as determined by *Lactobacillus casei* assay. Pure forms of folacin may be effective in doses less than ¼ of the RDA.

[b] Niacin equivalents include dietary sources of the vitamin itself plus 1 mg. equivalent for each 60 mg. of dietary tryptophan.

From the Food and Nutrition Board, National Academy of Sciences – National Research Council: Recommended Daily Dietary Allowances (1968).

During this period approximately 15 per cent of the total calories should be derived from protein so as to maintain a positive nitrogen balance. This means that the adolescent should receive up to 60 gm. of protein a day. This may be obtained from milk, eggs, meat and cheese. He needs a quart of milk to provide 1.3 gm. of calcium. He also needs about 400 International Units of vitamin D a day to absorb adequately and retain calcium in his body.

HEALTH SUPERVISION

Ephebiatrics (from the Greek *ephebos,* meaning youth, puberty) is a growing new specialty whose purpose is to help teenagers solve their problems. Adolescents as a group have special needs, and not all physicians are comfortable dealing with them. *Ephebiatrists,* then, are physicians who work with adolescents, many of them in adolescent clinics.

In recent years clinics for adolescents have been organized in several sections of this country. In these clinics all sorts of problems are seen and treated. They are general-practice clinics devoted to an age group instead of to a particular kind of illness or a specific problem. Specialists' help is available if the adolescent needs it.

Usually youths between twelve and twenty-one years of age are offered help regardless of their complaint, whether emotional, physical, social or intellectual. A physician interested in the total adolescent and his problems sees the young person and establishes a close relation with him. The parents may be interviewed initially and as necessary, but the primary relation is between the physician and the adolescent. The adolescent is expected to take the responsibility for his own health.

The care these adolescents need usually involves four concerns: physical growth and development, vigorous activity, school, and emotional factors in their development. Physicians in these clinics also see illnesses common to young people (see Chap. 25). The focus in management should be on the young person himself, not on the specific problem he presents.

Physicians trained in these clinics do not necessarily become specialists in the treatment of adolescents. They do, however, develop insights into the problems of this age group which will help them in their treatment of them, whether they are essentially pediatricians or internists.

Adolescents need someone to talk with about their problems. They also need measures to protect them against disease after their childhood immunizations have worn off (see the immunization schedule given in Chapter 12, p. 278).

Certain physical problems, however, may be prevented by proper care during adolescence. Because adolescents spend increasingly longer time at night studying, they need frequent reexamination of their eyes. Also, because boys are more athletic and subject to foot injuries and because girls are style-conscious and wear ill-fitting shoes, both sexes should be cautioned about the proper care of their feet. Both sexes also should have frequent dental examinations because caries, prevalent during the second decade of life partly because of a diet high in carbohydrate and erratic dental hygiene habits, should be treated promptly. The adolescent should assume responsibility both for his own general medical care and for his visits to the dentist.

Adolescents must develop a good attitude toward health so as to profit from factual information gained from various sources. Education about growth and development, accident prevention, nutrition, sex education and mental hygiene is of special interest to them. Facts about the effects of smoking on health should be given to adolescents, since many of them acquire this habit during this period of their lives. Older adolescent girls should be taught how to examine their breasts routinely by their physician or school nurse.

EFFECTS OF SEPARATION

The child during pubescence and the adolescent may be separated from their parents and home for long periods of time, with little problem if their emotional development has been sound. Young adolescents may spend a few nights at the homes of friends under the supervision of their parents. They may go to camp in summer for several weeks at a time. Others may spend the school year at boarding schools some distance from home. Although homesickness may be a complaint at the beginning of a separation, even when the young person goes to college, activities in the new environment quickly seize upon his interest.

*TEACHING AIDS AND OTHER INFORMATION**

American Medical Association
Lerrigo, M. O., and Southard, H.: Approaching Adulthood, 1966.

---

* Complete addresses are given in the Appendix.

Safeguarding the Health of the Athlete.
Smoking: Facts You Should Know.
The Look You Like.
Why Girls Menstruate.

American Social Health Association

Boys Want to Know.
Girls Want to Know.
Let's Tell the Whole Story About Sex.
Preparing for Your Marriage.

Association for the Aid of Crippled Children

Klein, D.: When Your Teen-Ager Starts to Drive.
McFarland, R. A., and Moore, R. C.: Youth and the Automobile.

Kimberly-Clark Corporation

Jones, M.: How to Tell the Retarded Girl About Menstruation.

Personal Products Company

Growing up and Liking It.
How Shall I Tell My Daughter?

Public Affairs Pamphlets

Black, A. D.: If I Marry Outside My Religion.
Duvall, E.: Building Your Marriage.
Duvall, E.: Keeping up with Teen-Agers.
Kirkendall, L. A.: Too Young to Marry?

Ross Laboratories

You and Your Adolescent.

The American Cancer Society, Inc.

The Nurse and Breast Self Examination.
Where There's Smoke . . . There's Danger.

United States Department of Health, Education, and Welfare

Age of Transition: Rural Youth in a Changing Society, 1967.
A Guide to Child-Labor Provisions of the Fair Labor Standards Act, 1966.
A Light on the Subject of Smoking, 1966.
Chilman, C. S.: Growing up Poor, 1966.
Dialogue on Adolescence, 1967.
Food for the Young Couple, 1967.
From School to Work, Federal Services to Help Communities Plan with Youth, 1965.
Moving into Adolescence, Your Child in His Pre-teens, 1966.
Pennywise Teenagers, 1966.
School or Else, 1965.
Smoking and Illness, 1967.
Smoking, Health, and You—Facts for Teenagers, 1965.
The Adolescent in Your Family, reprinted 1965.
What We Know About Children and Smoking, 1967.
When Teenagers Take Care of Children, A Guide for Baby Sitters, 1964.
Why Nick the Cigarette Is Nobody's Friend, 1966.
Young People Who Smoke, 1968.
Your Child in His Preteens, 1966.
Youth Physical Fitness, 1967.

REFERENCES

Publications

Adams, J. F.: *Understanding Adolescence: Current Developments in Adolescent Psychology.* Boston,
        Allyn and Bacon, Inc., 1968.
Breckenridge, M. E., and Vincent, E. L.: *Child Development. Physical and Psychologic Growth
        Through Adolescence.* 5th ed. Philadelphia, W. B. Saunders Company, 1965.
Child Study Association of America: *Sex Education and the New Morality—A Search for a Meaningful
        Social Ethic.* New York, Columbia University Press, 1967.

Committee on Adolescence: *Normal Adolescence: Its Dynamics and Impact.* New York, Group for The Advancement of Psychiatry, 1968.

Crow, L. D., and Crow, A.: *Adolescent Development and Adjustment.* 2nd ed. New York, McGraw-Hill Book Company, Inc., 1965.

Douvan, E., and Adelson, J.: *The Adolescent Experience.* New York, John Wiley and Sons, Inc., 1966.

Duvall, E. M., and Hill, R. L.: *When You Marry.* Boston, D. C. Heath and Company, 1967.

Erikson, E. H. (Ed.): *Youth: Change and Challenge.* New York, Basic Books, 1963.

Garrison, K. C.: *Psychology of Adolescence.* 6th ed. Englewood Cliffs, N.J., Prentice-Hall, Inc., 1965.

Havighurst, R. J., and Taba, H.: *Adolescent Character and Personality.* New York, John Wiley and Sons, Inc., 1963.

Hentoff, N.: *Our Children Are Dying.* New York, Viking Press, Inc., 1966.

Krause, M. V.: *Food, Nutrition and Diet Therapy.* 4th ed. Philadelphia, W. B. Saunders Company, 1966.

Landis, B. Y.: Religion and Youth; in E. Ginzberg (Ed.): *The Nation's Children.* 2. Development and Education. New York, Columbia University Press, 1960, p. 186.

Martin, A. R.: *Youth's Search for Identity.* New York, Boys' Clubs of America, 1965.

Mays, J. B.: *The Young Pretenders: A Study of Teen-Age Culture in Contemporary Society.* New York, Schocken Books, Inc., 1965.

Nash, R. C. (Ed.): *Rural Youth in a Changing Environment.* Washington, D.C., National Committee for Children and Youth, 1965.

Pike, J. A.: *Teen-Agers and Sex.* Englewood Cliffs, N.J., Prentice-Hall, Inc., 1965.

Recommended Dietary Allowances. Revised 1968. Washington, D.C., National Academy of Sciences – National Research Council.

Rosenberg, M.: *Society and the Adolescent Self-Image.* Princeton, N.J., Princeton University Press, 1965.

Sherif, M., and Sherif, C. W. (Eds.): *Problems of Youth: Transition to Adulthood in a Changing World.* Chicago, Aldine Publishing Company, 1965.

Usdin, G. L. (Ed.): *Adolescence: Care and Counseling.* Philadelphia, J. B. Lippincott Company, 1967.

Winnicott, D. W.: *The Family and Individual Development.* New York, Basic Books, Inc., 1965.

Witmer, H. L., and Kotinsky, R.: *Personality in the Making: The Fact-Finding Report of the Midcentury White House Conference on Children and Youth.* New York, Harper and Brothers, 1952.

World Health Organization: *Aspects of Family Mental Health in Europe.* New York, Columbia University Press, 1965.

Periodicals

A Guide to Understanding Teenagers. *Patient Care,* 1:23, August 1967.

Anderson, E.: Who Wants to Know What About Menstrual Health? *Nursing Outlook,* 13:47, September 1965.

Bauer, W. W.: Moving into Manhood: Boys and Girls Together. *Today's Health,* 41:54, September 1963.

Bealer, R. C., Willits, F. K., and Maida, P. R.: The Rebellious Youth Subculture – A Myth. *Children,* 11:43, 1964.

Berland, T., and Seyler, A. E.: Teeth Care for Teen-Agers. *Today's Health,* 46:66, March 1968.

Daly, M. J.: Physical and Psychological Development of the Adolescent Female. *Clin. Obst. Gynec.,* 9:711, 1966.

Daniels, A. M.: Training School Nurses to Work with Groups of Adolescents. *Children,* 13:210, 1966.

Eisenberg, L.: A Developmental Approach to Adolescence. *Children,* 12:131, 1965.

Francis, G. M.: How Do I Feel About Myself? *Am. J. Nursing,* 67:1244, 1967.

Freedman, M. K.: Perspectives in Youth Employment. *Children,* 12:75, 1965.

Golub, S.: How Nurses Reply to Questions About Sex. *RN,* 30:41, September 1967.

Hammar, S. L.: The Role of the Nutritionist in an Adolescent Clinic. *Children,* 13:217, 1966.

Higdon, R., and Higdon, H.: What Sports for Girls? *Today's Health,* 45:21, October 1967.

Irwin, T.: What Kind of Mates Will Our Teen-Agers Be? *Today's Health,* 45:21, September 1967.

Peckos, P. S., and Heald, F. P.: Nutrition of Adolescents. *Children,* 11:27, 1964.

Pratt, M. K., and Thompson, L. B.: Five Cared for Five Hundred. *Am. J. Nursing,* 67:1684, 1967.

PHS Heats up Warfare on Smoking. *Medical World News,* 8:29, September 8, 1967.

Roach, R. H.: Your Teen-Ager and Smoking. *Today's Health,* 46:68, January 1968.

Saxton, R. H.: Three Years of the Neighborhood Youth Corps. *Children,* 14:156, 1967.

Simon, H. M.: A Look at Secondary School Health Services. *Nursing Outlook,* 16:42, August 1968.

Spindler, E. B.: Better Diets for Teenagers. *Nursing Outlook,* 12:32, February 1964.

25

PROBLEMS OF PUBESCENCE AND ADOLESCENCE RELATED TO THE PROCESS OF GROWTH AND DEVELOPMENT

One of the common concerns of adolescents is the question, "Am I growing up the way I should?" This overconcern with themselves and their own bodies must be recognized and utilized to advantage by medical and nursing personnel if the adolescent is to be helped. Professional personnel must be more willing to listen to concerns than to advise and to show the young person respect as he approaches adulthood.

Since the adolescent is much more concerned than his parents usually are about the typical problems of adolescence such as acne, postural defects, fatigue, obesity or menstrual irregularities, it is he or she as an individual who should receive directly the guidance, medical assistance and directions for care needed from the physician or nurse. Although the parents should be informed of such actions, direct responsibility for following medical advice should belong to the young person himself. The experience of illness may thus help him not only to conquer present handicaps, but also to manage his future life better by himself. In this process many times

parents with guidance also learn that their job is to produce an adult, not a child.

The adolescent, in addition to seeking help with medical problems, may also need an adult who has no close ties with him such as his parents have, one who can discuss emotionally charged concerns such as sex, religion, death or school in an objective way. Such concerns or anxieties may result eventually in physical symptoms if they are not alleviated. If the physician or nurse has a warm, interested, neither disapproving nor approving manner, the confidence of the adolescent can be gained, and he can be helped with problems which concern him. If the adolescent does not receive such assistance and guidance when he needs it, he will probably be less able to accept it and profit from it as he grows older. If medical and nursing personnel refuse to recognize the adolescent as an individual in a particular stage of life, neither adult nor child, he will not continue treatment or will rebel and refuse to cooperate.

In summary, many of the symptoms of physical

distress complained of by pubescents and adolescents are the manifestations of normal physical and physiologic changes occurring in their bodies and of inner emotional turmoils they are experiencing. Treatment of these problems often requires the close cooperation of the patient, his parents, physician, teacher, counselor and the school, infirmary or public health nurse.

These problems cannot be clearly divided into physical or emotional groups, since each may be caused by a mixture of both.

Acne Vulgaris

Acne vulgaris is an inflammatory condition of the skin which occurs in and around sebaceous glands during adolescence especially. The condition results from a combination of hereditary factors and the production of hormones. The sebaceous glands become overactive. Not all the material formed can be eliminated to the skin surface. The glands become dilated, the pores become darkened from dirt accumulation, and bacteria thrive in the retained material.

Incidence and Clinical Manifestations. Acne occurs in both sexes so commonly that it can almost be called a normal manifestation of sexual development. At first blackheads or comedones form. These are followed by superficial and deep papules (see Plate 1, Figs. 5, 6). If no treatment is given, pustules and cysts are apt to form which later produce disfiguring scars.

The areas most commonly affected are the forehead, chin and cheeks. The back, shoulders and chest may also be involved. Itching may or may not be present. Acne may lead to the youth's withdrawal from social contact and ultimately to emotional problems.

Treatment and Prognosis. Acne should be treated as early as possible. The parents and the adolescent should be encouraged to seek medical attention if acne occurs, since this skin condition can produce permanent scars. The general health should be improved through dietary management, provision of adequate sleep, exposure to natural sunlight, reduction of emotional tension and anxiety, and adequate cleanliness. Chocolate, milk foods and especially foods with a very high carbohydrate or fat content (such as nuts or peanut butter) should be eliminated. Sports and exercise may be helpful, since profuse perspiration loosens blackheads plugging sebaceous glands and encourages the flow of sebum. The adolescent should bathe properly after perspiring.

The skin should be cleansed thoroughly at least twice a day with a washcloth, soap and hot water to remove bacteria and dirt. Soaps which contain hexachlorophene tend to reduce the severity of the lesions. Topical therapy may consist in the application of preparations containing sulfur, or sulfur and resorcin. Preparations which are cosmetically acceptable have been developed to hide the lesions. These preparations may prevent emotional upset in the adolescent by covering disfiguring lesions. If the skin is oily, 70 per cent alcohol or acetone may be applied before these preparations to encourage drying. The physician will probably warn the adolescent against picking or squeezing the pimples, since this practice may result in scarring.

Antibacterial creams are of value in the treatment of superficial, inflamed lesions. When a preparation new to the patient is used, it should be applied to one side of the face for several nights to determine whether it produces improvement in the condition of the skin.

In severe acne systemic antibiotic therapy may be advantageous. A broad-spectrum antibiotic should be used. Short courses of steroid therapy in low dosage may be given if the acne is persistent. Vitamin A may be given to reduce comedo formation.

If postacne scarring is severe, dermabrasion may be used; however, the results of this therapy are many times disappointing, and many physicians no longer utilize this type of treatment.

Acne vulgaris is usually relieved as adolescence is completed.

Postural Defects

The erect posture of the adult is usually attained during adolescence. There may be a period, however, during pubescence and early adolescence when posture is poor. There may be three reasons for this. Physically, since the bony structure of the body develops more rapidly than the muscles do, the child may appear clumsy and have poor posture. Another reason may be the emotional reaction of the youth who suddenly finds himself much taller than his peers. Since he does not want to appear different from them, he slumps so that he can be more nearly their size. Both boys and girls may have this difficulty. In addition, some girls may resent their developing breasts, and slump to hide this manifestation of sexual development.

If the cause of faulty posture is slow growth of muscles, a period of waiting until strength is gained may be all that is required for treatment. If faulty posture is due to embarrassment over rapid growth or sexual development, the problem should be discussed realistically with the adolescent. Ridicule, shaming or threatening should never be used.

Fatigue

Pubescents and adolescents frequently complain of being tired. They may be tired because

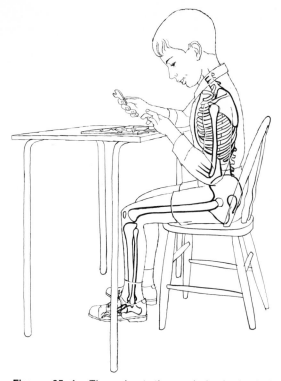

Figure 25–1. Throughout the period of physical growth the child, the pubescent and the adolescent need furniture that encourages them to maintain correct posture.

of extremely rapid physical growth, overactivity, lack of sleep, faulty nutrition, anemia or an emotional problem. If fatigue seems excessive or is prolonged, the underlying cause should be found and corrected.

Anemia

Before puberty the hemoglobin level is the same for both sexes. After puberty the level in girls is approximately 2 gm. below that in boys. Although the incidence of anemia is less than it was in the past, hypochromic anemia may occur and may be the cause of fatigue and fainting in this age group.

Obesity

Incidence. Obesity is a generalized and excessive accumulation of fat in subcutaneous tissue. It is relatively common during pubescence and adolescence. It occurs in both sexes. It is more frequent in the lower socioeconomic classes. Children with moderate obesity in the pubescent years usually require no treatment, since this may be considered normal. Many adolescents, however, who are obese because of overeating will continue to be obese as adults. This is un-

fortunate, since adolescence is a critical period for the possible development of a distorted body image.

Etiology, Clinical Manifestations and Diagnosis. The amount of food a person needs is determined by the energy needed for basal metabolism, growth and activity. The amount of food an adolescent requires and the amount he takes are influenced by a number of factors. Among the common causes of obesity are overeating with inactivity; hereditary, familial or racial factors; and emotional difficulties. An unhappy, withdrawn adolescent may develop an excessive appetite in order to try to escape from a difficult environment. Often the obesity makes the problem even more difficult, however. In other cases some overprotective mothers may force food upon their children. The children continue to be dependent upon their mothers and are likely to turn to eating as a comforting device for any deprivation.

Obesity due to endocrine problems such as hypothyroidism or hyperadenocorticism, which results in Cushing's syndrome, is rare.

Intracranial lesions may cause obesity as in Froelich's syndrome, but this too is rare.

The *clinical manifestations* are many. Obese adolescents are usually taller than the average for their age. The adolescent's appearance is a better criterion by which to judge obesity than is an arbitrary standard for normal and excess weight. These adolescents are usually inactive. Their facial features often appear fine or small. There may be collections of adipose tissue in the breast region, and they may have pendulous abdomens with striae. In boys the external genitalia may seem small, but this is only because they are buried in pubic fat.

The upper arms and the thighs may appear obese. These adolescents are often very clumsy and unable to take part successfully in competitive games. Slipping of the epiphysis of the head of the femur may occur. Flat feet and knock-knees are common.

Emotional disturbances are also common.

In making a *diagnosis* of the cause of obesity, the possibility of endocrine or other physical disturbance must be ruled out. The diet must be recorded to determine whether overeating is really present. Many of these adolescents eat normally at meals, but overeat between meals. An evaluation of the emotional status must be made.

Treatment and Prognosis. The cooperation of the adolescent and his family in the treatment of obesity is essential. If the cause is dietary, the diet should be reduced. Often the diet of the entire family must be adjusted. The diet should be based on nutritional needs, but the caloric intake may be reduced to 1000 to 1200 calories for children ten to fourteen years of age. The protein content should be high, and the fat and carbohydrate content low. The diet should contain as much bulk as possible. Vitamin concentrates, especially those containing vitamin D, for growth may also be given. Since adolescents often desire a midafternoon or an evening snack, these should be calculated in the diet. The energy output should be increased through exercise. The objective is burning of body fat to provide energy. A weight loss of 1 or 2 pounds a week is desirable.

If the child overeats because of emotional difficulties, the emphasis in treatment should not be on diet, but on the management of problem areas. The child should be helped to make a more adequate adjustment in his home, school and community. School personnel can often be of value in helping the child to form better relations with his peers. Psychotherapy may be necessary along with drug therapy.

The *prognosis* depends on the extent of cooperation among parents, child and physician. If even the best treatment ordered is not followed, there will be no weight reduction.

Menstrual Irregularities

Menstruation begins, on the average, at thirteen years of age, although the range is from eleven to fifteen years at onset. Since the cycles at first are anovulatory, irregularity in menstrual periods or a prolonged or scanty flow may be expected. If these symptoms continue to the second year, evaluation of the problem should be made. It is true that the normal cycle is more closely related to general health than to hormonal activity. If the girl is malnourished or obese, problems may be expected. Another frequent cause of menstrual difficulty during adolescence may be overactivity or underactivity. Improvement of diet and general hygiene is usually sufficient treatment.

Some adolescents who are emotionally disturbed, who may be striving too hard to achieve at school or who may be socially insecure may also have menstrual difficulties.

Less commonly, disturbance in thyroid functioning or organic lesions of the reproductive system may cause problems. Any young woman who continues to have difficulties despite improvement in her general well-being should have a determination of her basal metabolic rate and a gynecologic examination.

Hyperthyroidism

The basal metabolic rate generally decreases from early infancy to the end of the growth period. There is a relative increase, however, during the period of rapid growth preceding puberty. This temporarily elevated metabolic rate is probably related to the hyperthyroidism noted at this age.

Treatment includes a high caloric diet, reduction in school schedule and activity, and administration of iodine. This type of hyperthyroidism disappears when sexual maturity is reached.

Hyperthyroidism or exophthalmic goiter with excessive liberation of thyroid hormone is uncommon in children or adolescents.

Minor Neuroses

Mildly neurotic symptoms are present in many adolescents. These are usually short-lived and may result from some stress or challenge the youth has had. They persist only if he finds that the symptoms bring rewards from others in his environment.

The adolescent may show symptoms of tension over unpopularity, poor athletic ability or poor school work. Failure to participate in recreational activities or to gain a degree of independence from his parents, guilt about masturbation, and fear of sexual development or of being unsuccessful may cause neurotic manifestations.

The parents and the adolescent may complain specifically that he has insomnia, nightmares, headaches, difficulty in concentration, and gastrointestinal or menstrual problems.

Treatment of these mild neuroses consists in helping the adolescent to appreciate the basic cause of the problem. The physician should have good rapport with the parents and with the adolescent so that they will accept his plan of treatment and cooperate with him. The family physician or the pediatrician can usually treat these young people successfully. If there is a question of a deeper difficulty, however, consultation with a psychiatrist should be sought.

TEACHING AIDS AND OTHER INFORMATION*

American Medical Association

Aid for Acne.
Operation: Diet Right.
Something Can Be Done About Acne.
The Healthy Way to Weigh Less.

---

* Complete addresses are given in the Appendix.

Public Affairs Pamphlets

Irwin, M. H. K.: Overweight—A Problem for Millions, 1964.
King, C. G., and Lam, G.: Personality "Plus" Through Diet.
Landis, P. H.: Coming of Age: Problems of Teen-Agers.

United States Department of Health, Education, and Welfare

Food and Your Weight, 1967.
High School Dropouts: A 20th Century Tragedy.
Obesity and Health, 1966.

REFERENCES

Publications

Barness, L. A.: *Manual of Pediatric Physical Diagnosis.* 3rd ed. Chicago, Year Book Medical Publishers, Inc., 1966.
Gallagher, J. R.: *Medical Care of the Adolescent.* 2nd ed. New York, Appleton-Century-Crofts, 1966.
Hammer, S. L., and Eddy, J. K.: *Nursing Care of the Adolescent.* New York, Springer Publishing Company, 1966.
Heald, F. P. (Ed.): *Adolescent Gynecology.* Baltimore, Williams & Wilkins Company, 1966.
Lewis, G. M., and Wheeler, C. E.: *Practical Dermatology for Medical Students and General Practitioners.* 3rd ed. Philadelphia, W. B. Saunders Company, 1967.
Maibach, H. I., and Hildick-Smith, G. (Eds.): *Skin Bacteria and Their Role in Infection.* New York, Blakiston Division, McGraw-Hill Book Company, Inc., 1965.
Nelson, W. E. (Ed.): *Textbook of Pediatrics.* 8th ed. Philadelphia, W. B. Saunders Company, 1964.
Sauer, G. C.: *Manual of Skin Diseases.* 2nd ed. Philadelphia, J. B. Lippincott Company, 1966.
Schulman, J. L.: *Management of Emotional Disorders in Pediatric Practice: With a Focus on Techniques of Interviewing.* Chicago, Year Book Medical Publishers, Inc., 1967.
Silver, H. K., Kempe, C. H., and Bruyn, H. B.: *Handbook of Pediatrics.* 7th ed. Los Altos, California, Lange Medical Publications, 1967.
Sneddon, I. B., and Church, R. E.: *Practical Dermatology.* Baltimore, Williams & Wilkins Company, 1964.
Usdin, G. L. (Ed.): *Adolescence: Medical Care and Counseling.* Philadelphia, J. B. Lippincott Company, 1967.
World Health Organization: *Technical Report Series No. 308—Health Problem of Adolescence.* • *Report of a World Health Expert Committee.* Geneva, World Health Organization, 1965.

Periodicals

Anderson, E.: Who Wants to Know What About Menstrual Health? *Nursing Outlook,* 13:47, September 1965.
Barckley, V., and Stobo, E. C.: The Adolescent Who Smokes. *Nursing Outlook,* 12:25, February 1964.
Conway, E.: How a College Health Service Handles Menstrual Problems. *Nursing Outlook,* 13:51, September 1965.
Crawford, J. D., and Haessler, H. A.: Obesity—A Pediatric Viewpoint. *Medical Times,* 95:1269, 1967.
Dwyer, J. T., and others: Adolescent Dieters: Who Are They? *Am. J. Clin. Nutr.,* 20:1045, 1967.
Fay, A. B.: Dysmenorrhea: A School Nurse's Findings. *Am. J. Nursing,* 63:77, February 1963.
Gallagher, J. R.: A Clinic for Adolescents. *Children,* 1:165, 1954.
Hammar, S. L.: The Role of the Nutritionist in an Adolescent Clinic. *Children,* 13:217, 1966.
Hammar, S. L., and Eddy, J.: The Nurse and the Hospitalized Teen-Ager. *RN,* 29:68, December 1966.
Manning, M. L.: The Psychodynamics of Dietetics. *Nursing Outlook,* 13:57, April 1965.
Manthey, M. E.: A Guide for Interviewing. *Am. J. Nursing,* 67:2088, 1967.
Mayer, J.: Obesity Control. *Am. J. Nursing,* 65:112, June 1965.
Peckos, P. S., and Spargo, J. A.: For Overweight Teenage Girls. *Am. J. Nursing,* 64:85, May 1964.
Spindler, E. B.: Better Diets for Teenagers. *Nursing Outlook,* 12:32, February 1964.
Why Some Mothers Fatten Their Children. *Today's Health,* 45:56, November 1967.

26

LONG-TERM
CONDITIONS OF
THE ADOLESCENT

EFFECT OF ILLNESS ON ADOLESCENTS

Serious or prolonged illness during infancy or childhood may have negative effects on the personality of the adolescent unless special care has been taken to prevent this. Illness or accident may interfere with the child's sense of trust that his own body or the outside world is really dependable. Illness or accident may prove to the child that he is loved only when he is not well. Prolonged illness may lead the child whose sense of autonomy is not fully developed into over-dependency on others. Illness may also in later years so curb the development of a sense of initiative or of industry that the adolescent is unable to gain satisfaction from seeking the answers to questions or from starting or completing a project. Malnutrition occurring alone or in relation to a disease may result in apathy and listlessness.

Adolescence is difficult enough for normal young people, but more so for the handicapped person. Accepting his sex role, finding himself, emancipating himself from his family and selecting a career are difficult. The social aspects of his handicap are much greater during adolescence than they were earlier. If he did not accept the reality of his handicap earlier, he may be emotionally disturbed about it in adolescence.

The effects of a handicap such as impaired hearing, blindness, cardiac disease, diabetes or cerebral palsy tend to make children of any age overdependent on adults and to warp their personality development in several ways. Such conditions tend to limit both their social contacts with other children and their ability to relieve their pent-up emotions through physical activity, and to cause various degrees of rejection in themselves, their parents and peers. The adolescent, because of his feelings of guilt about his illness or handicap, may develop feelings of mistrust, self-doubt and inferiority. He may either give up in the battle for healthy personality development or may seek to punish others for his failure.

On the other hand, if handicapped or chronically ill children have been given the opportunity to master themselves and their environment within the limits of reality, to become independent, they will probably succeed in the battle of life. They must be given the opportunity to try; if they fail, they must be helped in their effort so that they can achieve success. If the adolescent cannot achieve success in the use of his legs, for instance, he can be helped to achieve by using his head or hands. Many people, even so-called normal people, have limitations which only they know. They have been able to use what they have to such advantage that the world is unaware of their handicap. They have developed a sense of security in their achievements with the help of their parents and other adults. Both they and their parents, facing the handicap realistically together, have been able to build parent-child relations which many normal children and parents might envy.

Long-term illness during adolescence may have disastrous effects. During illness the youth is unable to discover the kind of person he really is or what his role in the future will be, much less develop the sense of intimacy which is important to his later adjustment.

HOSPITAL CARE OF THE ILL ADOLESCENT

In the adult unit adolescents often annoy other patients with their noisy activities. Adolescents may also sustain considerable emotional damage because they are exposed to erroneous information given by adult patients or they may see sights or hear noises that may cause them to be terrified, since the adolescent has increased imagination and a tendency to introspection. In the children's unit adolescents may be annoyed with the crying of younger children, feel isolated because no other adolescents have been admitted, and become embarrassed because of their lack of privacy.

In recent years *adolescent units* have been opened in some hospitals. In these units adoles-

cents are comfortable with others in their own age group. Physicians and nurses are also likely to give more understanding care to their patients because they enjoy working with them. It is believed that adolescents need a continuing relation with their pediatricians until they reach maturity and find their place in the world.

In adolescent units the environment of the patients is very important. It should be as homelike and informal as possible. A phonograph in the lounge may provide a meeting place for all patients able to congregate together. A telephone beside each bed enables the adolescent to keep in contact with his friends at home. Certainly liberal visiting hours should be provided, since relations with peers are important at this age. Also, adolescents with their usually large appetites should be permitted to select their diets from menus provided unless they are on restricted diets. Snacks should be available as needed.

When adolescents are hospitalized, they are usually mature enough to admit that they are sick and to be aware of the adjustments required by their illness. They may protest, however, about restrictions such as special diets and the necessity for bed rest. They want information about their illnesses and procedures which must be done to them. They need reassurance about their medical progress and condition. Hospitalized adolescents need contact with their peers, diversion, and respect as individuals. The nurse is

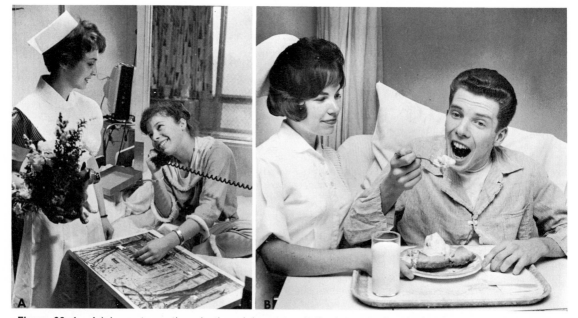

Figure 26–1. Adolescents continue in the adolescent unit the interests they had at home. *A*, The telephone provides diversion, but (*B*) so does eating! (*The Magazine of Lankenau Hospital*, Summer, 1962. Public Relations Department, Lankenau Hospital, Philadelphia, Pennsylvania.)

responsible, therefore, for providing the special type of care these young people need.

Role of the Nurse in Caring for Adolescents

The student nurse may find working with adolescents a difficult matter if she does not understand them and does not remember her professional role in working with them. The adolescent male may feel embarrassed when being given personal care by a student just a few years older than he. The adolescent female may be shy about exposing portions of her body to someone near her own age. Many times adolescents relate more easily to an older, more mature person; however, it is ultimately the responsibility of the student with the help of her instructor to work out her own feelings so that she can relate easily and provide professional care to these patients. The nurse, whatever her age, must help the adolescent to feel that he is important. The patient should be properly introduced to others and asked his opinions on matters that concern him.

The nurse must understand that adolescents are frequently unpredictable, that they may be emotionally unstable and torn between their desires to be dependent and independent. She must also remember their great need for security, to love and be loved, to be an accepted group member and to be approved. Sometimes these very needs make it difficult for them to verbalize their anxieties and feelings about illness and hospitalization to her. In addition, their language may be such that adults may not be able to understand the real meaning of what they say.

The nurse must be able to detect hostility and rejection in these patients. When such feelings are evident, she must often alter her approach completely in order to gain cooperation from them. She must remember not to argue with them, to avoid giving orders to them and to let them be as independent as possible. She should trust them and treat them as if they were grown up.

The nurse in the adolescent unit must provide the young person with freedom, but with guidance and restrictions when necessary. The limits on behavior that are established in the unit must be flexible, according to the capacity of the individual to handle situations. Restrictions must be related to privileges, and privileges must be related to responsibility. For example, although visiting hours may be over routinely in the adolescent unit at 9 p.m., if the friends of an adolescent patient who has a birthday wish to give her a party lasting until 9:30, they might be permitted to do so. They must realize, however, that excessive noise may disturb other patients; therefore they must assume the responsibility of remaining relatively quiet. They should also assume the responsibility of straightening up the area when the party is over.

If the nurse is aware of an adolescent's problem concerning acceptance of his newly developing body, she may be of great help to him at the time of a physical examination or when she carries out treatments. If she recognizes the fears characteristic of this phase of growth, she will sense the meaning behind some of his seemingly purposeless questions. She can help him by explaining that fears of this sort are common and are understandable to her. Adolescents need assurance that they are normal males or females. For a nurse to say to a pubescent girl, "Your genitalia must be abnormal, because I cannot locate the meatus," during a catheterization is inexcusable.

Adolescent girls are interested in making themselves as attractive as possible. Lipstick and other cosmetics are important to them. The nurse must understand that helping a young girl comb her hair in an attractive way, even though she is immobilized in a cast, is an important part of nursing care.

When adolescents are grouped together in one unit or part of a unit, the boys and girls have separate rooms and separate lavatories. These patients will form their own social group, much as they would if they were in their own communities. The nurse must be aware of the structure of such a group, its leader and its followers. She can do much to influence the group if she can convince the leader of the value of her ideas.

The nurse must also remember the emotional development of the persons involved. One of the greatest fears of adolescents is that of losing control of themselves in front of their peers. The nurse can see to it that this does not happen by handling them in a firm but fair manner. If a boy or a girl, but particularly a boy, is to face a painful treatment, it might be better to remove him from the group so that he can express his feelings openly rather than have him cry in the presence of others and be humiliated.

The young nurse may feel that simply because the patient is not a child he should understand that whatever is done is for his good, and she may fail to explain treatments to him. The adolescent, who is keenly interested in himself, his body and his illness, needs detailed explanations frequently. In giving such explanations the nurse must be willing to answer questions and to offer reassurance just as she does to younger children. She should be willing to spend time with the adolescent and to provide support when he needs it.

The adolescent should be helped to continue with his school work, even though he is hospitalized, so that he can join his group at school when he is discharged. The teenager's mind must be occupied with recreational interests when he is not doing school work. He will enjoy watching television, listening to the radio or helping with the care of younger children.

The physician and the nurse can help the adolescent by keeping the school teacher in the hospital and the school nurse in the community informed of the adolescent's disability and thereby help them to gain insight into his physical and psychologic needs in relation to his illness. They can also interpret to members of the community the fact that his basic needs are like those of normal adolescents.

In summary, if adolescents are given love, with limitations on their behavior, and with increasing amounts of responsibility for themselves and others in the hospital as well as at home, they will continue in their growth toward the goal of the independence of adulthood.

ILLNESS DURING ADOLESCENCE

The fact that children grow rapidly, physically and emotionally, during adolescence makes them particularly vulnerable to certain illnesses which may result in significant effects on the developmental process. Accidents, however, are the principal cause of death. The death rate from

Table 26–1. *Causes of Death*
(The Age Group from 15-24 Years, 1965)

RANK	CAUSE	NUMBER	RATE*
	Male, 15-24 Years		
	Total..	23,754	157.3
1	Accidents..	15,069	99.8
	Motor vehicle accidents...............	10,502	69.6
	Other accidents...........................	4,567	30.2
2	Homicide.......................................	1,609	10.7
3	Malignant neoplasms, including neoplasms of lymphatic and hematopoietic tissues..................	1,488	9.9
4	Suicide..	1,425	9.4
5	Diseases of heart...........................	508	3.4
	Female, 15-24 Years		
	Total...	9,339	61.5
1	Accidents.......................................	3,619	23.8
	Motor vehicle accidents...............	2,893	19.0
	Other accidents...........................	726	4.8
2	Malignant neoplasms, including neoplasms of lymphatic and hematopoietic tissues..................	997	6.6
3	Homicide.......................................	457	3.0
4	Suicide..	451	3.0
5	Diseases of heart...........................	425	2.8

* All rates are per 100,000 persons aged 15-24.
Department of Health, Education, and Welfare, United States Public Health Service, National Center for Health Statistics.

illness in this age group is relatively low. Although tuberculosis was at one time a leading cause of death, its incidence has been reduced in recent years. It is still true, however, that adolescents seem more susceptible to this disease than persons in other age groups.

Illnesses may also occur in adolescents which are more closely related to their *emotional* development than to their physical growth. Although some of these illnesses will be discussed in this chapter, it must be remembered that most adolescents reach normal levels of maturity for their age and ultimately become contributing members of their communities and positive models for their children, the next generation, to emulate.

Tuberculosis

Tuberculosis is a world-wide disease. Although its incidence has decreased in the more advanced countries, it is still prevalent in underdeveloped countries. The methods used to control tuberculosis in this country have brought excellent results, but they cannot be applied with equal success in other countries. Each country must find methods which can be utilized successfully with its own people in the areas of educational programs, better standards of living, earlier diagnosis and the best methods of treatment. The World Health Organization is working to help countries to bring this infection under control.

Incidence. The fact that adolescent girls seem to be more susceptible at an earlier age than boys may be related to their earlier maturation. The incidence is high in slum areas where overcrowding and poor health conditions are prevalent. There is also a higher incidence in areas with periods of flood or famine.

Early discovery and improved methods of treatment provide these young people with a good chance of cure.

Etiology and Epidemiology. Tuberculosis is caused by an acid-fast bacillus, *Mycobacterium tuberculosis.* Disease in man is produced by organisms causing either the bovine or the human form of the disease. A person may contract tuberculosis by drinking contaminated milk, although this method of infection has been almost completely eliminated in this country, owing to the practices of killing diseased cattle, forbidding the sale of contaminated milk, pasteurization of milk and testing milk handlers for tuberculosis.

The bacillus enters the body through the respiratory or the gastrointestinal tract. It is spread today chiefly by droplet infection or by direct contact with infected human beings. Entrance into the body may also take place by ingestion.

Children most frequently contract tuberculosis

from an infected adult in the home. This is the reason why newborn infants should be removed from mothers who have the disease; the mothers cannot then contaminate the children by breathing or coughing on them while feeding or caring for them. Older children and adolescents may contract the disease in their own homes or in the homes of friends or from close contact with their peer groups. Children of any age may put contaminated objects into their mouths. The unhygienic practice of sharing taffies, candy, or drinking or eating utensils may help spread the disease.

Predisposing Factors, Types of Infection and Pathology. Chronic illness, fatigue or undernutrition may predispose to tuberculosis.

A *primary infection* occurs when the tubercle bacillus enters the body, usually in the tissues of the lungs. Individual resistance and the number of organisms entering the body determine the extent of the disease. The reaction of the invaded tissue is basically one of inflammation and repair with later calcification, which may be noted on an x-ray film. The primary focus usually heals spontaneously.

The primary (Ghon) complex includes the initial lesion and lesions in the regional lymph nodes. The disease process may extend to other parts of the lung and to the gastrointestinal tract because of swallowed infected sputum. In some cases the organisms may produce symptoms of mild pneumonia. The organisms may enter the lymph nodes, lymph vessels and blood vessels. Foci of infection then occur in various organs and in serous membranes.

When widespread infection occurs, the child

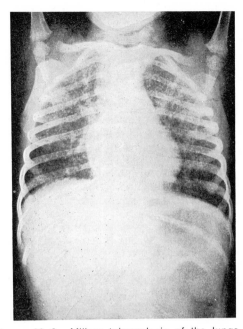

Figure 26-3. Miliary tuberculosis of the lungs in a white boy 3 years of age. His mother had pulmonary tuberculosis. The physical findings were fine, crackling rales throughout both lungs. Death occurred shortly after this roentgenogram was taken. The tuberculin reaction was positive. (R. H. High and W. E. Nelson in Nelson: *Textbook of Pediatrics.* 8th ed.)

is said to have *miliary tuberculosis.* This type generally occurs in the infant or very young child. Its onset is usually acute, with an irregular fever, rales in the chest, possibly an enlarged spleen, distended abdomen, prostration, dyspnea, cough and cyanosis. The mortality rate has been reduced through the use of newer drugs.

If the disease affects the meninges, *tuberculous meningitis* may result. Tuberculosis of the mesenteric or cervical lymph nodes, peritoneum, bones and joints may also occur. The bones most frequently involved include the head of the femur (*tuberculous coxitis*), fingers and toes (*tuberculous dactylitis*), and vertebrae (*tuberculous spondylitis* or *Pott's disease*).

If the child's resistance is good, healing of a primary lesion and calcification may take place. Later, because of lowered resistance, the latent lesion may again become active.

Secondary infections usually occur during adolescence or early in adult life either from the original focus or from reinfection. They differ from the primary type because of the allergic response of the body. Reinfection is a much more destructive process than the primary lesion. Secondary infection may include extensive inflammatory reaction with tissue destruction and cavitation. Healing in secondary infections is largely by means of scar tissue or fibrosis.

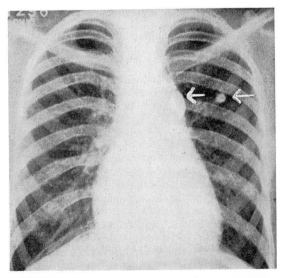

Figure 26-2. Calcified tuberculous focus (right arrow) and calcified tracheobronchial lymph node (left arrow) in a young girl. (R. H. High and W. E. Nelson in Nelson: *Textbook of Pediatrics.* 8th ed.)

The pulmonary lesion in a secondary infection is likely to be in the apex of the lung.

Clinical Manifestations and Diagnosis. In *primary* tuberculosis the *manifestations* of a pulmonary lesion may or may not be evident. The child may complain of malaise, fatigue and anorexia, have a weight loss and be irritable. If tuberculosis is suspected, but no symptoms are evident, the *diagnosis* may be made with a tuberculin test and an x-ray film of the chest.

The clinical manifestations of *secondary* tuberculosis may resemble those of infected adults. The disease may become chronic, progressive pulmonary tuberculosis with cough and expectoration, fever, hemoptysis, weight loss and night sweats.

For diagnostic testing two types of tuberculin are available: old tuberculin (O.T.) and purified protein derivative (P.P.D.). The tests used in the diagnosis of tuberculosis are the Mantoux test and the Heaf multiple puncture test or the tine test.

MANTOUX TEST. About six weeks after infection of a tuberculin-negative person the presence of allergy or hypersensitivity to tuberculoprotein may be observed by a positive skin test reaction to tuberculin. A known amount of tuberculin is injected intracutaneously. The test should be read in forty-eight to seventy-two hours. In a positive reaction an area of at least 5 mm. in diameter with erythema and definite induration occurs. The exact measurement of the reaction should be recorded. The larger the area of reaction, the greater is the risk that the child has a tuberculous infection. This is a most accurate test.

HEAF MULTIPLE PUNCTURE TEST (OR ITS MODIFICATION, THE TINE TEST). In the tine test a stainless steel disk with four prongs which are precoated with concentrated old tuberculin is pressed firmly against the cleansed (using alcohol or acetone) volar surface of the forearm. The tines penetrate the skin, depositing the tuberculin in the outer layer. The test should be read in forty-eight to seventy-two hours. The reaction is considered positive if the induration around one or more of the puncture sites is 2 mm. or more in diameter. Any persons having doubtful reactions should be tested with a Mantoux test.

MEANING OF REACTIONS. A positive tuberculin reaction is usually evidence that the person has been infected with the tubercle bacillus and is allergic or hypersensitive to its protein. It does not necessarily mean that the person has an active lesion at the time of testing. The size of the skin reaction indicates that the result is positive or negative.

Tuberculin tests should be done on the advice of the physician, depending on the risk of exposure of the child and the prevalence of tuberculosis in his geographic area. This would help in locating their source of infection.

Every child who shows a positive reaction to tuberculin should have a physical examination, have his temperature checked, and have a chest roentgenogram, blood cell count and sedimentation rate done. Contacts, whether parents, grandparents, siblings or friends, should be located and checked for tuberculosis.

A positive diagnosis of tuberculosis is made if the tubercle bacillus is found in the gastric contents or sputum. Young children seldom expectorate. Since sputum is swallowed, examination of the stomach contents obtained by gastric aspiration is of value.

Before breakfast a lavage tube is passed. After a few cubic centimeters of water have been injected a sample of the stomach contents is withdrawn by means of a syringe. The sediment in the return is examined for the tubercle bacillus by culture or guinea pig inoculation, or both. The test should be repeated three times before the result is considered negative.

Treatment and Nursing Care. Whether the patient is given care at home or in a hospital, the plan for his care depends on the total situation. If someone in his environment is infected, the patient should be removed from continued contact with this source of infection.

The patient should have mental and physical rest. Rest in bed may be necessary. A daily schedule to which he adheres is essential. Too much activity must be avoided. He must be kept out of school for his own sake and for the safety of other pupils. Adequate health supervision is essential.

The emotional attitude of the child and his family should be optimistic. The child should be isolated from close contact with other family members to prevent the spread of infection and also for his own protection from exposure to other infections which would tend further to drain his bodily resources. Measles is especially dangerous for a child with tuberculosis.

The patient requires an adequate diet, high in protein, calcium and vitamins, particularly B, C and D. Feeding should not be forced, but the child should be encouraged to eat sufficient food. Fresh air and sunshine may aid in his recovery and add to his sense of well-being.

The patient resumes his usual activities gradually as the lesion heals. He should be encouraged to do whatever he can for himself in order to prevent invalidism. He should be encouraged to plan with his parents and counselor for the future. The adolescent and even the older grade school child should be a member of the health team which plans for his care and rehabilitation. This team also includes his parents, physician, social worker, public school or visiting teacher, and nurse. Even during convalescence the child should be helped to keep in contact with his friends. A telephone near his bed and active correspondence with relatives and friends are of great value in helping him feel that he is still a part of his group and will return to them.

Several drugs have been used successfully in the treatment of tuberculosis, although no one specific drug will cure the disease. Prolonged treatment, from six months to a year, is usually necessary.

Isoniazid (INH) has a low toxicity, can control progressive lesions and is effective in preventing hematogenous dissemination. It may be given orally or parenterally.

Streptomycin is given intramuscularly. Long-term treatment may be complicated by damage to the eighth cranial nerve resulting in deafness. Streptomycin should not be used alone against tuberculosis, since streptomycin-resistant organisms rapidly emerge. Another tuberculostatic agent should be given at the same time.

Para-aminosalicylic acid (PAS) is given orally. It is not as effective as either streptomycin or isoniazid. The usual toxic reaction is gastric irritation. PAS is valuable because it inhibits the development of resistance by the bacilli to both streptomycin and isoniazid.

These drugs in various combinations have reduced the length of tuberculous infection and also certain secondary forms of the infection.

Other drugs which may be used include pyrizinamide, cycloserine, ethambutol and viomycin. Whether cortisone and corticotropin therapy is used depends on the type of lesion present.

Surgical treatment of tuberculous lesions other than bronchoscopy is rarely indicated in children.

Prognosis, Prevention and Methods of Control. In general the mortality rate is higher in infancy and adolescence than in childhood.

The primary lesion, usually benign, may become an extensive infection. The younger the child, the greater is the danger. During adolescence, however, there is an increased risk of development of chronic, progressive pulmonary tuberculosis, either from the primary focus or from reinfection. With secondary lesions the prognosis depends on the severity of the lesion, sex, age and environment of the child.

In recent years antimicrobial treatment has prevented the development of miliary tuberculosis and tuberculous meningitis in infants and toddlers who have been infected with tuberculosis. It has also prevented older children who have recently become tuberculin-positive from acquiring the disease. When isoniazid is given to such children for one year, the localized lesion usually does not progress, and hematogenous dissemination usually does not occur.

The only effective means to prevent tuberculosis is to avoid contact with infected persons. Widespread education of the public is essential. In order to build their resistance to the tubercle bacilli, persons should be taught to maintain adequate nutrition and to avoid fatigue and debilitating infections. They should be taught to drink only pasteurized milk from cows free of tuberculosis. They should be helped to understand the disease and the value of early diagnosis and treatment. Communities should organize tuberculin-testing and case-finding programs and also public health programs for control of the disease. These programs should include treatment of infectious patients, case-finding, examination of contacts, supervision of inactive cases, x-ray screening and measures to improve community health. Mobile x-ray units are used to locate patients who appear healthy, but are capable of spreading tuberculosis to others.

Ways to develop artificial immunity against tuberculosis have been attempted. Vaccination with BCG (bacillus of Calmette and Guérin) has been used. This vaccine may be given intradermally. With the aid of an ultrasonic nebulizer, BCG vaccination is a painless procedure. Children in classrooms can be immunized against tuberculosis by inhaling vaccine droplets floating in a man-made fog. The actual period of resistance to infection after the use of BCG is not known. Because BCG vaccine changes nonreactors to tuberculin tests into reactors, tests subsequent to its administration are of no value.

Infectious Mononucleosis

Definition, Etiology and Epidemiology. Infectious mononucleosis is an acute, world-wide illness, the cause of which is usually considered to be a virus. Recently a herpes-type virus known as the EB virus has appeared to be implicated in this disease. This condition occurs chiefly in older children and adolescents, although it may appear at any time in life. Although it is only mildly contagious, it may appear in epidemic form; however, sporadic cases are more commonly seen.

The incubation period is from one to two weeks. The period of communicability is not known. The mode of transmission is by direct contact with patients or by droplet infection. This disease is commonly believed to be spread by kissing and is therefore sometimes called the "kissing disease."

Pathology, Clinical Manifestations, Diagnosis and Differential Diagnosis. Infectious mononucleosis is a generalized disease which causes enlargement of lymphoid tissue throughout the body. *Clinical manifestations* vary markedly, but may include fever, pharyngitis, tonsillitis, generalized lymphadenopathy, especially of the

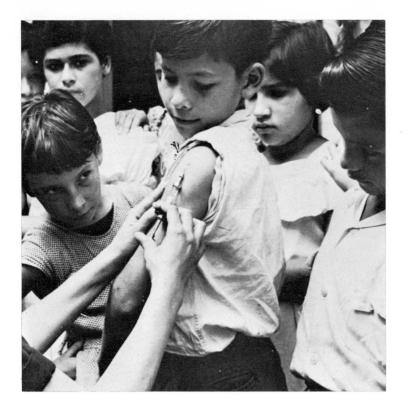

Figure 26–4. BCG vaccine is being used to vaccinate this child against tuberculosis. The World Health Organization has used BCG vaccination for the immunization of millions of children throughout the world in an effort to eliminate tuberculosis. (Byrd: *Health.* 4th ed. W. B. Saunders Co.)

cervical glands, splenomegaly, atypical lymphocytes, and the presence of heterophil antibodies. Anorexia and general malaise may occur. Skin rashes may occur early in the disease. Hepatitis with jaundice may be a common manifestation. Central nervous system manifestations may include a form of aseptic meningitis syndrome, encephalitis, or infectious polyneuritis (Guillain-Barré syndrome). Residual defects of the central nervous system may occur. Pneumonitis, pericarditis and thrombocytopenic purpura may also occur.

Diagnosis is based on laboratory findings: the peripheral blood smear reveals the presence of atypical lymphocytes, the leukocyte count may be normal or low, and the polymorphonuclear cells may increase initially. Lymphocytic leukocytosis develops which may reach leukemoid levels during the first days of the disease.

The heterophil antibody test is useful in the diagnosis, but positive results may or may not be obtained. Recently an accurate two-minute serologic slide test has been developed for the diagnosis of infectious mononucleosis. It is an extremely specific and sensitive test.

Other conditions which may be commonly confused with infectious mononucleosis include diphtheria, streptococcal or other forms of pharyngitis, leukemia, Hodgkin's disease, and other conditions which may cause aseptic meningitis, encephalitis or infectious polyneuritis, hepatitis,

scarlet fever, drug or allergic skin eruptions, and possibly appendicitis.

Treatment, Nursing Care, Prognosis and Prevention. *Treatment* is not specific and consists of symptomatic management, including bed rest and a high caloric diet. The patient must be observed for unusual manifestations of the disease. Steroid hormones as well as other drugs may be used to treat infectious mononucleosis.

The *prognosis* is usually good unless complications develop. Recovery is usually slow; complete return to full strength may not occur for several weeks.

There is no known means of *prevention* of infectious mononucleosis.

Scoliosis

Incidence and Types. Scoliosis is an S-shaped lateral curvature usually associated with rotation of the spine. Scoliosis is most frequent between the ages of twelve and sixteen years, a period of rapid growth.

There are two *types:* correctable or functional scoliosis and fixed or structural scoliosis. Correctable or *functional* scoliosis is usually caused by poor posture. It is seen especially in young persons who sit slumped over desks. Such persons can correct their scoliosis by bending toward the side of the curvature. If faulty posture is not corrected, structural changes may rarely occur, and the curvature is then not fully correctable.

Fixed or *structural* scoliosis is due to changes in the shape of the vertebrae or thorax. The patient cannot correct the deformity by bending.

Structural scoliosis most frequently is idiopathic and is usually found in young girls. Other causes may be congenital deformities (fusion of the ribs or vertebrae, hemivertebrae), infections of the vertebrae such as occur in Pott's disease caused by tuberculous infection, or paralytic diseases such as poliomyelitis.

Clinical Manifestations and Diagnosis. *Clinical manifestations* usually occur during periods of spinal growth such as at pubescence. The child or adolescent has no pain until the later stages of the disease. One shoulder is elevated, one hip may be prominent, or the spinal curve itself may be obvious.

The *diagnosis* is made on physical examination. An x-ray picture of the entire spine is taken with the patient in a standing position. Roentgenograms may also be taken with the patient bending as far as possible to the right and to the left.

Treatment. The child should receive a well balanced diet high in animal proteins, vitamins and minerals. Postural curves with no structural changes may be corrected by improving sitting habits and general health, by getting more rest and by doing appropriate exercises. The physiotherapist may teach the child exercises to correct the condition. The child can be appealed to through his desire to improve his appearance. If the scoliosis is not caused merely by faulty posture, the primary condition must be corrected before structural changes occur in the vertebrae.

Bracing is used to prevent the degree of curvature from increasing. A pressure brace known as the Milwaukee brace may be used as a conservative method of therapy. This brace may also be used for postoperative immobilization for those patients who require spinal fusion. A plaster cast with wedging may be used to obtain maximal correction. The scoliosis turnbuckle plaster jacket including the head and leg is designed in such a way that it can be cut at the apex of the primary curve and wedged to overcome the deformity. Application of such a cast is exhausting to the patient. In a few days the cast is cut, and the turnbuckle is placed on the side of the concavity. The turnbuckle is turned each day. The wedge-shaped opening on one side becomes smaller, and the opening on the side where the turnbuckle is becomes larger. The primary deforming curve is then fused.

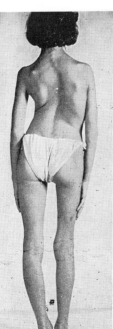

Figure 26–5. Scoliosis in a young girl, showing the tilt of the pelvis and shoulder and the deformity of the chest. (C. C. Chapple and J. R. Moore, in W. E. Nelson: *Textbook of Pediatrics.* 8th ed.)

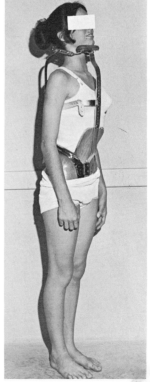

Figure 26–6. The Milwaukee brace. (Keiser in *Nurs. Clin. N. Am.*, Sept. 1967.)

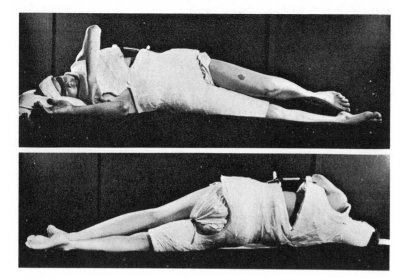

Figure 26–7. Turnbuckle cast. (From Wiebe: *Orthopedics in Nursing*.)

A newer device is the Risser localizer jacket. This is a lightweight cast in which the patient can walk. It is removed for operation, but must be reapplied afterwards. Spinal fusion may be done after maximum growth has occurred. For extensive surgery, fusion may have to be done in more than one stage. The orthopedist, the physiotherapist, the nurse, the parents and the patient must work closely together.

The use of Harrington rods is a method of internal instrumentation which consists of distraction and compression rods that assist in correcting the curves of scoliosis. This instrumentation or internal fixation is based on the

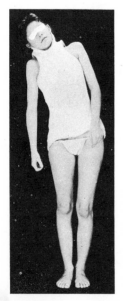

Figure 26–8. Localizer cast. (Courtesy of Orthopaedic Hospital, Los Angeles.)

principle of applying a distracting force on the concave side of the curve and a compression force on the convex side. A spinal fusion of the involved segment of the spine must be done at the time of application of the Harrington rods.

Nursing Care. The nurse assists with therapeutic exercises designed to promote realignment of the body, to increase the vital capacity and to improve muscle tone. Since these patients tire easily, periods of exercise should be alternated with periods of rest. Rest positions may be specified by the physician or physiotherapist and can be as valuable as exercises. The adolescent should be encouraged to sleep on a firm bed without a pillow. Breathing exercises may also be ordered. The nurse should know the exercises to be carried out so that she can supervise them properly.

The young patient in a thick, heavy type of turnbuckle or lighter cast requires comprehensive nursing care.

Skin care is important. Problems associated with the use of mechanical aids which forcefully correct scoliosis include the breakdown of skin around the edges of the cast and the creation of pressure areas beneath the cast. The nurse must observe and explore the skin with her fingers for pressure areas, especially over the ribs. She must check for the cause of all complaints of pain or discomfort. The nurse must not permit the adolescent to reach under his own cast to scratch, since in doing so he may injure his skin. Drug therapy may be used if the itching persists, but powder should not be applied.

All exposed edges of the cast must be covered with large adhesive petals (see p. 229) or stockinet should be pulled over the edges of the cast and securely fastened to it. The exposed skin should be rubbed frequently. Slight padding may be used to allay discomfort from pressure by the cast, but too much padding may cause extra pressure. The cast around the buttocks and genitalia must be protected with waterproof material. The skin should be cleansed thoroughly after soiling.

After spinal fusion, immobilization in casts or braces may be continued for six to twelve months. If a tibial graft has been taken, the limb should be handled carefully for at least eight weeks until healing has taken place.

Whenever the adolescent is examined, the nurse must be certain that he is adequately draped in order to avoid embarrassment.

Comprehensive nursing care is planned to meet the patient's needs during the long-term treatment of scoliosis. The patient may be cared for at home and taken to the outpatient department before and after hospitalization. The orthopedist, the physiotherapist and the nurse must work closely together. Crippled children's services in many states provide physiotherapy follow-up in the home. The child should continue exercises for months or years.

The public health nurse should give the child encouragement. An adolescent girl may not want to wear a brace because she is "too tired" or thinks that it ruins her appearance. She may not want to do her exercises because she is "too busy." Parents should be warned of such complaints and be given support in insisting that the physician's orders be carried out for the girl's future welfare.

If a cast or brace is worn by an adolescent for a prolonged time, the patient may isolate himself from his peer group. Parents may need assistance in helping the adolescent to maintain contact with his friends. Continuation in a school program may provide the contacts with peers that the adolescent needs.

If the adolescent exercises before a full-length mirror, he will become more conscious of his posture and be more able to see the correction which the use of his muscles creates. Dancing exercises are also of value for developing better balance. The adolescent should wear shoes that support him well.

Early recognition and treatment are vitally important to prevent serious deformity. The school or public health nurse should make observations on the posture of children. The tendency to postpone treatment while waiting to see whether the adolescent will outgrow the condition is dangerous.

Slipped Femoral Epiphysis

Etiology and Incidence. Epiphyseal closure, which marks the completion of skeletal growth, also coincides with the attainment of sexual maturity. This is related more to physiologic than to chronologic age. This fact of develop-ment is especially important in the occurrence of slipped epiphysis, which is one of the outstanding osseous disturbances of adolescence. Exactly why this condition occurs is not known, but trauma and hormonal changes may be factors.

The phase of maximum growth is, on the average, for girls twelve years and for boys between fourteen and fifteen years. Usually the adolescent in whom slipped femoral epiphysis occurs is tall and heavy, but not fat. Such a person needs larger than average amounts of calcium and vitamin D during the preadolescent growth spurt.

Clinical Manifestations, Diagnosis and Treatment. In the early stages, signs and symptoms of synovitis are present. The adolescent may have a slight limp to the affected side. Later the femoral portion of the epiphysis may slide farther upward. Finally the epiphysis may slip extensively upward with increased eversion of the limb. There is increased limitation of abduction and internal rotation. Pain in the hip causes the child to limp (the pain is sometimes referred to the knee). The symptoms are similar to those in Legg-Perthes disease in school children. The onset is insidious. The condition is frequently bilateral.

The *diagnosis* is based on roentgen examination, which shows that the femoral capital epiphysis has slipped posteriorly and inferiorly on a lateral view. The neck of the femur assumes a horseneck appearance. Early diagnosis and treatment are essential.

The main objective of *treatment* is to arrest slipping by internal fixation with a cast, followed by avoidance of weight bearing by use of crutches until healing occurs. In severe cases osteotomy or other operative procedures may be necessary.

Since this condition may be bilateral, the adolescent should be observed carefully for any indication of a problem with the other hip.

Malignant Tumors of Bone

The most frequent primary malignant bone tumors are osteosarcoma and Ewing's sarcoma. These occur most often between ten and twenty years of age and in boys more often than in girls.

The cause is unknown, but heredity may be a factor.

Roentgenographic features resemble those of non-neoplastic lesions of bone. Careful diagnosis must be made on the bases of roentgenographic examinations and surgical biopsy.

Osteosarcoma
(Osteogenic Sarcoma)

Clinical Manifestations, Diagnosis, Treatment and Prognosis. Osteosarcoma occurs more frequently than Ewing's sarcoma and usually involves the metaphyseal end of a long bone—the lower end of the femur or the upper end of the tibia or humerus. It may also occur in other locations. The *clinical manifestations* are pain and swelling of the affected part. The *diagnosis* is made on roentgenographic examination, which reveals destruction of bone and new bone formation. The only *treatment* is amputation of the affected extremity. The neoplasm may involve the medullary cavity, the cortex and the adjoining soft tissue. The sarcoma commonly metastasizes to the lungs, although other organs may be involved. The mortality rate is high.

Nursing care is similar to that of patients having Ewing's sarcoma.

Ewing's Sarcoma

Clinical Manifestations, Diagnosis, Treatment, Nursing Care and Prognosis. Ewing's sarcoma usually involves the shaft of a long bone. It may also involve the flat bones and ribs. The *clinical manifestations* are similar to those of osteosarcoma. Fever and leukocytosis may also be present. Usually at the time of diagnosis only one bone is involved, but other bones become affected. The *diagnosis* is made on roentgenographic examination and by histologic study of the tumor. *Treatment* is unsatisfactory. The neoplasm usually responds at first to roentgen therapy, but few young people are cured. Radiation therapy to the affected bone in addition to systemic chemotherapy (usually nitrogen mustard) has produced some measure of therapeutic success. Amputation is the only other treatment used.

When a nurse sees an adolescent with the symptoms of a malignant tumor of the bone, she should suggest a medical examination, without alarming him or his parents by telling them that she suspects a tumor of the bone.

As the disease progresses, the patient will become anemic and look pale and tired. The optimism the patient shows at the onset of the condition changes to depression. Parents, visitors and nurses should try to provide emotional support to help the patient face the probable outcome of the disease.

Since a pathologic fracture may occur at or near the site of the tumor, the nurse should be gentle with the extremity when making the bed or bathing the patient. If he is ambulatory, he should be protected from falling. Such fractures may be painless; therefore the nurse must observe carefully for evidence of fracture if the patient falls or otherwise sustains any trauma which could result in a fracture of the diseased bone.

The diet should be high in protein and vitamins to counteract the progressive anemia.

The nurse should watch for indications of lung involvement such as pain in the chest, coughing, and expectoration of blood, and report her findings immediately. As with osteogenic sarcoma, metastases to the lungs occur frequently.

Reticulum Cell Sarcoma

Ewing's sarcoma must be differentiated from reticulum cell sarcoma (medullary canal tumor), which is diagnosed by a biopsy, since its roentgen appearance may be variable. This tumor is sensitive to roentgen-ray therapy, which may be successful. Amputation may also be necessary. While the patient is undergoing roentgen therapy the limb should be protected by bracing or by a bivalved plaster cast in order to prevent fractures. After roentgen therapy the adolescent may experience problems with his skin, pain, nausea and vomiting. Intravenous therapy may be necessary to maintain hydration.

Failure of Sexual Development

Delayed puberty, like precocious puberty, may occur in both sexes. Parents may be much concerned when puberty is delayed in their son or daughter. The child may also be much concerned, since prolonged delay usually means that friends have outgrown him or her physically and emotionally.

Delayed Puberty in the Female

Etiology, Clinical Manifestations and Treatment. In *primary hypogonadism* there is ovarian agenesis or destruction. This may be due to surgical removal or destruction by roentgen therapy. *Secondary hypogonadism* may be due to destruction of or defect in the pituitary gland or in hypothalamic connections with the pituitary gland or to a severe systemic disease causing secondary pituitary deficiency, such as hypothyroidism (cretinism) (see p. 343), uncontrolled diabetes (see p. 585), fibrocystic disease (see p. 328) or tuberculosis (see p. 634).

At the normal age of puberty *clinical manifestations* become evident. There is failure of body hair growth and of the characteristic breast development. The genitalia remain infantile, and menstruation does not occur. There is retarded physical growth, and the epiphyses are late in closing. If the hypothalamus has been severely affected by a tumor, obesity may be seen occasionally in addition to sexual infantilism. This combination of clinical manifestations is termed *Froehlich's syndrome*.

Treatment for primary hypogonadism consists in administration of stilbestrol after the child has reached the age of puberty. Intermittent therapy with stilbestrol is continued indefinitely. Artificial menses occur without ovulation. These women are therefore sterile. There are positive psychologic benefits from therapy in addition to the fact that premature senility from lack of estrogen is prevented. In secondary hypogonadism the treatment of the underlying disorder may bring about normal sexual development.

Delayed Puberty in the Male

Etiology, Clinical Manifestations, Treatment and Prognosis. Failure of sexual development in the male is known as *eunuchoidism.* If the testes are missing or have been destroyed, there is no abnormality until puberty, when the genitalia fail to enlarge, pubic hair is sparse or absent, the voice remains childlike, and epiphyseal closure is slow. The 17-ketosteroid excretion is usually low. The *treatment* is by substitution therapy with testosterone given orally or intramuscularly. Prolonged effects may be obtained if pellets are implanted subcutaneously. Masculinization occurs with therapy, but the youths are sterile.

The Rebellious and Impulsive Adolescent

Rebellious and impulsive adolescents usually have parents who grew up in the years of economic depression and ultimately wanted only to achieve comfortable economic success. They wanted also that their children have minimal frustration and that they would be permitted to do what they desired without limits on their behavior. These parents wanted their children to have material advantages they never enjoyed themselves when they were young. At the same time they wanted their children to achieve in academic pursuits, personal beauty and social popularity. These children as they became older expected that they would be catered to by society since they had so few demands made on them as they were growing up at home. Certainly many of them were never required to work for remuneration, nor were they permitted to do so.

Many of these adolescents, then, wish to do nothing except sleep, eat and enjoy themselves. Their impulsive and rebellious behavior leads them to act solely as their whims dictate, many times recklessly and without any concern for others.

As one example of rebellious behavior, consider the current hair styles among adolescent males. Parents may protest the disheveled appearance of their sons, but in general meet with no response. If their sons do acquiesce in this instance, the ingenuity of youth will create new or bring back old themes of rebelliousness and add further to family disharmony.

This typical parent-child relationship is one of oversubmission by parents to their child's impulsiveness and then overcoercion by them in order for the child to achieve. Parents become more anxious, especially over scholastic performance, and the adolescent develops an even more pronounced "I don't care" attitude. The adolescent becomes oversubmissive to his own impulses and develops an impulsive desire for freedom. Without adequate self-control such a young person will give his impulses free rein as he becomes prematurely independent of parental control. He may display outward defiance and flaunt all authority, especially that of his parents.

Nursing Care. Nurses, because of their knowledge of normal growth and development, can many times observe rebellious behavior and assist parents who face the problem of having such an adolescent. These children may need professional help from their physicians or psychiatrists. Parents may need to separate themselves physically from their adolescent youth for a short time, to cease providing money and other luxuries without the youth's earning them through honest effort, and to discontinue doing those personal chores such as ironing his clothes which the adolescent can do for himself. Parents should not scold, lecture or criticize such an adolescent, because these will only produce more rebellion and family disharmony.

Unwed Adolescent Parents

It is unfortunate that in our society many thousands of unmarried adolescents are bearing children each year. For these young people the change from being an immature adolescent to being a parent may be overwhelming. Professional personnel of several disciplines can contribute to providing services and care for these teenagers in order to help them find solutions to their problems, the intensity of which may vary, depending upon the culture to which the adolescents belong.

Pregnancy out of wedlock occurs at every social, economic and intellectual level, although most often the teenager who is seen by a public health worker has been socially and economically deprived. Some of the underlying causes of pregnancy in the typical unwed adolescent may be conflict between her parents and herself, resulting in her feeling rejected and insecure at home, and lack of satisfactory adjustment in other areas of living. If the teenager has not received security or love at home, she may find a temporary source of fulfillment or a feeling of being wanted in casual intimacies. The unwed teenager is basically struggling with her desire for independence and her need for dependence on her parents.

A few reasons among others given for pregnancy out of wedlock include the presence of frustrations and pent-up emotions which seek an outlet, loss of inhibitions due to the use of alcohol or drugs, and a lack of knowledge about sex. These adolescents may also have been rebellious and impulsive prior to their pregnancies.

Some approaches to the prevention of pregnancy out of wedlock include the development in the female of a positive self-identity (see Chap. 24), the ability to postpone immediate desires in order to achieve long-range goals, and sufficient confidence in herself so that she does not have to conform to the wishes of her group. Parents can support their daughters in this regard by setting limits on their dating, by not forcing them to become "popular" at an early age, and by providing the kind of sex education that goes beyond the usual "facts of life."

The unmarried pregnant adolescent needs professional counseling. She needs help in dealing with her feelings of guilt, in planning for prenatal care and admission to a shelter or hospital, in planning for financial assistance, and in deciding whether to keep her infant or to relinquish him for adoption. The putative father also needs help in determining his role and, like the mother, needs guidance for the future.

Pregnancy at an early age carries significant medical risks such as increased infant mortality and prematurity, and increased susceptibility to toxemia of pregnancy for the mother. The unmarried adolescent many times has inadequate prenatal care and an unbalanced diet which contribute further to these risks. Although the dietary habits are many times poor, they may be worsened by eating compulsions arising from fears and anxiety which are associated with pregnancy. Instructions concerning diet given to these young women must be kept simple and practical in order for them to understand and to follow them properly.

The public health nurse, the school nurse or the nurse in the hospital may be the initial contact the unmarried pregnant girl may have with the community health services. This relation between the nurse and the unwed teenage mother is vital. The nurse must establish a relation of trust with the adolescent by being understanding and nonjudgmental and then help her to transfer this feeling of trust to the physician who will provide medical care for her. The nurse must know the resources in her particular community to care for such a patient. Interagency communication and cooperation are essential if the adolescent is to have continuity of care.

Most adolescent girls fear the birth process itself because of their lack of experience in coping with crisis situations. The nurse is many times the one to whom such an adolescent will turn for support. After the infant is born the nurse with other team members must support the mother in her decision as to whether or not she plans to keep the infant.

Attention has recently turned to the unmarried adolescent father and his needs in establishing his future relationships and goals. Male high school counselors and social workers are especially valuable in helping such young people.

If sufficient assistance and guidance are given to unmarried adolescent parents, much of the tragedy of broken lives, both those of the parents and the child, can be averted. If the decision is made not to keep the infant, he should be placed for adoption through a reputable agency instead of being placed on the black market.

The nurse is a vital member of the health team in both urban and rural areas and can with the physician and social worker assume leadership in the drive to provide unwed pregnant adolescents with good prenatal care and to help with their rehabilitation.

Venereal Diseases: Syphilis and Gonorrhea

Venereal disease is present to an alarming degree among adolescents, especially those fifteen to nineteen years old. These adolescents are from all socioeconomic groups. They engage in sexual intercourse because they are lonely or want status, not because they have a deep relation with their partners. Since adolescents are prone to worry about their bodies, their concern over subsequent venereal disease often prompts them to seek treatment. Some may not seek treatment, however, for fear that their behavior will become known.

Treatment must be undertaken by a large health team if success is to be achieved. Many of the aspects of adult treatment and control apply equally to adolescents, though special problems are present in the younger group.

The two most common venereal diseases are syphilis and gonorrhea. These diseases follow the adult pattern in adolescents. The medical aspects will not be discussed here, since they have already been discussed (see pp. 185, 184.)

Both diseases are contracted through sexual promiscuity. The important problems in adolescents are treatment of the disease, case-finding, and prevention by the health team. Early case-finding is especially important if the young girl is pregnant, in order that treatment may be completed before delivery of the infant.

Although the mortality rates from these diseases have decreased as a result of treatment, the infections persist and are being seen increasingly in the adolescent group. The social problem, a violation of sexual mores, is perhaps a greater problem than the morbidity.

The fact that adolescents turn to such an extent to promiscuous heterosexual relations may be a reflection of social maladjustment. Other indications of the same problem include increasing parenthood out of wedlock, juvenile deliquency and emotional problems.

Several members of the health team must work together to help control the problem of venereal disease: (a) the parents, who have contributed to the adolescent's forming a philosophy of life and his concept of other people, and have given approval to his selection of friends. Often it is the friends who initially lead the adolescent into this behavior. (b) The teacher, who helps to build proper attitudes toward these diseases through counseling, can disseminate information about venereal disease and help to guide troubled adolescents to appropriate sources for aid. (c) The clergyman, who appreciates the fact that religious motives have a great effect on the degree of inhibition exercised in subordinating unacceptable sexual expression, is an important team member. Apparently, the more active adolescents are in religion, the less they engage in promiscuity. (d) The social worker, working with nurses in helping these adolescents, can help the nurse appreciate the probable causes of such antisocial behavior and what disease means to the patient. (e) The family physician can teach his young patients about venereal disease, treat and report cases and locate their contacts. (f) The venereal disease investigator is a trained interviewer who interviews patients with an aim to locating contacts.

Role of the Nurse. The nurse cannot fully understand her own role without appreciating the roles of other members of the health team. One of her most important roles is assisting other members of the team in case-finding.

The school nurse should be aware of signs and symptoms of venereal disease as she is of other communicable diseases in students. She should be able to evaluate complaints and refer such adolescents to the physician. She should keep adequate health records on all students so that she knows their individual problems. She must have a nonjudgmental attitude about these diseases. She may also function as a teacher of health and as a counselor for the students on such matters.

The hospital nurse works in conjunction with the school nurse. Although syphilis and gonorrhea are usually treated on an outpatient basis, the nurse caring for adolescent patients in the hospital units must remember that because the incubation period of syphilis is about three weeks and of gonorrhea about five days, some adolescents recently admitted may manifest symptoms during the early part of a hospitalization period.

The primary chancre of syphilis and the pustular discharge of gonorrhea are highly infectious. Isolation technique to protect other patients as well as personnel is thus necessary.

The treatment of choice is penicillin. If the patient has gonorrhea, penicillin is given for a few days. If the patient has syphilis, penicillin is given for about two weeks. The nurse must watch for signs of untoward reaction to the drug during the course of therapy.

The clinic or office nurse can encourage the adolescent to return regularly for therapy. The nurse must know the diagnostic and therapeutic measures so that she can interpret these to the patients and reassure them. Adolescents want answers to their questions, especially those in relation to their own bodies. The nurse can also be active in case-finding.

The public health nurse can do a great deal in controlling venereal disease among adolescents by knowing her families well, by guidance, case-finding and by helping infected persons understand their responsibility in controlling the spread of infection to others.

The only way to control venereal disease in the adolescent group is by a multidisciplinary approach. The nurse should understand her responsibility as a cooperating member of the health team in order to reduce the incidence of this social tragedy of youth.

Juvenile Delinquency

Incidence and Etiology. A delinquent is one who does not behave in accordance with standards set by his society or community. Basically, delinquent behavior is antisocial, aggressive behavior usually due to anxiety and frustrations. Included under the category of delinquent behavior among others are shoplifting, which is almost becoming a national epidemic in persons under twenty-one years of age, truancy from school, running away from home, damage to and theft of property, especially automobiles, and violence, including sex offenses, against other persons. Juvenile delinquency in the United States has increased for more than twenty consecutive years.

There is usually a combination of causative factors in any one problem of delinquency.

DELINQUENCY DUE TO FORCE OF CIRCUMSTANCES. An example of this kind of delinquency is stealing so that the adolescent can have necessities, e.g. food. Spending money such as his friends have appears to many adolescents as a necessity. He may steal so that he can remain in the group. This sort of adolescent is essentially normal and dislikes stealing from others. He needs the help of the sociologist, the educator and the economist.

DELINQUENCY DUE TO POOR HOME AND COMMUNITY ENVIRONMENT. The adolescent whose insecurity at home, in his community and in society is very great may become delinquent. As a child he may have felt rejection or lack of understanding. As an adolescent he may engage in criminal activity such as robbery, sex orgies, addiction to narcotics or alcohol, and even apparently unmotivated murder. Actually, when he gets into trouble with the law, he harms his parents more than he does himself, because he gains a stronger position in his peer group by his delinquencies. He is thus likely to do anything the gang says so as not to be rejected by them. Treatment may be very difficult, since the basis of the insecurity is in the home and the community. Treatment lies in education and helping these adolescents to accept the mores of a new group.

A child who has been brought up according to one set of mores and then is transplanted to another society may be considered normal in his original society, but delinquent in the new one. In other words, the child who has been reared in a poor neighborhood may not be termed a delinquent when he steals an apple from a fruit stand, because this is fairly normal behavior. If he moves to a better neighborhood and

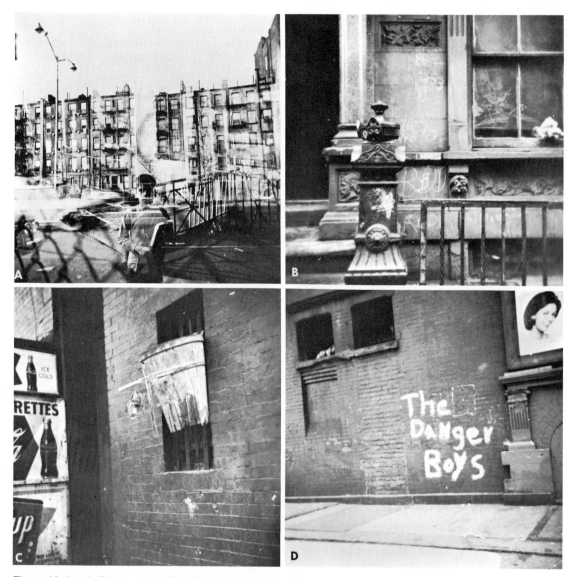

Figure 26–9. *A,* This is a lower East Side youth surrounded by urban problems: poverty, slum housing, physical and emotional neglect, lack of adequate educational opportunities and the endless lines of cars passing by his house. *B,* This is the place where he lives, *C,* this is the place where he plays, and *D,* this is what he may become—a danger to society. (From *T C Topics,* Vol. 12. Photograph by Joseph Deitch.)

steals fruit from a store, he is apprehended and held as a delinquent. The treatment again lies in education and helping the youth to accept the mores of his new group. At the same time his new social group should be helped to understand the adolescent's problem.

DELINQUENCY DUE TO MENTAL RETARDATION. A mentally retarded adolescent depends on other persons for emotional support and therefore is easily led by them. He is not able to distinguish clearly what property does not belong to him or what will happen to him as a result of asocial acts. Often he has not been able to develop a conscience, so that he does not know right from wrong. Since he probably has not received adequate love, he may develop an aggressive reaction pattern. He may be used by intelligent delinquents and many times is the one who is caught by the authorities. He needs protection, training and supervision.

DELINQUENCY DUE TO NEUROSIS. Some adolescents become delinquent because they have a need to be punished, since they feel guilty over something in the past. They carry out delinquent acts in order to be punished.

DELINQUENCY DUE TO CHARACTER DISORDER. Delinquents may have character disorders which result in behavior similar to that of adults who have psychopathic personalities. These adolescents seem to have weak characters. They cannot learn from experience. They cannot establish meaningful relations even with those persons who try to help them with their problems. They cannot control their desire to do exactly what they want without regard for the consequences to others or to themselves. They may require institutionalization and treatment in order to protect society from their acts. Many such delinquents could have been recognized in early childhood and given adequate treatment. Unfortunately, too often they are not given help until they come in conflict with the law, and then only if the court has facilities for treatment other than confinement in the outdated home for delinquents. Such institutions often have no psychiatrist or counselor, or so few in proportion to the number of inmates that individual treatment of only a small number of selected patients is possible.

DELINQUENCY DUE TO EMOTIONAL DISTURBANCES (PSYCHOSES). Emotionally disturbed or psychotic adolescents may become delinquent. Their behavior would be normal if the world of reality were like their world of delusions. This kind of delinquency is relatively rare in adolescence, but when it does occur, psychiatric treatment is necessary.

Treatment, Prevention and Role of the Nurse.
If the delinquent adolescent is to be given adequate *treatment*, emphasis should not be on the delinquent act alone, but must be placed on

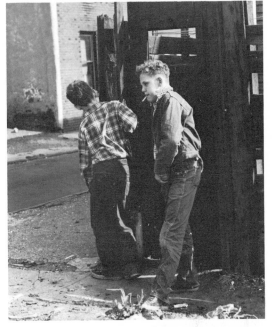

Figure 26–10. These young adolescents are members of a gang in a large urban area. They gain status from belonging to the gang, and emotional support from the other gang members. (H. Armstrong Roberts.)

the total individual in his home and community and on the reasons why he committed the act.

The delinquent adolescent can best be managed by personnel in the juvenile instead of the adult courts. The objectives of juvenile courts are basically diagnostic, protective and educational. After a study of the total individual, management is planned on the basis of his fundamental problem and what is best for him and for society.

Many suggestions for *prevention* have been made: more and better schools, playgrounds and recreational facilities and better housing. Authorities have also recommended that more attention be paid to children of minority groups (see p. 613) and to their economic and social status in their communities. The basic problem confronting all growing children in our society must be better understood if delinquency is to be prevented. If the living situation could be stabilized for all children, there would probably be less delinquency.

Broadly, prevention lies in relation not only to individual delinquents, but also to the causative factors operating in communities which lead adolescents into asocial acts. The sociologist, the educator, the economist, the psychologist and the psychiatrist must make efforts to alter customs and mores which our culture seems to have outgrown. Any preventive effort must combine the skills of many disciplines if it is to be successful.

The nurse may be called upon to care for delinquent adolescents. She must recognize that her patient is first of all an individual and must accept him as such without emphasis on his asocial acts. She must make accurate observations of his behavior, provide him with support and work closely with other members of the health team in his treatment.

The nurse must also use her professional insights in working with others in the community to help prevent the formation of personality traits which lead to delinquency.

Drug Dependence

Some adolescents or even younger children may become physically addicted to or psychologically dependent on drugs because in society today there is a general breakdown in communications among people. Even among family members who appear genuinely fond of each other, the youths may not feel really loved. They may therefore begin to take any drug for the comfort and pleasure it gives. Many have seen their parents become pleasure-seekers themselves who at the same time do not set limits on their children's behavior. Prevention of youthful drug addiction lies largely, therefore, in the improvement of family structure and in relations between parents and their children, the establishment of personal values, and the setting of limits on the behavior of the young. Adolescents especially must also be helped to find their own identity and purpose in life.

A broad definition of an addict is a person who abuses any drug because of its effect on his behavior or mood. The substances to which physical addiction or psychologic dependence may occur vary from nicotine, to glue, to Freon, to alcohol, and to drugs including amphetamines, barbiturates, marihuana, lysergic acid diethylamide (LSD), and narcotics.

Nicotine. Much publicity has been devoted recently to the dangers of smoking cigarettes, especially their potential effect on the health of the young person. Some children still, however, begin to smoke when they are students in elementary school or during their adolescent years. In addition to the widely distributed publicity both the schools and parents have a responsibility for educating children concerning the dangers of this habit.

Many schools and parents have cracked down hard on students who smoke. Some school administrators do not permit smoking on school grounds and require students to take courses on the harmful effects of smoking. Parents can best influence their child against smoking if they do not smoke themselves. If the child argues that, "If I don't smoke, I won't fit in with the gang," parents should point out that they have tried to

teach him to follow his own beliefs, to be independent, even though this requires strong will power. An adolescent who does not follow the advice of his parents may take such guidance more seriously if given by a respected teacher, physician, religious advisor, or nurse.

Glue-Sniffing. Some school-age children and adolescents have been known to become psychologically dependent on inhaling the toxic fumes from rubber cement and model airplane glue among other less commonly used products. Increased amounts are needed for the addict to get the response he desires. The use of large amounts of this substance may lead to intense exhilaration, intoxication, hallucinations, crime, and even death. Unfortunately, some adolescents in time turn from the use of glue to stronger drugs.

In order to attempt to prevent the adverse effects resulting from glue-sniffing, a type of glue is being developed which is vaporless and nontoxic to the human body. Until this product is more widely used, storekeepers should report any sudden increase in sales of glue to young people to the appropriate health department in his community. Parents should have a physician examine their child if they suspect that he has sniffed glue. Teachers should strongly suspect this habit if any of their students are irritable or inattentive, or become excessively drowsy in class. Also, community leaders should make intensive efforts to alert the public about the practice and hazards of glue-sniffing.

Freon-Sniffing. The sniffing or inhalation of a drinking glass-chilling gas which contains one of the Freons and is marketed in aerosol cans can produce a possible hazard to health. When the gas comes in contact with the skin, it can produce frostbite. When in contact with an open flame or a very hot surface, Freons can decompose into highly irritant and toxic gases. When inhaled in high concentrations, Freons have a narcotizing effect in addition to other reactions thought to be freezing damage to the lungs, laryngeal spasm or anoxia. Death may result from the inhalation of this substance.

Alcohol. Alcohol can become a problem for anyone using it if he has lost the ability to prevent himself from taking a drink or to control the amount he consumes. He develops a physiologic addiction along with a psychologic compulsion which destroys his ability to control his drinking. Alcoholism is a progressive and ultimately fatal disease if the addict does not learn to live without this drug.

Alcohol when consumed is absorbed rapidly into the bloodstream. Its most pronounced physiologic effects are on the brain, resulting, depending on the amount taken, in compulsiveness, loss of inhibitions, loss of control of the body as in walking, and ultimate stupor.

It is commonly believed that alcoholism can occur only after adult status has been achieved. This belief is a fallacy. It is not chronologic age, nor how many years the person has been drinking, that determines whether he is an alcoholic. The important point in making this decision is whether he can control his drinking or whether he is dependent on alcohol and cannot control the amount he consumes. A small percentage of alcoholics are alcoholic from their first drink. Loss of control or alcoholism may occur then as early as eighteen years of age. For the person who has lost control in his drinking, it is commonly believed that there is no compromise without abstinence.

For the alcoholic, alcohol is a drug rather than a beverage. He drinks because he is depressed, lonely, angry or nervous. Compulsive behavior in regard to the use of a chemical is a good indication of addiction. Continued excessive use of alcohol affects the person's power of reason, seriously impairs his ability to make critical judgments, and destroys his ability for self-evaluation.

In adolescence, recurrent drinking occurs more frequently among boys than among girls. Although excessive drinking occurs among adolescents in large metropolitan areas, it is occurring more frequently among adolescents in suburbia in the United States and in many countries throughout the world. It is true that the problem of excessive drinking, whether the person is an alcoholic or not, is responsible for many fatal highway accidents.

Guidance for therapy of alcoholics of any age may be obtained from the group known as Alcoholics Anonymous. Assistance for members of families of alcoholics may be obtained from Al-Anon, a group which helps relatives understand the scope of the problem. The National Council on Alcoholism, Inc., also provides the professions and the community with knowledge needed to prevent alcoholism and rehabilitate alcoholics.

The aim of modern alcohol education is to produce more intelligent approaches to the drinking experience itself. In a culture that generally approves of drinking, many young people will accept the prevailing pattern and use alcohol. Society is therefore concerned more with what kind of drinkers they will become, rather than with the simple fact of whether they do or do not drink. When alcohol is used as a beverage, an appetizer or as a religious or cultural symbol, its effects will probably be benign. When it is used as an intoxicant or drug as a means of escaping stress, it becomes a problem.

Amphetamines and Barbiturates. Amphetamines are drugs known for their ability to combat sleepiness and fatigue because they are stimulants to the central nervous system. They may also be used medically to suppress appetite. The amphetamines most commonly used are amphetamine (Benzadrine), methamphetamine (Methedrine) and dextroamphetamine (Dexedrine). To those persons who use slang terms for these drugs, they are called "pep pills," "speed" and "bennies."

Doses of amphetamines can produce a feeling of well-being and alertness, but overdoses can cause irritability and tension. These drugs cause tachycardia, increase in the blood pressure, rapid respirations, headache, diarrhea and increased perspiration. These effects are due to the fact that in the body these drugs stimulate the release of norepinephrine, a substance stored in nerve endings, and concentrate it in higher centers of the brain.

These stimulants may be misused by young people as well as those of all ages. Abusers may take them orally or intravenously; however, this practice is dangerous. Taking drugs intravenously is known as "speeding." As a result of injecting "speed" (Methedrine) into the vein, serum hepatitis, abscesses and long-term personality disorders or death may occur. A common saying in certain areas of the country is that "Speed kills."

Stimulant drugs do not produce physical dependence; however, the body can develop a tolerance to these drugs so that larger and larger doses are required to achieve the desired effect. Psychologic dependence on these drugs can occur.

Barbiturates are sedatives commonly used to relax the central nervous system. These drugs include the fast-acting phenobarbital (Nembutal) and secobarbital (Seconal) and the long-acting phenobarbital (Luminol), butabarbital (Butisol) and amobarbital (Amytal). Slang terms for the fast-acting barbiturates are "goof balls" and "barbs."

Barbiturates depress the action of the heart muscles, skeletal muscles, and nerves; thus they reduce the heart and respiratory rates and lower the blood pressure. Increased dosages of these drugs, however, cause confusion, slurred speech, staggering gait, and decreased ability to concentrate and work, and may ultimately produce anger, assaultive behavior or a deep sleep.

Barbiturates, especially when taken with alcohol, may be the cause of automobile accidents among adolescents as well as older persons. They are also, because they are readily obtained, one of the main ways people choose to commit suicide.

These drugs are physically addicting; thus increasingly higher doses are needed before the body can feel their effects. Rapid withdrawal from the use of these drugs may cause nausea, convulsions and death. Withdrawal under medical supervision may take several weeks or months on gradually reduced doses.

Both amphetamines and barbiturates are regulated nationally by the Food and Drug Administration. They may be obtained legally by prescription from a physician; however, all too often they are obtained illegally by adolescents. Research is currently being done to determine how young people learn to abuse drugs and what can be done once this occurs.

Marihuana. Marihuana is a drug found in the Indian hemp plant, *Cannabis sativa,* which grows in countries around the world having a mild climate. The flowers and leaves of this plant are dried and rolled and smoked in cigarettes or pipes. This substance can also be taken in food or sniffed. The cigarettes termed "joints," "sticks" or "reefers" have a sweetish odor when smoked.

The use of marihuana ("pot," "grass") has increased rapidly in the United States in recent years. When marihuana is smoked, it enters the bloodstream quickly and acts on the nervous system and brain. Physical reactions to the drug include tachycardia, reddening of the eyes, lowered body temperature, and an increase in appetite among other effects. Persons who use marihuana may become loud, very talkative, or drowsy with an inability to coordinate their movements. They may feel excited or depressed and have a distortion of their sense of distance, time, color and hearing ability. They may find it difficult to think clearly; thus they find it hard to make decisions.

In larger doses or higher strengths, marihuana may be termed a "hallucinogen" because it may cause visual hallucinations, illusions or delusions. Paranoia is the most common untoward reaction to this drug.

Marihuana at present is classified as a drug on which dependence develops rather than true addiction. It does not cause physical dependence as do narcotics. The body probably does not develop a tolerance to the drug, nor does withdrawal of the drug result in physical illness. Psychologic dependence, it is thought, may develop if it is used regularly.

Persons using marihuana may or may not ultimately use narcotics. Although no link has been found between these drugs, those who abuse one drug may abuse others or may be led to use them through their contacts with other users or sellers.

In the United States, possessing or selling marihuana is a felony under Federal law. If adolescents break the laws regarding this drug, their education may be interrupted and they may have a shadow cast on their future by having a police record. In addition to the legal aspects, a young person who experiments with drugs which may have an effect on his personality development may find it increasingly difficult to develop a sense of identity, to adjust to life as an adult and to develop a value system.

Lysergic Acid Diethylamide (LSD). Lysergic acid diethylamide is a man-made chemical which is classed as a "hallucinogen," a drug which affects the mind. It produces bizarre mental reactions in people, with severe distortions in their physical senses of seeing, smelling, hearing and touching. Other drugs which are also powerful hallucinogens, or psychedelic drugs, include mescaline, psilocylin, peyote, DMT and STP.

Although the use of LSD ("acid") is illegal in the United States except for government-approved use, it is used by many persons on either an experimental or regular basis. LSD may be taken on a sugar cube, cookie or other food, or it can be licked off a postage stamp on which the drug has been placed. The physical response to this drug includes tachycardia, irregular respirations, rise in blood pressure and temperature, shaking of the extremities, dilatation of the pupils, flushed or pale face, chills, nausea and anorexia. This drug is not physically addicting; therefore there is no physical illness when it is withdrawn.

The psychologic effects of this drug include changes in the physical senses, but it does not make people more creative, nor does it help them to find themselves. Colors may seem more brilliant, strange patterns may emerge before the eyes, and walls of rooms may appear to move. The senses of taste, smell, hearing and touch may seem more acute than usual. The sense of time may be disturbed, although consciousness is not lost. Users of this drug may feel happy and depressed at the same time. They may also lose the normal appreciation of the difference between their bodies and space; therefore they sometimes feel that they can fly or float through air. Individual users may explain, depending on their sensation, that they have had a "good" or a "bad" trip.

Long-continued use of this drug may impair the person's ability to concentrate, especially on a goal in life, and eventually cause him to leave what the usual person calls "society."

There are certain dangers involved in the use of LSD. The user may develop panic because he feels that he cannot stop the action of the drug once he has taken it, or he may develop paranoia. For the youthful users especially, the effect of this drug can be extremely frightening, since they are not yet mature in their emotional development. The user may have a recurrence of the effects of the drug long after he has taken it. He may become depressed or mentally deranged. The use of the drug may also contribute to acts of murder or suicide. Some persons may suffer acute or long-term mental illness after taking this drug.

The most important danger associated with the use of LSD is accidental death because the person under the effects of this drug may jump from a height, believing that he can float or fly, or jump in front of a moving vehicle, believing that no harm can come to him.

Of more serious consequence also is the possibility that the use of LSD may affect the chromosomes, causing chromosomal breakage and damage and possibly abnormalities in the children of those who have used this drug, or malignancy in the user of the drug. Research is being done to determine how these changes occur, since total genetic and psychologic damage caused by LSD to the human population may not be seen for some time to come.

There are strict penalties for anyone who illegally produces, sells or otherwise distributes LSD. Penalties may include imprisonment or fines and may be very severe.

Research is currently being done among other areas to determine the drug's action and value for human beings, the ways to treat those who suffer from the side effects of the drug, the extent of use of the drug, and the culture of those who use it.

Narcotics.   Narcotics is a term usually used to refer to opium, a product of the poppy flower, or drugs made from opium, including heroin and morphine. Cocaine made from cocoa leaves as well as other drugs may also be considered a narcotic. Heroin currently appears to be the most widely used narcotic, so that this is the drug which will be discussed more fully.

The person who becomes addicted ("hooked") to a narcotic craves repeated and larger doses of the drug because his body develops a tolerance for the substance taken. When the drug is withdrawn, physical illness occurs with symptoms of sweating, shaking, vomiting, diarrhea and severe abdominal pains. Psychologic dependence also occurs because the addict uses the drug as a means to escape facing the reality of life. If sufficient drug is taken, death may result.

When heroin is taken initially, the person may feel a reduction of his fears, a relief from his worries and a degree of inactivity which may result in stupor. The drug has the effect of depressing certain parts of the brain and nerves. It reduces thirst, hunger, the sex drive and feelings of pain. Malnutrition may result when this drug is used over a period of time. When the drug is discontinued, withdrawal symptoms appear in approximately eighteen hours.

Heroin addiction occurs chiefly among young men in large cities. Narcotic addiction unfortunately also occurs among young women who may also be pregnant. Infants born to these mothers may be narcotic addicts at birth who must go through a period of withdrawal during the neonatal period or who may die from their addiction.

Once a person is addicted, the main objective of his life is to obtain a continued supply of drugs.

His education and his working in gainful employment may be discontinued because he may be frequently ill from either withdrawal or overdosage of the drug. He may have difficulties with both his family and the law. Continuing his habit leads him into involvement with crime, chiefly thefts or other crimes against property, because his addiction is so costly. Illegal possession or sale of narcotics is punishable by fines or imprisonment.

Drug addiction is a medical illness, and therefore treatment is needed. After treatment resulting in withdrawal of the drug is successful, the person returns to his community, where he may find it difficult not to return to his use of drugs. Therapy, including physical, mental, social, and vocational rehabilitation efforts, has been attempted in order to prevent the person from returning to the drug and wasting his life.

Research is currently being done on the effects of narcotics, the users themselves, and on the antidotes which can be used for heroin addiction.

The Role of the Nurse.   The role of the nurse in relation to the adolescent who is taking drugs which may cause physical addiction or psychologic dependence is complex. Certainly her first obligation is to be alert to the possibility that addiction may exist in this age group and to be knowledgeable about the signs and symptoms of the various forms of addiction. She must be able to recognize certain personality or behavioral changes which occur with the use of certain drugs. The nurse must also be cognizant of the treatment of various forms of drug addiction, which is increasingly being considered a medical instead of a moral problem.

The nurse, whether in the hospital or in the community, must be prepared to answer questions about the use of drugs, whether these questions are asked by anxious parents or the adolescents themselves. She must know sources of help in her community to which she can refer such persons should the need arise. She should also know of educational materials such as those listed at the end of this chapter which can be used to educate the public.

The school nurse or the public health nurse may be asked to present classes in the school or in the community on the methods of identification of adolescents taking drugs, as well as on the dangerous aspects of the use of various drugs. Certainly she would need to be knowledgeable in this area if she were to accept such a challenge.

The nurse may also play an extremely important role in the prevention of addiction and in case-finding of adolescents who have become addicts. She must be sympathetic and understanding of the problems of these young people and not talk down to them or sit in judgment about them as individuals. She should listen to their comments attentively and try to help them, but when necessary, she should refer them to sources such as individual physicians or to clinics where further help can be obtained.

It is especially necessary for youth and their parents to recognize the fact that addiction to drugs except nicotine may result in rejection of an application for admission to a college, rejection by prospective employers, legal action against them for crimes committed under the influence of drugs, or ultimate death from the drug itself or from irresponsible actions while using the drug, such as careless driving of an automobile or motorcycle.

Since the actual therapy and nursing care of the adolescent who is addicted are not too different from those of the adult addict, details of rehabilitation will not be discussed in this text. The common denominator in the treatment and care of persons addicted to drugs is that of reducing anxiety through quiet, calm reassurance and support given in a controlled environment by a warm, understanding human being. A team approach to the rehabilitation of these young persons has been found helpful in many centers devoted to their care.

The nurse as a member of her community should be knowledgeable about the current laws relating to drugs in her area. She should actively strive to use her influence to have legislation passed to protect those too young to protect themselves from the possibility of physical addiction or psychologic dependence on drugs. If she suspects that drugs are being peddled in the schools or elsewhere in the area, she should notify the school authorities or the police. She should know also, however, that legal action is only part of the answer to the use of drugs by juveniles. The ultimate cure for the drug menace lies in the home and in the community, where many parents presently are not sufficiently concerned to provide guidance and control for their youth.

Severe Psychoneuroses

Adolescents may reveal manifestations of more severe neuroses similar to those seen in adults. They may show symptoms of severe depression, hysteria, anxiety or withdrawal. The patient usually has a mixture of these symptoms. Older adolescents may become anxious and show a deep concern about their physical health. Although this may be an extension of their normal concern about their health, they resist reassurance from their physician. They may also evidence highly organized compulsions and phobias. The physician and the nurse may need guidance from a psychiatrist in the care of such patients.

Adolescent Schizophrenic Reactions

Incidence and Etiology. Although schiz-

ophrenic reactions are not too common in children, they are the most important kind of mental illness during the adolescent years.

There are several theories about the causes of schizophrenic reactions. No one cause has been proved. It is not certain to what extent heredity is a factor. There may also be a basic biochemical or neurologic defect in schizophrenics. Environmental and developmental stresses may cause a defect in interpersonal relations. The schizophrenic has never in his life felt accepted by others or gained satisfaction from what he attempted to do. Usually, as a child he received too little love and affection. Too much was expected of him, and too little happiness or reward was given in return.

Clinical Manifestations and Diagnosis. The onset may seem acute, but personality changes have probably been going on for months or years. The following behavior may be shown: (a) Rigidity in adjustment to various persons or situations in the environment. The child cannot tolerate any kind of life other than his own. He abides by his rituals in his daily life and cannot change them quickly. (b) He begins to draw a curtain between himself and others. He becomes reserved and seems to have only brief periods of contact with reality. His personality becomes disorganized to a degree. (c) There is an emotional and intellectual split between the meaning of the act itself and his response to it. He may laugh when a tragedy occurs. He appears odd in his behavior. (d) He becomes careless, untidy and tardy and finally is satisfied just to sit alone. At last he retreats into his own world because the world of reality is intolerable. Delusions and hallucinations occur. Speech becomes irregular and illogical.

Mental illness is difficult to *diagnose* in adolescence because normal children and adoles-

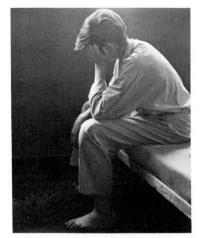

Figure 26–11. The schizophrenic prefers to sit alone, to withdraw from the world of reality to a world of his own making. (H. Armstrong Roberts.)

cents at one time or another in the developmental process may show similar manifestations of behavior. It is the degree to which abnormal behavior occurs that is important in making a diagnosis.

Treatment, Nursing Care and Prognosis. Psychiatric *treatment* should be given as promptly as possible. Care, to be effective, must be given by accepting, warm adults who give the young person their undivided attention. The adolescent must be provided with love and acceptance and recognition given to his need for appropriate experiences with gratification and mastery of frustration. His physical condition should be improved. Institutional care should be provided as necessary.

Before the age of twelve years it is difficult to be certain of the *prognosis*. Even with therapy and institutional care the prognosis has been poor. In recent years some success has been achieved with intensive therapy. Cure occurs rarely, but a satisfactory social adjustment can be made. More and more work is being done so that treatment of these adolescents can be more successful.

Suicide

Suicidal attempts and suicide are not rare in children and adolescents. The rate of these deaths has almost doubled in the last ten years. This problem is less common in school-age children than it is in adolescents; however, it may be seen in children as young as the early school years. Suicide is more common in males than females. Females, however, make more suicidal attempts than males. Suicide occurs most often in the spring of the year. It is surpassed in the age group from fifteen to nineteen years only by accidents, malignant neoplasms and homicides as a cause of death. Many suicides are disguised as accidents such as poisonings, falls, electrocutions, or motorcycle and automobile crashes.

Some physicians believe that the increased rate of suicide among adolescents can be blamed on the general permissiveness in modern society which, combined with a sexual revolution, results in the destruction rather than the strengthening of the egos of young people. More specifically, most children and adolescents who contemplate or commit suicide are "social isolates," come from disorganized homes and are under intolerable stress, having a sense of failure, feeling unloved, unwanted and bad. They react with anger, usually against their parents. These feelings produce guilt which leads to a suicidal effort and, in a way, results in their punishing their parents. Some adolescents who commit suicide may do so as a result of efforts to manipulate others, as a signal of distress, or because they are schizophrenic (see p. 652).

Adolescents who threaten or commit suicide are in general impulsive and immature persons who tend to overreact to even minor stresses. They are restless, bored, hyperactive persons who many times have a history of truancy from school, absence from the home, sexual promiscuity, and depression.

In the school-age and adolescent groups depression is often evidenced by disobedience, boredom, continued temper tantrums, restlessness, running away from home and school, and accident proneness. Many such adolescents act out their feelings through the use of drugs, alcohol and sexual promiscuity. They may evidence failure in school, inability to concentrate, isolation from others, weight loss due to anorexia, insomnia, and somatic complaints, a common one of which is overwhelming fatigue. They may also be preoccupied with the meaninglessness of their lives and a wish for death. The person's actual thought of death (see p. 76) depends on his age. This accounts in part for the lower incidence of suicide among children younger than adolescents.

Prior to a suicide attempt there is usually, but not always, a triggering event such as a major crisis involving discipline, punishment which the person considers unfair, jealousy in love, loss of a parent by divorce or death, or an illegitimate pregnancy. Suicidal attempts almost always occur when the person feels extremely lonely.

Adolescents who are depressed or who have threatened suicide require a thorough physical, neurologic and psychiatric evaluation. Often significant persons in the adolescent's life such as parents, teachers, religious advisors and Scout leaders can contribute observations which can be helpful in understanding his emotional adjustment. The adolescent should also be observed carefully for his behavior after admission to the hospital, especially for self-destructive behavior.

After a period of observation, both parents and the patient should be engaged in the process of therapy, given either by a pediatrician experienced in this clinical area or by a child psychiatrist. The physician must help the adolescent to build sufficient ego strength in order to face his serious emotional problems. If the adolescent does not trust his physician, he may resist therapy, deny his illness, and act out his feelings as a way of escaping from what he considers an intolerable situation. These patients should receive care and close observation for at least three months. The period of after-care is often more important than the immediate emergency therapy.

Nursing Care. Since adolescents commit suicide during an emotional crisis at a time when there is no one for them to talk to, the nurse who is in contact with this age group must be alert to changes in behavior evidenced by depression, disorientation, defiance and dissatisfaction with life which could lead to a suicidal act. The nurse must observe such behavior and take steps to obtain help for the person as soon as possible. This is especially true of those who give definite verbal warnings of suicidal intent. Nurses must also help parents to understand more about suicide and to spot presuicidal warning signs. Many suicide-prevention centers have been formed in cities across our country in order to provide assistance when needed.

Because of their extreme feelings of loneliness, many would-be suicides are easy to talk back to life. They are never totally certain that they want to die. If someone says, "Don't," they many times will not go through with the act. An interested person must answer the cry for help and assist the child or adolescent to cope with his loneliness and provide a hopeful, positive attitude toward life.

The responsible nurse when giving care to such a young person must respect and accept him as a person, and provide protection against self-destruction by reducing environmental hazards until he is able to assume this responsibility for himself. She must bolster his self-confidence and self-esteem. When he expresses feelings of worthlessness, the nurse can guide him into doing therapeutic tasks such as helping others. She can also provide diversional activities for him in order to help him express his feelings of aggression and hostility constructively and outwardly rather than destructively turning them inward on himself. The adolescent should be encouraged to participate in making plans for such activities and other aspects of his care.

Probably the most important factor for the nurse in helping the suicidal young person is in maintaining a therapeutic relation with him. The nurse must evidence her support and protection of him through her sincere interest, warmth and understanding until he can manage his self-destructive urges for himself.

CLINICAL SITUATIONS

Mrs. Horter brought her fourteen-year-old daughter, Barbara, to the adolescent clinic because she had "pimples on her face" which she persisted in picking. After an examination of the lesions the physician made the diagnosis of acne vulgaris. Barbara is a well developed and attractive adolescent whose menarche occurred when she was twelve years of age. Both Barbara and her mother appeared to be alert and interested in the activities of the clinic.

1. Acne vulgaris is caused primarily by
a. The erratic diet of the adolescent.
b. Changes in the skin during adolescence.
c. Irritation of the skin due to the habit of picking the face.
d. Allergy to foods containing chocolate.

2. Several weeks later the nurse, who had previously established a good relation with Barbara, met her in the clinic and commented on the improvement of her acne. During the conversation Barbara said, "I'm glad my mother didn't come with me today. She's always telling me what to do, and when I refuse to do what she says, she threatens to tell my father." In response to this expression of feeling the nurse would answer
a. "Your mother did seem to be a domineering type of woman. Perhaps if you do what she says, she won't bother you so much."
b. "If you would act your age, your mother wouldn't have to tell you what to do."
c. "Why don't you talk to your father about this situation and see how he feels about your mother?"
d. "Your mother may be having difficulty in remembering that you are almost grown up now. Perhaps if you would talk with her about this problem, you both would understand each other better."

3. Mrs. Horter confides in the nurse her deep concern because she has observed Barbara daydreaming on occasion. Some of the mothers of Barbara's friends are equally disturbed about this behavior in their adolescents. The nurse should realize in order to answer this comment that
a. Adolescents daydream because they want to evade doing their homework or helping with the housework.
b. They are showing early indications of becoming schizophrenics and should be examined by their physicians as soon as possible.
c. They need time to formulate their philosophies of life, to learn to know themselves and to plan for their futures.
d. They are growing rapidly and are too fatigued to engage in activities such as sports.

Fifteen-year-old Carmella Nignari has been admitted to the hospital with a diagnosis of pulmonary tuberculosis. Her father is a guard at a local warehouse, and her mother before Carmella's hospitalization worked as a waitress in the evenings and over the weekends to supplement the family income. When her mother worked, Carmella had cared for the six younger siblings. Now her mother must stay home from work to assume this responsibility.

4. As a result of Carmella's illness all the other members of her family had tuberculin tests and chest x-rays to determine whether they also had the infection. The infant and the toddler were examined thoroughly to determine the presence of
a. Miliary tuberculosis.
b. Pott's disease.
c. Tuberculosis of the cervical lymph nodes.
d. Tuberculous dactylitis.

5. A positive reaction to a tuberculin skin test indicates that the person
a. Has an active lesion of pulmonary tuberculosis.
b. Has never had tuberculosis or come in contact with the disease.
c. Has been infected with *Mycobacterium tuberculosis* and is hypersensitive to its protein.
d. Has not been infected with the disease, but is allergic to *Mycobacterium tuberculosis.*

6. Carmella is concerned about her health and asks

Hallan, M. B.: Attitudes Toward the Unwed Mother. *Nursing Clin. N. Amer.*, 2:775, 1967.

Herzog, E.: Unmarried Mothers—The Service Gap Revisited. *Children*, 14:105, 1967.

Howard, M.: Comprehensive Service Programs for School-Age Pregnant Girls. *Children*, 15:193, 1968.

Hustu, H. O., and others: Treatment of Ewing's Sarcoma with Concurrent Radiotherapy and Chemotherapy. *J. Pediat.*, 73:249, 1968.

Iungerich, Z.: High School for Unwed Mothers. *Am. J. Nursing*, 67:92, 1967.

Jacobziner, H.: Attempted Suicides in Adolescence. *J.A.M.A.*, 191:7, 1965.

Johnson, B. S., and Miller, L. C.: The Interpersonal Reflex in Psychiatric Nursing. *Nursing Outlook*, 15:60, May 1967.

Keeler, M. H.: Adverse Reaction to Marihuana. *Am. J. Psychiat.*, 124:674, 1967.

Keiser, R. P.: Treatment of Scoliosis. *Nursing Clin. N. Amer.*, 2:409, 1967.

Konopka, G.: Adolescent Delinquent Girls. *Children*, 11:21, 1964.

Kramer, J. C., and others: Amphetamine Abuse. *J.A.M.A.*, 201:305, 1967.

McPhetridge, L. M.: Nursing History: One Means to Personalize Care. *Am. J. Nursing*, 68:68, 1968.

Mellow, J.: Nursing Therapy as a Treatment and Clinical Investigative Approach to Emotional Illness. *Nursing Forum*, V:64, No. 3, 1966.

Nowlis, H. H.: Why Students Use Drugs. *Am. J. Nursing*, 68:1680, 1968.

Pannor, R.: Casework Service for Unmarried Fathers. *Children*, 10:65, 1963.

Polk, L. D.: UNWED Mother or Unwed MOTHER. *Nursing Outlook*, 12:38, February 1964.

Pollack, J. H.: Where *Unwed* Mothers Stay in School. *Today's Health*, 45:24, September 1967.

Ramirez, E.: Help for the Addict. *Am. J. Nursing*, 67:2348, 1967.

Redl, F.: A New Theory of Delinquency? It's About Time! *Children*, 13:119, 1966.

Reed, E. F.: Unmarried Mothers Who Kept Their Babies. *Children*, 12:118, 1965.

Rosenberg, M., and Gottlieb, R. P.: Current Approach to Tuberculosis in Childhood. *Pediat. Clin. N. Amer.*, 15:513, 1968.

Sankot, M., and Smith, D. E.: Drug Problems in the Haight-Ashbury. *Am. J. Nursing*, 68:1686, 1968.

Segal, A.: Some Observations About Mentally Retarded Adolescents. *Children*, 14:233, 1967.

Semmens, J. P.: Fourteen Thousand Teen-Age Pregnancies. *Am. J. Nursing*, 66:308, 1966.

South, J.: Impediments to TB Eradication. *Nursing Outlook*, 15:50, September 1967.

Stine, O. C., and others: School Leaving Due to Pregnancy in an Urban Adolescent Population. *Am. J. Pub. Health*, 54:1, 1964.

Thaler, O. F.: Grief and Depression. *Nursing Forum*, V:8, Spring 1966.

The Los Angeles Suicide Prevention Center. *Nursing Outlook*, 13:61, November 1965.

Townsend, J.: The Unmarried, Pregnant Adolescent's Use of Educational Literature. *Nursing Outlook*, 15:48, August 1967.

Vaccination Against TB Made Easy as Breathing. *Medical World News*, 8:38, December 8, 1967.

Weinberg, S., and others: Seminars in Nursing Care of the Adolescent. *Nursing Outlook*, 16:18, December 1968.

Wesseling, E.: The Adolescent Facing Amputation. *Am. J. Nursing*, 65:90, January 1965.

Where *Unwed* Mothers Stay in School. *Today's Health*, 45:24, September 1967.

Zellweger, H., and others: Is Lysergic-Acid Diethylamide a Teratogen? *Lancet*, 2:1066, 1967.

many questions about her condition. The nurse would

a. Ask the physician to talk with her about each question she asks.

b. Explain that worrying about her health is harmful for her. Assure her the physician knows how to care for persons having tuberculosis.

c. Ignore most of her questions because Carmella only wants attention.

d. Answer her questions to the best of her ability and refer those which she cannot answer to the physician.

7. Carmella asked why she could not be treated with only one kind of medication. To answer her question the nurse would need to know that streptomycin should not be used alone in the treatment of tuberculosis because

a. Streptomycin-resistant organisms emerge rapidly.

b. The eighth cranial nerve may be damaged.

c. The drug is not very effective against *Mycobacterium tuberculosis*.

d. Treatment with more than one drug hastens recovery.

8. The nurse who cared for Carmella had had a negative reaction to the Mantoux test when she entered the school of nursing. The physician had recommended that she be protected against *Mycobacterium tuberculosis* by

a. Bacillus of Calmette and Guérin vaccine.

b. Plague vaccine.

c. Salk vaccine.

d. Pertussis vaccine.

GUIDES TO FURTHER STUDY

1. Observe a group of adolescents in high school, a recreation center or a neighborhood meeting place.

Describe the general activity of the members of the group. Were any adolescents paired off in couples? What activity, if any, were the ones doing who did not mix with the others? Observe their posture when sitting and standing. Observe their manner of dress and their grooming. Compare your observations with your knowledge of the normal behavior patterns of adolescents.

2. What is your understanding of the function of a clinic for adolescents? How many adolescent clinics have been organized in your state or community?

3. A thirteen-year-old delinquent has been admitted to the pediatric unit with a diagnosis of tuberculosis. What would be your approach to this adolescent and his parents? What would be your role and responsibility as a member of the health team in providing care for this young person? Investigate the agencies in your community which could assist in his rehabilitation.

4. What are the most recent statistics in your state on the causes of mortality in the adolescent age group? What preventive measures could be taken to reduce these tragedies?

5. What rehabilitative services are available for physically and mentally handicapped adolescents in your hospital, your community and your state? Evaluate these services to determine whether they are adequately meeting the need.

6. What facilities are available in your state for the care of adolescents having a diagnosis of schizophrenia? Are these facilities adequately meeting the need?

7. Select the three experiences which were most disturbing to you and the three experiences which were most satisfying to you in providing care for children. State for each incident the age of the patient, his diagnosis and a description of the situation. Analyze each of these incidents to determine why they were disturbing or satisfying to you and discuss them in seminar.

TEACHING AIDS AND OTHER INFORMATION*

Alcoholics Anonymous, Inc.

Young People and A.A.

American Medical Association

How Teens Set the Stage for Alcoholism.
The Crutch That Cripples—Drug Dependence.
TB Control: Prospect for Eradication.
Why the Rise in Teenage Gonorrhea?
Why the Rise in Teenage Syphilis?

American Social Health Association

Deschin, C. S.: Teenagers and Venereal Disease.
Today's VD Control Problem, 1966.

Canadian Mental Health Association

The Juvenile Offender, 1967.

National Tuberculosis Association

South, J.: Tuberculosis Handbook for Public Health Nurses, 1965.
TB Through the Teens.

* Complete addresses are given in the Appendix.

Public Affairs Pamphlets

Brecher, R., and Brecher, E.: The Delinquent and the Law.
Butcher, R. L., and Robinson, M. O.: The Unmarried Mother.
Milt, H.: Serious Mental Illness in Children.
Ogg, E.: Psychotherapy—A Helping Process.
Saltman, J.: What We Can Do About Drug Abuse, 1966.
Shneidman, E. S., and Mandelkorn, P.: How to Prevent Suicide, 1967.

The National Council on Alcoholism, Inc.

Block, J. L.: Alcohol and the Adolescent.
Block, M. A.: Could Your Child Become an Alcoholic?
Lee, J. P.: What Shall We Tell Our Children About Drinking?
Oppenheim, G.: When Your Teen-Ager Starts Drinking.
Smith, A. J.: What I'd Teach My Children About Alcohol.
Strictly for Teenagers.

United States Department of Health, Education, and Welfare

A Child-Centered Program to Prevent Tuberculosis, 1965.
A New Look at School Dropouts, 1965.
Cancer of the Bone, 1967.
Drugs of Abuse, 1967.
Halfway House Programs for Delinquent Youth, 1965.
Herzog, E., and Bernstein, R.: Health Services for Unmarried Mothers, 1964.
"Hooked," 1967.
Hung on LSD . . . Stuck on Glue?, 1968.
Juvenile Delinquency—Facts, Facets, 1965.
Juvenile Delinquency Prevention in the United States, 1965.
Juvenile Gangs, 1965.
Lin-Fu, J. S.: Neonatal Narcotic Addiction, 1967.
Living Death—The Truth About Drug Addiction, 1965.
LSD: The False Illusion, 1967.
Savitz, R. A., McCann, M., and Stitt, P. G.: Childbearing in and Before the Years of Adolescence, 1966.
The Control and Treatment of Juvenile Delinquency in the United States, 1965.
The Culture of Youth, 1966.
Thinking About Drinking, 1968.
Trends in Illegitimacy: United States, 1940-1965.
Young People Who Smoke, 1968.

REFERENCES

Publications

Aguilera, D. C.: Use of Physical Contact (Touch) as a Technique of Non-verbal Communication with Psychiatric Patients; in Exploring Progress in Psychiatric Nursing Practice. Monograph 4, American Nurses' Association 1965 Regional Clinical Conferences. New York, American Nurses' Association, 1966, p. 33.
Child Study Association of America: Children of Poverty: Children of Affluence. New York, Child Study Association of America, 1967.
Cohen, A. C.: The Drug Treatment of Tuberculosis. Springfield, Ill., Charles C Thomas, 1966.
Deutsch, H.: Selected Problems of Adolescence. New York, International Universities Press, Inc., 1967.
Freedman, A. M., and Kaplan, H. I. (Eds.): Comprehensive Textbook of Psychiatry. Baltimore, Williams & Wilkins Company, 1967.
Friedman, A. S., and others: Psychotherapy for the Whole Family. New York, Springer Publishing Company, Inc., 1965.
Gallagher, J. R.: Medical Care of the Adolescent. 2nd ed. New York, Appleton-Century-Crofts, 1966.
Gallagher, J. R., and Harris, H. I.: Emotional Problems of Adolescents. 2nd ed. New York, Oxford University Press, 1964.
Giallombardo, R. (Ed.): Juvenile Delinquency. New York, John Wiley and Sons, Inc., 1966.
Hambling, J., and Hopkins, P. (Eds.): Psychosomatic Disorders in Adolescents and Young Adults. New York, Pergamon Press, Inc., 1965.
Harms, E. (Ed.): Drug Addiction in Youth. Long Island City, New York, Pergamon Press, 1965.
Hoagland, R. J.: Infectious Mononucleosis. New York, Grune & Stratton, Inc., 1967.
Hoch, P. H., and Zubin, J. (Eds.): Psychopathology of Schizophrenia. New York, Grune & Stratton, Inc., 1966.

Hofling, C. K., and Leininger, M. M.: Basic Psychiatric Concep... J. B. Lippincott Company, 1967.
Holmes, D. F.: The Adolescent in Psychotherapy. Boston, Little, B...
Jones, H. W., and Heller, R. H.: Pediatric and Adolescent Gynecolog... Company, 1966.
Kendig, E. L., Jr. (Ed.): Diseases of the Respiratory Tract in Children... Company, 1966.
Keniston, K.: The Uncommitted: Alienated Youth in American Society... and World, Inc., 1965.
Klein, M. W. (Ed.): Juvenile Gangs in Context. Englewood Cliffs, N.J., ...
Konopka, G.: The Adolescent Girl in Conflict. Englewood Cliffs, N.J., P...
MacLennan, B. W., and Felsenfeld, N.: Group Counseling and Psychotherapy... York, Columbia University Press, 1968.
Masterson, J. F.: The Psychiatric Dilemma of Adolescence. Boston, Little, Brown ...
National Association for Mental Health, Inc., in cooperation with the National ... Health, U.S. Public Health Service: Directory of Resources for Mentally I... United States. New York, National Association for Mental Health, 1964.
National Council on Illegitimacy: Directory of Maternity Homes and Residential F... married Mothers: A Guide for Use and Selection. New York, National Council o... 1966.
National Council on Illegitimacy: Unmarried Parenthood. New York, National Cou... gitimacy, 1967.
Podair, S., and Harris, W. D. M.: Venereal Disease: Man Against a Plague. Palo Alto, C... Fearon Publishers, 1966.
Roberts, R. W. (Ed.): The Unwed Mother. New York, Harper and Row Publishers, 1966.
Robins, L. N.: Deviant Children Grown Up. Baltimore, Williams & Wilkins Company, 1966.
Rubenfeld, S.: Family of Outcasts: A New Theory of Delinquency. New York, The Free Press, ...
Sauber, M., and Rubinstein, E.: Experiences of the Unwed Mother as a Parent; A Longitudinal Stu... of Unmarried Mothers Who Keep Their First-born. New York, Research Department, Co... munity Council of Greater New York, 1965.
Schlesinger, B.: Poverty in Canada and the United States. Toronto, Ontario, University of Toronto Press, 1966.
Semmens, J. P., and Lamers, W. M.: Teenage Pregnancy. Springfield, Ill., Charles C Thomas, 1967.
Shands, A. R., and Raney, R. B.: Handbook of Orthopaedic Surgery. 7th ed. St. Louis, C. V. Mosby Company, 1967.
Shaw, C. R.: The Psychiatric Disorders of Childhood. New York, Appleton-Century-Crofts, 1966.
Swanson, A.: The Self-Fulfilling Prophesy in Schizophrenia; in Exploring Progress in Psychiatric Nursing Practice. Monograph 4, American Nurses' Association 1965 Regional Clinical Conferences. New York, American Nurses' Association, 1966, p. 26.
Usdin, G. L. (Ed.): Psychoneurosis and Schizophrenia. Philadelphia, J. B. Lippincott Company, 1966.
Vermes, H., and Vermes, J.: Helping Youth Avoid Four Great Dangers: Smoking, Drinking, VD, Narcotics Addiction. Toronto, Ontario, G. R. Welch Company, 1965.
Wheeler, S., and Cottrell, L. S.: Juvenile Delinquency. New York, Russell Sage Foundation, 196...

Periodicals

A Guide for Collaboration of Physician, Social Worker, and Lawyer in Helping the Unma... Mother and Her Child. Children, 14:111, 1967.
Auerbach, A. B., and Rabinow, M.: Parent Education Groups for Unmarried Mothers. Nursi... look, 14:38, March 1966.
Blattner, R. J.: Isoniazid Prophylaxis in Tuberculin Reactors. J. Pediat., 72:131, 1968.
Boegli, E. H., and Steele, M. S.: Scoliosis: Spinal Instrumentation and Fusion. Am. J. N... 2399, 1968.
Burgess, L. C.: The Unmarried Father in Adoption Planning. Children, 15:71, 1968.
Burton, M., and Holter, I.: Health Education Classes for Unwed Mothers. Nursing O... March 1966.
Byers, M. L.: The Hospitalized Adolescent. Nursing Outlook, 15:32, August 1967.
Christ, A. E., and others: The Role of the Nurse in Child Psychiatry. Nursing Outloo... 1965.
Clark, A. L.: The Crisis of Adolescent Unwed Motherhood. Am. J. Nursing, 67:1...
Cochran, M. L., and Yeaworth, R. C.: Ward Meetings for Teen-Age Mothers. Am... 1967.
Cohen, S.: Pot, Acid and Speed. Medical Science, 19:30, February 1968.
Coles, R.: Violence in Ghetto Children. Children, 14:101, 1967.
Diagnosing Mononucleosis in Just Two Minutes. Medical World News, 8:36...
DiPalma, J. R.: A Hard Look at the Hallucinogens. RN, 31:55, July 1968.
Fleming, J. W.: Recognizing the Newborn Addict. Am. J. Nursing, 65:83, ...
Gimpel, H. S.: Group Work with Adolescent Girls. Nursing Outlook, 16:4...
Godeene, G. D.: A Psychiatrist's Techniques in Treating Adolescents. C...

APPENDIX

Abbott Laboratories: North Chicago, Ill. 60064.

Alcoholics Anonymous, Inc.: P.O. Box 459, Grand Central Station Post Office, New York, N.Y. 10017.

American Academy of Pediatrics: 1801 Hinman Ave., Evanston, Ill. 60204.

American Dental Association: 211 East Chicago Ave., Chicago, Ill. 60611.

American Diabetic Association, Inc.: 18 East 48th St., New York, N.Y. 10017.

American Foundation for the Blind, Inc.: 15 West 16th St., New York, N.Y. 10011.

American Heart Association: 44 East 23rd St., New York, N.Y. 10010.

American Medical Association: 535 North Dearborn St., Chicago, Ill. 60610.

American Nurses' Association: 10 Columbus Circle, New York, N.Y. 10019.

American Pharmaceutical Association: 2215 Constitution Ave., Northwest, Washington, D.C. 20037.

American Social Health Association: 1790 Broadway, New York, N.Y. 10019.

Association for the Aid of Crippled Children: 345 East 46th St., New York, N.Y. 10017.

Canadian Mental Health Association: 52 St. Clair Ave., East, Toronto 7, Ontario.

Charles Pfizer and Company, J. B. Roerig Division: 235 East 42nd St., New York, N.Y. 10017.

Children's Medical and Surgical Center, The Johns Hopkins Hospital: Wolfe & Monument Sts., Baltimore, Md. 21205.

Child Study Association of America: 9 East 89th St., New York, N.Y. 10028.

Evaporated Milk Association: 910 17th St., N.W., Washington, D.C. 20006.

Interdepartmental Committee on Children and Youth: U.S. Department of Health, Education and Welfare, 330 Independence Ave., S.W., Washington, D.C. 20201.

Joseph P. Kennedy, Jr. Foundation: 200 Park Ave., Rm. 3021, New York, N.Y. 10017.

Kimberly-Clark Corporation (Educational Department): Neenah, Wis. 54956.

Mead Johnson Laboratories: Evansville, Ind. 47721.

Medic Alert Foundation: Turlock, Calif. 95380.

Mental Health Division, Dept. of National Health and Welfare: Ottawa, Canada.

Mental Health Materials Center: 104 East 25th St., New York, N.Y. 10010.

National Association for Mental Health, Inc.: 10 Columbus Circle, New York, N.Y. 10019.

National Association for Retarded Children, Inc.: 420 Lexington Ave., New York, N.Y. 10017.

National Conference of Christians and Jews: 43 W. 57th St., New York, N.Y. 10019.

National Cystic Fibrosis Research Foundation: 202 E. 44th St., New York, N.Y. 10017.

National Society for Crippled Children and Adults, Inc.: 2023 West Ogden Ave., Chicago, Ill. 60612.

National Society for the Prevention of Blindness, Inc.: 79 Madison Ave., New York, N.Y. 10016.

National Tuberculosis Association: 1790 Broadway, New York, N.Y. 10019.

Personal Products Company: Box S-6, Milltown, N.J. 08850.

Play Schools Association: 120 West 57th St., New York, N.Y. 10019.

Project Head Start, Office of Economic Opportunity: 1200 19th St., N.W., Washington, D.C. 20006.

Public Affairs Committee, Inc.: 381 Park Ave. South, N.Y. 10016.

Ross Laboratories: Columbus, Ohio, 43216.

The American Cancer Society, Inc.: 219 East 42nd St., New York, N.Y. 10017.

The Children's Hospital Medical Center, Health Education: 300 Longwood Ave., Boston, Mass. 02115.

The Epilepsy Foundation: 1419 H St., N.W., Washington, D.C. 20005.

The National Council on Alcoholism, Inc.: New York Academy of Medicine Building, 2 East 103rd St., New York, N.Y. 10029.

The National Foundation-March of Dimes: 800 Second Ave., New York, N.Y. 10017.

United Cerebral Palsy Associations, Inc.: 321 West 44th St., New York, N.Y. 10036.

U.S. Department of Health, Education, and Welfare, Social Security Administration, Children's Bureau: U.S. Government Printing Office, Division of Public Documents, Washington, D.C. 20025.

INDEX

many questions about her condition. The nurse would

a. Ask the physician to talk with her about each question she asks.

b. Explain that worrying about her health is harmful for her. Assure her the physician knows how to care for persons having tuberculosis.

c. Ignore most of her questions because Carmella only wants attention.

d. Answer her questions to the best of her ability and refer those which she cannot answer to the physician.

7. Carmella asked why she could not be treated with only one kind of medication. To answer her question the nurse would need to know that streptomycin should not be used alone in the treatment of tuberculosis because

a. Streptomycin-resistant organisms emerge rapidly.

b. The eighth cranial nerve may be damaged.

c. The drug is not very effective against *Mycobacterium tuberculosis.*

d. Treatment with more than one drug hastens recovery.

8. The nurse who cared for Carmella had had a negative reaction to the Mantoux test when she entered the school of nursing. The physician had recommended that she be protected against *Mycobacterium tuberculosis* by

a. Bacillus of Calmette and Guérin vaccine.

b. Plague vaccine.

c. Salk vaccine.

d. Pertussis vaccine.

GUIDES TO FURTHER STUDY

1. Observe a group of adolescents in high school, a recreation center or a neighborhood meeting place. Describe the general activity of the members of the group. Were any adolescents paired off in couples? What activity, if any, were the ones doing who did not mix with the others? Observe their posture when sitting and standing. Observe their manner of dress and their grooming. Compare your observations with your knowledge of the normal behavior patterns of adolescents.

2. What is your understanding of the function of a clinic for adolescents? How many adolescent clinics have been organized in your state or community?

3. A thirteen-year-old delinquent has been admitted to the pediatric unit with a diagnosis of tuberculosis. What would be your approach to this adolescent and his parents? What would be your role and responsibility as a member of the health team in providing care for this young person? Investigate the agencies in your community which could assist in his rehabilitation.

4. What are the most recent statistics in your state on the causes of mortality in the adolescent age group? What preventive measures could be taken to reduce these tragedies?

5. What rehabilitative services are available for physically and mentally handicapped adolescents in your hospital, your community and your state? Evaluate these services to determine whether they are adequately meeting the need.

6. What facilities are available in your state for the care of adolescents having a diagnosis of schizophrenia? Are these facilities adequately meeting the need?

7. Select the three experiences which were most disturbing to you and the three experiences which were most satisfying to you in providing care for children. State for each incident the age of the patient, his diagnosis and a description of the situation. Analyze each of these incidents to determine why they were disturbing or satisfying to you and discuss them in seminar.

TEACHING AIDS AND OTHER INFORMATION*

Alcoholics Anonymous, Inc.

Young People and A.A.

American Medical Association

How Teens Set the Stage for Alcoholism.
The Crutch That Cripples—Drug Dependence.
TB Control: Prospect for Eradication.
Why the Rise in Teenage Gonorrhea?
Why the Rise in Teenage Syphilis?

American Social Health Association

Deschin, C. S.: Teenagers and Venereal Disease.
Today's VD Control Problem, 1966.

Canadian Mental Health Association

The Juvenile Offender, 1967.

National Tuberculosis Association

South, J.: Tuberculosis Handbook for Public Health Nurses, 1965.
TB Through the Teens.

* Complete addresses are given in the Appendix.

Public Affairs Pamphlets

Brecher, R., and Brecher, E.: The Delinquent and the Law.
Butcher, R. L., and Robinson, M. O.: The Unmarried Mother.
Milt, H.: Serious Mental Illness in Children.
Ogg, E.: Psychotherapy—A Helping Process.
Saltman, J.: What We Can Do About Drug Abuse, 1966.
Shneidman, E. S., and Mandelkorn, P.: How to Prevent Suicide, 1967.

The National Council on Alcoholism, Inc.

Block, J. L.: Alcohol and the Adolescent.
Block, M. A.: Could Your Child Become an Alcoholic?
Lee, J. P.: What Shall We Tell Our Children About Drinking?
Oppenheim, G.: When Your Teen-Ager Starts Drinking.
Smith, A. J.: What I'd Teach My Children About Alcohol.
Strictly for Teenagers.

United States Department of Health, Education, and Welfare

A Child-Centered Program to Prevent Tuberculosis, 1965.
A New Look at School Dropouts, 1965.
Cancer of the Bone, 1967.
Drugs of Abuse, 1967.
Halfway House Programs for Delinquent Youth, 1965.
Herzog, E., and Bernstein, R.: Health Services for Unmarried Mothers, 1964.
"Hooked," 1967.
Hung on LSD . . . Stuck on Glue?, 1968.
Juvenile Delinquency—Facts, Facets, 1965.
Juvenile Delinquency Prevention in the United States, 1965.
Juvenile Gangs, 1965.
Lin-Fu, J. S.: Neonatal Narcotic Addiction, 1967.
Living Death—The Truth About Drug Addiction, 1965.
LSD: The False Illusion, 1967.
Savitz, R. A., McCann, M., and Stitt, P. G.: Childbearing in and Before the Years of Adolescence, 1966.
The Control and Treatment of Juvenile Delinquency in the United States, 1965.
The Culture of Youth, 1966.
Thinking About Drinking, 1968.
Trends in Illegitimacy: United States, 1940-1965.
Young People Who Smoke, 1968.

REFERENCES

Publications

Aguilera, D. C.: Use of Physical Contact (Touch) as a Technique of Non-verbal Communication with Psychiatric Patients; in *Exploring Progress in Psychiatric Nursing Practice*. Monograph 4, American Nurses' Association 1965 Regional Clinical Conferences. New York, American Nurses' Association, 1966, p. 33.
Child Study Association of America: *Children of Poverty: Children of Affluence*. New York, Child Study Association of America, 1967.
Cohen, A. C.: *The Drug Treatment of Tuberculosis*. Springfield, Ill., Charles C Thomas, 1966.
Deutsch, H.: *Selected Problems of Adolescence*. New York, International Universities Press, Inc., 1967.
Freedman, A. M., and Kaplan, H. I. (Eds.): *Comprehensive Textbook of Psychiatry*. Baltimore, Williams & Wilkins Company, 1967.
Friedman, A. S., and others: *Psychotherapy for the Whole Family*. New York, Springer Publishing Company, Inc., 1965.
Gallagher, J. R.: *Medical Care of the Adolescent*. 2nd ed. New York, Appleton-Century-Crofts, 1966.
Gallagher, J. R., and Harris, H. I.: *Emotional Problems of Adolescents*. 2nd ed. New York, Oxford University Press, 1964.
Giallombardo, R. (Ed.): *Juvenile Delinquency*. New York, John Wiley and Sons, Inc., 1966.
Hambling, J., and Hopkins, P. (Eds.): *Psychosomatic Disorders in Adolescents and Young Adults*. New York, Pergamon Press, Inc., 1965.
Harms, E. (Ed.): *Drug Addiction in Youth*. Long Island City, New York, Pergamon Press, 1965.
Hoagland, R. J.: *Infectious Mononucleosis*. New York, Grune & Stratton, Inc., 1967.
Hoch, P. H., and Zubin, J. (Eds.): *Psychopathology of Schizophrenia*. New York, Grune & Stratton, Inc., 1966.

Hofling, C. K., and Leininger, M. M.: *Basic Psychiatric Concepts in Nursing.* 2nd ed. Philadelphia, J. B. Lippincott Company, 1967.

Holmes, D. F.: *The Adolescent in Psychotherapy.* Boston, Little, Brown and Company, 1964.

Jones, H. W., and Heller, R. H.: *Pediatric and Adolescent Gynecology.* Baltimore, Williams & Wilkins Company, 1966.

Kendig, E. L., Jr. (Ed.): *Diseases of the Respiratory Tract in Children.* Philadelphia, W. B. Saunders Company, 1966.

Keniston, K.: *The Uncommitted: Alienated Youth in American Society.* New York, Harcourt, Brace and World, Inc., 1965.

Klein, M. W. (Ed.): *Juvenile Gangs in Context.* Englewood Cliffs, N.J., Prentice-Hall, Inc., 1967.

Konopka, G.: *The Adolescent Girl in Conflict.* Englewood Cliffs, N.J., Prentice-Hall, Inc., 1966.

MacLennan, B. W., and Felsenfeld, N.: *Group Counseling and Psychotherapy with Adolescents.* New York, Columbia University Press, 1968.

Masterson, J. F.: *The Psychiatric Dilemma of Adolescence.* Boston, Little, Brown and Company, 1967.

National Association for Mental Health, Inc., in cooperation with the National Institute of Mental Health, U.S. Public Health Service: *Directory of Resources for Mentally Ill Children in the United States.* New York, National Association for Mental Health, 1964.

National Council on Illegitimacy: *Directory of Maternity Homes and Residential Facilities for Unmarried Mothers: A Guide for Use and Selection.* New York, National Council on Illegitimacy, 1966.

National Council on Illegitimacy: *Unmarried Parenthood.* New York, National Council on Illegitimacy, 1967.

Podair, S., and Harris, W. D. M.: *Venereal Disease: Man Against a Plague.* Palo Alto, California, Fearon Publishers, 1966.

Roberts, R. W. (Ed.): *The Unwed Mother.* New York, Harper and Row Publishers, 1966.

Robins, L. N.: *Deviant Children Grown Up.* Baltimore, Williams & Wilkins Company, 1966.

Rubenfeld, S.: *Family of Outcasts: A New Theory of Delinquency.* New York, The Free Press, 1965.

Sauber, M., and Rubinstein, E.: *Experiences of the Unwed Mother as a Parent; A Longitudinal Study of Unmarried Mothers Who Keep Their First-born.* New York, Research Department, Community Council of Greater New York, 1965.

Schlesinger, B.: *Poverty in Canada and the United States.* Toronto, Ontario, University of Toronto Press, 1966.

Semmens, J. P., and Lamers, W. M.: *Teenage Pregnancy.* Springfield, Ill., Charles C Thomas, 1967.

Shands, A. R., and Raney, R. B.: *Handbook of Orthopaedic Surgery.* 7th ed. St. Louis, C. V. Mosby Company, 1967.

Shaw, C. R.: *The Psychiatric Disorders of Childhood.* New York, Appleton-Century-Crofts, 1966.

Swanson, A.: The Self-Fulfilling Prophesy in Schizophrenia; in *Exploring Progress in Psychiatric Nursing Practice.* Monograph 4, American Nurses' Association 1965 Regional Clinical Conferences. New York, American Nurses' Association, 1966, p. 26.

Usdin, G. L. (Ed.): *Psychoneurosis and Schizophrenia.* Philadelphia, J. B. Lippincott Company, 1966.

Vermes, H., and Vermes, J.: *Helping Youth Avoid Four Great Dangers: Smoking, Drinking, VD, Narcotics Addiction.* Toronto, Ontario, G. R. Welch Company, 1965.

Wheeler, S., and Cottrell, L. S.: *Juvenile Delinquency.* New York, Russell Sage Foundation, 1966.

Periodicals

A Guide for Collaboration of Physician, Social Worker, and Lawyer in Helping the Unmarried Mother and Her Child. *Children,* 14:111, 1967.

Auerbach, A. B., and Rabinow, M.: Parent Education Groups for Unmarried Mothers. *Nursing Outlook,* 14:38, March 1966.

Blattner, R. J.: Isoniazid Prophylaxis in Tuberculin Reactors. *J. Pediat.,* 72:131, 1968.

Boegli, E. H., and Steele, M. S.: Scoliosis: Spinal Instrumentation and Fusion. *Am. J. Nursing,* 68:2399, 1968.

Burgess, L. C.: The Unmarried Father in Adoption Planning. *Children,* 15:71, 1968.

Burton, M., and Holter, I.: Health Education Classes for Unwed Mothers. *Nursing Outlook,* 14:35, March 1966.

Byers, M. L.: The Hospitalized Adolescent. *Nursing Outlook,* 15:32, August 1967.

Christ, A. E., and others: The Role of the Nurse in Child Psychiatry. *Nursing Outlook,* 13:30, January 1965.

Clark, A. L.: The Crisis of Adolescent Unwed Motherhood. *Am. J. Nursing,* 67:1465, 1967.

Cochran, M. L., and Yeaworth, R. C.: Ward Meetings for Teen-Age Mothers. *Am. J. Nursing,* 67:1044, 1967.

Cohen, S.: Pot, Acid and Speed. *Medical Science,* 19:30, February 1968.

Coles, R.: Violence in Ghetto Children. *Children,* 14:101, 1967.

Diagnosing Mononucleosis in Just Two Minutes. *Medical World News,* 8:36, October 6, 1967.

DiPalma, J. R.: A Hard Look at the Hallucinogens. *RN,* 31:55, July 1968.

Fleming, J. W.: Recognizing the Newborn Addict. *Am. J. Nursing,* 65:83, January 1965.

Gimpel, H. S.: Group Work with Adolescent Girls. *Nursing Outlook,* 16:46, April 1968.

Godeene, G. D.: A Psychiatrist's Techniques in Treating Adolescents. *Children,* 12:136, 1965.

Hallan, M. B.: Attitudes Toward the Unwed Mother. *Nursing Clin. N. Amer.*, 2:775, 1967.

Herzog, E.: Unmarried Mothers—The Service Gap Revisited. *Children*, 14:105, 1967.

Howard, M.: Comprehensive Service Programs for School-Age Pregnant Girls. *Children*, 15:193, 1968.

Hustu, H. O., and others: Treatment of Ewing's Sarcoma with Concurrent Radiotherapy and Chemotherapy. *J. Pediat.*, 73:249, 1968.

Iungerich, Z.: High School for Unwed Mothers. *Am. J. Nursing*, 67:92, 1967.

Jacobziner, H.: Attempted Suicides in Adolescence. *J.A.M.A.*, 191:7, 1965.

Johnson, B. S., and Miller, L. C.: The Interpersonal Reflex in Psychiatric Nursing. *Nursing Outlook*, 15:60, May 1967.

Keeler, M. H.: Adverse Reaction to Marihuana. *Am. J. Psychiat.*, 124:674, 1967.

Keiser, R. P.: Treatment of Scoliosis. *Nursing Clin. N. Amer.*, 2:409, 1967.

Konopka, G.: Adolescent Delinquent Girls. *Children*, 11:21, 1964.

Kramer, J. C., and others: Amphetamine Abuse. *J.A.M.A.*, 201:305, 1967.

McPhetridge, L. M.: Nursing History: One Means to Personalize Care. *Am. J. Nursing*, 68:68, 1968.

Mellow, J.: Nursing Therapy as a Treatment and Clinical Investigative Approach to Emotional Illness. *Nursing Forum*, V:64, No. 3, 1966.

Nowlis, H. H.: Why Students Use Drugs. *Am. J. Nursing*, 68:1680, 1968.

Pannor, R.: Casework Service for Unmarried Fathers. *Children*, 10:65, 1963.

Polk, L. D.: UNWED Mother or Unwed MOTHER. *Nursing Outlook*, 12:38, February 1964.

Pollack, J. H.: Where *Unwed* Mothers Stay in School. *Today's Health*, 45:24, September 1967.

Ramirez, E.: Help for the Addict. *Am. J. Nursing*, 67:2348, 1967.

Redl, F.: A New Theory of Delinquency? It's About Time! *Children*, 13:119, 1966.

Reed, E. F.: Unmarried Mothers Who Kept Their Babies. *Children*, 12:118, 1965.

Rosenberg, M., and Gottlieb, R. P.: Current Approach to Tuberculosis in Childhood. *Pediat. Clin. N. Amer.*, 15:513, 1968.

Sankot, M., and Smith, D. E.: Drug Problems in the Haight-Ashbury. *Am. J. Nursing*, 68:1686, 1968.

Segal, A.: Some Observations About Mentally Retarded Adolescents. *Children*, 14:233, 1967.

Semmens, J. P.: Fourteen Thousand Teen-Age Pregnancies. *Am. J. Nursing*, 66:308, 1966.

South, J.: Impediments to TB Eradication. *Nursing Outlook*, 15:50, September 1967.

Stine, O. C., and others: School Leaving Due to Pregnancy in an Urban Adolescent Population. *Am. J. Pub. Health*, 54:1, 1964.

Thaler, O. F.: Grief and Depression. *Nursing Forum*, V:8, Spring 1966.

The Los Angeles Suicide Prevention Center. *Nursing Outlook*, 13:61, November 1965.

Townsend, J.: The Unmarried, Pregnant Adolescent's Use of Educational Literature. *Nursing Outlook*, 15:48, August 1967.

Vaccination Against TB Made Easy as Breathing. *Medical World News*, 8:38, December 8, 1967.

Weinberg, S., and others: Seminars in Nursing Care of the Adolescent. *Nursing Outlook*, 16:18, December 1968.

Wesseling, E.: The Adolescent Facing Amputation. *Am. J. Nursing*, 65:90, January 1965.

Where *Unwed* Mothers Stay in School. *Today's Health*, 45:24, September 1967.

Zellweger, H., and others: Is Lysergic-Acid Diethylamide a Teratogen? *Lancet*, 2:1066, 1967.

APPENDIX

Addresses for Sources of Materials
Listed at the Ends of Chapters

Abbott Laboratories: North Chicago, Ill. 60064.

Alcoholics Anonymous, Inc.: P.O. Box 459, Grand Central Station Post Office, New York, N.Y. 10017.

American Academy of Pediatrics: 1801 Hinman Ave., Evanston, Ill. 60204.

American Dental Association: 211 East Chicago Ave., Chicago, Ill. 60611.

American Diabetic Association, Inc.: 18 East 48th St., New York, N.Y. 10017.

American Foundation for the Blind, Inc.: 15 West 16th St., New York, N.Y. 10011.

American Heart Association: 44 East 23rd St., New York, N.Y. 10010.

American Medical Association: 535 North Dearborn St., Chicago, Ill. 60610.

American Nurses' Association: 10 Columbus Circle, New York, N.Y. 10019.

American Pharmaceutical Association: 2215 Constitution Ave., Northwest, Washington, D.C. 20037.

American Social Health Association: 1790 Broadway, New York, N.Y. 10019.

Association for the Aid of Crippled Children: 345 East 46th St., New York, N.Y. 10017.

Canadian Mental Health Association: 52 St. Clair Ave., East, Toronto 7, Ontario.

Charles Pfizer and Company, J. B. Roerig Division: 235 East 42nd St., New York, N.Y. 10017.

Children's Medical and Surgical Center, The Johns Hopkins Hospital: Wolfe & Monument Sts., Baltimore, Md. 21205.

Child Study Association of America: 9 East 89th St., New York, N.Y. 10028.

Evaporated Milk Association: 910 17th St., N.W., Washington, D.C. 20006.

Interdepartmental Committee on Children and Youth: U.S. Department of Health, Education and Welfare, 330 Independence Ave., S.W., Washington, D.C. 20201.

Joseph P. Kennedy, Jr. Foundation: 200 Park Ave., Rm. 3021, New York, N.Y. 10017.

Kimberly-Clark Corporation (Educational Department): Neenah, Wis. 54956.

Mead Johnson Laboratories: Evansville, Ind. 47721.

Medic Alert Foundation: Turlock, Calif. 95380.

Mental Health Division, Dept. of National Health and Welfare: Ottawa, Canada.

Mental Health Materials Center: 104 East 25th St., New York, N.Y. 10010.

National Association for Mental Health, Inc.: 10 Columbus Circle, New York, N.Y. 10019.

National Association for Retarded Children, Inc.: 420 Lexington Ave., New York, N.Y. 10017.

National Conference of Christians and Jews: 43 W. 57th St., New York, N.Y. 10019.

National Cystic Fibrosis Research Foundation: 202 E. 44th St., New York, N.Y. 10017.

National Society for Crippled Children and Adults, Inc.: 2023 West Ogden Ave., Chicago, Ill. 60612.

National Society for the Prevention of Blindness, Inc.: 79 Madison Ave., New York, N.Y. 10016.

National Tuberculosis Association: 1790 Broadway, New York, N.Y. 10019.

Personal Products Company: Box S-6, Milltown, N.J. 08850.

Play Schools Association: 120 West 57th St., New York, N.Y. 10019.

Project Head Start, Office of Economic Opportunity: 1200 19th St., N.W., Washington, D.C. 20006.

Public Affairs Committee, Inc.: 381 Park Ave. South, N.Y. 10016.

Ross Laboratories: Columbus, Ohio, 43216.

The American Cancer Society, Inc.: 219 East 42nd St., New York, N.Y. 10017.

The Children's Hospital Medical Center, Health Education: 300 Longwood Ave., Boston, Mass. 02115.

The Epilepsy Foundation: 1419 H St., N.W., Washington, D.C. 20005.

The National Council on Alcoholism, Inc.: New York Academy of Medicine Building, 2 East 103rd St., New York, N.Y. 10029.

The National Foundation-March of Dimes: 800 Second Ave., New York, N.Y. 10017.

United Cerebral Palsy Associations, Inc.: 321 West 44th St., New York, N.Y. 10036.

U.S. Department of Health, Education, and Welfare, Social Security Administration, Children's Bureau: U.S. Government Printing Office, Division of Public Documents, Washington, D.C. 20025.

INDEX